CARDIAC PREEXCITATION SYNDROMES

CARDIAC PREEXCITATION SYNDROMES

Origins, Evaluation, and Treatment

edited by

David G. Benditt
D. Woodrow Benson, Jr.

Martinus Nijhoff Publishing
a member of the Kluwer Academic Publishers Group
BOSTON DORDRECHT LANCASTER

DISTRIBUTORS

for the United States and Canada: Kluwer Academic Publishers, 101 Philip Drive, Norwell, MA 02061, USA

for the UK and Ireland: Kluwer Academic Publishers, MTP Press Limited, Falcon House, Queen Square, Lancaster LA1 1RN, UK

for all other countries: Kluwer Academic Publishers Group, Distribution Centre, P.O. Box 322, 3300 AH Dordrecht, The Netherlands

Library of Congress Cataloging-in-Publication Data
Main entry under title:

Cardiac preexcitation syndromes.

Includes bibliographies and index.
1. Wolff-Parkinson-White syndrome. I. Benditt, David G. II. Benson, D. Woodrow. [DNLM: 1. Arrhythmia. WG 330 C2696]
RC685.W6C37 1985 616.1'2 85–25824
ISBN 978-1-4684-7528-9 ISBN 978-1-4684-7526-5 (eBook)
DOI 10.1007978-1-4684-7526-5

CONTENTS

CONTRIBUTING AUTHORS

Masood Akhtar
Professor of Medicine
University of Wisconsin-Milwaukee
Mount Sinai Medical Center
P.O. Box 342
Milwaukee, Wisconsin 53201

Adrian Almquist, M.D.
Assistant Professor of Medicine
Section of Cardiology
University of Minnesota Hospitals
Box 508 Mayo Memorial Building
Minneapolis, Minnesota 55455

Robert W. Anderson, M.D.
Professor of Surgery
Director of Cardiovascular and Thoracic Surgery
Evanston Hospital
2650 Ridge Avenue
Evanston, Illinois 60201

David G. Benditt, M.D.
Associate Professor of Medicine
Section of Cardiology
University of Minnesota Medical School
Box 341 Mayo Memorial Building
Minneapolis, Minnesota 55455

D. Woodrow Benson, Jr., M.D., Ph.D.
Professor of Pediatrics
Pediatric Cardiology
University of Minnesota Medical School
Box 94 Mayo Memorial Building
Minneapolis, Minnesota 55455

Elias Botvinick, M.D.
Associate Professor of Radiology and Medicine
University of California-San Francisco
3rd and Parnassus Avenues
San Francisco, California 94143

Jean-Paul Broustet, M.D.
Professor of Cardiology
University of Bordeaux
School of Medicine
Hospital Cardiologique, Haut-Leveque
Pessac, France

Howard B. Burchell, M.D.
Professor Emeritus of Medicine
University of Minnesota Medical School
260 Woodlawn Avenue
St. Paul, Minnesota 55105

Michael E. Cain, M.D.
Assistant Professor of Medicine
Washington University School of Medicine
4989 Barnes Hospital Plaza
Suite 4102 Queeny Tower
St. Louis, Missouri 63110

David C. Chung, M.D.
Associate Professor
Department of Anesthesia
University of Western Ontario
London, Ontario
Canada

Roland Cointe, M.D.
Fellow in Cardiology
University of Marseille
School of Medicine
Centre Cardiovasculaire J. Cantini
Marseille, France

James L. Cox, M.D.
Professor of Surgery
Washington University School of Medicine
Chief, Division of Cardiovascular Surgery
Barnes Hospital
4989 Barnes Hospital Plaza
Suite 3108 Queeny Tower
St. Louis, Missouri 63110

Giuseppe Critelli, M.D.
Department of Medicine
Section of Cardiology
University of Naples
Second Medical School
Naples, Italy

Michael W. Dae, M.D.
Assistant Professor of Radiology and Medicine
University of California-San Francisco
San Francisco, California 94143

Stephen Denker, M.D.
Assistant Professor of Medicine
University of Wisconsin-Milwaukee
Mount Sinai Medical Center
P.O. Box 342
Milwaukee, Wisconsin 534201

Anne Hamilton Dougherty, M.D.
Assistant Professor of Medicine
Director of Cardiac Pacing
The University of Texas Medical School at Houston
Division of Cardiology
P.O. Box 20708
Houston, Texas 77225–0708

David Dunbar, M.D.
Assistant Professor of Medicine
Hennepin County Medical Center
University of Minnesota Hospitals
701 Park Avenue
Minneapolis, Minnnesota 55415

Ann Dunnigan, M.D.
Assistant Professor of Pediatrics
Pediatric Cardiology
Box 94 Mayo Memorial Building
420 Delaware Street SE
University of Minnesota Hospitals
Minneapolis, Minnesota 55455

Gérard Faugère, M.D.
Assistant Professor of Medicine
University of Marseille
School of Medicine
Centre Cardiovasculaire J. Cantini
Marseille, France

Donald B. Faulkner, N.M.T.
Chief Imaging Technician
Department of Nuclear Medicine
University of California-San Francisco
San Francisco, California 94143

John J. Gallagher, M.D.
Consultant in Cardiology
Sanger Clinic
1960 Randolph Road
Charlotte, North Carolina 28207

Raymond Gérard, M.D.
Professor of Cardiology
Chairman, Division of Cardiology
University of Marseille
School of Medicine
Centre Cardiovasculaire J. Cantini
Marseille, France

Lawrence German, M.D.
Assistant Professor of Medicine
Director, Clinical Electrophysiology Laboratory
Duke University Medical Center
Box 3860
Durham, North Carolina 27710

Marcel R. Gilbert, M.D.
Assistant Professor of Medicine
Duke University Medical Center
Durham, North Carolina 27710

Charles C. Gornick, M.D.
Assistant Professor of Medicine
University of Minnesota Hospitals
Veterans Administration Medical Center
54th Street and 48th Avenue South
Minneapolis, Minnesota 55417

Gerard Guiraudon, M.D.
Associate Professor of Surgery
Department of Surgery
University Hospital
University of Western Ontario
London, Ontario, Canada

Donald Hackel, M.D.
Professor of Pathology
Duke University Medical Center
Durham, North Carolina 27710

David Holmes, Jr., M.D.
Associate Professor of Medicine
Department of Cardiovascular Diseases and Internal Medicine
Mayo Clinic and Mayo Foundation
Rochester, Minnesota 55901

Warren M. Jackman, M.D.
Assistant Professor of Medicine
Cardiology Section, Rm. 3E-204
University of Oklahoma Health Sciences Center
Oklahoma City, Oklahoma 73190

Douglas L. Jones, Ph.D.
University of Western Ontario
University Hospital
London, Ontario Canada

Jackie H. Kasell
Research Associate
Division of Cardiology
Department of Medicine
Duke University Medical Center
Durham, North Carolina 27710

Charles Kerr, M.D.
Associate Professor of Medicine
University of British Columbia
Division of Cardiology
Vancouver General Hospital
277 Heather Street
Vancouver, British Columbia, Canada

George J. Klein, M.D.
Cardiac Investigation Unit
University Hospital
University of Western Ontario
London, Ontario, Canada

John D. Kugler, M.D.
Associate Professor of Pediatrics
Department of Pediatrics
University of Nebraska Medical Center
42nd and Dewey Avenue
Omaha, Nebraska 68105

Michael H. Lehmann, M.D.
Assistant Professor of Medicine
University of Wisconsin-Milwaukee
Mount Sinai Medical Center
P.O. Box 342
Milwaukee, Wisconsin 53201

Samuel Levy, M.D.,
Professor of Cardiology
University of Marseille
School of Medicine
Director of Clinical Electrophysiology and Pacing Department
Centre Cardiovasculaire J. Cantini
8B, Avenue Vedrines
13009 Marseille, France

Rehan Mahmud, M.D.
Assistant Professor of Medicine
University of Wisconsin-Milwaukee,
Mount Sinai Medical Center
P.O. Box 342
Milwaukee, Wisconsin 53201

Marc Metge, M.D.
Assistant Professor of Medicine
University of Marseille
School of Medicine
Centre Cardiovasculaire J. Cantini
Marseille, France

Simon Milstein, M.D.
Fellow in Cardiology
Cardiac Investigation Unit
University of Western Ontario
London, Ontario, Canada

Fred Morady, M.D.
University of California-San Francisco
Room 573 Moffitt Hospital
San Francisco, California 94143

Gerald Naccarelli, M.D.
Assistant Professor of Medicine
Cardiology Division
University of Texas Medical School at Houston
P.O. Box 20708
Houston, Texas 77225–0708

J. William O'Connell, B.S.
Principal Programmer
Department of Radiology
University of California-San Francisco
San Francisco, California 94143

Robert Peters, M.D.
Associate Professor of Medicine
Division of Cardiology
VA Medical Center
3900 Loch Raven Blvd
Baltimore, Maryland 21218

Shanda Pool-Schneider, R.N.
Clinical Research Associate
University of Minnesota Hospital
Box 508 Mayo Memorial Building
Minneapolis, Minnesota 55455

Co-burn J. Porter, M.D.
Assistant Professor of Pediatrics
Section of Pediatric Cardiology
Mayo Clinic and Mayo Foundation
Rochester, Minnesota 55901

Edward L.C. Pritchett, M.D.
Associate Professor of Medicine
Division of Cardiology
Duke University Medical Center
Box 3477
Durham, North Carolina 27710

Eric M. Prystowsky, M.D.
Associate Professor of Medicine
Division of Cardiology
Krannert Institute of Cardiology
University of Indiana School of Medicine
1001 West Tenth Street
Indianapolis, Indiana 46202

W. Steves Ring, M.D.
Assistant Professor of Surgery
Department of Surgery
University of Minnesota Medical School

Box 331 Mayo Memorial Building
Minneapolis, Minnesota 55455

Lino Rossi, M.D.
Department of Medicine
Section of Cardiology
University of Milan
Milan, Italy

Melvin M. Scheinman, M.D.
Professor of Medicine
University of California-San Francisco
Room 312 Moffitt Hospital
San Francisco, California 94143

Arjun D. Sharma, M.D.
Assistant Professor of Medicine
Cardiac Investigation Unit
University Hospital University of Western Ontario
London, Ontario, Canada

Ruey J. Sung, M.D.
Professor of Medicine
University of California at San Francisco
Director, Section of Cardiac Electrophysiology
San Francisco General Hospital
San Francisco, California 94110

Der-Yan Tai, M.D.
Associate Professor of Medicine
Yang Ming Medical College
Director, Cardiac Electrophysiology Laboratory
Veterans General Hospital
Taipei, Taiwan

Gaetano Thiene, M.D.
Department of Medicine
Section of Cardiology
University of Padua
Padua, Italy

H. Gareth Tobler, M.D.
Research Fellow in Surgery
University of Minnesota Medical School
Box 469 Mayo Memorial Building
Minneapolis, Minnesota 55455

FOREWORD

The Wolff-Parkinson-White (WPW) syndrome, the most common variety of preexcitation, has for some time held a fascination for those interested in clinical electrophysiology because it seems to represent a naturally occurring event which, if adequately understood, would unmask answers to many fundamental questions concerning mechanisms and treatment of cardiac arrhythmias. Thus, it has been described by Scherf and Neufeld [1] as the "Rosetta Stone" of electrocardiography.

The historic overview of the preexcitation syndromes will be deferred to Dr. Burchell's authoritative chapter, but a few highlights deserve emphasis here because they graphically portray how elements of serendipity, courage, and luck played important roles in the unfolding of the mysteries of preexcitation.

Although Kent is forever linked to the literature of preexcitation by his description of a node-like structure [2] in the right lateral atrioventricular groove, it is now accepted that this structure bears little resemblance to the accessory atrioventricular connection known to form the basis of the WPW syndrome. Indeed, it is unlikely that Kent's "node" played any role in AV conduction, either in normal or abnormal hearts. Nevertheless, Kent succeeded in igniting a controversy which undoubtedly influenced Mines [3] to consider the possible role that such an "accessory pathway" might play in excitation of the human heart. Thus in 1914, Mines stated

> ... some instances of paroxysmal tachycardia observed in man where auricles and ventricles beat with the same frequency might conceivably be explained along somewhat similar lines (i.e., circulating excitations). I now repeat this suggestion in the light of the new histological demonstration by Stanley Kent that the muscular connexion between auricles and ventricles in the human heart is multiple.

Mines prophesized the possibility of surgical correction of such a reentry when he observed

> ... in a favourable experiment, the vigorous circulating wave and its instantaneous arrest by section of the ring is a sight not easily forgotten.

Courageous is the only way to describe the first attempt to surgically interrupt an accessory pathway. The immensity of the feat speaks for itself: Open heart surgery was performed to divide an invisible stream of electrons! This historic event was not anticipated. A fisherman from the coast of North Carolina presented to Duke University Medical Center in 1968 with refractory supraventricular tachycardia related to the WPW syndrome [2]. Attempts to control the tachycardia medically failed. Dr. Andrew Wallace (then Director of the Coronary Care Unit) had recently returned from the NIH where he had performed epicardial mapping studies on various forms of hypertrophy. He was continuing his mapping studies using facilities temporarily located in the laboratory of Dr. Will C. Sealy (Figure I–1), Chairman of the Department of Thoracic Surgery. Dr. Sealy in turn was known at the time to be interested in experimental surgical techniques to study car-

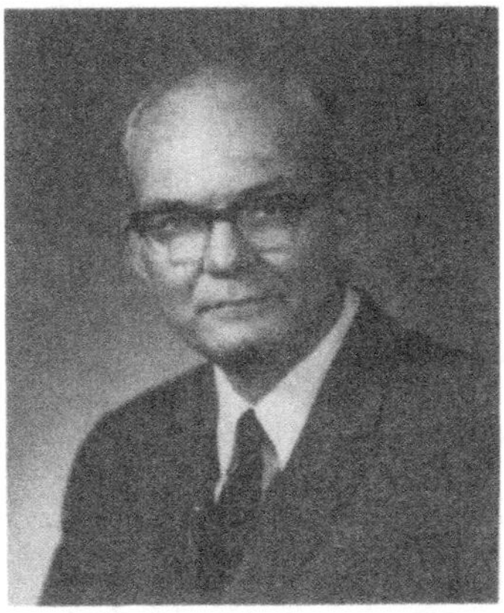

FIGURE I–1. Will C. Sealy, M.D., the first surgeon to divide an accessory AV pathway in man.

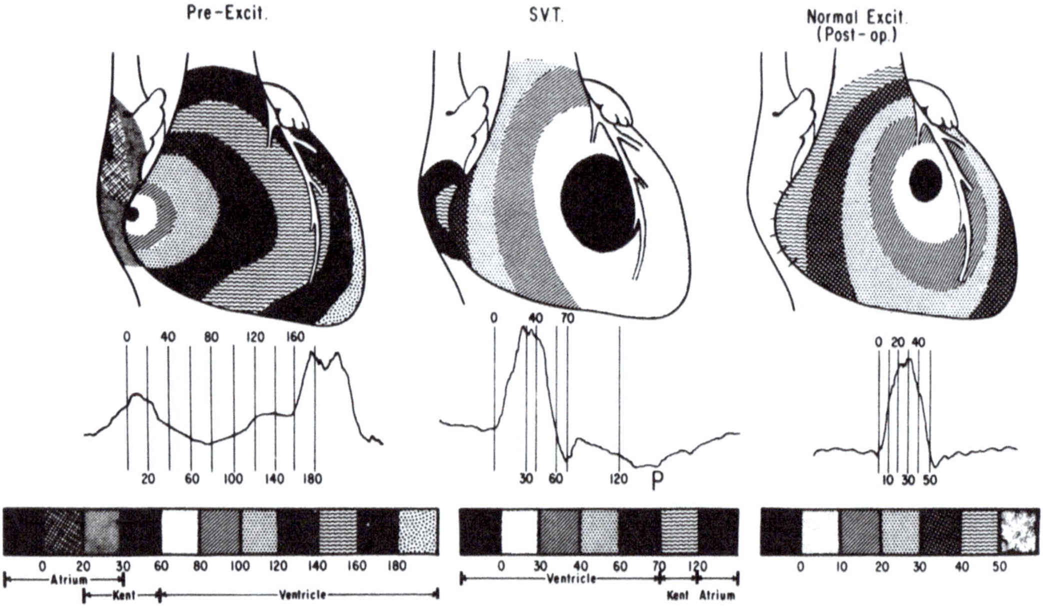

FIGURE I–2. Mapping of the first successful interruption of an accessory AV pathway maps are shown during preexcitation (*left panel*), supraventricular tachycardia (SVT) (*center panel*) and following dissection of the right AV groove (*right panel*). During preexcitation, the onset of the *p* wave was considered zero time. Early activation of the base of the lateral right ventricle is evident. During tachycardia, ventricular activation is normal, with earliest activity recorded over the midanterior right ventricle. Earliest retrograde atrial activity occurs on the lateral right atrium, contiguous with the previously demonstrated point of ventricular preexcitation. Following surgical dissection of the AV groove, ventricular activation is again normal and essentially identical to that observed during tachycardia.

diac rhythm disorders. Dr. Jack Boineau was extensively involved in body surface mapping in the Department of Pediatrics and was independently involved in his own animal mapping studies. The catalyst was a young medical resident, Dr. Fred Cobb, who brought this group together in the interest of providing a unique form of therapy for the ailing patient. Dr. Burchell's experience with transient block of an accessory pathway during surgery was fresh in everyone's mind and the decision was made to attempt a surgical cure. Luckily, the patient had a single free-wall accessory pathway (Figure I–2) [4,5]. If the accessory pathway in this index case had been located in the septum or multiple accessory pathways had been present, the promising venture might never have been repeated. Ultimately, dissection of the right AV groove in the vicinity of the pathway abolished the delta wave and no further tachycardia occurred.

This initial surgical success was a pivotal point in turning clinical investigation from a phenomenologic approach to one with therapeutic implications [6]. The simplicity of the demonstration seriously undermined other leading hypotheses of the day: that preexcitation was due to either an irritable focus or longitudinal dissociation of the normal conduction system. For his pioneering efforts in the field of surgical treatment of rhythm disorders, Dr. Sealy has been deservingly referred to as the "father of electrophysiologic surgery." Currently at the Sanger Clinic in Charlotte, North Carolina, he continues to work untiringly on new and improved techniques for surgically treating arrhythmias.

With the advent of intracardiac recording and stimulation, various types of preexcitation have been described with a wide spectrum of functional properties. The growth of information from laboratories all over the world has been exponential. Drs. Benditt and Benson have brought together in this volume a comprehensive accounting of the varied facets of the preexcitation syndromes. This volume thus joins the previous classics on the subject by Scherf and Neufeld [1], Laham [7], and Ferrer [8] and clearly defines the state of our knowledge of the preexcitation syndromes in 1986.

Much remains to be elucidated. Some areas which require further investigation are described below.

1. Despite the volume of electrophysiologic literature concerning the preexcitation syndromes, there is still a relative paucity of anatomic material with anatomicoelectrophysiologic correlation. This is especially true with regard to the variant forms of preexcitation.
2. The embryologic basis of accessory pathways, particularly the variant forms, needs to be more thoroughly defined. Why, for example, do accessory pathways of the atrioventricular type occur so often at the lateral margin of the left AV groove? Likewise, why are accessory pathways in this precise location so prone to develop unidirectional block with preservation of conduction in the retrograde direction?
3. Accessory pathways have been assumed to have fixed "all-or-none" properties of conduction. More recently, emphasis has been placed on autonomic nervous influences on properties of conduction and refractoriness. These concepts need to be further extended to include the possible effects of *physical* forces in the heart which may differ depending on the location of the accessory pathway. For example, it is quite likely that stress operative in the region of the posterior mitral annulus accounts not only for the known tendency of this area of the heart to calcify but also for the high incidence of unidirectional block in accessory pathways in this location. Furthermore, it seems reasonable to speculate that the dynamic changes of geometry which occur during tachycardia may directly affect conduction and refractoriness of the accessory pathway acutely and possibly chronically.
4. A long-term follow-up study of patients with preexcitation, preferably with randomized treatment groups, is sorely needed to establish whether high risk asymptomatic patients with preexcitation syndromes should be treated. Noninvasive techniques are needed to predict prognosis with greater sensitivity and specificity. Esophageal pacing and recording techniques appears promising and needs evaluation on a prospective basis.
5. It is now well accepted that accessory pathways can exhibit unidirectional block either in the anterograde or retrograde directions. Thus preexcitation need not be manifest on the surface ECG. In an analogous manner, nodoventricular or fasciculoventricular (Mahaim) connections may be capable of conducting only in the retrograde direction; if so, such fibers might be responsible for some forms of ventricular tachycardia apparently unassociated with organic heart disease [9].
6. Direct microelectrode studies of accessory pathway tissue would undoubtedly prove highly informative although logistically this would require block resection of portions of the AV groove, a procedure not required by currently accepted surgical techniques. Availability of such tissue, however, might permit further study of the possible existence of automaticity in fibers of the accessory pathway.

In closing, I am reminded of Hans Hecht's statement in 1970 while addressing an international symposium on Cardiac Arrhythmias held in Elsinore, Denmark [10]: "This (the WPW syndrome) has always been a very interesting syndrome, good for many publications. It always entertained us and will fortunately do so for quite some time more."

John J. Gallagher, M.D.,
August 1985

References

1. Scherf, L and Neufeld, HN: *The Preexcitation syndrome: facts and theories*. Yorke Medical Books. New York, 1978.
2. Kent, AFS: A conduction path between the right auricle and the external wall of the right ventricle in the heart of the mammal. *J. Physiol.* 48:57, 1914.
3. Mines, GR: On circulating excitations in heart muscles and their possible relation to tachycardia and fibrillation. *Proc. Roy. Soc. Canada* IV:43, 1914.
4. Cobb, FR, Blumenschein, SD, Sealy, WC, Boineau, JP, Wagner, GS and Wallace, AG: Successful surgical interruption of the bundle of

Kent in a patient with Wolff-Parkinson-White syndrome. *Circulation* 38:1018, 1968.
5. Sealy, WC, Hattler, BG, Blumenschein, SD, Cobb, FR: Surgical treatment of Wolff-Parkinson-White syndrome. *Ann. Thorac. Surg.* 8:1, 1969.
6. Sealy, WC: The Wolff-Parkinson-White syndrome and the beginnings of direct arrhythmia surgery. *Ann. Thor. Surg.* 38:176, 1984.
7. Latham, J: *Actualites electrocardiographiques. Le syndrome de Wolff-Parkinson-White.* Libraire Maloine, Paris, 1969.
8. Ferrer, IM: *Preexcitation including the Wolff-Parkinson-White syndrome and other related syndromes.* Futura Publ., Mount Kisco, N.Y., 1976.
9. German, LD, Packer, DL, Bardy, GH, Gallagher, JJ: Ventricular tachycardia induced by atrial stimulation in patients without symptomatic cardiac disease. *Am. J. Cardiol.* 52:1202, 1983.
10. Hecht, H: In *Symposium on cardiac arrhythmias.* Elsinore, Denmark. E Sandoe, E Flensted-Jensen, KH Olesen (eds.). AB Astra, Sweden, 1970, p. 375.

ACKNOWLEDGMENTS

We would like to thank the contributing authors not only for sharing their expertise within the individual chapters but also for valuable suggestions, which have been incorporated into the work "behind-the-scenes." We are very much aware of the disruption that writing book chapters introduced into the contributors' already busy schedule. We would especially like to thank our mentors Harold C. Strauss and Madison S. Spach and to specifically acknowledge John J. Gallagher, whose research, teaching, and criticism have played an important role in stimulating our own interest in the preexcitation syndromes. Howard B. Burchell, through his historic perspective insightful comments during numerous conversations, and capacity for asking unsettling questions, has had an enormous impact on our view and understanding of the subject material presented here. Special thanks is due to Frances Wallace for valuable assistance in organizing this book. We would also like to express our appreciation to Mary Beth Breitbach, Barry L.S. Detloff, Wendy Markuson, Sharon Ottomeyer, and Cheryl Yano for assistance in collating the manuscripts and preparing segments of the text, and to the publishers for their patience.

INTRODUCTION

The cardiac preexcitation syndromes provide physicians and physiologists the clearest insight into the basis of clinical cardiac arrhythmias and their potential for control by drugs, pacing systems, or surgery. The development of techniques for evaluating and treating patients with preexcitation syndromes has contributed importantly to progress in evaluation of the wide range of clinical tachyarrhythmias occurring in man, and represents one of the decade's major advances in the assessment and treatment of patients with cardiovascular disease.

Despite the passage of over 40 years since Ohnell [1] introduced the term *preexcitation* into the lexicon of cardiology, 70 years since electrocardiographic recordings compatible with ventricular preexcitation were first published [2,3], and almost 100 years since the landmark histologic observations of Kent raised the specter of accessory atrioventricular (AV) connections [4] (Table I–1), the fascination that preexcitation holds for physicians, physiologists, engineers, and other biomedical scientists continues unabated. This fascination is remark-

TABLE I–1. Preexcitation syndrome: A temporal view of key concepts

Era	Structure	Function
1890–1910	AV Bundle (His) Accessory AV connection (Kent, Paladino)	
1910–1920		Reentry (Mines, Erlanger) Initial ECG records (Cohn and Fraser, Wilson)
1930–1940		ECG-Clinical correlate (Wolff, Parkinson, White)
	Structure-Function correlate (Wood and Wolferth)	
1940–1950	Nodo and fasciculoventricular connections (Mahaim)	
	Structure-Function correlate, terminology: 'Preexcitation' (Ohnell)	
		ECG types (Rosenbaum in Wilson's laboratory)
1950–1960	A Period of "Fermentation"	
1960–1970	Intranodal (atrionodal) tracts (James)	Epicardial mapping, (Durrer, Burchell, Duke University Group [Boineau, Spach, Wallace]) His bundle recording (Scherlag in Damato's Laboratory, Castellanos)
1970–Present		Electrophysiology of accessory AV connections (Wellens, Gallagher)
	Atriofascicular tracts (Brechenmacher)	Surgical ablation techniques (Sealy) Electrophysiology of nodo and fasciculoventricular connections (Gallagher)
	Terminology (European Study Group)	

able given that the cardiac morphologic abnormalities and their associated functional disturbances comprising the preexcitation syndromes are relatively uncommon afflictions in man or animal.

Three factors may contribute to the abiding interest in the preexcitation syndromes. First, preexcitation syndromes provide unique natural models for the study of cardiac tachyarrhythmias and their response to therapeutic interventions. The development of methodologies for evaluating and treating affected patients has permitted the relationship between structure and function to be clearly delineated in some forms of the preexcitation syndromes (particularly those associated with accessory AV connections), and these morphologic-functional correlations have contributed importantly to general concepts of the genesis of tachyarrhythmias. In fact, reciprocating tachycardia utilizing the AV node–His bundle and an accessory AV connection (orthodromic reciprocating tachycardia) is the paradigm of reentrant arrhythmias. Second, preexcitation syndromes result from unique congenital cardiac anomalies. Clinical manifestations of these anomalies may first appear in utero or anytime after birth, sometimes delaying their appearance until the sixth or seventh decade. Symptoms in the preexcitation syndromes result from tachyarrhythmias; some only result in minimal symptoms and are not a serious threat to life, while others may be clearly life-threatening. On the other hand, preexcitation syndromes may never produce symptoms, and in many instances their presence is only detected serendipitiously during routine electrocardiographic recording. Third, unlike almost any other disorder of the cardiovascular system resulting in tachyarrhythmias, the most common form of the preexcitation syndromes, Wolff-Parkinson-White syndrome, is curable by ablation of the responsible accessory AV connection. The possibility for the less well defined forms of preexcitation syndromes to be similarly managed provides enticing opportunities for the years ahead.

This book provides a comprehensive and up-to-date survey of the preexcitation syndromes. Our understanding of the basis for these syndromes, and their electrocardiographic and electrophysiologic manifestations, is clearly and thoroughly reviewed. The techniques of intracardiac electrophysiologic evaluation of the wide spectrum of arrhythmias associated with these syndromes and approaches to their therapy are discussed in depth. Each chapter is written by well-recognized contributors to the recent literature on preexcitation syndromes. Consequently, the book provides the most authoritative, complete, and up-to-the minute assessment of this important topic available today.

Terminology

ANATOMIC SUBSTRATE

Given the prolonged period of time taken to formulate present concepts of the preexcitation syndromes, it is not surprising that its terminology has become complex. In particular, despite the value of eponyms in cementing our present thoughts with the names of important contributors of the past, it is time that the burden of these often inaccurately employed terms be removed. To this end, the contribution of the European Study Group for Preexcitation [5] has proved extremely valuable in establishing precise terminology for the structural components of the preexcitation syndrome. This terminology has been, in large measure, followed in this book (Table 1–1). In brief, this classification utilizes the term *tract* to describe accessory conduction tissue which inserts into the specialized conduction system of the heart (thus, "atriofascicular tracts"), and the term *connection* for accessory conduction tissue inserting into myocardium (thus, "accessory AV connection"). However, the reader will find a few author-dependent departures from this formula.

The most common divergence from the Study Group recommendations is retention of the term *pathway* instead of *connection* by some authors. The editors have also included the term *atrionodal* to describe the apparently ubiquitous fibers connecting the atria with the compact AV node (of the type described by James [6]), for which the Study Group prefers the term *intranodal.* In addition, the reader will find the term *nodofascicular* used in conjunction with the more widely accepted term *nodoventricular.* The latter reflects recent reevaluation of the site of insertion of these accessory conduction tissues [7].

TABLE I–2. Nomenclature for tachycardias associated with preexcitation syndrome

Preferred terminology	Definition or conventional terminology
1. Orthodromic reciprocating (reentrant) tachycardia	RT in which conduction in the antegrade (AV) direction uses the AV node–His bundle axis and conduction in the retrograde (VA) direction uses one or more accessory AV connections.
2. Antidromic reciprocating (reentrant) tachycardia	RT in which conduction in the antegrade (AV) direction uses an accessory AV connection and conduction in the retrograde (VA) direction uses either the AV node–His bundle or an additional accessory AV connection.
3. Reciprocating tachycardia due to reentry within the AV node	RT in which and "concealed" accessory AV connection has been excluded, the retrograde sequence of atrial activation is "midline", the critical elements of the reentry circuit appear to be restricted to the region of the AV junction.
4. "Incessant" AV reciprocating tachycardia	"Persistent" or "permanent" form of junctional reciprocating tachycardia (PJRT)
5. Preexcited QRS complex tachycardias	Tachycardias with a prolonged QRS complex in which ventricular activation appears to be primarily the result of conduction in the antegrade (AV) direction over an accessory connection or bypass tract.
6. Wide QRS complex tachycardias	Tachycardias with a prolonged QRS complex due to underlying or functional bundle-branch block, ventricular activation due to AV conduction over an accessory connection or bypass tract, or ventricular tachycardia.
7. Normal QRS complex tachycardias	Tachycardia in which the QRS complex is of normal duration.

Abbreviations: RT = reciprocating tachycardia; AV ‡ atrioventricular;
VA = ventriculoatrial.

ARRHYTHMIAS

A multitude of terms have been used to describe the most common arrhythmias associated with the preexcitation syndromes (e.g., orthodromic reciprocating tachycardia, PSVT, PAT, etc.) An attempt has been made to achieve a degree of uniformity of arrhythmia terminology within this volume, (Table I–2). Most of the preferred terms will be familiar to the reader. However, the usage "incessant AV reciprocating (reentry) tachycardia" has been introduced in parallel with, and as a suggested alternative to, the conventional but imprecise term *persistent* (or, "permanent form of") *junctional reciprocating tachycardia* (PJRT). It is hoped that the new term will be accepted and utilized since it emphasizes the role of AV reentry (versus reentry within the AV junction) in these cases, and avoids the confusing use of the letter "P" for *persistent* (or "permanent") in PJRT, and for *paroxysmal* in PSVT.

References

1. Ohnell RF: Preexcitation, a cardiac abnormality. *Acta Med. Scand.* (Suppl) 152:1, 1944.
2. Cohn AE, Fraser FR: Paroxysmal tachycardia and the effect of stimulation of the vagus nerves by pressure. *Heart* 5:93, 1913–1914.
3. Wilson FN: A case in which the vagus influenced the form of the ventricular complex of the electrocardiogram. *Arch. Int. Med.* 16:1008, 1915.
4. Kent AFS: Researches on the the structure and function of the mammalian heart. *J. Physiol.* 14:222, 1893.
5. Anderson RH, Becker AE, Brechenmacher C, Davies MJ, Rossi L: Ventricular preexcitation: A proposed nomenclature for its substrates. *Eur. J. Cardiol.* 3:27, 1975.
6. James TN: Morphology of the human atrioventricular node with remarks pertinent to its electrophysiology. *Am. Heart J.* 62:756, 1961.
7. Gallagher JJ: Variants of Preexcitation: Update 1984. In: Cardiac Electrophysiology and Arrhythmias. Zipes DP, Jalife J, eds., Orlando, Grune and Stratton, 1985, pp. 419–433.

I. BASIC CONCEPTS

1. VENTRICULAR PREEXCITATION: HISTORICAL OVERVIEW

Howard B. Burchell

"Nature is nowhere wont to reveal her innermost secrets more openly than where she shows faint traces of herself away from the beaten tract. . . ."

William Harvey[a]

"Year by year as the Twentieth Century rolls on, it becomes evident that the experimental sciences of Physiology, Pathology and Pharmacology are more and more directly influencing the practice of medicine."

Walter H. Gaskell[b]

"I am certain no great discovery can be made in the mechanism of the human body unless the problems suggested by a consideration of structure are resolved by the methods of experimental physiology."

Arthur Keith[c]

The advent of clinical electrocardiography and of detailed knowledge of the anatomy of the specialized conducting tissue in the heart were concurrent. The years 1903 to 1912 were particularly banner ones with many arrhythmias being defined, bundle branch function explored, and heart block explained. Indeed the first electrocardiographic abnormality attracting the attention of Einthoven [1] was a bundle branch block (in 1894), recorded by capillary electrometer — "a curve diverging from curves up till then recorded, which puzzled us." The authorities who dominated the scene in the beginning twentieth century taught that the "sole" conducting pathway between the mammalian atrium and the ventricle was the bundle described by His, Jr., and further reported upon by Tawara. The rigidity of the reigning dogma would seem to have inhibited imaginative concepts of multiple pathways.

Intermittent functional QRS aberration during supraventricular tachycardia was reported by Lewis in 1910 [2]. This case did *not* have atrioventricular (AV) nodal bypass preexcitation, but Lewis was troubled by the lack of a ready explanation, and at that time, prescient in his choice of phrases: "the explanation must be sought in a revision of our present ideas of the possible mode (or modes) of conduction from auricle to ventricle." This thought was not particularly relevant to his case, wherein bundle branch delays were operative, but prophetic in regard to the QRS aberration related to accessory atrioventricular (AV) corrections. How exhilarated Lewis would have been to hear the lecture named for him in 1981 when Anderson reviewed the fantastic variety of conduction tracts currently believed present between the atria and ventricles [3].

It was not until the 1930 paper of Wolff, Parkinson, and White [4] that curiosity was widely aroused concerning a syndrome characterized by intermittent QRS aberrancy and a short PR interval in young subjects prone to

[a] Harvey, W. "The Circulation of the Blood." Two anatomical lectures and nine letters written by him. Trans., K.J. Franklin, p. 97. Blackwell Scientific Publication, Oxford, 1958.

[b] Gaskell, W.H. Preface (First Issue), HEART, 1909.

[c] Keith A. From Cranefield, PF, "The Way In and Way Out," p. 1911. Correspondence reported in LANCET, Futura Publishing Company, New York, 1974.

paroxysmal tachycardia. They referred to the reports of other cases, including the early one with detailed observations on "vagal" effects by Wilson [5]. There is a prior paper with analogous data by Cohn and Fraser [6]. (Cohn had installed the first electrocardiograph in America; Fraser's later career has recently been outlined in a historical noted by Krikler [7].)

The term *preexcitation* utilized in this book was proposed by Öhnell [8] and has become a consensus preference to designate the presence of the anomalous ventricular excitation, whereby a portion of the ventricle is depolarized prior to any conduction through the AV (His) bundle. The phenomenon is essentially that of a fusion beat, with a short P-QRS interval and widened QRS, the latter being due to early potentials (or delta wave) in the latter part of the usual PR period. Wolff, Parkinson, and White had labelled the QRS aberration a functional bundle branch block, though noting that, theoretically, accelerated conduction through one of the bundle branches could produce the same effect.

The collaboration between Wolff, Parkinson, and White, insofar as publications reveal, was limited to the one paper, and the assignment of the principal credit for defining the syndrome initially is difficult. Though all beneficient, each had his own view of the role of his co-authors. Wolff [9] has ascribed to Parkinson a subsidiary role in the paper; in describing a trip taken by Paul White to Europe:

> In London, (Sir) John Parkinson's interest was aroused and he offered to look through his files in the hope of finding similar cases. He found three or four and graciously sent the material to be used for incorporation in our paper.

In 1939, when I was a student in London, I heard Dr. Parkinson say that he had already been interested in the syndrome and that Dr. White and he decided to collaborate rather than publish separately. He also had opined that others were aware of the syndrome and suggested prompt publication. Dr. Parkinson manifested delightful impish moments occasionally, and maybe he could have given me a minor distorted view of the events. However, it is no detraction from Dr. White's greatness to suggest he could also have pleasant self-inflationary periods.

The importance of the preexcitation syndrome with its associated tachycardia extends far beyond any challenges to the clinical electrocardiologist because it has constituted a natural model, wherein a circus movement, or macroreentry tachycardia, can be studied — with the physiological requirements to be defined and the response to pharmacological agents to be recorded. In this review, I have omitted discussion of the short PR interval with a QRS of normal duration although admitting the validity of a claim that this represents a form of early ("pre") excitation of the ventricle and that future studies may reveal the locus of the early activation.

One can identify ancient cases of preexcitation by reviewing papers having in their titles, the word "tachycardia." Some reports, indexed under "ventricular tachycardia" also, are clearly instances of atrial fibrillation with aberrant QRS complexes related to ventricular excitation over accessory pathways. For example, I believe Case IV of Gilchrist's series of paroxysmal ventricular tachycardia [10] had a wide QRS tachycardia related to an accessory pathway; likewise, the case of ventricular tachycardia and atrial fibrillation reported by Levine and Curtis [11]. I suspect also some of the cases reported by Wilson and associates [12] under the title of "A Clinical Type of Paroxysmal Tachycardia of Ventricular Origin in Which the Paroxysms Are Induced by Exertion" could have accessory pathways at the root of the problem. Cases of ventricular tachycardia (wide QRS with the same morphology of the preexcited QRS as when in sinus rhythm, and with intermittent AV dissociation in the sustained tachycardia) are extremely rare.

Morphological Basis

The study of preexcitation and associated arrhythmias mirrors the ages-old fascination with the relation between structure and function by scientists (or "natural philosophers"). Discoveries pertaining to the mechanisms of the animal body may either have their genesis in a study of structure or the observation of function. However, there has been always the compulsion to construct a structural model for any observed function; conversely, given the structure, there is a compulsion to determine the nature, if any, of its function.

The observations of Kent had an important bearing on the thinking of clinicians and electrophysiologists, some of whom have often used the eponym "Kent's bundle" for an accessory bundle which either caused anomalous early fractional ventricular excitation or completed the circus pathway in a tachycardia. Such mechanisms were first hypothesized and later documented electrophysiologically in selected cases.

I think that it is helpful to imagine oneself living before the turn of the century, confronted with the dilemma of how the mammalian ventricle regularly followed the atrial beat, despite there seeming to be a fibrous barrier separating the two. At this time also, the question of whether the heart beat was "neurogenic" or "myogenic" was still active. Two young men (born in the same year, 1863) were attracted by the problem and, in 1893, independently published their conclusions. The one, Stanley Kent [13,14] in England reported strands of muscle crossing the AV sulcus (he probably also saw part of the AV bundle); the other, Wilhelm His, Jr., a Swiss-born resident of Germany, gave a clear description of the AV bundle as we know it today [15]. The paper by His was more or less hidden in an obscure Leipzig journal and the findings were not well known until after Tawara's work on the AV node in Aschoff's laboratory, was published as a beautiful classic monograph, in 1906 [16]. Prior to the series of Kent's papers, Paladino had also reported atrial fibers descending over the AV values and ventricular fibers ascending into the same areas and making connections with the atria. The possible function of these fibers in AV valve closure and heart block was mentioned. Paladino has outlined his claim to priority and reviewed his earlier work in a subsequent paper which is readily available [17].

Kent's series of early reports to the Physiological Society were short and did not acquire high repute, particularly after Tawara's work on the AV node (1906) became widely known. A few years later, Keith and Flack re-examined the problem and published their observations on the connections between atria and ventricle in the mammal. Their report [18] was interpreted as giving the coup de grace to any physiologic importance of Kent's morphologic observations, and helped to establish the dogma that the AV bundle (of His) was the "sole" connection between these chambers. Kent, I suspect, was stung to return to study the connections again, seeming to focus on the assertion that the AV

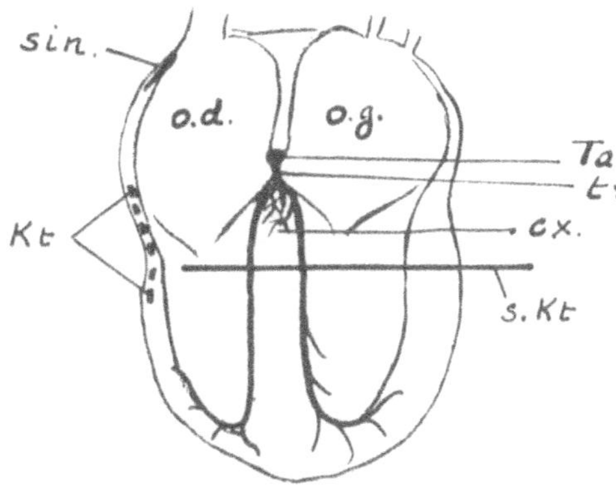

FIGURE 1–1. Schema of Mahaim, illustrating fibers from the lower His bundle and bundle branches entering the summit of the ventricular septum, Kt. Kent. SKT, experimental section described by Kent, with maintenance of AV conduction. Mahaim proposed that AV sequential beating was more likely to have been maintained by the central fibers than the proposed lateral bundle of Kent. By permission of the *Am. Heart J.*, 5: 297, 1932.

bundle was the "sole" connection. In a series of reports [19] to the Physiological Society in November, 1913, March and June, 1914, he made further claims for a "right lateral bundle" with a nodal structure at its atrial end, with results of experimentation on its conduction behavior. The illustration of this node appears in the June 27th abstract, and that such an anatomic structure can be seen is acknowledged by Anderson and Becker. Kent asserted that, in an experimental mammal, after a surgical incision resulting in a lateral band being the only connection remaining between atrial and ventricle, there could be conduction of the impulse in either direction, on electrical stimulation. This assertion strains one's credulity. [Curiously, Mahaim [20] suggested the results possibly were due to the incision being below early fibers being given off from the AV bundle to the top of the septum (Figure 1–1).]

Kent's name does not appear on the list of editorial collaborators when the journal HEART was launched in 1909, and this may reflect his status with Sir Thomas Lewis. Kent's work and reports have been critically reviewed by Mahaim [20], Öhnell [8], James [21], Lev [22], and Anderson and Becker [23] and found to be disappointing in anatomic detail. Despite these careful critiques, functioning AV connections at a distance from the AV node, conveniently called "Kent fibers," remained a popular explanation of preexcitation and an associated tachycardia. Morphologists were split into camps regarding the presence of "Kent fibers" in the human heart. Kent had emphasized that AV connections were more frequent in the hearts of newborns. This viewpoint was supported by the work of Truex, et al. [24] but not by that of Lev and Lerner [22].

A weakness in logic would seem present in the assertion of some authorities, viz., the equating of predictable consistent function with structure; when pointing out that fibers could be found *without* preexcitation and that preexcitation could be present *without* demonstrable muscular strands across the AV sulcus; ergo, such fasciculi could not be the cause of the preexcitation syndrome [25]. This view was later modified by these authors. The growth of knowledge concerning the role of accessory connections is reflected in the careful conclusions by Lev; in 1966 "The anatomic base of the Wolff-Parkinson-White syndrome is today unknown" [26], and 1973, "It would thus appear that from the morphologic standpoint there are two types of anatomic basis for the WPW syndrome" [27] (James, Mahaim, and Kent).

Wolff [9] has stated "the mechanism responsible for the abnormal electrocardiogram aroused our interest in 1928, and although the idea of a muscular bypass occurred to us, it seemed fanciful and unsupported by the facts available." I am emboldened to suggest that this viewpoint might be a concealed Lewis influence. The senior authors had both been long time acquaintances of Lewis, and knowledgeable regarding his work on QRS aberration and bundle branch block, and of his dismissal of Kent's observations as having any clinical importance. As a reflection on Kent's mature views, I suggest the reading of his lecture in 1914; "Some Problems in Cardiac Physiology" [28]. I think that it is regrettable that Kent did not show the courtesy to mention His by name in this review. There is also the second report of a committee of the British Association for the Advancement of Science, of Sherrington, Kent, and Buchanan, which endorses Kent's claims [29]. This would seem to have been prepared by Kent as secretary, a grave departure from scientific protocol, as already pointed out by others.

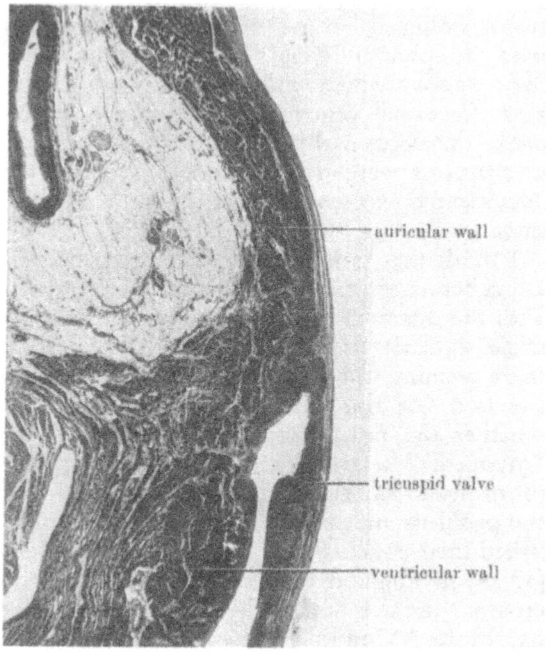

FIGURE 1–2. Illustration from Kent: observations on the auriculo-ventricular junction of the human heart, presumed to show continuity of myocardial fibers across the AV sulcus.

Kent's paper in the Quarterly Journal of Experimental Physiology in 1913 [30] is somewhat more definitive than the abstracts of his papers given to the Physiological Society and the illustration of the human heart (Figure 1–2) is supportive of his views. His first conclusion in this paper, "The muscular connection between the auricle and ventricle in the heart of man is not single and confined to the AV bundle but is multiple" is true. Wilhelm His, Jr., in his retirement, (a year or so before death from emphysema) wrote a review of the discovery of the AV bundle, acknowledging the work of Paladino and of Kent, giving the latter credit for having seen the AV bundle, or part of it. There is a scholarly translation of this paper and a biographical sketch of His by Bast and Gardner [31].

Kent's reports had given support to theoreticians searching for schema to explain anomalous preexcitation of the ventricle and for a basis for a circus movement of tachycardia. Independent of any preexcitation interests, Mines (32) had constructed a ring of atria and ventricle in the tortoise in which he could induce and stop a "circulating excitation" by electric stimuli (Figure 1–3). Proper credits to the background work of Garry and of Erlanger were given. Mines has written thus:

I ventured then to suggest that some instances of paroxysmal tachycardia observed in man where auricles and ventricles beat with the same frequency along somewhat similar lines ... Stanley Kent shows that an extensive muscular connexion is to be found at the right hand margin of the heart at the junction of the right auricle and right ventricle. Supposing for some reason, an impulse from the auricle reached the main AV bundle but failed to reach this "right" lateral connexion. It is possible that the ventricular end of this right lateral connexion not finding it refractory ... The wave spreading then to the auricle might be expected to circulate around the path indicated.

Years later (1927), in a review of the nature of "extrasystoles accumulies et des extrasystoles isolies," DeBoer [33] introduced the topic by mentioning two possible theories, that of the "circulating wave of excitation" and "parasystoles":

Pour expliquer chez l'homme la forme auriculoventriculaire de tachycardie parasystique, Mines and moi-meme avons attire l'attention sur le faisceau entra les orreilletes et les ventriculis.

The Wolff-Parkinson-White paper in 1930 was a challenge to electrocardiographers, stimulating them to reexamine the enigma with varied hypotheses offered to explain the syndrome. Some were immediately discomfited by the concept of a bundle branch block as a basic part of the syndrome; witness the reaction of Charles Wolferth, as recounted by Francis Wood in a recent letter to me:

Thanks for your letter of June 4th, the facts about the WPW are these: One morning I came to the office. Charlie Wolferth came over to my room full of excitement with the first paper of Wolff, Parkinson and White. He said, "Look ... Here is an EKG which is called Bundle Branch Block, and it can't be! When the EKG changes from the abnormal to normal, the distance from the beginning of P to the end of QRS doesn't change. It must be an early arrival of the impulse from the atrium and the ventricle." Then he said to me, "Go down to the library of the College of Physicians and see if you can find an article or two by A.F. Stanley Kent of Bristol who wrote about the time His described the AV bundle" ... "I found the articles by Kent, and Charlie put together the entire picture ... So it was Charlie's brain and my muscle." [Which resulted in the first paper by them (34).]

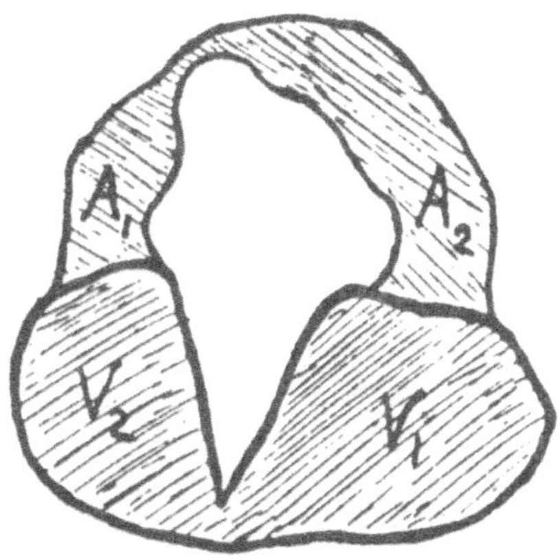

FIGURE 1–3. Reproduction of a drawing from Mines (1913), "On the Dynamic Equilibrium of the Heart," *J. Physiol.*, 46, page 372, (in the section on reciprocating rhythm and "circulating excitations.") "I devised another experiment which I carried out on the heart of a tortoise ... A longitudinal incision was then made extending through the anterior and posterior walls of the auricle and ventricle, so that the heart was converted into a ring ... A circulating excitation was observed ... The circumstances under which the phenomenon made its appearance was such as to produce slow conduction and a short refractory period. By its continuance, the circulating rhythm would tend to maintain these conditions, the conditions are easily upset by the occurrence of an extra systole and be reestablished by other extrasystoles."

In regard to the second paper [35], Wood states:

Later a physician friend of his (Wolferth's) from upstate had a patient with this EKG who died suddenly. I cut the AV sections and studied them ... and found three potential tracts along the right cardiac margin, again Charlie's brain and my muscle. ("A total of 2,897 sections were studied.")

In the paper the electrocardiogram includes one precordial lead. At that time this would be the "Wolferth lead" with large electrodes on the precordial and left scapular areas. The record would be the equivalent of "V_3" with reversal of polarity now generally used. The large delta wave is oriented to the left, upward and posteriorly and thus fits the location of the described accessory bundles (Figure 1–4).

David Scherf [36] had been shown tracings by Paul White during the latter's 1929 European trip and remembers that he had not recognized the phenomenon prior to this but that he remonstrated with Dr. White concerning a primary vagus action causation. Soon however, after careful study of a patient, he and Holzman [37], independently reached a conclusion akin to that of Wolferth, viz.:

Tätsachlich wurden von Kent Solche Muskelfaserzuge zwischen rechtem Vorhof und rechtem Ventrikel deschrieben, sie wurden von DeBoer zuer Erklarung paraxoysmaler auricularer Tachycardien herangezogen.

This paper appearing in the same year (1932) was appropriately referenced by Wolferth and Wood. The latters' illustration, reproduced here, shows the modern concept of the simplest form of preexcitation and of the associated circus movement tachycardia (Figure 1–5). In reply to a direct question by me, Wood has stated, "Yes, I drew those diagrams, but under Charlie Wolferth's careful direction."

The lucid explanations of Wood and Wolferth, and of Holzman and Scherf, were not convincing to everyone. I think this was partly because of the difficulties in finding further uniform morphological correlations, partly because some cases had tachycardia clearly of a different type and, partly because investigative data were offered supportive of another mechanism. In 1940, Parkinson with his senior registrar, Hunter, and a continental emigre, Papp [38], reviewed their accumulated cases and the varied hypotheses which had been offered to explain the syndrome. They were "inclined to think that the typical syndrome represented a double rhythm by two interfering pacemakers, one near the sinus and the other in one bundle branch."

Interfering also with the adoption of any unitarian hypothesis were the observations of Prinzmetal and associates [39] reporting at

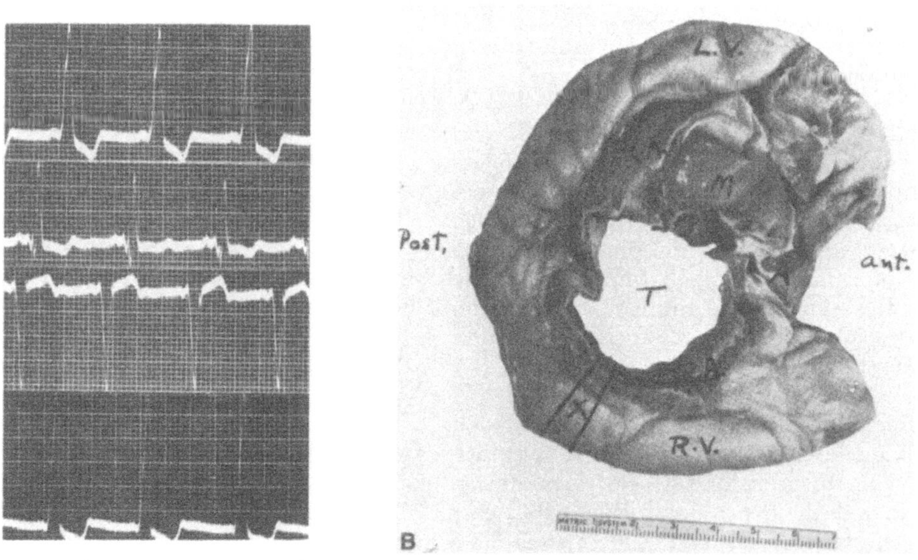

FIGURE 1–4. (A) Electrocardiogram of the patient, the victim of sudden death, in whom accessory bundles were found crossing the AV sulcus. (B) A sketch of the heart, to illustrate where the connections were found. The location of these connections fits with current predictive practices derived from the spatial orientation of delta wave. By permission of the *Am. Heart J.*

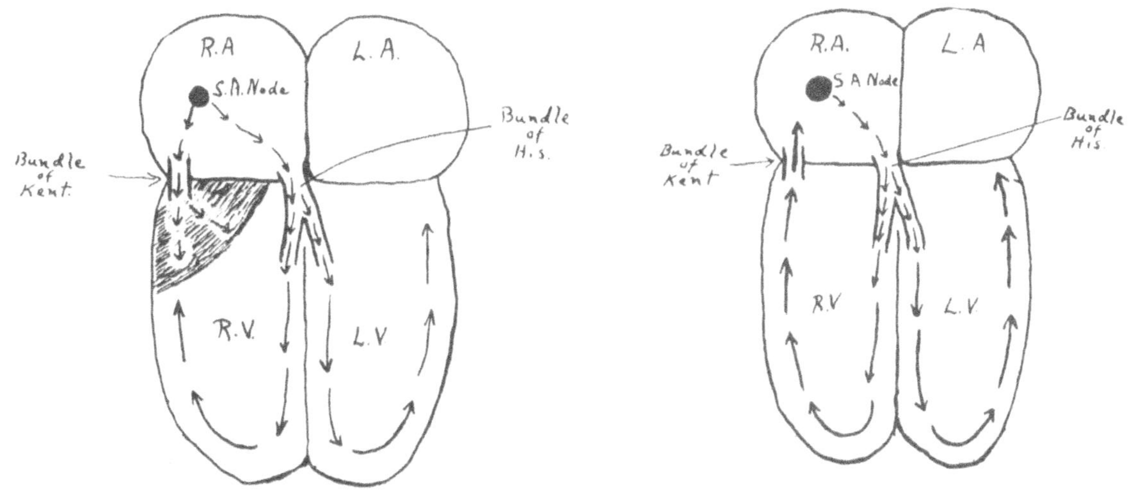

FIGURE 1–5. Diagrams drawn by Wood, reproduced from the paper of Wolferth's and Wood showing proposed mechanisms of preexcitation and of the circus movement tachycardia.
By permission of the *Am. Heart J.* and Dr. Wood.

length on the production of the preexcitation electrocardiogram experimentally; by mechanically, chemically, and electrically stimulating the summit of the ventricular septum. They espoused the view that there was accelerated conduction in one part of the AV node, which was expressed distally by a segmental contraction of the ventricle. In a seemingly analogous way, the appearance of aberrant QRS complexes immediately following the P wave, observed by Kossman et al. [40] and by many others, with a catheter in the right ventricle in the human heart, also supported the search for more than one etiologic substrate. Indeed, at this time, even in the isolated perfused dog heart, I observed intermittent preexcitation of the ventricle with the transient premature early activation of the right side of the septum [41].

Different varities of the preexcitation electrocardiograms, analyzed at the University of Michigan (1945) [42], engendered a classification of cases to A and B types, as derived from studies of unipolar body surface tracings. The classification was based mainly on the precordial leads; if delta and mean QRS vector were anteriorly oriented, "A"; if posteriorly oriented, "B." Esophageal records were particularly supportive to the concept of a posterior location of the accessory bundle in Type A. The large negative delta waves recorded in the esophageal lead just below the atrial border in some cases of the A type clearly reflected premature activation of the left ventricular basal area (Figure 1–6). As a beginning attempt to establish some order to the variety of electrocardiographic patterns, the 1945 report by Rosenbaum, et al. [42] represented a milestone, and it was soon followed by recordings of potentials within the heart (Figure 1–7) supporting the basic classification schema [43] (and later, 44,45).

Modern Electrophysiologic Beginnings

It was only after the introduction of sophisticated electrophysiologic mapping and programmed stimulation techniques that confidence in the explanations regarding the cause of the delta wave (preexcitation) and of the mechanisms of tachycardia evolved. The early accrued data were beautiful in their consistency and the measurements were often so precise and the localization of accessory pathways seemingly so exact, that any time-consuming morphologic confirmation seemed superfluous (even though still desirable). As years have passed, the realiza-

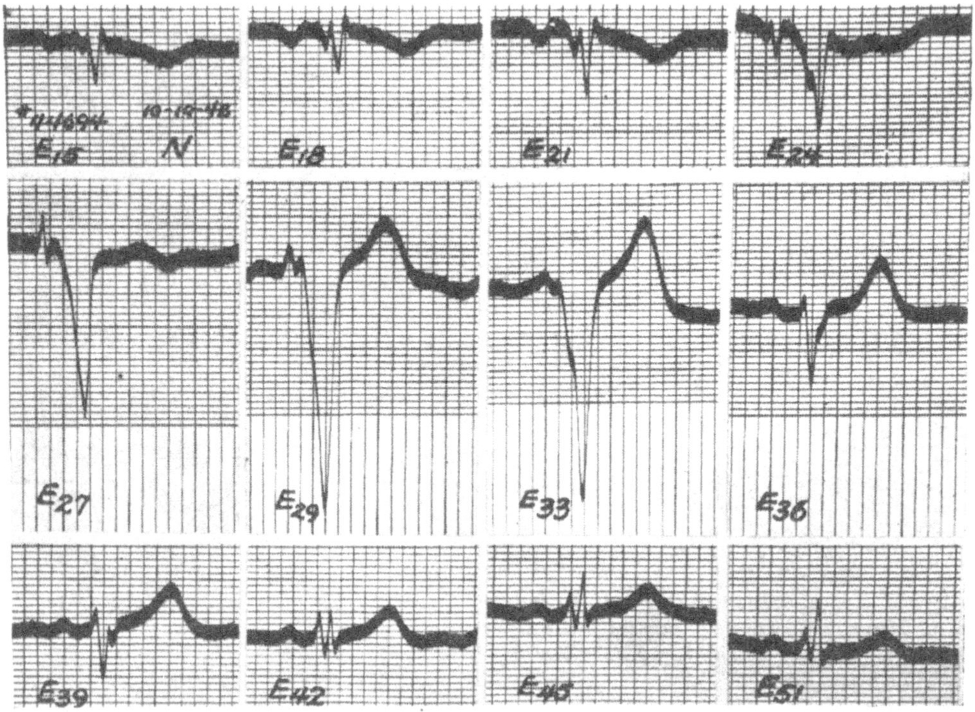

FIGURE 1–6. Reproduction of Figure 9 of the paper by Rosenbaum, et al. illustrating the large negative delta wave in the preexcitation syndrome in the type designated as A (see E_{29} in particular). By permission from the *Am. Heart J.*

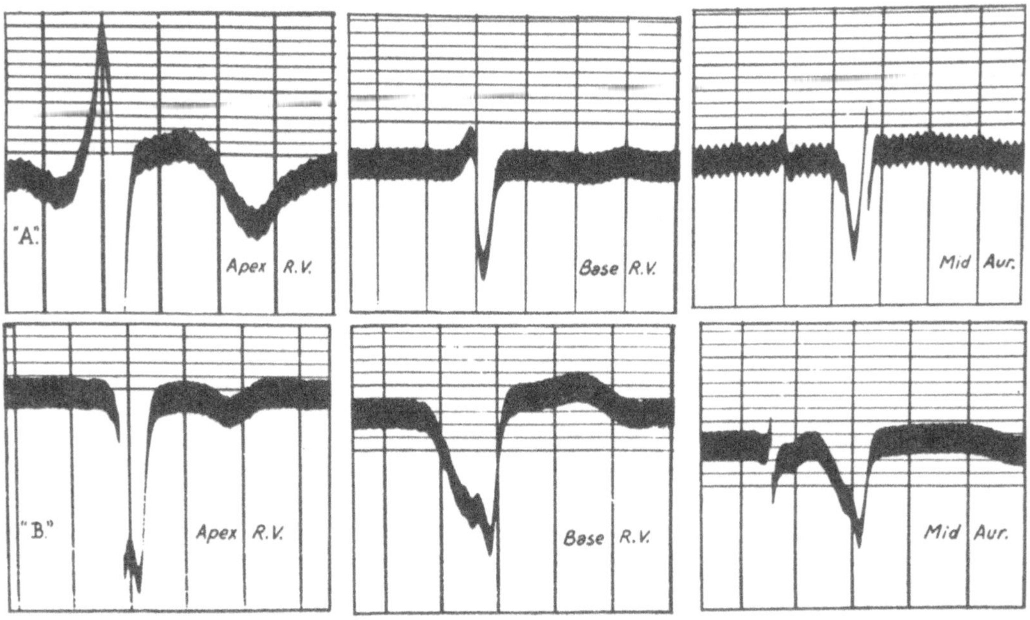

FIGURE 1–7. Early intracardiac leads in patients with preexcitation of two types: A and B. Hecht. H. By permission of the *Annals NY Acad. Sci.* 65:841, 1957.

tion that complex possibilities did exist has taught us to avoid any dogmatic posturing, particularly when varieties of septal pathways are suspect.

Pertinent to the teaching of a circus movement tachycardia, as conjured up with a lateral accessory connection, was a model built by Butterworth and Poindexter [46]. An "accessory pathway" was created by an electronic bridge from atrium to ventricle. By appropriate electronic delays, varied degrees of preexcitation, with delta waves in the animal's ECG were produced. Reversing the circuitry plan, the ventricular potential was used to stimulate the atrium; a tachycardia was produced with a normal QRS duration. This type of model was further developed, with advanced circuitry, by Moore and associates (1972) [47]. They demonstrated in the laboratory the potential risk of ventricular fibrillation, consequent to atrial fibrillation, with the appropriate conduction parameters across a bypass electronic tract.

Basic work with which I have been familiar occurred in the laboratory of Durrer in Amsterdam during the 1960s. Dirk Durrer's doctoral thesis in 1952 ("Experimenteel onderzack naar Het verloop van Het activate proces in der Hartspier") was on the activation of the heart, and mutual interests drew us together, establishing a friendship only terminated by his death in the past year. His work on ventricular excitation was early associated with explorations of the genesis of ventricular arrhythmias. He attracted dedicated young Dutchmen to work with him, and in the continuing elucidation of the preexcitation problem; Wellen's thesis [48] mirrors a milestone of progress. The key early papers from Durrer's laboratory pertaining to preexcitation, I suggest, are: "Epicardial Excitation of the Ventricles in a Patient with Wolff-Parkinson-White; Type B:" [49]. "The Role of Premature Beats in the Initiation and the Termination of Supraventricular Tachycardia in the Wolff-Parkinson-White syndrome" (1967) [50], and "Pre-Excitation Revisited" (1970) [51]. Having been shown some of these records prior to publication in 1967, I experienced a peak elation; the human heart with induced arrhythmias, behaving precisely as anticipated from theory, and in accord with the memories of the ancient experiments of Mines.

Concomitant with investigations of patients with arrhythmias associated with the preexcitation (WPW) syndrome, were advances in knowledge of how excitation and conduction were dependent upon transmembrane action potentials. The phenomena of reentry and slow conduction in isolated tissues, as explored by Cranefield, Wit, and Hoffman [52], in particular, afforded explanations for previously baffling clinical phenomena. Also, amongst the many physiologists with interest in the clinical implications of their research was Gordon Moe, my friend from his training period. His work on echo beats and parasystolic mechanisms has been a continuing stimulus and challenge to anyone who ever became satisfied with any status quo in our knowledge. His junior research associates have been many. An early key paper was entitled "Physiologic Evidence for a Dual AV Transmission" (1956) [53]. Pertinent to the preexcitation phenomena, de la Fuente, Sasyniuk, and he [54] presented electrophysiologic data on conduction through a narrow isthmus of atrial tissue, "A Model for the WPW Syndrome," which helped to explain the capricious nature of conduction through small accessory bundles. It also challenged any easy assumption that conduction characteristics might be used as absolute markers for different anatomic substrates of tissue.

Following the revolutionary electrophysiologic enlightenment from Durrer's laboratory, my associates and I had the opportunity to record at the right AV sulcus, with rather simple equipment, AV (when showing preexcitation) and, Ventriculoatrial (VA) (when in tachycardia with a normal QRS), rapid conduction [55]. The tachycardia repeatedly was stopped by pressure on a small area over the sulcus. The import of this study was, in particular, the rapid VA conduction during tachycardia. Further emphasis on the importance of mapping the atria during tachycardia in order to locate accessory connections soon came from many laboratories in increasingly more elegant studies. The field was wide open for the many investigators in the 1960s, and the popularization of the catheter technique for recording His Bundle activity in man (1969) from the report of Scherlag and associates [56] was overtly a boon for research teams. The "His Bundle Potential" gave a marker for the measurement of the AV node conduction time, and of the time of His bundle activation relative to the onset of the QRS. If a wide QRS complex had an onset prior to the recognizable "His Spike" some part of the ventricle must have been "preexcited" by some accessory connection bypassing the AV node–His route.

Many laboratories around the world took up the chase to define the varied mechanisms in reciprocating tachycardias. Early in solid accomplishments were those at Duke University, where the first successful cure of preexcitation with an associated life-threatening tachyarrhythmia was achieved by surgery [57]. The death of the second patient with arrhythmia in the early postoperative period must have had a chilling effect on the early program. The problems were reviewed after a five-year surgical experience [58]. In 1967, Dreifus, et al. [59] demonstrated that the paroxysms of tachycardia could be abolished by destruction of the AV nodal pathway with excitation of the ventricle possible over the accessory ("Kent") route. As they pointed out, this therapy would not prevent rapid ventricular rates with atrial flutter or fibrillation.

It has been a delight to observe how electrophysiological data fell neatly into place, to fit a schema of a macro reentry tachycardia when the accessory connections were across the AV sulcus at the free walls of the heart. The precise requirements for the initiation of tachycardia, dependent upon the relative refractory periods of the AV node–His and the accessory pathway, respectively, and timing of the electric stimulus within "the window" were particularly noteworthy. The rarer wide QRS tachycardia related to reversal of the usual direction of the circular excitation (antidromic in the His pathway) also soon became a documented event instead of an attractive hypothesis.

Special Problems Related to Central Accessory Connections

There can be no serious challenge to the authenticity of a gross circus movement tachycardia when there are accessory pathways on the right or left free wall of the heart. When, however, preexcitation and tachycardia are related to paranodal or septal accessory pathways, the mechanism is often not as neatly explainable and can engender controversy. It is not the failure of morphologists to come up with support for many types of bypass filaments in the septal area; indeed, when the electrophysiologist reaches out to diagram a tract which bypasses the AV node to enter the upper His bundle, or for one which bypasses the lower His bundle and main branches, he can find a profusion of possibilities in the anatomic reports [3].

In this volume, it was decided to minimize use of eponyms. While there is value in eponyms in giving credits to investigators, in stimulating students to read, and in facilitating scientific conversation when all are agreed on definitions, there are disadvantages as the communication may be inexact without it being realized. Thus, I espouse the recommendations of the Committee of the European Cardiologists on nomenclature [60]. However, I think the interested physician should remain facile in his cognition of "Kent's," "Mahaim's," "Öhnell's," "James'," and "Brechenmacher's" fibers.

Disease occurring in the complex nodal-His septal connections have been logically used to explain changing electrocardiographic patterns. One meticulous study correlating structure and function, changing with progressive disease, is that of Lev, et al. [61]. This study has been widely referenced, and the authors' interpretations generally accepted. However, one wonders what modern electrophysiologic studies at different stages of the conduction problem would have shown. I suspect that it may have been this careful study which primarily influenced James [62] as late as 1970, to caution the profession against any easy application of AV fibers of a "Kent" variety to explain preexcitation; viz., his concluding statement in his review:

> Based on present knowledge, it appears that most features of the W.P.W. syndrome in the most carefully studied cases can be best explained by abnormalities in structure and function of the AV node and His Bundle.

A further anatomic study supporting the role of Mahaim (nonventricular and fascicular-ventricular) fibers and James (intranodal bypass) fibers was published later from the same (Lev) laboratory [63], (18,600 sections being examined).

The many conundra related to septal pathways are covered in other chapters. From the historic viewpoint the connections described by Mahaim had been earlier noted also by His.

Although the latter's findings could not be confirmed by Cohn [69], they were readily identified by Lev [22]. The contention would be whether they established *functional* pathways into the top of the septum. It is now accepted that accessory bundles to the top of the ventricular septum do exist, as documented by anatomic, electrophysiologic, and surgical studies. When patients are studied by the usual electrodes to record His bundle potentials, there are also ventricular potentials recorded, which crudely reflect the time of activation of the ventricular septal summit. It has been long known that, normally, the summit of the septum is activated late relative to the lower septum. In most tracings showing preexcitation, the summit potentials begin at or before the time of RV apex activation, but in other instances these ventricular septal electrograms have shown large early deflections indicating preexcitation, though not indicative of its genesis [65–70]. These document an excitation pattern proposed by Durrer in his "Preexcitation Revisited" lecture [46]. In the one systematic retrospective analysis [70] of the ventricular septal summit potentials in cases at Stanford and the University of California wherein the location of the accessory bundle had been verified at surgery, it was concluded that in the occasional case the tracings could have good preoperative value for the location of the bundle. Similar records are readily discovered by review of the published records of patients with proven septal pathways, such as may be blocked mechanically by the cardiac catheter, as reported by Novick, et al. [66]. In a recent study, Prystowsky and associates [69] reported accessory pathway depolarization from a catheter electrode. The delta potentials are clearly illustrated to occur prior to activation of the right ventricular apex with a "spike" potential ("Kent") before the QRS onset. Prematurity of ventricular summit activation may be expected also in functioning His-ventricular or fasciculo-ventricular connections. It is noteworthy that the septal electrogram may be unaltered with the appearance and disappearance of a delta wave in the surface electrocardiograms, *when* there is a free wall accessory pathway, a splendid early example of which is in the paper by Castillo and Castellanos (their Figure 7) [71].

As yet we have few detailed studies of the complete pattern of ventricular activation in the varied preexcitation states, such as could be gathered by multiple contiguous plunge electrodes. The one study by Boineau and Moore [72] is an exception, showing right-sided ventricular *septal* activation with a right posterior pathway in a dog. The question whether in the human there is a "need to know" the minute details of activation arises; I think that interest in the topography of the preexcitation collision fronts would contribute to our knowledge and probably to our understanding of arrhythmias.

Observations on additional phenomena fitting theoretical predictions have been exciting events, such as the appropriate change in the cycle length of the tachycardia, with retrograde conduction in free wall accessory bundles, when ipsilateral bundle branch block developed [73]. The correlations between electrocardiographic analysis of preexcitation and mapping of atrial retrograde activation through the accessory pathway, with the surgical location of that pathway, have been reasonably good. Other observations of unique physiologic interest rapidly appeared such as recordings which supported a supranormal period of excitation of the accessory bundle [74], evidence of automaticity [75], and instances of slow conduction [76] or block [66] in the accessory bundle. Changes in the configuration of the P wave has long been noted to be occasionally associated with the appearance of a delta wave, now explained by a favored location of the atrial pacemaker affording early access to the accessory pathway. In one case of preexcitation with renal insufficiency, I have observed block in the accessory pathway whenever there was hyperkalemia. Concomitant with the floodtide of physiologic information, there has been a trickle of morphologic data, competing in uniqueness; for example, the accessory bundle found to be coursing over the mitral leaflet [77].

Mimicry, Pseudo-, and Acquired Preexcitation

Amongst the electrocardiographic records which simulate preexcitation QRS complexes are beats, sometimes in runs, of isochronic dissociation wherein the P wave immediately precedes an aberrant QRS. One variety is fairly frequently seen on the monitors in Coronary Care Units when there may be displayed a run of accelerated ventricular rhythm with a P wave just before the QRS. Examples of this phenomenon are illustrated in the monograph of Prinzmetal et al. [39]. This is a type of accrocharge in which, I believe, the atrial mechanical event "trips" the ventricular pacemaker. When a slowly developed delta wave does not characteristically initiate the QRS, one may require a number of tracings before one can be confident of the exact diagnosis.

In the routine reading of electrocardiograms, one encounters, on occasion, tracings with a short PR and grossly aberrant QRS, usually with a left bundle branch block configuration, which still engender perplexity. Particularly in the presence of overt ventricular disease and of premature ventricular contractions and/or ventricular tachycardia, one may not achieve certainity of diagnosis without an electrophysiologic study.

The question of whether preexcitation can be acquired is a moot one. I do not refer to the problem of a long latency before the expression of preexcitation. I do not believe that it can be claimed that preexcitation can be truly acquired, although mimicry can occur with left ventricular disease. Some cases of Fabry's disease have shortening of the PR interval over years (independent of rate or neurogenic effects) and if QRS aberration has developed, mimicry of the WPW complex can thus occur.

Electro-Mechanical Correlations

If a considerable portion of the ventricle is activated abnormally early, it has been long wondered whether this might be revealed in mechanical records. The initial approaches were guided by analogous studies on bundle branch blocks. Wilson [5] and Wolferth and Wood [34] in records of the jugular venous pulse revealed duplication of the C waves (Figure 1–8) con-

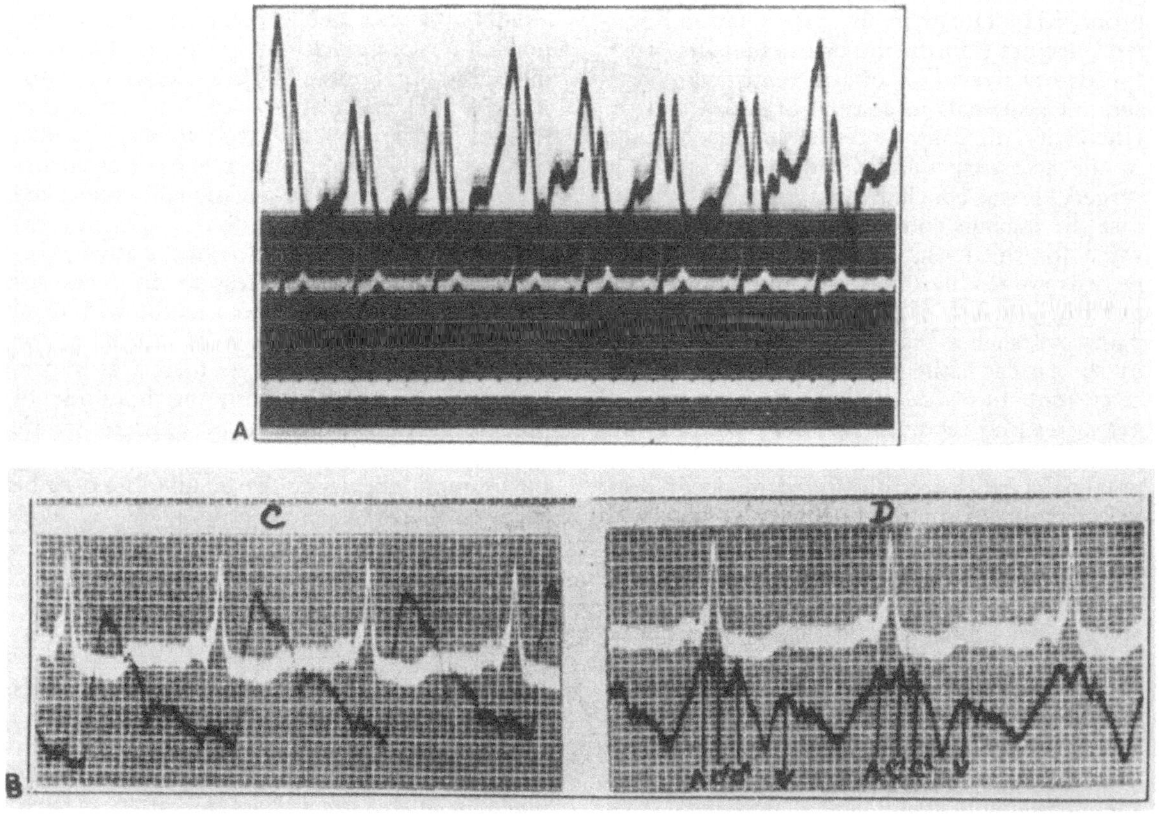

FIGURE 1–8. (A) Reproduction from a paper by Wilson et al. illustrating simultaneous jugular venous curves and electrocardiogram showing preexcitation. From *Arch. Int. Med.*, 16:1915. (B) A portion of an illustration from the paper of Wolferth and Wood showing the double "C" wave in the recording of the venous pulse with the electrocardiogram demonstrating preexcitation. By permission of the *Am. Heart J.*

sistent with ventricular asynchrony. Cardiac catheterization data such as published by Ferrer [78], Ishikawa [79], March, Selzer, and Hultgren [80] revealed different patterns dependent upon the preexcitation pattern. The data indicated that the electro-mechanical relationships were more complex than in bundle branch block; for instance, the left contraction parameters derived from noninvasive data in right-sided accessory pathway preexcitation differed from those of simple left bundle block.

The echocardiogram has allowed one to record local early movements of the ventricles in the preexcitation syndrome and a large body of literature is available. The findings based on M-Mode recordings are discussed in the texts on echocardiography. The nicest correlations are between posterior tracts and posterior left ventricular basal early twitches, and there may be associated early paradoxical septal movement. In the right free wall accessory pathways, early abnormal septal motion is not infrequently seen.

Association with Congenital Heart Defects

The earliest association clearly recognized of preexcitation with congenital heart disease was that with Ebstein's malformation, and the morphologic bases established [81]. One can make a strong case for electrophysiologic studies in any case prior to projected surgery for the hemodynamic faults. Preexcitation may be seen in patients with inversion of the ventricles (Corrected Transposition) and the anatomic substrate has been defined [82]. Other conditions where preexcitation is not uncommon is in hypertrophic cardiomyopathy and occasionally in mitral valve prolapse. In the latter instance, the click may be present with the preexcitaton complex, but not with the normal beat [83]. There is no reason to believe that the normal prevalence of preexcitation of an estimated 0.5% of the population would not pertain to the general spectrum of congenital and acquired heart disease. More extensive coverage of this aspect is presented in other chapters.

Management

The historic aspects of therapy with the use of drugs, new and old, by pacing techniques, by modern ablation techniques as well as direct surgical attack are discussed in other chapters. The algorithms which should guide the decision processes for care in different presentations of cases are important in order to develop uniformity of opinion regarding exact approaches, but complete agreement is not to be expected as yet. Amongst the exotica et curiosae of the syndrome is the report that a patient was able to control the heart rate and presence of preexcitation by biofeedback training [84]. There are also multiple problems of advising patients of insurance risks, evaluation, or the occupational hazards as with pilot training present over the decades [85,86].

Summary

The electrocardiographic abnormality of QRS aberration with a short P-QRS (PR) has occupied the attention of many investigators (physicians, surgeons, scientists, engineers) for the past fifty years. Brought to the attention of the profession by Wolff, Parkinson, and White in 1930, with an association of paroxysmal tachycardia, it was established as a definite syndrome. From what I distill from the literature and my acquaintance with them, Paul White was the ferment which just over a half a century ago, activated a life-long interest of Parkinson, of Wolferth, and of Scherf in the syndrome. That the condition was associated with an accessory connection, bypassing the AV node quickly became the favorite explanation of many investigators. A healthy controversy regarding the prevalence and locations of the connections has been of long duration, viz., those across the AV sulcus to the free wall of the right and left ventricle, or those proximate to the AV node and AV (His) bundle. The contributions of Kent afforded the early theoretical explanations and I believe they were helpful despite the vagueness of his descriptions and the exaggerated claims in his conclusions. While the free wall connections result in phenomena readily visualized, septal accessory connections are often less readily diagramed with exactitude and confidence, despite the sometimes clear conclusions reached from electrophysiologic studies. Each case of preexcitation, while readily fitted to a particular pattern, has usually some unique features, thus accounting in part for the plethora of the continuing reports. The basic scientific explanations should not become stagnant dogma, as Cranefield has implied in his foreword to Ferrer's book [87].

The preexcitation syndrome has afforded a model whereby tremendous strides have been made in the understanding of circus (reentry) tachycardias, and the responses of cardiac tissues to drugs. The cure of life-threatening conditions has been accomplished by surgical treatment or destruction of the accessory connection by less invasive means. The riddles of almost infinite expressions of preexcitation can be predicted to offer an ever-continuing opportunity for study for electrophysiologists and clinical investigators and challenges to their acumen as physicians.

References

1. Einthoven W: The string galvanometer and measurement of the action currents of the heart. Nobel Lecture – Physiology or Medicine, 1965. pp. 94–112. Elsevier Publication.
2. Lewis T: Paroxysmal tachycardia; the result of ectopic impulse formation. *Heart* 1:262, 1910.
3. Anderson RH, Becker AE, Tranum-Jensen J, Janse MJ: Anatomic electrophysiological correlations in the conduction system. *Br. Heart J.*, 45:67, 1981.
4. Wolff L, Parkinson J, White PD: Bundle branch block with short PR interval in healthy young people prone to paroxysmal tachycardia. *Am. Heart J.*, 5:685, 1930.
5. Wilson FN: A case in which the vagus influenced the form of the ventricular complex of the electrocardiogram. *Arch. Int. Med.* 16:1008, 1915.
6. Cohn AE and Fraser FR: Paroxysmal tachycardia and the effect of stimulating the vagus nerves by pressure. *Heart* 4:93, 1913–1914.
7. Krikler D: Wolff-Parkinson-White Syndrome. Long follow-up and an Anglo-American note. *J. Am. Coll. Cardiol.* 2:1216, 1983.
8. Öhnell RF: Pre-excitation — a cardiac abnormality. *Acta Med. Scand.* (Suppl) Vol. 152:1, 1944.
9. Wolff L: Anomalous atrioventricular excitation. The clinical entity. The electrophysiology of the heart. *Ann. N.Y. Acad. Sci.* 828, 1957.
10. Gilchrist AR: Paroxysmal ventricular tachycardia. *Am. Heart J.* 1:546, 1926.
11. Levine SA and Curtis AN: A case of ventricular tachycardia and atrial fibrillation. An unusual problem in therapy. *Am. Heart J.* 1:413, 1925–1926.
12. Wilson FN, Wishart SW, MacLeod AG, Barker PS: A clinical type of paroxysmal tachycardia of ventricular origin in which the paroxysms are induced by exertion. *Am. Heart J.* 8:155, 1932–1933.
13. Kent AFS: Researches on the structure and function of the mammalian heart. *J. Physiol.* 14:233, 1893.
14. Kent AFS. (as secretary): The structure and function of the mammalian heart. Committee: Shäfer, Sherrington, Kent. *Brit. Assoc. Adv. Sci.* 464, 1894.
15. His RJ: (Trans. Bast TH, Gardner WD) The activity of the embryonic human heart and its significance for the understanding of the heart movement in the adult. *J. Hist. Med. Allied Sci.* 4:289, 1949.
16. Tawara S: Des Reizleitung des Sangetierherzens Jena, Fischer. Eine anatomischhistologische studie über das atrioventrikular bundel und die Purkinjeschen Fäden. 1906.
17. Paladino G: Une question de priorite sur les rapports intimes entre 1a musculature des oreillettes et celle des ventricles du coeur. *Arch. Ital. Bul.* 53:47, 1910.
18. Keith A and Flack M: The form and nature of the muscular connections between the primary division of the vertebrate heart. *J. Anat. Physiol.* 41:172, 1907.
19. Kent AFS: The structure of cardiac tissues at the auricular ventricular junction. Proceedings of the Physiological Society. *J. Physiol.* 47:XVII, 48, IXII, 1913.
20. Mahaim I: Kent's fibers and AV paraspecific conduction through upper connections of the bundle of His-Tawara. *Am. Heart J.* 33:651, 1947.
21. James TN: The development of ideas concerning the conduction system of the heart. *Ulster Med. J.* 51:1982.
22. Lev M and Lerner R: The theory of Kent. A histological study of the normal atrioventricular communications of the human heart. *Circulation* 12:176, 1955.
23. Anderson RH and Becker AE: Stanley Kent and accessory atrioventricular connections. *J. Thorac. Cardiovasc. Surg.* 81:649, 1981.
24. Truex RC, Bishop JK, Hoffman EL: Accessory atrioventricular muscle bundles of the developing human heart. *Anat. Record.* 131:45, 1958.
25. Lev M, Kennamer R, Prinzmetal M, de Mesquite QH: A hisopathologic study of two hearts with the Wolff-Parkinson-White Syndrome. *Circulation* 24:41–50, 1961.
26. Lev M: Anatomic considerations of anomalous AV pathways. Mechanisms and Therapy of Cardiac Arrhythmias. Eds. Dreifus LS, Likoff W, Moyer JH. Grune and Stratton, New York, 1961, pp. 665–670.
27. Lev M: Anatomic considerations of the Wolff-Parkinson-White Syndrome. In: Cardiac

Arrhythmias. Eds. Dreifus LS, Likoff W. Grune and Stratton, New York, 1973, pp. 417–419.

28. Kent AFS: Some problems in cardiac physiology. *Brit. Med. J.* II:105, 1914.
29. Kent AFS: Committee Report (Sherrington, Kent, Buchanan). Report of British Association for Advancement of Science, 1915, p. 226.
30. Kent AFS: Observations on the auriculo-ventricular junction of the human heart. *Quart. J. Exp. Physiol.* 7:193, 1913.
31. His, Wilhelm, Jr: (Trans. by Bast and Gardner) The story of the atrioventricular bundle with remarks concerning embryonic heart activity. *J. Hist. Med. Allied Sci.* 4:319, 1919.
32. Mines GR (Trans., Third Series): On circulating excitations in heart muscle and their possible relations to tachycardia and fibrillation. *Royal Soc. Canad. Proc.* 8:43, 1914.
33. DeBoer S: Nature et origine des Extrasystoles accumulees et des extrasystolees. *Arch. Mal Coeur* 20:282, 1927.
34. Wolferth CC and Wood FC: The mechanism of production of short PR intervals and prolonged QRS complexes in patients with presumably undamaged hearts: Hypothesis of an accessory pathway of auriculoventricular conduction (Bundle of Kent). *Am. Heart J.* 8:297, 1932–1933.
35. Wood FC, Wolferth CC, Geckler CC: Histological demonstration of accessory muscular connection between auricle and ventricle in a case of short PR interval and prolonged QRS. *Am. Heart J.* 25:454, 1943.
36. Scherf D: A Cardiologist Remembers. *Persp Biol Med.* 11:614, 1967.
37. Holzman M and Scherf D: Über Elektrokardiogramme met verkürzter Vorhof-Kammer Distanz und positiven P Zachen. *Ztschr. Klin. Med.* 121:414, 1932.
38. Hunter A, Papp C, Parkinson J: The syndrome of short PR interval apparent bundle branch block and associated paroxysmal tachycardia. *Br. Heart J.* 2:107, 1940.
39. Prinzmetal M, Kennamer R, Corday E, Osbourne JA, Field J, Smith LA: Accelerated Conduction. The Wolff-Parkinson-White syndrome and related conditions. Mod Med Monographs. Grune and Stratton, New York, 1952.
40. Kossman CE, Berger AR, Rader B, Brumlick J, Donnelly JH: Anomalous atrioventricular excitation produced by catheterization of normal human hearts. *Circulation* 1:902, 1950.
41. Burchell HB: Ventricular pre-excitation in the isolated perfused heart. *Am. J. Physiol.* 169:721, 1952.
42. Rosenbaum FF, Hecht HH, Wilson FN, Johnson FD: The potential variation of the thorax and the esophagus in anomalous atrioventricular excitation. *Am. Heart J.* 29:281, 1945.
43. Hecht HH: Further observations on the spread of ventricular excitation. Anomalous atrioventricular excitation. The electrophysiology of the heart. *Ann. N.Y. Acad. Sci.* 65:841, 1957.
44. Sodi Pallares D, Soberon J, Thomsen P, Fishleder BL, Estandia A: Contribucion al estudio del Sindrome de WPW por las derivaciones intracavitarias. *Arch. Instit. Cardiol. Mex.* 8:1, 1948.
45. Castellanos A, Agha AS, Castillo CA, Myerburg RJ: Ventricular activation in the presence of the Wolff-Parkinson-White syndrome. In: Cardiac Arrhythmias. Eds. Dreifus LS, Likoff W. Grune and Stratton, New York, 1973, pp. 457–465.
46. Butterworth JS, Poindexter CA: Short PR interval associated with a prolonged QRS complex — a clinical and experimental study. *Arch. Int. Med.* 69:437, 1942.
47. Moore EN, Spear JR, Boineau JP: Electrophysiologic studies on preexcitation in the dog using an electronically simulated atrioventricular pathway. *Circ. Res.* 31:174, 1972.
48. Wellens HJJ: Electrical stimulation of the heart in the Study and Treatment of Tachycardias. University Park Press. Baltimore, Maryland, 1971.
49. Durrer D, Roos JP: Epicardial excitation of the ventricles in a patient with Wolff-Parkinson-White (Type B). *Circulation* 35:15, 1967.
50. Durrer D, Schoo L, Schuilenburg RM, Wellens HJJ: The role of premature beats in the initiation and the termination of supraventricular tachycardia in Wolff-Parkinson-White syndrome. *Circulation* 36:644, 1967.
51. Durrer D, Schuilenberg RM, Wellens HJJ: Pre-Excitation Revisited. *Am. J. Cardiol.* 25:690, 1970.
52. Wit AL, Hoffman BF, Cranefield PF: Slow conduction and reentry on the ventricular conduction system, I and II. *Circ. Res.* 30:1, 1972.
53. Moe GK, Preston JB, Burlington J: Physiologic evidence for dual AV transmission system. *Circ. Res.* 4:357, 1956.
54. de la Fuente D, Sasyniuk B, Moe G: Conduction through a narrow isthmus of isolated canine atrial tissue. A mode of the WPW syndrome. *Circulation* 44:803, 1971.
55. Burchell HB, Frye RL, Anderson MW, McGoon DC: Atrioventricular and ventriculoatrial excitation in Wolff-Parkinson-White syndrome. (Type B). *Circulation* 36:663, 1967.
56. Scherlag BJ, Lau SA, Helfant RH, Berkowtiz WD, Stein E, Damato AN: Catheter technique for recording His bundle activity in man. *Circulation* 39:13, 1969.
57. Cobb FR, Blumenschein SD, Sealy WC, Boineau JP, Wagner GS, Wallace AG: Successful surgical

interruption of the bundle of Kent in a patient with WPW syndrome. *Circulation* 38:1018, 1968.
58. Gallagher JJ, Gilbert M, Svenson RH, Sealy WC, Kasell J, Wallace AG: The problem, the evaluation and surgical correction. *Circulation* 51:767, 1975.
59. Dreifus LS, Nichols H, Morse D, Watanbe Y, Truex RC: Control of recurrent tachycardia of Wolff-Parkinson-White syndrome by surgical ligation of the AV bundle. *Circulation* 38:1030, 1968.
60. Anderson RH, Becker AE, Brechenmacher C, Davies MJ, Rossi L: Ventricular preexcitation, a proposed nomenclature for its substrates. *Eur. J. Cardiol.* 3:27, 1975.
61. Lev M, Leffler WB, Landendorf R, Pick A: Anatomic findings in a case of ventricular preexcitation (WPW) termination in complete atrioventricular block. *Circulation* 34:718, 1966.
62. James TN: The Wolff-Parkinson-White Syndrome — Evolving concepts of its pathogenesis. *Prog. Cardiovasc. Dis.* 13:159, 1970–1971.
63. Lev M, Fox SM, Bharati S, Greenfield JC, Rosen KM, Pick A: Mahaim and James fibers as a basis for a unique variety of ventricular preexcitation *Am. J. Cardiol.* 36:880, 1975.
64. Cohn AE: On the auriculo-nodal junction. *Heart*, 1:167, 1909.
65. Coumel P, Waynberger M, Fabiato A, Slama R, Aigueperse J, Bouvrain Y: Wolff-Parkinson-White Syndrome — Problems in the evaluation of multiple accessory pathway and surgical therapy. *Circulation* 45:1216, 1972.
66. Novick TL, Pritchett ELC, Campbell RWF, Rogers GC, Wallace AG, Gallagher JJ: Temporary catheter induced block in accessory pathways. *Circulation* 58:932, 1978.
67. Ward DE, Camm AS, Spurrell RAJ: Ventricular preexcitation due to anomalous nodal-ventricular pathways. Report of three patients. *Eur. J. Cardiol.* 9:111, 1979.
68. Gallagher JJ, Smith WM, Kasell JH, Benson DW, Sterba R, Grant AO: Role of Mahaim fibers in cardiac arrhythmias in man (see Figure 10). *Circulation* 64:176, 1981.
69. Prystowsky EN, Browne KF, Zipes DP: Intracardiac recording by catheter electrode of accessory pathway depolarization. *J. Am. Coll. Cardiol.* 1:468, 1983.
70. Mitchell LB, Mason JW, Scheinman MM, Winkle RA, Burchell HB: Recordings of basal ventricular pre-excitation from electrode catheters in patients with accessory atrioventricular connection. *Circulation* 69:233, 1984.
71. Castillo CA, Castellanos A: His bundle recordings in patients with reciprocating tachycardias and Wolff-Parkinson-White syndrome. *Circulation* 42:271, 1970.
72. Boineau JP, Moore EN: Evidences for propagation of activation across an accessory atrioventricular connection in Type A and B preexcitation. *Circulation* 41:375, 1970.
73. Broughton A, Gallagher JJ, German LD, Guarnieri T, Trantham JL: Differentiation of septal from free wall accessory pathway location: Observations during bundle branch block in reciprocating tachycardia in the presence of Type I antiarrhythmic drugs. *Am. J. Cardio.* 52:751, 1983.
74. McHenry PL, Knoebel SB, Fisch C: The Wolff-Parkinson-White syndrome with supranormal conduction through anomalous by-path. *Circulation* 34:734, 1966.
75. Przybyliski S, Chiale PA, Halpern S, Lazzari JO, Elizari MV, Rosenbaum MB: Existence of automaticity in anomalous bundle of Wolff-Parkinson-White. *Br. Heart J.* 40:672, 1978.
76. Rosen KM, Lopez-Arostigue F, Pouget JM: Preexcitation with normal PR intervals — a case secondary to slow Kent bundle conduction. *Chest* 62:581, 1972.
77. Gottlieb AL, Chan M, Palmer WH, Huang SN: Ventricular preexcitation syndrome accessory left AV connection and rhabdomyomatous myocardial fibers. *Arch. Pathol. Lab. Med.* 101:486, 1977.
78. Ferrer MI, Harvey RM, Weiner HM, Cathcart RT, Cournand A: Hemodynamic studies in two cases of Wolff-Parkinson-White syndrome with paroxysmal AV nodal tachycardia. *Am. J. Med.* 6:725, 1949.
79. Ishikawa H, Kagoshima T, Hasegawa S, Hoshika Y, Hiroshige Y, Takeshi Y, Yamamoto T, Kigawa Y: Wolff Parkinson-White syndrome mechano-cardiographic study on the mechanical consequences of ventricular preexcitation. *Am. Heart J.* 90:35, 1975.
80. March H, Selzer A, Hultgren HN: Mechanical consequences of anomalous atrioventricular excitation (WPW syndrome). *Circulation* 23:582, 1961.
81. Lev M, Gibson S, Miller RA: Ebstein's disease with Wolff-Parkinson-White syndrome. *Am. Heart J.* 49:729, 1955.
82. Bharati S, Rosen K, Steinfield L, Miller RA, Lev M: Anatomic substrate for preexcitation in corrected transposition. *Circulation* 62:831, 1980.
83. Bjerregaard P, Peterson EL: Letter to Editor. *Circulation* 56:137, 1977.
84. Bleeker EF, Engel BT: Learned control of cardiac rate and cardiac conduction in the Wolff-Parkinson-White syndrome. *New Engl. J. Med.* 288:560, 1973.
85. Averill KH, Fosmoe RJ, Lamb LE: Electrocardiographic findings in 67,375 asymptomatic individuals. Part IV. The Wolff-Parkinson-White

syndrome. First International Symposium on Cardiology in Aviation. School of Aviation Medicine. Brooks Air Force Base, Texas, 1959, p. 205.
86. Ward D: Ventricular preexcitation. The First United Kingdom Workshop in Aviation Cardiology. *Eur. Heart. J.* 5 (Suppl A):119, 1984.
87. Cranfield P (Foreword): In: Ferrer ML, *Pre-Excitation* (including Wolff-Parkinson-White and other related syndrome, pp. VII–XI). Futura Publishing Company, 1976. New York.

2. DEVELOPMENTAL ASPECTS AND NATURAL HISTORY OF PREEXCITATION SYNDROMES

Ann Dunnigan

As reviewed in the preceding chapter by Howard Burchell, our knowledge of preexcitation syndromes began retrospectively with the anatomic descriptions of Kent [1]. However, many years passed before a clinical application [2] and even longer before a functional–morphologic correlation [3–5] was made for these structures. Subsequently, morphologic descriptions of other potential substrates (i.e. nodoventricular connections, atriofascicular tracts, etc.) for ventricular preexcitation have also been made (Figure 2–1) [6–10].

Following the observation that critically timed electrical stimulation could initiate reentrant tachycardia, and with the advent of intracardiac catheter studies, our understanding of the functional characteristics of structures resulting in preexcitation has increased rapidly. Additionally, there has been an effort to explain electrophysiologic abnormalities in some patients based on anatomic structures observed in other patients. In only a few reports have ECG or electrophysiologic observations and cardiac morphology been compared in the same patient, and it is important to note that with one exception [11] all of these patients had accessory atrioventricular (AV) connections [3–5, 11–16]. No similar functional–morphologic studies exist for the less common types of accessory connections or bypass tracts illustrated in Figure 2–1.

From the Department of Pediatrics (Pediatric Cardiology), Variety Club Heart Hospital, University of Minnesota, Minneapolis, Minnesota. This work supported in part by the Dwan Family Fund.

The paucity of structural–functional correlation in patients with preexcitation syndromes has made extrapolation from developmental anatomic observations to electrophysiologic (functional) findings more tenuous. Thus, our understanding of the developmental and natural history aspects of accessory connections is incomplete. Several factors may account for our limited understanding of the embryology and natural history of preexcitation syndromes. Perhaps the most important of these factors is the lack of a readily available, naturally occurring animal model. Although Boineau and Moore [17] and Boineau et al. [18] reported electrophysiologic and anatomic observations in both a dog and a squirrel monkey with preexcitation, the occurrence of preexcitation in animals appears to be rare. Second, the meticulous, time-consuming examination necessary to locate accessory connections microscopically [19] has limited this analysis to only a few specialized centers. Third, since morphologic assessment of accessory connections cannot be performed serially in the same patient, present understanding is based almost exclusively upon studies assessing the presence or absence of accessory connections in fetuses, infants, children, and adults at a single point in time. Fourth, longitudinal clinical studies have

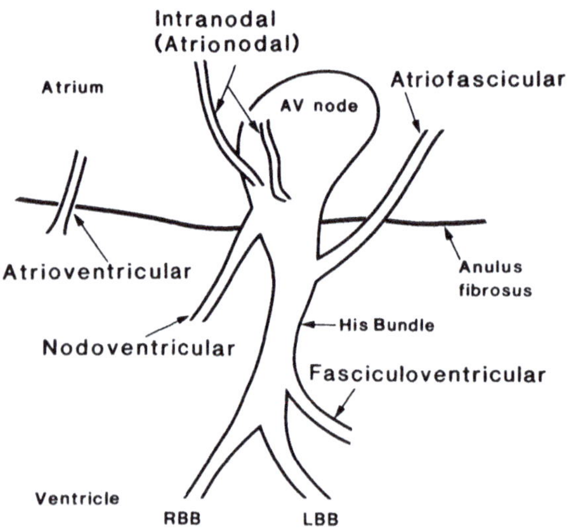

FIGURE 2-1. Diagrammatic representation of accessory connections and bypass tracts discussed in this chapter and elsewhere in this volume. Terminology is modified from Anderson et al. [7].

usually restricted themselves to evaluation of the presence or absence of either preexcitation in sinus rhythm on serial ECGs or clinically apparent tachycardia, over a relatively short (less than 10 year) period of time. Only rarely have serial electrophysiologic studies been performed to assess functional capabilities of accessory connections in patients [20,21]. Thus, a fundamental question is: What happens to accessory connections following birth? While some studies have supported the view that accessory connections may become nonfunctional over time, results in many cases have suggested that in certain patients the accessory connections maintain their functional capacity over decades [22].

Given the limitations of available studies, this chapter will review present concepts of the development of accessory connections and their natural history. Accessory AV connections will be the principal focus of attention because their functional-morphologic features have been most extensively defined.

Embryology of Normal and Accessory Cardiac Conduction Tissue

Details of the embryologic development of the normal fetal cardiac conduction system have been well described by Anderson et al. [23]. During early cardiac development, there is direct physical continuity between the atrial and ventricular myocardium. This physical continuity, and, by implication, electrical continuity, is normally lost along the lateral cardiac aspects by ingrowth of AV sulcus tissue and formation of the anulus fibrosus (Figure 2-2). During atrial and ventricular septal development, AV muscular continuity is also lost by formation of the anulus fibrosus, except in the region of the His bundle.

Defects in the anulus fibrosus are frequently present in term infants [23,24]. This observation has led to the concept that persistance of these defects permits AV continuity and thereby provides the anatomic basis of preexcitation [25]. Additionally, remnants of conducting tissue connecting the AV node to the ventricular myocardium may be present in the term infant or adult heart [23]; anatomically, they are referred to as accessory nodoventricular (nodofascicular) connections. However, the temptation to assume every anatomic structure has electrophysiologic function must be resisted, as demonstrated by Janse et al. [26], who argued the importance of establishing functional correlation for anatomic or pathologic observations. These authors studied electrophysiologic properties and anatomic appearance of AV conduction in a fetus of 12 weeks' gestation. Using programmed electrical stimulation, they demonstrated normal (mature) AV nodal, atrial, and ventricular refractory periods in the fetal heart. However, histologically there were defects in the anulus fibrosus, suggesting the presence of accessory AV connections, and multiple insertions from the AV node into the ventricular myocardium, compatible with accessory nodoventricular connections. Thus, anatomically present accessory connections had no functional significance. Therefore, the importance of utilizing caution in extrapolating from morphologic findings to functional characteristics cannot be overemphasized.

Morphologic Observations

With an awareness in mind of the potential shortcomings of anatomic studies, a review of the available morphologic data for accessory AV connections is appropriate. In 1958, Truex and co-workers [27] evaluated serial sections through the AV junctions in six fetuses (age

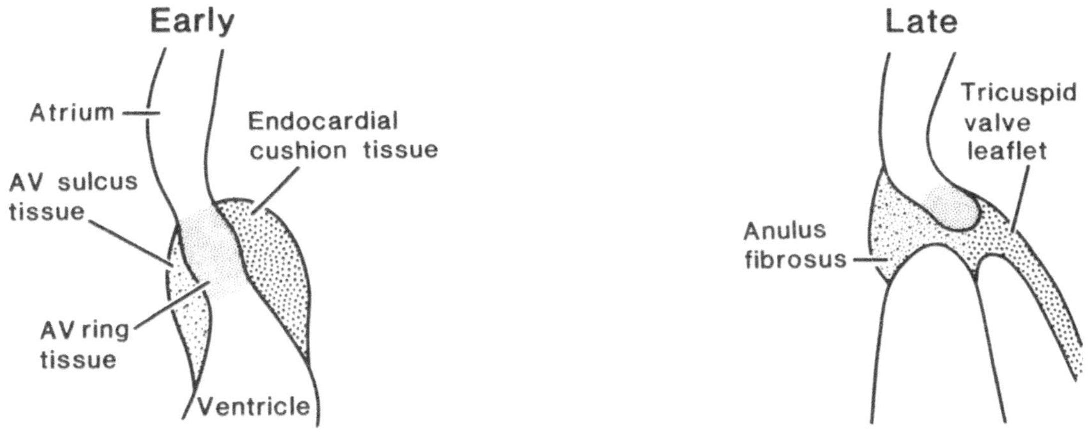

FIGURE 2–2. Proposed sequence of AV separation and development of the anulus fibrosus. On the *left*, during early cardiogenesis, there is physical, and by implication electrical, continuity between the primitive atria and ventricles. The *right* panel illustrates a later phase of cardiogenesis, following formation of the anulus fibrosus by ingrowth of AV sulcus tissue. At this time, the atria and ventricles are electrically isolated except for the His bundle.

four to nine months' gestation) and nine infants (age two days to three years). These workers demonstrated accessory muscular connections between the right atrium and either the anterior or posterior right ventricle in both prenatal and postnatal specimens. All accessory AV connections demonstrated were in infants less than six months of postnatal age, suggesting that final separation of the right atrium from the right ventricle may occur as part of normal post-natal development.

Defects in the anulus fibrosus may explain the subendocardial position of accessory AV connections around the tricuspid valve. However, accessory AV connections on the left side of the heart (i.e., around the mitral valve) have not usually been associated with defects in the anulus fibrosus [11]. The latter observation and the fact that left-sided connections are usually subepicardial, rather than subendocardial, support the view that their origin differs from right-sided accessory connections [11] (Figure 2–3).

Most accessory AV connections are thought to be composed of ordinary myocardium [19], but Anderson et al. [6] have demonstrated the presence of histologically distinct, cholinesterase-positive specialized AV ring tissue in fetuses, infants and adult hearts, and they have proposed that this may represent conduction tissue. In the fetuses, this specialized tissue was in contact with the ventricular myocardium, while in the infants and adults, remnants of this specialized tissue were still present around both the mitral and tricuspid valves, but contact with the ventricular myocardium and presumably any possible functional significance had been lost. These authors postulate that in some situations the persistance of specialized AV ring tissue in contact with ventricular myocardium might be capable of ventricular preexcitation [6]. What has been clearly demonstrated by Anderson et al. [6] is that during cardiac development, connections between atrium and ventricle, other than the His bundle, normally regress.

Accessory AV connections are very common in certain congenital heart defects (see Chapter 14). For example, accessory AV connections have been demonstrated both morphologically [13,14] as well as functionally [13,28] in patients with Ebstein's anomaly of the tricuspid valve with both normal and inverted ventricles (corrected or L-transposition). The unexpectedly high occurrence rate of accessory AV connections in patients with Ebstein's anomaly lends indirect support for their being associated with abnormalities occurring during separation of atria and ventricles in early cardiogenesis.

The role of embryologic abnormalities in the occurrence of other accessory conduction tissue illustrated in Figure 2–1 is unknown; for

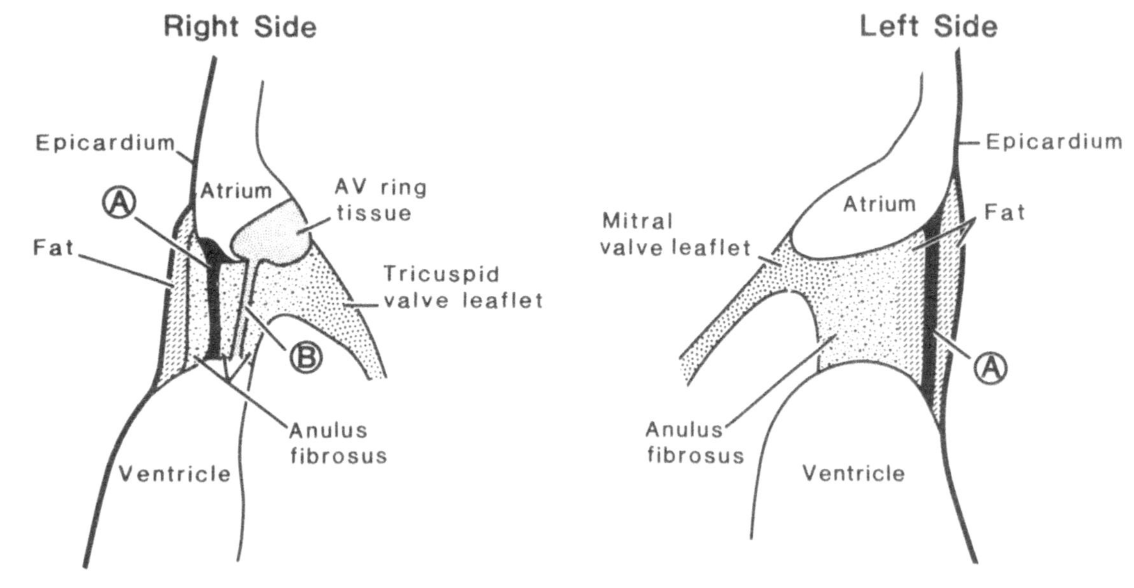

FIGURE 2–3. Diagrammatic representation of relative positions of right and left-sided accessory AV connection. In the *left* panel accessory muscular connections (A) and specialized tissue (B) connections are present as defects in the anulus fibrosus around the tricuspid valve. In the *right* panel, the accessory muscular connection (A) is present in a subepicardial position. On both the right and left side, the atria and ventricles are electrically isolated by the anulus fibrosus.

atriofascicular (atrio-Hisian) [8] or atrionodal (intranodal) [9] bypass tracts, nodoventricular [10] or fasciculoventricular [29] connections, only occasional morphologic descriptions exist.

To summarize available morphologic observations, AV connections appear to occur during normal cardiogenesis and may be composed of specialized or ordinary myocardium. Findings also suggest that accessory AV connections are uncommon in normal infants (i.e., greater than six months of age), and that they are not present in asymptomatic adults. It has been postulated that failure to lose accessory AV connections during development is the basis of the most common form of ventricular preexcitation. The development of other forms of accessory connections is much less well understood.

Functional Observations

While comparative morphologic studies have provided insight into the developmental aspects of accessory AV connections, serial study of functional characteristics of accessory connections in patients has provided most of our understanding of their natural history. However, all previously reported natural history studies have been in patients with accessory AV connections, since they are most frequently recognized among patients with preexcitation syndromes.

In a series of 107 patients with WPW syndrome age eight to 76 years, Wellens [30] demonstrated the relative constancy of the effective refractory period of the accessory AV connections with respect to age. However, electrophysiologic studies have added little additional information to our knowledge of the natural history of these connections, since serial studies are rarely performed. Further, many patients undergoing electrophysiologic study are treated (by drugs or surgical ablation of the accessory connection) for symptoms associated with the preexcitation syndromes. Thus, little is known of the natural history of accessory connections as defined by electrophysiologic measurements.

Two aspects of the functional characteristics of accessory connections have been the basis of serial ECG studies: the occurrence of clinically apparent paroxysms of tachycardia and the occurrence of preexcitation during sinus rhythm. The natural history of recurrences of paroxysmal tachycardia has been the subject of many reports [3,31–38], but length of follow-up in most reports has been short. The relevance of such studies to the natural history is open to some doubt since cessation of spontaneous tachycardia recurrences may result from changes in initiating events [39] rather than to changes in the accessory AV connections. In other studies, the continued presence, or conversely, disappearance of ECG evidence of preexcitation during sinus rhythm has been frequently used to describe the natural history of Wolff-Parkinson-White (WPW) syndrome in patients with or without tachycardia. However, this natural history description is limited due to the recognition that ECG evidence of preexcitation may be intermittent or in some instances may not appear for years after tachycardia is first noted [34,37] (see also Chapters 8 by Klein et al. and 15 by Levy et al.). The extent to which these changes in preexcitation reflect age-related changes in autonomic innervation or AV node function rather than changes in accessory AV connections is unknown.

The manifestations of the preexcitation syndrome in an individual patient may be influenced by changes in the normal conduction system. For example, in a study of 40 children ages seven months to 15 years [40], it was noted that atrial and AV node refractory periods were shorter than those in adults. Additionally, it is well recognized that normal ECG intervals are age-related, with normal PR intervals and QRS durations being shorter in young children [41]. Thus, postnatal changes occur in the normal conduction system, and these may play a role in the apparent presence or absence of preexcitation syndromes and may in part determine whether associated arrhythmias become manifest (see also Chapter 7 by Akhtar et al.). With these cautions in mind, natural history studies in patients with preexcitation syndromes are reviewed in this section.

OBSERVATIONS ON TACHYCARDIA RECURRENCE

The term *paroxysmal atrial tachycardia* continues to be used to describe tachycardias in infancy, and is defined as a regular tachycardia of rate 180 to 320 beats per minute, with a normal QRS duration, absence of AV dissociation, and abrupt onset and termination. It has been proposed that paroxysmal atrial tachycardia in infants is a reentrant tachycardia which utilizes an accessory AV connection for retrograde atrial activation, even when preexcitation is absent in sinus rhythm [33,42]. Thus, paroxysmal atrial tachycardia in infants represents orthodromic reciprocating tachycardia; consequently, cessation of tachycardia in some infants has been hypothesized to relate to changes in retrograde conduction in the accessory AV connection [42]. However, assessment of retrograde conduction characteristics has not been extensively evaluated because of the infrequent need for serial invasive catheter studies in infants. Other factors, including maturational changes in autonomic function [33] or changes in the initiating events for tachycardia onset [39] have been proposed as possibly important factors for observed variations in tachycardia episodes over time. Little information is available regarding the influence of these factors in children or adults with preexcitation syndromes.

Although paroxysmal tachycardia in fetuses has in some cases been associated with fetal death [43–46], inability to record intrauterine ECGs has been a barrier to obtaining information about the presence of preexcitation in utero. Thus, during the first seven months following cardiogenesis, functional data regarding accessory connections in the absence of tachycardia are not available. The observation that intrauterine tachycardia is not usually reported before 24 weeks' gestation may be related to either technical limitations of monitoring intrauterine heart rate or the lack of a functional anatomic circuit for reentrant tachycardia prior to that time. However, the transient nature of the ECG evidence of preexcitation associated with bouts of paroxysmal tachycardia which occurred in utero has been well documented [43,47].

Studies of tachycardia recurrences have evaluated differences in recurrences between various age patients or between patients with or without preexcitation in sinus rhythm. For example, 20 to 40% of infants with WPW syndrome have been reported to have tachycardia recurrence after one year of age [31–35]. Although some authors noted tachycardia recurrence to be more likely in infants with ECG evidence of preexcitation in sinus rhythm [31], this has not been a universal finding [35].

The observation that paroxysmal tachycardia tends to recur more often in children with ECG evidence of preexcitation than in those without preexcitation was reported by Nadas et al. [31]. These authors also noticed that infants under four months of age at first tachycardia occurrence were less likely to have tachycardia recurrence than older infants. In follow-up exceeding 12 months, there was a 22% chance of recurrence of tachycardia when the first episode occurred prior to four months of age, compared to an 83% recurrence rate in infants and children older than 4 months at first episode of tachycardia. Lubbers et al. [36] reported 24 infants with supraventricular tachycardia followed for an average of four years. In contrast to the report by Nadas et al. [31], significant tachycardia recurrences were common in Lubbers report, whether or not preexcitation was present in sinus rhythm [36].

In an impressive study reported by Lundberg [37], 40 patients who had had paroxysmal atrial tachycardia in infancy were followed for an average of 24 years. Recurrences of tachycardia varied with patient age and the presence or absence of preexcitation. During infancy, tachycardia recurrence was 65% for infants with ventricular preexcitation and 46% for those without. Between age one and ten years, 46% of patients with ventricular preexcitation and 6% without had recurrent tachycardia. After age ten, 53% of children with preexcitation and 9% without had recurrences. However, by the third decade, 50% with preexcitation had recurrences, compared to 25% without.

Orinious [38] reported the long-term follow-up (21 years) of 50 patients (age 29 to 84 years) with paroxysmal tachycardia and ventricular preexcitation originally reported by Ohnell [3]. Of these 50 patients, six were already dead at the time of Ohnell's report, and 11 died during the follow-up period, a mortality rate not statistically different than that predicted for similarly aged patients in the Swedish population. One patient, however, died during an episode of tachycardia. Two patients were lost to follow-up, leaving 31 patients who were evaluated 21 years later. Seventeen of 31 patients reported that attacks of tachycardia had decreased in frequency over the follow-up period, while five thought they had more episodes of tachycardia; four patients reported no change in clinical status, and five patients were uncertain. Fourteen of the 31 patients (45%) had had no episodes of tachycardia for several years, but 49% had at least a few attacks each year.

OBSERVATIONS ON ECG MANIFESTATIONS OF PREEXCITATION

Evaluation of the natural history of antegrade conduction in the accessory AV connection has been performed by follow-up studies evaluating the presence or absence of preexcitation on the ECG in sinus rhythm. These studies have usually demonstrated loss of preexcitation in some patients [33,34,37,38,48] during the follow-up period, whether infants or adults were evaluated. Most of these studies, however, also included reports of patients who acquired ECG evidence of ventricular preexcitation in sinus rhythm. For example, Swiderski et al. [34] reported two infants who acquired ECG evidence of preexcitation nine months and 12 months following their first ECG. Four of 22 patients in their report had intermittent preexcitation. This study emphasizes the inability of one ECG recording to categorically state that accessory connections have "disappeared."

Lundberg [37] reported long-term follow-up (average 24 years) in 23 patients who had WPW syndrome in infancy. ECG evidence of preexcitation persisted between age two and age ten years in 13 of 23 patients, and continued to be present after age ten in these 13 patients. One additional patient was noted to have ECG evidence of preexcitation only after age ten, and in two patients with WPW syndrome in infancy and normal ECGs between age two and age ten years, preexcitation recurred after age ten years. Similar results were found in older patients by Orinious [38] who reported the 21 year follow-up of 31 patients age 29 to 64 years with WPW syndrome. He noted that 15 of the 31 patients continued to have ECG evidence of preexcitation in sinus rhythm.

Occasionally, provocative maneuvers (isoproterenol infusion, carotid sinus massage, exercise, hyperventilation) have been employed to unmask or demonstrate preexcitation in patients with a normal ECG during sinus rhythm [20,21,38,49], but these studies have not been commonly performed on infants and children. For example, Przybylski et al. [21] evaluated 21 adult patients who had lost the previously demonstrated ECG finding of ventricular preexcitation. Ten patients were receiving no drug treatment, and 11 patients were receiving amiodarone. In 9 of 21 patients, bradycardia resulting from carotid sinus massage resulted in reappearance of ventricular preexcitation, while in 5 of 12 patients a graded isoproterenol infusion resulted in reappearance of ventricular preexcitation. This study further illustrates the difficulty in evaluating the presence or absence of accessory connections based on a single ECG recording.

OBSERVATIONS BASED ON STIMULATION STUDIES

In addition to the follow-up studies based on tachycardia recurrence or presence of preexcitation in sinus rhythm, stimulation studies reported by Benson et al. [20] and Przybylski et al. [21], have provided additional insight into the natural history of accessory connections.

In the report by Benson et al. [20] findings during follow-up in 12 patients with tachycardia utilizing an accessory AV connection in infancy were presented. Only 3 of 12 patients had persistance of spontaneous tachycardia at greater than seven months of age, but 6 of 12 patients had inducible tachycardia. These results suggest that in the 6 of 12 infants without inducible tachycardia, a functional accessory AV connection had disappeared, perhaps as part of a normal maturational process. Further, since of 6 patients with inducible tachycardia only 3 had had spontaneous recurrences, these findings indicate that absence of spontaneous tachycardia does not mean that the AV connections are absent. Changes in conduction characteristics of the accessory connection in both the antegrade (disappearance of preexcitation in 2 of 4 patients), and the retrograde (increase in the ventriculoatrial interval by 80 ms compared to initial study in one patient) directions, support the concept that developmental changes do occur in accessory connections.

In the study by Przybylski et al. [21], four patients who had lost ECG evidence of preexcitation underwent catheter electrophysiologic studies to assess conduction characteristics of the previously demonstrated accessory AV connection in the retrograde direction. In three of four patients, these authors demonstrated retrograde conduction utilizing an accessory AV connection; all three patients had eccentric atrial activation during ventricular pacing, although only one patient had inducible tachycardia.

Summary

A precise assessment of the natural history of accessory connections cannot be provided until more follow-up studies, including serial studies employing electrical stimulation techniques with larger numbers of patients, are available. Ohnell [3] recognized that death could occur during an episode of tachycardia; additionally, patients could die suddenly without an episode of tachycardia being recognized. Similarly, Gallagher et al. [50] noted that many patients referred for electrophysiologic evaluation had had a catastrophic event associated with their first tachycardia episode. However, the denominator (total number of patients with accessory connections) is difficult to determine, since a noninvasive screening method for diagnosis of functional accessory connections is not available. Additionally, spontaneous variation in tachycardia frequency frustrates interpretation of the natural history of accessory connections based on the presence or absence of tachycardia, as demonstrated by Pritchett et al. [51]. Nonetheless, available morphologic and functional studies have demonstrated that accessory connections occur during cardiac development but are not present in the hearts of normal adults. Based on available information, it appears that the functional characteristics of accessory connections change in some, but not all, patients over time.

References

1. Kent AFS: Research on the structure and function of the mammalian heart. *J. Physiol.* 14:233, 1893.
2. Wolff L, Parkinson J, White PD: Bundle branch block with short P-R interval in healthy young people prone to paroxysmal tachycardia. *Am. Heart J.* 5:685, 1930.
3. Ohnell RF: Pre-excitation. A cardiac abnormality. *Acta Med. Scand. Suppl.* 152:9, 1944.
4. Lev M, Gibson S, Miller RA: Ebstein's disease with Wolff-Parkinson-White syndrome. Report of a case with histopathologic study of possible conduction pathways. *Am. Heart J.* 49:724, 1955.
5. Wood FC, Wolferth CC, Geckeler GD: Histologic demonstrations of accessory muscular connections between auricle and ventricle in a case of short P-R interval and prolonged QRS complex. *Am. Heart J.* 25:454, 1943.
6. Anderson RH, Davies MJ, Becker AE: Atrioventricular ring specialized tissue in the normal heart. *Eur. J. Cardiol.* 2:219, 1974.
7. Anderson RH, Becker AE, Brechenmacher C, Davies MJ, Rossi L: Ventricular preexcitation. A proposed nomenclature for its substrates. *Eur. J. Cardiol.* 3:27, 1975.

8. Brechenmacher C: Atrio-His bundle tracts. *Br. Heart J.* 37:853, 1975.
9. James TN: Morphology of the human atrioventricular node, with remarks pertinent to its electrophysiology. *Am. Heart J.* 62:756, 1961.
10. Mahaim I, Benatt A: Nouvelles recherches sur les connexions superieures de la branche gauche du faisceau de His-Tawara avec la cloison interventriculaire. *Cardiologia* 1:61, 1938.
11. Becker AE, Anderson RH, Durrer D, Wellens HJJ: The anatomical substrates of Wolff-Parkinson-White syndrome: A clinicopathologic correlation in seven patients. *Circulation* 57:870, 1978.
12. Klein GJ, Hackel DB, Gallagher JJ: Anatomic substrate of impaired antegrade conduction over an accessory atrioventricular pathway in the Wolff-Parkinson-White syndrome. *Circulation* 61:1249, 1980.
13. Rossi L, Thiene G: Mild Ebstein's anomaly associated with supraventricular tachycardia and sudden death: Clinicomorphologic features in 3 patients. *Am. J. Cardiol.* 53:332, 1984.
14. Bharati S, Rosen K, Steinfield L, Miller RA, Lev M: The anatomic substrate for preexcitation in corrected transposition. 62:831, 1980.
15. Brechenmacher C, Coumel P, Fauchier J-P, Cachera J-P, James TN: De subitaneis mortibus. XXII. Intractable paroxysmal tachycardias which proved fatal in type A Wolff-Parkinson-White syndrome. *Circulation* 55:408, 1977.
16. Truex RC, Bishof JK, Downing DF: Accessory atrioventricular muscle bundles. II. Cardiac conduction system in a human specimen with Wolff-Parkinson-White syndrome. *Anat. Rec.* 137:417, 1960.
17. Boineau JP, Moore EN: Evidence for propagation of activation across an accessory atrioventricular connection in types A and B preexcitation. *Circulation* 41:375, 1970.
18. Boineau JP, Moore EN, Spear JF, Sealy WC: Basis of static and dynamic electrocardiographic variations in Wolff-Parkinson-White syndrome. Anatomic and electrophysiologic observations in right and left ventricular preexcitation. *Am. J. Cardiol.* 32:32, 1973.
19. Anderson RH, Ho SY, Smith A, Wilkinson JL, Becker AE: Study of the cardiac conduction tissues in the paediatric age group. *Diagn. Histopathol.* 4:3, 1981.
20. Benson DW Jr, Dunnigan A, Schneider SP, Schiff J, Johnson W: Follow-up of infant paroxysmal atrial tachycardia: Transesophageal study. (Abstr) *Circulation* 70:II–206, 1984.
21. Przybylski J, Chiale PA, Halpern MS, Nau GJ, Elizari MV, Rosenbaum MB: Unmasking of ventricular preexcitation by vagal stimulation or isoproterenol administration. *Circulation* 61: 1030, 1980.
22. Krikler DM: Wolff-Parkinson-White Syndrome: Long follow-up and an Anglo-American historical note. *J. Am. Coll. Cardiol.* 2:1216, 1983.
23. Anderson RH, Becker AE, Wenink ACG, Janse MJ: The development of the caridac specialized tissue. In *The Conduction System of the Heart: Structure, Function, and Clinical Implications.* Wellens HJJ, Lie KE, Janse MJ (eds.). Philadelphia, Lea and Febiger, 1976, pp. 3–28.
24. Robb JS, Kaylor CT, Turman WG: A study of specialized heart tissue at various stages of development of the human fetal heart. *Am. J. Med.* 5:324, 1948.
25. Lunel AAW: Significance of annulus fibrosus of heart in relation to AV conduction and ventricular activation in cases of Wolff-Parkinson-White syndrome. *Br. Heart J.* 34:1263, 1972.
26. Janse MJ, Anderson RH, van Capelle FJL, Durrer D: A combined electrophysiological and anatomical study of the human fetal heart. *Am. Heart J.* 91:556, 1976.
27. Truex RC, Bishof JK, Hoffman EL: Accessory atrioventricular muscle bundles of the developing human heart. *Anat. Rec.* 131:45, 1958.
28. Smith WM, Gallagher JJ, Kerr CR, Sealy WC, Kasell JH, Benson DW Jr, Reiter MJ, Sterba R, Grant AO: The electrophysiologic basis and management of symptomatic recurrent tachycardia in patients with Ebstein's anomaly of the tricuspid valve. *Am. J. Cardiol.* 49:1223, 1982.
29. Gallagher JJ, Smith WM, Kasell JH, Benson DW Jr, Sterba R, Grant AO: Role of Mahaim fibers in cardiac arrhythmias in man. *Circulation* 64:176, 1981.
30. Wellens HJJ: The electrophysiologic properties of the accessory pathway in the Wolff-Parkinson-White syndrome. In: *The Conduction System of the Heart: Structure, Function, and Clinical Implications.* Wellens JHH, Lie KE, Janse MJ (eds.) Philadelphia, Lea and Febiger, 1976, pp. 567–587.
31. Nadas AS, Daeschner CW, Roth A, Blumenthal SL: Paroxysmal tachycardia in infants and children: Study of 41 cases. *Pediatrics* 9:167, 1952.
32. Mantakas ME, McCue CM, Miller WW: Natural history of Wolff-Parkinson-White syndrome discovered in infancy. *Am. J. Cardiol.* 41:1097, 1978.
33. Wolff GS, Han J, Curran J: Wolff-Parkinson-White syndrome in the neonate. *Am. J. Cardiol.* 41:559, 1978.
34. Swiderski J, Lees MH, Nadas AS: The Wolff-Parkinson-White syndrome in infancy and childhood. *Br. Heart J.* 24:561, 1962.
35. Deal BJ, Keane JF, Gillette PC, Garson A Jr: Wolff-Parkinson-White syndrome and supraventricular tachycardia during infancy: Management and follow-up. *J. Am. Coll. Cardiol.* 5:130, 1985.

36. Lubbers WJ, Losekoot TG, Anderson RH, Wellens HJJ: Paroxysmal supraventricular tachycardia in infancy and childhood. *Eur. J. Cardiol.* 2:91, 1974.
37. Lundberg A: Paroxysmal atrial tachycardia in infancy: Long-term follow-up study of 49 subjects. *Pediatrics* 70:638, 1982.
38. Orinious E: Pre-excitation: studies on criteria, prognosis, and heredity. *Acta Med. Scand. Suppl.* 465:1, 1966.
39. Dunnigan A, Benditt DG, Benson DW Jr: Modes of spontaneous onset of paroxysmal atrial tachycardia in infants and children. *J. Am. Coll. Cardiol.* 5:497, 1985.
40. DuBrow IW, Fisher EA, Amat-y-Leon F, Denes P, Wu D, Rosen K, Hastreiter AR: Comparison of cardiac refractory periods in children and adults. *Circulation* 51:485, 1975.
41. Davignon A, Rautaharju P, Boisselle E, Soumis F, Magelas M, Choquette A: Normal ECG standards for infants and children. *Pediatr. Cardiol.* 1:123, 1979/80.
42. Benson DW Jr, Dunnigan A, Benditt DG, Pritzker MR, Thompson TR: Transesophageal study of infant supraventricular tachycardia: Electrophysiologic characteristics. *Am. J. Cardiol.* 52:1002, 1983.
43. Belhassen B, Pauzner D, Blieden L, Sherez J, Zinger A, David M, Muhlbauer B, Laniado S: Intrauterine and postnatal atrial fibrillation in the Wolff-Parkinson-White syndrome. *Circulation* 66:1124, 1982.
44. Kleinman CS, Donnerstein RL, Jaffe CC, DeVore GR, Weinstein EM, Lynch DC, Talner NS, Bukowitz RL, Hobbins JC: Fetal echocardiography. A tool for evaluation of in utero cardiac arrhythmias and monitoring of in utero therapy: analysis of 71 patients. *Am. J. Cardiol.* 51:237, 1983.
45. Kleinman CS, Donnerstein RL, DeVore GR, Jaffe CC, Lynch DC, Berkowitz RL, Talner NS, Hobbins JC: Fetal echocardiography for evaluation of in utero congestive heart failure. A technique for study of nonimmune fetal hydrops. *N. Engl. J. Med.* 306:568, 1982.
46. Given BD, Phillippe M, Sanders SP, Dzau VJ: Procainamide cardioversion of fetal supraventricular tachyarrhythmia. *Am. J. Cardiol.* 53:1460, 1984.
47. Moene RJ, Roos JP: Transient Wolff-Parkinson-White syndrome and neonatal reciprocating tachycardia. *Circulation* 48:443, 1973.
48. Berkman NL, Lamb LE: The Wolff-Parkinson-White electrocardiogram. A follow-up study of five to twenty-eight years. *N. Engl. J. Med.* 278:492, 1968.
49. Lamb LE: Respiratory maneuvers in converting WPW syndrome to normal conduction and converting normal conduction to WPW syndrome. *Am. Heart J.* 55:174, 1958.
50. Gallagher JJ, Gilbert M, Svenson RH, Sealy WC, Kasell J, Wallace AG: Wolff-Parkinson-White syndrome. The problem, evaluation, and surgical correction. *Circulation* 51:767, 1975.
51. Pritchett ELC, Hammill SC, Reiter MJ, Lee KL, McCarthy EA, Zimmerman JM, Shand DG: Life-table methods for evaluating antiarrhythmic drug efficacy in patients with paroxysmal atrial tachycardia. *Am. J. Cardiol.* 52:1007, 1983.

3. ANATOMIC BASIS FOR PREEXCITATION SYNDROMES

Donald B. Hackel

The usual and normal route to ventricular excitation is via the sino-auricular node–atrioventricular (AV) node–His bundle–bundle branch system. The AV node is a region in which impulse conduction is normally delayed. Although the mechanism for the this delay is not agreed upon, it is an important feature of the AV node which helps to maintain an orderly sequence of atrial and ventricular contraction. However, there are several potential routes, by which the normal AV node–common bundle pathway may be bypassed, and which are, for the most part, made up of morphologically normal myocytes which often permit initiation of ventricular depolarization prior to that anticipated from activation via the normal conduction system. The main contribution of this chapter will be to describe these various potential bypass pathways which provide an anatomical basis for the occurrence of preexcitation. The terminology used will, for the most part, be that recommended by the European Study Group for Preexcitation [1].

Atrioventricular Conduction in Historical Perspective

Several important contributions to the knowledge of the anatomy of the heart were made during the latter part of the nineteenth century,

Dr. Hackel is supported by a Research Career Award (HLB–K6–14188) and by a research grant (HLB–17670) from the US Public Health Service.

and some of the anatomic structures of the conducting system were described, although understanding of the functional aspects of the described structures was limited. As early as 1845 Purkinje had described the large clear cells of the right and left bundle branches, but he did not relate them to a conduction system [2].

In 1893 Kent described lateral AV connections [3], and in the same year His described the common bundle [4]; neither observed a connection of these structures with the distal bundle branch conducting system. In recent years the term *bundle of Kent* has been applied to potential accessory pathways of conduction between the atria and ventricles, and the term *bundle of His* has been applied to the common bundle.

Despite these perceptive anatomic observations, however, it was not until 1906 that Tawara described the AV conduction system in continuity from the AV node to the common bundle extending on to the right and left bundle branches [5]. Keith and Flack endorsed these findings of Tawara [6] and the next year, they described the sinus node [7] which was recognized as the pacemaker of the heart [8].

Substrates of Preexcitation

There are several possible routes by which the cardiac electrical impulse can bypass the usual common bundle route (Figure 3–1), including:

1. *Accessory AV Connections.* The accessory atrioventricular connections of the so-called bundle of Kent type have been described in patients with the Wolff-Parkinson-White (WPW) syndrome [9], but may also be found in occasional "normal" hearts [10]. The bundles

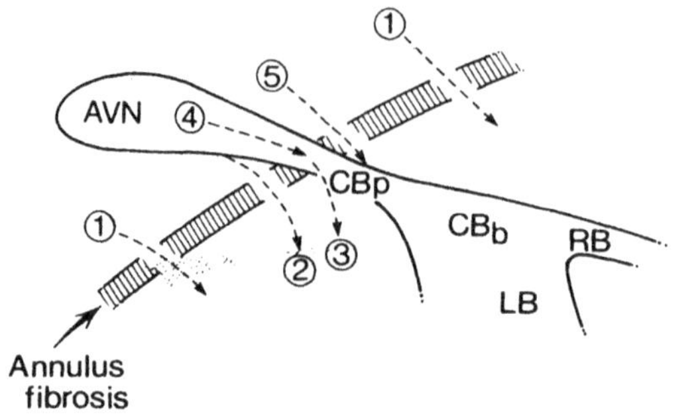

FIGURE 3–1. Diagram illustrating the various possible routes of accessory pathways of conduction, including: 1. Accessory AV Pathway free wall and septal; 2. Accessory Nodo-ventricular Connection; 3. Fasciculo-ventricular Connection; 4. Intranodal Bypass Tract; 5. Atriofascicular Bypass Tract. AVN = atrioventricular node, CB_b = branching common bundle, CB_p = penetrating common bundle, LB = left bundle, RB = right bundle.

originate and insert into ordinary myocardium, and can involve either the septal (anterior or posterior) or parietal walls (free wall, right or left) of the heart [11]. The parietal accessory AV connection is the type that was first successfully treated by a surgical approach [12]. Thus, in a patient with a life-threatening tachyarrhythmia that has been identified as involving preexcitation, the heart can be explored at surgery by the use of surface electrodes, the point of earliest epicardial activation can be determined and the accessory pathway can be eliminated [13].

The anatomic appearance of accessory AV pathways of this type is illustrated in Figures 3–2 and 3–3. In both of these pictures the accessory pathway consists of a thin strand of morphologically normal myocardium that bridges that fibro-fatty epicardial gap between the left atrium and left ventricle and permits both the occurrence of preexcitation and of a reentrant tachycardia with circus movement. The pathway may, however, be in a subendocardial position; this location is rare overall, but is most common in the right lateral AV position [14] (Figure 3–4). Because of the position of the accessory pathway deep in the AV groove, Sealy et al. recommended an extensive surgical incision with dissection of all the fat and vessels away from the ventricular surface and separation of the atrium from the ventricle followed by their reanastomosis, since an incomplete incision risks missing the bypass tract [15]. An alternate approach using cryosurgery has been described by Klein et al. [16].

Accessory AV pathways have been described in otherwise normal fetal hearts [10] and in the hearts of children up to (but not over) 6 months of age [17] although Lev has reported their absence in the hearts of normal fetuses and newborns [18]. Accessory AV pathways are not usually found in the hearts of adults without the occurrence of the WPW syndrome or of supraventricular tachycardia.

2. *Nodoventricular and Fasciculoventricular Connections.* Fibers of this type pass directly from the AV node into the upper interventricular septum inserting into either ordinary myocardium (nodoventricular) or into the specialized cardiac conduction or pass from the common bundle to ordinary ventricular myocardium (fasciculoventricular). Thus these accessory connections bypass the bundle branches, all or part of the common bundle, and sometimes the distal part of the AV node (Figure 3–5). They have been described in normal hearts [17,18], in the hearts of patients with WPW syndrome [19], and in the hearts of patients with atypical features of preexcitation (e.g., with a normal PR interval and an abnormal QRS complex) [20]. Nodoventricular and fasciculoventricular fibers have been described in the fetus and in children [18] and in some normal adult hearts [17].

3. *Intranodal and Atriofascicular Bypass Tracts.* James described an accessory AV pathway consisting of the myofibers that are normally present between the AV node and the right atrial endocardium (Figure 3–6). Such fibers may join the distal fibers of the AV node (atrionodal) or the common bundle (atriofascicular), may terminate in the AV ring, or may penetrate the valve ring to enter the upper interventricular septum [21,22]. Intranodal bypass tracts (atrionodal) are said to exist in all hearts, whereas atriofascicular tracts are rare, occurring in only 2 out of 687 hearts that were studied by Brechenmacher [28].

It has been suggested that distinct dual pathways can exist within the AV node itself, which may be of fast and slow conducting varieties [1,20,23,24]. No actual anatomical demonstration of such pathways has been accomplished, however, so that this intranodal type of dual pathway is only hypothetical.

4. *Nodal Malformations.* It was suggested by Caracta et al. that abnormally shaped or sized

AV nodes might result in abnormal conduction through the AV node, with a small node not being able to produce the usual delay [25]. This is a reasonable suggestion but it is no more than an unproven hypothesis at the present time, and there is some reason to believe that it may not be valid (see Chapter 12 by Benditt et al.).

Other Variants of Preexcitation Syndromes

There are several other variants of preexcitation syndromes.

1. *Associated with Other Congenital Heart Disease*. The WPW syndrome usually occurs in an otherwise normal heart. However, in about 20% of patients with the WPW syndrome there are other accompanying congenital anomalies [23]. Ebsteins' anomaly of the tricuspid valve is one of the most common anomalies that accompanies right sided or posteroseptal accessory pathways [26]. This is apparently related to the abnormal downward displacement of the tricuspid valve ring with severe loss of definition of the AV junction. Other congenital anomalies that are associated with the WPW syndrome include: ventricular septal defect, atrial septal defect, idiopathic hypertrophic subaortic stenosis, aortic stenosis, cardiomyopathy, and corrected transposition of the great vessels with Ebstein's anomaly of the left AV valve (see Chapter 14 by Porter and Holmes this volume).

2. *Lown-Ganong-Levine Syndrome*. This syndrome in which rapid heart beating is associated with a short PR interval, no delta wave and a normal QRS morphology [27] has been postulated to result from one of the following possible conducting system situations: (1) short AV node, (2) of a rapidly conducting intranodal bypass tract, or (3) atriofascicular bypass pathway [28].

3. *Concealed Accessory AV Pathways*. Some pathways permit conduction only in the retrograde direction are associated with no ECG manifestations of ventricular preexcitation, and are referred to as "concealed." Delta waves and short PR intervals are absent although reentrant tachycardia orthodromic reciprocating tachycardia can occur [29,30]. It is not known whether these concealed conduction pathways have morphological features which differentiate the unidirectional from the bidirectional bypass pathways.

Fibrotic Changes in Bypass Pathways

Klein et al. reported their observation of partial or complete fibrosis of three separate, but closely spaced, left lateral AV pathways in a patient with WPW syndrome (Figure 3–2). Electrophysiologic study during life had demonstrated the presence of a single left lateral AV free wall accessory pathway that sustained conduction well in the retrograde direction, but only intermittently in the antegrade direction. It was suggested that the fibrosis could be the anatomic basis for the impaired antegrade conduction [31]. Degenerative changes have been reported at the base of the ventricles in association with calcification of the cardiac skeleton. This aging change could involve the slender accessory connections traversing the AV groove, since they would be susceptible to the mechanical stresses that have been described as the basis for the occurrence of heart block in aged persons [32].

Comments on Methodology

Sections of the conducting tissues of the heart are not routinely taken by most pathologists. As a result they may not be familiar with the pertinent anatomy and so do not often study the region even when there are good indications to do so. It is really not a difficult procedure, however, and could be easily done by any pathologist who has had some instruction in the technique. It is usually adequate to take multiple step sections through the crista terminalis region of the right atrium so as to include the SA node; step sections can also be taken through the AV node-common bundle-bundle branch structures. Cuts are made perpendicular to and just above the tricuspid valve ring starting anterior to the coronary sinus orifice and continuing to just anterior to the membranous septum so as to include the base of the papillary muscle of the IV septum. This will produce 8–12 blocks of 2–3 mm thickness which are then embedded in paraffin, sectioned, and stained with a connective tissue stain such as Masson's. The remainder of each block is retained so that it can be cut more completely as needed. In this way, with a little practice, adequate sections of the major structures of the conducting tissue of the heart can be obtained. However, it is sometimes necessary to obtain serial sections of the complete region so as not to miss a small focal involvement. The techni-

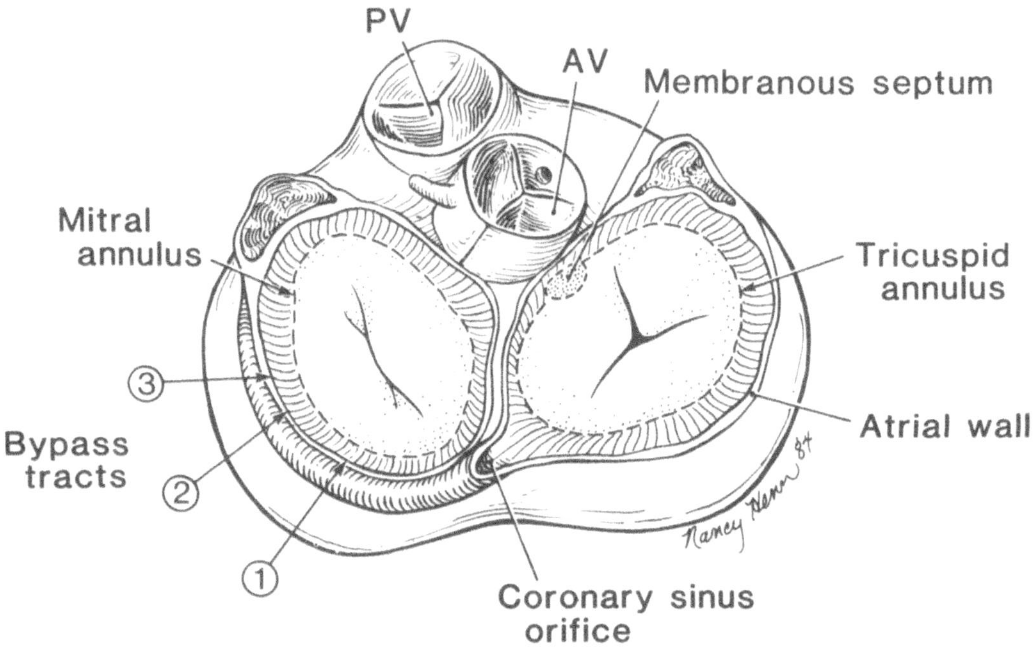
PV
AV
Membranous septum
Mitral annulus
Tricuspid annulus
③
Bypass tracts
②
①
Atrial wall
Coronary sinus orifice

A

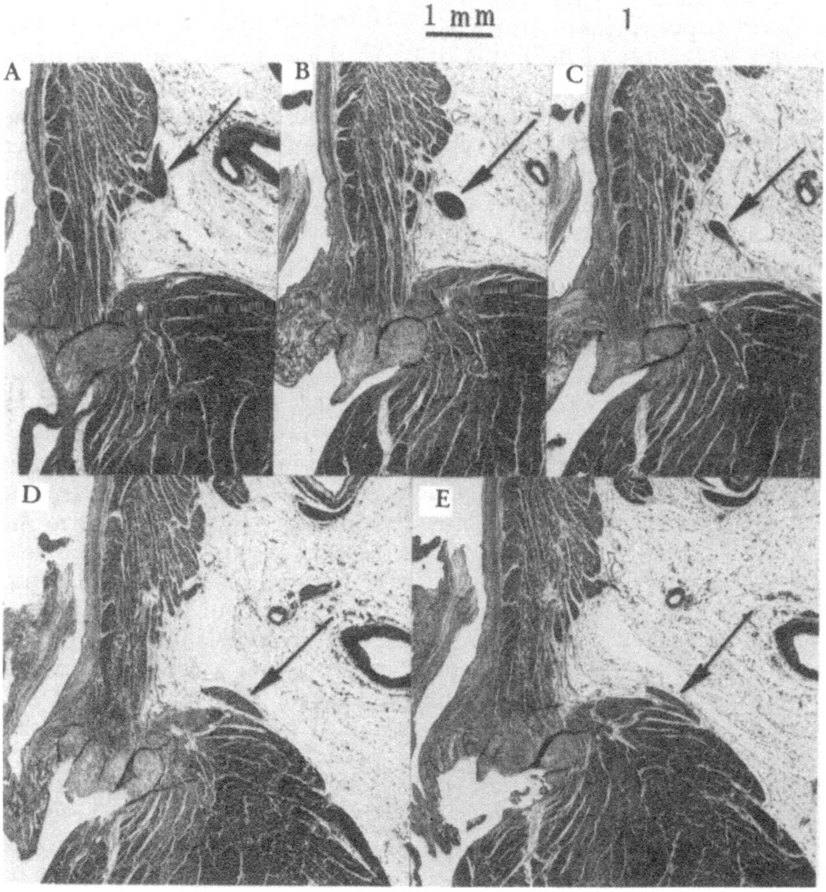
1 mm
1
A
B
C
D
E

B

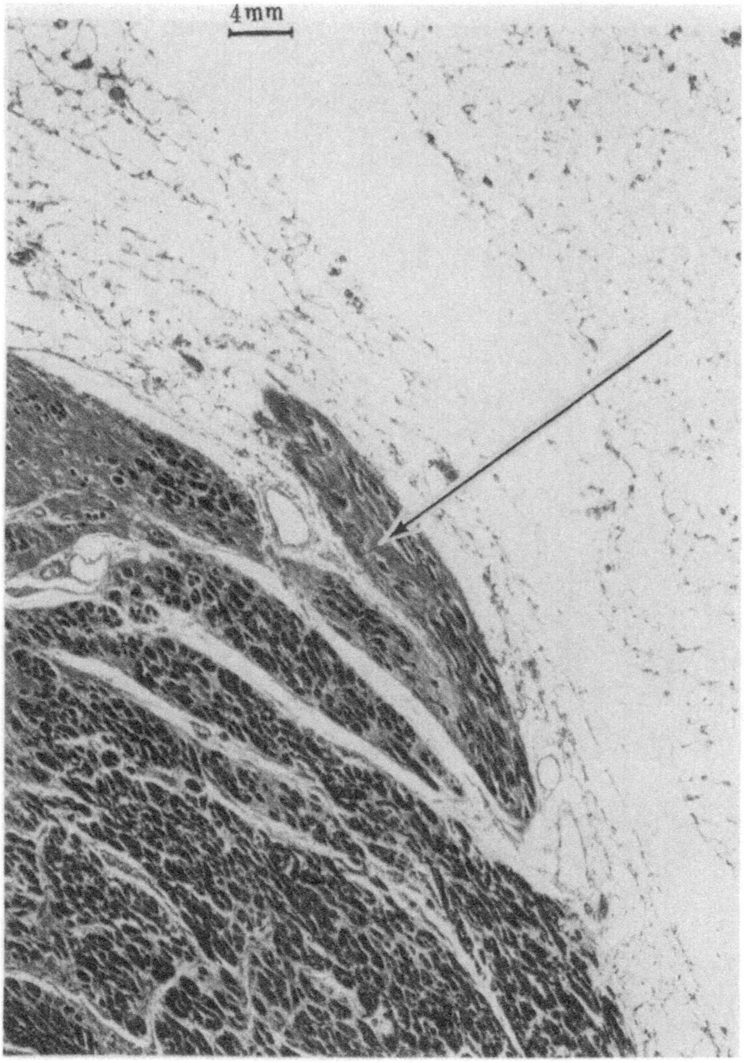

C

FIGURE 3–2. (A) Diagram of the AV rings showing the position of 3 accessory AV pathways indicated by the arrows. PV = pulmonary valve. (B) Sequential steps taken through the left AV junction showing bypass tract number 1. Note the bridge passing from left atrium in A, across epicardial fat in B, C, and D, and joining with the left ventricle in E. Masson's stain. X9.5. (C) Higher power view of the ventricular insertion of the muscular bridge shown in 2E. Arrow points to collagen (pale), the muscle fibers are dark. Masson's stain. X40. (Note: figs. 2a, 2b, and 2c reprinted with permission from the *Am. Heart Assoc.* with revisions, from ref. #31.)

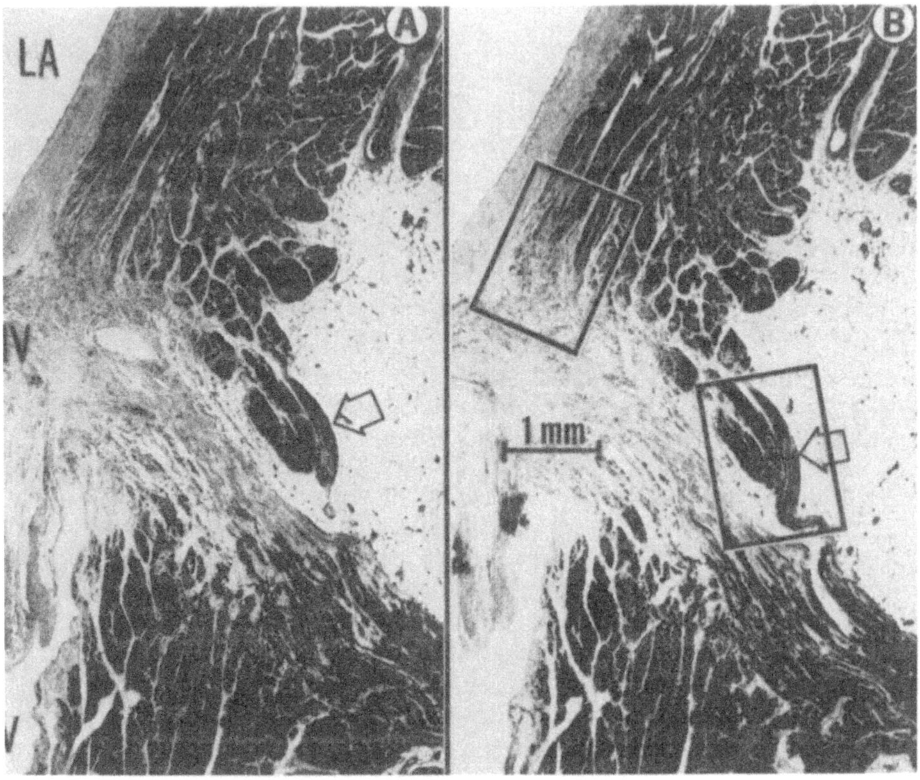
A
B
LA
1 mm

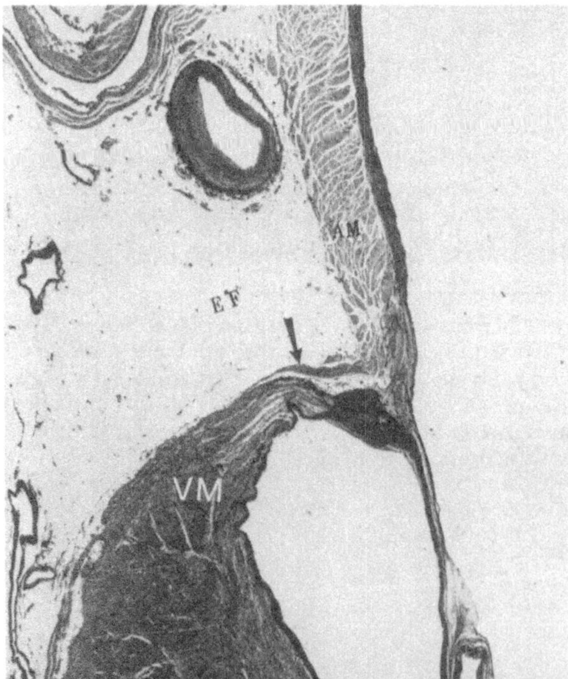
AM
EF
VM

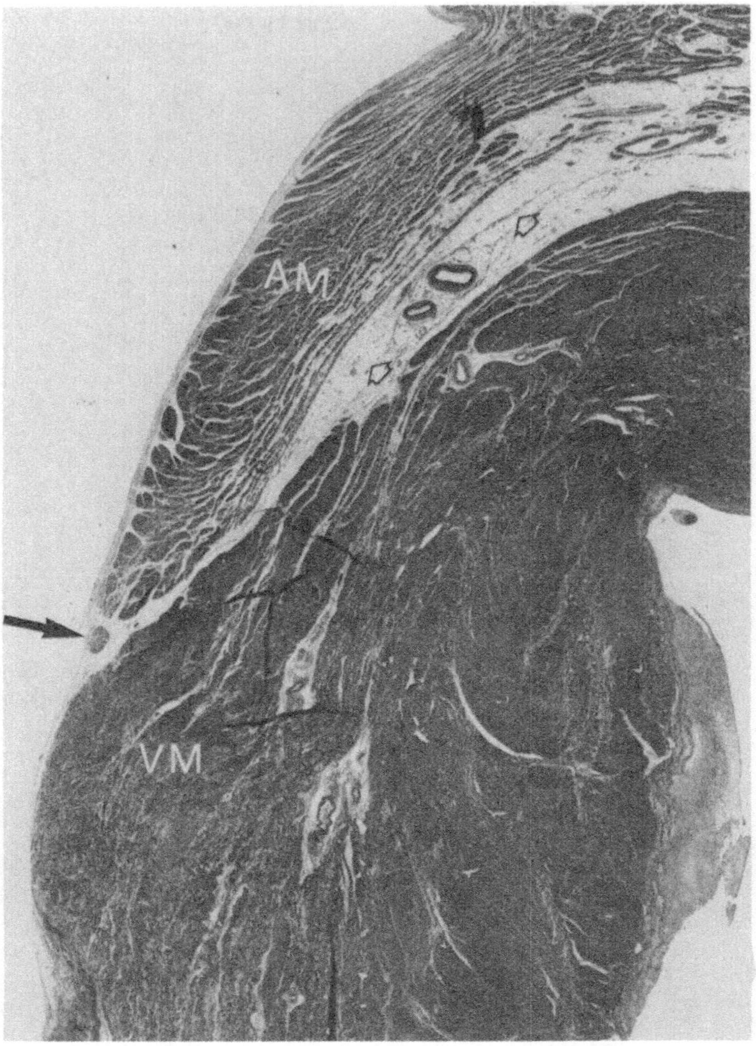

FIGURE 3–4. Septal accessory pathway (*arrow*) which connects the atrial (AM) muscle and ventricular muscle (VM) in a subendocardial position. Note that the interatrial and interventricular septa are separated only by the epicardial fat (*open arrows*), the anulus fibrosus being deficient in this area. Sections just anterior and posterior to the one shown demonstrate the connection with the atrial and ventricular muscle. (Reprinted with permission from *Am. Heart Assoc.*, ref. #15.)

FIGURE 3–3. (A and B) Low-power microscopic views of a left lateral accessory AV pathway. Course of the AV connection is indicated by open arrows. Mitral valve (MV) is to the *left*, epicardial fat is to *right*. (Photograph reprinted with permission from the *Am. Heart Assoc.* from ref. #33.) (C) Accessory pathway (*arrow*) in left lateral position; note that it skirts a well formed anulus fibrosus and extends through the epicardial fat (EF) to join atrial muscle (AM) and ventricular muscle (VM). (Reprinted with permission from *Am. Heart Assoc.*, ref. #15.)

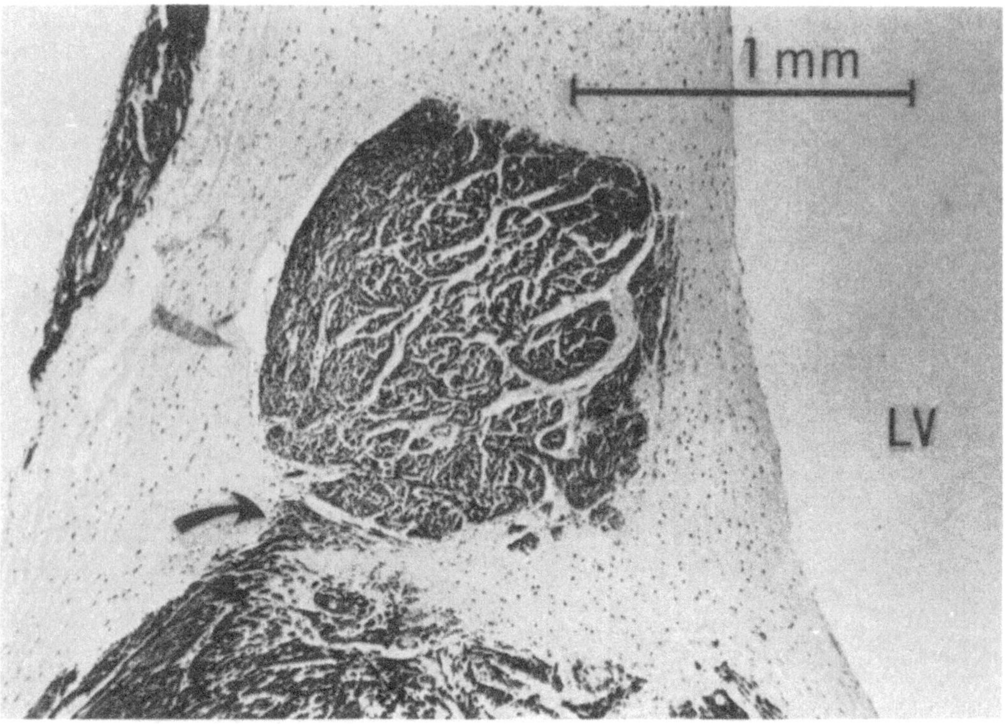

FIGURE 3–5. Microscopic section showing common bundle and a fasciculo ventricular connection (*black curved arrow*) between the common bundle and the interventricular septum. (Photograph supplied by Dr. Thomas N James.)

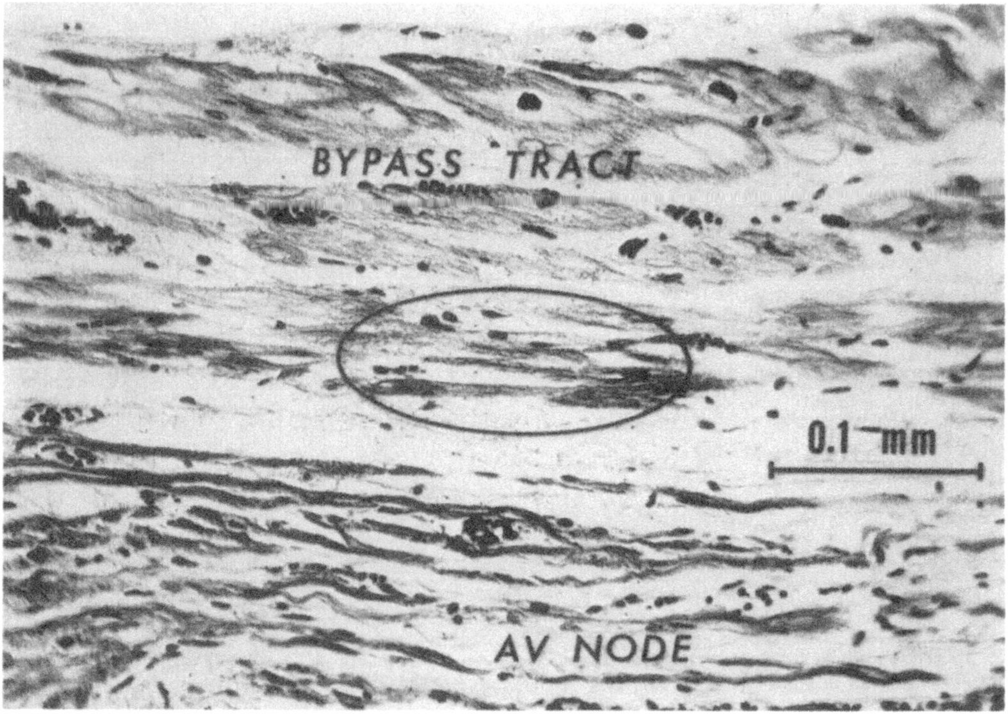

FIGURE 3–6. Microscopic view of right side of interatrial septum showing a James type bypass tract (atrionodal or intranodal) (*above*), and the slender AV nodal cells (*below*), with the oval enclosing fibers that provide direct connections between the two regions. (Photograph supplied by Dr. Thomas N James.)

que that we have previously described is uniquely suitable for this type of study; it involves the complete sectioning of the blocks containing the conducting tissues, mounting the sections on 35 mm mylar tape, and staining the tape as a unit [34,35]. It is much more difficult and time consuming to study adequately the AV ring region for accessory pathways. It is thus desirable to obtain any available antemortem clues as to the position of the accessory pathway that might be known by the clinician. This would permit the selective examination of a small region of the AV ring. Without a clue of this sort, it is necessary to serially section the entire AV ring, which can be a huge, time-consuming task.

References

1. Anderson RH, Becker AE, Brechenmacher C, Davies MJ, Rossi L: Ventricular preexcitation A proposed nomenclature for its substrates. *Eur. J. Cardiol.* 31:27, 1975.
2. Purkinje JE: Microsckopisch neurologische Beobachtungen. *Arch fur Anat. Physiol.* Wissenschaftliche Medecin 12:281, 1845.
3. Kent AFS: Researches on the structure and function of the mammalian heart. *J. Physiol.* 14:233, 1893.
4. His W Jr: Die Tatigkeit des embryonalen Herzens and deren Bedeutung fur die Lehre von der Herzbewegung beim Erwachsenen. Arbeit a.d. medicin Klinik zu Leipzig xx: pp. 14–49, 1893.
5. Tawara S: Das reizleitungssystem des Saugetierherzens. Jena. Gustav Fischer, 1906.
6. Keith A, Flack M: The auriculo-ventricular bundle of the human heart. *Lancet* 2:359, 1906.
7. Keith A, Flack M: The form and nature of the muscular connections between the primary divisions of the vertebrate heart. *J. Anat. Physiol.* 41:172, 1907.
8. Wenckebach KF: Beitrage zur Kenntnis der mennschlichen Herztatigkeit. *Arch Anat. Physiol.* 2:1, 1907.
9. Wood FC, Wolferth CC, Geckeler GD: Histologic demonstration of accessory muscular connections between auricle and ventricle in a case of short PR interval and prolonged QRS complex. *Am. Heart J.* 25:454, 1943.
10. Robb JS, Kaylor CT, Turman WG: A study of specialized heart tissue at various stages of development of the human fetal heart. *Am. J. Med.* 5:324, 1948.
11. Sealy WC: Effectiveness of surgical management of the Wolff-Parkinson-White syndrome. *Am. J. Surg.* 145:756, 1983.
12. Cobb FR, Blumenschein SD, Sealy WC, Boineau JP, Wagner GS, Wallace AG: Successful surgical interruption of the bundle of Kent in a patient with Wolff-Parkinson-White syndrome. *Circulation* 38:1018, 1968.
13. Gallagher JJ, Gilbert M, Svenson RH, Sealy WC, Kasell J, Wallace AG: Wolff-Parkinson-White syndrome. The problem, evaluation, and surgical correction. *Circulation* 51:767, 1975.
14. Becker AG, Anderson RW, Durrer D, Wellens HJ: The anatomical substrates of Wolff-Parkinson-White syndrome. A clinicopathological condition seen in patients. *Circulation* 57:870, 1978.
15. Sealy WC, Gallagher JJ, Wallace AG: The surgical treatment of Wolff-Parkinson-White syndrome. Evaluation of improved methods for identification and interruption of the Kent bundle. *Ann. Thorac. Surg.* 22:443, 1976.
16. Klein G, Guiraudon GM, Perkins DG, Jones DL, Yee R, Jarvis E: Surgical correction of the Wolff-Parkinson-White syndrome in the closed heart using cryosurgery. *JACC* 3:405, 1984.
17. Truex RC, Bishof JK, Hoffman EL: Accessory atrioventricular muscle bundles of the developing human heart. *Anat. Rec.* 131:45, 1958.
18. Lev M, Lerner R: The theory of Kent. A histologic study of the normal AV communications of the human heart. *Circulation* 12:176, 1955.
19. Lev M, Fox SM, Bharati S, Greenfield JC, Rosen KM, Pick A: Mahaim and James fibers as a basis for a unique variety of ventricular preexcitation. *Am. J. Cardiol.* 36:880, 1975.
20. Ferrer MI: New concepts relating to the preexcitation syndrome *JAMA* 201:1038, 1967.
21. James TN: Morphology of the human AV node, with remarks pertinent to its electrophysiology. *Am. Heart J.* 62:756, 1961.
22. Rossi L, Rovelli F: Anomalia del sistema atrioventricolare in un caso di sindrome di WPW. *Riv. Anat. Patol. Oncol.* 9:160, 1955.
23. Greene HL: Accessory AV conduction syndrome. *J. Hopkins Med. J.* 139:13, 1976.
24. Rosen KM, Mehta A, Miller RA: Demonstration of dual atrioventricular nodal pathways in man. *Am. J. Cardiol.* 33:291, 1974.
25. Caracta AR, Damato AN, Callagher JJ, Josephson ME, Varghese PJ, Lua SH, Westura EE: Electrophysiologic studies in the syndrome of short PR interval, normal QRS complex. *Am. J. Cardiol.* 31:245, 1973.
26. Lev M, Gibson S, Miller RA: Ebstein's disease with WPW syndrome. *Am. Heart J.* 49:724, 1958.
27. Lown B, Ganong WF, Levine SA: The syndrome of short PR interval, normal QRS complex and paroxysmal rapid heart action, *Circulation* 5:693, 1952.
28. Brechenmacher C: Atrio-His bundle tracts. *Brit. Heart J.* 37:853, 1975.

29. Narula OS: Retrograde preexcitation. Comparison of antegrade and retrograde conduction intervals in man. *Circulation* 50:1129, 1974.
30. Gillette PC: Concealed anomalous cardiac conduction pathways: a frequent cause of supraventricular tachycardia. *Am. J. Cardiol.* 40:848, 1977.
31. Klein GJ, Hackel DB, Gallagher JJ: Anatomic substrate of impaired antegrade conduction over an accessory AV pathway in the Wolff-Parkinson-White syndrome. *Circulation* 61: 1249, 1980.
32. Lev M: Normal anatomy of the conduction system in man and its pathology in AV block. *Ann. N.Y. Acad. Sci.* 111:817, 1964.
33. Brechenmacher C, Coumel P, Fauchier JP, Cachera JP, James TN: Di Subitaneis Mortibus XXII. *Circulation* 55:404, 1977.
34. Harper JR, Harley A, Hackel DB, Estes EF: Coronary artery disease and major conduction disturbances. *Am. Heart J.* 77:411, 1969.
35. Pickett JP, Sommer JR. Thirty five mm film as a mounting base and plastic spray as cover glass for histologic sections. *Arch. Pathol.* 69:239, 1960.

II. ELECTROCARDIOGRAPHIC AND ELECTROPHYSIOLOGIC MANIFESTATIONS

4. ELECTROCARDIOGRAPHIC ASPECTS OF THE PREEXCITATION SYNDROMES

Charles C. Gornick
D. Woodrow Benson, Jr.

The preexcitation syndromes are characterized by the existence of abnormal propagation of depolarization from the heart's atrium to its ventricles which results in early excitation of the ventricles and can result in deformation of the QRS complex. This unusual excitatory sequence coined "anomalous atrioventricular excitation" [1] or "preexcitation" [2] interested early electrocardiographers and was reported in isolated cases or small series by Cohn and Fraser in 1913 [3], Wilson in 1915 [4], Wedd in 1924 [5], Bain and Hamilton in 1926 [6], Bach in 1929 [7], and Hamburger in 1929 [8]. In 1930, Wolff, Parkinson, and White described in 11 patients a syndrome with the ECG features of "bundle branch block with short PR interval in healthy young people prone to paroxysmal tachycardia" [9]. Subsequently, the Wolff-Parkinson-White (WPW) syndrome eponym describing the most frequently observed of the preexcitation syndromes, has become established in the lexicon of cardiology.

The incidence of the ECG abnormalities resulting from ventricular preexcitation is estimated to occur in 1 to 3 out of every 1,000 persons [10]. According to the type of population analyzed, 4.3% to 90% of all patients with ECG evidence of preexcitation experience tachyarrhythmias of some kind [10–13]. In the past 50 years, the volume of literature written about this syndrome far exceeds that which would be expected based on this low incidence. Reasons for this interest include the recognized morbidity and mortality associated with preexcitation syndromes in otherwise healthy young people; the unique model providing functional and anatomic features of a reentrant circuit which establishes atrioventricular (AV) reentry as the paradigm of reentrant rhythms; and finally the potential for "cure" by anomalous pathway ablation which has become available since 1968 [14].

This chapter's intention will be to describe the major ECG features of the preexcitation syndromes including pertinent historical perspectives. Obviously all possible ECG patterns cannot be presented. Rather, by utilizing descriptive examples and focusing on the underlying physiologic mechanisms (when known), an attempt will be made to foster a premonitory understanding of potential ECG manifestations of the preexcitation syndromes including the ECG appearance of arrhythmias associated with these syndromes. Additionally, explanations will be provided for the varying extent of the

The authors express their sincere appreciation to Camille L. Quaglio and Frances Wallace for their secretarial assistance in preparation of this manuscript; to Bettimae Richmond of Biomedical Graphics for preparing the illustrations; and Dr. Howard Burchell for his appreciated reviewing of the manuscript.

ECG features of preexcitation in individual patients as may be seen in association with alterations in autonomic tone, exercise, and age. Finally, the use of electrocardiographic techniques (electrocardiography, vectorcardiography, and body surface potential mapping) in characterizing the location of anomalous conduction pathways will be discussed.

Definitions and Origins of Terms

Preexcitation, a term first proposed by Ohnell in 1944 [2] and later redefined by Durrer in 1970 [15] is said to be present "if in the relation to atrial events, the whole or some part of the ventricular muscle is activated earlier by the impulse originating from the atrium than would be expected if the impulse reached the ventricles by way of the normal specific conduction system only" [15]. That, in fact, early ventricular activation was occurring was confirmed in 1970 by Castellanos [16]. Using catheter techniques, His bundle activation was demonstrated to occur either simultaneously with or after ventricular activation had begun in preexcited beats [16]. The abnormally slurred initial upstroke of the QRS on the ECG representing ventricular preexcitation was termed the *delta wave* by Segers in 1944 [17].

In view of the variety of anomalous conduction pathways known to exist anatomically [18], it is reasonable to extend this original functional definition of preexcitation to any case in which activation (either in the antegrade or retrograde direction) arrives earlier at any site than can be explained by conduction over the specialized cardiac conduction system [19]. The ECG features and clinical syndromes resulting from the various anomalous conduction pathways make up the preexcitation syndromes [20–24].

When possible, because of its descriptive qualities, the proposed anatomic nomenclature of the European Study Group for preexcitation will be used in conjunction with the ECG descriptions provided [18]. Hence, the term *accessory connection* is used to describe anomalous conduction pathways that terminate in ordinary, nonspecialized myocardium regardless of their origin [18]. The term *tract* is used to describe anomalous conduction pathways that insert into the specialized conduction system regardless of their origin [18]. The structures of current clinical interest are described in Table 4–1, which contains the anatomic descriptive terminology and the previous historic terminology.

TABLE 4–1. Anatomic terminology describing substrates in the preexcitation syndromes

Anatomic terminology	Previous terminology
Accessory AV connection	Kent bundle (in septum Paladino tract)
Atriofascicular bypass tract	Atrio-Hisian fiber
Nodoventricular/fascicular connection (fiber)	Mahaim fiber
Fasciculoventricular connection (fiber)	Mahaim fiber

Electrocardiographic Manifestations of Preexcitation

The ECG manifestations of the preexcitation syndromes can be divided into three major groups:

1. short PR intervals and anomalous QRS complexes;
2. normal (conceivably even prolonged) PR intervals with anomalous QRS complexes;
3. short PR intervals with normal QRS complexes.

The classic configurations presumed responsible for the observed ECG patterns are depicted in Figure 4–1.

SHORT PR INTERVAL, ANOMALOUS QRS COMPLEXES

The most common variety of preexcitation is that associated with an accessory AV connection [18] which have also been referred to as a "Kent bundle" [25] (Figure 4–2). Connections arising in the septum either from atrial myocardium or the transitional zone of the AV node and inserting in ventricular muscle have also been referred to as "Paladino Tracts" [26]. The typical ECG features of accessory AV connections have been well described and include:

1. a shortened PR interval for age [27] (less than 0.12 seconds in adults)
2. prolonged QRS duration for age [27] (greater

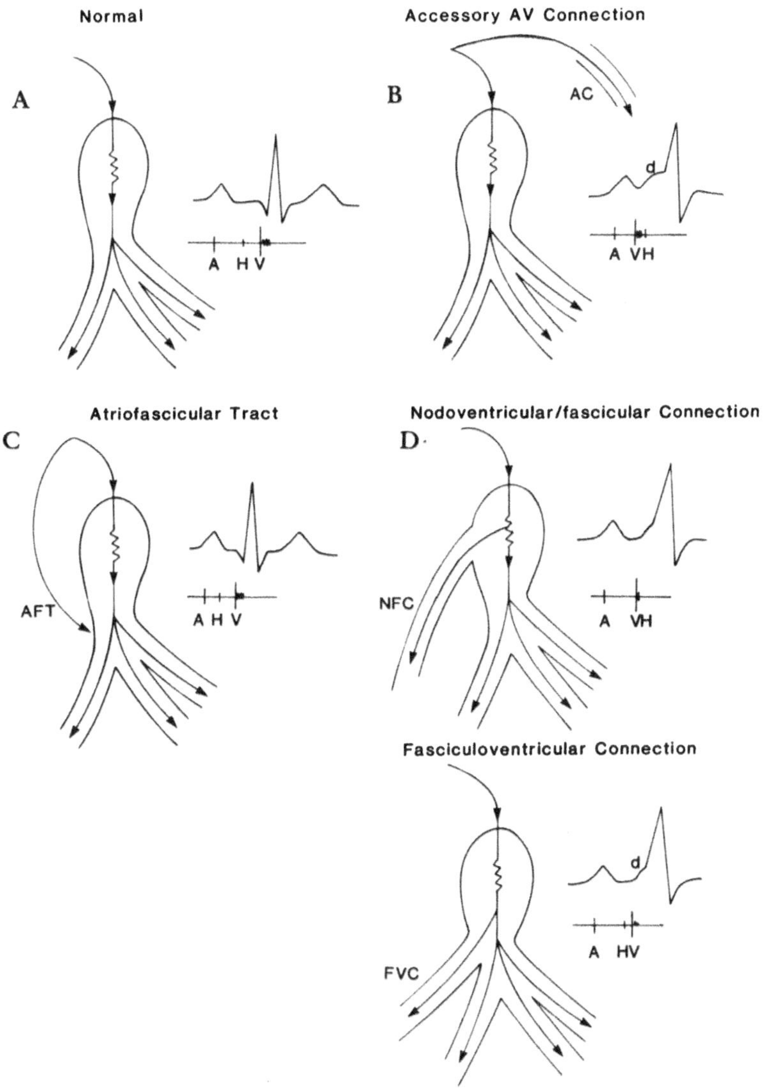

FIGURE 4–1. Configurations presumed responsible for the observed ECG patterns in preexcitation. The electrocardiogram, His bundle electrogram, and schematic of the conduction system as occurs normally (A), with an accessory AV connection (B), an atriofascicular tract (C), and nodoventricular/fascicular and fasciculo-ventricular connections (D). A, atrial electrogram; H, His bundle electrogram; V, ventricular electrogram; and d, delta wave; AC, accessory AV connection; AFT, atriofascicular tract; NFC, nodoventricular/fascicular connection; and FVC, fasciculoventricular connection.

than 0.12 seconds for adults) with a slurred slow-rising onset of the R wave upstroke (delta wave) consistent with preexcitation of the base of the heart;

3. secondary ST-T wave changes which are directed opposite to the major delta and QRS vectors.

Figure 4–3 provides a schematic illustration of the alterations in the ECG induced by preexcitation. The ECG abnormalities are the result of fusion of ventricular activation via the normal conduction system and the accessory connection. Notably, PR interval shortening is the result of early ventricular activation over the

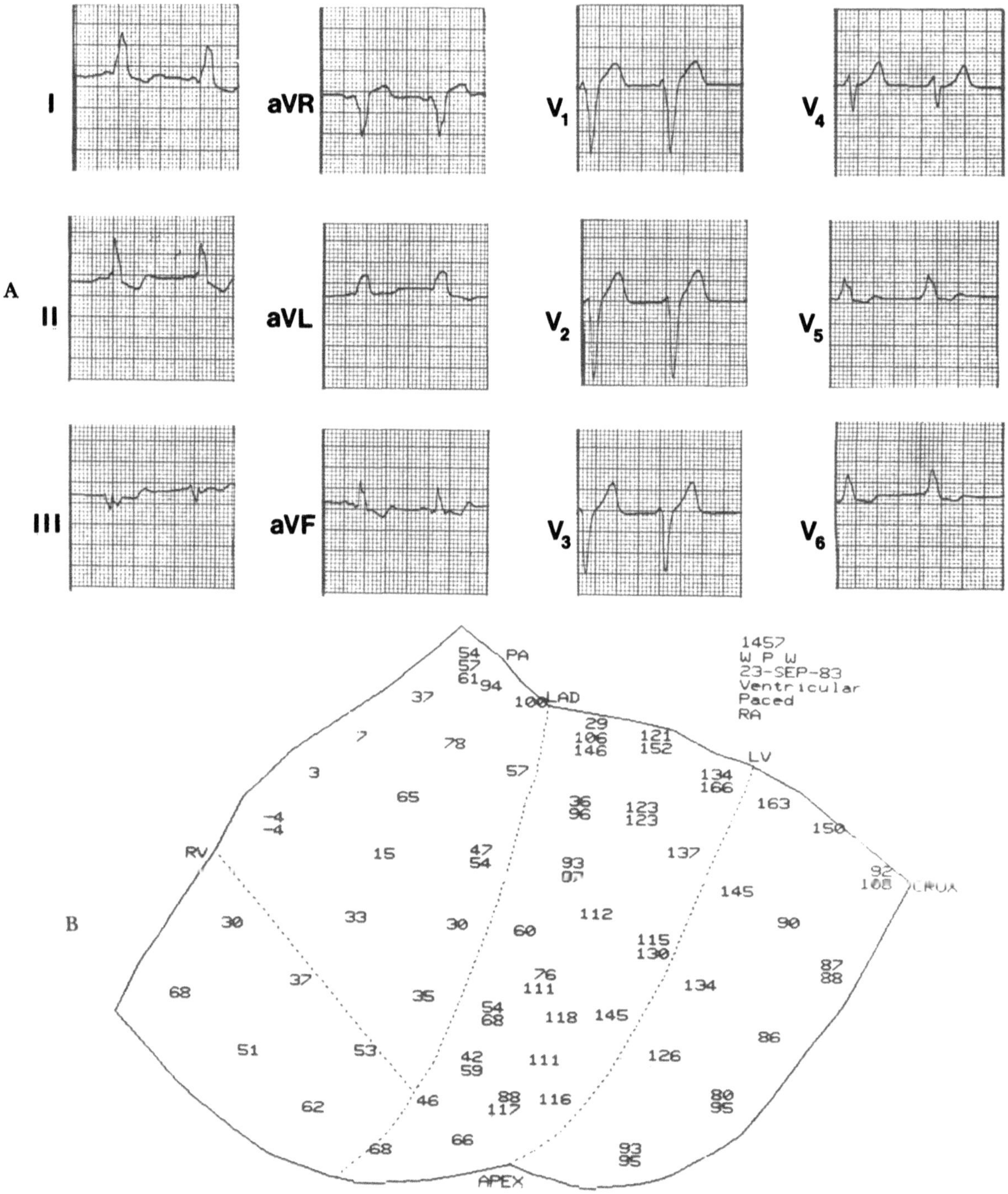

FIGURE 4–2. (A) Standard ECG with typical features of a right lateral accessory AV connection including short PR interval and evidence of obvious ventricular preexcitation (delta waves). Note delta waves are + in leads I, AVL, II, V_{1-6}, and – in AVR, III, AVF. (B) Ventricular epicardial activation timing at operation obtained with right atrial pacing (recorded times are in ms referenced to onset of QRS on surface ECG). Notably earliest ventricular activation occurs just over the right lateral AV groove. RV, right ventricle; PA, pulmonary artery; LAD, left anterior descending coronary artery; and LV, left ventricle.

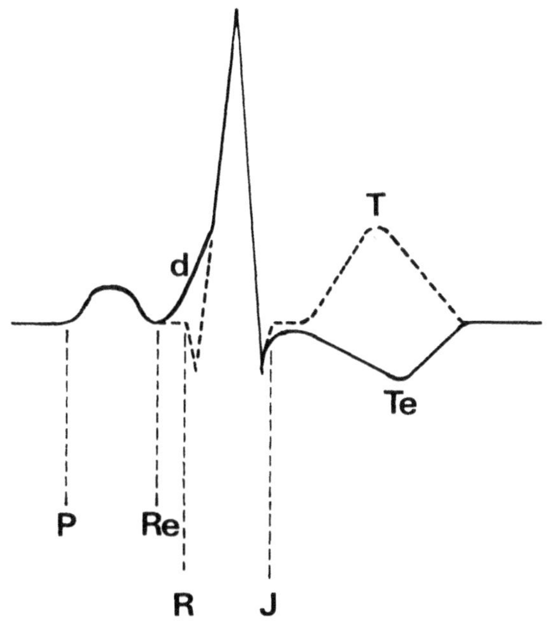

FIGURE 4–3. Schematic representation of alterations in the ECG Induced by preexcitation. The solid line indicates ventricular depolarization initiated by an accessory AV connection, while the dotted line indicates ventricular depolarization initiated via the specialized conduction system. PRe and PR intervals represent AV conduction associated with and without preexcitation, respectively. The PRe interval is shorter because of early ventricular activation by the accessory connection. Note the PJ intervals are unchanged indicating the time to complete ventricular depolarization is unchanged. Te of preexcited complexes is directed in the opposite direction to that of depolarization (see text) (after Chung [83]).

accessory connection with the PJ interval being the same in preexcited and normal beats, suggesting that the time to complete ventricular depolarization is unchanged.

With the advent of His bundle recordings in man [28], it was noted that the His deflection occurred after onset of earliest recorded ventricular activation in maximally preexcited beats and before ventricular activation in beats which had a more normal QRS appearance (less preexcitation) [16] (Figure 4–1). Electrograms thought to represent depolarization in the accessory connection have been recorded prior to His bundle activation in preexcited beats from the epicardial surface of the heart [19,20] and with intracardiac catheters [29,30].

That the preexcited QRS is a fusion complex resulting from colliding wave fronts originating by way of the normal AV conduction system and an accessory AV muscle bundle was suggested by Holzmann and Scherf [31] and independently by Wolferth and Wood [32] in 1932–1933. In 1942, Butterworth and Poindexter [33] passed currents picked up from the atrial surface through a vacuum tube amplifier and utilized the output to stimulate the ventricles. In this way, they were able to mimic ECGs seen in patients with preexcitation. By reversing the connections and applying amplified ventricular currents to the atrium, they were also able to produce paroxysms of tachycardia with a normal QRS simulating those seen in patients with preexcitation.

Histologic proof of the existence of accessory connections in patients with ECG evidence of preexcitation was provided in 1941 by Ohnell (left–sided accessory AV connection) [34] and in 1943 by Wood et al. (right–sided accessory AV connection) [35]. Boineau and Moore [36] and Boineau et al. [37] provided final proof of the relationship between accessory AV connections and preexcitation by combining both anatomic evidence and functional demonstration of propagation across accessory AV connections in a dog and monkey both with naturally occurring preexcitation. In man, direct epicardial excitation timing recorded during cardiac surgery [38,39] and successful surgical division of suspected accessory AV connections [14] with disappearance of preexcitation, substantiated the nature of the preexcited QRS.

Studies of the electrophysiologic basis of ventricular preexcitation have evaluated depolarization almost exclusively, and the ST-T wave changes exhibited during preexcited beats have rarely been investigated. However, Spach et al. [40] showed that for similar sequences of ventricular activation, there is a similarity of epicardial events throughout excitation and repolarization, the latter having potential distributions that essentially mirror image the former. Thus, when a significant portion of ventricular activation occurs by way of an accessory AV connection (maximal preexcitation) the ST-T waves have a polarity opposite to the delta wave and QRS.

A short PR interval is one manifestation of preexcitation and may result from early ventricular activation via an accessory AV connection. Alternate origins of a short PR interval include any situation in which normal conduction delay in the AV node is abbreviated, thus shortening the PR interval [41]. The combination of accelerated AV node conduction with earlier ventricular activation than would be expected over the normal ventricular conduction system has been recognized clinically in several patients with enhanced AV node conduction [20] in association with fasciculoventricular connections [18,20, 42–45]. Fasciculoventricular connections arise from the His bundle or bundle branches and insert into the ventricular myocardium [18]. Their functional significance is unknown but may depend on the site of take-off from the distal conduction system, the number and size of the fibers, their conduction velocity, and distal insertion site [18]. Generally, the PR interval would be expected to be normal in association with isolated fasciculoventricular connections [24,45]; however, in previously described cases [43,44,45], the PR interval is frequently short. Thus, the principal electrophysiologic features mimic ventricular preexcitation as seen with accessory AV connections.

The QRS complex associated with fasciculoventricular connections are usually slightly prolonged with slurring of the initial forces suggesting a delta wave [45]. Anomalous QRS morphology resembling right as well as left bundle branch block has been described [45]. The QRS morphology should be reasonably constant since fusion does not vary [24]. Extrasystoles arising in the His bundle or pacing of the His bundle should not normalize the QRS unless the extrasystoles arise below the take-off of the fasciculoventricular connection [46].

NORMAL PR INTERVAL WITH ANOMALOUS QRS COMPLEXES

The presence of ventricular preexcitation depends on the location of the accessory connection and conduction properties of the atrium, ventricle, accessory connection, AV node, and His-Purkinje system. Since the delta wave results from depolarization of ventricular muscle by an atrial impulse conducted over the accessory connection, situations in which conduction throughout the specialized cardiac conduction system is delayed can result in a normal or prolonged PR interval with preexcitation of the ventricle occurring by means of the accessory connection. This concept is illustrated in a patient with a left posterior AV connection (Figure 4–4). When preexcitation was not evident, the PR interval was greater than 0.20 seconds. With preexcitation, the PR interval was greater than 0.12 seconds. Thus, the length of the PR interval alone does not exclude an accessory AV muscle connection as the etiology of preexcitation.

Figure 4–5 illustrates ECGs with findings characteristic of a left lateral accessory AV connection. In panel A, subtle findings of preexcitation are present. However, atrial pacing at faster rates produces very obvious ventricular preexcitation with PR interval shortening on the surface ECG (panel B). During pacing, AV nodal conduction may slow sufficiently to allow for more obvious preexcitation to occur. Pacing the coronary sinus in close proximity to the connection increases the extent of preexcitation (panel C).

Although accessory connections arising within the AV node and inserting into ventricular myocardium (nodoventricular) were first described anatomically by Mahaim [47,48] in the 1940s, it was not until 1971 that Wellens [49] reported the electrophysiologic findings in a patient with a nodoventricular connection. Only a single case report is available which correlates anatomic and electrophysiologic findings in a patient with a nodoventricular connection [50].

Nodoventricular/fascicular connections arise in the AV node and insert into the right ventricular specialized conduction system and/or ventricular myocardium [19]. To date, no example of a left ventricular insertion site has been shown [19,24,45]. Depending on the level of take-off from the AV node relative to the area of physiologic delay, the PR interval may be abbreviated or, more commonly, normal [51,52]. The electrocardiogram during sinus rhythm is usually normal [51,52], but may show evidence of early right ventricular activation.

Typically in patients with nodoventricular/fascicular connections, atrial pacing or premature atrial stimulation results in PR interval prolongation and the QRS complex assumes a left bundle branch block morphology with left axis deviation. Despite the appearance of a preexcited QRS, the PR interval remains normal or prolongs in contrast to accessory AV connections. Frequently patients with nodoventricular/fascicular connections have associated Ebstein's anomaly [19,45]. Thus intermittent left bundle branch block (related to ventricular preexcitation via a nodoventricular connection)

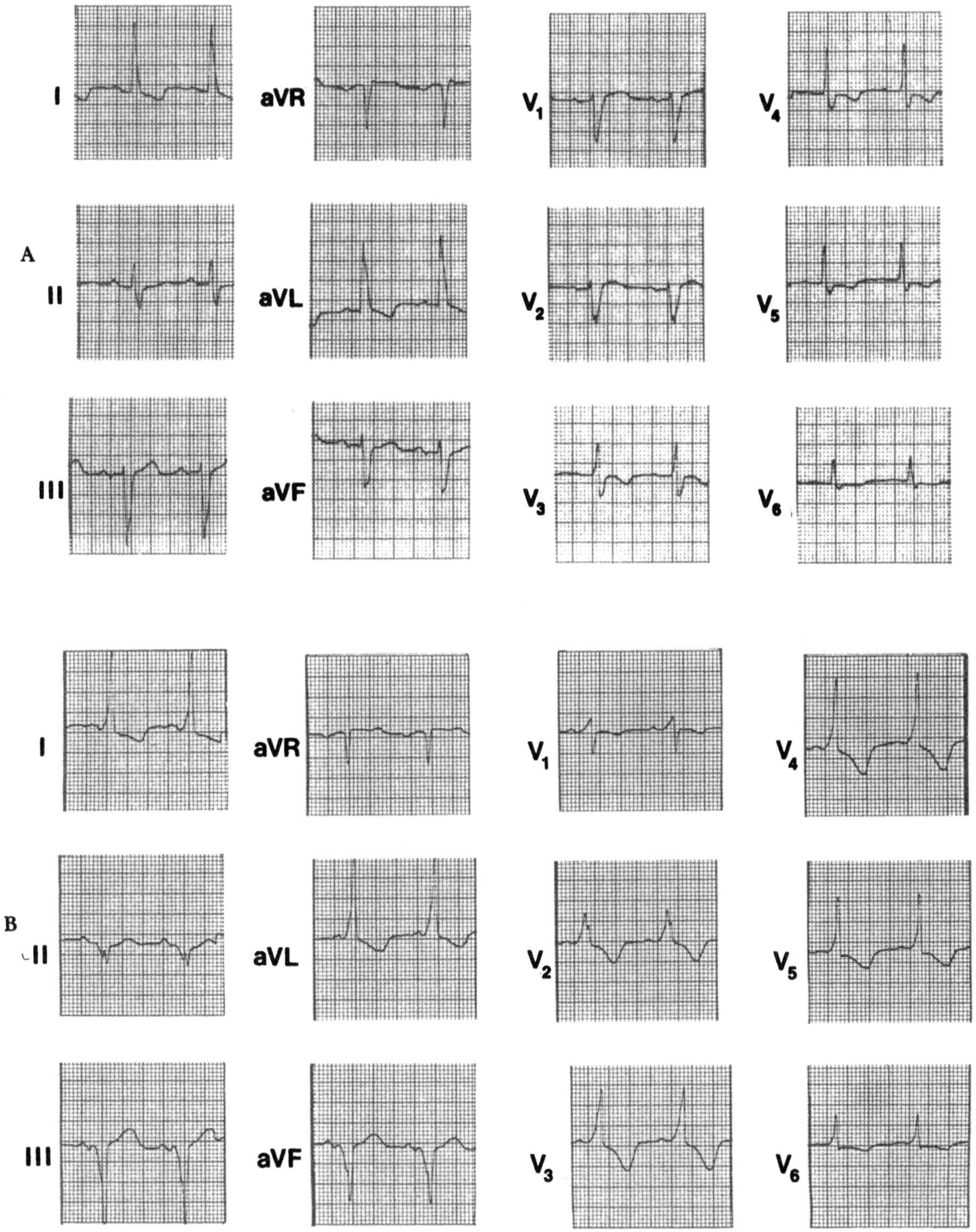

FIGURE 4–4. Standard ECGs in a patient with a left posterolateral accessory AV connection and known ischemic heart disease. (A) Without evident ventricular preexcitation, the PR interval is greater than 0.20 sec. (B) With ventricular preexcitation, the PR interval remains >0.12 sec.

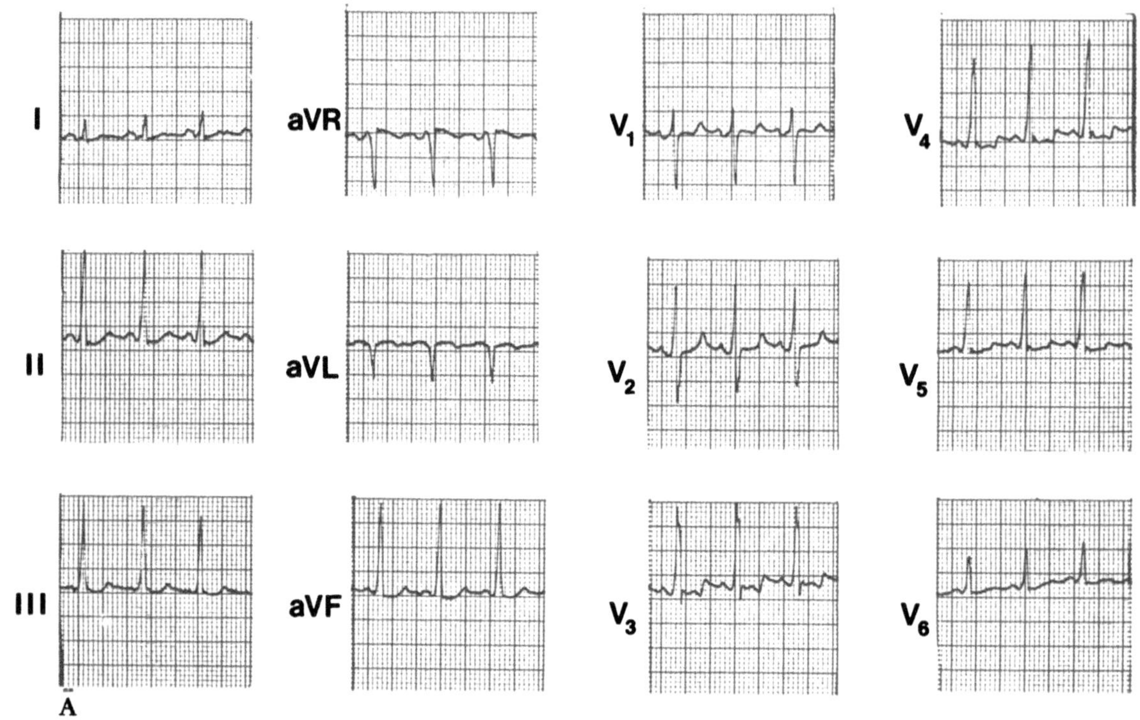
I
aVR
V1
V4
II
aVL
V2
V5
III
aVF
V3
V6

A

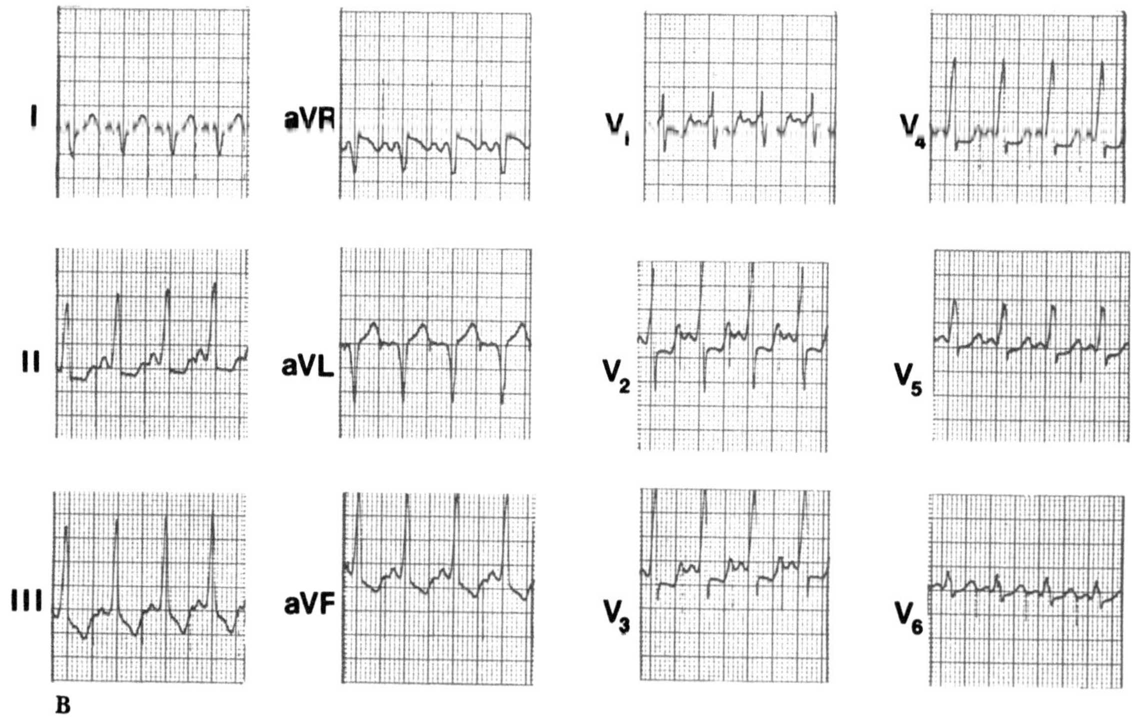
I
aVR
V1
V4
II
aVL
V2
V5
III
aVF
V3
V6

B

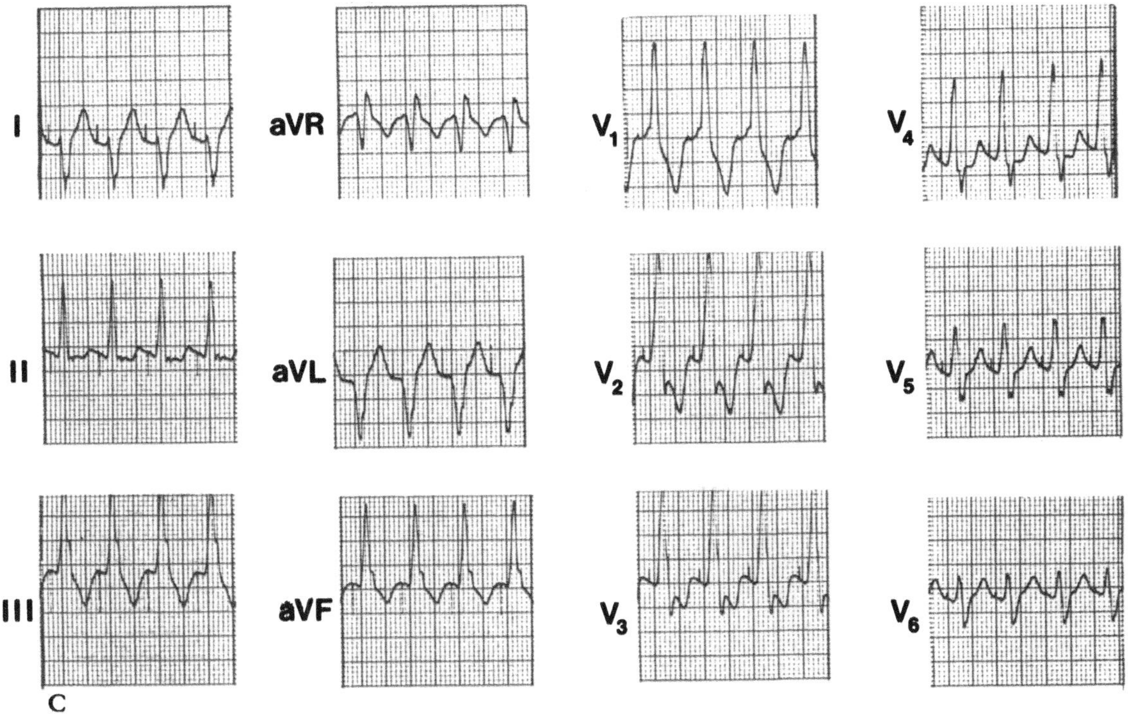

FIGURE 4–5. Standard ECGs demonstrating the variability in preexcitation obtained by varying pacing rate and site in a left lateral accessory connection. (A) Sinus rhythm (CL-490 ms). (B) Right atrial pacing (CL 400 ms). (C) Coronary sinus pacing (CL 400 ms). Note the increasing degree of ventricular preexcitation on each subsequent tracing.

and right bundle branch block (related to the Ebstein's anomaly) can be seen [19]. Figure 4–6 is an example of recordings from a patient with a nodoventricular/fascicular connection demonstrated during sinus rhythm and atrial pacing.

SHORT PR INTERVAL, NORMAL QRS COMPLEXES

Patients with short PR interval, normal QRS complex, and palpitations were described by Clerc and colleagues in 1938 [53] and later further characterized by Lown, Ganong, and Levine [54] in 1952. The latter authors described the occurrence of paroxysmal tachycardia in 19 of 184 patients (>10 years of age) demonstrating short PR intervals (<0.12 sec) with suggestive symptoms in an additional 15 cases. In contrast, in a control group of 200 patients with normal PR intervals (>0.12 sec), only one case of documented tachycardia and 7 suggestive histories were obtained. The cases described by Lown et al. [54] were obtained by reviewing retrospectively 13,500 consecutive electrocardiograms performed on a hospital population. Thus, the incidence of short PR intervals is low, but in affected patients, there may be a predisposition to have tachycardia.

The important issues to be addressed in individuals with short PR intervals are the mechanisms of the short PR interval and whether a short PR interval predisposes one to tachyarrhythmias. The PR interval represents the sum of conduction times through the atrium (PA interval), AV node (AH interval), and His-Purkinje system (HV interval). In most instances, differences in PR intervals between patients with normal QRS complexes can be explained by differences in AH intervals with little change in PA or HV intervals. In patients with short PR intervals, relatively short AH intervals have been recorded [55–58]. The abbreviated AH (PR) could be related to conduction over an atriofascicular bypass tract (44, 59, 60), but these occur only rarely. Additionally, the concept of "enhanced" AV nodal conduction (EAVN) has been proposed [20,41]. In

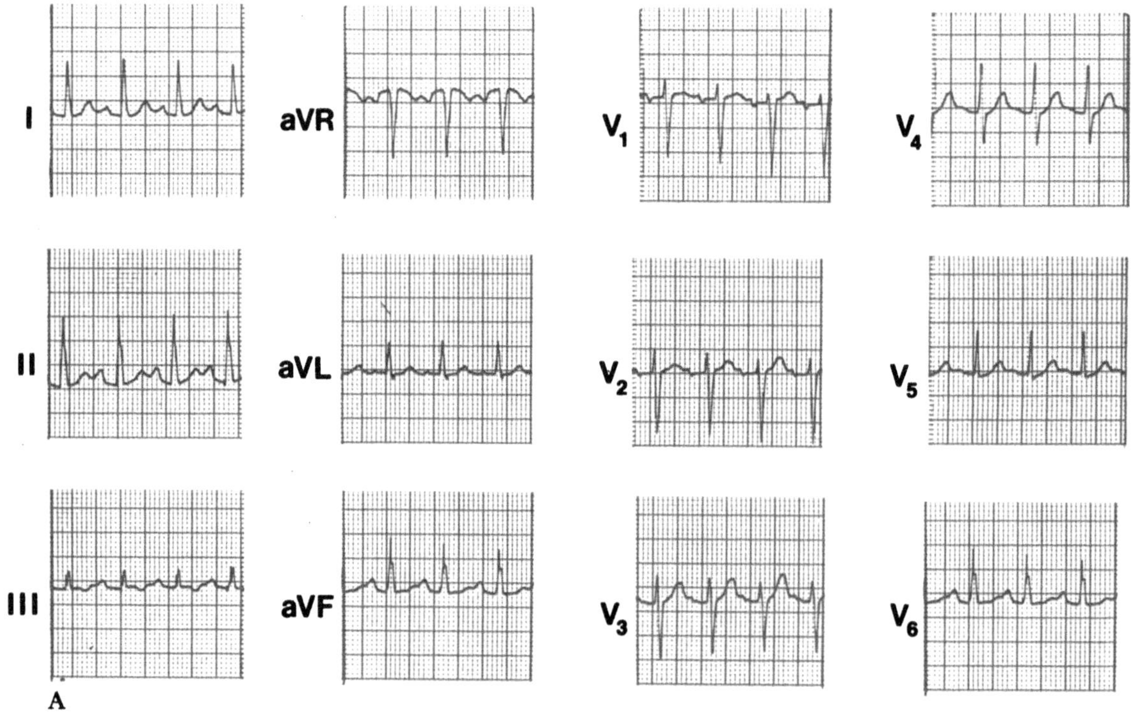
I
aVR
V_1
V_4
II
aVL
V_2
V_5
III
aVF
V_3
V_6

A

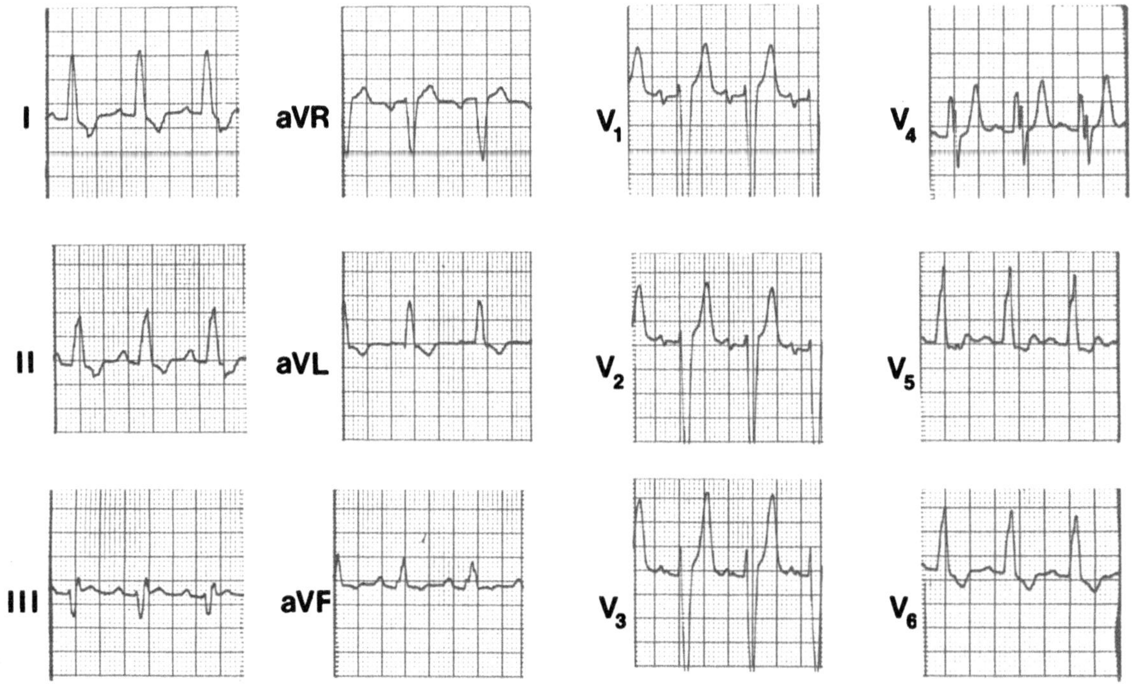
I
aVR
V_1
V_4
II
aVL
V_2
V_5
III
aVF
V_3
V_6

B

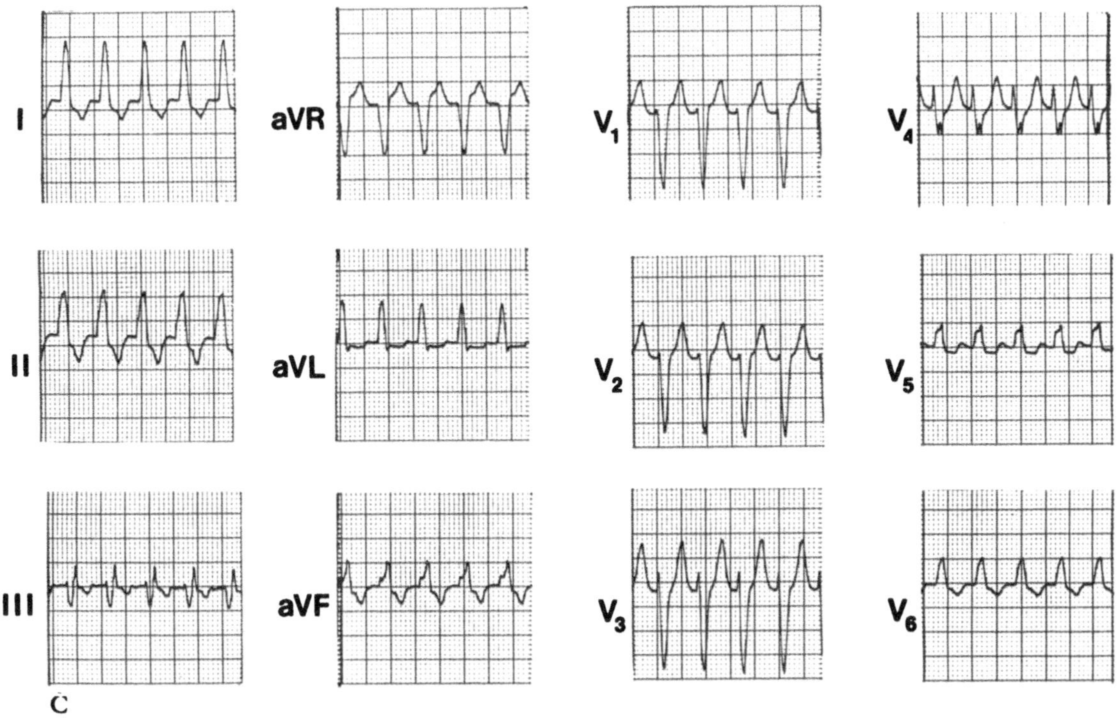

FIGURE 4–6. Standard ECGs from a patient with a nodoventricular/fascicular connection. (A) Sinus rhythm without evident ventricular preexcitation. (B) Sinus rhythm with ventricular preexcitation. ECG demonstrates characteristic left bundle branch features of preexcitation through a nodoventricular/fascicular connection (see text). (C) Tachycardia demonstrating identical QRS morphology to sinus rhythm ECG in (B).

short, EAVN describes an AV node lacking normal delay producing characteristics, thus allowing rapid AV signal transmission. Benditt, et al. [55] demonstrated an increased incidence (7 of 12, 58%) of EAVN in patients with short PR intervals and documented arrhythmias with a lesser incidence (7 of 28, 25%) in a group of patients with normal PR intervals referred for evaluation of regular narrow QRS tachycardias or atrial fibrillation-flutter.

Explanations provided for a shortened PR interval do not demonstrate a causal relationship to the initiation or maintenance of supraventricular tachycardias. It is possible that the relatively short AH intervals recorded represent conduction over the "fast" pathway in some patients with dual AV nodal physiology with or without reentry within the AV node [61]. Unidirectional antegrade block in this "fast" pathway could allow conduction over the "slow" AV nodal pathway with the initiation of tachycardia due to reentry within the AV node. However, most patients with tachycardia due to reentry within the AV node have normal PR intervals with only a minority having shortened or prolonged PR intervals [62].

The types of arrhythmias reported in patients with short PR intervals include reciprocating tachycardia using an accessory AV connection with conduction only in the retrograde direction, tachycardia due to reentry within the AV node, primary atrial tachycardia (i.e., atrial fibrillation-flutter) with rapid ventricular response rates, and ventricular tachycardia/fibrillation [55]. Tachyarrhythmias which traverse the AV node (primary atrial or AV reentrant tachycardias) associated with EAVN tend to result in more rapid ventricular rates [55,63,64] than similar tachyarrhythmias in patients without EAVN. In contrast in patients with tachycardia due to reentry within the AV node combined with EAVN, the cycle length of tachycardia is not significantly affected [64,65]. The association of ventricular dysrhythmias in patients with a short PR interval is poorly defined. Sudden death has been reported in patients with short PR intervals and a history of atrial fibrillation [54,55]. In one case R-on-T phenomena during atrial fibrillation was suggested as a potential etiology [66]. In other instances ventricular dysrhythmias were likely due to concomitant organic heart disease [62].

Thus, although there clearly is a group of patients in whom short PR intervals are associated with tachydysrhythmias, the nature of this apparent relationship remains ill-defined. Hence, the significance of an isolated short PR interval on a routine ECG without a history of dysrhythmias has unknown significance.

DYNAMIC ELECTROCARDIOGRAPHIC VARIATIONS IN ATRIOVENTRICULAR PREEXCITATION

Early electrocardiographers observed the dynamic variability of the ECG recordings in patients having anomalous AV conduction. In 1915, in one of the first cases described, Wilson [4] hypothesized an important role was played by the vagus on influencing the form of the ventricular complex. In 1930, Wolff, Parkinson, and White [9] observed intermittent preexcitation in some of their cases. For example, after recording an ECG that demonstrated preexcitation at rest, and given the history of symptoms of palpitations appearing with exercise, one patient was instructed to run up and down four flights of stairs in hopes of provoking an attack of tachycardia. The response to exercise was unexpected as the ventricular complexes became normal and the PR interval increased from 0.10 seconds to 0.16 seconds despite the fact that the heart rate rose to levels of 120 to 140 beats/minute. On a subsequent visit to Dr. White's laboratory, the abnormal ECG was again observed. Following subcutaneous injection of 2 mg atropine, the recording again normalized as it had with exercise previously. In 1944, Ohnell [2] described what he termed the *concertina effect* or the dynamic variability in beat to beat magnitude of the delta wave (Figure 4–7), which he correctly attributed to variation in the extent of fusion of ventricular depolarization

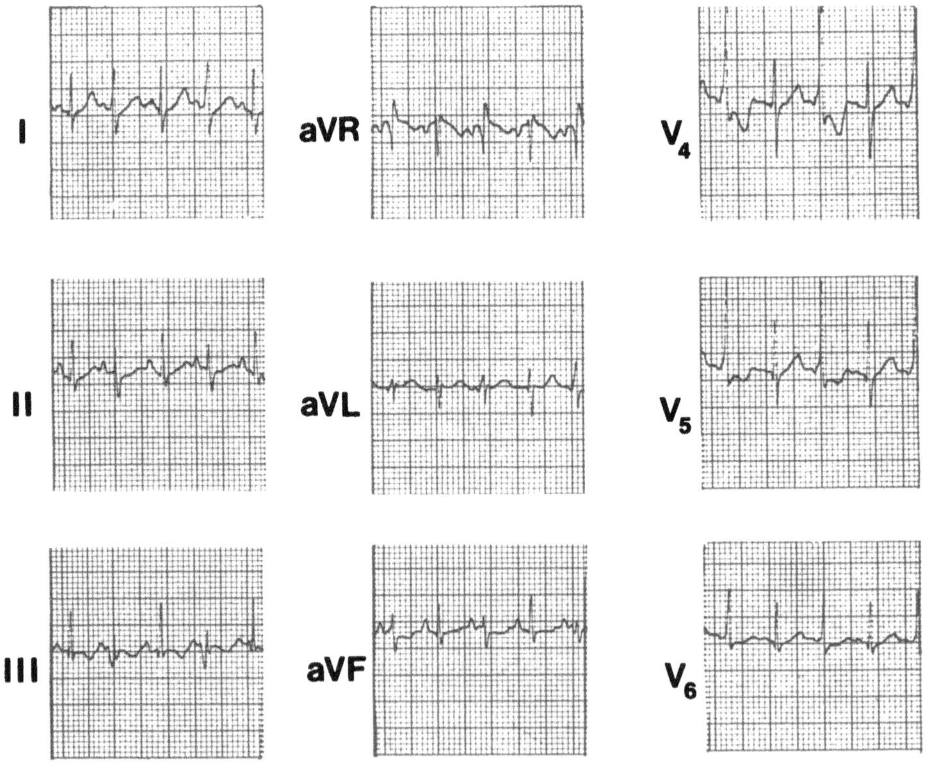

FIGURE 4–7. ECG demonstrating dynamic beat to beat preexcitation.

occurring via the AV node and that occurring via an anomalous connection.

Reflex vagal stimulation, such as may be achieved by carotid sinus massage, may favor the occurrence of preexcitation in some patients with accessory AV connection by slowing AV nodal conduction thereby favoring ventricular activation via the accessory connection [22]. In other instances, the fact that a critical cycle length separates conduction from block supports the interpretation that vagal stimulation acts by prolonging cycle length beyond the end of a long refractory period of some accessory connections [68]. A direct vagal effect on the accessory connection must also be considered. De la Fuente et al. [69], working with an isthmus of isolated canine atrial tissue simulating some of the features of preexcitation, showed that acetylcholine could improve conduction within the model of an accessory AV connection under certain conditions. Additionally, vagal stimulation may enhance intraatrial conduction or shift the site of impulse formation from the sinus node to an ectopic atrial site, and as a consequence produce a change in the mode and/or site of entry into the accessory connection and AV node [68]. Muscarinic blockade with atropine can result in QRS normalization presumably by improving AV nodal conduction [9].

Catecholamines have been demonstrated to improve conduction and shorten refractoriness in normal cardiac tissue [70,71]. Consequently, it is not surprising that Wellens et al. [72] have been able to show that isoproterenol shortens the refractory period of accessory connections in the antegrade direction. Further, by administering isoproterenol in combination with carotid sinus massage, Przbylski et al. [68] was able to reinduce ECG evidence of preexcitation in 5 of 12 patients in which carotid sinus massage alone failed.

The site of the accessory connection also determines the extent of preexcitation. For example, during sinus rhythm, right sided connections usually manifest more obvious preexcitation than those on the left side of the heart (Figure 4–2 vs. Figure 4–8). Boineau et al. [37], using epicardial activation mapping, demonstrated QRS duration during preexcitation to be dependent on collision of wave fronts conducted over the normal and accessory connections in subjects with preexcitation. The greater distance from the sinus node to the atrial input of the accessory connection in left ventricular versus right ventricular forms of preexcitation resulted in later activation of the accessory connection and allowed more time for ventricular activation to be initiated by the normal conduction system. Additionally, dynamic QRS changes which were induced by a slight shift of the spontaneous atrial pacemaker resulted in a change in atrial activation and hence the degree of ventricular preexcitation (Figure 4–5).

Geometric considerations or "impedance mismatch" may be important in determining the ability of an accessory connection to preexcite ventricular muscle [69]. De la Fuente et al. [69], using isolated blocks of canine atrial tissue dissected to provide a narrow isthmus connecting two broader areas, demonstrated undirectional block at the junctions of the narrow band with the larger areas. Thus, although the isthmus could conduct quite effectively, the geometry of the insertion of a narrow band into a larger mass of muscle appeared to provide only a narrow margin of safety for propagation [69].

Exercise may be associated with variation in preexcitation (see Chapter 8 by Lévy et al.). Responsible mechanisms may include release of vagal tone with an increase in sympathetic activity. Resulting improved AV nodal conduction (evidenced by the shortened PR interval) would lessen the opportunity for preexcitation. Alternatively, in other instances, increased circulating catecholamines might enhance conduction in the antegrade direction over accessory AV connections, thereby accentuating the degree of preexcitation.

Several investigators have reported the disappearance of evidence of preexcitation for years both in children and adults [68,73]. In children, especially neonates, the disappearance of delta waves has been thought to be related to postnatal shaping and molding of the AV node and His bundle with increasing age such that the final form of these structures in some way influences the appearance of delta waves [74,75]. Developmental changes may also occur in the accessory connections themselves; causing loss of preexcitation [76]. Additionally, age-related changes in autonomic input to the heart may be responsible for variable preexcitation. In adults, accessory connection conduction and/or refractory characteristics may be prolonged sufficiently to alter preexcitation [68]. Conversely,

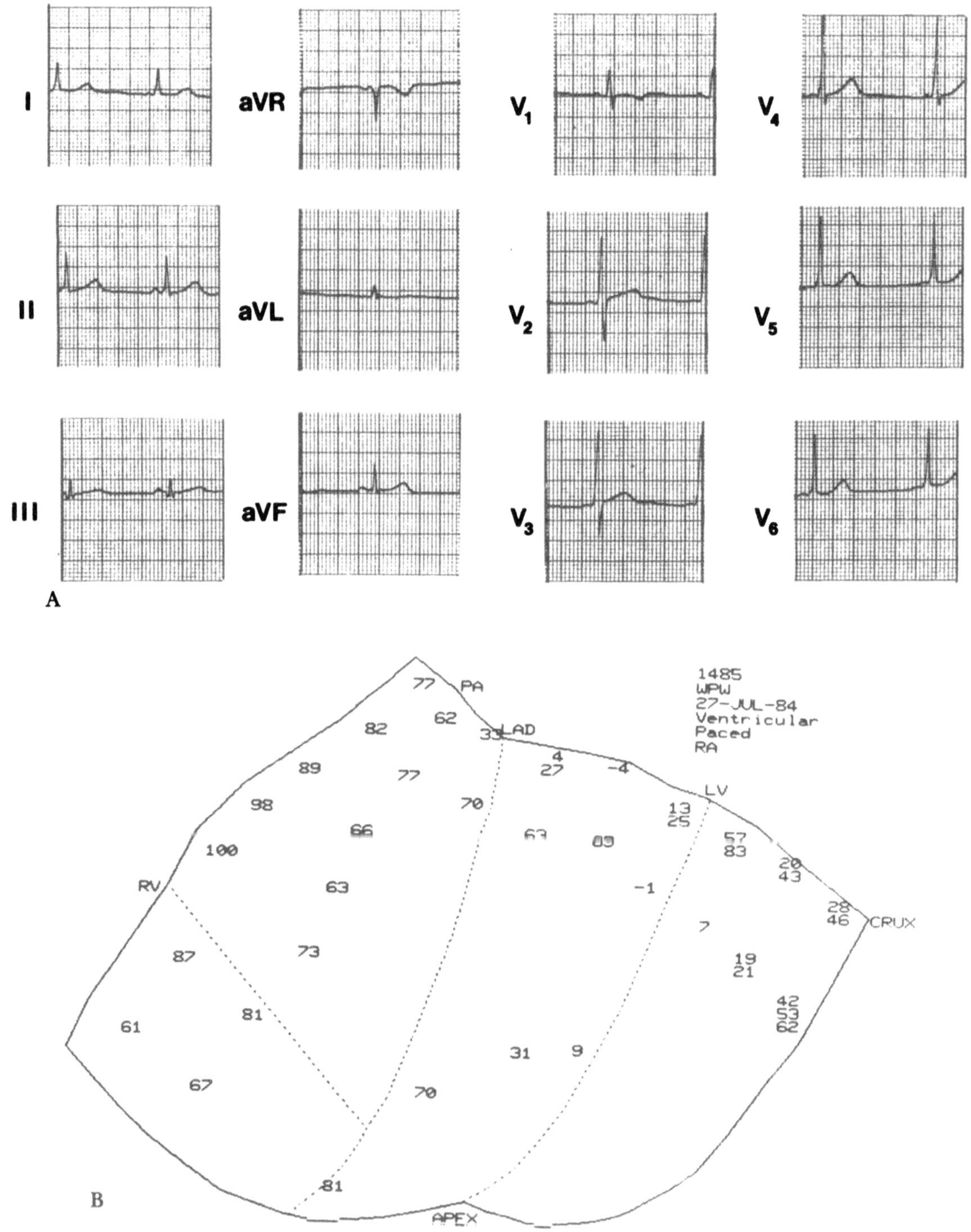

FIGURE 4–8. (A) standard ECG from a patient with a left lateral accessory AV connection. Note + delta waves in I, AVL, II, V_{1-6} and – in III, AVR, AVF. (B) Ventricular epicardial activation timing recorded during right atrial pacing (recorded times are in ms referenced to onset of QRS on surface ECG). Notably ventricular activation occurs earliest just across the left lateral AV groove. (Abbreviations as in Figure 4–2.)

alterations occurring with age or as a result of disease processes may influence the normal specialized conduction system enough to enable more manifest preexcitation [24].

USE OF ECG TECHNIQUES IN THE LOCATION OF THE SITE OF PREEXCITATION

In 1933, just three years after the description of the WPW syndrome, Wolferth and Wood suggested that intrapatient differences in the morphology of the initial QRS deflection might be due to variations in the location of accessory connections [32]. In 1945, Rosenbaum et al. [1], while working in Wilson's laboratory, reported on ten cases of preexcitation in detail. In Rosenbaum's series, leads from the left side of the precordium (V4 through V6) were always dominated by a large R wave with the ascending limb of the QRS slurred in a positive direction by the delta wave. In most instances, a small S wave was noted, but a Q wave was never present. Thus, depending on the variability of QRS configuration in leads from the right precordium, (V1 and V2) and the esophageal lead (V_E), two types of preexcitation were described. In Type A, the R wave is the only dominant deflection in leads V1, V2, V_E and in Type B, an S (rS-current terminology) or QS deflection predominated in at least one of the right precordial leads. Rosenbaum et al. [1] concluded that the dorsal wall of the ventricles was activated prematurely and the differences between Type A and B cases was due, at least in part, to differences in the order of ventricular activation. Subsequently, Giraud et al. [77] speculated that Type A was related to left posterior basilar preexcitation and Type B was the result of right lateral ventricular preexcitation. Laham [23] has reviewed various other systems of classification in detail. Most of the early classifications, however, failed to suggest the possibility of septal connections.

As described, Rosenbaum's classification was based on the polarity of the major deflection in the right precordial leads and not specifically on the vectorial direction of the delta vector. Later investigators tried to classify ventricular preexcitation by the use of both delta and QRS vectors in all three planes as utilized in standard Frank vectorcardiography [78,79]. However, what was lacking was a "gold standard" technique to precisely locate accessory connections in order to test ECG methods. By the late 1960s and early 1970s, direct atrial and ventricular epicardial activation mapping at surgery provided insight into the basis of variations observed in the surface ECG [14,38,39].

The group at Duke University correlated the initial delta wave polarity on the 12-lead ECG with the site of the accessory connection determined at surgery by epicardial mapping [20,79] (Figure 4–9). Their technique involves: (1) recording simultaneous ECG leads to allow careful identification of isoelectric portions of the delta wave; (2) minimizing the influence of fusion with the normal conduction system by examining only maximally preexcited beats with a QRS duration greater than 0.14 seconds; and (3) basing classification on the analysis of the vector of the first 40 ms [20] following onset of ventricular depolarization (QRS) as recorded by the standard ECG. Final conformation of connection location was provided by ablation of preexcitation by a relatively localized surgical incision through the adjacent AV valve anulus.

As can be seen in the table in Figure 4–9, simple designation of the polarity of the delta wave in V_1 does not permit identification of the possible existence of septal accessory connections. In fact, septal accessory connections can have a variable appearance in V_1 with either an isoelectric or positive delta wave (Figure 4–10). Further, in contrast to Rosenbaum's initial classification scheme, a form of preexcitation in which negative delta waves are observed in V_5 and V_6 simulating Q waves has been described [23,79]. Invariably, these patients are found to have left posterolateral accessory connections (sites 7,8).

Although as many as 10 sites have been described (Figure 4–9), correlation of delta wave polarity with accessory AV connection location demonstrates that considerable overlap exists among the multiple sites. A more practicable approach consists in locating accessory AV connections according to general areas along the AV groove. Septal/paraseptal connections can be divided into either anterior (site 1) or posterior (sites 5,6) locations. Free wall connections can be grouped into either right anterior (site 2), right or left lateral (site 3 on right; sites 9,10 on left), or right or left posterolateral (site 4 on right; sites 7,8 on left) areas. The surgical approach to AV connection disruption follows this more generalized AV groove area location scheme by utilizing AV ring exploration on both sides of a "site" localized connection.

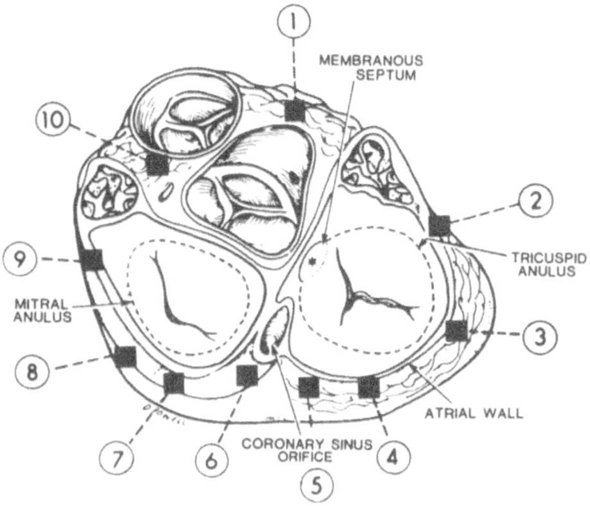

1. RIGHT ANTERIOR PARASEPTAL
2. RIGHT ANTERIOR
3. RIGHT LATERAL
4. RIGHT POSTERIOR
5. RIGHT PARASEPTAL
6. LEFT POSTERIOR PARASEPTAL
7. LEFT POSTERIOR
8. LEFT LATERAL
9. LEFT ANTERIOR
10. LEFT ANTERIOR PARASEPTAL

DELTA WAVE POLARITY

	I	II	III	AVR	AVL	AVF	V_1	V_2	V_3	V_4	V_5	V_6
①	+	+	+(±)	-	±(+)	+	±	±	+(±)	+	+	+
②	+	+	-(±)	-	+(±)	±(-)	±	+(±)	+(±)	+	+	+
③	+	±(-)	-	-	+	-(±)	±	±	±	+	+	+
④	+	-	-	-	+	-	±(+)	±	+	+	+	+
⑤	+	-	-	-(+)	+	-	±	+	+	+	+	+
⑥	+	-	-	-	+	-	+	+	+	+	+	+
⑦	+	-	-	±(+)	+	-	+	+	+	+	+	-(±)
⑧	-(±)	±	±	±(+)	-(±)	±	+	+	+	+	-(±)	-(±)
⑨	-(±)	+	+	-	-(±)	+	+	+	+	+	+	+
⑩	+	+	+(±)	-	±	+	±(+)	+	+	+	+	+

± = Initial 40 msec delta wave isoelectric
+ = Initial 40 msec delta wave positive
- = Initial 40 msec delta wave negative

FIGURE 4–9. Electrocardiographic classification of the Wolff-Parkinson-White syndrome. Ten representative sites of epicardial preexcitation are depicted on a schematic cross-section of the ventricles at the level of the atrioventricular rings. The expected polarity of the delta wave resulting from preexcitation at these sites is indicated for each of the 12 standard ECG leads. (Reproduced with permission [20].)

A previous comparison was made between site localization provided by the 20 msec delta wave vector from the ECG and the 10 msec vector from the vectorcardiogram [79]. The additional information that the vectorcardiogram supplied was twofold. It seemed to be a crude discriminator between septal and free wall connections. In eight patients with septal accessory connections, the vector was superiorly directed while in seven patients with either left or right free wall connections, the direction was inferior. Secondly, the early QRS forces in the great majority of patients were partially directed anteriorly regardless of the location of the accessory connection. This was felt related to the relative posterior location of the base of the heart, the site where preexcitation was initially occurring.

Isopotential body surface maps have been used to localize the site of ventricular preexcitation [80,81,82]. In this technique, ECGs are recorded at multiple sites over the anterior and posterior torso. Rather than viewing the scalar tracings (voltage-time variation) as done in standard electrocardiography, the maps display the potentials on the torso (voltage-space variation) at specific time instants. Spach et al. [40] modeled WPW syndrome in chimpanzees and evaluated the effect of ventricular preexcitation on epicardial and body surface distributions. The major manifestations on the body surface of selective epicardial events were changes in distant low-level potentials while there was no change in the potential distributions near the maximum or minimum potentials. The ST-T wave body surface potential distributions were as useful as the QRS patterns for localizing the site of ventricular preexcitation.

The presence of significant fusion of ventricular activation initiated via a single accessory connection and the normal conduction system or via multiple accessory connections complicates interpretation of any ECG technique including body surface maps. However, when fusion is minimized and ventricular activation is controlled primarily by a single accessory connection (ectopic site), the distribution of positive and negative potentials on the anterior and posterior torso during QRS and the ST segment provide an excellent index of the location of the accessory connection to one of six sites (posterior septal or anterior; lateral, posterior locations on the right or left). The localization of the site of the accessory connection using distributions too early in the QRS (before 40 ms) was unreliable because the early distributions varied from patient to patient for the same preexcitation site; however, the potential distributions during the ST segment were both stable and consistent from patient to patient for the same preexcitation site [82]. An example of an ST-T wave body surface map in a chimpanzee (Panel A) and a WPW syndrome patient (Panel B) is contained in Figure 4–11. In both the experimental and patient maps, the distribution of positive and negative potentials on the anterior and posterior torso during the ST-T wave are similar. The map in panel A was obtained from a chimpanzee following depolarization of the posterior right ventricle near the AV groove, whereas the map in panel B was obtained from a patient with a right posterior accessory AV connection. The corresponding measured epicardial potential distribution is shown for the chimpanzee; for the patient a calculated inverse epicardial potential distribution is shown.

Any ECG mapping technique has important limitations for localization of preexcitation sites [20,82]. These include: (1) possible existence of multiple accessory connections; (2) variable and often unknown degree of fusion of ventricular excitation due to conduction over both the normal and accessory connection, especially in situations where only minimal preexcitation is evident; and (3) superimposition of the terminal portion of the P wave on the initial aspect of the delta wave. Age, size, and associated heart disease appear to have little influence on the ECG when maximal preexcitation is present [82]. The utility of ECG techniques for localizing preexcitation sites can be enhanced by pharmacologic or pacing manuevers which tend to enhance preexcitation. Obviously, the ECG techniques of connection location have little or no utility in the assessment of connections with limited or no evident ventricular preexcitation. Thus, ECG localization techniques can be useful to supplement, not replace, the information gained by invasive intracardiac stimulation and recording studies.

PREEXCITATION — ELECTROCARDIOGRAPHIC MIMICRY

A clinically relevant feature of the preexcitation syndromes is their ability to mimic other entities electrocardiographically [20,83]. Depending on the site of insertion of accessory AV connections, preexcitation has been most commonly confused with either bundle branch block or myocardial infarction. Techniques which normalize the QRS including atrial pacing [85] or pharmacologic maneuvers may clarify the presence of the absence of preexcitation.

Right ventricular preexcitation can mimic left bundle branch (Figure 4–2), left ventricular hypertrophy, and/or anterior wall myocardial infarction. Septal connections which result in preexcitation of the diaphragmatic surface of the heart have superiorly directed electrical forces which can be misinterpreted as representing inferior wall infarction (see Figure 4–10). Left ventricular preexcitation can be misdiagnosed as right bundle branch block, right ventricular hypertrophy, and/or true posterior or lateral myocardial infarction. Generally, confusion with left bundle branch block can be avoided by recognizing the characteristic slurring of the QRS (delta wave) as opposed to the late intrinsicoid deflection resulting from the bundle branch block. RBBB has a rapid initial intrinsicoid deflection, especially in V_1, making misinterpretation less likely.

Delta waves misdiagnosed as Q waves representing infarction has been reported to occur in approximately one-third of cases with ventricular preexcitation due to accessory AV connections [84] (see Figure 4–4 — lower panel). In most instances, the appearance of the delta wave in multiple leads combined with large R or QS complexes should clarify the ECG interpretation. False positive exercise tests (i.e., exercise tests suggestive of myocardial ischemia) have been described in association with preexcitation [85,86]. If preexcitation persists with exercise, the ST-T waves which are directed opposite to the delta-QRS vector can demonstrate further ST depression making interpretation impossible. If preexcitation is not present or disappears with exercise, the ST-T changes should normalize with the QRS and not result in a false positive interpretation.

Other cardiac abnormalities with their associated ECG features can occur in patients with the preexcitation syndromes. The association of preexcitation with Ebstein's anomaly creates special problems for ECG interpretation [19,20]. An accessory AV connection resulting in right ventricular preexcitation can mask the often present late right ventricular activation seen in association with Ebstein's anomaly. Further, alternating left and right bundle branch block QRS morphologies may occur when

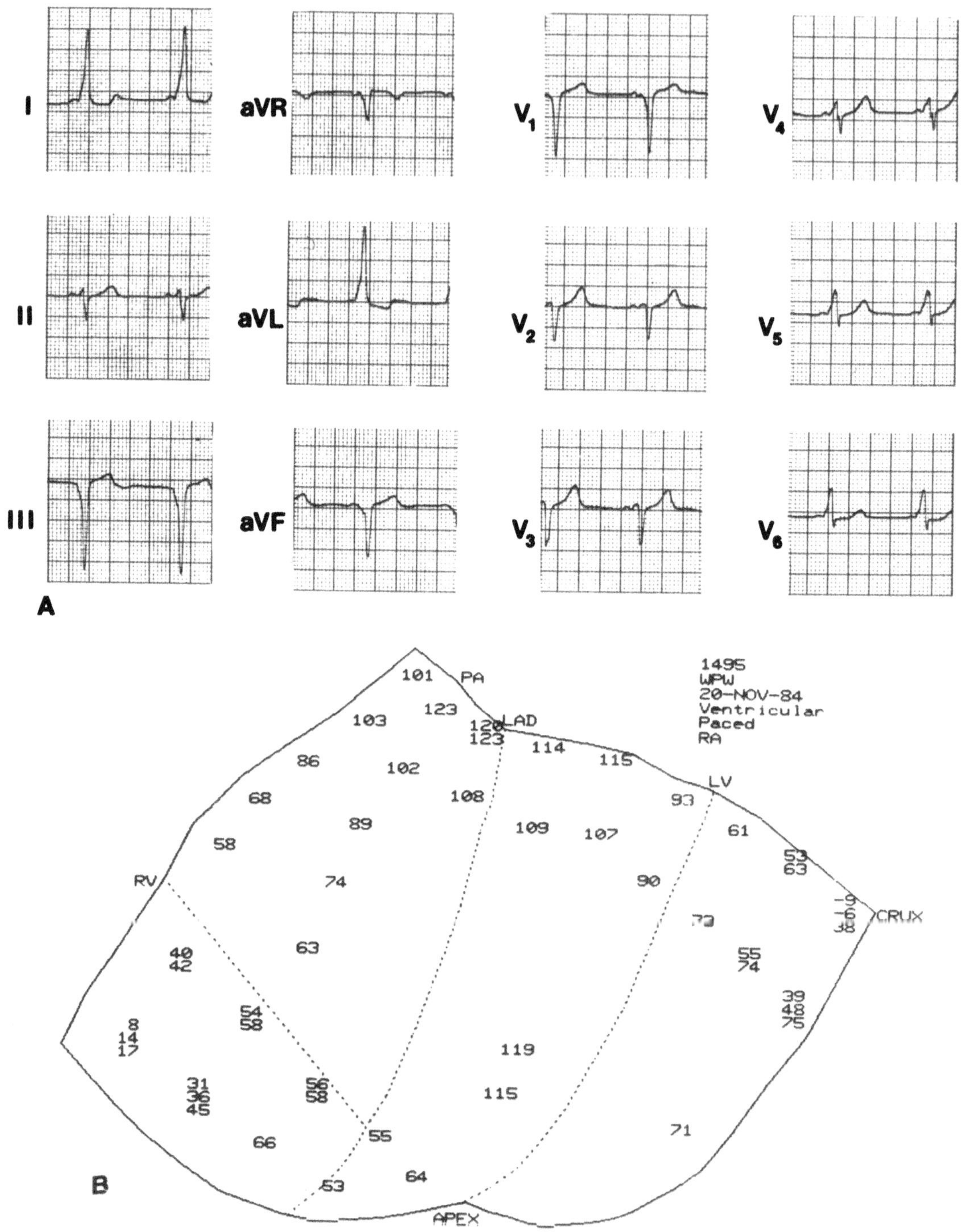

FIGURE 4–10. (A) Standard ECG from a patient with a posterior paraseptal accessory AV connection. Note + delta waves in I, AVL, V_{2-6}; isoelectric in V_1, II, and – in III, AVR, AVF. Comparing the delta wave polarity with Gallagher's proposed "site" classification system (Figure 4–9), would lead one to classify this connection as being on the right side of the septum. (B) However, epicardial activation timing recorded during right atrial pacing at surgery (recorded times are in ms referenced to the onset of the QRS on surface ECG) confirms a left posterior paraseptal area location of the connection (abbreviations as in Figure 4–2). Thus, ECG techniques can help localize posterior septal connections, but are probable not specific enough to locate these connections as being on either the right or left side of the septum.

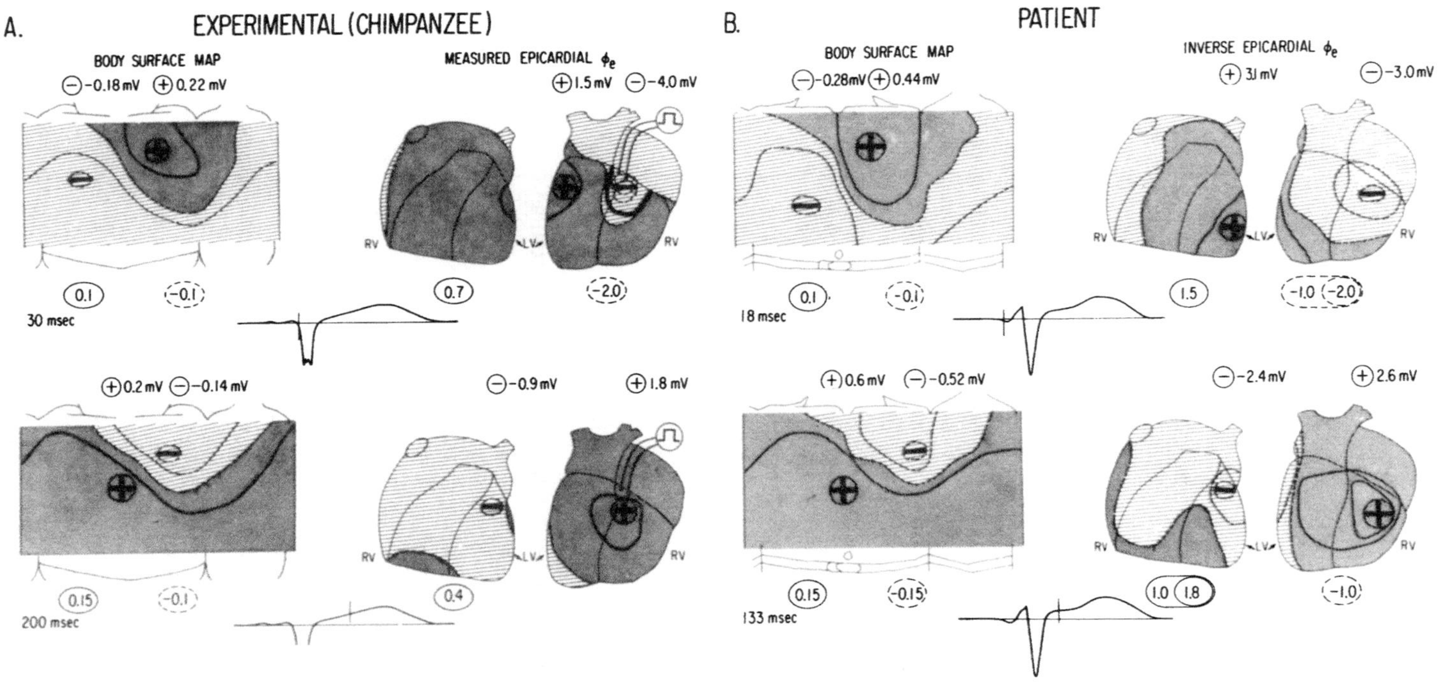

FIGURE 4–11. Comparison of isopotential body surface and epicardial measured maps in an intact chimpanzee and the maps of our 10-month-old patient. (A) Measured epicardial and body surface maps are shown for the chimpanzee following premature stimulation on the posterior right ventricle near the AV ring. (B) The infant's body surface maps were measured and the inverse epicardial potential distributions shown were computed from the body surface maps. The epicardial outlines of the heart show the anterior surface of the heart on the left and diaphragmatic surface on the right. A vertical marker is shown on a scalar reference trace below each map. The reference trace is not in the same location for the chimpanzee as for the patient. The shaded area represents positive potentials and the lined area represents negative potentials. The values of the maxima and the minima are indicated above each map. The exact times of comparison are not identical since the major features of the body surface and epicardial distributions are quite stable. RV = Right ventricle; LV = Left ventricle; Φ_e = potentials. (Reproduced with permission [105].)

Ebstein's anomaly is associated with a nodoventricular/fascicular connection. Apparent left bundle branch block QRS morphology occurs when ventricular activation is due primarily to conduction over the nodoventricular/fascicular connection whereas conduction restricted to the specialized conduction system results in a right bundle branch block pattern.

Electrocardiographic Features of Tachycardia

This section will discuss certain ECG characteristics which can be of diagnostic value in determining if an accessory connection participates in an observed arrhythmia and provides a differential diagnosis of arrhythmias seen in association with the preexcitation syndromes.

DIAGNOSTIC CLUES SUGGESTING PARTICIPATION OF AN ACCESSORY CONNECTION

Tachycardia rate [87] has been suggested as a means of separating normal QRS tachycardias related to accessory connections, AV node reentry, or mechanisms confined to the atria (primary atrial tachycardias). Generally, tachycardia rate exceeding 200 beats/minute suggests participation of an accessory connection. Tachycardias with rates less than 200 beats/minute, however, can occur by any of the above mechanisms. For the most part, tachycardia rate alone is not a sufficiently specific diagnostic clue to permit distinction of the various forms of tachycardia associated with a normal QRS.

The occurrence of bundle block can be helpful. Functional bundle branch block occurring during tachycardia with a normal QRS may result in tachycardia slowing [88] if the tachycardia utilizes an accessory AV connection ipsilateral to the bundle-branch block (Figure 4–12). In contrast, bundle branch block associated with tachycardia due to reentry within the AV node or primary atrial tachycardia usually occurs at faster tachycardia rates than when a normal QRS is present during tachycardia (i.e., rate related bundle branch block). Irrespective of rate, functional left bundle branch block suggests participation of an accessory AV connection [89] since left bundle branch block occurs uncommonly in association with tachycardia due to reentry within the AV node or primary atrial tachycardias.

QRS alternans (Figure 4–13) in tachycardias with an otherwise normal QRS is suggestive of a orthodromic reciprocating tachycardia [90]. However, although relatively specific, QRS alternans was noted in only 22% of patients with normal QRS complex tachycardia related to an accessory connection [90].

Mode of onset of tachycardia, although infrequently observed, can provide some clue to participation of an accessory connection in the tachycardia. If preexcitation is evident on the resting ECG, the initiating beat of tachycardia, frequently a premature atrial beat, will show loss of delta wave with onset of narrow QRS complex tachycardia. Upon termination of tachycardia such as with carotid sinus massage, the delta wave will reappear suggesting the presence of an accessory connection. The suggestion has been made that initiation of tachycardia during the course of a gradual increase in sinus rate without prolongation of the PR interval is suggestive of the presence of a concealed accessory AV connection [91].

Discernible P waves may not be apparent on an ECG during tachycardia. However, when they are visible, P-wave axis can be an important diagnostic clue to the type of tachycardia [92]. When atrial depolarization is not readily apparent, use of an esophageal electrode can be very helpful in defining the temporal relationship between atrial and ventricular depolarization (Figure 4–14). With recordings of atrial and ventricular depolarizations, regular tachycardias with a normal QRS can be divided into those with "short" R-P intervals, "intermediate" R-P intervals, or "long" R-P intervals.

In its most common form, tachycardia due to reentry within the AV node is characterized by near simultaneous atrial and ventricular depolarization. Benditt et al. [93] demonstrated that the interval between the onset of ventricular activation and the earliest recorded atrial activity to be on the average 51 ms in patients with tachycardia due to reentry within the AV node. Thus, the absence of a discernable P wave on the surface ECG (Figure 4–15) or the presence of near simultaneous or very short R-P interval during esophageal recording suggest reentry within the AV node as the etiology of the tachycardia. (To avoid confusion in determining simultaneous AV activation, it may be necessary to record from the esophageal lead after tachycardia termination to insure the recording of separate A and V electrograms.)

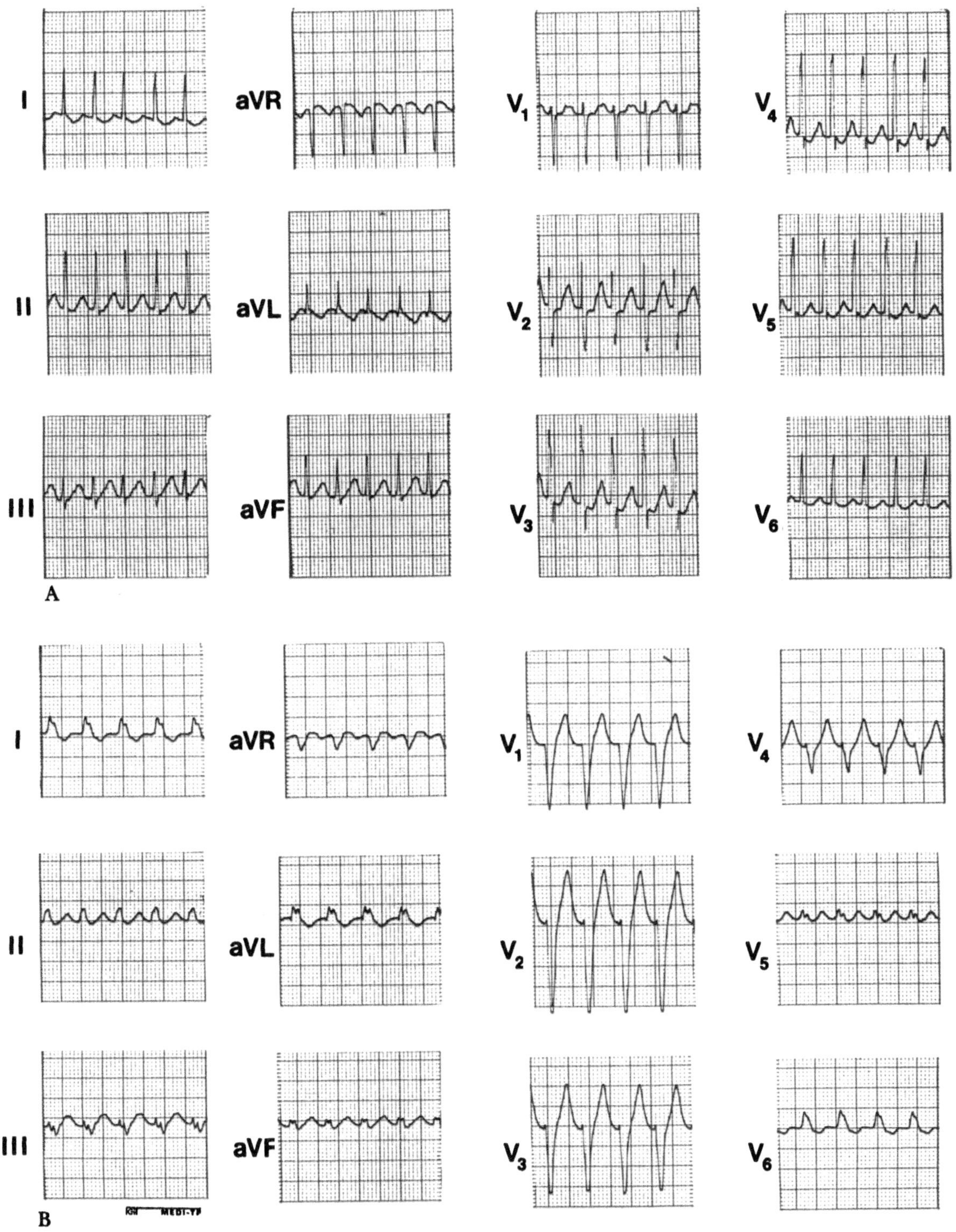

FIGURE 4–12. (A) Standard ECG from a patient with a left lateral accessory AV connection during an episode of narrow complex tachycardia (CL 310 ms). (B) 12 lead ECG obtained moments later in the same patient during LBBB tachycardia (CL 360 ms). The 50 ms slowing in tachycardia cycle length with BBB is consistent with an ipsilateral accessory connection.

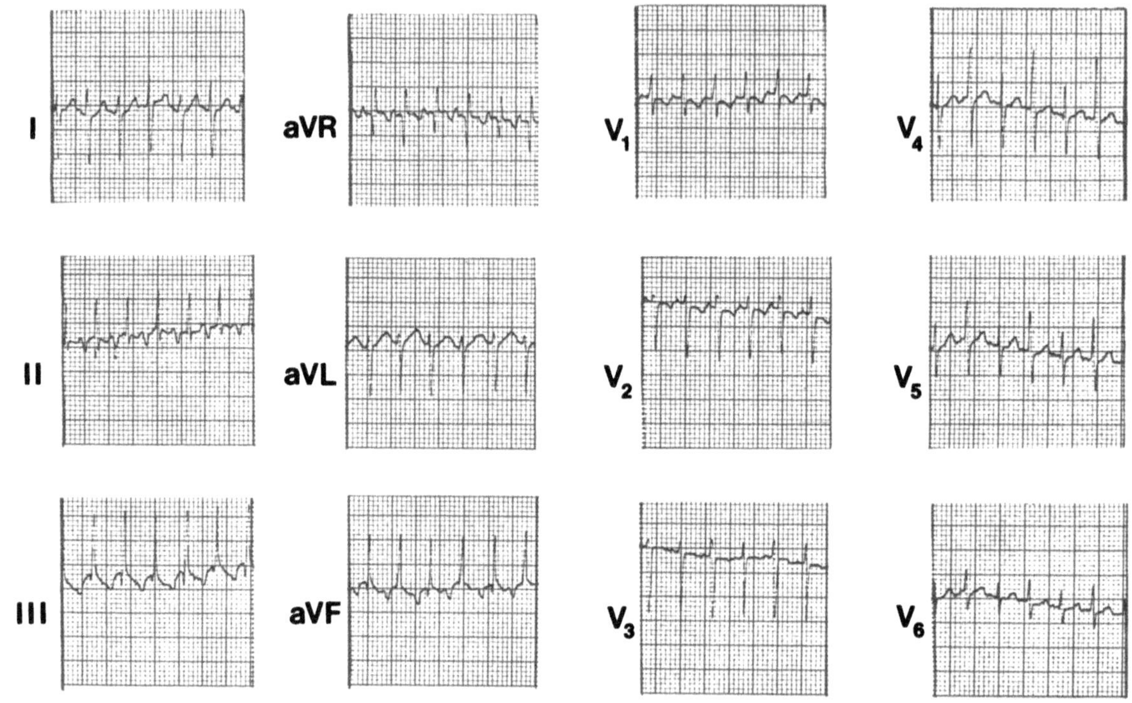

FIGURE 4–13. Standard ECG demonstrating QRS alternans from a patient with an accessory AV connection.

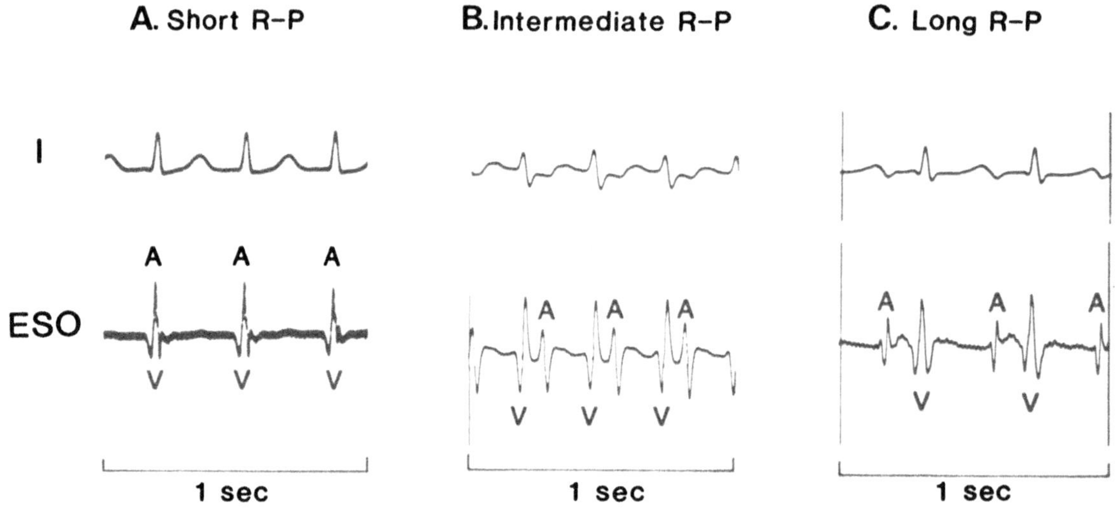

FIGURE 4–14. Surface ECG lead I and recordings from an esophageal lead (ESO) obtained during normal QRS tachycardia are shown. (A) Short RP tachycardia is associated with simultaneous atrial (A) and ventricular (V) activation as demonstrated on the ESO. (B) Intermediate RP tachycardia is characterized by distinct A and V components on the ESO with the VA (RP) being greater than 70 ms. (C) Long RP tachycardia is characterized by a long VA. The VA timing is longer than the subsequent AV interval.

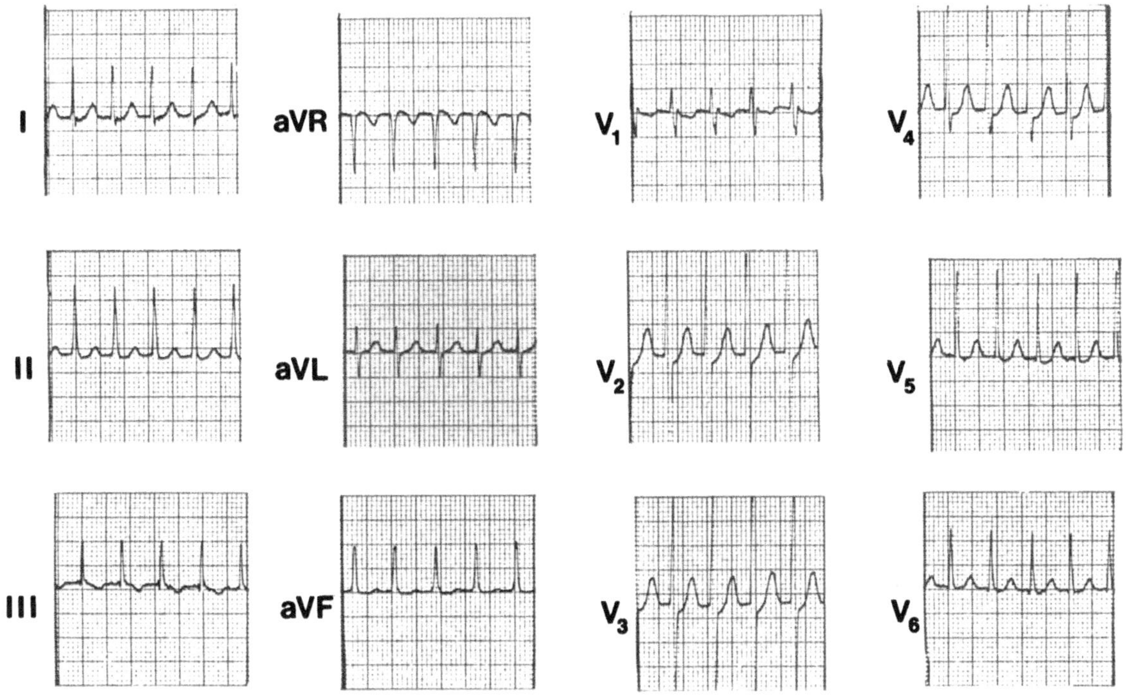

FIGURE 4–15. Standard ECG from a patient with tachycardia due to reentry within the AV node. The absence of discernable P waves on ECG is characteristic of this tachycardia.

Orthodromic reciprocating tachycardias usually have intermediate R-P intervals (approximate range 70–130 ms) (Figure 4–16). In 50 patients with accessory AV connections, Benditt, et al. [93] demonstrated a mean ventriculoatrial conduction time of 106 ms and never recorded a conduction time of less than 70 ms. Thus, the recording of an R-P interval of less than 70 ms effectively excludes participation of an accéssory connection in the tachycardia. Primary atrial tachycardias with prolonged PR interval may also exhibit apparent R-P intervals of intermediate duration.

Tachycardias associated with long R-P intervals (approximate range 130–250 ms) include the so-called permanent form of junctional reciprocating tachycardia or incessant AV reciprocating tachycardia (IAVRT) (Figure 4–17), primary atrial tachycardias, the rare form of "fast-slow" reentry within the AV node, and accessory A-V connections with prolonged A-V conduction (particularly those associated with Ebstein's anomaly). In 36 cases of long R-P tachycardia undergoing electrophysiologic study, occurrence, Gallagher et al. [19] described the following etiologies: IAVRT — 7 cases, primary atrial tachycardia — 3 cases, "fast-slow" AV node reentry — 2 cases, accessory AV connections associated with Ebstein's anomaly — 21 cases, and isolated accessory AV connections — 3 cases.

DIFFERENTIAL DIAGNOSIS OF ARRHYTHMIAS ASSOCIATED WITH THE PREEXCITATION SYNDROMES

The most common normal QRS complex tachycardia – orthodromic reciprocating tachycardia in patients with accessory AV connections utilizes the AV node as the antegrade limb and the accessory AV connection as the retrograde limb of the reentry circuit. However, other mechanisms are possible (Figure 4–18). Primary atrial tachycardias or tachycardia due to reentry with the AV node may be associated with normal QRS complexes even in patients with accessory connections if ventricular activation occurs primarily via the normal specialized conduction system during tachycardia [94,95].

There are multiple mechanisms for tachycardia with a prolonged or wide QRS in patients

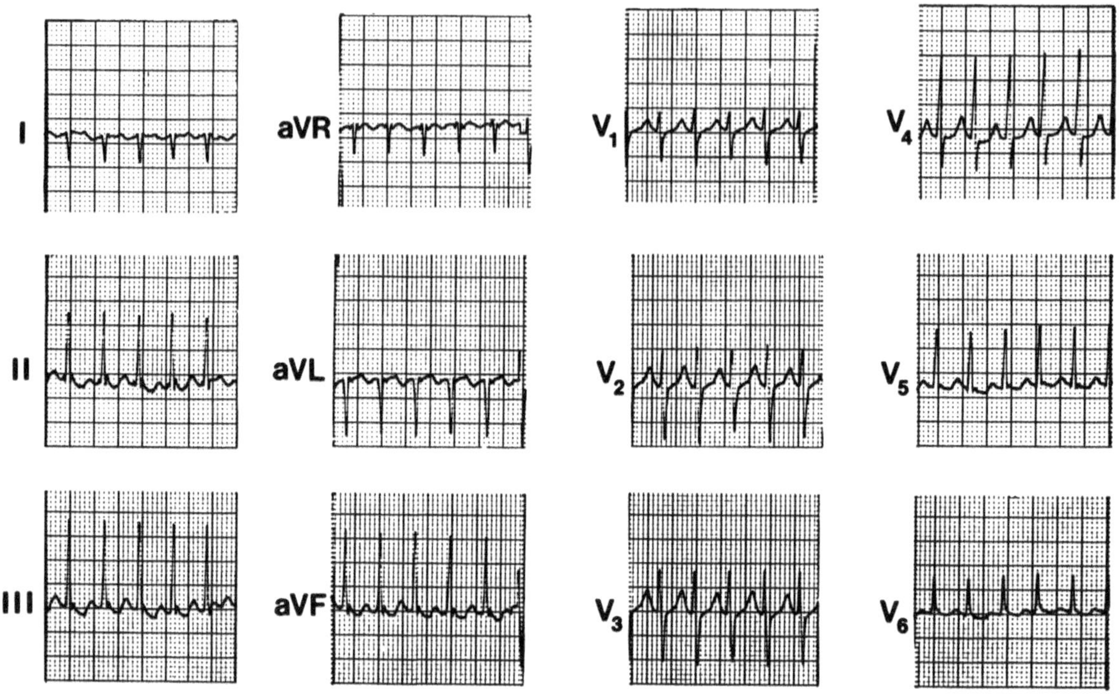

FIRURE 4–16. Standard ECG from a patient with orthodromic reciprocating tachy-cardia. Distortion of the ST-T wave especially in the inferior leads is suggestive of retrograde P waves (intermediate RP tachycardia).

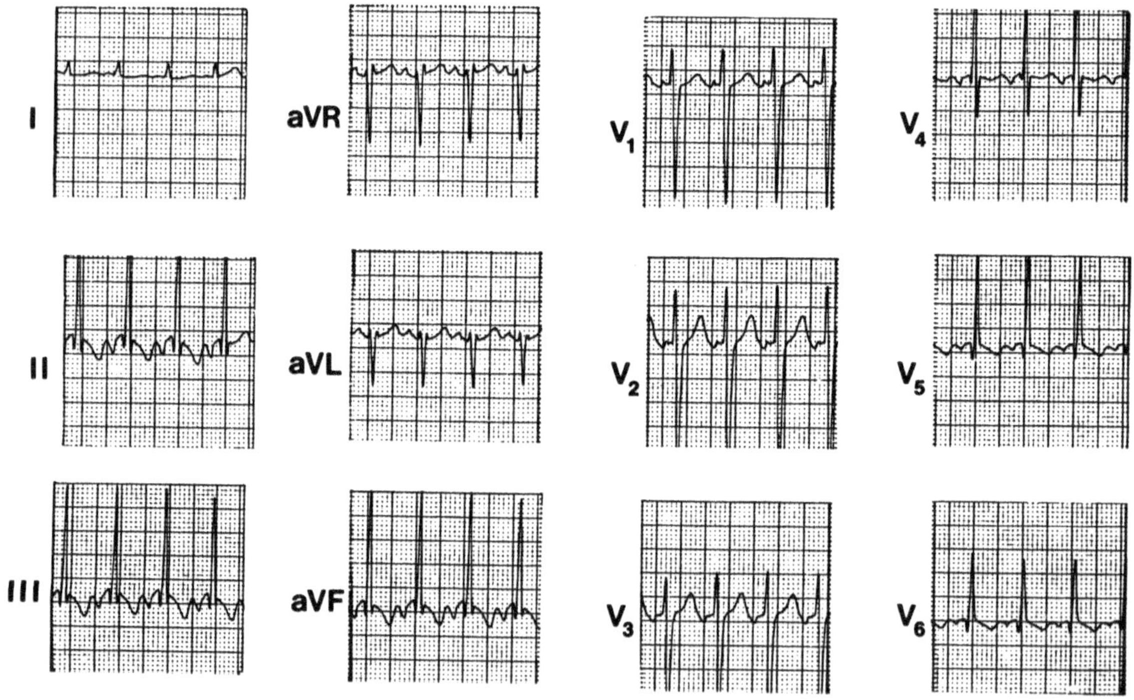

FIGURE 4–17. Standard ECG from a patient with incessant AV reciprocating tachycardia (IAVRT). Negative P waves in leads II, III, AVF which occur closer to the succeeding QRS than the preceding one are characteristic (one form of long RP tachycardia).

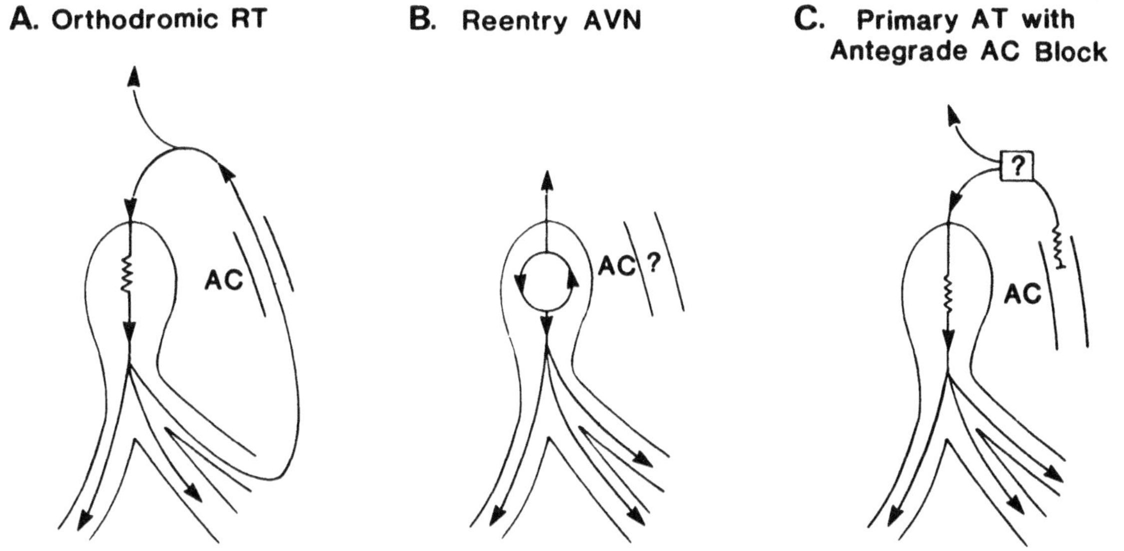

FIGURE 4–18. Schematic representation of mechanisms of normal QRS tachycardia in patients with accessory connections. RT, reciprocating tachycardia; AT, atrial tachycardia; AVN, atrioventricular node; AC, accessory AV connection; and NFC, nodoventricular/fascicular connection.

with accessory AV connections (Figure 4–19). Orthodromic reciprocating tachycardia with functional bundle branch block is common. Less commonly, the tachycardia circuit utilizes the accessory connection for antegrade conduction and the specialized conduction system for retrograde conduction (antidromic reciprocating tachycardia). In this situation, the ECG will reveal a similarity between the preexcited QRS during sinus rhythm and the QRS during tachycardia. However, a similar finding may occur if a primary atrial tachycardia or tachycardia due to reentry within the AV node results in conduction or a "bystander" accessory connection. The primary atrial tachycardia may be benign conducting at a slow rate such as sinus node reentry or potentially life-threatening such as atrial fibrillation with a rapid preexcited ventricular response [96,97]. The latter arrhythmia has been the primary reason for referral in the small group of patients with accessory AV connections that conduct only in the antegrade direction [98,99].

Patients with accessory AV connections may have tachycardia due to reentry within the AV node [95]. During tachycardia, the QRS complexes can be wide with activation of the ventricle occurring partially via the accessory connection. Since the accessory AV connection does not specifically play a role in maintaining the tachycardia, it is termed a *bystander* [100].

Multiple accessory connections may exist in the same patient [20,63]. In this situation, an unusual form of tachycardia can occur which uses one accessory pathway for antegrade conduction and the other accessory pathway and/or the specialized conduction system for retrograde conduction. Electrophysiologic study is necessary to identify these reentrant circuits.

Finally, ventricular tachycardia can occur in patients with the preexcitation syndromes and may be the cause of syncope [99]. Thus, it is important in patients with preexcitation to obtain ECG documentation during symptoms so that appropriate therapy can be initiated.

ARRHYTHMIAS ASSOCIATED WITH NODOVENTRICULAR/ FASCICULAR CONNECTION

The characteristic ECG features associated with maximal preexcitation over a nodoventricular/fascicular connection has been a QRS morphology resembling left bundle branch block with left axis deviation. Bardy et al. [52] analyzed 87

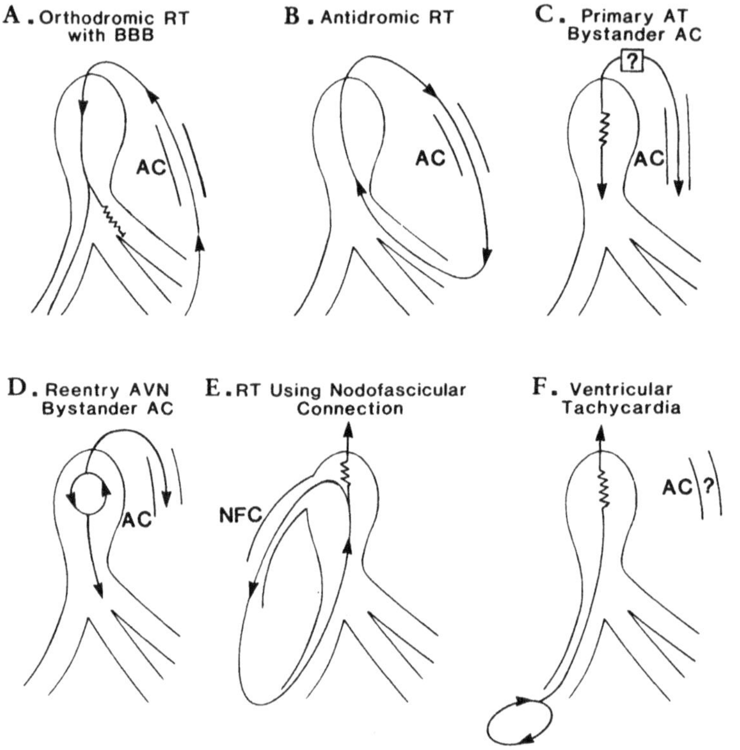

FIGURE 4–19. Schematic representation of mechanisms of tachycardia with a prolonged or wide QRS in patients with accessory connections. RT, reciprocating tachycardia; AVN, atrioventricular node; AT, atrial tachycardia; and AC, accessory connection.

consecutive patients with tachycardia of left bundle branch block QRS morphology for features that might be suggestive of tachycardia using a nodoventricular/fascicular connection. The study group consisted of 13 patients with tachycardia related to a nodoventricular/fascicular connection, 34 patients with orthodromic tachycardia with functional left bundle branch block, 22 patients with ventricular tachycardia, and 18 patients with antidromic tachycardia using a right-sided accessory AV connection. Six variables were found predictive of a nodoventricular/fascicular connection: cycle length between 220 and 450 msec, QRS axis of 0 to −75°, QRS duration of 0.15 seconds or less, R wave in lead I, rS in precordial lead V_1, and a precordial transition from a predominantly negative to a predominantly positive QRS complex after V_4. Overall, in the group studied, 12 of 13 patients with tachycardia using a nodoventricular/fascicular connection were correctly identified along with 4 false positive ECG's.

Two distinct mechanisms have been advanced to explain the genesis of reciprocating tachycardia observed in patients with nodoventricular/fascicular connections [19] (Figure 4–20). The first involves antegrade conduction over the connection to the right ventricle with retrograde conduction over the specialized conduction system and completion of the reentrant circuit within the AV node. The second suggests that tachycardia is due to reentry confined to the AV node with the nodoventricular/fascicular connection functioning as a bystander [101]. Probably both mechanisms exist [19].

INCESSANT AV RECIPROCATING TACHYCARDIA (IAVRT)

The "permanent or recurring form of junctional reciprocating tachycardia" (PJRT) or more descriptively, incessant AV reciprocating tachy-

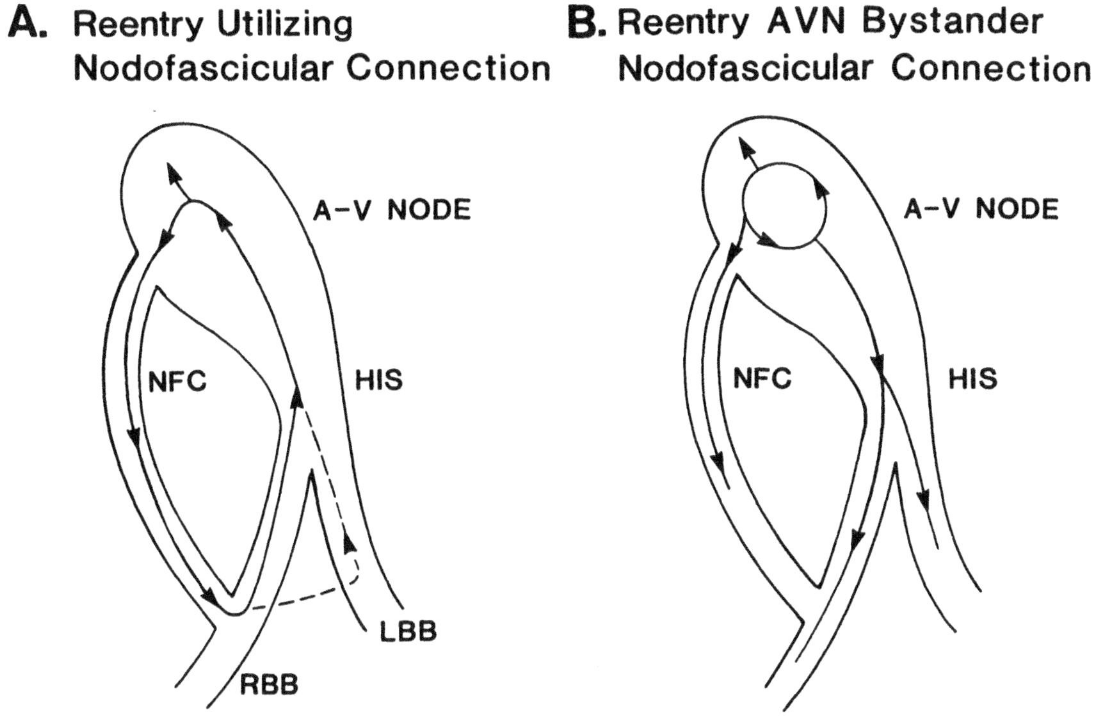

FIGURE 4–20. Schematic representation of the two proposed mechanisms of tachycardia associated with nodoventricular/fascicular connection (NFC). (A) Reentry circuit utilizes the NFC in the antegrade direction with the retrograde loop completed by either of the bundle branches (RBB or LBB), His–Purkinje system, and AV node. (B) Reentry is confined to the AV node with ventricular activation occurring over both the NFC and His–Purkinje system.

cardia (IAVRT) was first reported by Gallavardin and Veil in 1927 [102]. However, it was not until 1967 that Coumel [103,104] described the ECG features of the tachycardia. A distinctive feature of this tachycardia is repetitive terminations, with either a P wave or QRS, only to recur after a few beats (often preceded by acceleration of sinus rate) without prolongation of the P-R interval. A pecularity of the tachycardia is the pattern and timing of the P waves, which demonstrate negativity in leads II, III, and AVF and occur closer to the succeeding QRS than the preceding one leading to classification of this tachycardia with those associated with a long R–P (see Figure 4–20).

Conclusions

Analysis of surface potentials (ECGs) remains a useful tool in diagnosing and evaluating the preexcitation syndromes. It is clear that careful analysis of ECGs during both sinus rhythm and tachycardia provides important clues in the diagnosis of preexcitation syndromes.

References

1. Rosenbaum FF, Hecht HH, Wilson FN, Johnston FD: The potential variations of the thorax and the esophagus in anomalous atrioventricular excitation (Wolff-Parkinson-White Syndrome). *Am. Heart J.* 29:281, 1945.
2. Öhnell RF: Preexcitation, a cardiac abnormality. *Acta Med. Scand.* (Suppl) 152:1, 1944.
3. Cohn AE, Fraser FR: Paroxysmal tachycardia and the effect of stimulation of the vagus nerves by pressure. *Heart* 5:93, 1913–1914.
4. Wilson FN: A case in which the vagus influenced the form of the ventricular complex of the electrocardiogram. *Arch. Int. Med.* 16:1008, 1915.
5. Wedd AM: Paroxysmal tachycardia: With reference to nomotopic tachycardia and the role

of the extrinsic cardiac nerves. Asch *Int. Med.* 27:571, 1921.
6. Bain CWC, Hemilton CK: Electrocardiographic changes in rheumatic carditis. *Lancet* 1:807, 1926.
7. Bach F: Paroxysmal tachycardia of forty-eight years' duration and right bundle branch block. *Proc. Roy. Soc. Med.* 22:412, 1928–1929.
8. Hamburger WW: Bundle branch block: Four cases of intraventricular block showing some interesting and unusual clinical features. *Med. Clin. North Am.* 13:343, 1929.
9. Wolff L, Parkinson J, White PD: Bundle branch block with short PR interval in healthy young people prone to paroxysmal tachycardia. *Am. Heart J.* 5:685, 1930.
10. Chung KY, Walsh TJ, Massie E: Wolff-Parkinson-White syndrome. *Am. Heart J.* 69:116, 1965.
11. Sears GA, Manning GW: Wolff-Parkinson-White pattern in routine electrocardiography. *Can. Med. Assoc. J.* 87:1213, 1962.
12. Newman BJ, Donoso E, Friedberg CK: Arrhythmias in the Wolff-Parkinson-White syndrome. *Prog. Cardiovasc. Dis.* 9:147, 1966.
13. Berkman NL, Lamb LE: The Wolff-Parkinson-White electrocardiogram. A follow-up study of five to twenty-eight years. *N. Engl. J. Med.* 278:492, 1968.
14. Cobb FR, Blumenschein SD, Sealy WC, Boineau JP, Wagner GS, Wallace AG: Successful surgical interruption of the bundle of Kent in a patient with Wolff-Parkinson-White syndrome. *Circulation* 38:1018, 1968.
15. Durrer D, Schuilenberg RM, Wellens HJJ: Preexcitation revisited. *Am. J. Cardiol.* 25:690, 1970.
16. Castellanos A, Chapunoff E, Castillo C, Mayton O, Lemberg L: His bundle electrograms in two cases of Wolff-Parkinson-White (Preexcitation) syndrome. *Circulation* 41:399, 1970.
17. Segers M, Lequime J, Denolin H: L'activation ventriculaire precoce de certains coeurs hyperexcitables: Etude de l'onde delta de l'electrocardiogramme. *Cardiologia* 8:113, 1944.
18. Anderson RH, Becker AE, Breckenmacher C, Davies MJ, Rossi L: Ventricular preexcitation: A proposed nomenclature for its substrates. *Eur. J. Cardiol.* 3:27, 1975.
19. Gallagher JJ: Variants of preexcitation: Update 1984, in Zipes DP, Jalife J (eds.): Cardiac Electrophysiology and Arrhythmias. Grune and Stratton, 1984, pp. 419–433.
20. Gallagher JJ, Pritchett ELC, Sealy WC, Kasell J, Wallace AG: The preexcitation syndromes. *Prog. Cardiovasc. Dis.* 20:285, 1978.
21. Scherf L, Neufeld HN: The Preexcitation Syndrome: Facts and Theories. New York, Yorke Medical Books, 1978.
22. Ferrer I: Preexcitation. Mount Kisco, New York, Futura Publishing, 1976.
23. Laham J: Actualités electrocardiographiques 1969: Le syndrome de Wolff-Parkinson-White. Paris, Librarie Malone SA, 1969.
24. Prystowsky EN, Miles WM, Heger JJ, Zipes DP: Preexcitation syndromes. *Med. Clin. North Am.* 68:831, 1984.
25. Kent AFS: Researches on the structure and function of the mammalian heart. *J. Physiol.* 14:222, 1983.
26. Paladino G: Contribuzione ali anatomia, istologia e fisiologia del cuore. *Movimento Napoli* 8:428, 1896.
27. Davignon A, Rautaharju P, Boiselle E, Megelas M, Choquette A: Normal ECG standards for infants and children. *Pediatr. Cardiol.* 1:123, 1979–1980.
28. Scherlag BJ, Lau SH, Helfant RH, Berkowitz WO, Stein E, Damato AW: Catheter technique for recording His bundle activity in man. *Circulation* 39:13, 1969.
29. Prystowsky EN, Browne KF, Zipes DP: Intracardiac recording by catheter electrode of accessory pathway depolarization. *J. Am. Coll. Cardiol.* 1:468, 1983.
30. Jackman W, Beck B, Aliot K, Friday K, Lazzara R: Basis for concealed accessory AV pathways. *Circulation* II 70:337 (Abst), 1984.
31. Holzmann M, Sherf D: Uber electrocardiogramme mit verkurzter Vorhof-Kammer-Distanz und positiven P-Zacken. *Z. Klin. Med.* 121:404, 1932.
32. Wolferth CC, Wood FC: Mechanism of production of short PR intervals and prolonged QRS complexes in patients with presumably damaged hearts: Hypothesis of an accessory pathway of auriculoventricular conduction (bundle of Kent). *Am. Heart J.* 8:297, 1933.
33. Butterworth JS, Poindexter CA: Short P-R interval associated with a prolonged QRS complex. A clinical and experimental study. *Arch. Intern.* Med 69:437, 1942.
34. Ohnell RF: Lecture in Svesha Foren. f. inv. med., October 4, 1941. (Printed in Swedish in Nord Medicine 14:1827, 1942.)
35. Wood FC, Wolferth CC, Geckeler GD: Histologic demonstration of accessory muscular connections between auricle and ventricle in a case of short P-R interval and prolonged QRS complex. *Am. Heart J.* 25:454, 1943.
36. Boineau JP, Moore EN: Evidence for propagation of activation across an accessory atrioventricular connection in types A and B preexcitation. *Circulation* 41:375–397, 1970.
37. Boineau JP, Moore EN, Spear JF, Sealy WC: Basis of static and dynamic electrocardiographic variations in Wolff-Parkinson-White syn-

drome. Anatomic and electrophysiologic observations in right and left ventricular preexcitation. *Am. J. Cardiol.* 32:32, 1973.
38. Durrer D, Roos JP: Epicardial excitation of the ventricles in a patient with Wolff-Parkinson-White syndrome (Type B). *Circulation* 35:15, 1967.
39. Burchell HB, Frye RL, Anderson MW, McGoon DC: Atrioventricular and ventriculoatrial excitation in Wolff-Parkinson-White syndrome (Type B). *Circulation* 36:663, 1967.
40. Spach MS, Barr RC, Lanning CF: Experimental basis for QRS and T wave potentials in the WPW syndrome. *Circulation* 42:103, 1978.
41. Caracta AR, Damato AN, Gallagher JJ, Josephson ME, Varghese PJ, Lau SH, Westura EE: Electrophysiologic studies in the syndrome of short PR interval, normal QRS complex. *Am. J. Cardiol.* 31:245, 1973.
42. Mahaim I, Benatt A: Nouvelles recherches sur les connexions superieures de la branch gauche du faisceau de His Tawara avec la cloison interventriculaire. *Cardiologia* 1:61, 1937.
43. Lev M, Leffler WB, Langendorf R, Pick A: Anatomic findings in a case of ventricular preexcitation (WPW) terminating in complete atrioventricular block. *Circulation* 34:718, 1966.
44. Brechenmacher C, Courtadon M, Jourde M, Yermia JC, Cheynel J, Voegtlin R: Syndrome de Wolff-Parkinson-White par association de fibres atriohissienes et de fibres de Mahaim: Confrontation entre l'electrophysiologic et l'histologic. *Arch. Mal Coeur* 69:1275–1283, 1976.
45. Gallagher JJ, Smith WM, Kasell J, Benson DW Jr, Sterba R, Grant AO: Role of Mahaim fibers in cardiac arrhythmias in man. *Circulation* 64:176, 1981.
46. Pick A, Katz LN: Disturbance of impulse formation and conduction in the preexcitation syndrome: Their bearing on its mechanism. *Am. J. Med.* 19:759, 1955.
47. Mahaim I, Winston MR: Recherches d'anatomie comparee et de pathologie experimantale sur les connexions hautes du faisceau de His Tawara. *Cardiologia* 5:189, 1941.
48. Mahaim I: Kent's fibers and the A-V paraspecific conduction through the upper connections of the bundle of His-Tawara. *Am. Heart J.* 33:651, 1947.
49. Wellens HJJ: Electrical stimulation of the heart in the study and treatment of tachycardias. Baltimore, University Park Press, pp. 97–109, 1971.
50. Motte G, Brechenmacher C, Davy JM, Belhassen B: Association de fibers nodoventriculaires et atrioventriculaires a l'origine de tachycardies reciproques. *Arch. Mal Coeur* 73:737, 1980.
51. Gallagher JJ, German LD, Broughton A, Guarnieri T, Trantham JL: Variants of the preexcitation syndrome, in Rosenbaum MB, Elizari MV (eds.): Frontiers of cardiac electrophysiology. The Hague, Martinus Nijhoff, pp. 724–772, 1982.
52. Bardy GH, Fedor JM, German LD, Packer DL, Gallagher JJ: Surface electrocardiographic clues suggesting the presence of a nodofascicular Mahaim fiber. *JACC* 3:1161, 1984.
53. Clerc A, Levy R, Cristesco C: A propos du raccourcissement permanent du lespace P-R de l'electrocardiogramme sans deformation du complexe ventriculaire. *Arch. Mal Coeur* 31:569, 1938.
54. Lown B, Ganong WF, Levine SA: The syndrome of short P-R interval, normal QRS complex and paroxysmal rapid heart action. *Circulation* 5:693, 1952.
55. Benditt DG, Pritchett ELC, Smith WM, Wallace AG, Gallagher JJ: Characteristics of atrioventricular conduction and the spectrum of arrhythmias in Lown-Ganong-Levine syndrome. *Circulation* 57:454, 1978.
56. Bisset JK, de Soyza N, Kane JJ, Murphy ML: Altered refractory periods in patients with short P-R intervals and normal QRS complex. *Am. J. Cardiol.* 35:487, 1975.
57. Castellanos A, Jr, Castillo CA, Agha AS, Tessler M: His bundle electrograms in patients with short P-R intervals, narrow QRS complexes, and paroxysmal tachycardias. *Circulation* 43:667, 1971.
58. Iannone LA: Electrophysiology of atrial pacing in patients with short PR interval, normal QRS complex. *Am. Heart J.* 89:74, 1975.
59. Brechenmacher C: Atrio-His bundle tracts. *Br. Heart J.* 37:853, 1975.
60. Brechenmacher C, Laham J, Iris L, Gerbaux A, Lenegre J: Etude histologique des voies anormales de conduction dans un syndrome de Wolff-Parkinson-White et dans un syndrome de Lown-Ganong-Levine. *Arch, Mal Coeur* 67:507, 1974.
61. Denes P, Wu D, Rosen KM: Demonstration of dual A-V pathways in a patient with Lown-Ganong-Levine syndrome. *Chest* 65:343, 1974.
62. Akhtar M: Atrioventricular nodal reentrant tachycardia. *Med. Clin. North Am.* 68:819, 1984.
63. Gallagher JJ, Sealy WC, Kasell J, Wallace AG: Multiple accessory pathways in patients with the preexcitation syndrome. *Circulation* 54:571, 1976.
64. Benditt DG, Epstein ML, Arentzen CE, Kriett JM, Klein GJ: Enhanced atrioventricular conduction in patients without preexcitation syndrome: Relation to heart rate in paroxysmal reciprocating tachycardia. *Circulation* 65:1474, 1982.

65. Bauernfeind RA, Ayers BF, Wyndham CC, Dhingra RC, Surryn SP, Strasberg B, Rosen KM: Cycle length in atrioventricular nodal reentrant paroxysmal tachycardia with observations in the Lown-Ganong-Levine syndrome. *Am. J. Cardiol.* 45:1148, 1980.
66. Castellanos A, Vagueiro MC, Befeler B, Myerburg RJ: Syndrome of short P-R, narrow QRS, and repetitive supraventricular tachyarrhythmias: The possible occurrence of the R-on-T phenomena and the limits of this syndrome. *Eur. J. Cardiol.* 3:337, 1975.
67. Castellanos A, Zaman L, Moleiro F, Aranda JM, Myerburg RJ: The Lown-Ganong-Levine syndrome. *Pace* 5:715–740, 1982.
68. Przybylski J, Chiale PA, Halpern S, Nau GJ, Elizari MV, Rosenbaum MB: Unmasking of ventricular preexcitation by vagal stimulation or isoproterenol administration. *Circulation* 61:1030, 1980.
69. De la Fuente D, Sasyniuk B, Moe GK: Conduction through a narrow isthmus in isolated canine atrial tissue. A model of the WPW syndrome. *Circulation* 44:803, 1971.
70. Wallace AG, Sarnoff SJ: Effects of cardiac sympathetic nerve stimulation on conduction in the heart. *Circ. Res.* 14:86, 1964.
71. Dhingra RC, Winslow E, Pouget JM, Rahimtoola SH, Rosen KM: The effects of isoproterenol on atrioventricular and intraventricular conduction. *Am. J. Cardiol.* 32:629, 1973.
72. Wellens HJJ, Brugada P, Roy D, Weiss J, Bar FW: Effects of isoproterenol on the antegrade refractory period of the accessory pathway in patients with the Wolff-Parkinson-White syndrome. *Am. J. Cardiol.* 50:180, 1982.
73. Giardina ACV, Ehlers KH, Engle MA: Wolff-Parkinson-White syndrome in infants and children. A long-term follow-up study. *Br. Heart J.* 34:839 1972.
74. James TN: Cardiac conduction system: Fetal and postnatal development. *Am. J. Cardiol.* 25:213, 1970.
75. James TN: The Wolff-Parkinson-White syndrome: Evolving concepts of its pathogenesis. *Prog. Cardiovasc. Dis.* 13:159, 1970.
76. Benson DW, Jr, Dunnigan A, Schneider SP, Schiff J, Johnson W: Follow-up of infant paroxysmal atrial tachycardia: Transesophageal study. *Circulation* 70:1II–206 (Abstract), 1984.
77. Giraud G, Latour H, Puech P, Roujon J: Les troubles de rhythme du syndrome de Wolff-Parkinson-White. Analyse electrocardiographique endocavitaire. *Arch. Mal Coeur* 49:101, 1956.
78. Lowe KG, Emslie-Smith D, Ward C, Watson H: Classification of ventricular preexcitation. Vectorcardiographic study. *Br. Heart J.* 37:9, 1975.
79. Tonkin AM, Wagner GS, Gallagher JJ, Cope GD, Kasell J, Wallace AG: Initial forces of ventricular depolarization in the Wolff-Parkinson-White syndrome. Analysis based upon localization of the accessory pathway by epicardial mapping. *Circulation* 52:1030, 1975.
80. Yamada K, Toyama J, Wada M, Sugiyama S, Sugenoga J, Toyoshima H, Mizuro Y, Sotohata I, Kobayashi T, Okajima M: Body surface isopotential mapping in Wolff-Parkinson-White syndrome: Noninvasive method to determine the localization of the accessory atrioventricular pathway. *Am. Heart J.* 90:721, 1975.
81. De Ambroggi L, Taccardi B, Macchi E: Body surface maps of heart potentials. Tentative localization of pre-excited areas in forty-two Wolff-Parkinson-White patients. *Circulation* 54:251, 1976.
82. Benson DW, Jr, Sterba R, Gallagher JJ, Watson A, Spach MS: Localization of the site of ventricular preexcitation with body surface maps in patients with Wolff-Parkinson-White syndrome. *Circulation* 65:1259, 1982.
83. Chung EK: Wolff-Parkinson-White syndrome — Current Views. *Am. J. Med.* 62:252, 1977.
84. Ruskin JN, Akhtar M, Damato AN, Ticzon AR, Lau Sh, Caracta AR: Abnormal Q waves in Wolff-Parkinson-White syndrome. Incidence and clinical significance. *JAMA* 235:2727, 1976.
85. Gayes DC: False positive exercise test in the presence of Wolff-Parkinson-White syndrome. *Am. Heart J.* 78:13, 1969.
86. Greenland P, Kauffman R, Weir EK: Profound exercise-induced ST depression in a patient with W-P-W syndrome and normal coronary arteriograms. *Thorax* 35:559, 1980.
87. Wu D, Denes P, Amat-y-Leon F, Wyndham C, Ramesh D, Rosen K: Clinical, electrocardiographic, and electrophysiologic observations in patients with paroxysmal supraventricular tachycardia. *Am. J. Cardiol.* 39:264 (Abstract), 1977.
88. Coumel P, Attuel P: Reciprocating tachycardia in overt and latent preexcitation. Influence of functional bundle branch block on the rate of tachycardia. *Eur. J. Cardiol.* 1:423, 1974.
89. Farshidi A, Josephson ME, Horowitz LN: Electrophysiologic characteristics of concealed bypass tracts: Clinical and electrocardiographic correlates. *Am. J. Cardiol.* 41:1052, 1978.
90. Green M, Heddle B, Dassen W, Wehr M, Abdollah H, Brugada P, Wellens HJJ: Value of QRS alternation in determining the site of origin of narrow QRS supraventricular tachycardia. *Circulation* 68:368, 1983.
91. Sung RJ, Gelband H, Castellanos A, Aranda JM, Myerburg RJ: Clinical and electrophysiologic observations in patients with concealed

accessory atrioventricular bypass tracts. *Am. J. Cardiol.* 40:839, 1977.
92. Wu D, Denes P, Amat-y-Leon F, Dhingra R, Wyndham CRC, Bauernfeind R, Latif P, Rosen KM: Clinical electrocardiographic and electrophysiologic observations in patients with paroxysmal supraventricular tachycardia. *Am. J. Cardiol.* 41:1045, 1978.
93. Benditt DG, Pritchett ELC, Smith WM, Gallagher JJ: Ventriculoatrial intervals: Diagnostic use in paroxysmal supraventricular tachycardia. *Ann. Int. Med.* 91:161, 1979.
94. Benditt DG, Pritchett ELC, Gallagher JJ: Spectrum of regular tachycardias with wide QRS complexes in patients with accessory atrioventricular pathways. *Am. J. Cardiol.* 42:828, 1978.
95. Sung RJ, Styperek JL: Electrophysiologic identification of dual atrioventricular nodal pathway conduction in patients with reciprocating tachycardia using anomalous bypass tracts. *Circulation* 60:1464, 1979.
96. Dreifus LS, Haiat R, Watanabe Y, Arrioga J, Reitman N: Ventricular fibrillation: A possible mechanism of sudden death in patients with Wolff-Parkinson-White syndrome. *Circulation* 43:520, 1971
97. Sellers TD, Bashore TM, Gallagher JJ: Digitalis in the preexcitation syndrome: Analysis during atrial fibrillation. *Circulation* 56:260, 1970.
98. Hammill SC, Pritchett ELC, Klein GJ, Smith WM, Gallagher JJ: Accessory atrioventricular pathways that conduct only in the antegrade direction. *Circulation* 62:1335, 1980.
99. Lloyd EA, Hauer RN, Zipes DP, Heger JJ, Prystowsky EN: Syncope and ventricular tachycardia in patients with ventricular preexcitation. *Am. J. Cardiol.* 52:79, 1983.
100. Smith WM, Broughton A, Reiter MJ, Benson DW Jr, Grant HO, Gallagher JJ: Bystander accessory pathway during AV node re-entrant tachycardia. *Pace* 6:537, 1983.
101. Kerr CR, Benson DW, Gallagher JJ: Role of specialized conducting fibers in the genesis of "AV nodal" reentry tachycardia. *Pace* 6:171, 1983.
102. Gallavardin L, Veil P: Tachycardies auriculaires en slaves. *Arch. Mal Couer* 20:1, 1927.
103. Coumel P, Cabrol C, Fabiato A, Gourgon R, Slawa R: Tachycardie permanent par rhythm reciproque. 1. Preuves ou diagnostic par stimulation auriculaire et ventriculaire. *Arch. Mal Couer* 60:1830, 1967.
104. Coumel P, Attuel P, Mugica J: Junctional reciprocating tachycardia. The permanent form, in Kulbertus H. (ed.). Reentrant Arrhythmias. Lancaster, England, MTP Press, 1977, pp. 170–183.
105. Benson DW Jr, Gallagher JJ, Spach MS, Barr RC, Edwards SB, Oldham HN, Kasell J: Accessory atrioventricular pathway in an infant: Prediction of location with body surface maps and ablation with cryosurgery. *J. Pediatr.* 96:41, 1980.

5. FIRST HARMONIC FOURIER (PHASE) ANALYSIS OF BLOOD POOL SCINTIGRAMS FOR THE ANALYSIS OF CARDIAC CONDUCTION ABNORMALITIES

Elias H. Botvinick, Melvin M. Scheinman, Michael W. Dae,
J. William O'Connell, Donald B. Faulkner

In recent years there has been a burgeoning of noninvasive imaging techniques for the evaluation of cardiac structure, perfusion, and function. Prominent among these methods and widely used owing to their important clinical impact are cardiac scintigraphic methods [1–3]. Here, a minute intravenous dose of a radiopharmaceutical permits image characterization and often, quantification of some quality of the cardiac whole. The radiation dose is small (generally less than that related to a flat and upright X-ray of the abdomen) and requires only a single peripheral injection of the radionuclide. In addition to its noninvasive nature, primary advantages of the scintigraphic method include its ability to analyze pathophysiologic markers, its quantitative nature, and its extreme amenability to computer analysis.

The Equilibrium Blood Pool Method

A good example of these features is equilibrium blood pool scintigraphy [4–6]. A well-established method for accurate and reproducible determinations of global ventricular function and wall motion [7], the technique provides the basic data to permit the extraction of a multitude of derived global and regional functional parameters and provide images of their distribution. Red blood cells are labled with Technetium-99m and allowed to mix thoroughly. We generally employ the modified in vivo tagging method [8] where unlabled stannous ions, in the form of stannous pyrophosphate, are administered intravenously and allowed to mix for approximately 20 minutes. The stannous ions prepare the red cell membrane, making it receptive to the technetium ion. Twenty to 25 mCi of the latter is combined as the pertechnetate with 10 cc of extracted red cells. The labeled cells are then readministered and allowed to come to equilibrium, 5–10 minutes after radionuclide administration, when each cubic centimeter of blood has the same radioactivity. A scintillation camera then obtains image data in sequence with the cardiac cycle in multiple projections; anterior, 70° left anterior oblique [9], and "best septal" left anterior oblique which best separates the ventricles.

Triggered by or "gated" to the R wave, frame mode acquisition serially images predetermined fractions of the cardiac cycle and is best em-

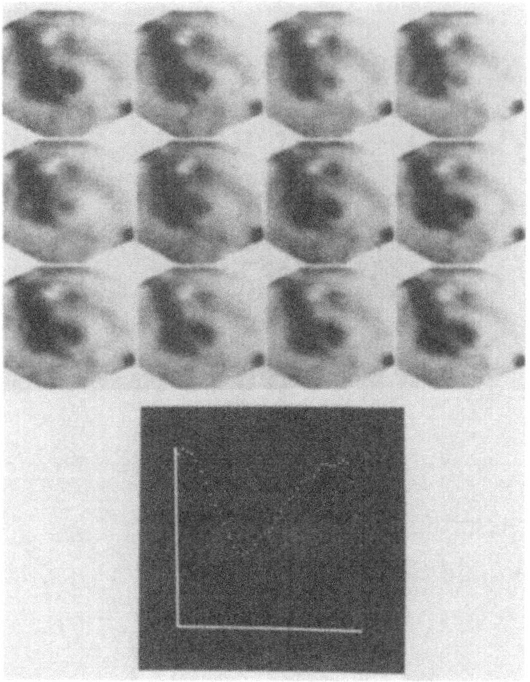

FIGURE 5–1. Equilibrium blood pool scintigraphy. Shown are 12 frames from the blood pool scintigram of a patient with left ventricular hypertrophy and excellent left ventricular function. Serial changes in projected size of the ventricular regions of interest and counts within them can be traced from the upper left frame at end systole. Excellent ventricular emptying can be seen and the clear halo surrounding the left ventricle is consistent with hypertrophy. Subsequent frames demonstrate ventricular diastolic filling. Below, computer counts within the left ventricular region of interest are plotted on the ordinate versus time for each of the acquired frames. The curve closely parallels the left ventricular time versus volume curve. Note the terminal count fall off related to slight irregularities in the R-R interval. (From Schiller, NB and Botvinick, EB: Noninvasive Quantitation of the Left Heart by Echocardiography and Scintigraphy; *Cardiovasc. Clinics* 1985, [in press].)

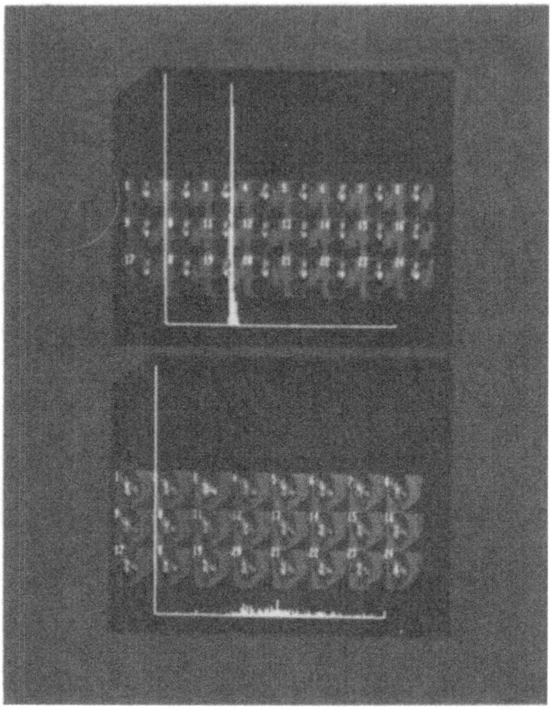

FIGURE 5–2. List Mode Acquisition. Shown are histograms plotting R-R interval on the abscissa versus interval frequency on the ordinate obtained by list mode acquisition in a patient in sinus rhythm (*above*) and in atrial fibrillation (*below*). While the former can more efficiently be acquired in frame mode, the latter may be subsequently formated in frame mode to assess ventricular function at any desired R-R interval.

ployed with regular rhythms. In each fraction, temporal interval, or frame, image data is combined to yield a summed picture. Depending on the computer capability, acquisition can be made in 16, 28, or more frames. Frame duration can also be expressed or acquired in milliseconds (msec), where generally frames of less than 50 msec are required to provide an acquisition frequency rapid enough to capture volume changes during the cardiac cycle. Data from each frame are combined in subsequent cycles with that of the preceding cycle until each frame holds adequate information to permit the generation of well-resolved images and the statistical analysis of counts within background corrected cavitary regions of interest. In our laboratory the sum of all counts in all 28 frames must equal 7,000,000 (Figure 5–1). Alternatively, with irregular, or intermittent, rhythms, scintigraphic data can be acquired in list mode. Although reliable average values can be obtained in frame mode [10], list mode acquisition permits all events to be individually and serially acquired, identified spatially, and temporally related to the R wave signal without pooling sequential data. Subsequently, an R-R histogram can be generated and data framed for the cycle length desired (Figure 5–2).

Each method yields sequential images of the

central blood pool over a typical averaged cycle of given duration. In each region of the blood pool a background subtracted time versus radioactivity curve can be generated which is proportional to a time versus volume curve [11]. From these curves relative parameters, as left and right ventricular ejection fractions, can be accurately, reproducibly, and serially assessed, relative volumes can be followed, or, with calibration, absolute ventricular volumes can be calculated [12]. While frame mode acquisition is simpler, less computer intensive, and more widely performed, it often yields a decline of counts in the terminal frames owing to irregularities in the R-R interval included in the analysis. This decline can seriously influence the measurement of some functional parameters and must be addressed (see below).

Functional or Parametric Images

Since counts in blood pool images are proportional to volume, regional counts and their serial alterations can be compared to yield information relating to regional stroke volume, ejection fraction, and regional and global ventricular emptying and filling rates (Figure 5–3). Counts can be expressed in absolute volumes to yield important quantitative information related to functional measurements made serially at rest, with exercise or with pharmacologic or surgical intervention. Ventricular stroke volumes can be compared to yield accurate, reproducible, regurgitant fractions [13]. Additionally, relatively simple mathematical manipulation of the equilibrium time versus radioactivity curve can be performed to derive parameters relating to the degree and sequence of ventricular (and atrial) emptying. First harmonic Fourier analysis, yielding phase and amplitude measurements, is such an example [14]. When the equilibrium study is reconstructed to yield an image which spatially displays one of these derived parameters, in grey shades or colors, a functional or parametric image is produced. These are powerful tools which can simply and rapidly display, in a condensed, easily interpretable form, the regional distribution of often complex but clinically useful functional measurements. Frequently, these measurements can be neither made nor displayed conveniently in any other way, and occasionally, they cannot be made using other modalities even with difficulty.

Goris notes [15] that the term *parametric* implies images which display a function that can be mathematically defined. Alternatively, the term has been applied to images demonstrating an aspect of a larger physiologic category. In this way, parametric and functional images are the same and indicate that "the mapped [parameter] is related to, or descriptive of, a known physiological phenomenon under study ...", as stroke volume [16] or ejection fraction images [17]. We agree with Dr. Goris in these aspects and believe the phase and amplitude images approach his criteria for parametric image utility:

They appear to have clinical utility.
They are relatively insensitive to error.
Their mathematics are well based.

We will here consider, in depth, only the amplitude and the phase images. Other derived images which aid the objective evaluation of ventricular function, as the stroke volume and ejection fraction images, will be reviewed briefly to contrast them with amplitude and phase images. Only the latter have been extensively and successfully applied to the noninvasive evaluation of the sequence of ventricular contraction and conduction which forms the subject of this chapter.

Stroke Volume and Ejection Fraction Images

The stroke volume image is a parametric image which codes, in relative grey shades or colors, regional stroke volume, the volume ejected with each cycle (Figure 5–3). It is the graphic representation of the pixel by pixel difference between background corrected end-diastolic and end-systolic counts and is obtained by subtracting the end-systolic from the end-diastrolic image. Unlike the amplitude image, the stroke volume image recognizes sign and sets to zero or black, pixels where the stroke volume is negative, where end-systolic counts exceed end-diastrolic counts. Thus, atrial regions and regions of apparent paradoxical motion are not visualized. Nevertheless, the stroke volume image provides an excellent objective map of regional ventricular emptying and has additionally proven useful to quantitate the degree of valvular regurgitation.

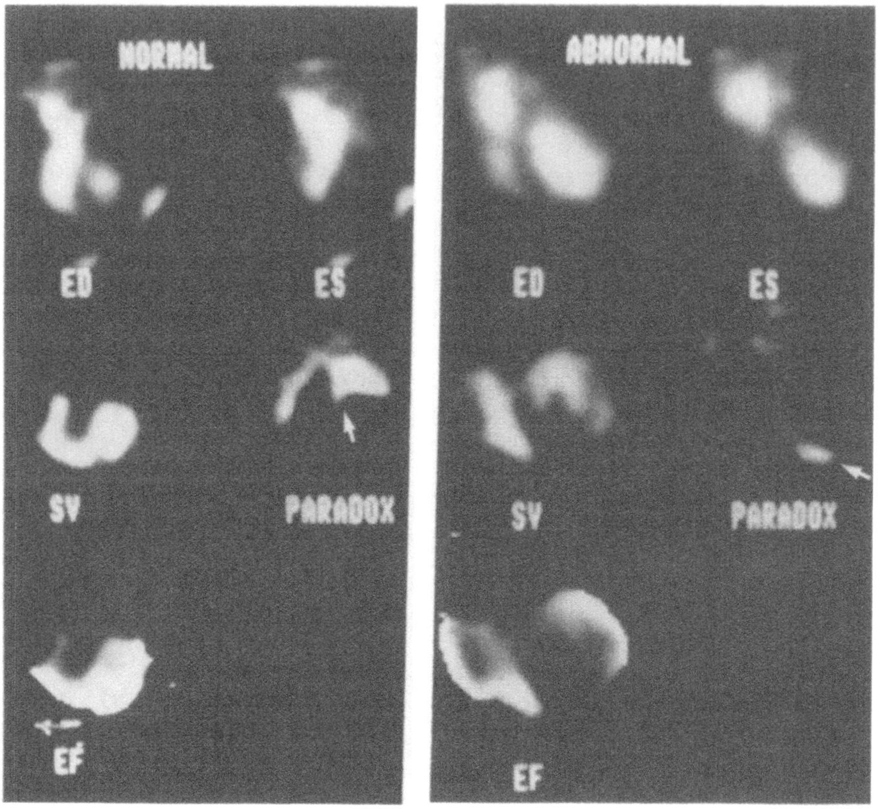

FIGURE 5–3. Functional Images. Shown are end diastolic (ED) and end systolic (ES) frames from a gated equilibrium study in a patient with normal function (NORMAL) and a patient with a left ventricular aneurysm (ABNORMAL). Symbols: EF = ejection fraction image (increased intensity corresponds to increased ejection fraction); paradox = paradox image; SV = stroke volume image (arrow in NORMAL indicates atrial stroke volume, arrow in ABNORMAL indicates dyskinesis in the left ventricle). (From Dae M et al.: Parametric Imaging in Cardiovascular Nuclear Medicine. *Cardiovasc. Rev. Reports* 16:16, 1985.)

Similarly, the ejection fraction image codes regional ejection fraction and represents the graphic display of the quotient derived from the stroke volume and end-diastolic images [17]. It is derived by dividing, pixel by pixel, the stroke volume value by the background corrected end-diastolic value (see Figure 5–3). The ejection fraction image can be an important supplement to scintigraphic functional data since global ventricular performance and ejection fraction may be well maintained in the presence of regional dysfunction. Further, the qualitative assessment of wall motion from the dynamic blood pool display may not be sufficient for accurate, objective detection of regional dysfunction, particularly when abnormally contracting segments are viewed an face. The converse of the stroke volume image, the paradox image, reveals the difference between endsystolic and end-diastolic images, accentuating atrial regions and dyskinetic ventricular segments [18] (see Figure 5–3).

Both stroke volume and ejection fraction images provide objective evidence of relative regional ventricular function and can effectively do so in a single "best septal" projection owing to the dependence of scintigraphic data on counts data rather than geometry. They can be further analyzed to yield quantitative measures of regional stroke volume and ejection fraction. We routinely produce a color coded ejection fraction image in the "best septal" projection in association with all blood pool studies.

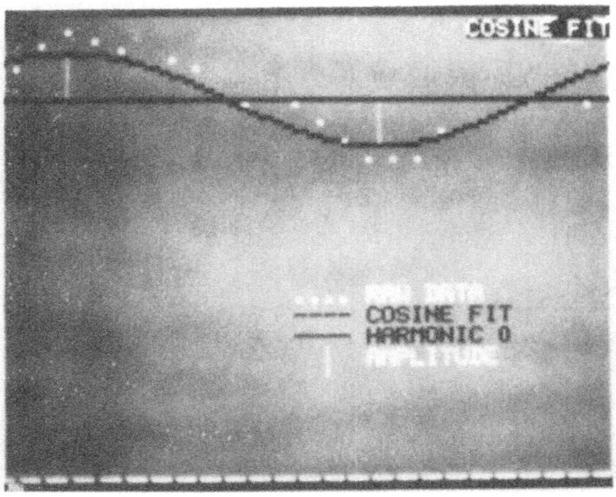

FIGURE 5–4. Curve Fit. Superimposed on the raw time versus radioactivity curve obtained from a single pixel location in the left ventricular region of interest of a multiple gated blood pool scintigram is the fitted first Fourier harmonic transform. The phase angle marked in the diagram relates to the point where the curve begins to lose amplitude or when the ventricle begins to lose counts, the onset of contraction. The amplitude of the curve is another variable that helps to characterize it. Curve amplitude is measured at the phase angle. Its magnitude is generally related to the stroke volume but, unlike that variable, does not consider sign. (From Frais MA et al.: Phase Characterization of Ventricular Contraction in Left and Right Bundle Branch Block. *Am. J. Cardiol*, 50:95, 1982.)

First Fourier Harmonic Transformation

THE AMPLITUDE AND PHASE IMAGES – DEFINITION

The phase image is a computer derived parametric image assembled from an analysis of the time versus radioactivity curve in each pixel location of the blood pool scintigram. Here, each curve is fitted with its first harmonic Fourier transform, equivalent to a symmetric cosine curve (Figure 5–4). Such a curve undergoes one complete sequence during each cardiac cycle from the onset of the electrocardiographic R wave, or 0°, to the following R wave, or 360°. If ventricular contraction began immediately with the R wave and the time versus radioactivity curve was completely symmetrical, it would mirror a cosine curve that began with the cardiac cycle — at the R wave and ended with the subsequent R wave. However, owing to a finite delay related to electrical conduction and a period of isovolumetric contraction, neither regional nor global systole begin exactly with the R wave. As a result, the peak of the true time versus radioactivity curve and that of the fitted curve are displaced. Because it remains symmetric with the periodicity of a cosine curve, regardless of its time of onset, the fitted curve, unlike the asymmetric raw curve, can be characterized by two features, its amplitude or height, and a single number, the phase angle, representing the angular location of its time of onset in the cardiac cycle.

With reference to the ventricles, the phase angle is expressed in degrees beginning at the initiating R wave, from 0° to 360° over the R-R interval, or one complete cycle. In this way a pixel location with fitted curve peak one-eighth through the cardiac cycle would have a designated phase angle of 45° while a region with its fitted curve peak one-quarter through the cycle would have a designated phase angle of 90° (Figure 5–5). Each pixel so characterized can be grey scale or color coded with reference to phase angle to present a functional image of such data, the phase image. Although derived from all points in the time versus radioactivity curve and representative of all points in the fitted curve, the phase angle may be viewed as a relative measure of the timing of the loss of regional counts, chamber emptying, or contraction. Phase analysis may be roughly interpreted to demonstrate the pattern of ventricular contraction, but is importantly influenced by both the temporal sequence and magnitude of such motion. To the degree that contraction follows conduction, the grey scale coded display of phase angle appears to portray, quite faithfully, the pattern of inter- and intraventricular conduction in the absence of marked contraction abnormalities. Conversely, in the absence of conduction abnormalities, the pattern of phase progression relates to the sequence and extent of ventricular emptying or contraction.

Method of Derivation

First implemented approximately 10 years ago by Geffers, Adam, Bitter, and coworkers [19], the method was advanced and refined by Deconninck [20]. Introduced in the U.S. by Verba and coworkers [21], its clinical implications were realized early and have been applied

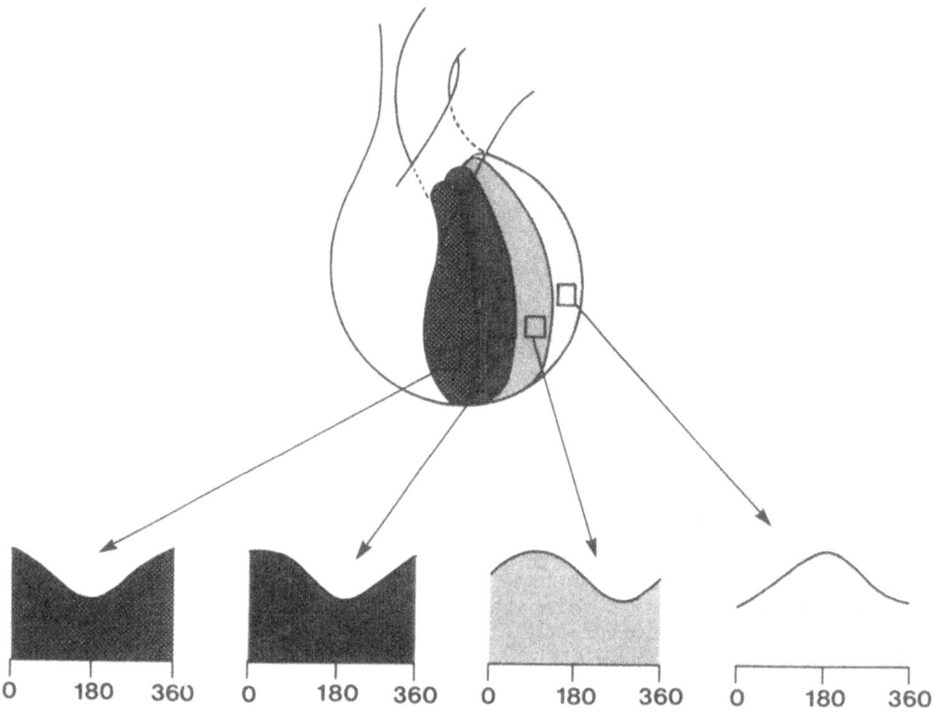

FIGURE 5–5. Phase Image Analysis. Shown is a diagrammatic sketch of the right and left ventricles and great vessels in the "best septal" left anterior oblique projections. The left ventricle has been divided into 4 regions characterized by varying time of contraction onset and phase angle. Each region has been grey scale coded according to the time of contraction onset and phase angle, where pixels in the darkest region near the septum begin contraction at the electrocardiographic R wave gating signal with a phase angle of 0°. Contiguous segments with progressively lighter grey shades are related to progressively delayed contraction, conduction and more delayed phase angles. Moving from the septum toward the lateral left ventricular wall, pixels in progressive segments demonstrate contraction onset one eighth, one quarter and one half of the way through the cardiac cycle with related phase angles of 45°, 90°, and 180°. Below the cardiac diagram are the first harmonic Fourier transforms related to each of the ventricular contraction segments. Each curve is grey scale coded as its related ventricular region. From left to right, the curves demonstrate a 0° phase angle, with curve onset at the R wave gating signal, a 45° phase angle, with contraction onset one eighth through the cardiac cycle, a 90° phase angle, with contraction onset one quarter through the cardiac cycle and a 180 phase angle, with contraction onset half way through the cardiac cycle. (From Frais MA et al.: Phase Image Characterization of Ventricular Contraction in Left Bundle Branch Block. *Am. J. Cardiol*, 50:95, 1982.)

widely by Pavel [22] and coworkers and other advocates of the method.

Any periodic function, as the time versus radioactivity (volume) relation, can be described by the sum of sine and cosine curves of varying frequencies, a Fourier series. The Fourier series may be described as a sequence of harmonic or periodic functions which each add an increasing level of resolution when used to describe a more complex function. The amplitude and phase images are parametric images derived by fitting this first Fourier harmonic to the time versus radioactivity curve generated on a pixel by pixel basis. The resultant fitted curve is of the form:

$$f(t) = A_o + A_1 \cos(t - \omega)$$

where t takes values between 0° and 360°, $f(t)$ is the fitted function ($\sum_{k=1}^{N} f(k)/N$), where N is the number of study frames, A_1 is the first harmonic amplitude, A_0 is the mean time versus radioactivity curve value, and is ω the first harmonic phase, the angular delay of the cosine maximum. The amplitude may be viewed conceptually as an approximate proportionate measure of stroke counts or stroke volume. Phase angle is influenced by curve symmetry, here a measure of the symmetry of the time versus radioactivity curve, and describes the relative position of the peak of the fitted curve with respect to the gating trigger, generally the electrocardiographic R wave.

Phase is a periodic function and attempts to use it in association with first pass, noncyclic phenomenon should be assessed with caution [23]. Also, the degree of asymmetry varies from area to area with first pass flow studies. This reduces the usefulness of related amplitude images since amplitude is strongly dependent on the degree of curve asymmetry.

Phase Image Analysis and Display

In each study phase image analysis is currently performed using the fundamental Fourier harmonic to fit the first 25 frames of the blood pool study. The last 3 frames of the frame mode study are not fitted if found to have reduced data content owing to the variability of the included R–R interval in normals. Alternatively, a narrow window of beat selection by frame or list mode provides technically optimal curves. Forward-background compilation may be employed to eliminate irregular terminal frame date drop off in list mode acquisition. Images are acquired in a 64 by 64 matrix and interpolated to 128 by 128.

The phase image is displayed and analyzed in steps. Each pixel in each projection of the phase image is initially coded in 256 grey shades or 64 colors. In this image pixels demonstrating the same phase angle, with simultaneous counts reduction or contraction onset, demonstrate the same color. The fitted volume curve is assessed at each location and pixels coded black (green) if the curve in that region demostrates ventricular contraction to progress immediately after the R wave peak at 0°. Increasingly lighter grey shades or varying colors are assigned to pixels where the fitted curve demonstrates increasingly delayed phase angle. Because previous experience has shown that imperfect curve fitting methods may result in normal ventricular phase angles of less than 0°, the grey scale is rotated through −90° in order to prevent a black–white interface in an otherwise normal ventricular region of interest. This rotation is not needed for the continuous color wheel. Atrial regions, which actually fill when ventricular contraction occurs, appear in light (blue) shades with approximately 180° phase angle delay. Uncoordinated contraction or random variations, as seen in regions of background, appear as a "salt and pepper" distribution of varying grey shades or colors. This display is visually reviewed to provide an overview of phase relations in preparation for the quantitative assessment that follows (Figures 5–6, 5–7).

Next, the borders of each ventricle are outlined on the phase image. Border localization of regions of interest is aided by the simultaneous superimposition of outlines on the ungated blood pool image. Phase histograms of each ventricle or atrium are constructed from data in these respective regions, in the "best septal" projection. The histogram relates phase angle, on the abscissa, to the number of pixels at any given phase angle on the ordinate. From these histograms, the mean phase angle and standard deviation of phase for each region of interest is calculated. Moveable cursors placed on the histogram are than used to designate any selected range of phase angle as small as 2.8°. Pixels in the phase image within the designated range of phase angle are coded white and by selective, serial, progressive movement of the cursor window to higher phase angles, the

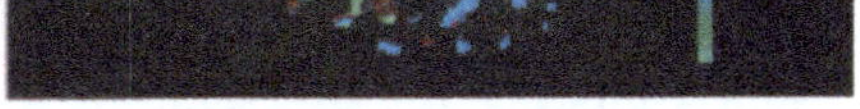

FIGURE 5–6. Normal Phase Image. Shown is a color coded phase image in the "best septal" projection in a patient with normal contraction and conduction. Earliest contraction and smallest phase angle is seen in the septum (green) with early, homogeneous phase angle (blue) in both ventricles. The atrial regions are marked in red, with much delayed phase angle with reference to the R wave gating signal. Background has been suppressed by an amplitude threshold.

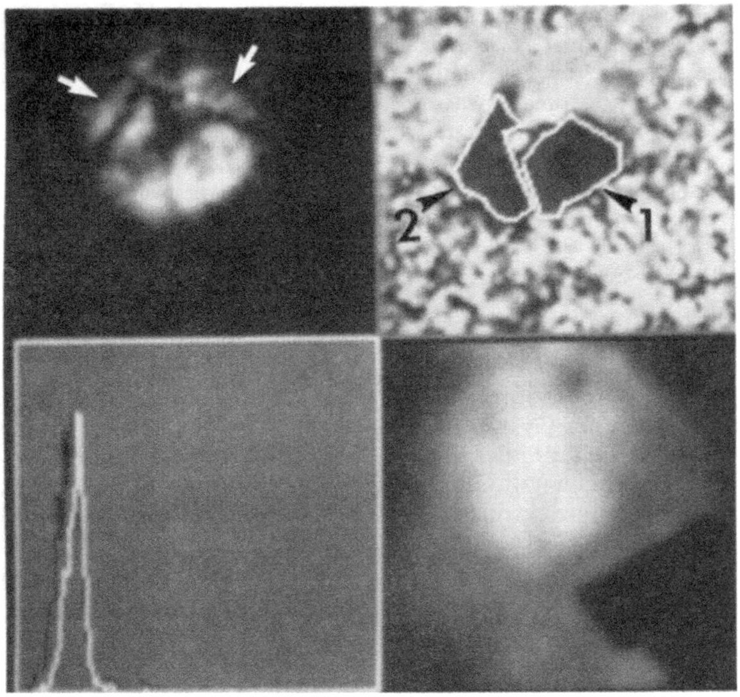

FIGURE 5–7. Normal Image and Histogram. Shown are normal amplitude (*upper left*), and phase (*upper right*) images in a patient without contraction or conduction abnormalities. The composite blood pool image (*lower right*) guides left (arrow points 1) and right (arrow points 2) ventricular region of interest identification. The phase histograms generated from right (black) and left (white) ventricular regions are shown at lower left. Dark grey homogeneous coloration in ventricular regions indicate early, coordinate contraction. Note the position of the histograms early and nearly superimposed, consistent with early symmetrical ventricular contraction, and the atrial region (white arrows, upper left) out of phase with the ventricles. Histograms shown here and many through this presentation are normalized to peak values within the respective region of interest.

sequential pattern of ventricular "contraction" was mapped. Histograms may conveniently be normalized to the most frequent phase angle. In each study, regions of earliest and latest phase angle in each ventricle were those which appeared first and last as the moveable cursors were advanced across the phase range in small increments. The earliest phase angle for each region, its standard deviation, and differences between regional values "for" earliest phase angle could be calculated (see Figures 5–7, 5–8, 5–9). When looking for the sight of earliest phase angle we seek to exclude random regions of varying phase angles from the histogram. We can exclude areas of late or extremely delayed phase angle with impunity regardless of amplitude, but we do not want to exclude areas of reduced amplitude and early phase angle. When looking at the phase sequence we wish to include all regions and assess phase angle without excluding low amplitude pixels. An empirical noise correction is introduced by applying a 5% frequency threshold in the regions of interest and accepting data only from regions with at least three adjacent pixels in spatial and temporal concordance. An amplitude threshold may be applied outside the regions of interest in an effort to simply suppress background and is routinely used only for the cine display (see below).

This sequential phase progression is also displayed in a dynamic 16-frame movie version of the grey scale coded image. Here again sequential frames, each representing an equal range of phase angle, are coded white in regions with phase angle and onset of ventricular contraction occurring within that range. The dynamic display permits an appreciation of the gross phase relations and sequential contraction pattern, but is not used in quantitative aspects of phase

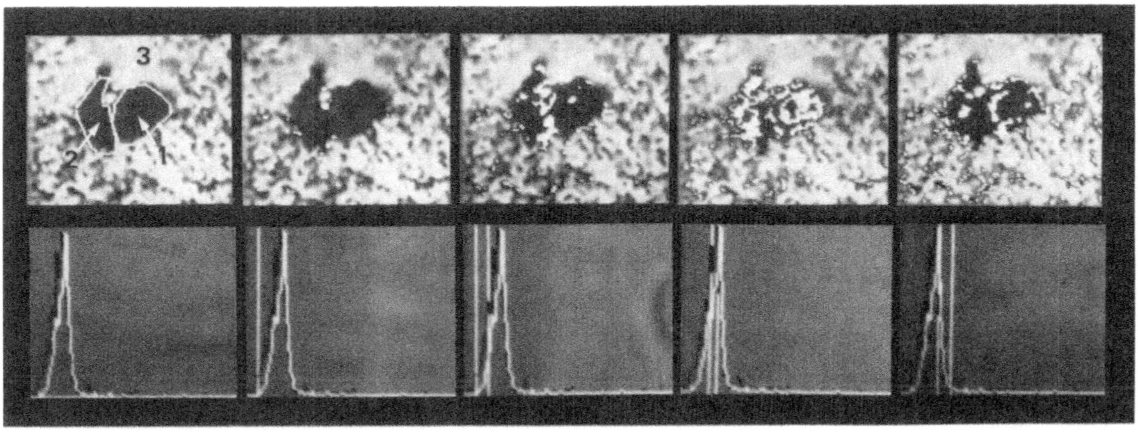

A

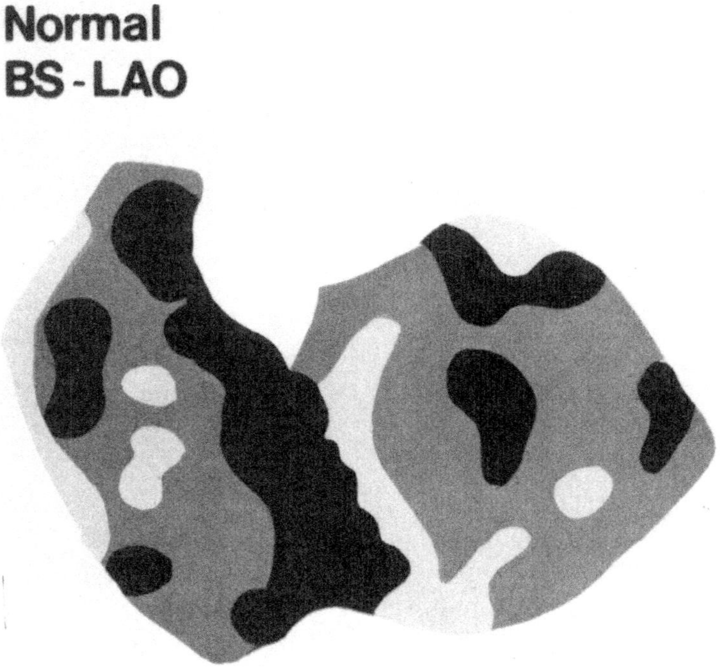

B

FIGURE 5–8. Normal Phase Image Analysis. (A) shown is the phase image in a normal patient in the "best septal" left anterior oblique projection. Ventricular regions of interest have been outlined and appear in homogeneous dark grey, indicating an early phase angle characteristic of normal ventricles. Above the ventricular regions, the homogeneous light areas represent the atrial regions, out of phase with the ventricles. The background, lacking any relation to the cardiac cycle, appears as a random "salt and pepper" distribution of grey shades. Below, normalized right (*black*) and, left (*white*) ventricular phase histograms are seen as in Figure 5–7. In sequential panels, individual pixels in the phase image, which correspond to the serial windows marked on the phase histograms, are enhanced in white. The sequence, from left to right, again indicates early septal phase angle with relatively symmetric involvement of both ventricles. (B) Shown is a sketch of serial phase angles plotted regionally in the "best septal" left anterior oblique projection for the image shown in Figure 5–8A. Again earliest phase angle is depicted in darkest shades. (From Frais, M et al.: Phase Image Characterization of Localized and Generalized Left Ventricular Contraction Abnormalities. *J. Am. Coll. Cardiol*, 4:987, 1984.)

A

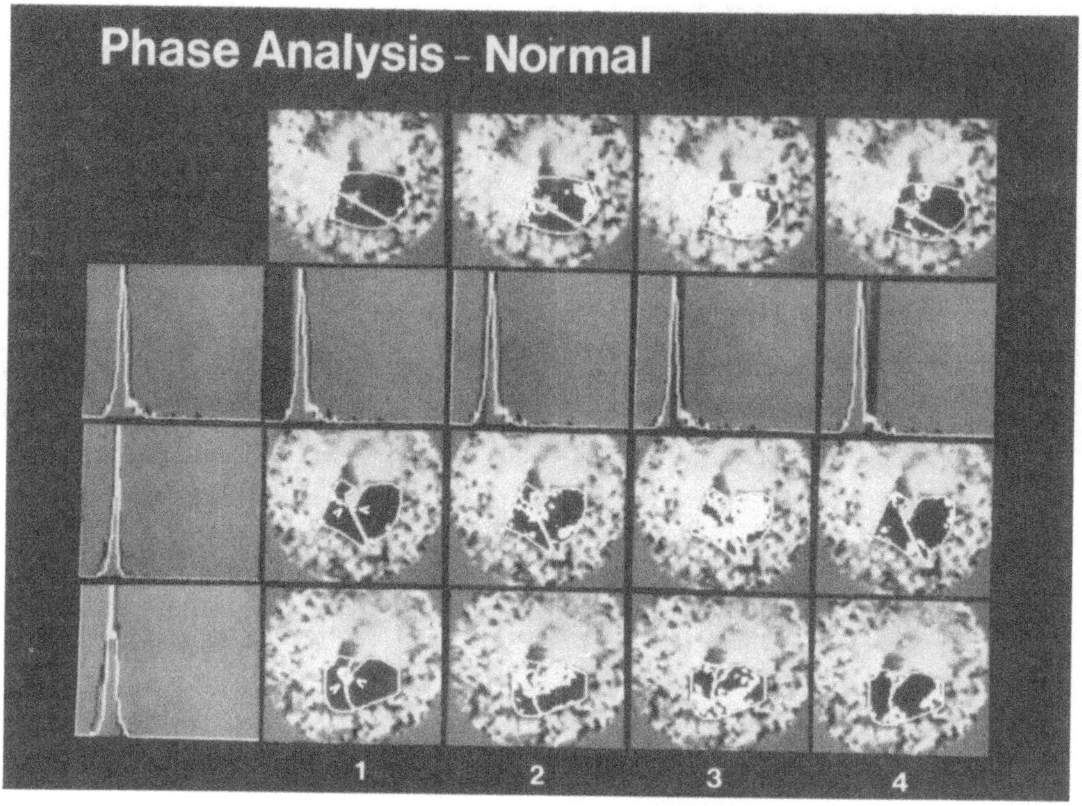

B

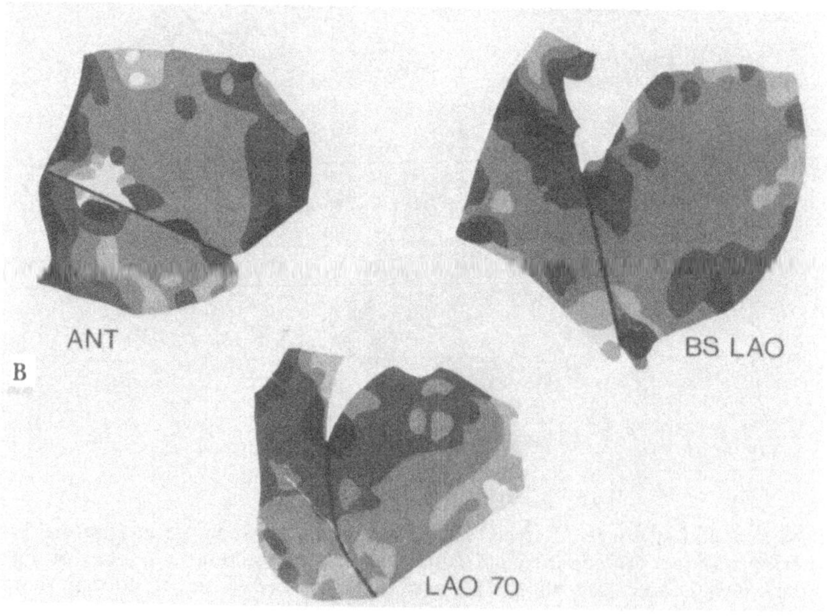

FIGURE 5–9. Phase Analysis in Multiple Projections. (A) Shown in the top row are sequential phase images performed in the anterior projection in a normal patient. In each panel the estimated left and right ventricular regions of interest are outlined. Phase angle is indicated by the grey scale in which increasingly lighter shades represent increasing phase angle. Here, both ventricles appear as homogeneous dark grey shades. Again, the atria appear in light shades superior and to the left of the ventricles while the background is a random "salt and pepper" pattern and the ventricular histograms (row 2) are nearly superimposed. Similar findings are noted in relation to "best septal" (row 3) and 70° left anterior oblique (bottom row) projections. In each case serial sampling of regional phase angles demonstrates earliest septal phase angle and symmetrical biventricular phase progression (*arrow points*). (B) Shown are diagrammatic representations of the same phase images where regions of earliest phase angle are shown in black.

analysis. Again, isolated phase changes in pixels that showed no contiguity to subsequent changes were considered noise and an amplitude threshold was generally applied.

Technical Considerations

Pavel and coworkers [24] note that stroke volume and ejection fraction images depend on single frame statistics, cardiac motion and anatomy, and on accurate selection of end-diastolic and end-systolic frames. Like these images, phase and amplitude images are also affected by adjacent structures but they are not dependent on frame selection, use data from the entire cardiac cycle, are unaffected by the normal cardiac morphology, are not anatomy modulated, delineate functional borders, and are easy to interpret. They are based on simple mathematics and the phase angle provides far better temporal resolution than frames.

Although the phase image may be considered to portray the graphic representation of sequential ventricular contraction, its true derivation must always be kept in mind. The phase angle is as much influenced by diastolic as by systolic events and is thus influenced by the symmetry of the fitted function or the time versus radioactivity curve.

Since first harmonic analysis seeks to fit a symmetrical function to the generally asymmetric ventricular time versus radioactivity curve, the duration of diastole and therefore heart rate will importantly affect phase angle. The latter may best be approached by forcing a mathematical fit of both diastolic and systolic data. Others have demonstrated an improvement in the error corrected phase distribution function when diastasis frames are excluded. We generally address the problem by processing only the initial 25 of the 28 acquired frames.

Pavel [24] notes the inherent dangers in curve correction methods. Squeezed and amputated diastole makes the curve symmetrical but presents errors and artifacts. Yet, although not as technically pure, methodological compromises have been applied successfully. As might be expected, the accuracy of phase angle assessment suffers in the setting of reduced amplitude, ejection fraction, and count density. Statistical reliability must be used as the criterion for including or excluding a pixel within the distribution function. Bacharach and coworkers [25] developed an objective method for evaluation of functional images based on the calculated regional error in curve analysis and fit.

A number of workers have sought to apply higher harmonics in order to optimize the curve fit [26]. However, these do not necessarily appear advantageous. Alternatively, one may avoid the problems of the fitted curve and seek true parameters related to the excursion and time of onset of the time versus radioactivity curve itself. In this way a parametric image depicting the time of onset of regional emptying may be derived and compared to its counterpart, the phase image. While the distribution of data is similar in the two images, the phase image demonstrates less statistical variation (Figure 5–10). This relates to the fact that parameters and images derived from fitted curves are statistically supported by all points in the acquired data rather than victimized by the significant statistical variation related to each individual point in the time versus radioactivity curve. Probably owing to this statistical advantage we have generally obtained easily legible phase images after as little as one minute of acquisition. Brevity of data acquisition may be critical when seeking to map the contraction sequence in the setting of a poorly tolerated arrhythmia, as ventricular tachycardia. In order to perform detailed analysis of phase progression, phase images are analyzed in multiple projections seeking to triangulate generated patterns and overcome difficulties arising from structural overlap (see Figure 5–9 and below).

Recently, Bacharach and coworkers [27] have sought to improve the sensitivity of phase detection of ventricular dysfunction by integrating amplitude information with it. In processing our first harmonic images we generally produce a display, color coded for phase angle and intensity coded for amplitude. This has the advantage of providing extensive information in one image and again automatically provides thresholding. However, when we want to assess serial phase angle, or when the site of earliest phase angle appears to be a region of reduced amplitude, separate amplitude and phase images must be generated. The dual coded images are particularly helpful in aiding objectivity in serial study or before and after interventions (Figure 5–11).

Regardless of these technical and, in cases, theoretical considerations, we and others have noted the relationship between phase angle and patterns of contraction and conduction.

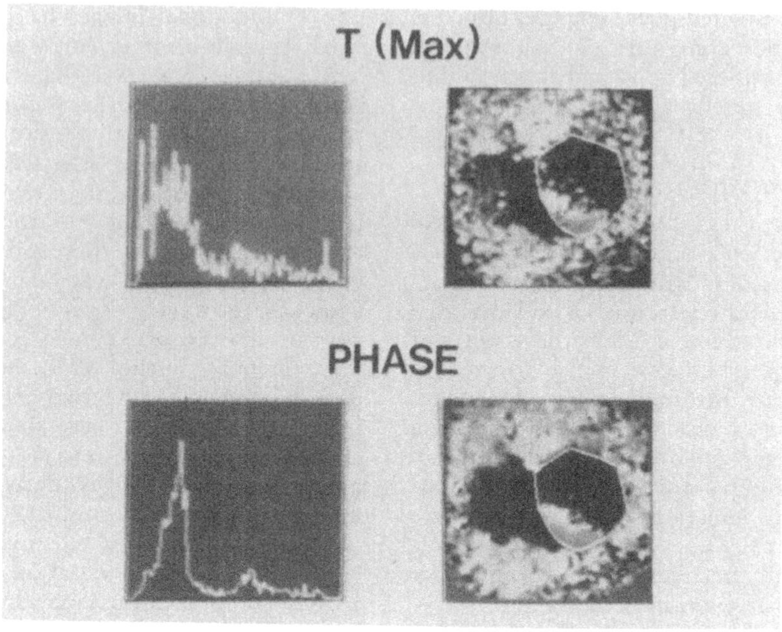

FIGURE 5–10. Direct Curve Sampling. Shown above (*left*) is the global left ventricular time versus radioactivity curve in a patient with an aneurysm. At right is the derived T (max) image, where each pixel is grey scale coded for the relative time of maximum counts or contraction onset. This is to be compared to the ventricular phase histogram and derived phase image in the same patient. Although phase image and T (max) image look similar, the phase image is more noise free owing to its improved statistics related to the anchoring of the phase angle parameter by all points in the time versus radioactivity curve rather than a single point, as the time to maximum counts.

Regarding the former, it is dangerous to draw a parallel between prolonged phase angle and "tardokinesis" unless the rate of systolic emptying is specifically analyzed. Rather, it should simply be noted that regions of the ventricle with reduced wall motion appear to have prolonged phase angle. Regarding this relationship, it would appear that since the sight of the focus represents the onset of excitation and the phase angle is a derived mechanical parameter, the correspondence between the sight of electrical focus and the sight of earliest phase angle indicates electromechanical coupling. While care must be taken in making such conclusions, the general relationships between phase angle and measurements of regional ventricular contraction and excitation do exist, are clinically important and will be examined. However, since both contraction and conduction patterns will produce alterations in phase and amplitude data, we will first evaluate their applications to the assessment of regional ventricular function.

The Normal Amplitude and Phase Image

The amplitude image in a normal patient simply presents, in relative intensities, the regional amplitude of the cardiac chambers. It will closely resemble the stroke volume image but will differ in several respects. Amplitude is not synonymous with stroke volume but is generated from a curve fitting method which does not depend on the precise localization of global systolic or diastolic frames. Thus, if regional emptying were everywhere simultaneous and the proper frames were chosen, amplitude patterns would mirror those of stroke volume. To the extent that the timing of regional systole does not parallel that of global systole, the amplitude distribution will likely demonstrate a better estimate of true regional emptying, independent of time constraints (See-Phase Analysis for Assessment of Contraction Abnormalities-below). Also, since the amplitude measurement is independent of time, it recognizes no func-

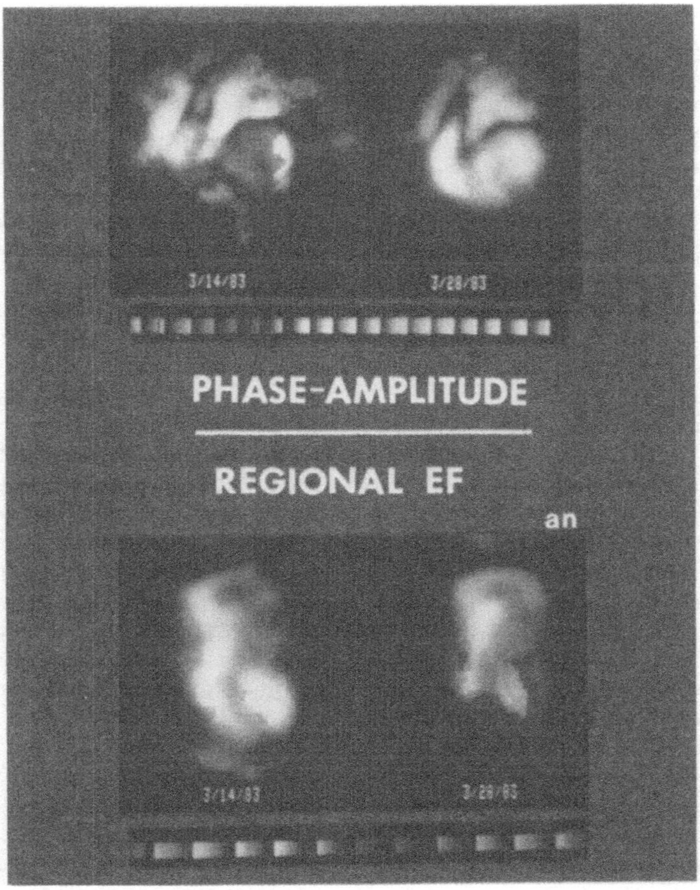

FIGURE 5–11. Functional Images. Shown above are functional images coded by shading for phase angle and intensity coded for amplitude in a patient with severe ventricular dysfunction at rest (*left*) but much improved when subsequently studied after treatment (*right*). The alteration in shade coding indicates the presence of earlier phase angles, and the increased intensity indicates increased amplitude or ventricular stroke volume in the post treatment study. Shown below are the regional ejection fraction maps corresponding to the same serial scintigraphic acquisitions illustrated above. Typically, these images are presented in a color-coded fashion and provide vivid visual evidence of regional functional improvement following treatment. (From Dae, M et al: Parametric Imaging in Cardiovascular Nuclear Medicine. Cardiovasc. Rev. Rep 16:16, 1985.)

tional differences and no ventricular systolic emptying, "dyskinetic" ventricular motion and atrial changes will all be registered similarly. While the paradoxical nature of some regions of the amplitude image may not be appreciated, regional correlation with phase will clarify this issue. Such an interaction between amplitude and phase angle is employed to correct amplitude for the contraction pattern when utilizing amplitude ratios to assess the degree of valvular regurgitation. Lastly, it must again be realized that amplitude is a derived parameter depending strongly on the ability of the fitted curve to reflect the full excursion of the regional time versus radioactivity and representing one-half that value. To the extent that this is not true, the parameter will err. Regions of reduced ventricular amplitude generally correspond to contraction abnormalities assessed on a counts, not a geometric, basis. Such defects in the amplitude image, when peripherally located, may be unappreciated if not compared to the ventricular silhouette in the blood pool image. The image serves as a useful objective indicator of regional motion abnormalities.

Assessment of the phase movie and quantitative analysis of the static phase image employing phase histograms with moveable cursors reveals the sequence of phase variation [28]. Within the temporal constraints of the analytic method, multiple sites of phase onset and termination are sometimes seen. The sequence of phase variation in normal subjects shows an orderly progression across both ventricles with minor irregularities. The site of earliest left ventricular phase is always in the proximal septum but is also noted at the left ventricular base, in the inferoapical region, and in the distal septum in some patients. The sequence of phase variation spread concentrically in an inferoapical and lateral direction, with late phase angle occurring at inferoapical, proximal septal, posterolateral, and distal septal sites. The regions of earliest right ventricular phase angle were also in the proximal septum, basal, and inferoapical regions with spread in a superolateral direction and latest phase angle at the outflow tract, base, and, rarely, in the inferoapical region. The mean left ventricular phase angle was 7.2 ± 11.5° while that for the right ventricle was 8.8 ± 11.5°. The mean standard deviation of left ventricular phase angle was 21.6 ± 10.0°, and of the right ventricle, 29.5 ± 10.7°. The difference between these values was significant, indicating a somewhat greater phase range in the normal right than in the normal left ventricle. See Figures 5–6 through 5–9.

Phase Analysis for the Assessment of Contraction Abnormalities

While the specific cause for the relationship remains somewhat unclear, numerous authors have noted increased phase angle in regions with contraction abnormalities. Even in our primitive initial work [29], akinetic and dyskinetic segments demonstrated impressive phase delay compared to normals. However, hypokinetic segments were often related to a less impressive phase alteration and often overlapped with the normal range of phase angle. Subsequently, phase angle, standard deviation of phase angle, and phase histogram skewness, taken as a measure of contraction asynchrony, were all related to abnormal contraction. Although there is an expected generalized and rate related increase in phase angle, segmental phase prolongation, and the other parameters noted, were shown in a number of studies, to relate to stress induced contraction abnormalities. Turner and coworkers [30] noted exaggerated histogram skewness at maximum stress to be equally sensitive and more specific than the presence of ischemia as determined from conventional stress scintigraphic parameters. Mancini and coworkers [31] found curve skewness to be the best phase parameter for identifying functional abnormalities at rest, but sensitivity was poor and Norris et al. [32] noted only a marginally increased sensitivity for detection of coronary disease during supine bicycle exercise, when phase measurements were added to changes in global ejection fraction values. However, Ratib and coworkers [33] found the standard deviation of phase to be the abnormal in 95% of 37 coronary patients during exercise, while only 86% had a pathological ejection fraction response. They found such phase abnormalities in only 2 of 11 patients with pathologic ejection fraction responses in the setting of valvular disease and claimed that although induced phase abnormalities are not totally specific, they are indeed sensitive and adequately specific for the diagnosis of coronary disease. However, this was not well substantiated by other investigators although these same initial workers [34], again subsequently demonstrated that the exercise related standard deviation of left ventricular phase angle was highly specific for ischemia in patients with normal or mildly reduced left ventricular ejection fraction. While remaining sensitive in patients with severe resting contraction abnormalities, specificities seemed reduced and others have shown that the standard deviation of left ventricular phase angle is a sensitive index for the detection of transient left ventricular dysfunction associated with ischemia at rest.

In our initial study [29] relating phase angle to regional motion, we were frame limited and could not express phase angle in degrees but only in terms of frame intervals. This crude estimate in fact parallels our later, more refined analysis [28] of normal phase histograms where mean left ventricular phase angle varied from −12.5 to 28.7° (mean 8.5°) with a S.D. of 11.8° and a mean right ventricular phase angle of 13.6 ± 12.9°. Repeated subsequently in a group of patients with normal electrocardiogram and normal wall motion using the more strenuous noise suppression methods discussed above [35], mean left and right ventricular phase angle varied around similar narrow limits with mean ventricular phase angles previously noted. In each case the phase image revealed a homogeneous ventricular pattern of dark grey shade, corresponding to early phase angle without regions of gross phase delay, but with a small significant difference in mean ventricular phase angle. The phase histogram of each ventricle approximated a narrow Gaussian distribution with their earliest onset of contraction occurring almost simultaneously. Although earliest phase angle of the right ventricle frequently preceded that of the left ventricle, the mean intrapatient difference between the onset of left and right ventricular phase was not significant, 1.9 ± 6.5°. Since earliest phase angle was always seen in the septal region, assignment of the location to right or left ventricular regions of interest was occasionally affected by the somewhat variable localization of the septal division. However, the mean standard deviation of right ventricular phase angle, the duration of right ventricular activation, an index of asynchrony, was significantly greater than that of the left ventricle. Overall, these results are consistent with the known temporal relationship between right and left ventricular conduction and contraction [36] and parallel the documented pattern of myocardial activation.

Phase analysis may be particularly helpful in the assessment of aneurysms, with akinetic or apparently dyskinetic segments in an otherwise normal ventricle. In this setting, corresponding well defined phase abnormalities are noted with increased phase angle, standard deviation of phase angle, and a peculiar but characteristic discrete secondary histogram peak [37] (Figures 5–12, 5–13). The progression of phase angle is discontinuous but orderly and the region of phase abnormalities can be superimposed on the end-diastolic frame to determine the percentage of end-diastolic volume involved in the aneurysm. This parameter correlates well with the percent akinetic segment measured angiographically and is of potential clinical significance. This pattern is well differentiated from that of ventricles with generalized contraction abnormalities which reveal yet greater mean phase angle, a grossly irregular histogram and a disorderly spatial progression of phase angle. Jones and coworkers [38] used the phase image to identify and localize left ventricular aneurysms and Yiannikes et al. [39] reported that the preoperative first harmonic blood pool assessment of aneurysm size and contribution correlated well with left ventricular ejection fraction measured after aneurysm resection in 18 patients.

Atrial Phase Analysis

While the atrial volume and related time versus radioactivity curve is not as simple, as predictable, or as easily extracted from the blood pool image, atrial amplitude and phase can be characterized. Generally reflecting the period of atrial emptying, the phase angle likely relates to the period of atrioventricular valve opening at the end of systole. It is also probably tempered somewhat by the component of active atrial contraction. In normal phase images the atrial regions are generally well seen and demonstrate extreme phase delay similar to that observed in paradoxical ventricular segments. This is not unexpected owing to the opposition of atrial and ventricular emptying patterns. Normally, the atrial regions are well identified proximal to the ventricles in the "best septal" left anterior oblique projection. Earlier atrial phase can be seen when the atrium is paced and triggering occurs from the atrial pacemaker spike (Figure 5–14). In such cases regional phase angles are altered yet the sequence appears to be preserved. Atrial phase angle may be difficult to evaluate in those conditions associated with reduced atrial amplitude. This can be seen in association with the loss of active atrial contraction in atrial fibrillation, and has been noted in cases of atrial flutter with 2:1 atrioventricular (AV) conduction [40]. Similarly, atrial amplitude may fall precipitously in ventricular tachycardia when there is no retrograde AV conduction or when the mechanical effects of retrograde AV conduction are blunted by closure of the AV valves. This may explain the difficulty in identifying the site of accessory connections when seeking to assess the site of earliest atrial phase angle with ventricular pacing or the difficulty in identification of retrograde atrial activity during ventricular tachycardia. Electrophysiologic assessment is easily performed in these settings but phase analysis depends on a mechanical atrial counterpart which may be blunted by atrial stimulation immediately after. Yet phase image documentation of ventriculoatrial conduction in the presence of ventricular pacing has been demon-

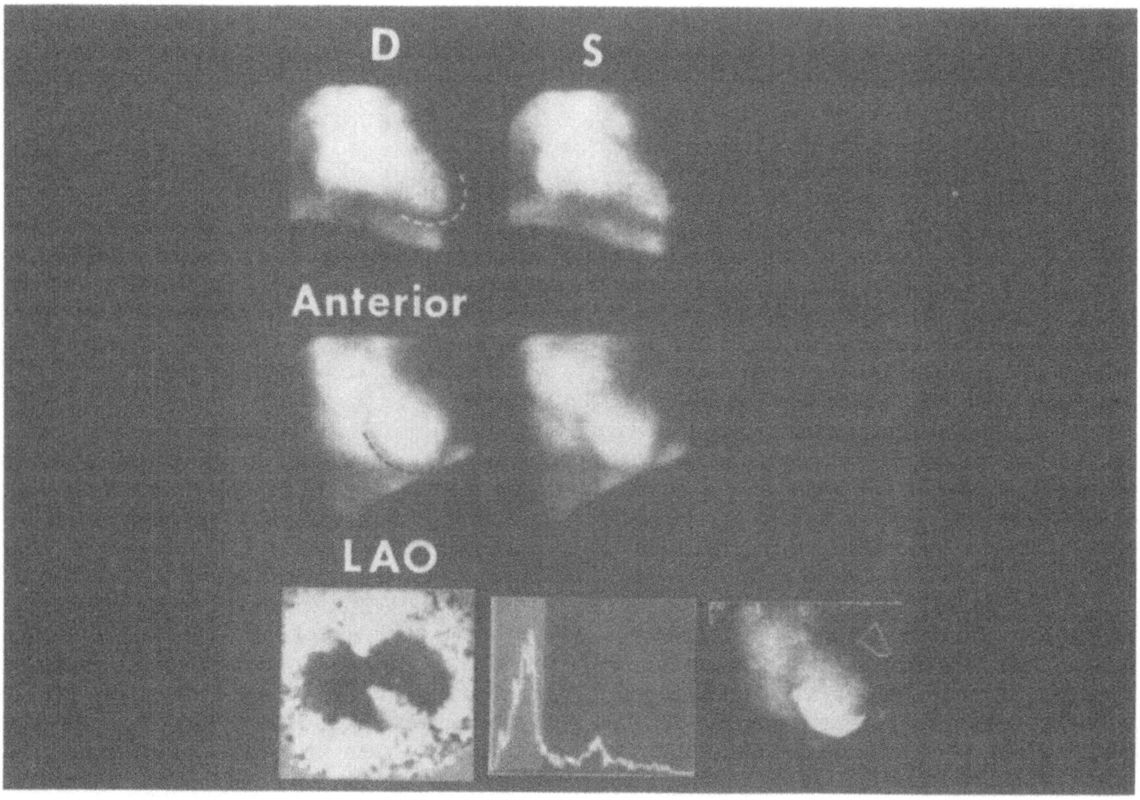

FIGURE 5–12. Phase Analysis Versus Wall Motion Analysis. In the four upper images in anterior and "best septal" left anterior oblique (LAO) projections are the diastolic (D) and systolic (S) frames from the equilibrium blood pool scintigram in a patient with a well defined apicoseptal aneurysm. The akinetic regions have been highlighted with a dotted line on the diastolic image in each projection. In the lower row is the phase image generated from the LAO projection in this patient (*left*) and the phase histogram generated from the left ventricular region of interest in this same phase image (*middle*). Examination of the phase image reveals the left ventricle to be divided into two sharply defined componens, a larger, more proximal region (*dark grey*) corresponding to an early phase angle component, and an apical region (*light grey*) corresponding to the location of dyskinesia in this projection. The phase histogram in this patient with a segmental contraction abnormality again reveals two peaks and was divided at that phase angle equal to the normal left ventricular mean value plus two standard deviations. In the right panel of the bottom row pixels corresponding to phase angles beyond this cutoff have been highlighted in white and superimposed on the end diastolic frame. The close correspondence between the akinetic segment, the region of grossly abnormal phase angle and the objectively superimposed region of abnormal phase angle is clearly evident. From such an analysis, the percent of the end diastolic volume involved in the severe segmental contraction abnormality or aneurysm can be simply and objectively calculated. (From Frais, M et al.: Phase Image Characterization of Localized and Generalized Left Ventricular Contraction Abnormalities. *J. Am. Coll. Cardiol.* 4:987, 1984.)

strated [41] and accessory connections are well seen by phase image analysis when conduction occurs antegrade down the bypass pathway. Attempts to map foci of supraventricular tachycardias may be possible in the setting of a regular AV relationship, although higher harmonics would be required when AV conduction is greater than unity. However, problems relating to the irregularity of the atrial time-volume curve, inability to fully view atrial regions of interest and the cyclic pathway of intraatrial conduction make atrial mapping problematic at this point. Nevertheless, atrial phase can often be evaluated and one of the advantages of the

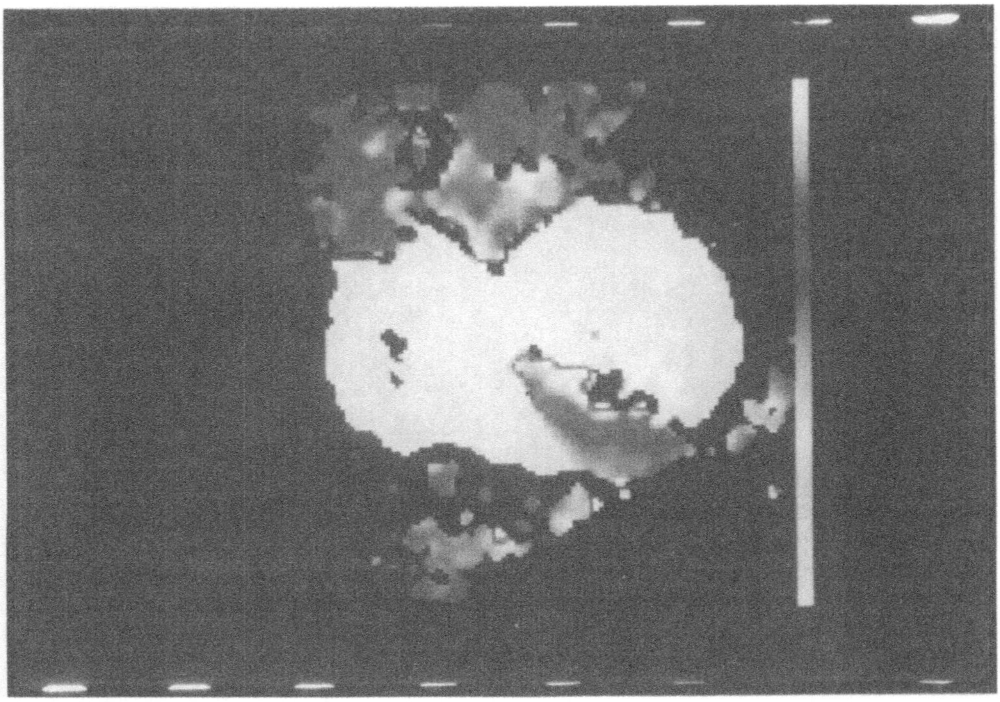

FIGURE 5–13. Phase Image of an Aneurysm. Shown is the phase image in the patient with an apicoseptal aneurysm. Earliest phase angles are seen in the region of the right ventricle and septum in this patient with a left bundle branch block. The aneurysm, with "paradoxical" wall motion is shaded, similar to that of the atrial regions at the top of the figure. The region of segmental phase delay, corresponding to the aneurysm, can be superimposed on the end diastolic image from which it was generated and the percentage of the left ventricle involvement can be assessed. (From Schiller, NB, and Botvinick, EH: Noninvasive Quantitation of the Left Heart by Echocardiography and Scintigraphy. *Cardiovasc. Clin.* 1985 [in press].)

phase method relates to its ability to seperate cardiac chambers with varying functional characteristics not otherwise separable on conventional blood pool images.

A region of well-defined "paradoxical" atrial phase over the region of the liver in the area of the inferior vena cava has been shown by Handler and coworkers [42] to relate to significant tricuspid regurgitation in patients with a systolic murmur. Atrial regions have been identified in paradox images and analyzed to determine a fractional emptying parameter [18,21]. We have utilized the atrial amplitude assessment to correct ventricular amplitude ratios for atrial overlap in the right ventricular region of interest (see above). Unfortunately, the difficulties noted above prevent a more complete assessment of atrial amplitude, phase, and overall function by scintigraphic methods.

Noninvasive Imaging Methods to Analyze Ventricular Conduction Abnormalities

Even the early cinematic displays of Verba [21] demonstrated a pattern of serial progression of phase angle which is extremely reminiscent of the wave of electrical activation. Verba's method, however, employed the total Fourier transform of each pixel and multiplied the transform by a filter function. This required a larger computer.

Although the phase angle is determined by the first Fourier harmonic fit of all points in the time versus radioactivity curve, there nevertheless seems to be a relatively good relationship between the phase angle and the timing of onset of ventricular systole. That is, the phase angle has been correlated with the onset and sequence

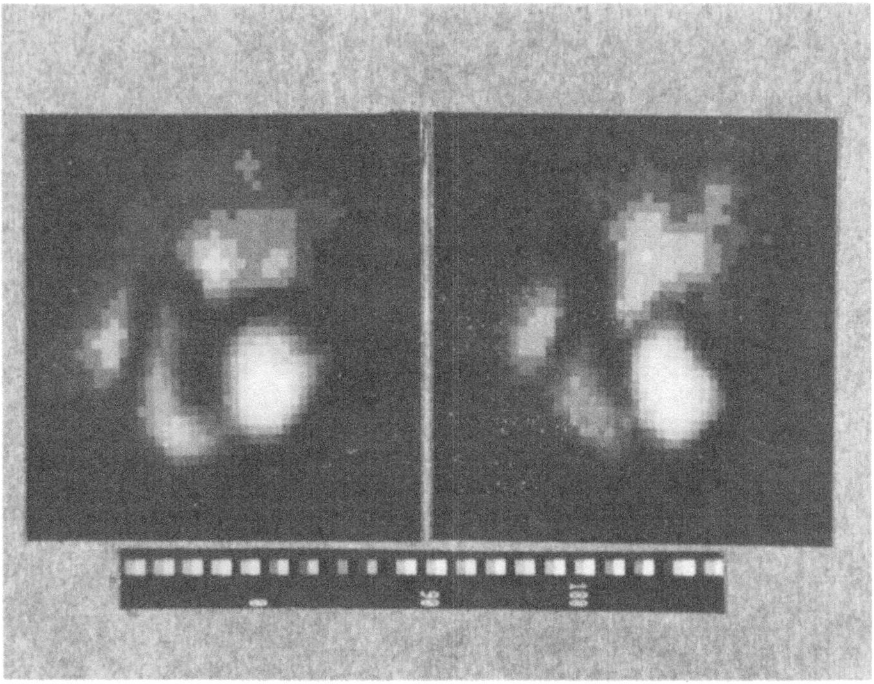

FIGURE 5–14. Effects of Atrial Pacing. Shown are phase images in the "best septal" left anterior oblique projection, acquired both at rest (*left*) and with rapid atrial pacing (*right*) in a patient with preexcitation syndrome and a left lateral AV connection. (See text for description of the technique. Typically, these images are presented in a color-coded fashion, thereby simplifying their interpretation.)

of regional emptying. This is, in fact, a very difficult parameter to measure as other methods (even angiography) do not have the ability to view global ventricular contraction pattern and objectively discern the earliest and sequential contraction sites. Angiography is a silhouette method, limited in temporal resolution by the framing rate, generally unable to assess both ventricles simultaneously, and without the appropriate edge detection software to automate motion analysis. Echocardiography has again a limited sampling window, is observer dependent, and lacks the application of computerized methods to objectively and readily extract sequential wall motion data [43]. Yet it has been applied to the identification of contraction patterns in preexcitation with atrioventricular connections [44]. Of course, both digital angiography and new computerized two-dimensional echocardiographic methods promise to bring such analysis to the practical realm. Yet the ability to assess serial motion over the body of the ventricles, the extreme ease of digitization and computer analysis, and its ability to evaluate all of the central blood pool simultaneously overcomes the nonselective nature of the method and presents significant advantages for the application of scintigraphic phase analysis to the assessment of ventricular contraction sequence. Owing to the insufficiency of other methods, much of the documentation and corroboration of the scintigraphic method has come from correlations of phase maps with expected contraction patterns based on known patterns of electrical activation. Conversely, since evidence suggests that excitation and contraction are generally linked [45], the scintigraphic map has been used to assess patterns of electrophysiologic activation and has been extensively correlated with surface ECG and electrophysiologic data. This relationship between sequential phase angle and the sequence of ventricular contraction and activation, has been confirmed in a number of studies relating the site of earliest phase angle to the site of initial activation, and the pattern of phase progression to the pattern of activation.

Of course, since phase analysis deals primarily with the time versus radioactivity curve, a measurement of mechanical activity, all such studies depend for their success on the linkage of electrical activation and mechanical contraction. If these events were not spatially and temporally linked, phase analysis could not comment on patterns of electrical activation and conduction. This, however, is seemingly not a problem or controversy except possibly in patients with scarred ventricles and ventricular tachycardia, where uncoupling of these events has been said to explain occasional image ambiguities or errors. It must also be realized that phase analysis cannot provide actual time markers for cardiac events. However, owing to displacement of the fitted curve from the real data, at best a relative map of sequential contraction can be provided.

Phase Characterization of Electrical Activation and Conduction

POTENTIAL METHODOLOGIC DIFFICULTIES

Since the phase angle appears to parallel the timing and extent of regional contraction, the earliest phase angle could theoretically be correlated with the localization of artificial pacemakers (Figure 5–15) and applied to the identification of accessory connections and ectopic foci. If mechanical activity parallels electrical, then the phase map could also serve to define the sequence of contraction and, by implication, activation. However, since contraction abnormalities bring phase angle delay, these could potentially alter the apparent progression of phase angle and influence phase prolongation unrelated to a conduction delay. In fact, the phase pattern of bundle branch block can be well appreciated even in the setting of a gross aneurysm (see Figure 5–13). When applying the method to the identification and localization of accessory connections or other sites of ventricular activation, the contraction pattern should not influence the results unless the earliest region of electrical activation occurs in a poorly contracting segment with relatively delayed phase angle in the presence of electromechanical dissociation. From our experience and that of others, it appears that this is uncommon, as the site of earliest phase angle corresponds well to the documented site of earliest electrical activation, or close enough to make resolving the difference impossible by scintigraphic techniques whose intrinsic resolution is approximately .5–1.0 cm. Further, in patients with ventricular tachycardia, it is not uncommon for the site of earliest phase angle to be located in a region which has suppressed ventricular function. The region with the best ventricular function need not be the area of earliest phase angle. Were this not the case, there would be little hope of localizing ventricular tachycardia foci and other abnormalities which might reasonably originate in or near abnormal myocardium. Thus, the phase angle need not always parallel amplitude. Yet, with blunted or absent amplitude the possibility of accurate phase assessment is lost. To the extent that these abnormalities of contraction prevent proper identification of the site of earliest conduction, phase analysis will be faulted and could only localize the focus to the next nearest site of mechanical influence. However, more often, the focus is both electrophysiologically and scintigraphically localized to a region adjacent to an aneurysm. Other difficulties which may affect evaluation of the contraction and conduction sequence from phase maps is the presence of a wide QRS complex, as seen in ventricular tachycardia. This can displace the gating signal due to its slow, ill-defined electrical upslope, but can be adjusted in evaluation provided one knows the relationship between gating signal and QRS complex. Similarly, curve fitting of a time versus radioactivity curve with a prolonged systolic component in the presence of incoordinate contraction and ventricular tachycardia can yield an ambiguous phase map of continuous cyclical activity. While this parallels the electrophysiologic findings, it nevertheless stands as an occasional obstacle to focus localization and may be aided by a more exacting method which reflects absolute timing rather than just the sequence of contraction.

Applications of the Phase Method

BUNDLE BRANCH BLOCK

Links and coworkers [46], simply employed the phase angle of the fundamental frequency and a small computer to perform a preliminary analy-

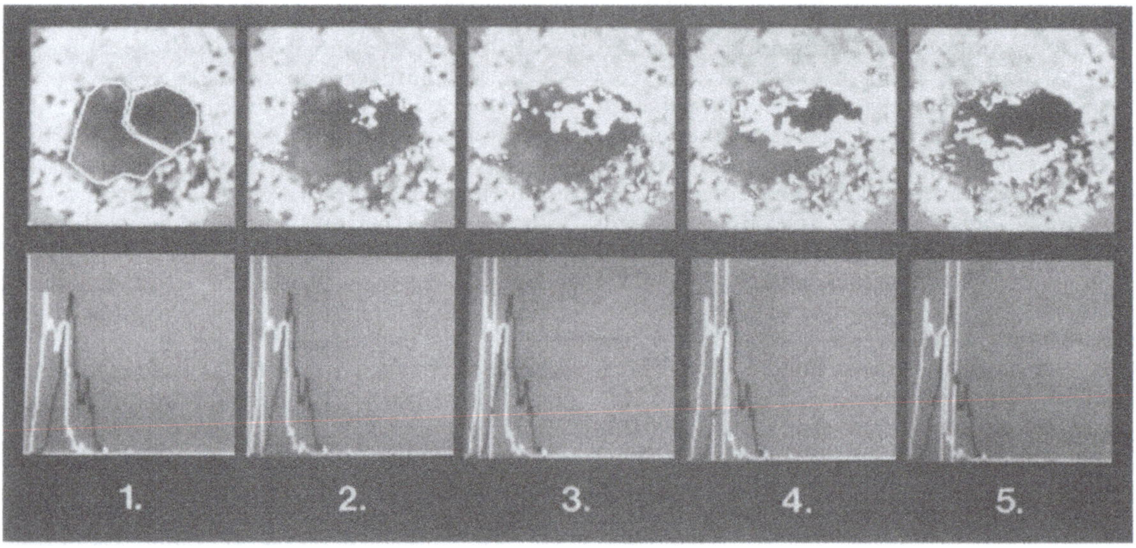

FIGURE 5–15. Epicardial Pacemaker. Shown are sequential phase images and associated ventricular phase histograms. In contrast to the pattern in patients with normal conduction, or those with a right ventricular pacemaker (see Figure 5–18), the left ventricular region of interest is represented by a darker grey shade than that of the right ventricle. The site of earliest phase angle is in the left ventricular lateral wall and the right ventricular phase histogram has a later onset and peak than that of the left ventricle. The highlighted sequence of phase change is correspondingly later in the right ventricle than that of the left ventricle. (Botvinick, EH et al.: An Accurate Means of Detecting and Characterizing Abnormal Patterns of Ventricular Activation by Phase Analysis. *Am. J. Cardiol.* 50:289, 1982.)

sis of the relationship between the phase image and the conduction pattern in normals, patients with bundle branch block and a single patient with an implanted ventricular pacemaker. The pattern and distribution of phase angles paralleled the expected pattern of contraction and conduction in each case. Additionally, the patient with the ventricular pacemaker demonstrated a close relationship between the site of earliest phase angle and the pacemaker site. The authors concluded that "temporal Fourier analysis permits visualization of the pattern of ventricular emptying".

Subsequently, the relationship between the pattern of phase angle progression and the apparent pattern of ventricular excitation was more specifically evaluated in patients with left and right bundle branch block [47,48]. In all areas the phase image of each ventricle demonstrated homogeneous phase progression across both ventricles. The site of earliest phase angle in bundle branch block was generally septal or paraseptal, similar to that noted in normal patients and consistent with the normal conduction pattern proximal to the bundle branch bifurcation. Ventricular phase histograms were again Gaussian, but that of the affected side always followed that of the contralateral ventricle. Interestingly, the mean phase angle of the right ventricle in patients with right bundle branch block and of the left ventricle in those with left bundle branch block was delayed compared with that in patients with normal conduction. Further, the mean intrapatient difference between left and right ventricular mean phase angle in patients with normal conduction ($-5.2 \pm 6.8°$) was significantly different from that in patients with right ($-21.8 \pm 10.3°$) or left ($21.8 \pm 6.8°$) bundle branch block consistent with the known relative delay in ventricular excitation and related contraction on the side of the affected ventricle. In parallel fashion, the mean intrapatient difference between onset of left and right ventricular phase angle was also significantly different from normal in patients with right ($-10.6 \pm 7.5°$) or left ($18.7 \pm 8.3°$) bundle branch block (Figure 5–16). These findings are in agreement with others, demon-

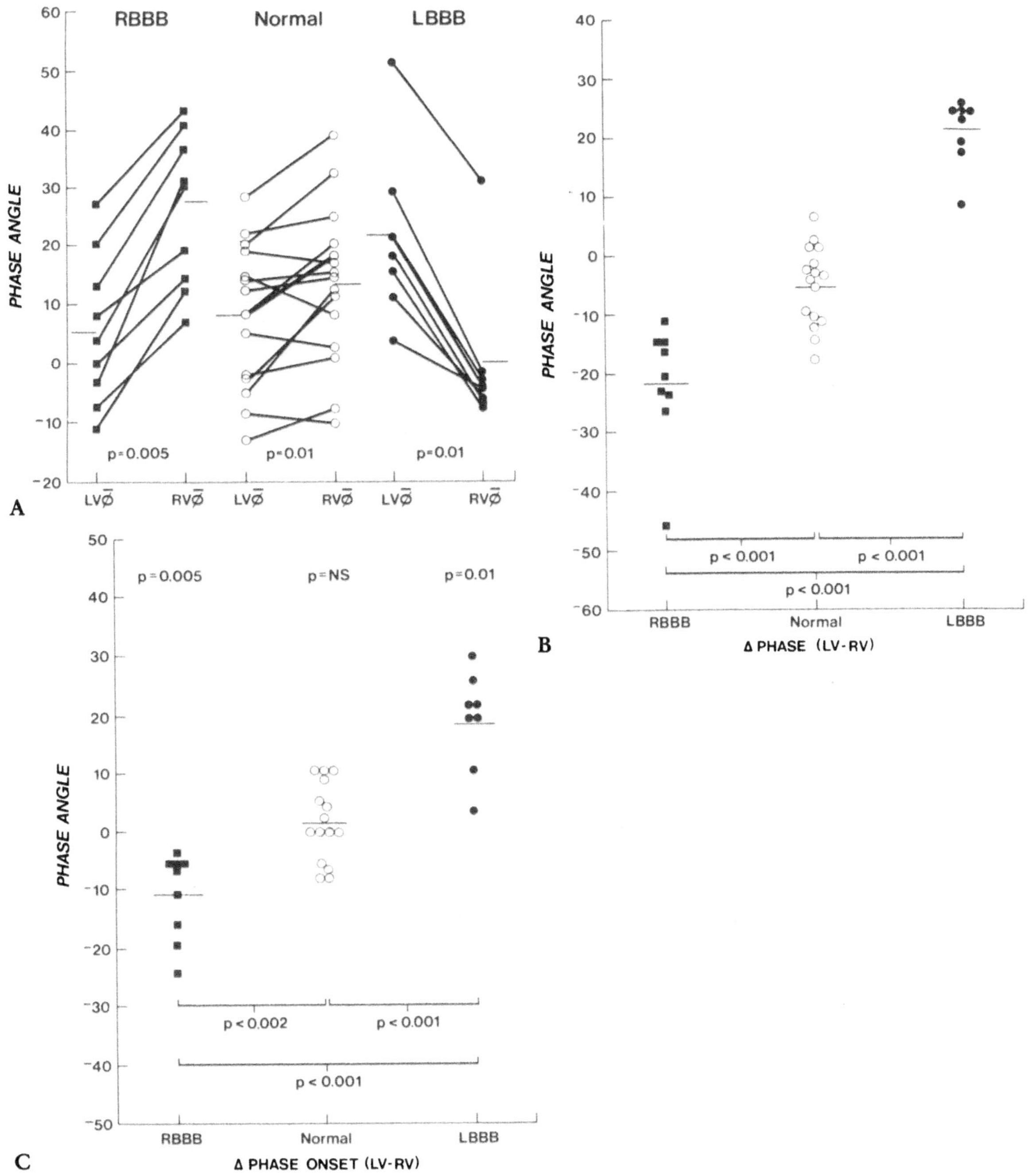

FIGURE 5–16. Bundle Branch Block. (A) Mean Ventricular Phase Angle. Shown are the relationships between mean left and right ventricular phase angles (LVφ and RVφ, respectively) in patients with right bundle branch block (RBBB), normal conduction, and left bundle branch block (LBBB). (B) Intrapatient differences. Shown are intrapatient differences between left and right ventricular phase angle, Δφ(LV-RV) in patients with RBBB, normal conduction and LBBB. (C) Phase Onset. Shown are differences in left and right ventricular phase onset (Δφ onset [LV-RV]) in patients with RBBB and LBBB. (From Frais, MA et al.: Phase Image Characterization of Ventricular Contraction in Left and Right Bundle Branch Block. *Am. J. Cardiol.* 50:95, 1982.)

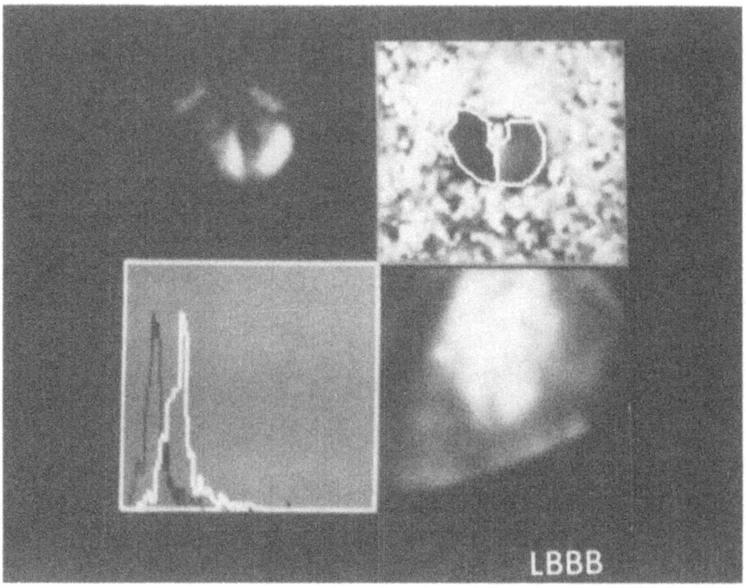

A

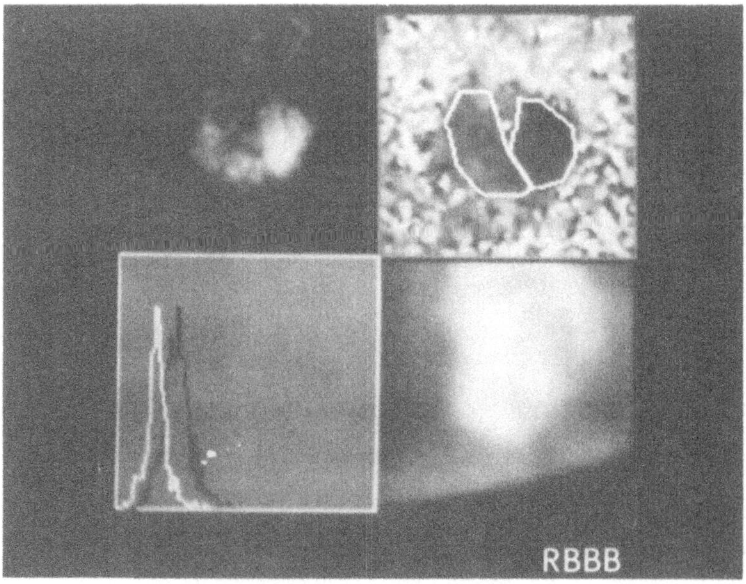

B

FIGURE 5–17. Phase Analysis in Bundle Branch Block. (A) Left Bundle Branch Block (LBBB). Shown are amplitude (*upper left*), and phase (*upper right*) images in a patient with normal wall motion and LBBB. At lower right is the ungated blood pool image which is employed to aid identification of the ventricular regions of interest. At the lower left are the respective ventricular phase histograms. Note the broad, delayed left ventricular histogram (*black*) characteristic of LBBB, in this "best septal" left anterior oblique projection. (B) Right Bundle Branch Block (RBBB). Shown according to the same format are amplitude, phase, and ungated blood pool images in a patient with normal wall motion and RBBB. Note the broad, delayed left ventricular histogram (*white*) characteristic of RBBB.

strating that the phase image could characterize familiar conduction abnormalities. Additionally, Machac and coworkers [49] demonstrated similar asynchrony and phase difference in artificial ventricular pacemaker rhythms and showed the method to permit assessment of asynchrony within as well as between the ventricles (Figures 5–16, 5–17).

LEFT ANTERIOR FASCICULAR BLOCK

Owing to the frequent ambiguity of scalar ECG interpretation and the potential clinical significance of the pattern of left anterior fascicular block, especially in the setting of prior infarction, we sought to assess the phase image in a group of 12 of these patients defined objectively by Warner criteria [50]. Seeking best to separate anterior from inferior left ventricular segments, we analyzed phase images in the 70° left anterior oblique projection. Left ventricular contraction patterns were assessed by examining the sequence of phase angles. Segmental histograms were assessed for their relative contraction onset via the difference between anterior and inferior segment mean phase angle, and relative duration of contraction from segmental histogram width. Relative stroke volume was assessed on the amplitude image.

Eighteen controls with normal ECG and ventricular function demonstrated normal amplitude with earlier phase angle (contraction) of the anterior segment. As previously, theirs was a narrow histogram width. However, among 12 patients with ECG criteria for left anterior fascicular block, 7 were concordant with phase analysis demonstrating an appropriate contraction (phase) delay. Two of these 7 had minor differences between segments with a narrow histogram and a normal amplitude image and were compatible with a pure anterior conduction delay. However, 5 of these 7 patients had a large difference between the mean phase angle of anterior and inferior segment, a broad ventricular histogram and reduced amplitude with anterior infarction. Phase analysis was discordant with the diagnosis of left anterior fascicular block in 5 patients. Three of these had broad segmental phase angle differences, a broad left ventricular histogram and reduced inferior amplitude compatible with prior inferior infarction without the scintgraphic pattern of left anterior fascicular block. The remaining 2 had otherwise normal phase and amplitude maps. Phase patterns appear characteristic in left anterior fascicular block with or without associated infarction. Together, phase angle and amplitude analysis show promise to aid clarification of the surface ECG interpretation and provide etiologic insight into the left anterior fascicular block ECG pattern. Here again it appeared as though not only the site of initial phase angle, but also the pattern of phase progression paralleled the expected course of electrophysiologic activation.

Phase Characterization of the Conduction Sequence

As a preliminary study [51], we evaluated 12 activation sequences during atrial and right and left ventricular pacing in 4 normal dogs. For each sequence, phase maps, generated in multiple projections, were compared to epicardial maps obtained from a roving bipolar electrode after thoracotomy. Thirty-four sites were recorded and referenced to 2 intracardiac and 2 surface electrograms for each sequence. Pacing catheters were kept stationary during phase and epicardial mapping. In 11 of 12 sequences, epicardial breakthrough and the same region. Areas with secondary breakthrough showed islands of early contraction or phase angle. Sequences were comparable in direction, speed of spread, and location of terminal activity. Regions with synchronous excitation were comparable in distribution to regions with homogeneous contraction. The study demonstrated the close correlation between phase sequences and activation patterns in normal hearts. It supported the potential of the method as a noninvasive tool to delineate the spatial sequence of altered excitation in terms of a functional parameter.

Phase Assessment of the Activation Site

In an initial effort [28], we compared the pattern of phase distribution and sequential phase changes over both right and left ventricles in 16 patients with normal electrical activation to that of 8 patients with an artificial ventricular pacemaker and 4 patients with normal contraction and accessory atrioventricular connections. Compared to normals, the site of earliest phase angle was located at the right ventricular apex in 7 patients with a right ventricular endocardial

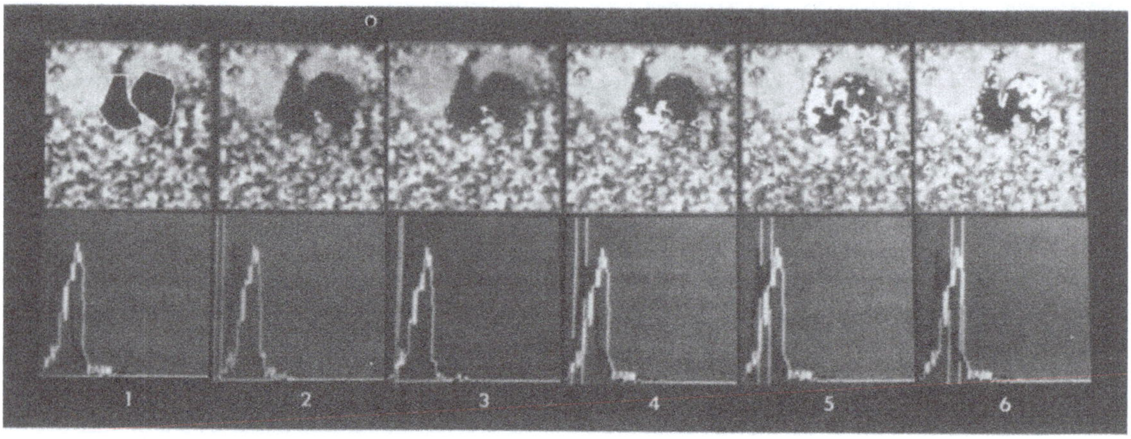

FIGURE 5–18. Phase Analysis in Association with a Right Ventricular Pacemaker. Shown as in previous figures are sequential phase images and associated ventricular histograms in a patient with a right ventricular endocardial pacemaker. In contrast to the pattern in normal patients, the right ventricle, particularly in its apical and septal segments, is represented by a darker grey shade then that of the left ventricle. The sites are earliest phase angle are localized to the right ventricular apex and distal septum. Owing to the pacemaker effect on the septum, the phase histograms of each ventricle have a simultaneous onset. However, the left ventricular phase histogram demonstrates delayed upstroke and peak compared with that of the right ventricle owing to delayed left ventricular activation. The highlighted sequence of phase changes again demonstrates initial right ventricular apical and septal changes. The subsequent phase sequence involves the right ventricular body with subsequent involvement of the right ventricular base and left ventricle. (From Botvinick, EH et al.: An Accurate Means of Detecting and Characterizing Abnormal Patterns of Ventricular Activation by Phase Image Analysis. *Am. J. Cardiol.* 50:289, 1982.)

pacemaker (Figure 5–18) and in the lateral left ventricular wall in 1 patient with a left ventricular epicardial pacemaker (see Figure 5–15). In each case the site corresponded to the exact position of the pacing electrode as seen on the patient's radiograph, and sequential phase changes spread from the initial focus through both ventricles. In those with preexcitation, the site of earliest phase angle corresponded exactly to the site of the accessory connections determined by endocardial mapping, in posterior left paraseptal, left lateral and right lateral locations.

Similarly, Turner and coworkers [52], using least square phase analysis, demonstrated the sequence of inward ventricular movement to parallel the sequence of depolarization in 14 patients with pacemakers and 3 with ventricular tachycardia. Further, the duration of spread of contraction onset or standard deviation of phase angle related well to the QRS duration. Bashore [53] later supported these findings and demonstrated the method sensitivity with the report that phase image patterns accurately localized all of 35 right and 21 of 25 left ventricular pacing and premature ventricular contraction sites regardless of the presence of wall motion or contraction abnormalities. Sites as close as 1.5 cm were identified, whereas the surface electrocardiogram was both insensitive and nonspecific. They concluded that the method could define both sites of pacing and intermittent ventricular stimulation. Rolfe and coworkers [54] went on to employ the method to show that the effect of premature ventricular contractions are independent of the site of origin, baseline contraction abnormalities or the coupling interval in a select population. While these conclusions may find controversy, they demonstrated the use of the imaging method to the analysis of pathophysiologic questions. Links [55] again confirmed this work, demonstrating in 40 studies the agreement between ventricular pacing site and site of earliest phase angle over 48 sites in 12 patients at varying pacing rates. Sequential variations may also be noted in the pacing sequence, and we have seen a patient with a right ventricular demand pacemaker and left sided phase delay, convert to sinus conduction at high heart rates exposing the underlying right bundle branch block, with right sided phase delay (Figure 5–19).

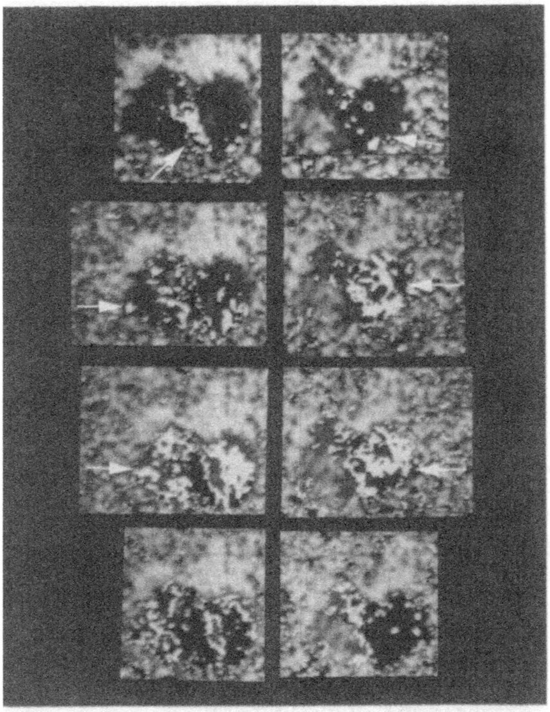

FIGURE 5–19. Phase Image at Rest and with Stress. Shown are serial phase images in the "best septal" left anterior oblique projection performed at rest (*left*) and during maximal reclining bicycle exercise (*right*), in a patient with a right ventricular endocardial pacemaker. The sequential samples of phase progression here illustrated, advance from above downward. At rest, initial "activation" begins in the septum and right ventricular apex (*arrow*), top frame. Activation proceeds from the inferoapical region to the base, simultaneously involving elements of both ventricles thereafter. The white arrows in successive panels indicate the right ventricle. This pattern of activation is abnormal since it begins at the apex and primarily involves elements of the right ventricle, spreading proximally in both ventricles. At this time, the electrocardiogram showed a right ventricular pacemaker rhythm. At maximal exercise (*right*), initial activation again involves elements of the septum as well as the left ventricular apex and lateral wall (*arrows*), but without early right ventricular activation. Phase angle progresses to involve the right ventricle. This pattern was different from that seen at rest and was consistent with the electrocardiographic pattern, which at maximum stress, revealed a right bundle branch block configuration. (From Botvinick, EH et al.: The Phase Image: Its Relationship to Patterns of Contraction and Conduction. *Circulation* 65:551, 1982.)

Phase Analysis in Preexcitation with Accessory AV Connections

Phase image analysis has been widely applied to the identification of the accessory connection and characterization of the conduction pattern in patients with preexcitation syndromes. In an initial examination [35], the site of earliest ventricular phase angle correlated closely with the location of the accessory connection, documented at electrophysiologic study in 17 patients preexcited at rest. This site could be objectively separated from normals in each of 8 subjects with an active left sided connection (Figure 5–20) and in 2 with a right sided connection (Figure 5–21). Those with septal connection revealed earliest septal phase angle, but could not be separated from normals. In the 8 patients with a left sided connections, the onset, upstroke and peak of the left ventricular histogram preceded those of the right ventricular histogram. Here, the mean left ventricular phase angle, difference between mean left and mean right ventricular phase angle, and the difference between earliest left and right ventricular phase angles were significantly less than that in normal subjects. These variables presented converse characteristics in those with right sided connections (Figure 5–22). The focus could at times by localized in some patients, not obviously preexcited on the surface ECG (Figure 5–23). Sequential phase changes in 10 studies suggested "fusion" of normal septal and lateral bypass fronts. Further, atrial pacing, performed in 2 patients, brought augmented preexcitation, relatively earlier phase angle at the accessory connection, and a shift in the site, of "phase" fusion away from the preexcitation focus (Figure 5–24). That is, with increased preexcitation the phase image was able to reflect the electrical dominance of the accessory connection and the fact that, owing to its increased prematurity, it activates a greater proportion of adjacent myocardium. In a recent study we noted such consistent image evidence of augmented preexcitation during atrial pacing among 11 patients with right and left lateral connections who were also studied during sinus rhythm. In 5 of these, only the pacing study could accurately localize the accessory connections (see below).

Subsequently, we have studied more than 40 patients during preexcitation with excellent ability to identify the site of the pathway. There

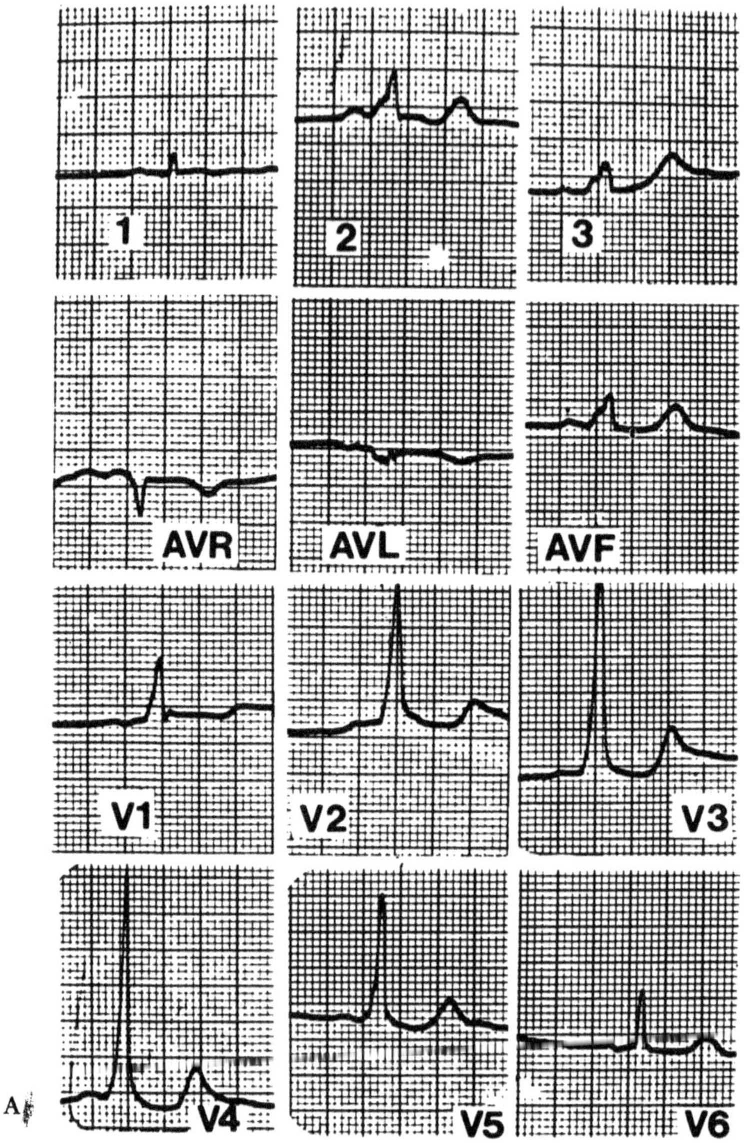

FIGURE 5–20. Phase Image in Preexcitation. (A) Electrocardiogram. Shown is the surface 12 lead ECG in a patient with a left accessory AV connection. Although a clear delta wave is apparent, the location of the delta wave is more consistent with a left anterior rather than a left lateral pathway. (B) Anterior Projection. Shown is the phase image and right (*black*) and left (*white*) ventricular histograms in this same patient. Serial sampling of the spatial distribution of phase angle reveals the site of earliest phase angle at the high lateral left ventricular base. (C) (D) Left Anterior Oblique Projections. Shown is the phase image and ventricular histograms in the same patient in the "best septal" left anterior oblique projection (C). Again, sequential phase sampling indicates a left lateral basal focus as confirmed by the same analysis in the 70° Left anterior oblique projection (D). Note the early occurance of the left ventricular histogram (*white*). (E) Diagrams. Shown are diagrammatic sketches of sequential phase angles in anterior (Ant.), "best septal" (BS) and 70° left anterior oblique (LAO) projections. Earliest phase angle is shown in black. The changes summarize those illustrated above in the actual phase images and show the site of earliest phase angle in each projection to be located at the lateral left ventricular base. In spite of the nonselective nature of the method and problems arising from structural overlap, triangulation is possible and often helpful. (F) Electrophysiologic Assessment. Shown are simultaneous surface leads V1 and 1 together with recordings from the high right atrium (HRA), distal coronary sinus (CSd), low atrial septum and the His bundle electrogram (HBE) are shown during orthodromic atrioventricular reentrant tachycardia. The sequence of retrograde atrial activation can be determined by noting the ventricular (V) – atrial (A) conduction time. During tachycardia, the atrial electrogram recorded from the distal coronary sinus preceded all othe recorded atrial positions, confirming the presence of a left lateral AV accessory connection. VA conduction times are noted. (G) Cross Section. Shown is the diagrammatic cross section of the heart at the level of the AV

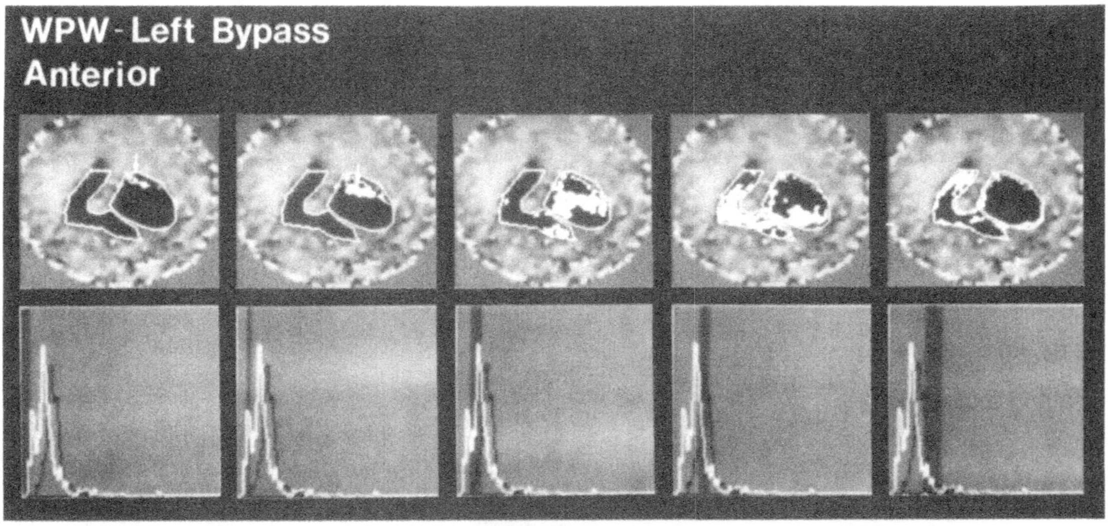

B

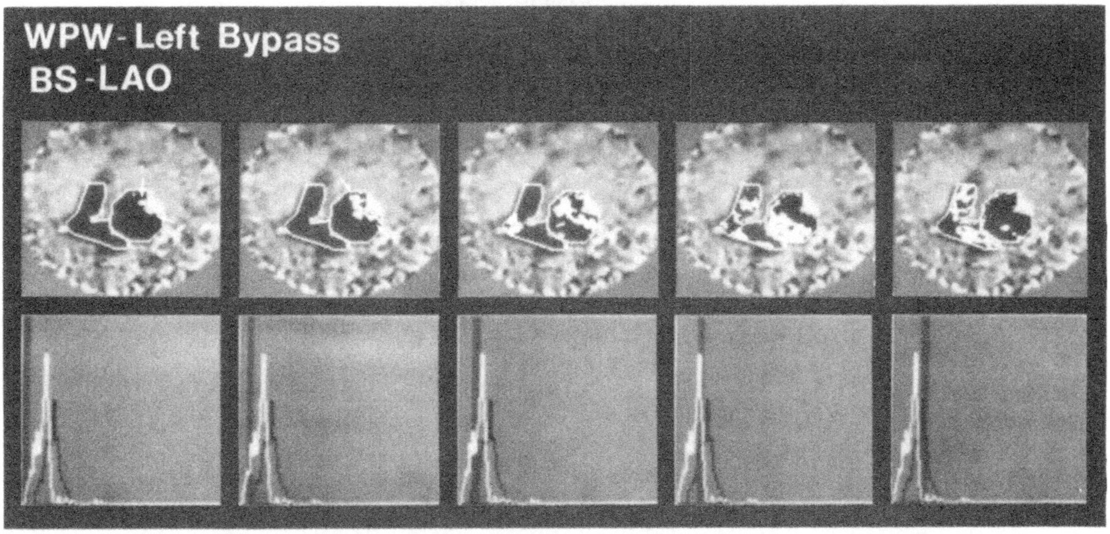

C

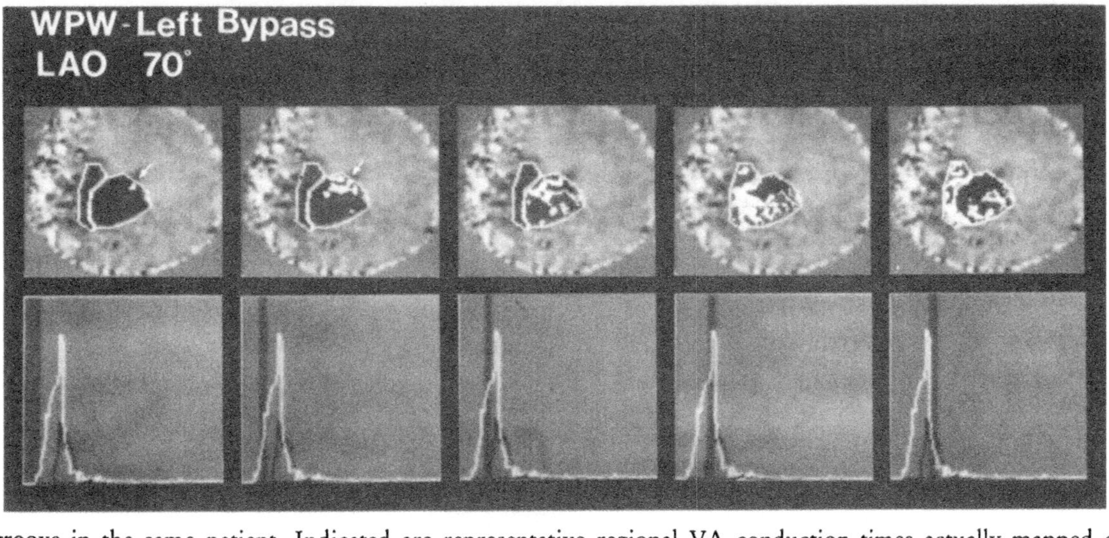

D

groove in the same patient. Indicated are representative regional VA conduction times actually mapped at electrophysiologic study. The shortest interval, 100 ms, corresponds to the lateral left ventricular location determined above. (From Botvinick, EH et al.: Phase Image Evaluation of Patients with Ventricular Preexcitation Syndromes. *J. Am. Coll. Cardiol.* 3:799, 1984.)

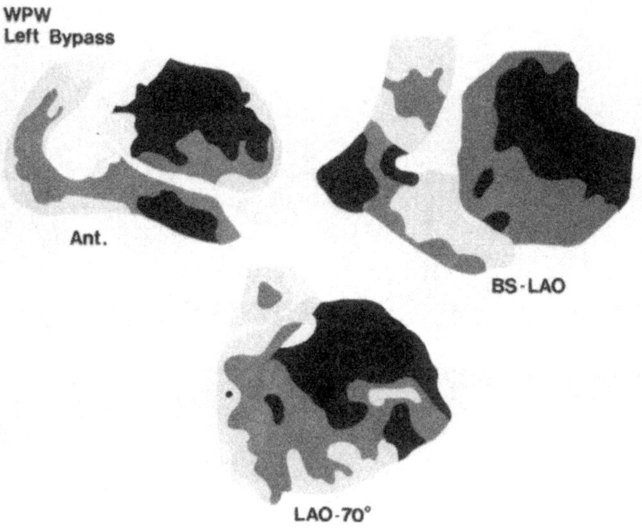

E

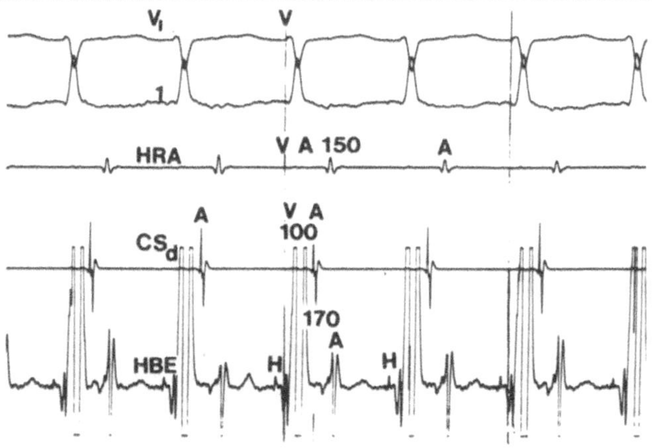

F

G

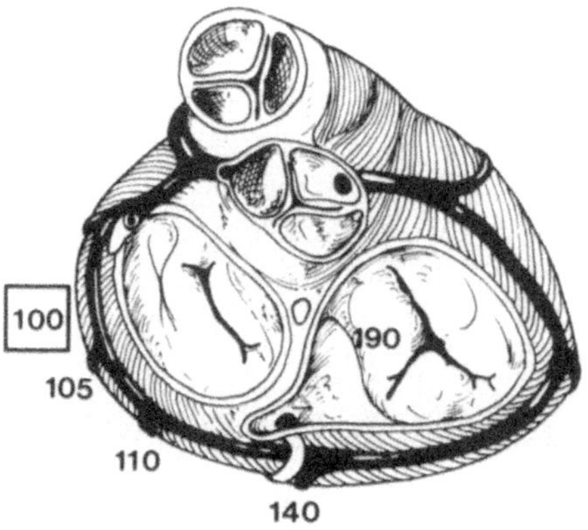

FIGURE 5–20. Continued

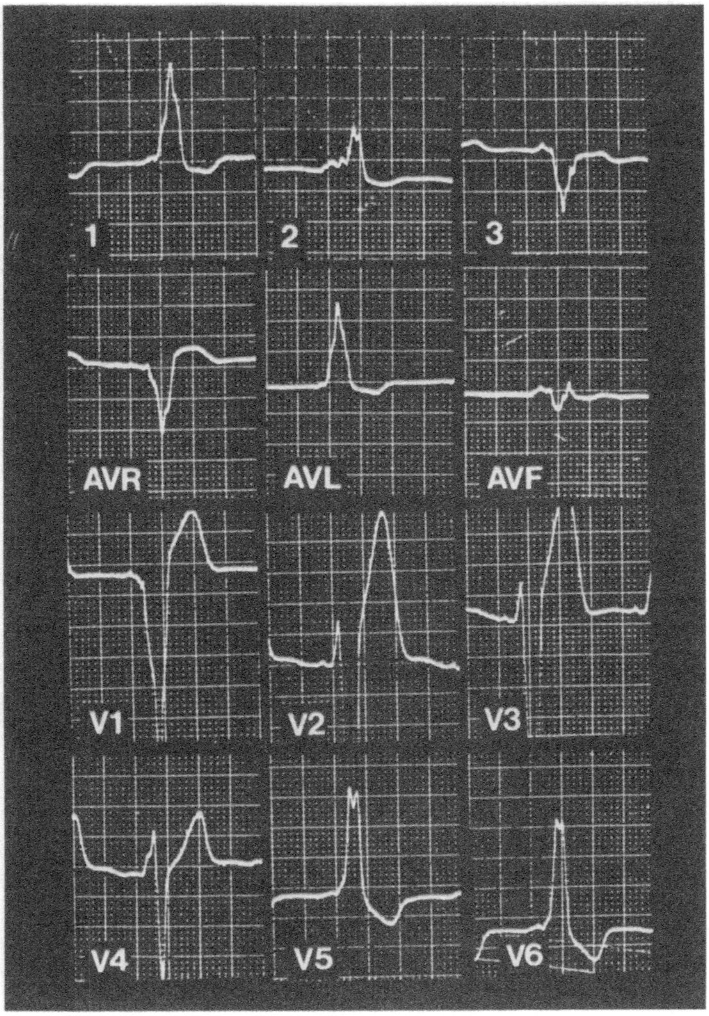

A

FIGURE 5–21. Right-Sided Accessory AV Connection. (A) Electrocardiogram — Shown is the ECG in a patient with a right-sided accessory AV connection. Note the short PR interval and prolonged QRS. (B) Phase Images. Shown is the phase image and ventricular histograms, as previously formated, in this patient with a right sided pathway. Note the earlier occurance of the right (*black*) histogram and the site of earliest phase angle in the basal right ventricular wall in this "best septal" left anterior oblique projection. (C) Sketches. Shown are diagrammatic sketches of the phase images in this same patient in anterior (ANT) and "best septal" left anterior oblique (LAO) projections. Earliest phase angle, in black, is seen again at the right anterior base, near the atrioventricular groove. (D) Electrophysiologic Study. Shown are simultaneous surface ECG leads V1, 1, and 3 together with recordings from the lateral right atrium (Lat RA), coronary sinus ostium (CSos), distal coronary sinus (CSd) and the His bundle electrogram (HBE) during orthodromic AV reentrant tachycardia. The sequence of retrograde atrial activation can again be noted with reference to the ventriculo (V) – atrial (A) conduction time. During tachycardia, the atrial electrogram recorded from the lateral right atrium preceded those from all other recorded positions in the atria, confirming the presence of a right anterior or lateral AV accessory connection.

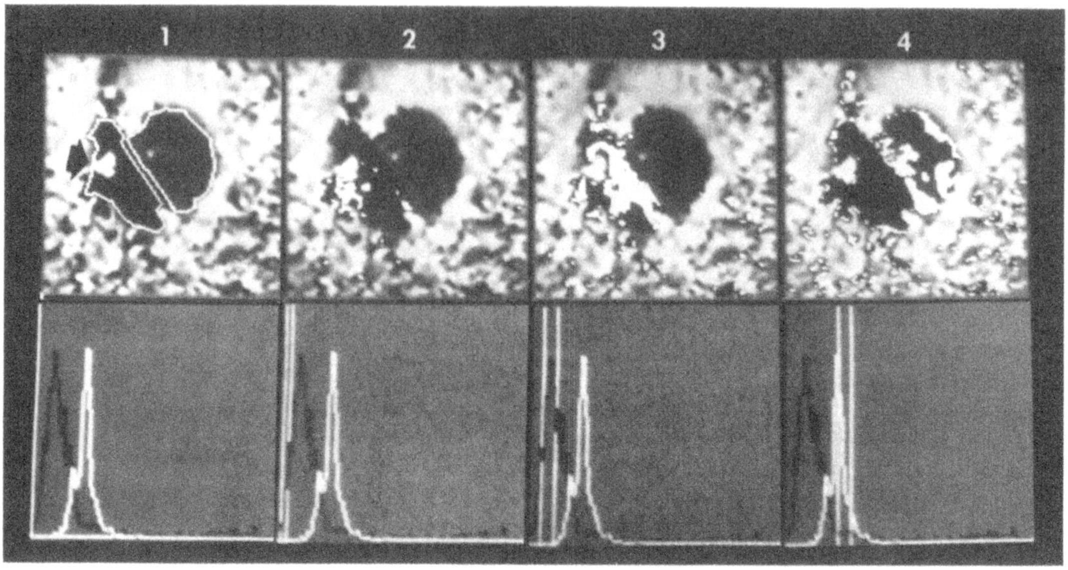
1
2
3
4

B

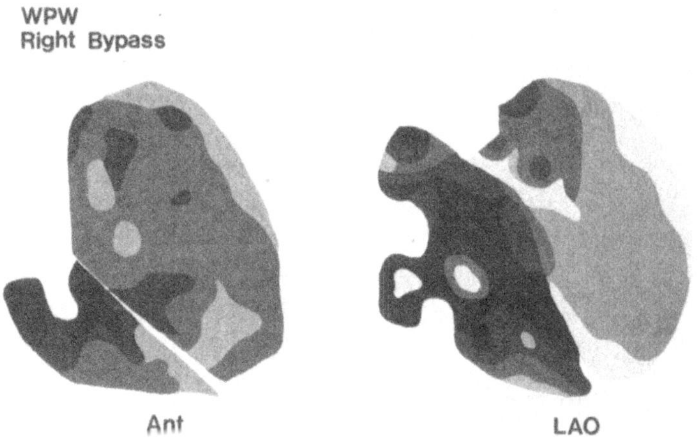
WPW
Right Bypass
Ant
LAO

C

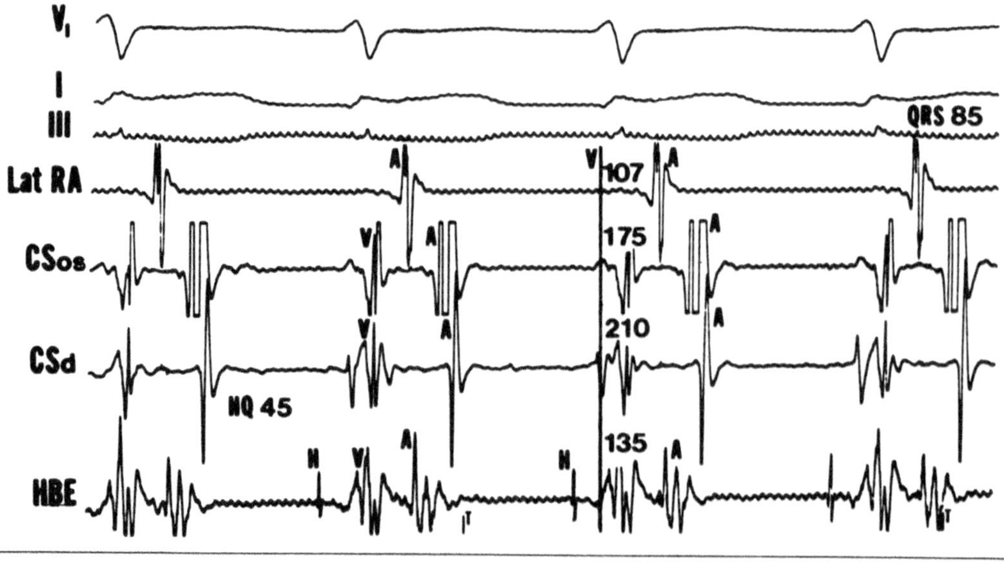
V1
I
III
QRS 85
Lat RA
CSos
CSd
HBE
V
A
107
175
210
135
HQ 45
H

D

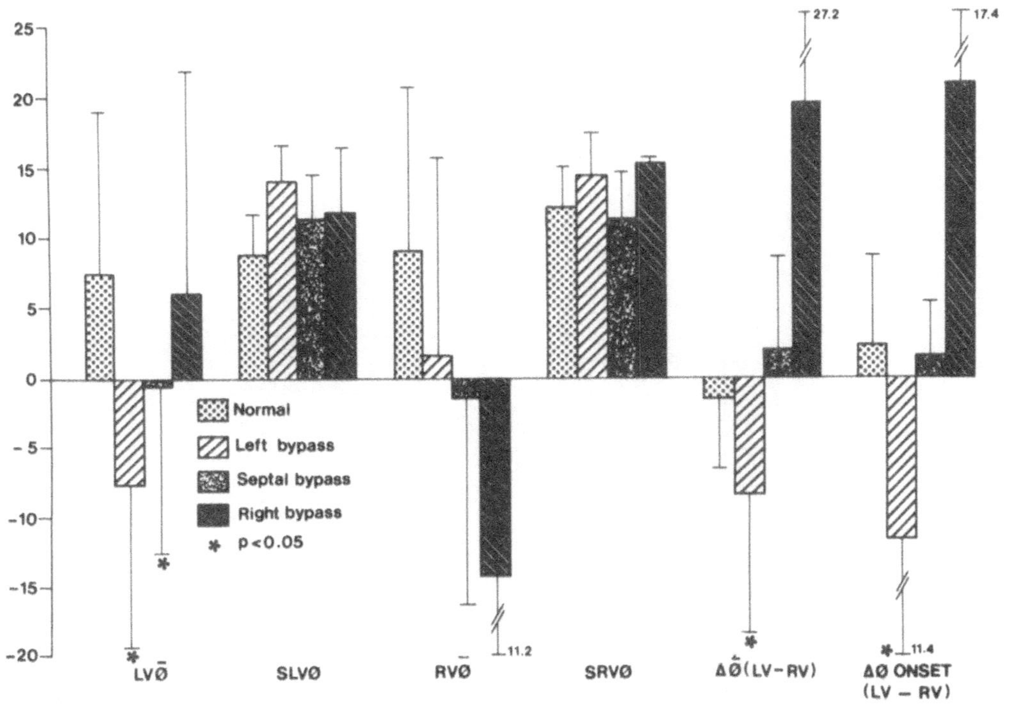

FIGURE 5–22. Phase Data in Preexcitation. Shown is a summary of phase data in patients with normal conduction and in those with a left, septal or right-sided accessory connections. Abbreviation: Δϕ(LV-RV) = difference between mean left and right ventricular phase angle; Δϕ onset (LV-RV) = difference between the earliest left and right ventricular phase angles, LVϕ = mean left ventricular phase angle, RVϕ = mean right ventricular phase angle, SLVϕ = standard deviation of mean left ventricular phase angle, SRVϕ = standard deviation of mean right ventricular phase angle. (From Botvinick EH et al.: Phase Image Evaluation of Patients with Ventricular Preexcitation Syndromes. *J. Am. Coll. Cardiol.* 3:799, 1984.)

have been only 7 patients where image and electrophysiologic assessment grossly disagreed. These not infrequently occurred in patients with 2 accessory connections: one identified on electrophysiologic testing, the other seen on the phase image. On other occasions, ambiguities at catheter study were clarified by image evaluation while in other cases, differences were related to a lack of preexcitation at image evaluation. In other cases, full endocardial mapping was unsuccessful. Difficult for the imaging method is the specific resolution and differentiation of septal and paraseptal accessory connections. Problems also arise owing to the difficulties related to triangulation in this nonselective imaging method. However, these can generally be overcome with primary reliance on the phase pattern in the "best septal" projection for right-left localization, and utilization of anterior and 70° left anterior oblique projections for localization in the anterior–posterior plane. The method appears to be especially helpful, not to diagnose the condition, but to aid clarification of ambiguities at electrophysiologic study and provide increased security and accuracy of localization in patients who are to undergo catheter ablation or surgical resection of accessory connections. As with ventricular tachycardia foci, the image can identify the focus prior to invasive evaluation and indicate by its location the feasibility of the catheter ablation approach.

When currently evaluating patients with known or suspected preexcitation a 12 lead is always obtained in order to identify the pattern at baseline rest image acquisition, compare it to the 12 lead study at electrophysiologic assessment, and clarify any ambiguities or differences

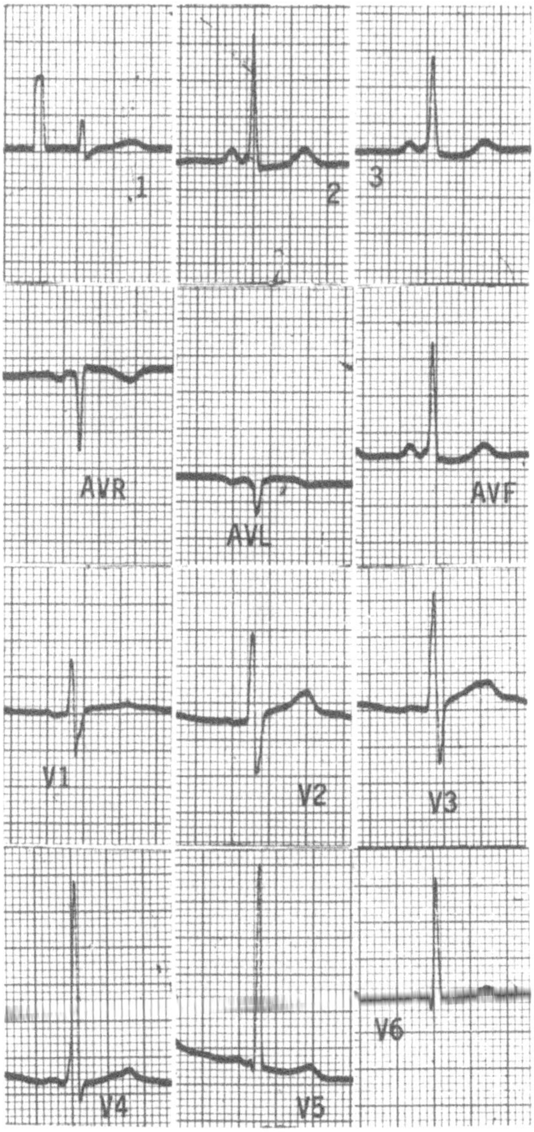

A

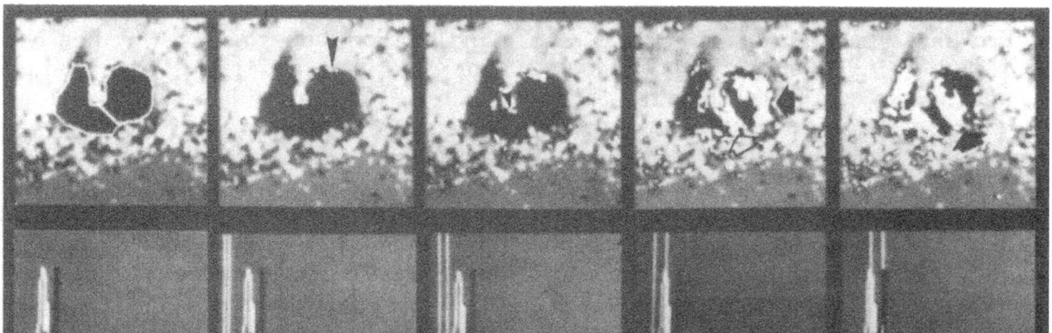

B

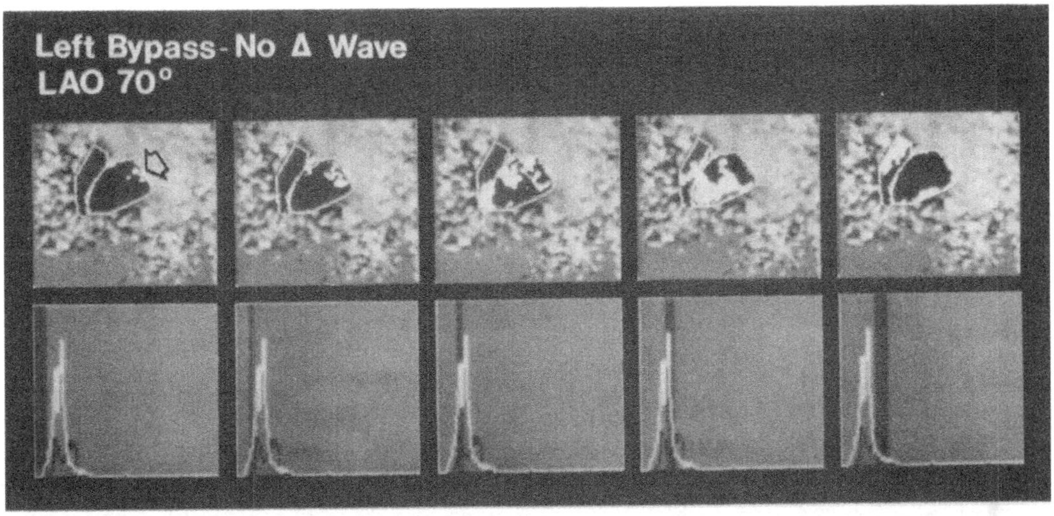

C

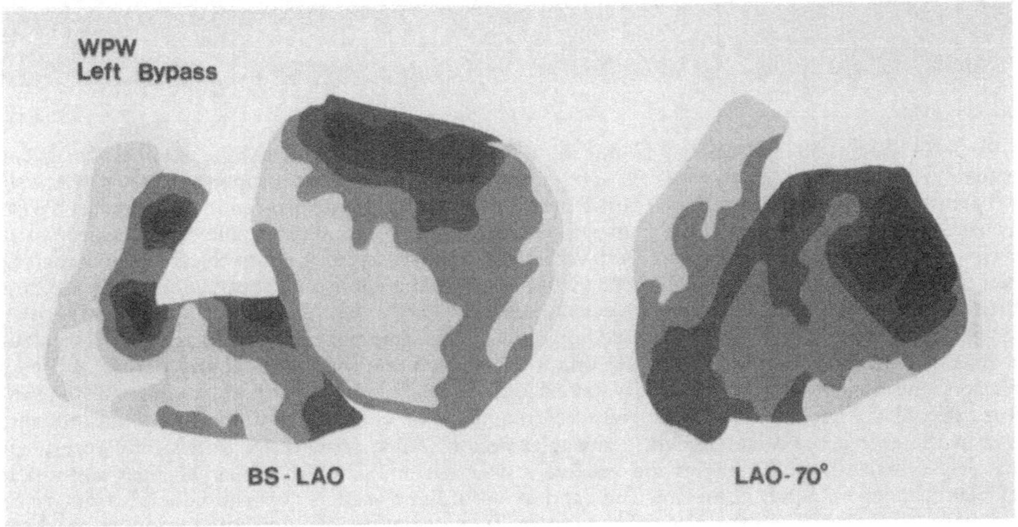

D

FIGURE 5–23. Phase Analysis, Preexcitation, No Delta Wave. (A) Electrocardiogram. Shown is the 12 lead ECG in a patient without obvious delta wave. Although the R wave appears slurred in lead V4 and the PR interval appears short in some leads, independent blinded evaluation failed to identify a delta wave in this patient with a left lateral accessory connection documented on electrophysiologic study. (B) (C) Phase Images — Shown are phase images and associated phase histograms (*right, black and left, white*) in "best septal" (B) and 70° left anterior oblique (C) projections in the same patient. Slightly darker shades are seen in the left ventricular region of interest with the left ventricular histogram slightly preceding the right. Histograms have not been normalized. Sequential histogram sampling revealed the earliest site of phase angle in the left ventricular lateral basal region followed closely by the septum. The last panel, in the "best septal" projection, demonstrates regions with the greatest phase angle. Merger of such coherent phase fronts, originating from normal and bypass pathways, could represent the image parallel of electrophysiologic fusion. The pattern is similar in the 70° left anterior oblique projection. (D) Diagram. Shown are diagrammatic sketches of the phase changes in "best septal" (BS – LAO) and 70° left anterior oblique (LAO – 70°) projections. Again, the darkest grey shades, representing the sites of earliest phase angle, are seen to localize in the lateral and basal left ventricular walls. Sometimes phase imaging can localize the accessory connection in the absence of a delta wave. (From Botvinick, EH et al.: Phase Image Evaluation of Patients with Ventricular Preexcitation Syndromes. *J. Am. Coll. Cardiol.* 3:799, 1984.)

A

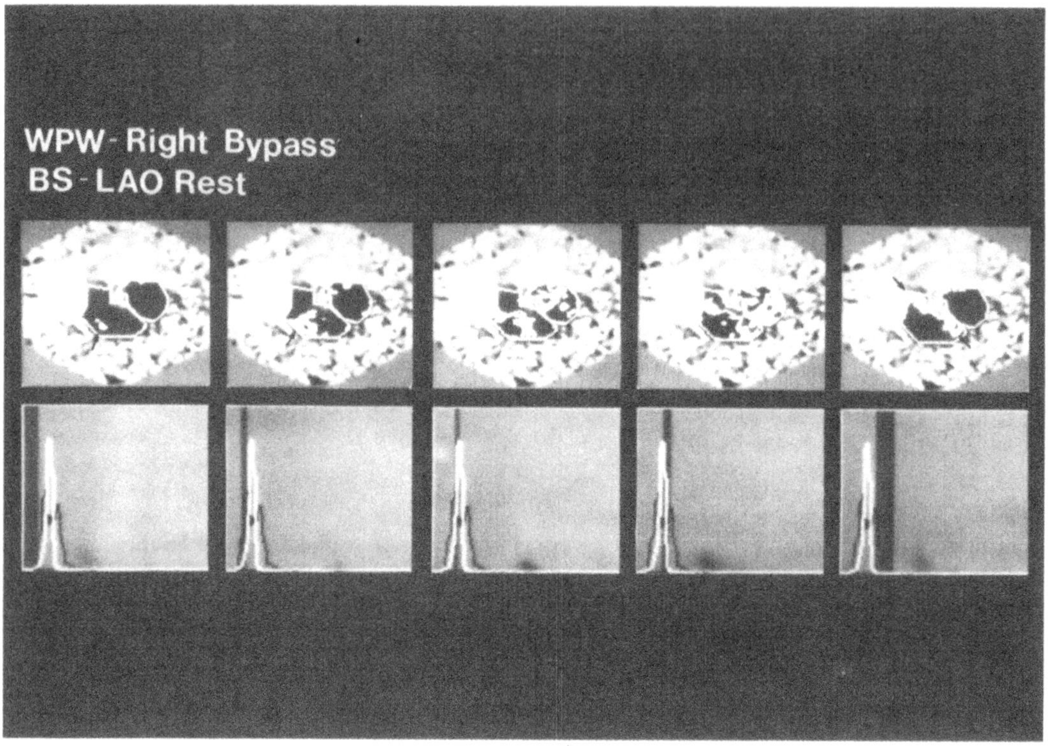

FIGURE 5–24. Right-Sided Accessory Connection, Rest and Pacing. (A) Shown is the phase image and phase histograms (*right ventricle, black and left, white*) with progressive phase sampling, in a patient with a right bypass pathway, evaluated at rest in the "best septal" left anterior oblique projection. Histograms have not been normalized. The site of earliest phase angle is seen localized to the anterior and lateral aspect of the right ventricle (*arrows, left panel*). However, left ventricular changes ar seen relatively early, and the regions of greatest phase angle, representing the last ventricular regions to demonstrate contraction onset, are localized to paraseptal and right basal areas in this projection (*arrow, right panel*). (B) Shown in the same format are the phase image, histograms and serial phase progression in the same patient and projection in association with rapid atrial pacing at a rate of 140 beats per minute. Owing to the shorter refractory period of the accessory connection, the patient is now maximally preexcited. Here, the right ventricular phase histogram greatly precedes that of the left ventricle, as do right ventricular phase angles. Again, the site of earliest phase angle appears in the anterior and lateral right ventricular region (*black arrows, left panels*). However, with atrial pacing, left ventricular phase angles are relatively delayed, and left ventricular changes occur after right ventricular changes are nearly complete. The band of latest phase angle is now shifted left (*arrow, right panel*). This pattern corresponds to the electrophysiologic documentation of augmented conduction through the accessory connection with increased relative prematurity of electrical events on the right side. (C) Diagrams. Shown are sketches of sequential phase changes in the "best septal" left anterior oblique projection at rest (*left*) and with atrial pacing (*right*). Again, darker shades represent earlier phase angle. As noted in the preceding phase images from which these drawings are derived, the anterior and lateral aspects of the right ventricle demonstrate earliest phase angle both at rest and with atrial pacing. However, right-sided phase angles are relatively earlier that their left sided counterparts with atrial pacing as conduction through the accessory connection predominates. As would be expected by such augmentation to the accessory connection, the region of latest phase angle is seen to shift leftward with atrial pacing. The smaller size of the projected ventricular silhouette during atrial pacing is consistent with the diminution in ventricular volumes which occur. (D) (E) Electrophysiology. Shown for the same patient are electrophysiologic records obtained during atrial pacing at 120 (D) and 140 (E) beats per minute. Each figure demonstrates simultaneous surface leads V1, 1 and 3, as well as recordings from the high right atrium (HRA), low atrial septum and the His bundle electrogram (HBE). Time lines representing 1 second intervals are indicated as are the intervals between atrial pacing stimuli. An increase in atrial pacing rate produced augmentation of conduction through the right-sided accessory connection. Such predominance of conduction through the accessory connection is reflected by a progressive widening of the QRS complex and increased prematurity of ventricular activation (V) as the HV interval moves from 20 to −10. Ventricular activation actually preceded His bundle activation at the more rapid pacing rate and enhanced preexcitation. Such sequential electrophysiologic changes directly parallel image findings in each case. (From Botvinick, EH et al.: Phase Image Evaluation of Patients with Ventricular Preexcitation Syndromes. *J. Am. Coll. Cardiol.* 3:799, 1984.)

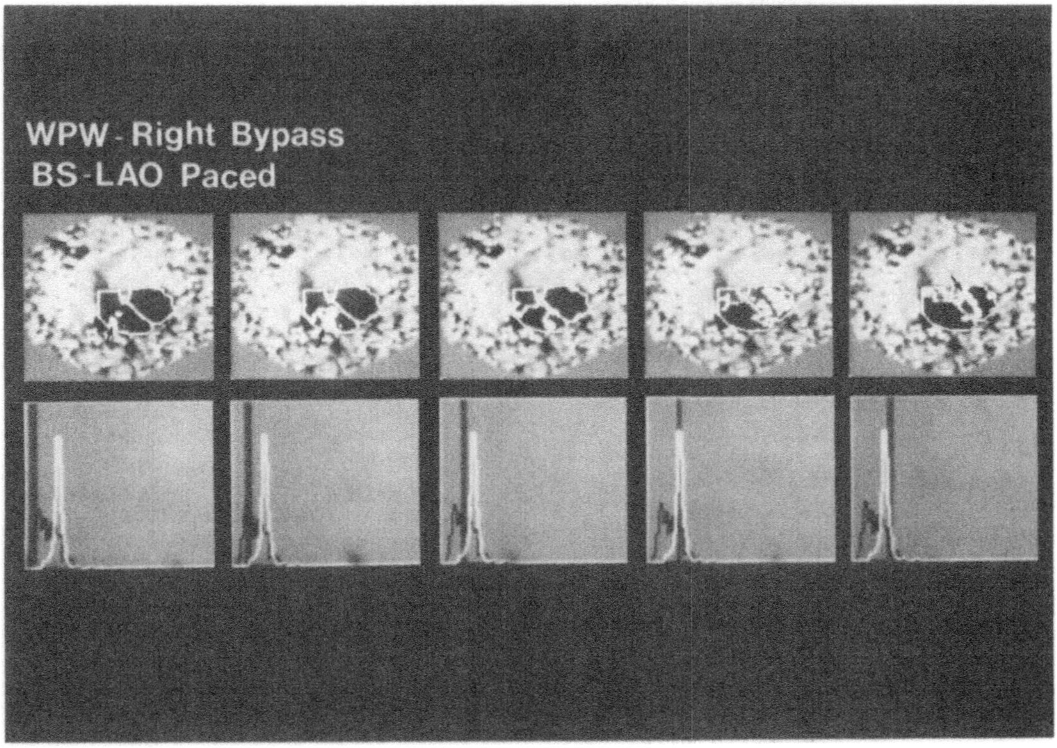
WPW - Right Bypass
BS-LAO Paced

B

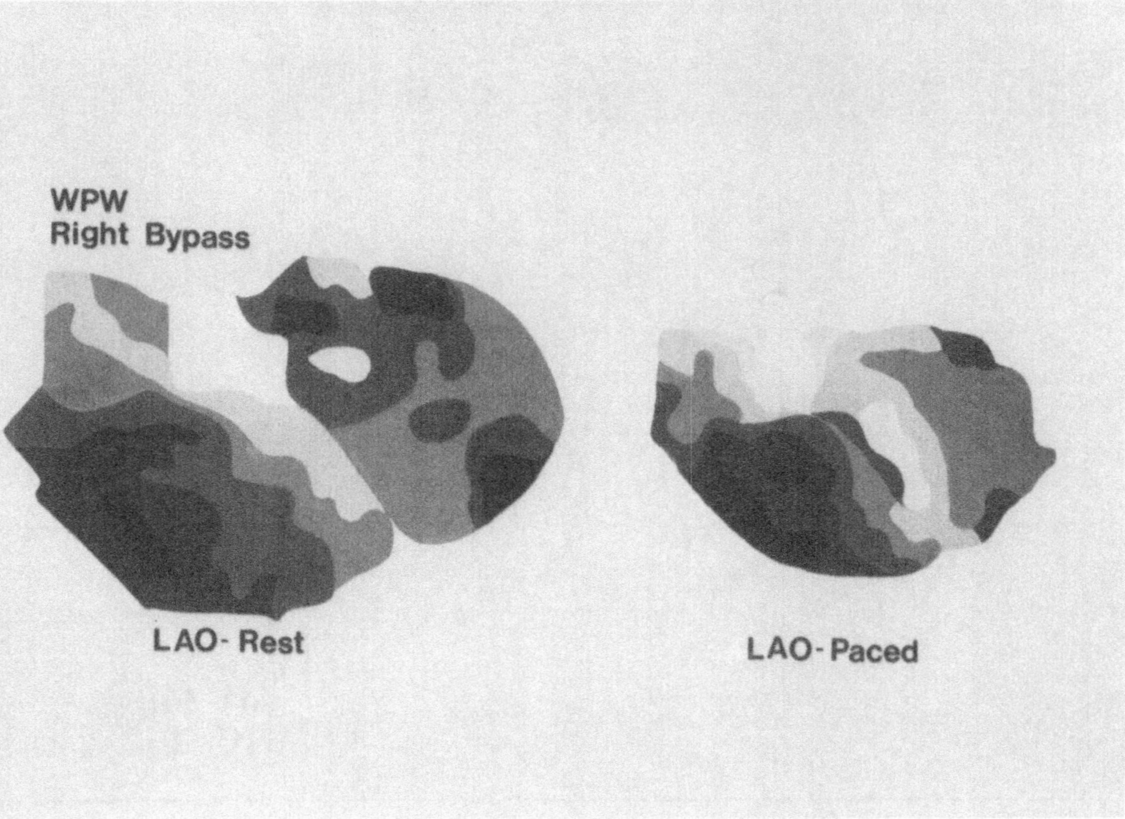
WPW
Right Bypass
LAO- Rest
LAO- Paced

C

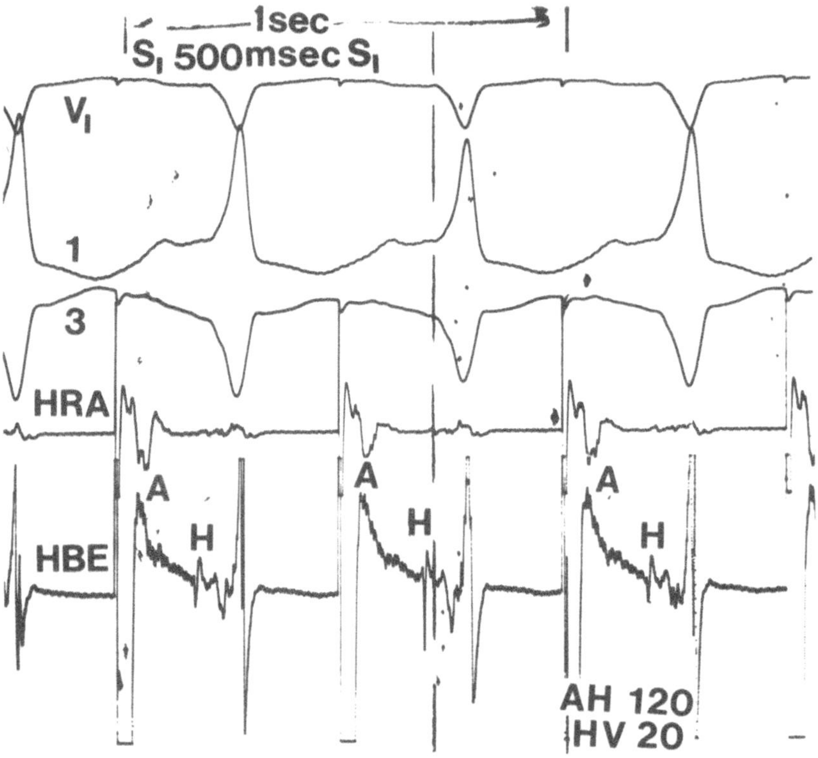

D

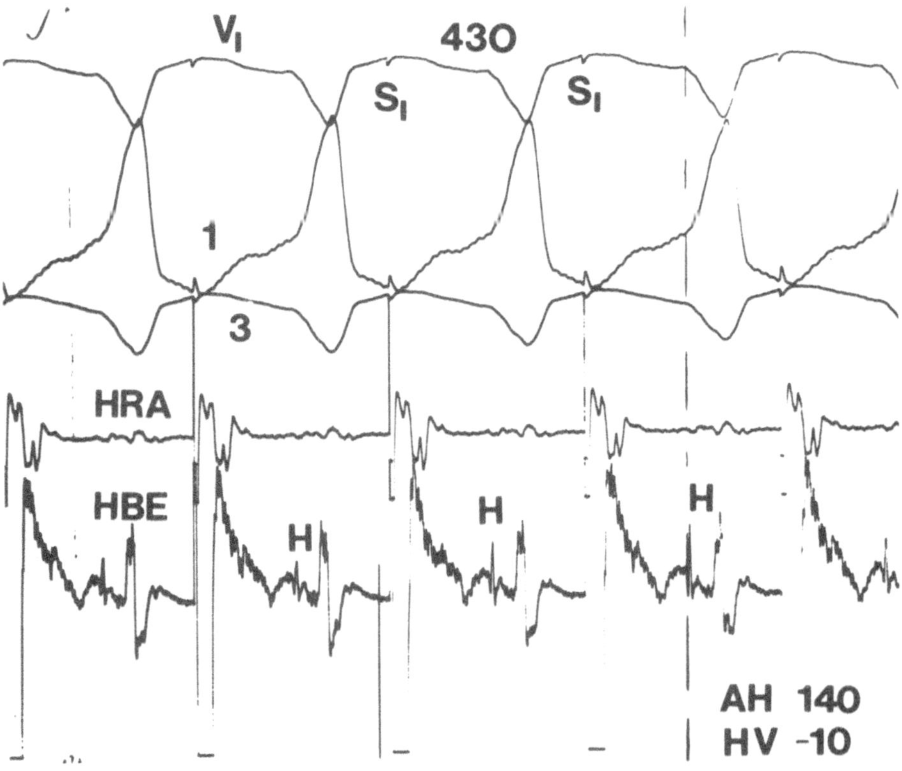

E

FIGURE 5-24. continued

between findings. Further, imaging will be performed in the Nuclear Medicine Section or at the bedside during atrial pacing in any patient not grossly preexcited in the rest tracing. The absence of a delta wave does not exclude preexcitation via accessory AV connections, as these could be concealed in an apparent nonspecific conduction abnormality or may be entirely absent in the presence of accessory atriohisian or atrionodal connections. The latter present essentially normal phase maps. Owing to its ability only to map the pathway when conducting antegrade, difficulties should be expected when seeking to apply the phase method to the localization of accessory connections which appear to conduct only in the retrograde direction.

Nishimura [56] could confirm the location of the accessory connection in 19 of 20 patients preexcited with AV connections using multiple projections. In 8 patients localization was supported and apparently simplified by the application of single photon emission computer tomography. Several patients demonstrated a return to normal phase patterns with the application of procainamide or surgery. Their claim to the identification of 2 accessory connections in each of 3 phase images could be hard to support objectively. Chan and coworkers [57] also showed complete agreement between phase and electrophysiologic maps and excellent correlation with changes induced at atrial pacing. Nakajima and coworkers [58] demonstrated the potential superiority of tomographic reconstruction when the method correctly identified the site of the pathway in 12 of 14 patients with preexcitation compared with only 8 of 14 using conventional planar methods. While such tomographic methods may help, the technical problems they present may bring ambiguities in analysis, the computer memory they require may exceed the capabilities of many laboratories, and processing time may obstruct its effective clinical applications.

The Effects of Atrial Pacing

We went on to assess the effects of atrial pacing on phase image evaluation in 11 patients with left or right lateral accessory AV connections and normal ventricular function [59] (see Figure 5–24, above). In 6 patients with minimal preexcitation at rest, ventricular phase patterns were normal. The site of earliest phase angle occurred at the site of the accessory connection in the remaining patients. With atrial pacing, phase analysis was abnormal in all patients. Earliest phase angle always occurred at the site of the bypass pathway and that of the preexcited ventricle preceded the earliest phase angle of the contralateral ventricle by 27, while the difference in mean ventricular phase angle increased to 20.2 — significantly different from these values in the group at rest, 3.8, and 5.0 respectively. Again these measurements simply indicate that pacing made image abnormalities more obvious as preexcitation was augmented. The latter was again supported by the observation that atrial pacing moved the site of latest phase angle, the site of "fusion," away from the accessory connection and brought a widening of the QRS complex from a mean of .09 to .13 seconds. These findings were confirmed by a shortening of the H-Q interval in all patients during atrial pacing at electrophysiologic study.

Preexcitation via Nodoventricular and Fasciculoventricular Connections

Accessory nodoventricular and fasciculoventricular connections [60,61] may also present with ECG abnormalities and nodoventricular pathways have been documented to play a significant role in sustained reentrant tachycardias. Additionally, they may add to the ambiguities of electrophysiologic and phase analysis.

We characterized the scintigraphic pattern in 9 patients with preexcitation due to either nodoventricular (5 patients) or fasciculoventricular (4 patients) connections confirmed on electrophysiologic study. Images were compared with those of 15 normal patients, 14 with bundle branch block, 18 with right or left lateral and 12 with septal accessory AV connections. In 5 patients with nodoventricular and 2 with fasciculoventricular connections, the site of earliest phase angle was septal or paraseptal with an obvious delay in left ventricular phase angle (Figure 5–25). Remaining patients with fasciculoventricular connections revealed septal or left paraseptal sites of earliest phase angle with a gross phase delay over the right ventricular region of interest. In both groups the absolute mean difference in right and left ventricular phase angle significantly exceeded the normal

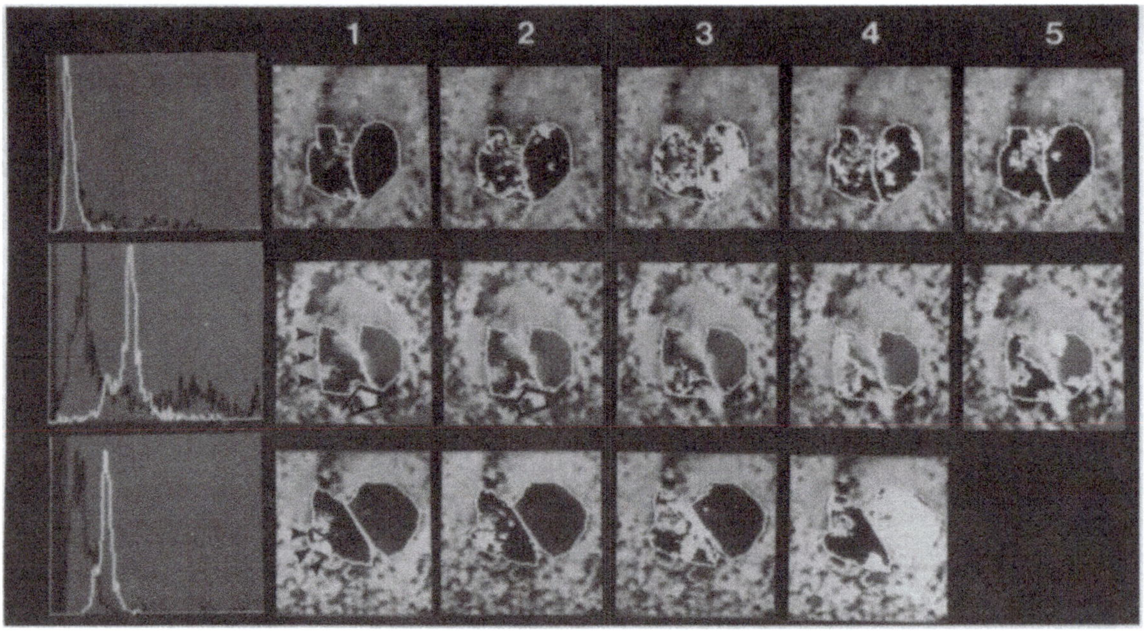

A

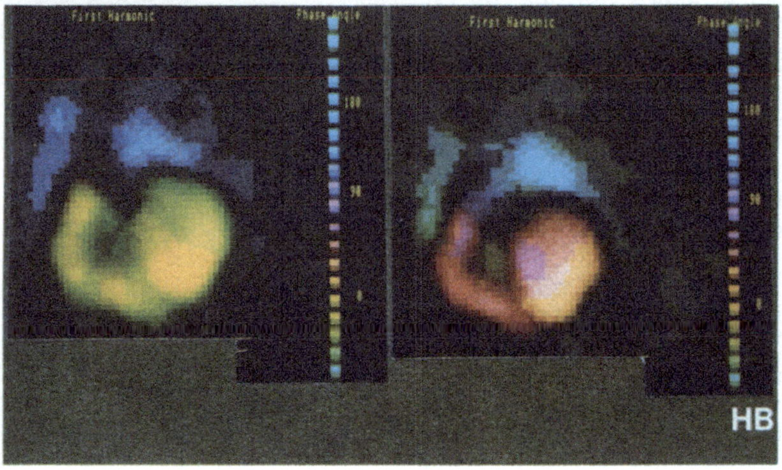

B

FIGURE 5–25. Phase Analysis in Nodoventricular and Fasciculoventricular (Mahaim) connections. (A) Phase Image Comparison. In the left panel of each row are phase histograms for left (*white*) and right (*black*) ventricular regions of interest, obtained, in the "best septal" left anterior oblique projection from the related phase image at right. These demonstrate the sequential phase angle progression superimposed on the phase image of a patient with normal conduction (*top*), a patient with a documented nodoventricular accessory connection, (*middle*), and a patient with a right-sided accessory AV connection (*bottom*). Compared to the pattern noted with normal and accessory AV connections, the pattern of phase progression in the patient with the nodoventricular connection takes onset relatively low in the septum and progresses toward the right ventricle with late left ventricular activation. This pattern also differs from the conventional patern in septal preexcitation where the site of earliest phase angle is high in the base of the septum, with near simultaneous phase progression through both ventricles. (From Bhandari, A et al.: Catheter Induced His Bundle Ablation in a Patient with Reentrant Tachycardia Associated with a Nodoventricular Tract. *J. Am. Coll. Cardiol.* 4:611, 1984.) (B) Color Analysis. Shown are color phase images obtained in the same patient with a nodoventricular accessory connections, conducting normally at rest (*left*) and, during rapid atrial pacing, through the bypass pathway (*right*). Note the symmetric pattern of ventricular phase angle at rest (*yellow*) compared to the early focus at the right septum (*brown*) and delayed right ventricular phase angle (*red*) during preexcitation. Note the endless loop nature of the color code. The rapid rate shifts the phase angle designation and codes the earliest phase angle in brown with the left atrial region, the site of the triggering atrial spikes, is seen in blue.

value. These patterns paralleled the known activation sequence and could be differentiated from normals, those with septal accessory AV connections, with symmetric right and left ventricular phase variation, and from lateral right and left ventricular accessory AV pathways, with earliest phase angle in the lateral basal aspect of the affected ventricle. Yet, these patterns did not differ from those in right or left bundle branch block without preexcitation. The strength of the imaging method was well demonstrated in 2 patients with both left lateral accessory AV and fasciculoventricular connections. Their respective phase images showed alterations in the typical phase patterns associated first with the left lateral connection and, subsequent to ablation, the pattern of right sided phase delay consistent with the fasciculoventricular connection. The study extended the scope of the technique and demonstrated the ability of scintigraphic phase parameters to sensitively suggest the presence of nodoventricular and fasciculoventricular connections, aiding electrophysiologic study when patients are evaluated during preexcitation.

Phase Analysis in Ventricular Tachycardia

Recent work has documented the importance of sudden arrhythmic death and much effort has been directed at its diagnosis, characterization, suppression, and cure. Particularly, ventricular stimulation studies performed for diagnotic and therapeutic assessment may be conveniently combined with endocardial mapping procedures. The latter are increasingly important to differentiate among multiple foci and accurately localize the focus. Such localization permits the best possibility of catheter ablation while facilitating epicardial mapping at surgery allowing precise resection of the ectopic focus and the best opportunity of cure. Blood pool study and phase mapping promises to provide an accurate noninvasive tool for the localization of these foci, aiding often complex, arduous, and sometimes ambiguous electrophysiologic evaluation while providing quantitative evaluation of ventricular size and function.

While patient stability is a requirement for such image analysis, so too is it required for catheter assessment. In fact, owing to the statistical advantage of the parametric method, we have been able to provide accurate maps of the ventricular tachycardia focus with less than 1 minute of acquisition time as consecutive frame mode or summed list mode studies. Studies have been performed at the bedside or in the catheterization laboratory during tachycardia induction. While multiple projections are helpful for localization, the "best septal," 70° left anterior oblique and anterior are obtained in that priority, and even a single projection can alone provide much assistance to the electrophysiologist.

Swiryn and coworkers [62] first studied six patients with clinical ventricular tachycardia during sinus rhythm and during spontaneous or induced sustained ventricular tachycardia. Their phase map, correlated with QRS morphology and axis in most, but (not unexpectedly) not all, tachycardias. The site of earliest phase angle usually demonstrated the tachycardia origin to lie at the border of a severe contraction abnormality and to correlate closely with the site of the focus at endocardial mapping in one patient. In one patient imaged during two tachycardia morphologies, the phase map revealed different ectopic foci at opposing borders of the contraction abnormality.

Thus far we have studied 25 patients during ventricular tachycardia with 28 different foci. Each underwent electrophysiologic study but owing to difficulties encountered and patient intolerance, only 18 foci were mapped successfully. Several of these had to be studied sequentially to obtain the full body of electrophysiologic data. The phase image localized 5 right ventricular, 10 septal and 13 left ventricular foci [24] which corresponded to the same or adjacent endocardial sites in 14 and matched ECG findings in 10 others including 2 patients with multiple foci. Again the image foci often corresponded to the borders of discrete contraction abnormalities. When compared to the blood pool study in 19 of these patients [63] obtained at rest in sinus rhythm, hemodynamic deterioration during ventricular tachycardia in 8 patients related to a higher mean ventricular rate (159), and a greater relative fall in end diastolic volume (.74), stroke volume (.31), and cardiac output (.62) compared to these values in patients tolerant to ventricular tachycardia during scintigraphy (127), to greater dysynchrony in wall motion and a lower ventricular tachycardia ejection fraction (.28 compared with .13).

McCarthy and coworkers [64] confirmed the tachycardia site to be located at the border of localized contraction abnormalities in coronary patients but found difficulty in applying phase analysis to the localization of the tachycardia focus. While correlating well in some patients, the site of earliest phase angle was often adjacent to the endocardial site mapped at catheterization. Since a number of technical factors might influence their analysis, it remains to be proven that electromechanical dissociation is the cause of the disparity. While the latter would make correlation of electrical and phase maps impossible, it is not a likely source of error as the focus is often on the periphery of a scar, rather than imbedded in it as would be expected with dissociation. Rather, problems with triangulation, gating, and gross, often paradoxical, wall motion can lead to phase localization ambiguities as it has in four patients we have thus far studied. The technique promises too great an advantage to institutions attempting the evaluation of these extremely complex and sick individuals for it to be put aside because of initial difficulties especially in view of success at many centers.

Phase image localization of preexcitation pathways and ventricular tachycardia foci have been confirmed as well from epicardial maps generated at surgery. Such confirmation was provided by Nakajima and coworkers [65] in 16 of 20 patients with accessory atrioventricular pathways undergoing surgical resection. We have demonstrated a close correlation between the site of earliest phase angle and the ectopic focus mapped at surgery in 8 patients with preexcitation from accessory AV connections and 4 patients with ventricular tachycardia [66]. In each case resection of the site led to amelioration and termination of related arrhythmias. We believe phase mapping, a more global assessment of the "conduction" pattern, could provide an inclusive guide to the localization of ectopic foci. This could potentially permit the performance of a more limited and targeted, yet equally accurate, endocardial or epicardial mapping procedure, saving time, discomfort and possibly risk, while actually adding to the security of results.

Other noninvasive imaging methods offer little to the evaluation of sequential contraction patterns. Particularly echocardiography, widely used to qualitatively and, with difficulty, quantitatively, assess ventricular volume, presents problems for the accurate, serial, quantitative, and reproducible evaluation of regional ventricular function and wall motion. There are greater difficulties encountered, related to its selective sampling window, its limited capability for digital analysis, and its anatomic and geometric dependence, when one seeks to apply it to the assessment of sequential contraction patterns. Only limited studies have defined echocardiographic patterns during preexcitation [43,44].

The advantages of phase analysis for the localization of the site of bypass pathways in the setting of preexcitation, and for the identification of the ventricular tachycardia focus, are multiple. While the surface electrocardiogram is extremely helpful in localization of the bypass pathway, it is less helpful in the setting of ventricular tachycardia. Here, in fact the same focus can produce divergent electrocardiographic patterns as the conduction pathway is altered. Similarly, the exact location of the bypass pathway is frequently sought, rather than the general ECG description. The phase map tends to provide better localizing information even when not maximally preexcited and can be helpful in the setting of multiple pathways, conditions which cloud ECG assessment. Such localization is especially important when consideration is given to catheter ablation, a method of treatment which can only be applied to accessory connections or ectopic foci of specific, generally septal location.

Multiple foci present an additional problem and scintigraphic study has been extremely useful in drawing attention to accessory connections or ventricular tachycardia foci not appreciated or only suspected after electrophysiologic assessment. Phase analysis of the ventricular tachycardia focus has been increasingly requested to differentiate between a single focus with multiple conduction pathways and multiple foci.

The scintigraphic method is often valuable in confirming foci in the presence of insecure or incomplete electrophysiologic mapping. Not infrequently, patient inolerance or other difficulties prevent electrical mapping altogether and phase localization could shorten the time while increasing the security of performing endocardial catheter mapping or epicardial mapping in the operating room. In such cases and generally, when surgical incision or catheter ablation are contemplated, confirmation of ECG and electrophysiologic localizing data from a totally independent source, based on a totally independent mechanism, seems to be a valuable and useful measurement.

Conclusion

It is not intended here to present data relating to a completely evolved method of parametric image analysis. Rather, we simply seek to present the current method and applications of first Fourier harmonic analysis of blood pool studies. While the resulting amplitude and phase images have already documented unexpected capabilities and utility from a relatively simple mathematical computation, they need not represent the final form. Rather, they are likely simply a step in the evolution of methods to express information relating to the extent and sequence of cardiac contraction. Already, amplitude and phase images provide a useful, objective guide to the evaluation of regional contraction abnormalities which appear most valuable in serial function assessment. Some evidence suggests they may even surpass more conventional indicators of ventricular dysfunction and Fourier analysis may itself be useful to aid measurement of emptying and filling rate indices. These images permit quantitative aneurysm analysis, aid atrioventricular separation and facilitate quantitation of regurgitant valvular and shunt lesions. Again, as a tool to assess serial contraction, and indirectly, conduction patterns, phase analysis has already exceeded its expected potential. Reflective of conventional conduction abnormalities, it has been used to clarify ambiguous ECG patterns, seems well capable of mapping preexcitation foci from a variety of sources and can probably localize the ventricular tachycardia focus as well. Results of preliminary animal studies support assumptions regarding a parallel between the full pattern of phase progression and the sequence of electrical activation. Yet phase maps present only derived relative data, subject to the ambiguities, assumptions, and errors intrinsic to the method. There is yet much to do.

Acknowledgment

This work was supported in part by a grant from the Fannie Rippel Foundation, Madison, New Jersey. Dr. Botrinick is an Established Investigator of the American Heart Association, and is supported in part by a grant from the George D Smith Fund, San Francisco, California.

Reference

1. Patterson RE, Eng C, Horowitz SF: Practical diagnosis of coronary artery disease: A Bayes' theorem nomogram to correlate clinical data with noninvasive exercise tests. *Am. J. Cardiol.* 53:253, 1984.
2. Werner JA, Botvinick E, Shames D, Parmley W: Acute myocardial infarction imaging: The clinical application of technetium-99 m stannous pyrophosphate infarct scintigraphy. *West. J. Med.* 127:464, 1977.
3. Botvinick EH, Schiller NB: The complementary roles of m-mode echocardiography and scintigraphy in the evaluation of adults with suspected left-to-right shunts. *Circulation* 62:1070, 1980.
4. Ashburn WL, Schelbert HR, Verba JW: Left ventricular ejection fraction — a review of several radionuclide angiographic approaches using the scintilation camera. *Prog. Cardiorasc. Dis.* 20:267, 1978.
5. Botvinick EH, Glazer HB, Shosa DW: What is the reliability and the utility of scintigraphic methods for the assessment of ventricular function? In Rahimtoola SH (ed.): Controversies in Coronary Artery Disease, Philadelphia, FA Davis Co., 1982.
6. Schiller NB, Botvinick EH: Noninvasive quantitation of the left heart by echocardiography and scintigraphy. *Cardiovasc. Clin.* 1985 (in press).
7. Okada RD, Kirschenbaum HD, Kushner FG, Strauss HW, Dinsmore R, Newall J, Boucher C, Block P, Pohost G: Observer variance in the qualitative evaluation of left ventricular wall motion and quantitation of left ventricular ejection fraction using rest and exercise multigated blood pool imaging. *Circulation* 61:128, 1980.
8. Pavel DG, Zimmer M, Patterson VN: In vivo labeling of red blood cells with 99 m-technetium: A new approach to blood pool visualization. *J. Nucl. Med.* 18:305, 1977.
9. Freeman M, Berman D, Staniloff H, Waxman AD, Maddahi J, Buchbinder NA, Forrester JS, Swan HJC: Improved assessment of inferior segmental wall motion by the addition of the 70° left anterior oblique view in multiple gated scintigraphy. *Am. Heart J.* 101:169, 1981.
10. Bacharach SL, Green MV, Bonow RO, Findley SL, Ostrow H, Johnston GS: Measurements of ventricular function by ECG gated blood pool scintigraphy during atrial fibrilation. *J. Nucl. Med.* 22:226, 1981.
11. Green MV, Ostrow HG, Scott RN, Douglas MA, Bailey JT, Johnston GS: A comparison of simultaneous measurements of systolic function

in the baboon by electromagnetic flow meter and high frame rate ECG gated blood pool scintigraphy. *Circulation* 60:312, 1979.
12. Links JM, Becker LS, Shindledecker JG, Guzman P, Burow RD, Nickeloff EL, Alderson PO, Wagner HN: Measurement of absolute left ventricular volume from gated blood pool studies. *Circulation* 65:82, 1982.
13. Rigo P, Alderson PO, Robertson RM, Becker LC, Wagner HN: Measurement of aortic and mitral regurgitation by gated cardiac blood pool scans. *Circulation* 60:306, 1979.
14. Champeney DC: Fourier transforms and their physical applications. New York, Academic Press, 1973, p. 8.
15. Goris ML: Functional or parametric images. *J. Nucl. Med.* 23:360, 1982.
16. Gandsman EJ, North DL, Shulman RS, Bough EW: Measurement of the ventricular stroke volume ratio by gated radionuclide angiography. *Radiology* 138:161, 1980.
17. Maddox DE, Holman BL, Wynne J, Idoine J, Parker AJ, Uren R, Neill JM, Cohn PF: Ejection fraction image: A noninvasive index of regional left ventricular wall motion. *Am. J. Cardiol.* 41:1230, 1978.
18. Holman BL, Wynne J, Idoine J, Zielonka J, Neill J: The paradox image: Noninvasive index of regional left ventricular dyskinesis (abstract). *J. Nucl. Med.* 20:P661, 1979.
19. Geffers H, Adam WE, Bitter F, et al.: Data processing and functional imaging in radionuclide ventriculography In Information in Medical Processing, Oakridge, Biological Computing Technology Information Center, 1977, p. 332.
20. Deconinck F, Bossuyt A, Hermanne A: A cyclic color cycle as an essential requirement in functional imaging of periodic phenomena. *Med. Phys.* 6:331, 1979.
21. Verba JW, Bornstein I, Alazraki NP, Taylor A, Bhargava V, Shabetai R, LeWinter M: Onset and progression of mechanical systole derived from gated radionuclide techniques and displayed in cine format. *J. Nucl. Med.* 20:625, 1979 (abstract).
22. Pavel DC, Swiryn S. Byrom E, Lam W: Ventricular phase analysis of radionuclide gated studies. (Abstract.) *Am. J. Cardiol.* 45:398, 1980.
23. Walton S, Jell P, Jarritt PH, Swanton RH: Phase analysis of the first pass radionuclide angiogram. *Br. Heart J.* 48:441, 1982.
24. Pavel BG, Briandet PA: Quo vadis phase analysis. *Clin. Nucl. Med.* 8:564, 1983.
25. Bacharach S, Green M, Bonow R, DeGraaf CN, Johnston GS: A method for objective evaluation of functional images. *J. Nucl. Med.* 23:285, 1982.
26. Miller TR, Goldman KJ, Kondapuram SS, Biello DR, Ludbrook PA, Sobel BE: Analysis of cardiac diastolic function: Application in coronary artery disease. *J. Nucl. Med.* 24:2, 1983.
27. Bacharach SL, Green MV, Bonow RO, Pace L, Bennetti A, Larson SM: Detection of cardiac wall motion defects with combined amplitude/phase analysis. (Abstract.) *J. Nucl. Med.* 26:P86, 1985.
28. Botvinick E, Frais M, Shosa D, O'Connell W, Pacheco-Alvarez JA, Scheinman M, Hattner R, Morady F, Faulkner D: An accurate means of detecting and characterizing abnormal patterns of ventricular activation by phase image analysis. *Am. J. Cardiol.* 50:289, 1982.
29. Botvinick E, Dunn R, O'Connell W, Shosa D, Herfkens R, Scheinman M: The phase image, its relationship to patterns of contraction and conduction. *Circulation* 65:551, 1982.
30. Turner DA, Shuma MA, Ruggie N, VonBehron PL, Jarosky MJ, Ali A, Grotch MW, Messer JV, Fordham EW: Coronary artery disease: Detection by phase analysis of rest/exercise radionuclide angiograms. *Radiology* 148:539, 1983.
31. Mancini GBJ, Peck WW, Slutsky RA: Analysis of phase angle histograms from equilibrium radionuclide studies: Correlation with semiquantitative grading of wall motion. *Am. J. Cardiol.* 55:535, 1985.
32. Norris SL, Slutsky RA, Gerber KH, Geiss KR, Ashburn WL, Higgins CB: Sensitivity and specificity of nuclear phase analysis vs. ejection fraction in coronary artery disease. *Am. J. Cardiol.* 53:1547, 1984.
33. Ratib O, Henze E, Schon H, Schelbert H: Phase analysis of radionuclide ventriculograms for the detection of coronary artery disease. *Am. Heart J.* 104:1, 1982.
34. Schwaiger M, Ratib O, Henze E, Schelbert HR: Limitations of quantitative phase analysis of radionuclide angiograms for detecting coronary artery disease in patients with impaired left ventricular function. *Am. Heart J.* 108:942, 1984.
35. Botvinick E, Frais M, O'Connell W, Faulkner D, Scheinman M, Morady F, Sung R, Shosa D, Dae M: Phase image evaluation of patients with ventricular preexcitation syndromes. *J. Am. Coll. Cardiol.* 3:799, 1984.
36. Clayton PD, Bulawa WF, Klausner SC, Urie PM, Marshall HW, Warner HR: The characteristics sequence for the onset of contraction in the normal left ventricle. *Circulation* 59:671, 1979.
37. Frais M, Botvinick E, Shosa D, O'Connell W, Pacheco-Alvarez J, Dae M, Hattner R, Faulkner D: Phase image characterization of localized and generalized left ventricular contraction abnormalities. *J. Am. Coll. Cardiol.* 4:987, 1984.
38. Jones L Jr, Weber PM, Schurr DA: Phase imaging of the left ventricular ECG gated equilibrium blood pool radionuclide scan as a noninvasive method for detecting aneurysms. *Circulation*

63:III, P229, 1980 (abstract).
39. Yiannikes J, MacIntyre W, Underwood D, Cook S, Go R, Loop F: Prediction of improvement in left ventricular function following ventricular aneurysmectomy using Fourier phase and amplitude analysis. (Abstract.) *Am. J. Cardiol.* 49:1045, 1982.
40. Bough EW, Gandsman EJ, Schulman RS: Measurement of normal left atrial function with gated radionuclide angiography. *Am. J. Cardiol.* 48:473, 1981.
41. Rabinovitch MA, Stewart J, Chan W, Dunlap TE, Kalff V, Clare J, Thrall JH, Pitt B: Scintigraphic demonstration of ventriculo-atrial conduction in the ventricular pacemaker syndrome. *J. Nucl. Med.* 23:795, 1982.
42. Handler B, Pavel B, Pietras R, Swiryn S, Byrom E, Lam W, Rosen K: Equilibrium radionuclide gated angiography in patients with tricuspid regurgitation. *Am. J. Cardiol.* 51:305, 1983.
43. DeMaria AN, Mason DT: Echocardiographic evaluation of disturbances of cardiac rhythm and conduction (editorial). *Chest* 71:439, 1977.
44. DeMaria AN, Vera Z, Neumann A, Mason DT: Alterations in ventricular contraction pattern in the Wolff-Parkinson-White Syndrome: Detection by echocardiography. *Circulation* 53:249, 1976.
45. Wyndham CR, Meeran MK, Smith T, Saxena A, Engelman R, Levitsky S, Rosen K: Epicardial activation of the intact human heart without conduction defects. *Circulation* 59:161, 1979.
46. Links JM, Douglass KH, Wagner HN: Patterns of ventricular emptying by Fourier analysis of gated blood studies. *J. Nucl. Med.* 21:978, 1980.
47. Swiryn S, Pavel D, Byrom E, Witham D, Meyer-Powel C, Wyndham C, Handler B, Rosen K: Sequential regional phase mapping of radionuclide gated biventriculograms in patients with left bundle branch block. *Am. Heart J.* 102:1000, 1982.
48. Frais M, Botvinick E, Shosa D, O'Connell WJ, Scheinman MM, Hattner RS, Morady F: Phase image characterization of ventricular contraction in left and right bundle branch block. *Am. J. Cardiol.* 50:95, 1982.
49. Machac J, Horowitz SF, Mielli K, Pollack B, Lee K, Goldman ME, Goldsmith SJ, Teichholz LE: Quantification of cardiac conduction abnormalities using segmental vector Fourier analysis of radionuclide gated blood pool scintigrams. *J. Am. Coll. Cardiol.* 2:1099, 1983.
50. Dae M, Wen YM, Botvinick E, Scheinman M: Assessment of left anterior fascicular block by scintigraphic phase analysis. (Abstract.) *J. Am. Coll. Cardiol.* 3:591, 1984.
51. Dae M, Davis J, Botvinick E, Matsubura T, Scheinman M, Faulkner D: Comparison of scintigraphic phase maps through epicardial activation maps in dogs. (Abstract.) *J. Nucl. Med.* 26:p57, 1985.
52. Turner DA, VonBehren PL, Ruggie NT, Hauser RG, Denes P, Ali A, Messer JV, Forham EW, Groch MW: Noninvasive identification of the initial site of abnormal ventricular activation by least square phase analysis of radionuclide cineangiograms. *Circulation* 65:1511, 1982.
53. Bashore TM, Sterne RA, Schaffer PB, Bush CA, Lier CV, Shaal SF: The noninvasive localization of ventricular pacing sites by radionuclide phase imaging. *Circulation* 70:681, 1984.
54. Rolfe SJ, Rasor T, Schaffer PA, Sanitate PA, Bashore TM: Relation between premature ventricular contraction site of origin defined by radionuclide phase analysis and subsequent left ventricular function. *Am. J. Cardiol.* 53:1028, 1984.
55. Links JM, Raichlin JS, Wagner HN Jr, Reed PR: Assessment of the site of ventricular activation by Fourier analysis of gated blood pool studies. *J. Nucl. Med.* 26:27, 1985.
56. Nishimura Y, Yamamuro M, Komishi T, Nakano T, Tahizawa H: Visualization of Kent bundle position in WPW syndrome using phase analysis. (Abstract.) *J. Nucl. Med.* 26:P58, 1985.
57. Chan WWC, Kalff V, McDonald D II, Rabinovitch MH, Thrall JH, Pitt B: Topography of pre-emptying ventricular segments in patients with Wolff-Parkinson-White Syndrome using scintigraphic phase mapping and esophageal pacing. *Circulation* 67:1139, 1983.
58. Nakajima K, Bunko H, Tada A, Tonami N, Hisada K, Misaki T, Iwa T: Nuclear tomographic phase analysis: Localization of accessory conduction pathways in patients with Wolff-Parkinson-White Syndrome. *Am. Heart J.* 109:809, 1985.
59. Botvinick E, Dae MW, Scheinman M, Davis J, Schechtman N, O'Connell W, Faulkner D, Iskanian J: Augmented pre-excitation assessed by scintigraphic phase analysis during atrial pacing. (Abstract.) *J. Nucl. Med.* 26:p58, 1985.
60. Bhandari A, Moradi F, Shen EN, Schwartz AB, Botvinick E, Scheinman MM: Catheter-induced His bundle ablation in a patient with reentrant tachycardia associated with a nodoventricular tract. *J. Am. Coll. Cardiol.* 4:611, 1984.
61. Schechtmann N, Scheinman M, Botvinick E, Davis J, Winston S, Schwartz A, Dae M: The phase characterization of ventricular preexcitation via Mahaim pathways. (Abstract.) *J. Nucl. Med.* 26:58, 1985.
62. Swiryn S, Pavel D, Byrom E, et al.: Sequential regional phase mapping of radionuclide gated biventriculograms in patients with ventricular tachycardia: Close correlation with electrophysiologic characteristics. *Am. Heart J.* 103:319, 1982.

63. Botvinick E, Scheinman M, Morady F, Sung R, Lanzer P, O'Connell W, Faulkner D: The scintigraphic assessment of sequential changes in ventricular tachycardia. (Abstract.) *J. Am. Coll. Cardiol.* 1:711, 1983.
64. McCarthy DM, Makler PT, Waxman HL: Fourier phase image during ventricular tachycardia: Relationship to endocardial site of origin. (Abstract.) *J. Am. Coll. Cardiol.* 1:712, 1983.
65. Nakajima K, Bunko H, Tada A, Taki J, Tonami N, Hisada K, Misaki T, Iwa T: Phase analysis in patients with Wolff-Parkinson-White Syndrome with surgically proven accessory conduction pathways. *J. Nucl. Med.* 25:7, 1984.
66. Dae M, Botvinick E, Schechtman N, O'Connell W, Faulkner D: Correlation of scintigraphic phase maps with intraoperative epicardial/endocardial maps and surgical results in patients with activation disturbances. (Abstract.) *Circulation* 70, suppl II:371, 1984.

6. THE SPECTRUM OF TACHYARRHYTHMIAS IN PREEXCITATION SYNDROMES

Fred Morady

A variety of tachyarrhythmias may occur in patients with preexcitation syndromes. These tachyarrhythmias are usually associated with symptoms, ranging in severity from mild to life-threatening. Therefore, many patients with preexcitation syndromes and tachyarrhythmias will require treatment. The most appropriate form of therapy for these patients will depend upon the particular mechanism of the tachyarrhythmia. Although invasive electrophysiologic testing is often required to establish the mechanism of a tachyarrhythmia, in many patients the electrocardiogram may provide important clues to the type of tachycardia [1,2]. This chapter reviews the spectrum of tachyarrhythmias in preexcitation syndromes and highlights the value and limitations of the electrocardiogram in the diagnosis of these tachyarrhythmias.

Tachyarrhythmias Involving an Accessory Atrioventricular Connection

ORTHODROMIC RECIPROCATING TACHYCARDIA

The most common type of tachyarrhythmia in patients who have an accessory atrioventricular (AV) connection is referred to as *orthodromic reciprocating tachycardia*. This tachycardia utilizes the AV node as the anterograde limb of the reentry circuit and the accessory AV connection as the retrograde limb. The portions of the atrium and ventricle which intervene between the AV node and the accessory AV connection are necessarily also a part of the reentry circuit (Figure 6–1). The accessory AV connection may be of the type that conducts both in the anterograde and retrograde directions during sinus rhythm or may be of the type which appears to conduct only in the retrograde direction ("concealed"). It is therefore important to note that the absence of ventricular preexcitation on the electrocardiogram during sinus rhythm by no means rules out the possibility that a tachyarrhythmia circuit involves an accessory AV connection.

In orthodromic reciprocating tachycardia, ventricular activation occurs solely via the AV node-His bundle axis. Therefore the QRS duration is usually normal. When there is aberration of the QRS complexes during orthodromic reciprocating tachycardia, this is due to an underlying or functional bundle branch block and not preexcitation (Figure 6–2).

Tachycardia rate. The rate of orthodromic reciprocating tachycardia is age-related, and in adults is usually between 150 and 240/min. In fact a regular narrow complex tachycardia with a rate greater than 200/min should raise the suspicion of orthodromic reciprocating tachycardia.

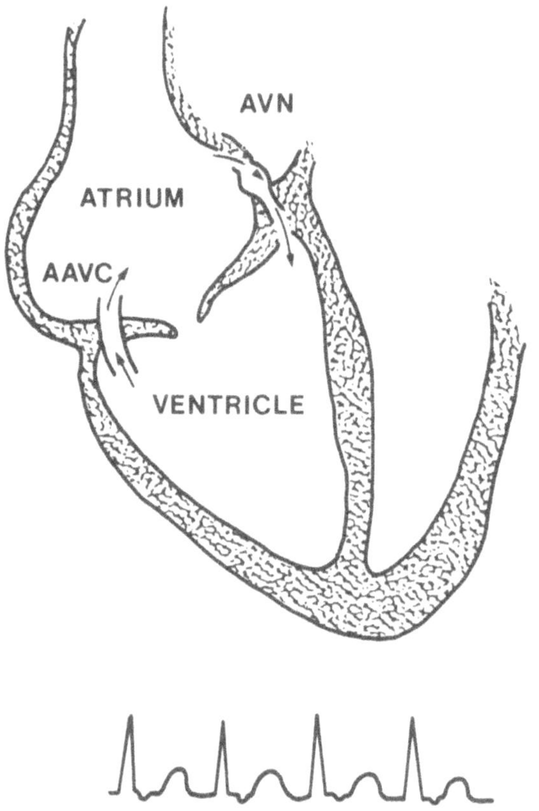

FIGURE 6–1. A schematic representation of the reentry circuit in orthodromic reciprocating tachycardia. The atrioventricular node (AVN) serves as the anterograde "slow" limb of the reentry circuit and an accessory atrioventricular connection (AAVC) as the retrograde "fast" limb. The intervening atrium and ventricle are also necessary components of the reentry circuit.

Because retrograde conduction through the accessory AV connection is usually rapid compared to anterograde conduction in the AV node during orthodromic reciprocating tachycardia and because retrograde activation of the atrium through the accessory AV connection can occur only after ventricular activation, the P wave is usually inscribed shortly after the QRS complex, with the RP interval being shorter than the PR interval (Figure 6–3). Whenever the P wave occurs in the left half of the RR cycle during a narrow complex tachycardia, this suggests the possibility of orthodromic reciprocating tachycardia.

P wave. Other types of narrow complex tachycardia in which the P wave may occur shortly after the QRS include atrial tachycardia in association with first degree AV block (Figure 6–4), and reciprocating tachycardia due to reentry within the AV node. However, in the latter type of tachyarrhythmia, the P waves are more commonly buried within the QRS complexes and are therefore usually not apparent on the electrocardiogram (Figure 6–5).

In some patients with orthodromic reciprocating tachycardia, the P waves may be of low amplitude and buried within the ST segment; in these patients orthodromic reciprocating tachycardia may be impossible to distinguish from reciprocating tachycardia due to reentry within the AV node (Figure 6–6). However, although upon first glance P waves may not be apparent, careful inspection of all 12 leads of the electrocardiogram and comparison of the ST segments during tachycardia with the ST segments in each lead during sinus rhythm may reveal evidence of a P wave in the left half of the RR cycle, suggesting the possibility of orthodromic reciprocating tachycardia (Figure 6–7).

In patients with orthodromic reciprocating tachycardia, inspection of the retrograde P wave polarity in the electrocardiogram may provide a clue to the location of the accessory AV connection. It has been reported that in patients with orthodromic reciprocating tachycardia utilizing a left lateral accessory AV connection, the retrograde P wave is usually negative in lead 1 [3]. In contrast, when orthodromic reciprocating venticular tachycardia utilizes a right lateral accessory AV connection, the P wave is usually positive in lead 1. However, because retrograde P wave polarity can often not be accurately determined by inspection of the electrocardiogram during tachycardia, this clue is often of limited value.

Bundle-branch block. An electrocardiographic finding which may be very helpful in distinguishing orthodromic reciprocating tachycardia from other types of narrow-complex tachycardia is the change in the tachycardia rate which occurs when there is functional bundle branch block. In patients with an atrial tachycardia or reciprocating tachycardia due to reentry within the AV node, aberration of the QRS complex due to functional bundle branch block is usually associated with a faster tachycardia rate than when the QRS complexes are narrow. In con-

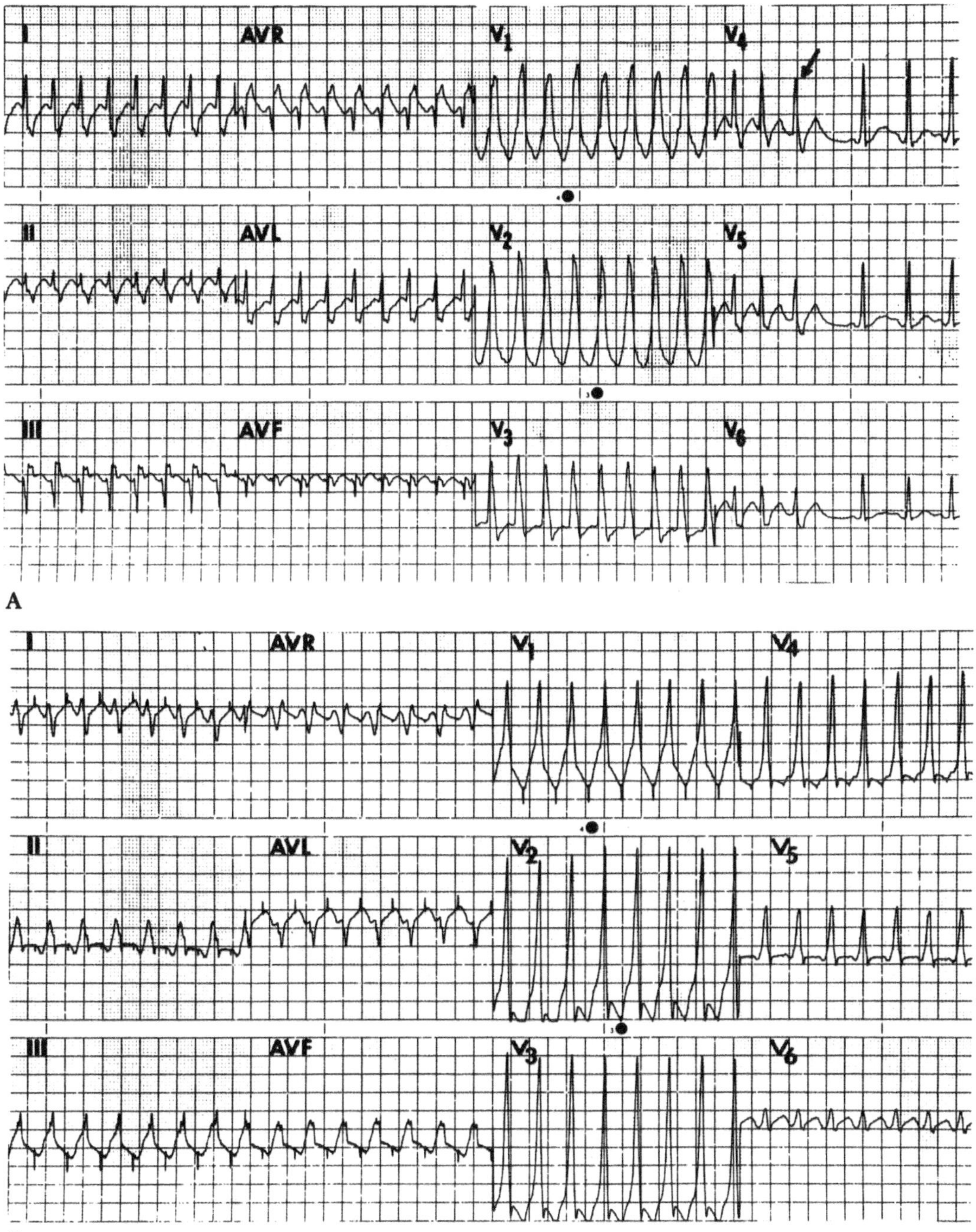

FIGURE 6–2. (A) A 3-channel, 12-lead electrocardiogram of orthodromic reciprocating tachycardia, rate 200/minute, in a patient with a left lateral accessory atrioventricular connection. There is a functional right bundle branch block. The arrow points to the last beat of the tachycardia. During sinus rhythm there is a PR interval of 0.10 seconds, small delta waves in leads V_4, V_5, and V_6, and no evidence of an underlying right bundle branch block. In this and all subsequent figures (except Figure 6–8), the mechanism of the tachycardia was established by electrophysiologic testing. (B) Atrial pacing, rate 170/minute, in the same patient as in Figure 2A. There is again a right bundle branch block configuration, however, in this case due to preexcitation of the left ventricle. Note the slurred upstroke of the QRS complexes in this figure, as opposed to Figure 6–2A, in which the QRS complexes during the tachycardia have a brisk upstroke and a terminal conduction delay typical of a functional right bundle branch block. Aberration of the QRS complexes during orthodromic reciprocating tachycardia is due to a functional or underlying bundle branch block and not preexcitation.

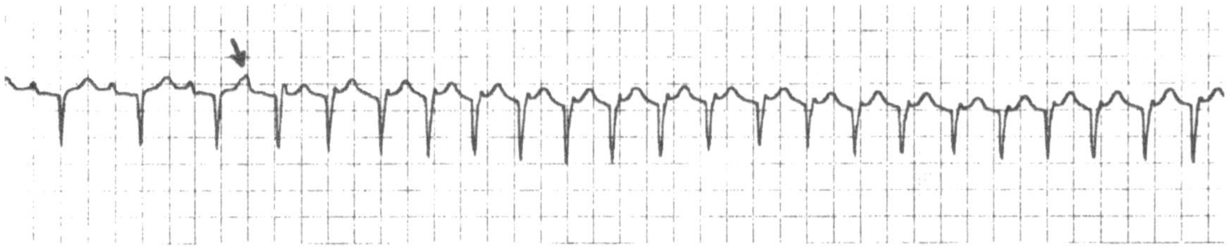

FIGURE 6–3. A typical example of orthodromic reciprocating tachycardia, rate 170/minute, initiated by an atrial premature depolarization (*arrow*). Note that during the tachycardia there is a *p* wave buried in the ST segment. Whenever the *p* waves occur in the left half of the RR cycle during a narrow-complex tachycardia, this should suggest the possibility of orthodromic reciprocating tachycardia. Shown is lead V_1.

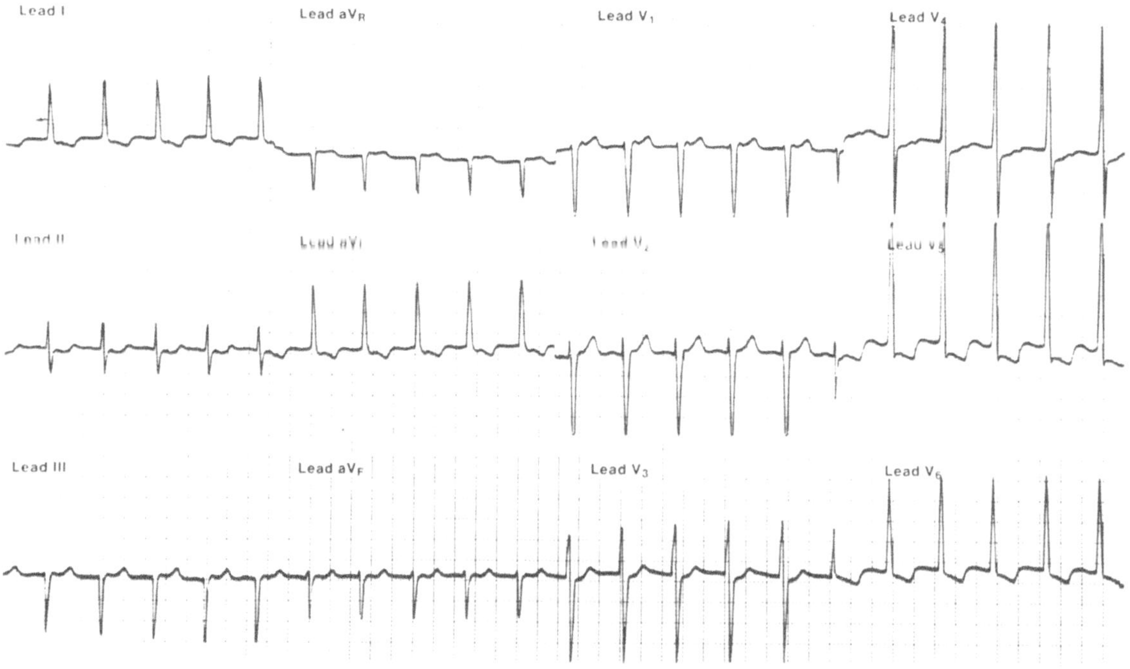

FIGURE 6–4. A narrow-complex tachycardia, rate 120/minute, in which the P wave occurs in the left half of the RR cycle. This is an atrial tachycardia with a first degree AV block. The rate of 120/minute is slower than typically seen in orthodromic reciprocating tachycardia (150–240/minute). When the *p* wave follows shortly after the QRS complex in a narrow-complex tachycardia, this is not necessarily diagnostic of orthodromic reciprocating tachycardia.

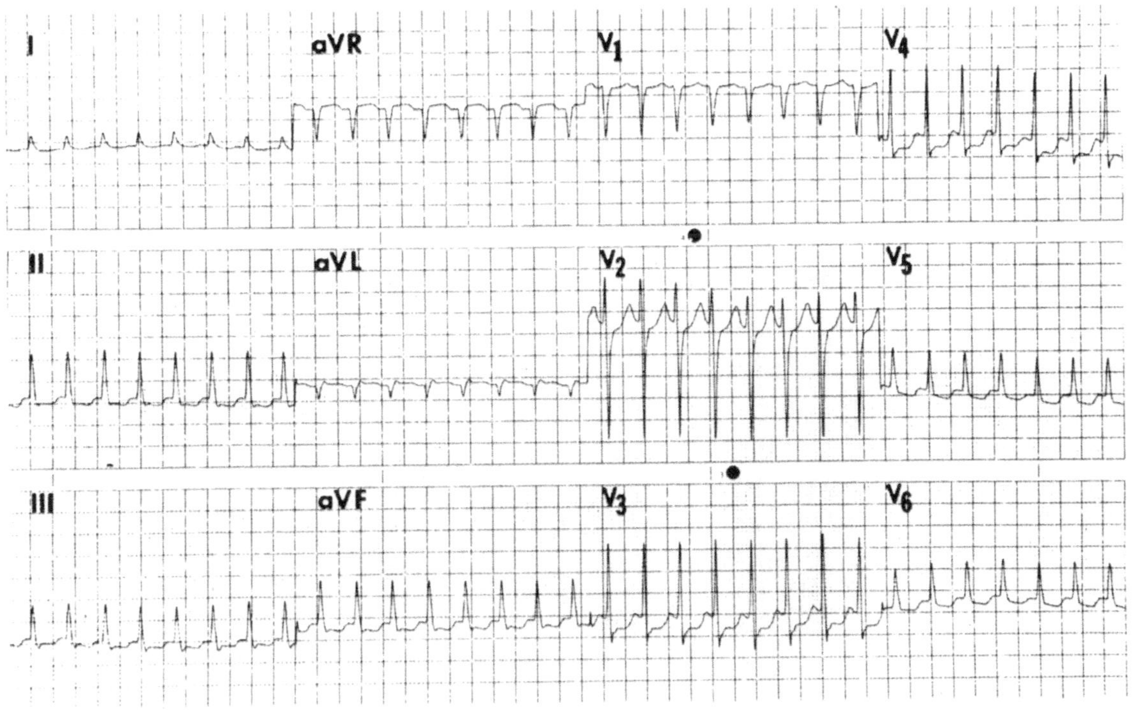

FIGURE 6–5. Reciprocating tachycardia due to reentry within the atrioventricular node. The rate of the tachycardia is 180/minute. The predominant electrocardiographic feature that distinguishes this type of tachycardia from orthodromic reciprocating tachycardia is the absence of visible *p* waves. In reciprocating tachycardia due to reentry within the atrioventricular node, the atria and ventricles are usually depolarized simultaneously. In contrast, in orthodromic reciprocating tachycardia, depolarization of the atria follows depolarization of the ventricles.

trast, in patients with orthodromic reciprocating tachycardia, if the bundle branch block during tachycardia occurs on the same side (i.e., ipsilateral) as a free wall accessory AV connection, the rate of the tachycardia may be slower when there is aberration compared to when the QRS complexes are narrow [4] (Figure 6–8). Tachycardia slowing occurs because a bundle branch block ipsilateral to the accessory AV connection lengthens the reentrant circuit responsible for the orthodromic reciprocating tachycardia. In other types of narrow-complex tachycardia, functional bundle branch block would not be associated with a slowing of the heart rate unless there was marked prolongation of the infranodal conduction time (HV interval). A slowing of the tachycardia rate in association with the occurrence of functional bundle branch block is therefore highly suggestive of orthodromic reciprocating tachycardia, and also provides information on the location of the accessory AV connection. However, electrophysiologic study is required to confirm that the slowing of the tachycardia rate is not due to prolongation in the HV interval.

If there is not a decrease in the tachycardia rate when functional bundle branch block occurs, this does not rule out the possibility of orthodromic reciprocating tachycardia. The accessory AV connection may be contralateral to the bundle branch block (Figure 6–9). Even when the bundle branch block is ipsilateral to the accessory AV connection, a shortening of the AV nodal conduction time (i.e., AH interval) may compensate for the effects of the bundle branch block, resulting in little or no change in the tachycardia rate [4]. In addition, functional bundle branch block during ortho-

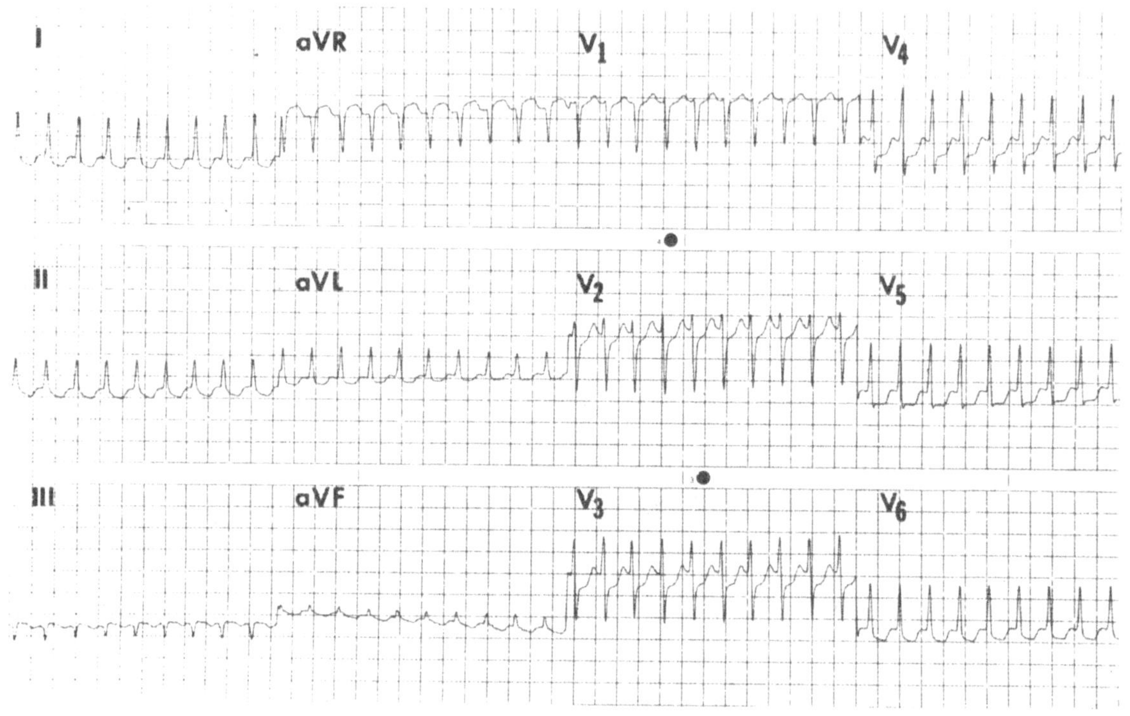

FIGURE 6–6. Orthodromic reciprocating tachycardia, rate 220/minute. The absence of discernible *p* waves following the QRS complexes could easily lead to the incorrect conclusion that this tachycardia is due to reentry within the atrioventricular node. The only clue that suggests the possibility of orthodromic reciprocating tachycardia is that the rate is greater than 200/minute.

dromic reciprocating tachycardia in patients with a septal accessory AV connection may be associated with little or no change in the tachycardia rate [4].

Irrespective of changes in the tachycardia rate, the occurrence of functional left bundle branch block by itself is suggestive of orthodromic reciprocating tachycardia. A functional left bundle branch block has been reported to occur only rarely with atrial tachycardias or reciprocating tachycardias due to reentry within the AV node, and more commonly with orthodromic reciprocating tachycardia [5]. Persistent complete or incomplete right bundle branch block during tachycardia is commonly associated with Ebstein's anomaly, and this association should be considered especially in the presence of a long RP interval [6].

An additional electrocardiographic feature which, when present, is helpful in distinguishing orthodromic reciprocating tachycardia from other types of narrow complex tachycardia is QRS alternans (Figure 6–10). Although not a sensitive indicator of orthodromic reciprocating tachycardia, QRS alternans appears to be fairly specific for this type of tachycardia. QRS alternans was reported to be present in 37% of orthodromic reciprocating tachycardias, compared to only 4% of atrial tachycardias or reciprocating tachycardias due to reentry within the AV node [7].

Other electrocardiographic findings. It should be noted that orthodromic reciprocating tachycardia may at times have an alternating pattern of long and short RR cycles. This usually indicates alternation between two different anterograde limbs of the reentry circuit. For example, in patients with dual AV nodal pathways and an accessory AV connection, orthodromic reciprocating tachycardia may utilize in alternating fashion the fast and slow AV nodal pathways as the anterograde limb of the tachycardia circuit [8] (Figure 6–11).

Mention should be made of a type of incessant AV reentrant tachycardia which may

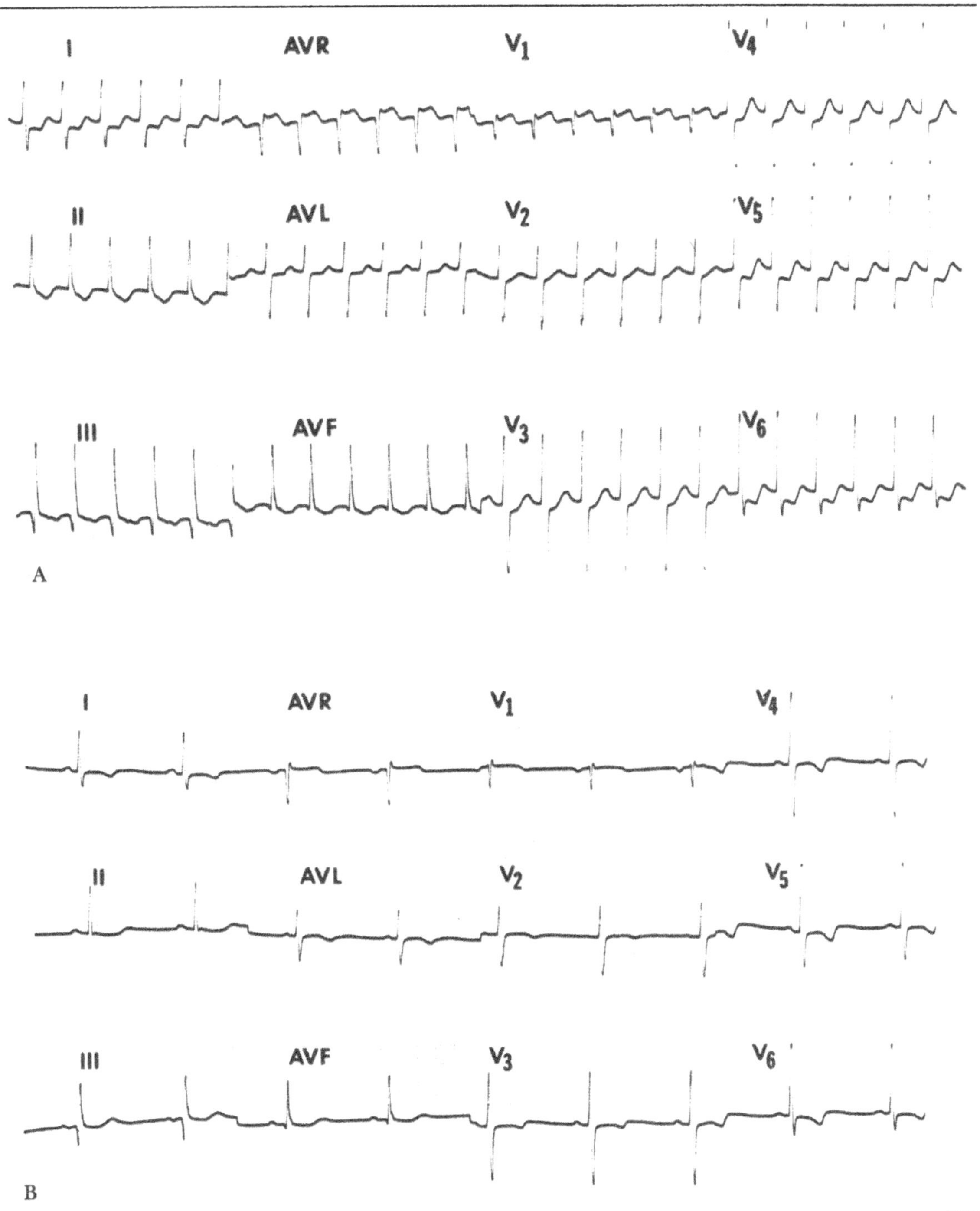

FIGURE 6–7. (A) Orthodromic reciprocating tachycardia, rate 150/minute. Upon first glance, it may not be apparent that there are P waves in the left half of the RR cycle. More careful inspection of the electrocardiogram reveals a notch in the ST segments in lead III which may be a *p* wave. (B) During sinus rhythm, in the same patient, there is no notching of the ST segment in lead III. This suggests that lead III during the tachycardia in Figure 6–8A does demonstrate a *p* wave following the QRS. Careful inspection and comparison with an electrocardiographic recording of sinus rhythm may be required to discern the *p* wave – QRS relationship during a tachycardia.

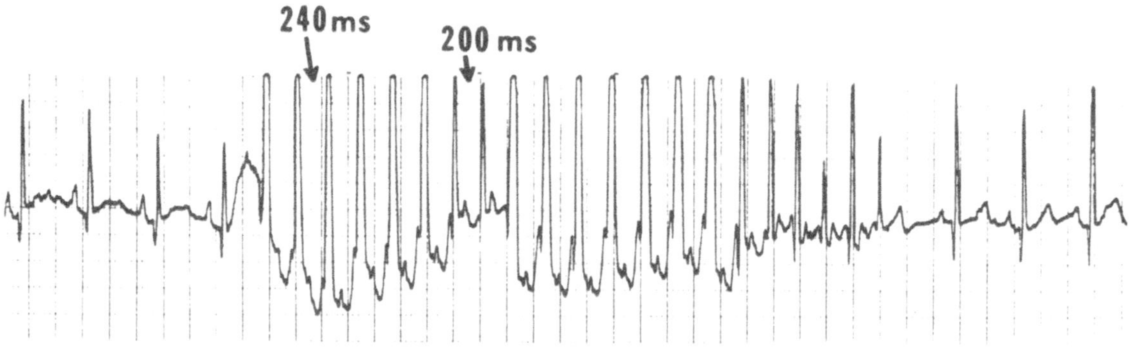

FIGURE 6–8. A wide-complex tachycardia, rate approximately 250/minute, recorded in lead V_6. There is left bundle branch block aberration and intermittently narrow QRS complexes. The tachycardia cycle length is 240 msec when the QRS complexes are wide, and 200 ms when the QRS complexes are narrow. A lengthening of the tachycardia cycle length (or slowing of the rate) in association with left bundle branch block aberration is highly suggestive of orthodromic reciprocating tachycardia utilizing a left-sided accessory atrioventricular connection as the retrograde limb of the reentry circuit. When the functional bundle branch block is ipsilateral to the accessory atrioventricular connection, the length of the reentry circuit increases. This tachycardia occurred in an infant and has a more rapid rate than would usually occur in an adult with orthodromic reciprocating tachycardia. (Electrocardiogram courtesy of Dr. Paul Stanger.)

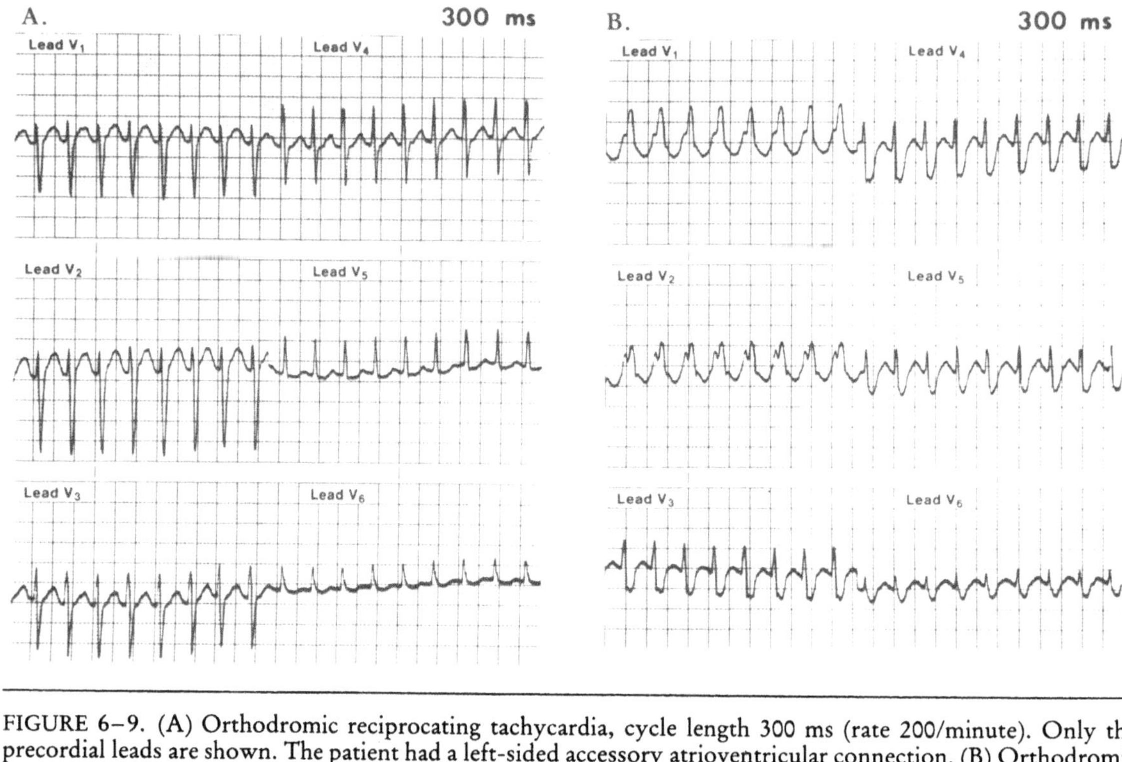

FIGURE 6–9. (A) Orthodromic reciprocating tachycardia, cycle length 300 ms (rate 200/minute). Only the precordial leads are shown. The patient had a left-sided accessory atrioventricular connection. (B) Orthodromic reciprocating tachycardia, in the same patient as in Figure 6–10A. There is now a functional right bundle branch block, but the cycle length of the tachycardia is unchanged. This is because the length of the reentry circuit in orthodromic reciprocating tachycardia is not affected when the bundle branch block is contralateral to the accessory atrioventricular connection.

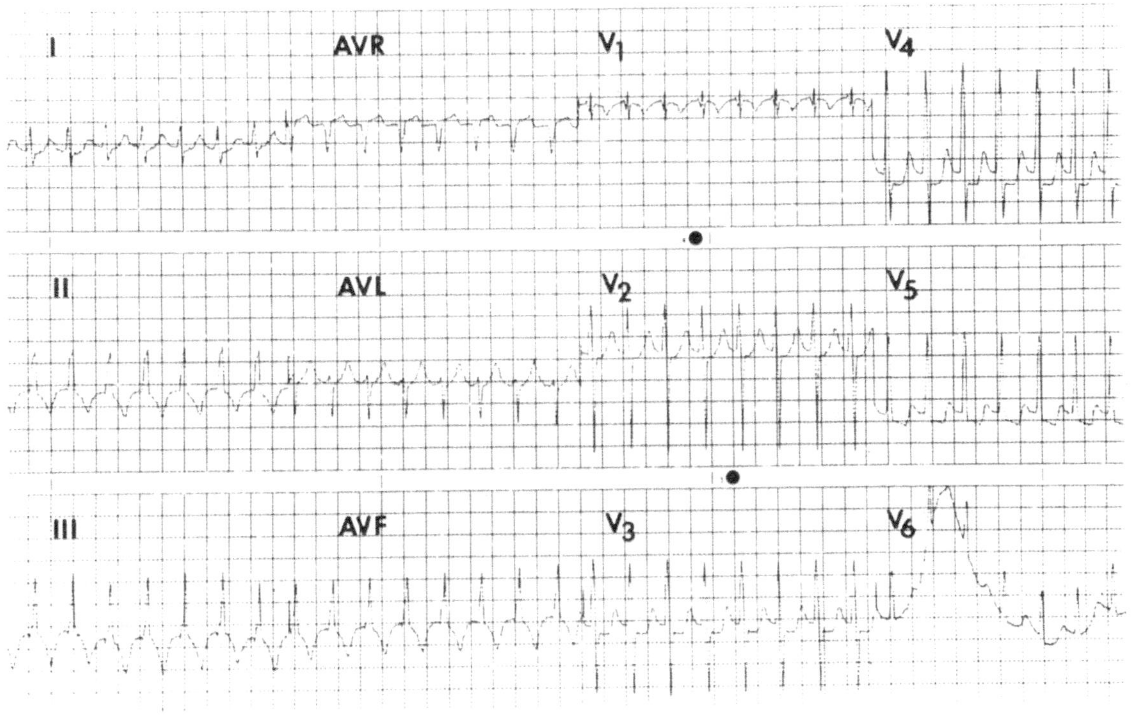

FIGURE 6–10. Orthodromic reciprocating tachycardia, rate 175/minute. The most helpful clue as to the mechanism of this tachycardia is QRS alternans, seen in leads V_2 and V_3. Because definite *p* waves are not apparent, this tachycardia could easily by mistaken for reciprocating tachycardia due to reentry within the atrioventricular node. However, QRS alternans has a high degree of specificity for orthodromic reciprocating tachycardia.

represent a variant of orthodromic reciprocating tachycardia: namely the so-called permanent form of junctional reciprocating tachycardia [9]. The electrocardiographic features of this type of narrow complex tachycardia are: (1) rate usually between 130 and 200/minute; (2) inverted P waves in the inferior leads; and (3) the P wave occurs in the right half of the R-R cycle (i.e., the PR interval is shorter than the RP interval) (Figure 6–12). As in typical orthodromic reciprocating tachycardia, the anterograde limb of the reentry circuit in the permanent form of junctional reciprocating tachycardia is the AV node–His bundle axis. Although the retrograde limb of this tachycardia has been thought by some to be within the AV node, anatomic and electrophysiologic data have been presented suggesting that the retrograde limb may be an accessory pathway with a long conduction time [10].

Table 6–1 summarizes the electrocardiographic findings suggestive of orthodromic reciprocating tachycardia. It should be emphasized that these electrocardiographic findings are only clues, and not the basis for a definitive diagnosis of the mechanism of a tachycardia. Even when several features suggestive of orthodromic reciprocating tachycardia are present, the tachycardia may in fact be due to a different mechanism (Figure 6–13). The definitive diagnosis of orthodromic reciprocating tachycardia usually requires invasive electrophysiologic evaluation.

TABLE 6–1. Electrocardiographic findings suggestive of orthodromic reciprocating tachycardia

Rate greater than 200/min
P wave in left half of RR cycle
Slowing of the tachycardia rate during functional bundle branch block
Functional left bundle branch block
QRS alternans

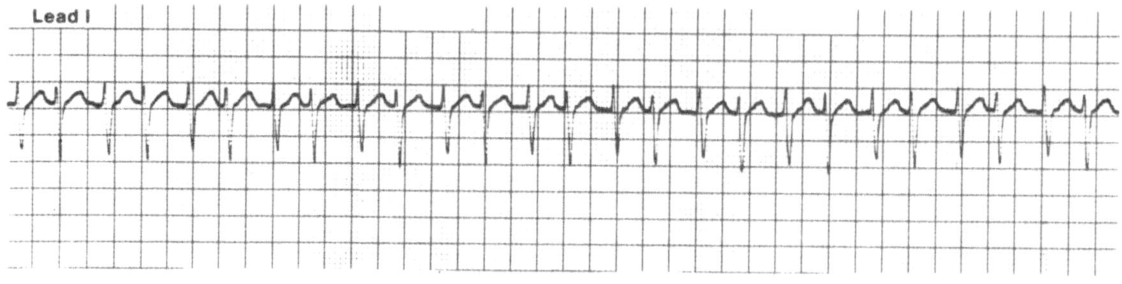

FIGURE 6–11. Orthodromic reciprocating tachycardia with an alternating pattern of long and short cycle lengths. The patient had a left-sided accessory atrioventricular connection and dual atrioventricular nodal pathways. The anterograde limb of the reentry circuit consisted of the "fast" and "slow" atrioventricular nodal pathways, in alternating fashion. The retrograde limb of the reentry circuit was always the accessory atrioventricular connection. Alternating long and short cycle lengths during a tachycardia may be a manifestation of "triple pathways", i.e., two atrioventricular nodal pathways and an accessory atrioventricular connection.

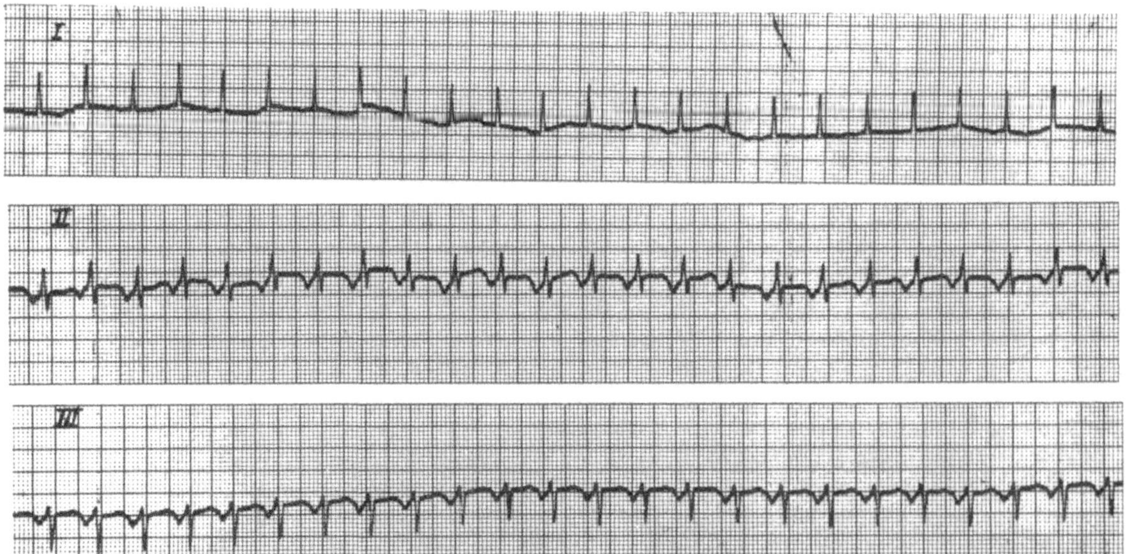

FIGURE 6–12. An example of the permanent form of junctional reciprocating tachycardia. Shown are leads I, II, and III. The rate of the tachycardia is 145/minute. Characteristic features of this type of tachycardia are an inverted P wave in the inferior leads and a PR interval shorter than the RP interval.

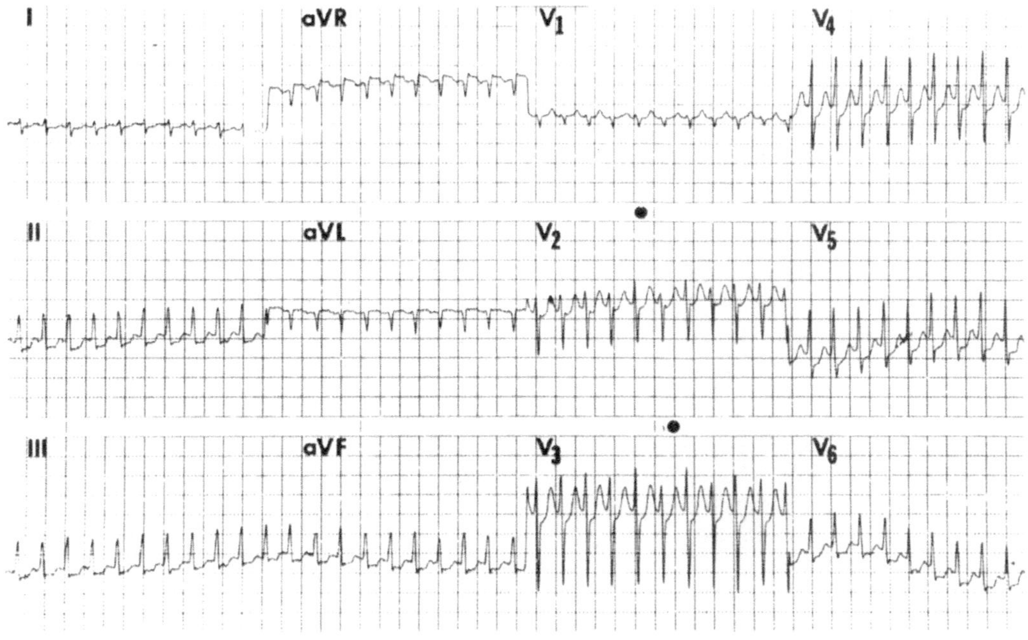

A

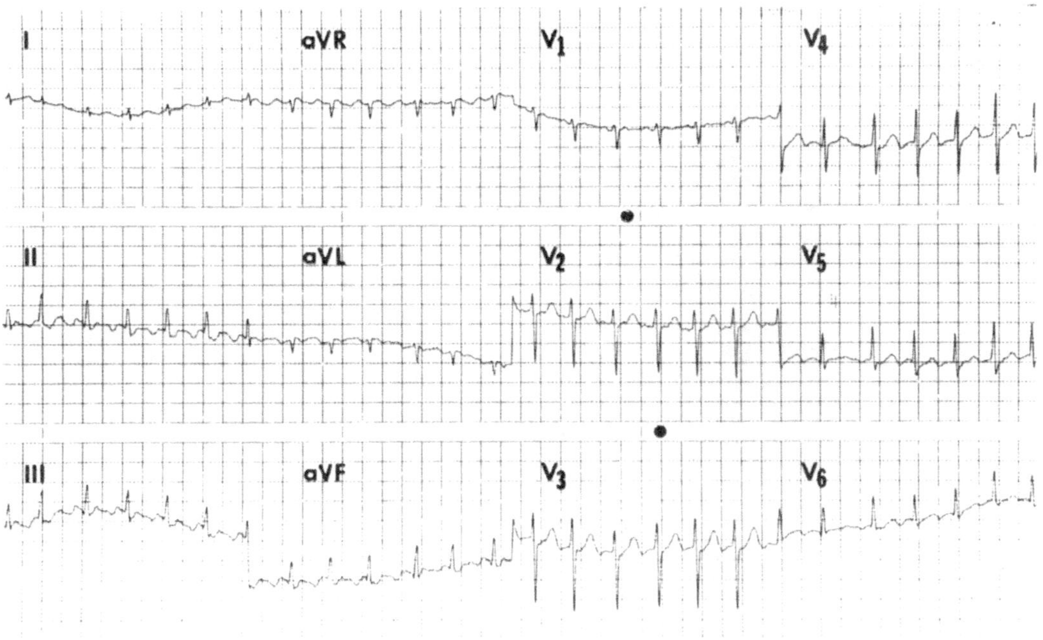

B

FIGURE 6–13. (A) This tachycardia has three features which suggest that it is an orthodromic reciprocating tachycardia: a rate greater than 200/minute, apparent *p* waves following the QRS complexes, and QRS alternans (most readily seen in lead V_4). (B) The tachycardia was actually atrial flutter with one-to-one conduction. This electrocardiogram shows the same tachycardia after spontaneous 2:1 or variable atrioventricular block occurred. Flutter waves are apparent in the inferior leads. This example demonstrates that there are no electrocardiographic findings which are absolutely diagnostic of a particular tachycardia mechanism.

ANTIDROMIC RECIPROCATING TACHYCARDIA

Antidromic reciprocating tachycardia occurs much less commonly than orthodromic reciprocating tachycardia. The reentry circuit which underlies antidromic reciprocating tachycardia consists of the same components as in orthodromic reciprocating tachycardia, however in antidromic reciprocating tachycardia the accessory AV connection serves as the anterograde limb of the reentry circuit, and the AV node–His bundle axis as the retrograde limb (Figure 6–14). In some cases, the retrograde limb of the tachycardia circuit may be a second accessory AV connection [10–14]. Because ventricular activation occurs only through the accessory AV connection, the QRS complexes during antidromic reciprocating tachycardia are always wide and maximally preexcited.

The rate of antidromic reciprocating tachycardia is usually in the range of 150 to 240/min [14]. Because retrograde conduction from the ventricle to the atrium through the AV node–His bundle axis is usually slow relative to anterograde conduction through the accessory AV connection, the PR interval during antidromic reciprocating tachycardia is shorter than the RP interval. However, from a practical standpoint, this electrocardiographic feature of antidromic reciprocating tachycardia is often of little diagnostic value, because the rapid rate of the tachycardia and the maximally preexcited QRS complexes often result in indiscernible P waves (Figure 6–15).

Using the electrocardiogram alone, antidromic reciprocating tachycardia may be impossible to distinguish from atrial flutter or ventricular tachycardia. Atrial flutter with 1:1 conduction through an accessory AV connection, or with 1:1 conduction through the AV node with underlying or functional bundle branch block, may have an appearance identical to that of antidromic reciprocating tachycardia. It has been reported that among 15 patients who had an accessory AV connection and atrial flutter with 1:1 conduction, 11 patients had a heart rate greater than 250/min [11]. In contrast, among 7 patients who had antidromic reciprocating tachycardia, the rate of the tachycardia was greater than 250/min in only 1 [11]. Therefore, a tachycardia rate greater than 250/min favors the diagnosis of atrial flutter with 1:1 conduction rather than antidromic reciprocating tachycardia. However, because of overlap in the range of tachycardia rates, the tachycardia rate cannot be used as an absolute diagnostic feature.

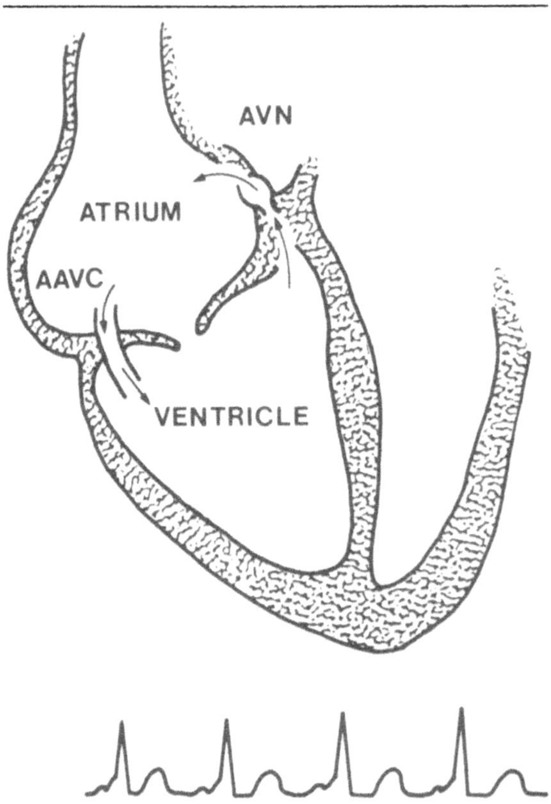

FIGURE 6–14. A schematic representation of the reentry circuit in antidromic reciprocating tachycardia. The accessory atrioventricular connection serves as the anterograde "fast" limb of the reentry circuit, and the atrioventricular node as the "retrograde" slow limb. As is the case in orthodromic reciprocating tachycardia, the intervening atrium and ventricle are also direct participants in the reentry circuit. Because ventricular activation occurs solely via the accessory atrioventricular connection, the QRS complexes have a maximally preexcited configuration during the tachycardia.

Ventricular tachycardia may also be impossible to distinguish from antidromic reciprocating tachycardia using the electrocardiogram alone. Although the presence of delta waves on the electrocardiogram during sinus rhythm suggests that a regular wide complex tachycardia involves an accessory AV connection as either an active or passive participant in the tachycardia,

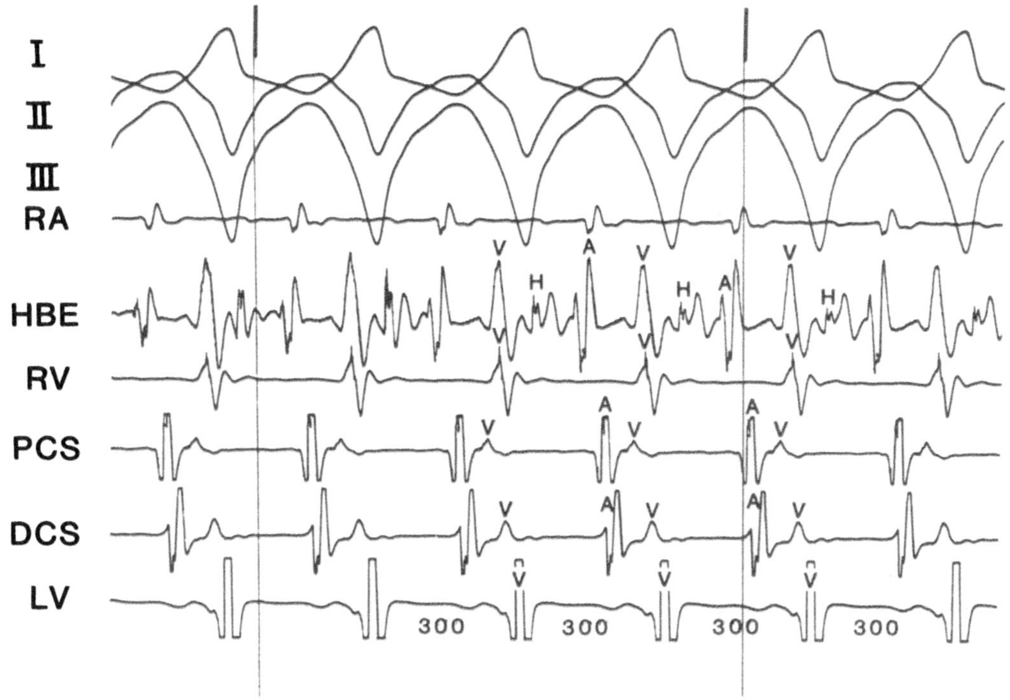

FIGURE 6–15. An example of antidromic reciprocating tachycardia, rate 200/minute (cycle length 300 ms). From top to bottom are leads I, II, and III, a right atrial electrogram (RA), His bundle electrogram (HBE), and intracardiac electrograms recorded in the right ventricle (RV), proximal coronary sinus (PCS), distal coronary sinus (DCS), and left ventricle (LV). Because ventricular activation occurs through an accessory atrioventricular connection the QRS complexes have a preexcited configuration. Atrial activation occurs by retrograde conduction through the atrioventricular node. Note that a retrograde His bundle depolarization (H) occurs after the ventricular electrograms (V). Although the atrial electrograms (A) occur between the QRS complexes, *p* waves are not apparent on the surface electrocardiogram. The time lines in this figure represent one-second intervals. (Illustration courtesy of Dr. David G Benditt.)

it should be noted that wide complex tachycardia in a patient with an accessory AV connection may be ventricular in origin [15]. The presence of AV dissociation or fusion beats on the electrocardiogram suggests that a wide complex tachycardia is ventricular rather than antidromic reciprocating tachycardia. However, these electrocardigraphic findings are often not present.

An electrocardiographic feature of antidromic reciprocating tachycardia which may be helpful in distinguishing this tachyarrhythmia from others types of regular wide complex tachycardia is an abrupt change in the tachycardia rate. It has been reported that five of five patients with antidromic reciprocating tachycardia demonstrated a sudden increase or decrease in the tachycardia rate [16]. This was thought to be due to sudden changes in the bundle branch being used as the retrograde limb of the tachycardia circuit. Abrupt changes in rate are less likely to occur in ventricular tachycardia. However, in most cases electrophysiologic study is required to establish the diagnosis of antidromic reciprocating tachycardia.

ATRIAL FIBRILLATION AND FLUTTER

Atrial fibrillation and flutter have been reported to occur in up to 32% of adult patients who have an accessory AV connection and symptomatic tachyarrhythmias [17]. It is not clear why the incidence of atrial fibrillation and flut-

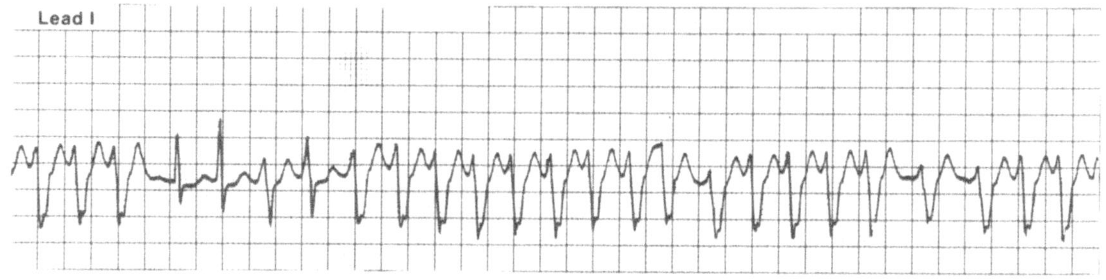

FIGURE 6–16. Atrial fibrillation, average ventricular rate 190/minute, in a patient with a left-sided accessory atrioventricular connection. Most of the QRS complexes have a preexcited configuration, however, the fourth and fifth complexes are narrow indicating that ventricular activation occurred via the His–Purkinje axis. The next two complexes are fusion beats which have a configuration intermediate between that of the narrow and wide QRS complexes. The irregularly irregular ventricular response and the presence of fusion beats are chracteristic of atrial fibrillation in a patient with an accessory atrioventricular connection.

ter is higher in patients with an accessory AV connection than in the general population. It is possible that the accessory AV connection plays an indirect role in the initiation of these arrhythmias by allowing an orthodromic or antidromic reciprocating tachycardia to occur; in some patients, a spontaneous atrial premature depolarization during orthodromic reciprocating tachycardia appears to be the mechanism by which atrial fibrillation is initiated [17–19]. Another possibility is that the accessory AV connection allows a ventricular premature depolarization to conduct rapidly to the atrium, resulting in an atrial depolarization which initiates atrial fibrillation during the atrial vulnerable period.

The determinants of the ventricular rate during atrial fibrillation consist of the refractory periods of the accessory AV connection and the AV node–His bundle axis, the extent of retrograde penetration of the accessory AV connection, and the ventricular effective refractory period [20]. Adrenergic tone also plays an important role; an increase in sympathetic tone, as may occur during exercise, may cause the accessory AV connection to conduct impulses more rapidly [21,22].

Depending on the relative refractoriness and conduction properties of the accessory AV connection and the AV node, the electrocardiogram may demonstrate QRS complexes that are narrow, wide due to functional or underlying bundle branch block, or wide due to ventricular preexcitation. Often the electrocardiogram during atrial fibrillation demonstrates various degrees of fusion between preexcited complexes and narrow complexes resulting from normal ventricular activation (Figure 6–16).

The hallmark of atrial fibrillation is an "irregularly irregular" ventricular response. In patients with an accessory AV connection the ventricular rate may be as high as 350/min. Because of this rapid rate, atrial fibrillation may at times appear to be regular rather than irregular, and may mimic atrial flutter with one-to-one conduction, antidromic reciprocating tachycardia, or ventricular tachycardia (Figure 6–17). The extremely rapid ventricular rate which may occur during atrial fibrillation in patients with an accessory AV connection may result in ventricular fibrillation [23,24]. The propensity for ventricular fibrillation has been reported to be higher when the shortest interval between two preexcited QRS complexes during atrial fibrillation is less than 250 msec [23,24].

When atrial flutter occurs in a patient with an accessory AV connection which is not capable of rapid conduction of impulses, the QRS complexes may or may not demonstrate preexcitation and the ventricular rate is usually not excessively rapid. However, many patients with an accessory AV connection have 1:1 conduction during atrial flutter and have ventricular rates between 250 and 350/minute (Figure 6–18). As stated earlier, atrial flutter with 1:1 conduction may be difficult or impossible to distinguish from antidromic reciprocating tachycardia, although a ventricular rate greater

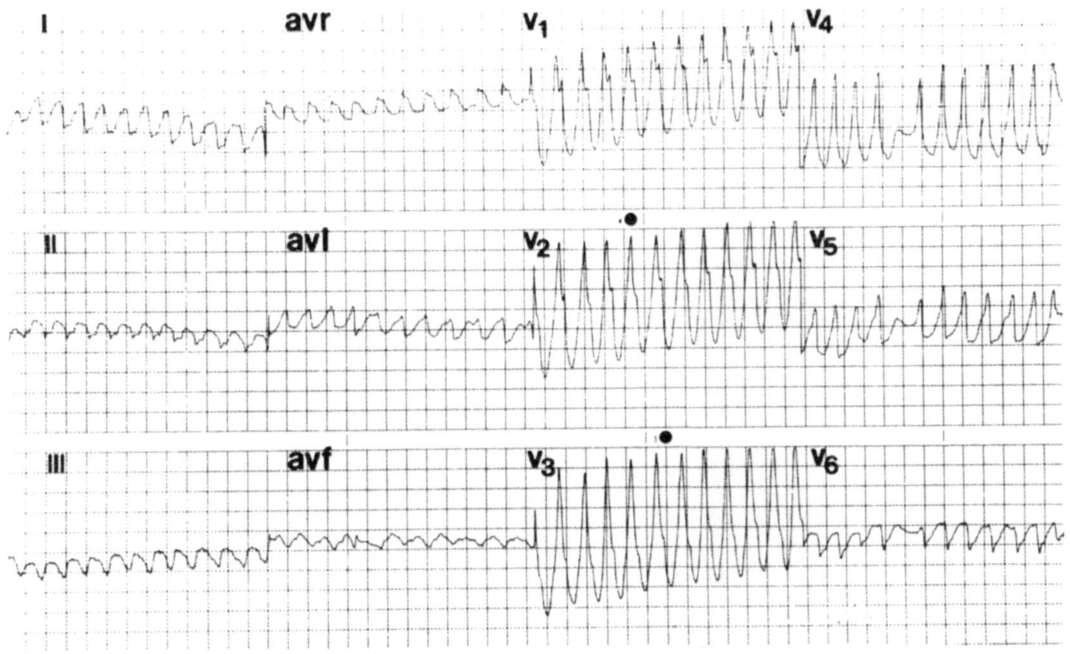

FIGURE 6–17. Atrial fibrillation, average ventricular rate 260/minute, in a patient with a left-sided accessory atrioventricular connection. The rapidity of the ventricular rate results in little variation in the RR cycle lengths. The regular appearance of the tachycardia in the frontal plane leads and V_1–V_3 is consistent with antidromic reciprocating tachycardia, atrial flutter with one-to-one conduction, or ventricular flutter. However, the brief period of irregularity seen in leads V_4–V_6 is more consistent with atrial fibrillation.

than 250/min favors the former [11]. Rapid ventricular tachycardia may also be impossible to distinguish from atrial flutter with 1:1 conduction. If spontaneous episodes of 2:1 or 3:1 AV block occur during atrial flutter, this is very helpful in uncovering atrial flutter waves and ruling out antidromic reciprocating tachycardia and ventricular tachycardia.

OTHER TACHYARRHYTHMIAS IN PATIENTS WITH AN ACCESSORY AV CONNECTION

Patients with an accessory AV connection may at times have more than one type of tachyarrhythmia. For example, a patient with an accessory AV connection was reported to have both a typical orthodromic reciprocating tachycardia and a primary atrial tachycardia due to either atrial reentry or an ectopic atrial rhythm [11]. Some patients with an accessory AV connection may have dual AV nodal pathways [8] and may have reciprocating tachycardia due to reentry within the AV node. In the latter tachyarrhythmia, the QRS complexes may be narrow or preexcited, depending on whether impulses originating in the AV junction activate the ventricles primarily via the normal His–Purkinje axis or via the accessory AV connection [25].

TACHYARRHYTHMIAS IN PATIENTS WITH AN ACCESSORY NODOVENTRICULAR OR FASCICULOVENTRICULAR CONNECTIONS

Since clinically apparent accessory nodoventricular connections insert into the right ventricle (or possibly into the specialized conduction system within the right ventricle, there is preexcitation of the right ventricle during tachycardias involving an accessory nodoventricular connection, and the QRS complexes have a left bundle branch block configuration [26]. Two types of tachycardia have been described in patients with an accessory nodoventricular connection: (1) a reentrant

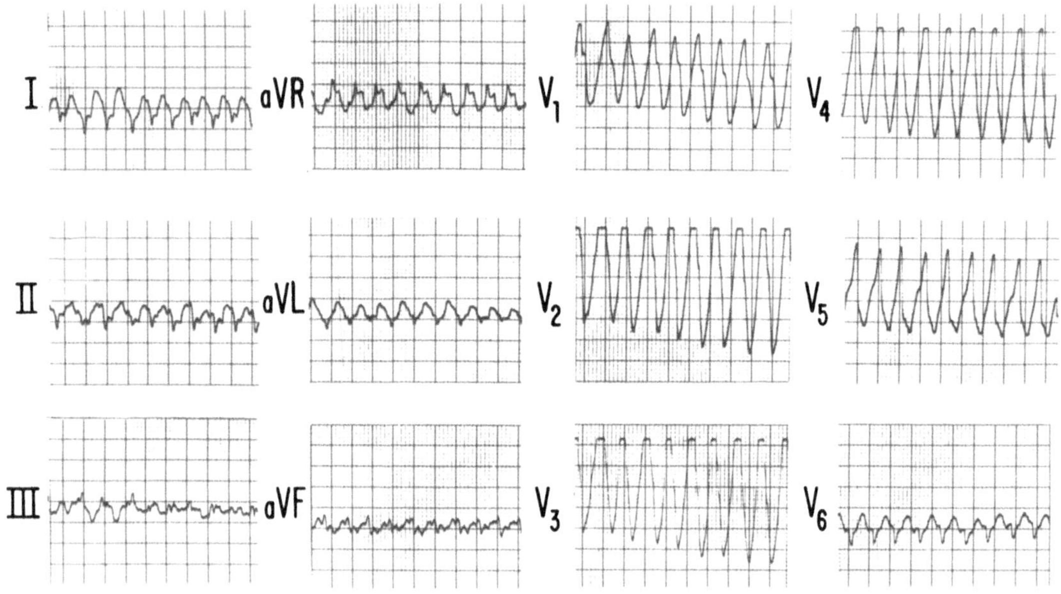

FIGURE 6–18. Atrial flutter, rate 300/minute, with one-to-one conduction in a patient with an accessory atrioventricular connection; this tachycardia may be impossible to distinguish from antidromic reciprocating tachycardia or ventricular tachycardia by analysis of the electrocardiogram alone. (Electrocardiogram courtesy of Dr. David G Benditt.)

tachycardia which utilizes the accessory nodoventricular connection as the anterograde limb of the circuit and the His–Purkinje system or an accessory AV connection as the retrograde limb [26]; and (2) reciprocating tachycardia due to reentry within the AV node, in which the accessory nodoventricular connection is a passive bystander [27].

The electrocardiogram during sinus rhythm in patients with an accessory nodoventricular connection may demonstrate no specific abnormalities; the PR interval is normal and although the QRS complexes may at times have varying degrees of a left bundle branch block configuration, they often have a normal configuration [28,29] (Figure 6–19).

Tachycardias involving an accessory nodoventricular connection usually have the following features (Figure 6–20): (1) a rate between 140 and 260/minute; (2) a frontal plane axis between 0 and −75 degrees; (3) a QRS width between 0.12 and 0.15 seconds; (4) an R wave in lead 1; (5) an rS wave in lead V_1; and (6) a precordial transition from a negative to a positive QRS complex after lead V_4 [29]. Although tachycardias involving an accessory nodoventricular connection may mimic ventricular tachycardia with a left bundle branch block configuration, supraventricular tachycardia with left bundle branch block aberration, or antidromic tachycardia utilizing a right sided accessory AV connection as the anterograde limb of the reentry circuit, it is uncommon for the above six findings to all be present in these other types of tachycardia. These six findings were all present in 12 of 13 patients (92%) with a tachycardia involving an accessory nodoventricular connection; in contrast, they were all present in 0 of 22 patients with ventricular tachycardia having a left bundle branch block configuration, 3 of 34 patients (9%) with supraventricular tachycardia and left bundle branch block aberration, and only 1 of 18 patients (6%) with antidromic tachycardia [29]. Although there are no electrocardiographic findings which are diagnostic of a tachycardia involving an accessory nodoventricular connection, the electrocardiogram may provide clues very suggestive of this type of tachycardia.

VA dissociation during a wide complex

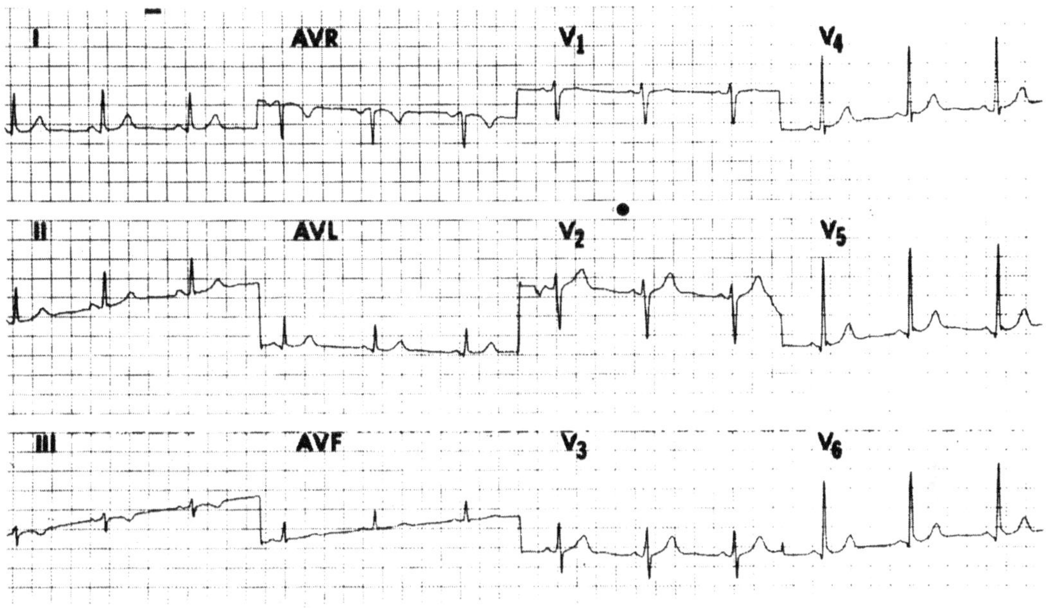

FIGURE 6–19. The 12-lead electrocardiogram during sinus rhythm in a patient who had an accessory nodoventricular connection and recurrent tachycardia (see Figure 6–20). Note that the PR interval is normal and that the QRS complexes are also normal. A normal electrocardiogram during sinus rhythm is common in patients with an accessory nodoventricular connection.

tachycardia is a finding strongly suggestive of ventricular tachycardia as opposed to supraventricular tachycardia with aberration. However, it is important to note that VA dissociation may also occur in tachycardias involving an accessory nodoventricular connection. Among seven patients who had a tachycardia involving an accessory nodoventricular connection, VA dissociation was present during the tachycardia in three [28].

When atrial fibrillation occurs in patients with an accessory nodoventricular connection, the ventricular rate is usually not excessively rapid unless there is also enhanced AV nodal conduction. The QRS complexes may have varying degrees of a left bundle branch block configuration (Figure 6–21). If there is an underlying right bundle branch block, atrial fibrillation in a patient with an accessory nodoventricular connection may mimic alternating bundle branch block.

Accessory fasciculoventricular connections have to date not been reported to be directly involved in the generation of tachyarrhythmias.

TACHYARRHYTHMIAS IN PATIENTS WITH ATRIONODAL OR ATRIOFASCICULAR CONNECTIONS

Patients with an atrionodal or atriohisian connection have a short PR interval during sinus rhythm, and no delta waves or specific QRS abnormalities. Along with patients who may have a congentially small AV node or rapid conduction through the AV node because of autonomic neural influence, patients with an atrionodal or atriofascicular connection may exhibit "enhanced AV conduction" [30–32]. Among patients with manifestations of enhanced AV conduction, it is not possible to distinguish unequivocally those who have an atrionodal or atriofascicular connection do not.

There are no tachyarrhythmias which are specific to patients with an atrionodal or atriofascicular connection. These patients may have reciprocating tachycardia due to reentry within the AV node, or orthodromic reciprocating tachycardia. The latter tachyarrhythmia tends to have a more rapid rate in patients with "enhanced AV conduction" [30–32] compared

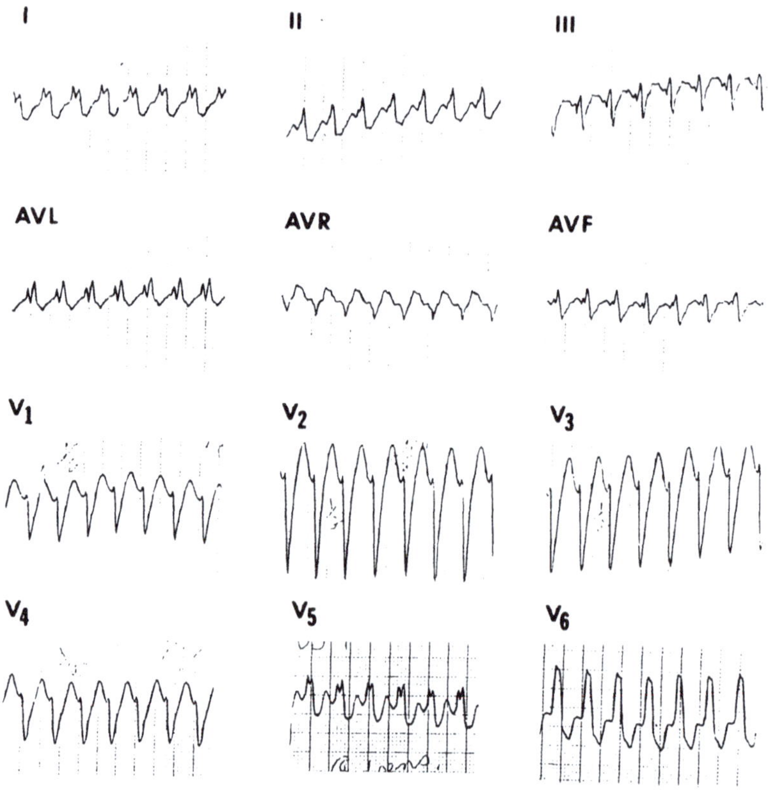

FIGURE 6–20. A typical example of tachycardia in a patient with an accessory nodoventricular connection. In this patient, the mechanism of the tachycardia was reentry within the atrioventricular node, and the accessory nodoventricular connection was a passive bystander. The other type of tachycardia which occurs in patients with an accessory nodoventricular connection is a reentrant tachycardia utilizing the accessory nodoventricular connection as the anterograde limb and the His Purkinje system as the retrograde limb. Both types of tachycardia have a similar electrocardiographic appearance. Note the following typical features: rate between 140 and 260/minute (200/minute in this case); QRS axis between 0 and −75° (−30° in this case); QRS width between 0.12 and 0.15 seconds (0.14 seconds in this case); an R wave in lead I; an rS wave in V_1; and a precordial transition from a negative to a positive QRS complex after V_4.

to patients with normal AV node conduction. Atrial fibrillation usually has a ventricular rate of 160 to 200/minute when it occurs in patients with enhanced AV conduction (Figure 6–22), while the occurrence of 1:1 conduction with narrow QRS complexes during atrial flutter also suggests the presence of "enhanced AV conduction."

Conclusion

In conclusion, the spectrum of tachyarrhythmias which may occur in patients with preexcitation syndromes is wide, and includes tachyarrhythmias which occur only in patients who have an accessory connection (e.g., orthodromic or antidromic reciprocating tachycardia), in addition to tachyarrhythmias which are not specific to patients with an accessory connection (e.g., atrial fibrillation or flutter). This chapter has described the electrocardiographic findings which provide clues as to the particular mechanism of a tachycardia in the patient with a preexcitation syndrome. However, it must be emphasized that the electrocardiographic findings, although often suggestive of a tachycardia mechanism, are usually not diagnostic. In most cases, detailed electrophysiologic studies

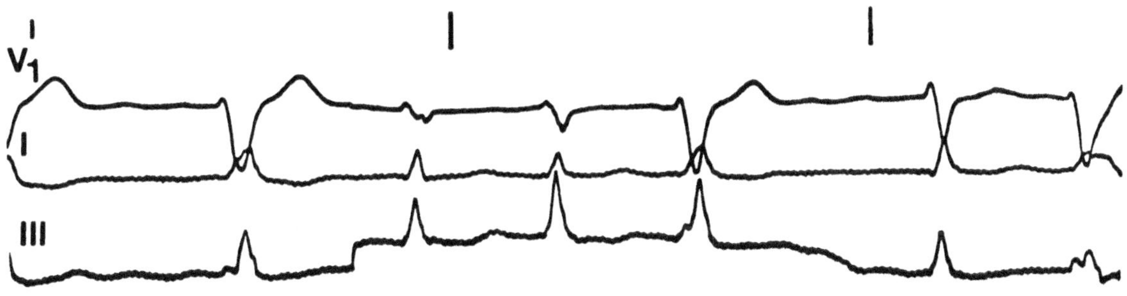

FIGURE 6–21. Atrial fibrillation in a patient with an accessory nodoventricular connection. From top to bottom are leads V_1, I, and III. The average rate is 150/minute. Note that the QRS complexes have varying degrees of a left bundle branch block configuration. This is due to varying degrees of fusion between impulses conducted over the accessory nodoventricular connection and the His–Purkinje axis. Because clinically apparent accessory nodoventricular connections insert into the right ventricle, ventricular preexcitation due to this type of accessory connection always results in QRS complexes which have a left bundle branch block configuration. The time lines in this figure represent one-second intervals.

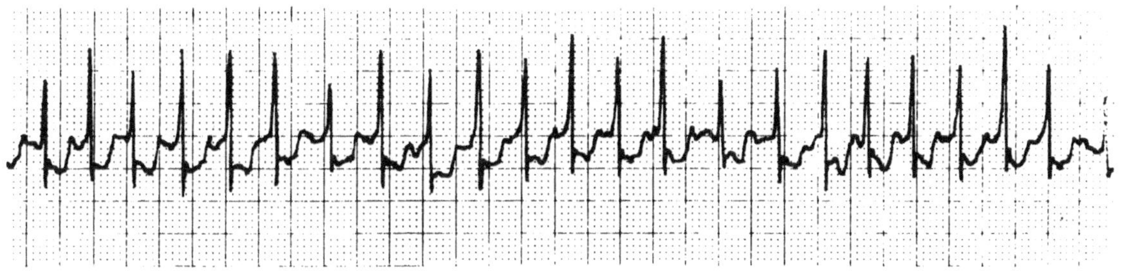

FIGURE 6–22. Atrial fibrillation, ventricular rate 190/minute. The rapid ventricular rate and narrow QRS complexes are typical of atrial fibrillation in a patient with an atrionodal connection. If the QRS complexes are wide in a patient with an atrionodal connection, this is due to a functional bundle branch block and not ventricular preexcitation.

are needed to establish the tachyarrhythmia mechanism in patients with preexcitation syndromes.

References

1. Wellens HJJ, Brugada P, Heddle WF: Value of the 12 lead electrocardiogram in diagnosing type and mechanism of a tachycardia: A survey among 22 cardiologists. *J. Am. Coll. Cardiol.* 4:176, 1984.
2. Bar FW, Brugada P, Dassen WRM, Wellens HJJ: Differential diagnosis of tachycardia with narrow QRS complex (shorter than 0.12 second). *Am. J. Cardiol.* 54:555, 1984.
3. Civera RC, Ferrero JA, Sanjuan R, Insa L, Rodriguez M, Segui J, Merino VL, Llavador J: Retrograde P wave polarity in reciprocating tachycardia utilizing lateral bypass tracts. *Eur. Heart J.* 1:137, 1980.
4. Kerr CR, Gallagher JJ, German LD: Changes in ventriculoatrial intervals with bundle branch block aberration during reciprocating tachycardia in patients with accessory atrioventricular pathways. *Circulation* 66:196, 1982.
5. Farshidi A, Josephson ME, Horowitz LN: Electrophysiologic characteristics of concealed

bypass tracts: Clinical and electrocardiographic correlates. *Am. J. Cardiol.* 41:1052, 1978.
6. Smith WM, Gallagher JJ, Kerr CR, Sealy WC, Kasell JH, Benson DW Jr, Reiter MJ, Sterba R, Grant AO: The electrophysiologic basis and management of symptomatic recurrent tachycardia in patients with Ebstein's anomaly of the tricuspid valve. *Am. J. Cardiol.* 49:1223, 1982.
7. Green M, Heddle B, Dassen W, Wehr M, Abdollah H, Brugada P, Wellens HJJ: Value of QRS alternation in determining the site of origin of narrow QRS supraventricular tachycardia. *Circulation* 68:368, 1983.
8. Sung RJ, Styperek JL: Electrophysiologic identification of dual atrioventricular nodal pathway conduction in patients with reciprocating tachycardia using anomalous bypass tracts. *Circulation* 60:1464, 1979.
9. Guarnieri T, Sealy WC, Kasell JH, German LD, Gallagher JJ: The nonpharmacologic management of the permanent form of junctional reciprocating tachycardia. *Circulation* 69:269, 1984.
10. Critelli G, Gallagher JJ, Monda V, Coltorti F, Scherillo M, Rossi L: 1984. Anatomic and electrophysiologic substrate of the permanent form of junctional reciprocating tachycardia. *J. Am. Coll. Cardiol.* 4:601, 1984.
11. Benditt DG, Pritchett ELC, Gallagher JJ: Spectrum of regular tachycardias with wide QRS complexes in patients with accessory atrioventricular pathways. *Am. J. Cardiol.* 42:828, 1978.
12. Cinca J, Valle V, Gutierrez L, Figueras J, Rius J: Reciprocating tachycardia using bilateral anomalous pathways: Electrophysiologic and clinical implications. *Circulation* 62:657, 1980.
13. Heddle WF, Brugada P, Wellens HJJ: Multiple circus movement tachycardias with multiple accessory pathways. *J. Am. Coll. Cardiol.* 4:168, 1980.
14. Bardy GH, Packer DL, German LD, Gallagher JJ: Preexcited reciprocating tachycardia in patients with Wolff-Parkinson-White syndrome: incidence and mechanisms. *Circulation* 70:377, 1984.
15. Lloyd EA, Hauer RN, Zipes DP, Heger JJ, Prystowsky EN: Syncope and ventricular tachycardia in patients with ventricular preexcitation. *Am. J. Cardiol.* 52:79, 1983.
16. Kuck KH, Brugada P, Wellens HJJ: Observations on the antidromic type of circus movement tachycardia in the Wolff-Parkinson-White syndrome. *J. Am. Coll. Cardiol.* 2:1003, 1983.
17. Campbell RWF, Smith RA, Gallagher JJ, Pritchett ELC, Wallace AG: Atrial fibrillation in the preexcitation syndrome. *Am. J. Cardiol.* 40:514, 1977.
18. Bauernfeind RA, Wyndham CR, Swiryn SP, Palileo EV, Strasberg B, Lam W, Westveer D, Rosen KM: Paroxysmal atrial fibrillation in the Wolff-Parkinson-White Syndrome. *Am. J. Cardiol.* 47:562, 1981.
19. Cosio FG, Benson DW, Jr, Anderson RW, Hession WT, Pritzker MR, Kriett JM, Benditt DG: Onset of atrial fibrillation during antidromic tachycardia: Association with sudden cardiac arrest and ventricular fibrillation in a patient with Wolff-Parkinson-White syndrome. *Am. J. Cardiol.* 50:353, 1982.
20. Wellens HJ, Durrer D: Wolff-Parkinson-White Syndrome and atrial fibrillation. Relation between refractory period of accessory pathway and ventricular rate during atrial fibrillation. *Am. J. Cardiol.* 34:777, 1974.
21. Wellens HJJ, Brugada P, Roy D, Weiss J, Bar FW: Effect of isoproterenol on the anterograde refractory period of the accessory pathway in patients with the Wolff-Parkinson-White syndrome. *Am. J. Cardiol.* 50:180, 1982.
22. German LD, Gallagher JJ Broughton A, Guarnieri T, Trantham JL: Effects of exercise and isoproterenol during atrial fibrillation in patients with Wolff-Parkinson-White syndrome. *Am. J. Cardiol.* 51:1203, 1983.
23. Sellers TD, Bashore TM, Gallagher JJ: Digitalis in the pre-excitation syndrome. Analysis during atrial fibrillation. *Circulation* 56:260, 1977.
24. Klein GJ, Bashore TM, Sellers TD, Pritchett ELC, Smith WM, Gallagher JJ: Ventricular fibrillation in the Wolff-Parkinson-White syndrome. *N. Engl. J. Med.* 301:1080, 1979.
25. Smith WM, Broughton A, Reiter MJ, Benson DW Jr, Grant AO, Gallagher JJ: Bystander accessory pathway during AV node re-entrant tachycardia. *PACE* 6:537, 1983.
26. Gallagher JJ, Smith WM, Kasell JH, Benson DW Jr, Sterba R, Grant AO: Role of Mahaim fibers in cardiac arrhythmias in man. *Circulation* 64:176, 1981.
27. Morady F, Scheinman MM, Gonzalez R, Hess D: His-ventricular dissociation in a patient with reciprocating tachycardia and a nodoventricular bypass tract. *Circulation* 64:839, 1981.
28. Reiter MJ, Smith WM, Gallagher JJ: Clinical spectrum of ventricular tachycardia with left bundle branch morphology. *Am. J. Cardiol.* 51:113, 1983.
29. Bardy GH, Fedor JM, German LD, Packer DL, Gallagher JJ: Surface electrocardiographic clues suggesting presence of a nodofascicular Mahaim fiber. *J. Am. Coll. Cardiol.* 3:1161, 1984.
30. Gallagher JJ, Sealy WC, Kasell J, Wallace AG: Multiple accessory pathways in patients with pre-excitation syndrome. *Circulation* 54:571, 1976.
31. Benditt DG, Pritchett ELC, Smith WM, Wallace AG, Gallagher JJ: Characteristics of atrioventricular conduction and the spectrum of arrhythmias in Lown-Ganong-Levine syndrome. *Cir-*

culation 57:454, 1978.
32. Holmes DR Jr, Hartzler GO, Maloney JD: Concealed retrograde bypass tracts and enhanced atrioventricular nodal conduction. An unusual subset of patients with refractory paroxysmal supraventricular tachycardia. *Am. J. Cardiol.* 45:1053, 1980.

7. ROLE OF HIS–PURKINJE SYSTEM IN THE INITIATION OF ORTHODROMIC TACHYCARDIA IN WOLFF-PARKINSON-WHITE SYNDROME

Masood Akhtar
Michael H. Lehmann
Stephen Denker
Rehan Mahmud

With the introduction of intracardiac recording techniques and programmed electrical stimulation, the tachyarrhythmias in Wolff-Parkinson-White (WPW) have been extensively studied [1–10]. The most common arrhythmia in this patient population is the reciprocating tachycardia utilizing the normal pathway in one direction and the accessory pathway in the other. Less commonly, the accessory pathway may constitute both the anterograde and retrograde limbs of the reentry circuit [8,10]. Depending upon the site and method of stimulation, presence of multiple accessory pathways, as well as the electrophysiologic properties of the accessory and normal pathways in both directions, reciprocating tachycardia of either the orthodromic or antidromic variety can be initiated. With the usual pacing techniques (incremental and extrastimulus method) from the atrial and ventricular sites the orthodromic reciprocating tachycardia is induced more frequently and consistently than the antidromic type [2]. Since orthodromic reciprocating tachycardia is also the more common clinical arrhythmia and its electrophysiology is more clearly understood, it will be the primary subject of this review [2].

Benditt, D.G. and Benson, D.W., Cardiac Preexcitation Syndromes.

It is widely appreciated that block in the accessory pathway or normal pathway during atrial or ventricular pacing is essential to initiate this arrhythmia. From the two stimulation sites, however, the normal pathway and its two components (i.e., the atrioventricular (AV) node and the His–Purkinje system) play a different and specific role in the induction of tachycardia. During atrial pacing, for example, an effective propagation of the impulse through the His–Purkinje system is a prerequisite for tachycardia initiation, whereas with ventricular stimulation effective conduction along the His–Purkinje system will prevent tachycardia initiation. Since the His–Purkinje system makes a different contribution to tachycardia induction depending on whether activation results from atrial versus ventricular stunulation, the two are presented separately.

Initiation of Tachycardia with Atrial Stimulation

With overt ventricular preexcitation during atrial pacing tachycardia cannot be induced until a block is achieved in the accessory pathway. Following a block of atrial impulse in the accessory pathway with concomitant AV conduction via the normal conduction system, tachycardia initiation is primarily dependent upon the recovery properties of the accessory pathway for conduction in the retrograde direction. Although refractoriness of the atrial myocardium has been cited as a possible mechanism limiting initiation of tachycardia, this has to be an exception rather than the rule [11,12]. Accessory pathway excitability after a block of atrial impulse depends upon two main factors: (1) inherent recovery properties of the pathway; and (2) the interval which elapses between the point of deepest pathway penetration and arrival of impulse in the pathway from the opposite direction. This critical interval is a composite of intraatrial, AV node and His–Purkinje conduction (i.e., the AV interval) and the conduction time within the ventricular myocardium [3,11]. The last of these four components is the most difficult to quantitate. The contribution of intraatrial conduction times to the overall AV interval is a function of stimulation site (relative to the AV node) and the degree of intraatrial delays. The latter is only of significant magnitude when the relative refractory period of the atrium exceeds the effective refractory period of the accessory pathway. Regardless, however, during atrial pacing the intraatrial conduction times generally remain constant and when the tachycardia starts seldom a change in the intraatrial conduction is considered a causative mechanism. On the other hand, increasing delays in the AV node and/or His–Purkinje system with atrial pacing are the usual determinants of tachycardia initiation.

Anterograde His–Purkinje System Delays and Tachycardia Initiation

Even though the role of critical AV delays in the initiation of orthodromic reciprocating tachycardia is widely recognized, the relative contribution of AH vs. HV interval has not been carefully dissected [13]. Since in most cases the induced His–Purkinje system conduction delays are functional in nature, the method of pacing (i.e., incremental vs. extrastimulus technique) and the duration of basic cycle length chosen can affect the incidence of functional His–Purkinje system delays. Another parameter which indirectly influences the role of His–Purkinje system in tachycardia initiation is the effective refractory period of the accessory pathway, as explained below. During overt ventricular preexcitation delays in the His–Purkinje system cannot be assessed until a block is encountered in the accessory pathway. For this reason, patients with accessory pathways functioning only in the retrograde direction provide a better subset to study the contribution of the His–Purkinje system in tachycardia initiation. In our own experience in patients with tachycardia unassociated with ventricular preexcitation, an HV interval prolongation of greater magnitude (as compared to AH increase) is not uncommon at the outer end of the tachycardia zone (i.e., the longest A_1A_2 interval where the tachycardia is induced). As the atrial coupling intervals are shortened the resulting H_1H_2 intervals prolong to values which often exceed the relative refractory period of the His–Purkinje system and therefore, HV prolongation or bundle branch block is no longer seen [14]. Within the usual basic cycle length ranges (i.e., 400–700 ms), the A_1A_2 intervals which initiate tachycardia without His–Purkinje system delays are generally short (i.e., ≤300 ms) and fall along the ascending limb of the AV node functional refractory period curve. It would, therefore, seem that in patients with ventricular preexcitation and a relatively short effective refractory period of the accessory pathway, His–Purkinje system delays may not be encountered at the outer end of the tachycardia zone. At short A_1A_2 intervals when accessory pathway block is initially noted, corresponding AV node delays may already be of significant magnitude such that the resultant H_1H_2 values exceed the relative refractory period of the His–Purkinje system.

It should be pointed out that most of the available literature deals with initiation of tachycardia at paced atrial cycle length which are often significantly shorter than the spontaneous sinus cycle length. The longer sinus cycle length could permit the occurrence of His–Purkinje system delays by prolonging the relative refractory period of the His–Purkinje system and/or the effective refractory period of the accessory pathway, without significantly affecting the functional refractory period of the AV node. It is conceivable, therefore, that at sinus rates the His–Purkinje system delays may contribute to tachycardia initiation more often than at paced cycle lengths generally utilized. The onset of tachycardia in the setting of sinus rhythm is obviously more relevant to the occurrence of spontaneous clinical arrhythmia than paced rhythm. This effect of longer cycle length on the relative refractory period of the His–Purkinje system may be further exaggerated in the setting of sudden cycle length change such as atrial bigeminy [15]. On the other hand, at short cycle length (≥400 ms with extrastimulus technique) and during incremental atrial pacing, His–Purkinje system delays are less commonly encountered and AV node conduction is generally responsible providing the critical delays for tachycardia initiation.

In addition to HV interval lengthening which contributes toward tachycardia initiation by adding to the overall AV interval, the occurrence of bundle branch block per se can facilitate tachycardia induction [11]. Such a facilitation is only noted when the accessory pathway is ipsilateral to the bundle branch showing the block (Figure 7–1). The amount of additional time provided by the ipsilateral bundle branch block causing the delays in the arrival of impulse to the retrograde end of the accessory pathway is difficult to quantitate but can exceed 30 msec as depicted in Figure 7–1.

Initiation of Tachycardia with Ventricular Stimulation

Right ventricular pacing is generally at least as effective in inducing tachycardia as atrial stimulation if the effective refractory period of the accessory pathway exceeds that of the normal conduction system [16]. Whenever a block is encountered along the normal conduction system, the potential for tachycardia initiation exists [3,6,7,17]. However, the consequences of a retrograde block in the His–Purkinje system vs the AV node could be quite different. Due to the inability to identify a retrograde His bundle deflection during constant cycle length pacing the determination of the site of retrograde block has been difficult during incremental ventricular pacing [18]. With the ventricular extrastimulus technique, the various parameters of His–Purkinje system refractoriness are easier to measure and it is evident that compared to the AV node, the refractoriness of the His–Purkinje system plays a more direct and important role in tachycardia initiation and this is detailed below [17].

Retrograde His–Purkinje System Block and Tachycardia Initiation

As pointed out earlier, a block of retrograde impulse in the normal conduction system with comcomitant atrial activation via the accessory pathway provides the essential combination to initiate tachycardia during ventricular pacing. Convincing data illustrating the site of retrograde block along the specialized ventriculo-atrial conduction system in patients with WPW syndrome is not always available. Difficulty in identifying the exact site of retrograde block in the normal conduction system is compounded by the fact that the location of retrograde block may not be the same during different pacing methods (i.e., extrastimulus vs. incremental pacing even in the same patient) [18]. This is primarily related to the electrophysiologic properties of the two components of the normal conduction system which may respond differently to the two methods of stimulation. Since the extrastimulus [V_2] method provides a clearer comprehension of His–Purkinje system conduction, we undertook a study to address the mechanism of tachycardia initiation with V_2 technique in 14 consecutive patient with WPW syndrome in whom the tachycardia could be induced during right ventricular pacing [17]. The findings presented in Figure 7–2 show the typical response in these cases during scanning of a basic ventricular cycle length. The V_2A_2 response suggests intra-atrial fusion until a V_1V_2 of 380 msec and from then on atrial activation is exclusively via the accessory pathway which is closer to the catheter positioned in the coronary sinus. The retrograde His bundle activation is seen at a V_1V_2 of 360 ms and precedes A_2 recordings from all atrial sites. A sudden jump in V_2H_2 occurs at a V_1V_2 of 340 ms such that the His bundle activation now follows the A_2 deflections and this occurrence coincides with the onset of tachycardia. The abrupt increase in VH interval represents the onset of retrograde block in the His–Purkinje system and a shift from retrograde His bundle activation via the bundle branches to its antegrade depolarization from the atrial impulse (A_2). Interestingly, when retrograde V_2H_2 conduction resumes at shorter V_1V_2 interval (retrograde gap phenomenon in the His–Purkinje system [19] the tachycardia is no longer initiated. This suggests that whereas a block of V_2 in the His–Purkinje facilitates tachycardia

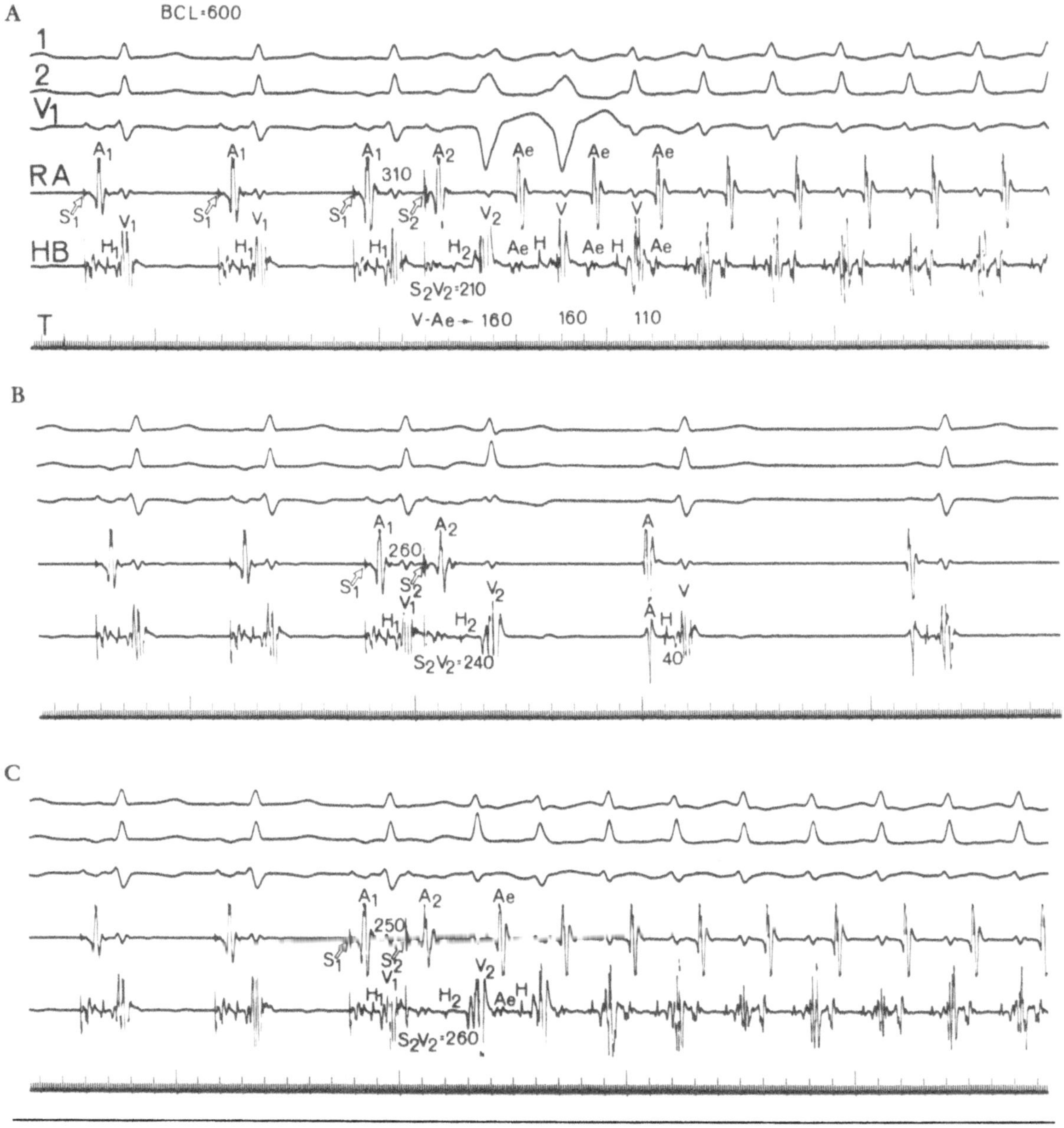

FIGURE 7–1. Role of intraventricular conduction delay in the initiation of orthodromic reciprocating tachycardia.

Tracings in each panel from top to bottom are ECG leads 1, 2, V_1, right atrial (RA) and His bundle (HB) electrograms. T denotes time lines at 10 and 100 ms.

During pacing from coronary sinus at a basic cycle length of 600 ms and an atrial coupling interval (S_1S_2) of 310 ms (*Panel A*) the S_2 conducts with an S_2V_2 interval of 210 ms and a left bundle branch block (LBBB) pattern to initiate tachycardia. Note the V-A interval decrease from 160 to 100 ms with normalization of QRS complex suggesting a left free wall accessory pathway. At a shorter S_1S_2 of 260 ms (*Panel B*) the S_2 conducts with right bundle branch block pattern and tachycardia is not initiated despite the fact that the S_2 V_2 interval is 30 ms longer than Panel A. This observation suggests that additional intra left ventricular conduction delay during LBBB facilitates the onset of tachycardia. Panel C depicts that during normal intraventricular conduction longer S_2V_2 of 260 ms is associated with induction of tachycardia. Although a small amount of latency is noted between the S_2 and A_2 response in Panels B and C, the A_2 V_2 intervals in these two panels nonetheless exceed those in Panel A. Th H_2V_2 interval in all panels is significantly longer than H_1V_1 interval and His–Purkinje conduction times therefore make a substantial contribution to the overall A_2V_2 delays.

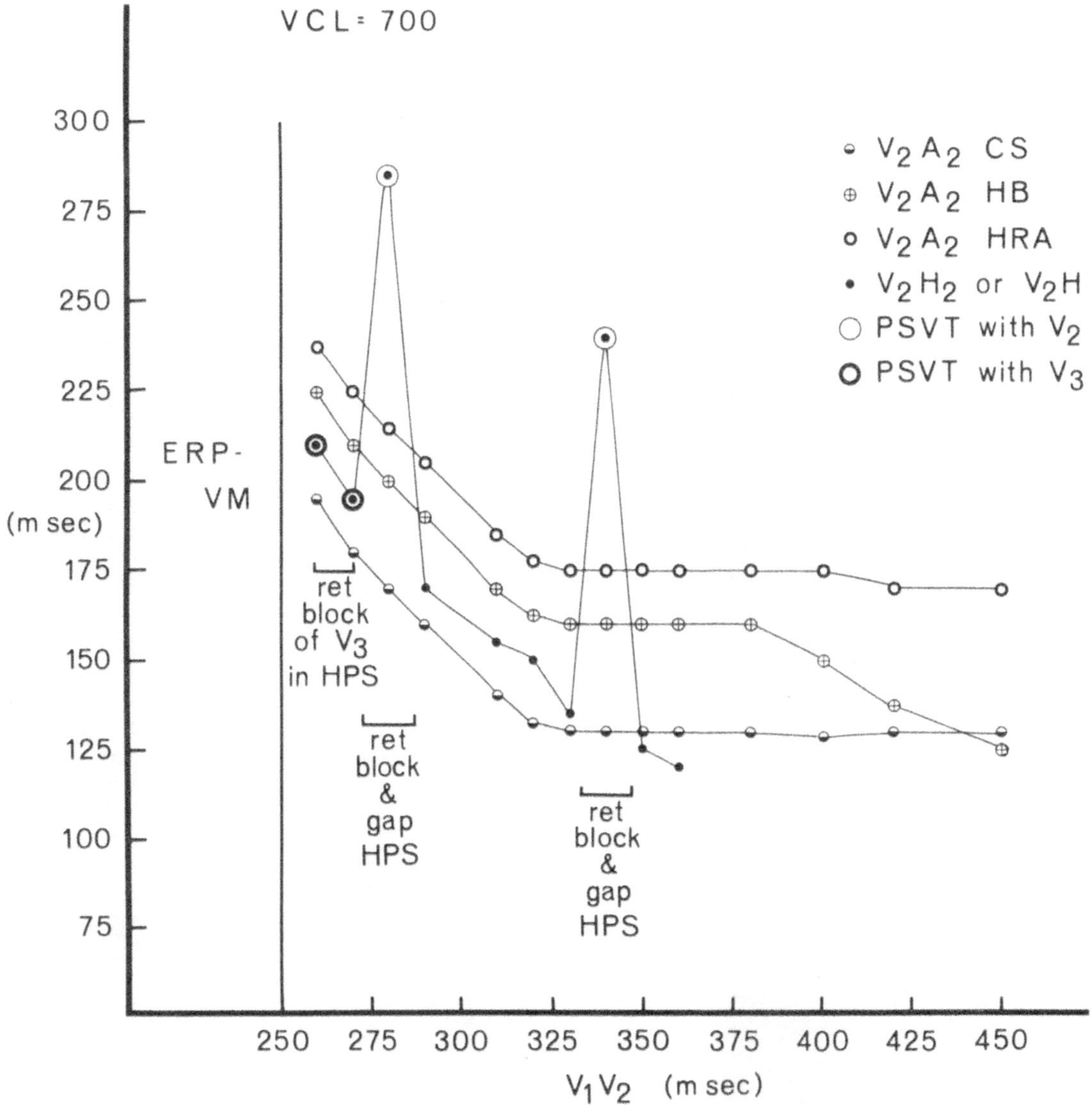

FIGURE 7–2. Retrograde His–Purkinje block and tachycardia initiation. The figure depicts the sequence of events during the scanning of a basic ventricular cycle length of 700 ms with progressively shorter coupling intervals (V_1V_2). All intervals are in ms and the various parameters measured are shown. (See text for details.) Abbreviations: ERP-VM — effective refractory period ventricular myocardium electrogram sites. PSVT — paroxysmal supraventricular tachycardia. CS — coronary sinus. HB — His bundle. HRA — high right atrium. Reproduced with permission from Akhtar et al. Figure 4. *J. Clin. Invest.* 67:1047–1055, 1981.

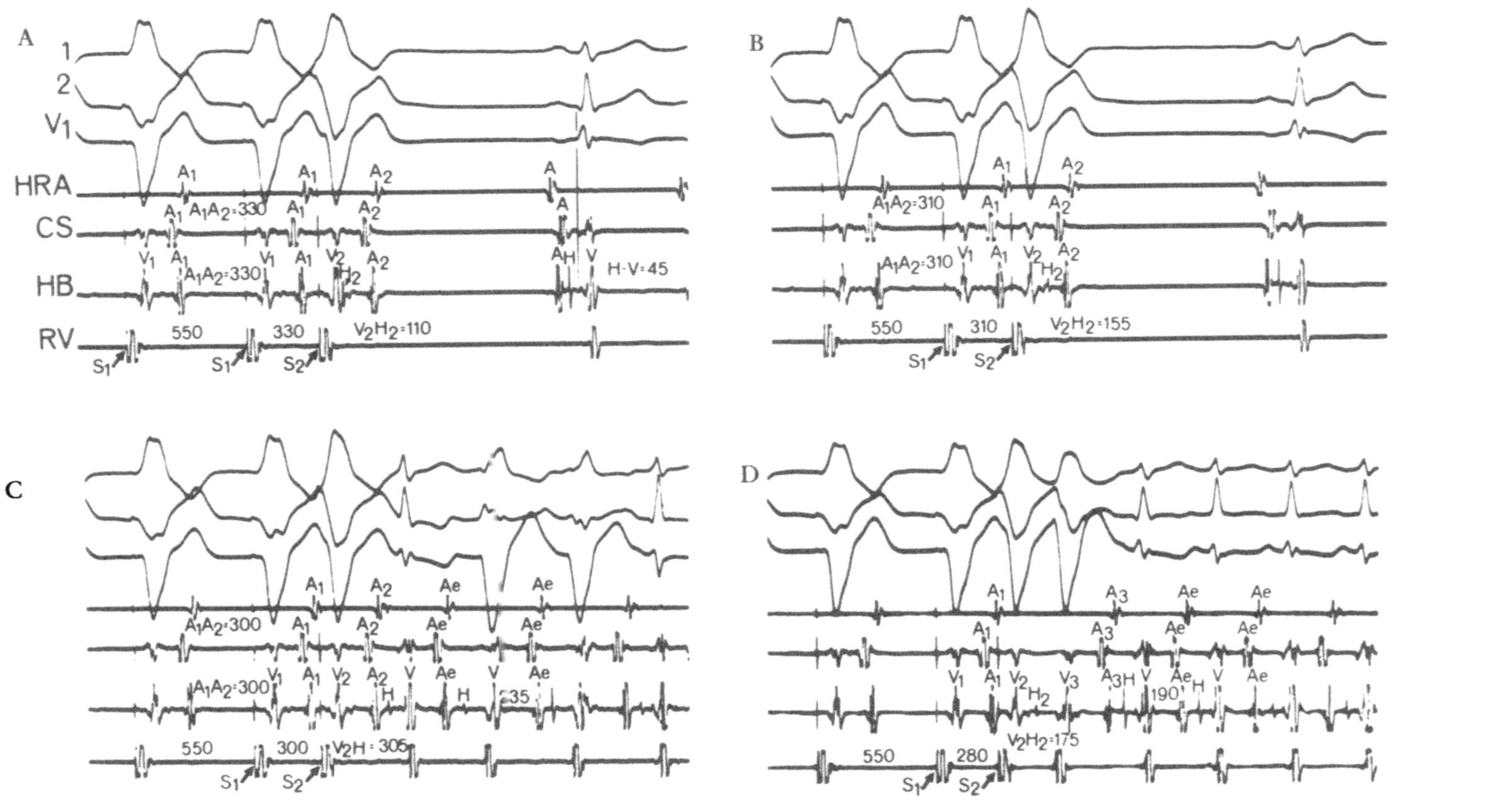

FIGURE 7–3. Retrograde His–Purkinje block of V_2 and V_3 and the initiation of tachycardia. The basic ventricular cycle length is 550 ms in all panels. During right ventricular pacing VA conduction occurs exclusively via a left side accessory pathway and the activation of coronary sinus (CS) precedes that on the HB and high right atrial (HRA) electrogram. At an S_1S_2 of 330 ms (*Panel A*) the V_2 conducts to the His bundle (H_2) via the bundle branches but activates the atria (A_2) via the accessory pathway. At a closer V_1V_2 of 310 ms a further increase in V_2H_2 from 110 ms to 155 ms is noted but the V_2A_2 shows no prolongation such that the corresponding A_1A_2 interval equals V_1V_2. In Panel C the V_2 blocks in the His–Purkinje system, conducts to the atria via the accessory pathway and then anterogradely activates the His bundle to initiate tachycardia. Note the VA interval during LBBB is 235 ms which is 45 ms longer than seen without LBBB (*Panel D*) suggesting a left free wall AV accessory pathway. In Panel D retrograde conduction to the H_2 resumes at shorter V_1V_2 of 280 but V_2 blocks in the accessory pathway (i.e., no A_2). However, V_2 is followed by V_3 due to macroreentry in the His–Purkinje system, which in turn blocks in the His–Purkinje system, conducts via the accessory pathway and starts the tachycardia. Pertinent intervals are labelled. RV — right ventricular electrogram. Reproduced with permission from Akhtar et al. Figure 3. *J. Clin. Invest.* 67:1047–1055, 1981.

induction and a retrograde intranodal penetration of V_2 (i.e., whenever V_2 reaches the His bundle (H_2) and AV node thereafter) abolishes such an initiation. If V_2 produces the H_2 response via the bundle branches the tachycardia occurs only if H_2 is followed by another ventricular response (V_3) which is due to macroreentry in the His–Purkinje system [20,21]. This occurs because V_3 in turn blocks in the His–Purkinje system and conducts to the atria via the accessory pathway to start the tachycardia.

Figure 7–3 shows the tracings taken from another patient demonstrating the onset of tachycardia initiation with a retrograde block of V_2 (Panel C) or V_3 (Panel D) in the His–Purkinje system. It should be noted again that whenever the retrograde H_2 activation occurs (and intranodal penetration follows) tachycardia is not inducible (i.e., Panels A, B and D). The ventricular impulses (V_2 in Panel C and V_3 in Panel D) of necessity must block in the His–Purkinje system for tachycardia to start in the tracings shown.

The observations depicted in Figures 7–2 and 7–3 represent the usual manner by which the tachycardia is initiated during programmed ventricular premature stimulation at the usual basic cycle length routinely tested in the electrophysiology laboratory. We have not encountered a single patient where the onset of tachycardia could be conclusively ascribed to a retrograde block of V_2 in the AV node. We offer the following interpretation of this consistent finding. When the V_2 or V_3 blocks in the His–Purkinje system, the atrial impulse (i.e., A_2 via the accessory pathway) finds the AV node recovered since it is not penetrated by the V_2 impulse and its passage through the AV node is relatively rapid. As the anterograde impulse approaches the His–Purkinje system several phenomena are possible: (1) If the arrival is too early such that the His–Purkinje system has not recovered excitability from V_2 impulse, ventricular excitation will fail to occur and will not be initiated; (2) when one of the bundle branches has not recovered excitability (usually the left due to delayed penetration from paced V_2 delivered in the right ventricle) the anterograde impulse will conduct with a bundle branch block pattern; and (3) if the His–Purkinje system is completely recovered tachycardia will start with the first beat showing no HV interval prolongation or bundle branch block.

Our own experience is that initiation of tachycardia following a retrograde block of V_2 in the AV node is a distinctly rare phenomenon. It is logical to assume that effective anterograde propagation of impulse through the AV node is made difficult by prior intranodal penetration of the V_2 impulse via the His bundle (H_2). A set of circumstances would be required to initiate tachycardia by this mechanism which include: (1) relatively distal block in the AV node to provide longer time for recovery; (2) long V_2A_2 conduction times along the accessory pathway; (3) initiation of intranodal reciprocation producing the first ventricular echo response. It is clear from the data available that such settings indeed are seldom encountered and, hence, one would expect that tachycardia initiation following a retrograde intranodal block will be rare during ventricular extrastimulus technique.

During incremental ventricular pacing it is conceivable that tachycardia may be initiated with retrograde AV node block since a retrograde block in the His–Purkinje system during constant cycle length pacing is presumably not common [3,13,18]. Unfortunately, however, the exact mechanism of tachycardia initiation during incremental ventricular pacing has not undergone a beat to beat scrutiny either. Our preliminary observations indicate that the underlying mechanism of tachycardia onset during ventricular pacing is a function of many factors, the two most important being: (1) pacing cycle length, and (2) temporal relationship between the onset of ventricular pacing and the beginning of tachycardia. When the pacing cycle length is short ($\leq$400 ms) a retrograde block in the His–Purkinje system can occur with the onset of pacing at the prevailing sinus rates if the paced cycle length approaches a value 50% of the sinus cycle length [22]. Retrograde block in the His–Purkinje system typically occurs within the first 3–4 beats and continuation of ventricular pacing after a block in the His–Purkinje system is already established simply maintains this block by intra His–Purkinje interference between the paced ventricular impulse and the anterograde conduction of the entrained atrial impulse (Figure 7–4, Panel B) [23]. At a given paced cycle length a distal migration of the point of interference between the two impulses can result in tachycardia initiation (Figure 7–4, Panel C) [23,24]. If a block in the His–Purkinje system does not occur within three to four paced ventricular

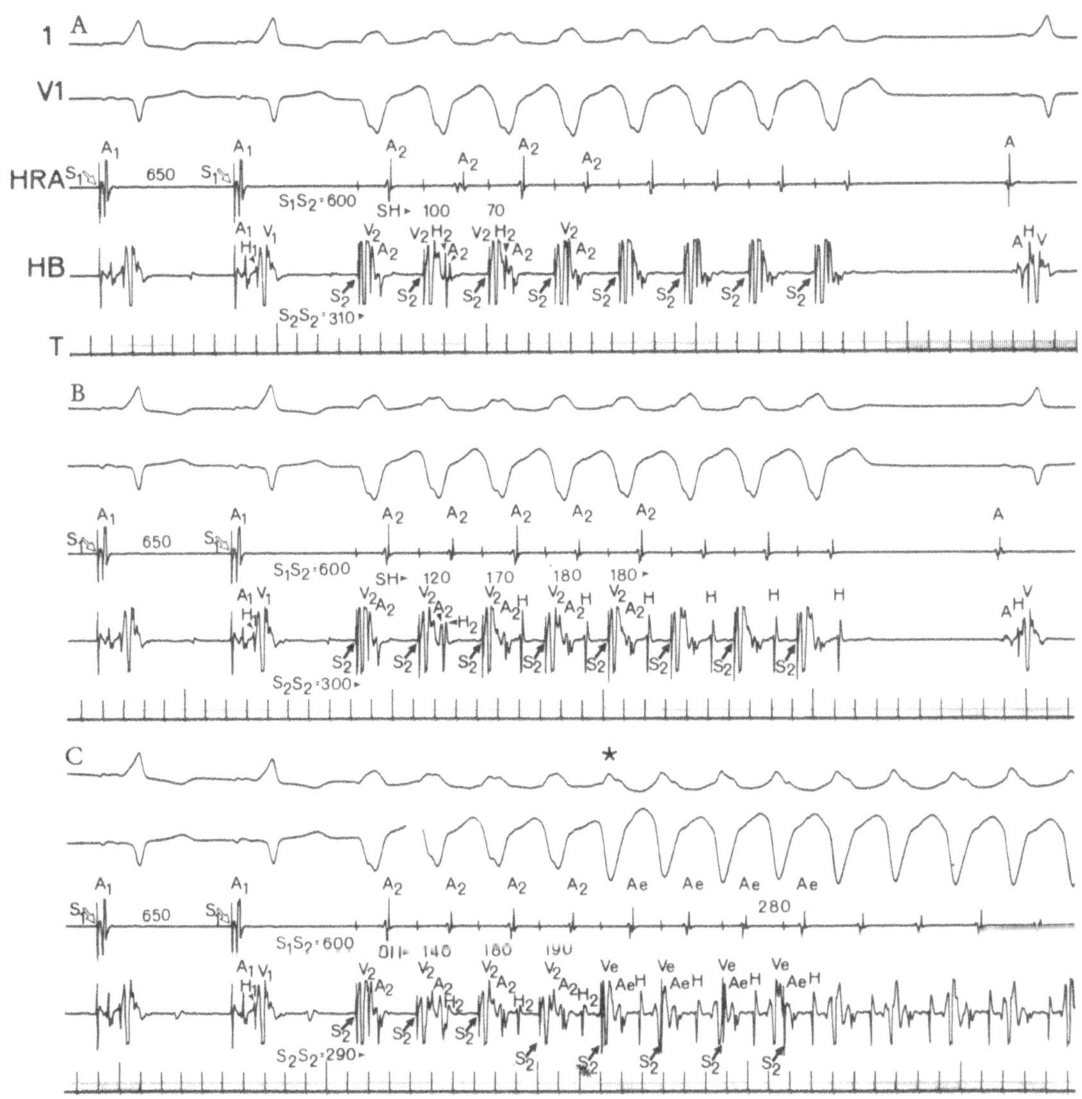

FIGURE 7–4. His–Purkinje system block and tachycardia initiation during constant cycle length pacing. The tracing illustrates a beat to beat analysis of the sequence of events during constant cycle length pacing where prior atrial rhythm (S_1S_1 *white arrow*) and of ventricular pacing (S_2S_2 *black arrow*) and the pause between the last atrial beat and the first ventricular paced beat (S_1-S_2) are all programmed. The S_1-S_1 and S_1-S_2 are constant in all panels and only S_2-S_2 are progressively shortened from Panels A and C. In Panel A slight degree of His–Purkinje system delay is encountered after the 2nd and 3rd paced beat and the H2 deflection can be identified at the end of the local V_2 electrogram. With subsequent His–Purkinje system accommodation the H2 activation merges into V_2 electrogram and can no longer be identified. Panel B shows the onset of retrograde block with the third paced ventricular beat and concomitant retrograde atrial activation via the accessory pathway with subsequent anterograde His bundle activation. From then on interference occurs within the His–Purkinje system between successive anterograde and retrograde impulses. At a shorter cycle length of pacing (*Panel C*) a retrograde block in the His–Purkinje system (3rd ventricular paced beat) is followed by anterograde His bundle activation and with the next paced impulse the interference point migrates downstream along the right bundle and orthodromic reciprocating tachycardia is initiated (*asterisk*) showing a LBBB. Reproduced with permission from Lehmann, et al. *Circulation* 71:254–265, 1985.

beats, His–Purkinje system conduction accommodates and retrograde block is unlikely with the subsequent paced beats [22]. If tachycardia initiation takes place after His–Purkinje system accommodation, the site of retrograde block is generally the AV node.

Relationship Between the Type of Bundle Branch Block and Stimulation Site at the Onset of Tachycardia

Since production of bundle branch block has diagnostic importance and the presence of intraventricular conduction per se can facilitate the occurrence of tachycardia, it would be of interest to learn if there is a predictable relationship between the site of pacing and the type of bundle branch block induced. We recently examined this in 20 consecutive patients with WPW syndrome in all of whom orthodromic reciprocating tachycardia was induced with atrial and/or ventricular extrastimulus method [16]. The overall incidence of bundle branch block was greater with ventricular as compared to atrial extrastimulus technique (79% vs. 39%) at the basic cycle length tested. During atrial pacing right bundle branch block (RBBB) occurred in 4/13 and left bundle branch block (LBBB) in only 1/13. On the other hand, during ventricular stimulation LBBB was noted in 11/14 while a RBBB was observed in one of these 11 cases on one occasion.

The more frequent occurrence of RBBB with atrial premature stimulation is in line with observations in patients without preexcitation syndrome. Higher incidence of RBBB is primarily related to the longer refractoriness of RBBB at the usual cycle length and this incidence can be further increased with abrupt short to long cycle length change and induced atrial bigeminy [15,25].

The high incidence of LBBB following a block of either V_2 or V_3 in the His–Purkinje is easy to explain and is related to delayed recovery of left versus right bundle branch following right ventricular impulses [26]. Retrograde bilateral His–Purkinje block is associated with concealed penetration of both the right, as well as the left bundle branch. The manifestation of this concealed conduction during propagation of subsequent atrial impulse is a function of the proximity of anterograde His activation to the preceding His–Purkinje system penetration which can be roughly estimated by the interval from the initiating V_2 (or V_3) impulse to the next anterograde His bundle activation (i.e., the VH interval) [16]. When the anterograde AV node conduction (i.e., the AH interval) is normal, the VH intervals are generally within the ranges where LBBB is quite likely with the first tachycardia beat. Occasionally the recovery of the right exceeds the left bundle branch and a RBBB may be observed at the tachycardia onset [16]. Longer refractoriness of the left compared to right bundle branch has been previously documented in some patients without WPW syndrome during right ventricular premature stimulation and obviously could also occur in patients with preexcitation syndrome [27].

Conclusion

It can be concluded from the above discussion that His–Purkinje system block plays a major role in the initiation of tachycardia with programmed electrical stimulation. This is particularly true in regard to ventricular pacing where the onset of retrograde His–Purkinje system block is easily achieved and coincides with tachycardia induction. In fact, with ventricular extrastimulus method the induction of retrograde block in the His–Purkinje system is the most common underlying mechanism of tachycardia initiation.

References

1. Durrer D, and Schoo L, Schuilenburg RM, Wellens HJJ: Role of premature beats in the initiation and the termination of supraventricular tachycardia in the Wolff-Parkinson-White syndrome. *Circulation* 36:644, 1967.
2. Gallagher JJ, Pritchett ELC, Sealy WC, Kasell J, Wallace AG: The preexcitation syndromes. *Prog. Cardiovasc. Dis.* 20:285, 1978.
3. Denes P, Wu D, Amat-Y-Leon F, Dhingra R, Bauernfeind R, Kehoe R, Rosen KM: Determinants of atrioventricular reentrant paroxysmal tachycardia in patients with Wolff-Parkinson-White syndrome. *Circulation* 58:415, 1978.
4. Wellens HJJ, Durrer D: The role of an accessory atrio-ventricular pathway in reciprocating tachycardia. Observations in patients with and without the Wolff-Parkinson-White syndrome. *Circulation* 52:58, 1975.
5. Svenson RH, Miller HC, Gallagher JJ, Wallace AG: Electrophysiological evaluation of the Wolff-Parkinson-White syndrome: problems in

assessing anterograde and retrograde conduction over the accessory pathway. *Circulation* 52:552, 1975.

6. Wellens HJ: Modes of initiation of circus movement tachycardia in 139 patients with the Wolff-Parkinson-White syndrome studied by programmed electrical stimulation. In Kulbertus HE, (ed.): Re-entrant arrhythmias. Mechanisms and Treatment. Lancaster, 1977, MTP Press Limited, p. 153.
7. Sung RJ, Castellanos A, Mallon SM, Gelband H, Mendoza I, Myerburg RJ: Mode of initiation of reciprocating tachycardia during programmed ventricular stimulation in the Wolff-Parkinson-White syndrome with reference to various patterns of ventricular conduction. *Am. J. Cardiol.* 40:24, 1977.
8. Benditt DG, Pritchett ELC, Gallagher JJ: Spectrum of regular tachycardias with wide QRS complexes in patients with accessory atrioventricular pathways. *Am. J. Cardiol.* 42:828, 1978.
9. Akhtar M: Electrophysiologic basis for wide QRS complex tachycardia. *PACE* 6:81, 1983.
10. Bardy GH, Packer DL, German LD, Gallagher JJ: Preexcited reciprocating tachycardia in patients with Wolff-Parkinson-White syndrome: incidence and mechanisms. *Circulation* 70:377, 1984.
11. Pritchett ELC, Gallagher JJ, Scheinman M, Smith WM: Determinants of antegrade echo zone in the Wolff-Parkinson-White syndrome. *Circulation* 57:671, 1978.
12. Ohe T, Kamakura S, Matsuhisa M, Hirata Y, Sato I, Shimomura K: Limiting factor for the initiation of reentrant tachycardia in concealed Wolff-Parkinson-White syndrome. *Intern. J. Cardiol.* 3:207, 1983.
13. Akhtar M, Damato AN, Ruskin JN, Batsford WP, Reddy CP, Ticzon AR, Dhatt MS, Gomes JAC, Calon AH: Antegrade and retrograde conduction characteristics in three patterns of paroxysmal atrioventricular junctional reentrant tachycardia. *Am. Heart. J.* 95:22, 1978.
14. Akhtar M, Damato AN, Batsford WP, Caracta AR, Vargas G, Lau SH: Unmasking and conversion of gap phenomenon in the human heart. *Circulation* 49:624, 1974.
15. Denker S, Lehmann M, Mahmud R, Gilbert C, Akhtar M: Effects of alternating cycle lengths on refractoriness of the His–Purkinje system. *J. Clin. Invest.* 74:559, 1984.
16. Lehmann, MH, Denker S, Mahmud R, Tchou P, Dongas J, Akhtar M: Electrophysiologic mechanisms of functional bundle branch block at onset of induced orthodromic tachycardia in the Wolff-Parkinson-White syndrome: role of stimulation method *J. Clin. Invest.* 76:1566, 1985.
17. Akhtar M, Shenasa M, Schmidt DH: Role of retrograde His Purkinje block in the initiation of supraventriclar tachycardia by ventricular premuture stimulation in the Wolff-Parkinson-White syndrome. *J. Clin. Invest.* 67:1047, 1981.
18. Akhtar M, Damato AN, Batsford WP, Ruskin JN, Ogunkelu JB: A comparative analysis of antegrade and retrograde conduction patterns in man. *Circulation* 52:766, 1975.
19. Akhtar M, Damato AN, Caracta AR, Batsford WP, Lau S: The gap phenomena during retrograde conduction in man. *Circulation* 49:811, 1974.
20. Akhtar M, Damato AN, Batsford WP, Ogunkelu JB, Ruskin JN: Demonstration of re-entry within the His–Purkinje system in man. *Circulation* 50:1150, 1974.
21. Akhtar M, Gilbert C, Wolf F, Schmidt, D: Reentry within the His Purkinje system. Elucidation of reentrant circuit utilizing right bundle branch and His bundle recordings. *Circulation* 58: 295, 1978.
22. Lehmann MH, Denker ST, Mahmud R, Akhtar M: Functional His–Purkinje system behavior during sudden ventricular rate acceleration in man. *Circulation* 68:767, 1983.
23. Lehmann, MH, Denker S, Mahmud R, Addas A, Akhtar M: Linking: a dynamic electrophysiologic phenomenon in macroreentry circuits. *Circulation* 71:254, 1985.
24. Charleson H, Estrada A, Denker S, Lehmann M, Mahmud R, Akhtar M: Mechanisms of orthodromic tachycardia initiation during incremental ventricular pacing in Wolff-Parkinson-White syndrome (Abstract.) *Circulation* 68 (Suppl III):III–10, 1983.
25. Denker ST, Gilbert CJ, Shenasa M, Akhtar M: An electrocardiographic-electrophysiologic correlation of aberrant ventricular conduction in man. *J. Electrocardiol.* 16:269, 1983.
26. Dongas, J, Charleson H, Lehmann M, Mahmud R, Denker S, Akhtar M: Electrophysiologic manifestations of retrograde concealed conduction in the human His–Purkinje system. (Abstract.) *Circulation* 68 (Suppl III): III–424, 1983.
27. Akhtar M, Gilbert CJ, Wolf FG, Schmidt D: Retrograde conduction in the His–Purkinje system: analysis of the routes of impulse propagation using His and right bundle branch recordings. *Circulation* 59:1252, 1979.

8. RESPONSE OF ACCESSORY AV PATHWAYS TO EXERCISE AND CATECHOLAMINES

Samuel Lévy
Jean-Paul Broustet
Marc Metge
Roland Cointe
Gérard Faugère
Raymond Gérard

There has been increasing interest in the last decade in the role played by the autonomic nervous system in tachycardia induction and termination [1–3]. Furthermore, recent reports have provided evidence that accessory pathway properties may be influenced by exercise and catecholamines [4–8]. Most of the data available concern atrioventricular (AV) pathways, and we shall focus our discussion on this type of accessory connection which is associated with the Wolff-Parkinson-White (WPW) syndrome. As developed elsewhere in this volume, tachyarrhythmias associated with WPW syndrome include both reciprocating tachycardias and atrial flutter-fibrillation. The changes induced by exercise and catecholamines on both normal pathway and accessory pathway may affect both types of tachyarrhythmias.

Exercise testing in the Wolff-Parkinson-White syndrome

In their initial description of the syndrome, Wolff, Parkinson, and White [9] observed that the typical ECG pattern of preexcitation may disappear during exercise. They stated that "following release of vagal tone by exercise or atropinization, there is a transition from aberrant ventricular complexes to perfectly normal ones." This is well illustrated in their case 1. Isolated case reports [10,11] have also mentioned such possibilities. Sandberg et al. [12] reported findings in a series of patients studied to assess the effect of exercise on the preexcitation pattern. They found disappearance of the preexcitation pattern in 8 of 26 patients (30%), but it is not clear from their report the type of exercise used, or the heart rates achieved. The absence of systematic study using graded exercise testing prompted us to undertake a prospective study both to evaluate the incidence of QRS complex normalization in a series of subjects with WPW syndrome and to establish correlation with electrophysiologic findings.

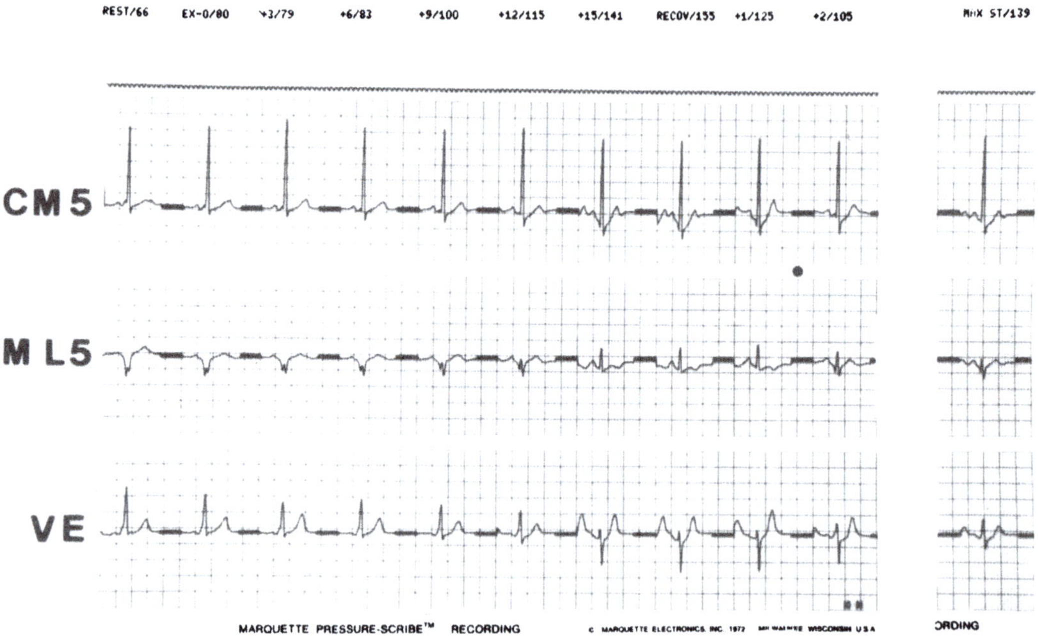

FIGURE 8–1. Exercise-test using the Marquette computerized system and 3 leads CM5, ML5, and VE. Top line indicate time/cardiac rate. Progressive and complete normalization of the QRS complex is shown. As the QRS complex gets gradually narrow and the delta wave disappears, QRS configuration changes. In lead ML5 the QRS complex, exclusively negative, becomes predominantly positive. The reverse in seen in lead VE. Note in lead CM5 prolongation of PR interval and a distinct *q* wave.

INCIDENCE OF NORMALIZATION OF THE QRS COMPLEX DURING EXERCISE TESTING

Normalization of the QRS complex is best defined as the disappearance of the delta wave replaced by a Q wave indicating normal septal activation (i.e., direction of the initial vector). It is associated with normal QRS complexes (in the absence of bundle branch block) and increase in PR duration. Changes in frontal plane QRS axis and changes in ventricular repolarization may also be observed. In our laboratory we have used the following three criteria to indicate "complete" normalization of the QRS complex: (1) clearly defined "septal Q waves," (2) normal QRS duration (3) normal PR interval. When (2) and (3) are present, but (1) is absent, normalization of the QRS complex is said to be "incomplete." A certain degree of QRS complex narrowing together with a decrease in the amplitude of the delta wave may be observed in those patients in whom the preexcitation pattern persists throughout the exercise test.

In our series of 40 cases including 10 asymptomatic subjects, with typical preexcitation, who underwent maximal predicted heart rate or symptom limited exercise-test, 21 (52.5%) had normalization of the QRS complex. A similar incidence was reported by Strasberg et al. [6] who found normalization of the QRS complex in 18 out of their 36 patients (50%).

Table 8–1 shows the results of exercise testing in our series [4] and the series of Strasberg et al. [6]. Different modes of normalization of the QRS complex are illustrated in Figures 8–1 to 8–3. Progressive normalization of the QRS complex is shown in Figure 8–1. The QRS complex gradually narrowed until complete normalization at 12 minutes of exercise. Simultaneously, the delta wave diminished whereas the PR interval lengthened. Sudden normalization of the QRS complex is shown in Figure

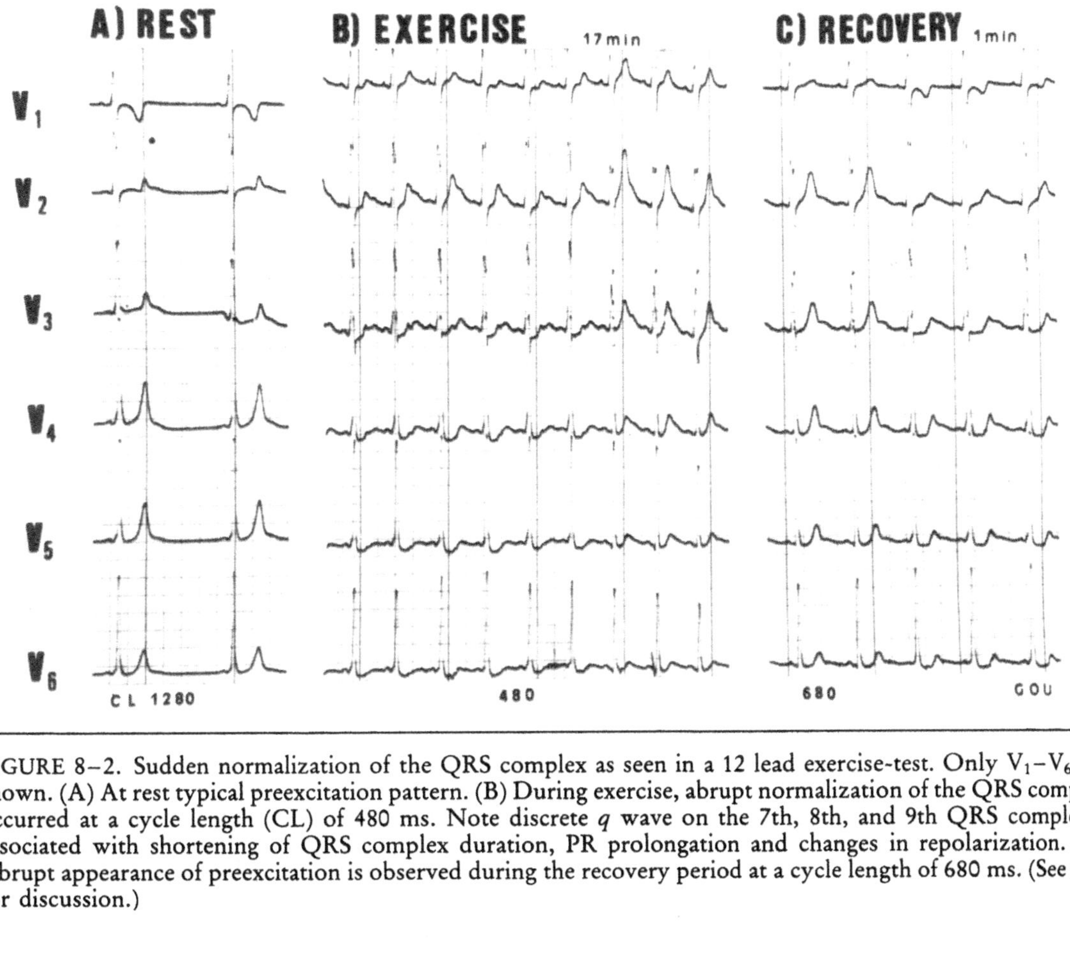

FIGURE 8–2. Sudden normalization of the QRS complex as seen in a 12 lead exercise-test. Only V_1–V_6 are shown. (A) At rest typical preexcitation pattern. (B) During exercise, abrupt normalization of the QRS complex occurred at a cycle length (CL) of 480 ms. Note discrete *q* wave on the 7th, 8th, and 9th QRS complexes associated with shortening of QRS complex duration, PR prolongation and changes in repolarization. (C) Abrupt appearance of preexcitation is observed during the recovery period at a cycle length of 680 ms. (See text for discussion.)

TABLE 8–1. Exercise testing in the WPW syndrome: Incidence of the normalization of the QRS complex in two reported series

	Broustet et al. [4]	Strasberg et al. [6]
Total N° of patients	40	36
Persistent preexcitation	19	18
Normalization of the QRS complex	21 (52.5%)	18 (50%)
Progressive	12	14
Abrupt	4	4
Alternate	2	0
"Incomplete"	3	0

8–2. It may be preceded by a certain degree of QRS narrowing. Disappearance of the delta wave may occur on alternate QRS complexes with 2: 1 block over the accessory pathway before giving way to complete normalization of the QRS complex. Reappearance of preexcitation may follow the same pattern as the disappearance of preexcitation or may be dissimilar. When normalization of the QRS complex is sudden, the cycle length at which the preexcitation pattern reappears is usually longer than that at which it occurs as shown in Figure 8–2. The latter observation suggests catecholamine mediated shortening of the anterograde refractory period of the accessory pathway during exercise [13]. Occasionally, the pattern of disappearance and reappearance of preexcitation pattern may differ at a repeat exercise test (Figure 8–3).

EXERCISE TESTING IN UNMASKING PREEXCITATION

Preexcitation may be exposed by exercise in patients with intermittent or latent preexcita-

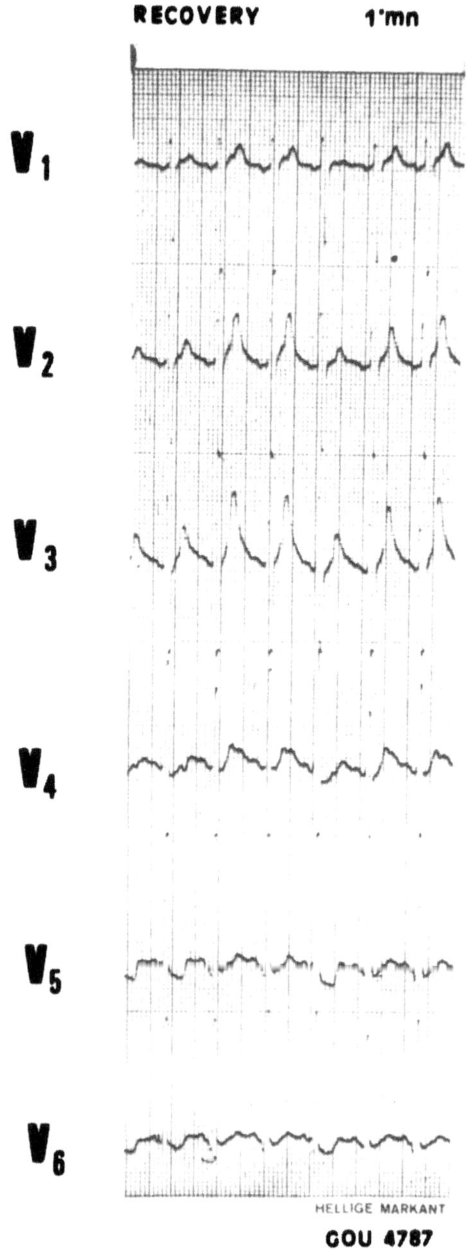

FIGURE 8–3. Reapparance of preexcitation on alternate cycles. (Same patient as Figure 8–2, repeat exercise test.) Preexcitation is present on 1st and 4th QRS complexes. 3:1 block over the accessory pathway occurred before 1:1 conduction over the normal pathway.

tion. Such phenomenon may be explained by facilitation of conduction over the accessory pathway due to catecholamines. An alternate explanation lies in the possibility that the accessory pathway may conduct only within a particular range of heart rates calling in the concept of phase 3 or/and phase 4 block in the accessory pathway. Both mechanisms may play a role. An example of exercise-induced preexcitation is shown in Figure 8–4. Normal QRS complexes were present at rest. During exercise preexcitation appeared on alternate beats before becoming permanent and persisted until the recovery period. Note that the cycle length at which the preexcitation disappeared during the recovery period is shorter than that at which the preexcitation appeared and became permanent, suggesting the role played by catecholamines on accessory pathway properties. Another example of exercise-induced preexcitation is shown in Figure 8–5. Preexcited QRS complexes were present every other beat when the cardiac rate reached 110 beats/min (cycle length 545 ms). The exercise test was interrupted as the preexcited QRS complexes were erroneously interpreted by the operator as premature ventricular complexes. During the recovery period, preexcitation disappeared at a cycle length longer than that at which it appeared. During electrophysiologic study to evaluate the basis of paroxysmal tachycardia, preexcitation with 2:1 block in the accessory pathway was elicited by atrial pacing at a cycle length of 550 ms. Preexcitation was not observed at longer and shorter cycle lengths. Findings in this demonstrate the critical role of cycle length in determining occurrence of preexcitation.

Response of the accessory atrioventricular pathway to exercise

Since little information has been available until recently on the effect of exercise on the anterograde refractory period of accessory pathway in patients with the WPW syndrome, we undertook such a study. The anterograde refractory period of the accessory pathway was measured during sinus rhythm and at the same paced cycle length before and immediately after maximal exercise in 8 patients. Although the maximal amount of shortening was found during sinus rhythm, the variation in cycle length could have accounted in part for such effect (40–180 ms). At the same paced cycle length, exercise

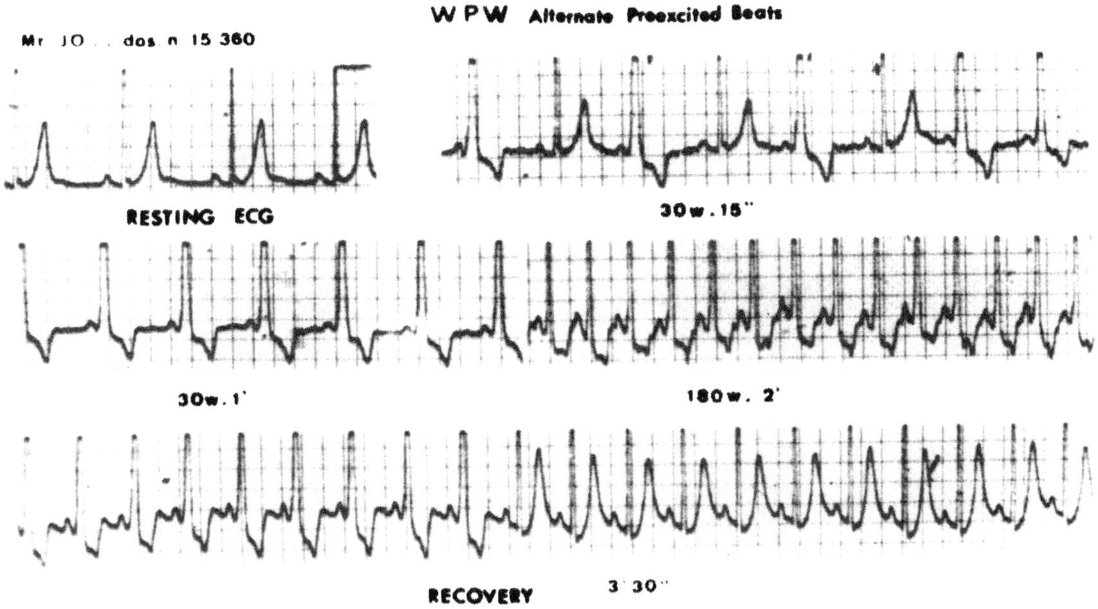

FIGURE 8–4. Exercise-induced preexcitation in a patient with intermittent WPW syndrome. Exclusive conduction over the normal pathway is seen at rest. During exercise, preexcitation of alternate beats preceeds 1:1 conduction over the accessory pathway at a cycle length of 760 ms. Abrupt normalization of the QRS complex was observed at a shorter cycle length of 520 ms. (Taken from Broustet et al. [4] with permission of the publisher.)

shortens initial values by 20 to 105 ms (7 to 35%). As shown in Figure 8–6, our findings suggest a more rapid preexcited ventricular response during exercise should atrial fibrillation occur. Crick et al. [14] studied the effect of exercise in 5 patients and found that the preexcited ventricular response during atrial fibrillation was faster following exercise. The increase in rate ranged 11 to 54% and in 2 patients the rate exceeded 300 beats/min. In contrast, German et al. [15] found that exercise resulted in a significantly lower percentage of preexcited QRS complexes during atrial fibrillation and shortened the mean RR interval. However, exercise did not affect the shortest RR interval between preexcited complexes during atrial fibrillation which is in contrast with our observations and those of others [14].

EXERCISE-INDUCED TACHYARRHYTHMIAS

Although exercise testing is part of the routine evaluation of patients with supraventricular tachyarrhythmias, it is generally accepted that its use in unmasking such arrhythmia is of limited value. In our study of 42 patients with the WPW syndrome, tachyarrhythmias occurred in only 4 (9.5%).

We recently observed [16] in a patient with concealed preexcitation a reciprocating tachycardia reproducibly induced by exercise as shown in Figure 8–7. Electrophysiologic study revealed the existence of a concealed septal accessory AV pathway. The tachycardia could be induced by isoproterenol infusion (Figure 8–8) whereas the latter could not be provoked by overdrive atrial pacing at rate similar to those at which it occurred during exercise suggesting that the role played by catecholamines was essential.

Using programmed electrical stimulation we have been able to induce reciprocating tachycardia following exercise in about 50% of our patients in whom tachycardia was not inducible during the control state. In addition tachycardia cycle length was significantly shorter following maximal exercise compared to control values in patients in whom tachycardia was inducible at

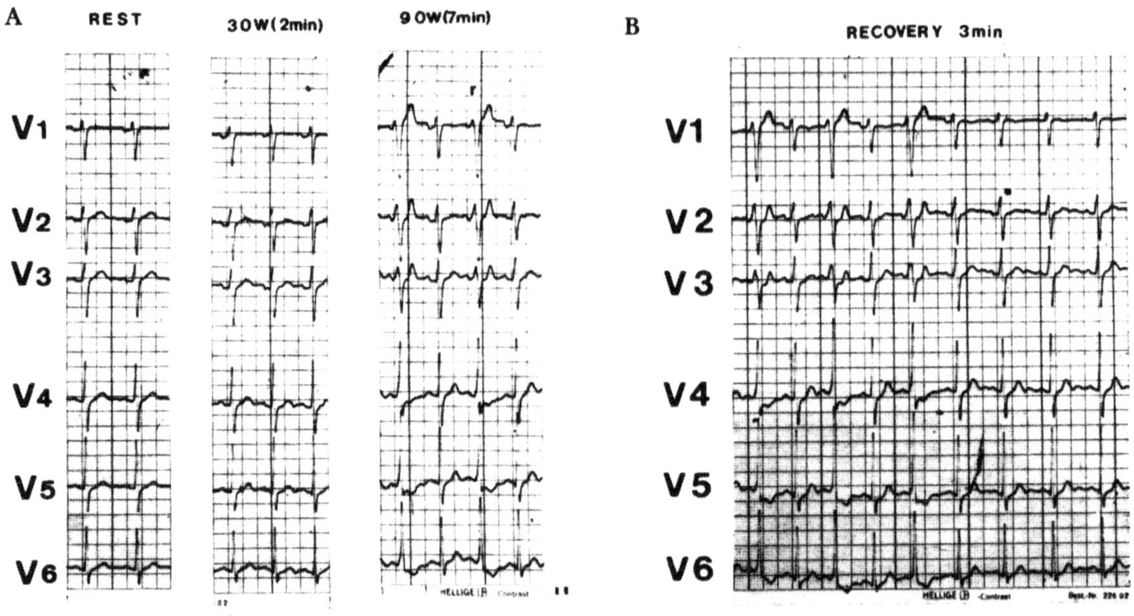

FIGURE 8–5. Exercise-induced preexcitation. (A) Normal conduction is seen on resting electrocardiogram and during exercise (30 Watts 2 min). At the seventh minute of exercise, when the cycle length reached 550 ms preexcitation of alternate beats occurred. (B) As the cycle length lengthened to 640 ms preexcitation disappeared (recovery period). However, the PP interval of preexcited beats (1080 ms) is the same during exercise as during the recovery period suggesting that the accessory pathway is operating at a given cycle length only.

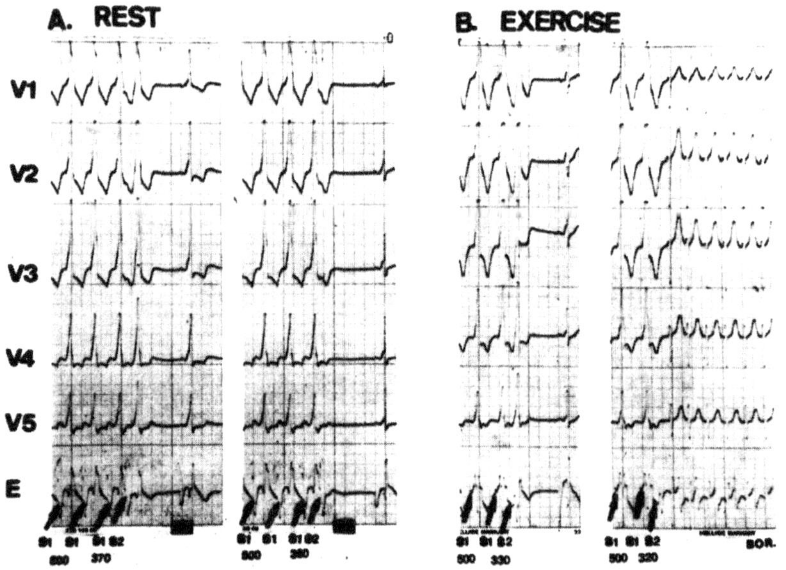

FIGURE 8–6. Effect of exercise on anterograde refractory period of the accessory pathway. From top to bottom peripheral leads V_1–V_5 and endocavitary recording of the left atrium (coronary sinus). Pacing is performed through the proximal coronary sinus at a basic cycle length of 500 ms. A) At rest, a premature stimulus delivered at a coupling interval of 370 ms was conducted through the accessory pathway. At a slightly shorter coupling interval of 360 ms the refractory period of the accessory pathway was reached. Immediately after exercise the refractory period shortened to 320 and orthodromic tachycardia was induced (see text for discussion).

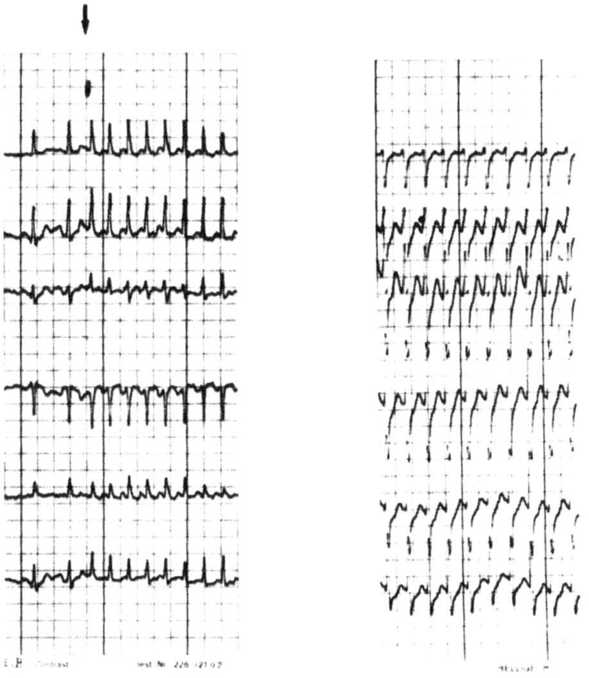

FIGURE 8–7. Exercise-induced paroxysmal reciprocating tachycardia in a patient with a concealed AV accessory pathway. It is difficult to determine if the tachycardia is induced by a premature atrial beat or by facilitation of conduction through the AV node and shortening of retrograde refractory period due to catecholamine discharge allowing a sinus impulse to reach the ventricle outside the retrograde refractory period of the accessory pathway and to induce a reciprocating tachycardia. *P* wave morphology in lead I leads us to favor the latter explanation. (From Lévy et al. [16] with permission of the publisher.)

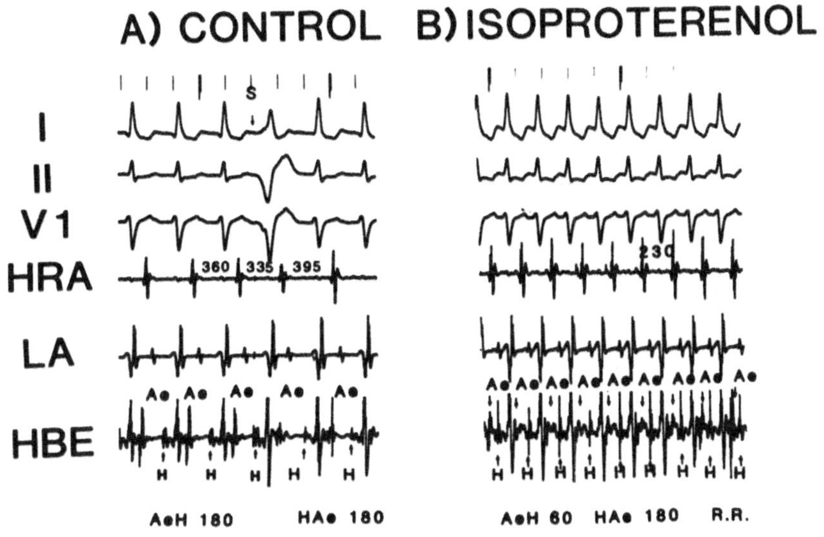

FIGURE 8–8. (Same patient as Figure 8–7.) Effect of isoproterenol on reciprocating tachycardia. From top to bottom are displayed peripheral leads I, II, V_1, and endocavitary high right atrium (HRA) left atrium (LA) recorded through the distal coronary sinus and His bundle electrogram (HBE). (A) Pacing-induced tachycardia during the control state. Septal atrium on the HBE lead is first activated. However, a ventricular extrastimulus S delivered when the His bundle is refractory resulted in atrial preexcitation most likely through a concealed Kent bundle. (B) Isoproterenol induced tachycardia. Note that the cycle length is 230 ms (130 ms shorter than control). Cycle length shortening is due to facilitation of conduction through the AV node whereas retrograde conduction is not affected.

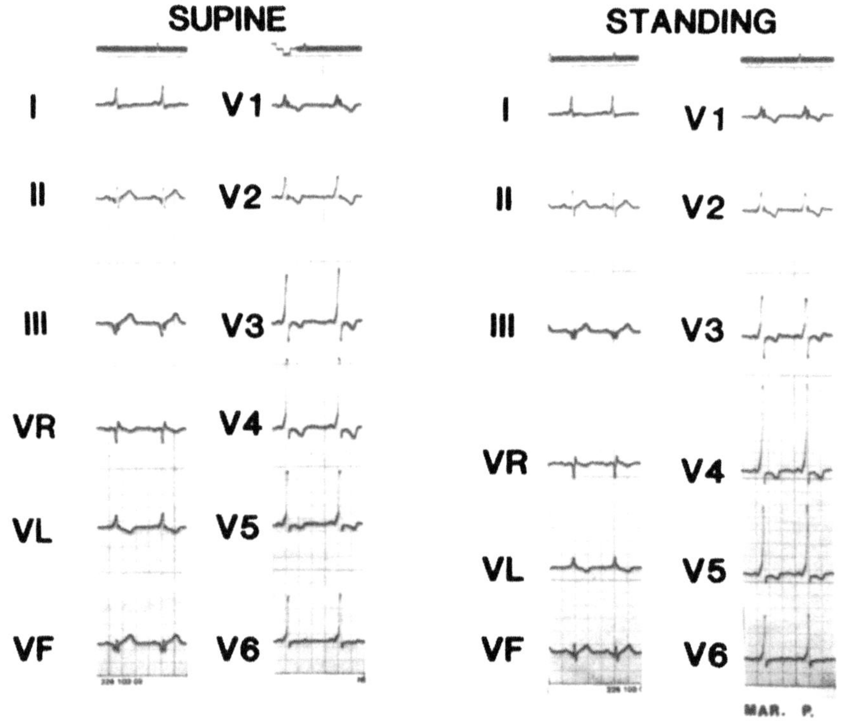

FIGURE 8–9. Effect of posture on the 12 lead electrocardiogram. Note that the QRS complex is 0.15s in lead II during supine position and 0.13 in the standing position. Significant changes of QRS morphology are seen in lead III and VF related in part to changes in heart position in the thorax. Higher voltage of QRS complexes are observed in V_5 and V_6. The cycle length shortened from 720 to 640 ms.

rest. Our findings are consistent with those of Butrous et al. [17] and Franck et al. [18]. Shortening of the tachycardia cycle length is mainly related to the effect of exercise on the AV node whereas VA conduction is apparently not affected.

EFFECT OF POSTURE ON ACCESSORY AV PATHWAY PROPERTIES

In our experience, posture may induce subtle but significant changes in the electrocardiographic features of preexcitation. The QRS complex may become narrower during upright or sitting position as opposed to the supine position as shown in Figure 8–9. The changes are likely related to cycle length variation and to isometric contraction during upright position.

The effect of posture on accessory AV pathway properties has been recently studied by Butrous et al. [17]. They found that standing caused a maximum shortening of 18% of the anterograde refractory period and 35% in retrograde refractory period in patients with refractory periods longer than 240 and 270 ms respectively. No significant change was detectable in patients with refractory periods shorter than these values.

EFFECT OF VAGAL MANEUVERS

It is well known that vagal maneuvers in some patients with the WPW syndrome result in an increase in the degree of preexcitation by prolonging conduction over the AV node–His bundle and by slowing heart rate. In some patients with apparently concealed accessory AV pathway, the preexcitation pattern may be elicited by carotid sinus massage or oculocardiac reflex [19] leading to the concept that concealed bypass tracts may be accessory pathways with very long effective refractory period.

Occasionally, vagal maneuvers may be useful in detecting multiple accessory pathway as shown in Figure 8–10.

ACCESSORY ATRIOVENTRICULAR PATHWAY RESPONSE TO EXOGENOUS CATECHOLAMINES

The effect of isoproterenol on the duration of the effective refractory period of the accessory AV pathway has been studied by Wellens et al. [8] in 7 patients with the WPW syndrome. Using an initial dose of 0.25 μg and an infusion in order to obtain a cardiac "rate" 20 to 30% higher than that immediately before isoproterenol administration, they found in patients with an effective refractory period longer than 290 ms, a decrease ranging from 30 to 80 ms. Of interest is the fact that the amount of shortening was dependent on the control value: the longer the initial value, the greater the shortening. Using a different protocol, based on computation of the amount of isoproterenol according to patient body weight, and pacing at the same basic rate in order to avoid the effect of cycle length variation, we found a decrease of the anterograde effective refractory period of the accessory pathway of 30–90 ms (10–34% of the control values) as shown in Figure 8–11.

Another way of evaluating the effect of catecholamines on the anterograde refractory period of the accessory pathway is to measure the effect of isoproterenol on the shortest RR between preexcited complexes during atrial fibrillation. German et al. [15] observed a significant shortening of the mean cycle length during atrial fibrillation, and a shortening of the shortest RR between preexcited complexes as well as the shortest RR between normal complexes.

SIGNIFICANCE OF THE NORMALIZATION OF THE QRS COMPLEX DURING EXERCISE TESTING

A good correlation has been established between the duration of the effective refractory period of the accessory AV pathway and the ventricular rate during atrial fibrillation in patients with the WPW syndrome [13,20]. The relationship between the duration of the effective refractory period of the accessory pathway as opposed to that of the AV node–His bundle is even more critical as it will, at least in part, determine the ventricular rate should atrial fibrillation develop. Exercise may modify QRS morphology by altering both conduction and refractory periods of both anomalous and normal pathways (Figure 8–12). The influence of exercise may be related to the effect of cycle length shortening and to the direct effect of catecholamines on both conduction and refractoriness of both pathways. Exercise enhances conduction of the normal pathway as shown by shortening of the PR interval in patients without preexcitation. The effect of cycle length shortening on the effective refractory period of the normal pathway varies according to the technique utilized. Denes et al. [21] found that the effective refractory period of the AV node increases when the pacing cycle length shortens. In our laboratory we have observed that exercise shortens the effective refractory period of the AV node independently of its effect on cycle length shortening. The effective refractory period of the AV node was measured before and immediately following maximal or symptom limited exercise. Our preliminary data showed that exercise shortens the effective refractory period of the AV node, by a mean of 60 ms as compared to control values. Normalization of the QRS complex may result from exercise-induced facilitation of conduction through the AV node. This is probably the mechanism taking place in cases with progressive gradual normalization of the QRS complex. Abrupt normalization of the QRS complex suggests rate-dependent block of the accessory pathway. As normalization of the QRS complex occurs in approximately 50% of the patients with the Wolff-Parkinson-White syndrome we postulated that such finding could be indicative of an effective refractory period of the accessory pathway longer than that of the normal pathway. Therefore, the normal pathway could play a role in case of atrial fibrillation. The effective refractory of the accessory pathway and the effective refractory period of the AV node were measured in 14 patients who underwent maximal predicted heart rate exercise test. Our working hypothesis was verified in 12 of 14 patients (85.8%) as total normalization of the QRS complex was observed in 8 out 9 patients with effective refractory period of the accessory pathway longer than that of the normal pathway and persisted in 4 out of 5 patients in whom the effective refractory period of the accessory pathway was shorter than that of the normal pathway. Consequently, normalization of the QRS complex during exercise may detect those

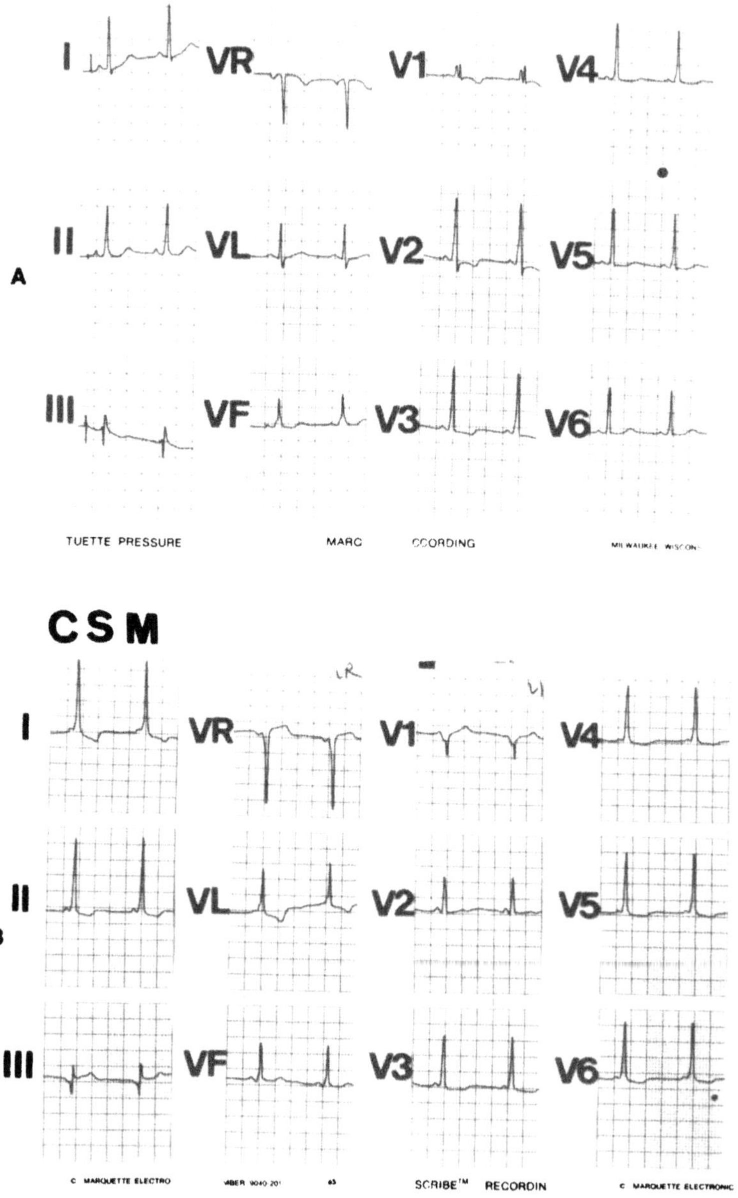

FIGURE 8–10. Top tracing. Twelve lead electrocardiogram of a 15-year-old girl with the WPW syndrome. The delta wave polarity is consistent with a left sided accessory pathway. Following carotid sinus massage or spontaneously the tracing recorded (bottom tracing) is significantly different and consistent with a right anterior accessory pathway. Electrophysiologic study confirmed the existence of two pathways.

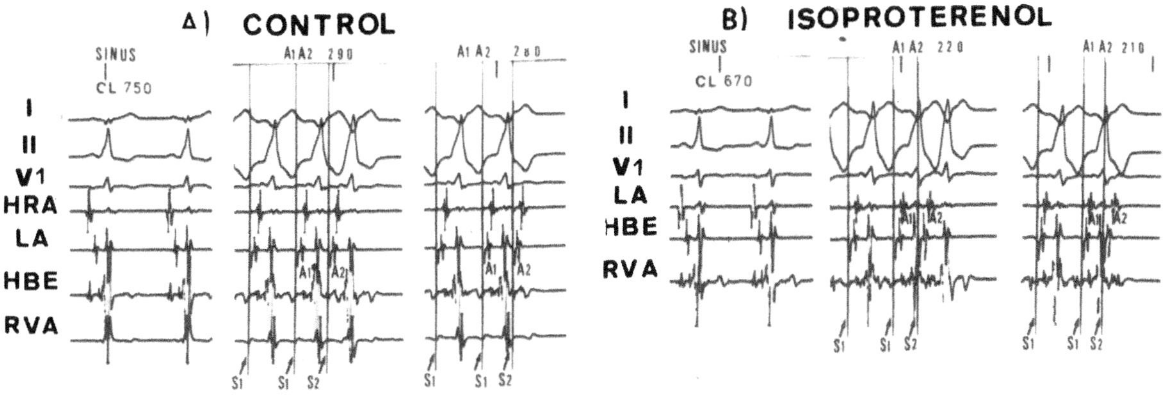

FIGURE 8–11. Effect of isoproterenol infusion on antegrade refractory period of accessory pathway. From top to bottom leads I, II, V_1, HRA, LA, HBE (same abbreviations as Figure 8–8) and right ventricular apex (RVA). (A) Control. The effective refractory period of the accessory pathway measured by pacing the left atrium via coronary sinus at a basic cycle length of 450 ms in a 27-year-old man with a left sided accessory pathway was 280 ms. (B) Isoproterenol. Using the same basic cycle length the anterograde effective refractory period shortened to 210 ms.

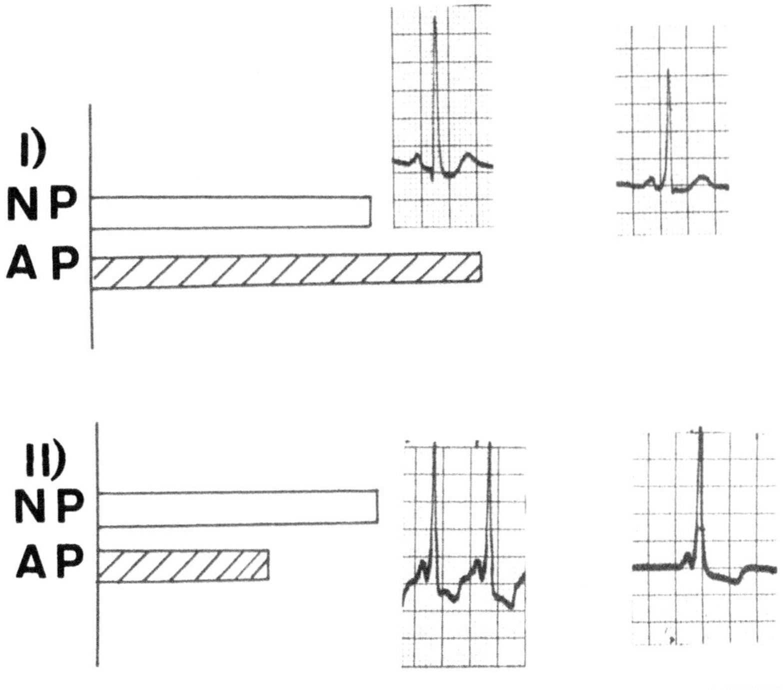

FIGURE 8–12. Working hypothesis on the effect of exercise testing on the electrocardiographic pattern of preexcitation. (I) In patients with anterograde effective refractory period of the accessory pathway (AP) longer than of the normal pathway (NP) normalization of the QRS complex should occur. (II) In contrast in patients with anterograde effective refractory period of the AP shorter than that of the NP the preexcitation pattern should virtually persist. (See text for discussion. From Lévy et al. [5] with permission of the publisher.)

patients with effective refractory period of the accessory pathway longer than that of the normal pathway virtually less prone to fast ventricular rates during atrial fibrillation. Exercise-testing appears therefore a useful non invasive technique providing important information on the properties of the accessory pathway responsible for the electrocardiographic pattern of preexcitation.

Conclusion

The preliminary data on the effect of exercise on accessory pathway properties have improved our understanding of changes in QRS configuration, tachycardia induction, and heart rates during spontaneous as opposed to pacing-induced tachyarrhythmias (reciprocating tachycardias and atrial fibrillation). Further studies are still needed in order to clarify the mechanism of exercise or catecholamine induced tachyarrhythmias.

References

1. Krikler D, Curry P: Atypical initiation of reciprocating tachycardia in the Wolff-Parkinson-White syndrome. In *Reentrant Arrhythmias. Mechanisms and Treatment.* Kulbertus H. (ed.), University Park Press, Baltimore, 1976, p. 144.
2. Waxman MB, Wald RW, Sharma AD, Huerta F, Cameron DA: Vagal techniques for termination of paroxysmal supraventricular tachycardia. *Am. J. Cardiol.* 46:655, 1980.
3. Benson DW Jr, Gallagher JJ, Sterba R, Klein GJ, Armstrong BE: Catecholamine-induced double tachycardia: case report in a child. *PACE* 3:96, 1980.
4. Broustet JP, Lévy S, Vircoulon B, Guern P, Clementy J, Choussat A: Syndrome de Wolff-Parkinson-White. Comportement au cours de l'épreuve d'effort limitée par les symptômes. *Arch. Mal Coeur* 72:625, 1979.
5. Lévy S, Broustet JP, Clémenty J, Vircoulon B, Guern P, Bricaud H: Syndrome de Wolff-Parkinson-White. Corrélations entre l'exploration électrophysiologique et l'effet de l'épreuve d'effort sur l'aspect électrocardiographique de préexcitation. *Arch. Mal Coeur* 72:634, 1979.
6. Strasberg B, Ashley WW, Wyndham CRC, Bauernfeind RA, Swiryn SP, Dhingra RC, Rosen KM: Treadmill exercise testing in the Wolff-Parkinson-White syndrome. *Am. J. Cardiol.* 45:742, 1980.
7. Lévy S, Broustet JP: Exercise testing in the Wolff-Parkinson-White syndrome. *Am. J. Cardiol.* 48:976, 1981.
8. Wellens HJJ, Brugada P, Roy D, Weiss J, Bär FW: Effect of isoproterenol on the anterograde refractory period of the accessory pathway in patients with the Wolff-Parkinson-White syndrome. *Am. J. Cardiol.* 50:180, 1982.
9. Wolff L, Parkinson J, White PD: Bundle branch block with short PR interval in healthy young people prone to paroxysmal tachycardia. *Am. Heart J.* 5:685, 1930.
10. Lamb LE: Multiple variations of Wolff-Parkinson-White conduction in one subject. Intermittent normal conduction and a false positive exercise tolerance test. *Am. J. Cardiol.* 4:346, 1959.
11. S'jongers JJ, Dirix A, Jolie P, Borms J, Segers M: Wolff-Parkinson-White syndrome and sports aptitude. *J. Sports Med.* 16:6, 1976.
12. Sandberg L: The effect of exercise on the electrocardiogram of preexcitation. *Acta Med. Scand.* Suppl 169 (Supp 365):88, 1961.
13. Wellens HJJ: Wolff-Parkinson-White syndrome. In Cardiac Arrhythmias: From diagnosis to therapy. Levy S, Scheinman M (eds.), Futura Publishing, New-York, 1984, p. 287.
14. Crick JCP, Davies DW, Holt P, Curry PVL, Sowton E: Effect of exercise on the accessory atrio-ventricular pathway. (Abstract.) Presented at the International Symposium on Cardiac Arrhythmias. Marseille. 1982, p. 22.
15. German LD, Gallagher JJ, Broughton A, Guarnieri T, Trantham JL: Effects of exercise and isoproterenol during atrial fibrillation in patients with Wolff-Parkinson-White Syndrome. *Am. J. Cardiol.* 51:1205, 1983.
16. Lévy S, Pierron JP, Eisinger JF, Franchi J, Faugère G, Valeix B, Marion J, Gérard R: Tachycardie supraventriculaire induite par l'effort et les catécholamines. *Arch. Mal Coeur.* 78:1431, 1985.
17. Butrous GS, Nathan AW, Bexton RS, Hellestrand KJ, Camm AJ: The effect of posture and exercise on the electrophysiological properties of direct atrioventricular accessory pathways. (Abstract.) *J. Am. Coll. Cardiol.* 3:612, 1984.
18. Frank R, Fontaine G, Tonet JL, Grosggeat Y: Effect of exercise on orthodromic tachycardia induction and termination by pacing. (Abstract.) *JACC* 3:611, 1984.
19. Przybyliski J, Chiale PA, Halpern MS, Nau GJ, Elizari MV, Rosenbaum MB: Unmasking of ventricular preexcitation by vagal stimulation or isoproterenol administration. *Circulation* 61:1030, 1980.
20. Castellanos A, Lévy S, Befeler B, Myerburg RJ: Mechanism determining the ventricular rate in Wolff-Parkinson-White arrhythmias. *Adv. Cardiol.* 14:221, 1975.
21. Denes P, Wu D, Dhingra R, Pietras R, Rosen KM: The effects of cycle length on cardiac refractory periods in man. *Circulation* 49:32, 1974.

III. SPECTRUM OF PREEXCITATION SYNDROMES

9. ELECTROPHYSIOLOGIC CHARACTERISTICS OF ACCESSORY CONNECTIONS: AN OVERVIEW

Ruey J. Sung
Der-Yan Tai

In a fully developed human heart, the atrial and ventricular myocardium are separated by fibrous atrioventricular (AV) rings (anulus fibrosus) which are insulated to cardiac impulses. An atrial impulse is conveyed to the ventricles by way of the normal AV conduction pathway – the AV node–His–Purkinje system [1,2]. The AV node possesses two unique electrophysiologic properties and functions as a protective barrier [3]: (1) delaying intranodal conduction, and (2) serving as a filter to prevent an excessive number of atrial impulses from reaching the ventricle.

When there is an accessory connection bypassing or short-circuiting the normal AV conduction pathway, the ventricle may be excited earlier than would be normally expected. This electrophysiologic phenomenon is referred to as "ventricular preexcitation." Under this circumstance, the protective barrier usually provided by the AV node may be breached and the presence of two AV conduction pathways (normal and accessory) may provide an anatomic substrate for the occurrence of AV reciprocating (circus movement) tachycardia. Based on the findings in anatomic and electrophysiologic studies, Anderson and his coworkers of the European Study Group on Preexcitation classified accessory connections into several forms [4]: (1) accessory AV muscle bundles; (2) accessory nodoventricular muscle bundles; (3) atriofascicular bypass tracts; (4) intranodal bypass tracts; (5) nodal malformations, and (6) fasciculoventricular accessory connections. Some of these accessory connections have been demonstrated to exist only anatomically or electrophysiologically, a few have been demonstrated both anatomically and electrophysiologically, but others are only hypothetical and remain very much debatable.

Electrophysiologic properties of these accessory connections are usually different from those of the normal AV conduction pathway. Due to this electrophysiologic disparity between the two AV conduction pathways (normal and accessory), a bizarre electrocardiographic pattern may occur, and there is a high frequency of cardiac arrhythmias. The electrophysiologic properties of accessory connections vary greatly among patients and are influenced by age, heart rate, autonomic tone, pharmacologic agents, and their anatomic locations. Using the technique of programmed electrical stimulation along with intracardiac recordings, some of the electrophysiologic properties of these accessory connections can be elucidated and characterized. This presentation updates our understanding of the electrophysiologic characteristics of some of these accessory connections.

Benditt, D.G. and Benson, D.W., Cardiac Preexcitation Syndromes.

Accessory AV Connections

Accessory AV connections consist of working atrial or ventricular myocardium bridging the atria and the ventricle. [5–7] These accessory AV connections totally bypass the normal AV conduction pathway and are often called "bundles of Kent." [8] Conduction over most accessory AV connections reveals an all-or-none pattern as conduction is fast and exhibits no refractory-dependent delay [9,10]. In the presence of two AV conduction pathways (normal and accessory), ventricular activation may occur simultaneously over these two pathways resulting in a ventricular fusion beat following an atrial impulse. Fast conduction over the accessory AV connection bypassing the AV node accounts for the short P-R interval and subsequent ventricular preexcitation for slurring of the initial portion (delta wave) of the QRS complex [11–13]. The duration of the QRS complex is usually wide as determined by the degree of ventricular preexcitation. The occurrence of paroxysms of tachycardia associated with this electrocardiographic pattern is referred to as the Wolff-Parkinson-White syndrome [14] — the most common form of ventricular preexcitation.

DEGREE OF VENTRICULAR PREEXCITATION

Varying degrees of ventricular preexcitation with dynamic variations in the QRS configuration can be observed at different times in the same patient. The degree of ventricular preexcitation is determined by the time relation of the two different wavefronts from the normal and accessory AV conduction pathways arriving at the ventricle [15–17].

Ventricular preexcitation during sinus rhythm is often more pronounced in association with right-sided than with left-sided accessory AV connections, since right-sided accessory AV connection are relatively closer to the sinus node, thereby diminishing the time available for fusion via the AV node–His bundle axis to occur. A shift in the location of atrial pacemaker or atrial pacing site can also change the degree of ventricular preexcitation. The nearer the site of an atrial impulse to the accessory AV connection, the greater will be the degree of ventricular preexcitation. A change in the cardiac cycle length may also cause variation in the degree of ventricular preexcitation. Before reaching the anterograde effective refractory period of an accessory AV connection, atrial pacing at faster rates and atrial premature stimulation with progressively shorter coupling intervals increase the degree of ventricular preexcitation (Figure 9–1). This is because progressive lengthening of AV nodal conduction time consequent upon shortening of the cardiac cycle length allows more ventricular excitation to occur via the accessory AV connection. Despite increasing degree of ventricular preexcitation, the atrial stimulus-to-delta wave (P–R interval) remains constant, characteristic of conduction over an accessory AV connection. Finally, vagal stimulation may also be expected to increase the degree of ventricular preexcitation by prolonging AV nodal conduction time, thereby promoting contribution to ventricular excitation via the accessory AV connection. On the other hand, releasing vagal tone by exercise or following administration of atropine facilitates AV nodal conduction and may thus normalize the QRS complex (with disappearance of ventricular preexcitation) followed by prolongation of the P–R interval. These paradoxical effects of vagal influence on the P–R interval in patients with accessory AV connections have been noted since the original description of the Wolff-Parkinson-White (WPW) syndrome [14].

Normalization of the QRS complex with disappearance of ventricular preexcitation may also occur in a variety of situations [15–18]: (1) late activation of the accessory AV connection relative to the normal AV conduction pathway: (2) ineffective atrial conduction over the entrance of the accessory AV connection; (3) enhanced AV nodal conduction (Figure 9–2) and (4) within the cycle lengths at which the accessory AV connection exhibits rate-dependent conduction block [19].

DOUBLE VENTRICULAR RESPONSES

Rarely, an atrial impulse with simultaneous conduction over two AV conduction pathways (normal and accessory) may produce double ventricular responses (1:2 AV conduction) [20,21]. This phenomenon may also occur in patients with dual AV nodal pathways [22] and those possibly with an atriofascicular tract [23]. By the marked difference in conduction time between the two AV conduction pathways, an atrial impulse is able to first activate the ventricle through then accessory AV connection and then reactivate the ventricle through then AV node–His–Purkinje system.

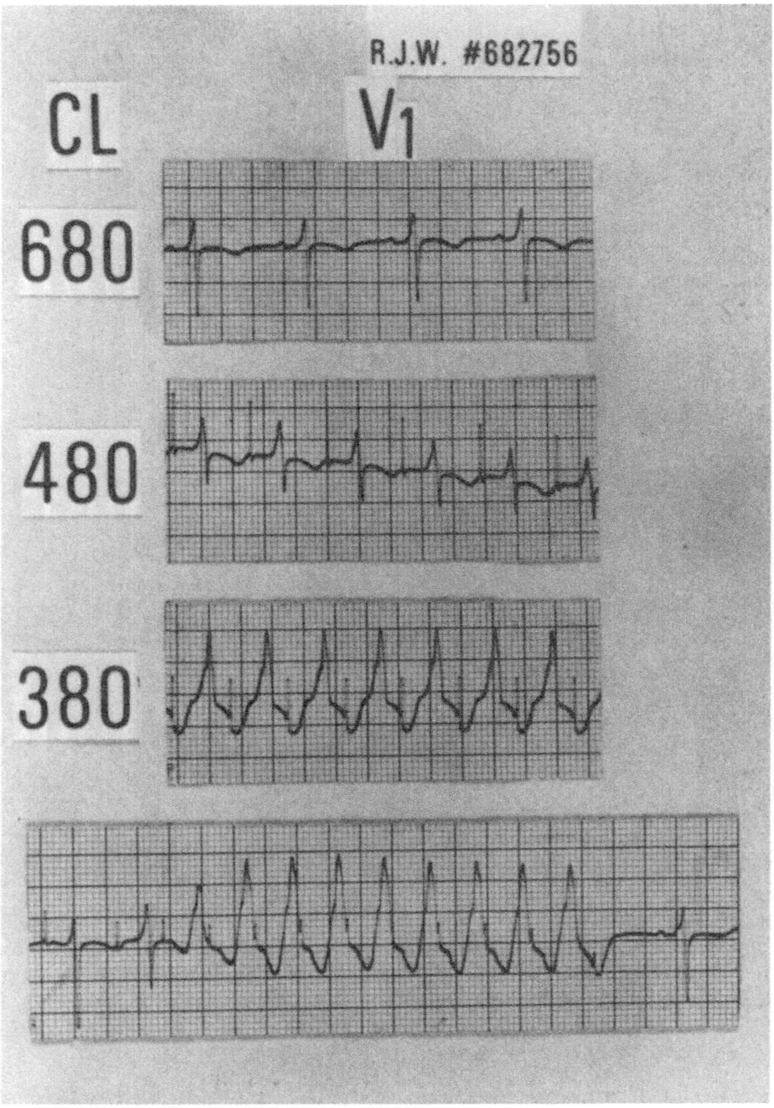

FIGURE 9–1. Increasing degree of ventricular preexcitation during incremental atrial pacing in a patient with a left-sided accessory AV connection. CL = cycle length of atrial pacing. A burst of rapid atrial pacing produces 1:1AV conduction over the accessory AV connection mimicking ventricular tachycardia (*bottom tracing*). Electrocardiographic lead V_1 is recorded.

The difference in conduction time between the two AV conduction pathways must be, therefore, longer than the effective refractory period of His–Purkinje system and the ventricle. Slow conduction in the AV node, minimal degree of retrograde concealed conduction of the His–Purkinje system, and short effective refractory period of the ventricle favor the occurrence of this phenomenon. Repetition of double ventricular responses during sinus rhythm or an atrial arrhythmia may theoretically generate a non-reentrant form of supraventricular tachycardia [24].

ATRIAL FLUTTER-FIBRILLATION

The genesis of atrial flutter-fibrillation is believed to be related to the presence of atrial vulnerability in a diseased atrium, although this

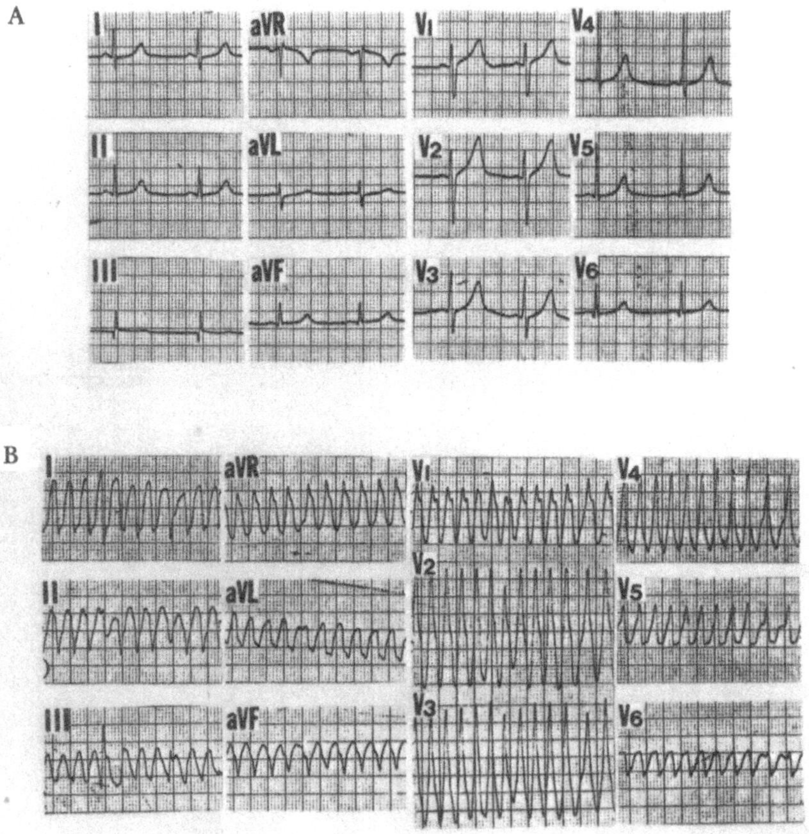

FIGURE 9–2. 12-lead electrocardiograms of a 23-year-old man with a left-sided accessory AV connection. A. During sinus rhythm, ventricular preexcitation is not evident because of enhanced AV nodal conduction [18] (PR interval: 0.12 seconds) confirmed by electrophysiologic studies. B. Same patient as in A. During atrial fibrillation, ventricular preexcitation becomes evident.

may not be the case in young patients with preexcitation syndrome. Electrophysiologically, atrial vulnerability is defined as the occurrence of repetitive atrial responses or a paroxysm of atrial flutter-fibrillation when an atrial premature stimulus is delivered close to the functional refractory period of the atrium (Figure 9–3A) [25,26]. During atrial flutter-fibrillation, three types of AV conduction pattern may be observed: (1) exclusive conduction through the accessory AV connection with a maximal preexcited QRS complex; (2) exclusive conduction through the normal AV conduction pathway with a normal QRS complex and (3) fusion beat resulting from conduction through both AV conduction pathways (normal and accessory).

The rate of ventricular response during atrial flutter-fibrillation is determined by the electrophysiologic properties of both AV conduction pathways (normal and accessory), the interplay between AV conduction over these two pathways, the electrophysiologic properties of the ventricle, and the state of autonomic tone [27–30]. Generally, if the accessory AV connection has a very short anterograde refractory period, exceedingly rapid ventricular responses can develop during atrial flutter-fibrillation, and in some instances ventricular fibrillation may ensue [31]. Clinical studies have demonstrated that the duration of anterograde effective refractory period of the accessory AV connection is of value in identifying patients at risk of developing life-threatening fast ventricular

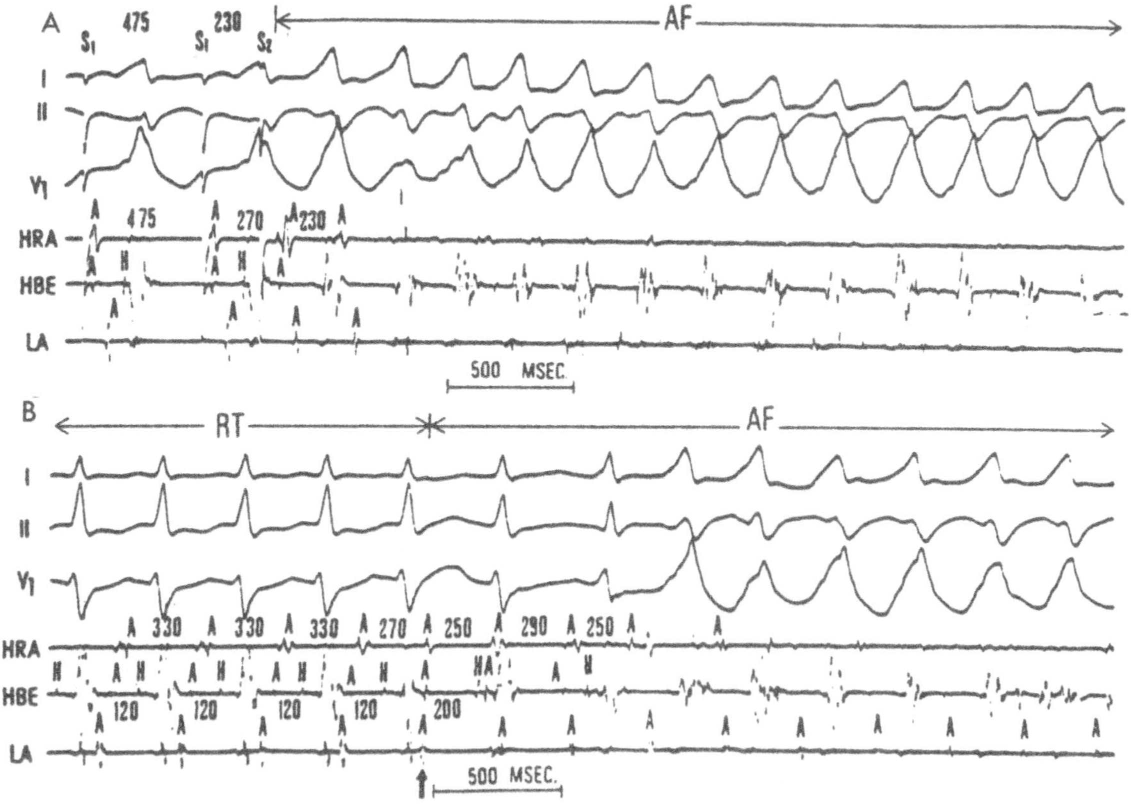

FIGURE 9–3. (A) Initiation of atrial flutter-fibrillation (AF) with atrial premature stimulation during the atrial vulnerable phase. ECG leads I, II, and V_1 are simultaneously recorded with high right atrial (HRA), His bundle (HBE), and left atrial (LA) electrographic leads. The high right atrium is driven at a cycle length (S_1-S_1) of 475 ms; an atrial premature beat (S_2) with a premature coupling interval (S_1-S_2) of 230 ms initiates an onset of atrial flutter-fibrillation (AF) with a mean cycle length of 210 ms. During atrial flutter-fibrillation, the accessory AV connection maintains anterograde conduction for all propagated beats. The corresponding ventricular rate is approximately 290 beats per minute. (B) Spontaneous conversion of AV reciprocating tachycardia (RT) to atrial flutter-fibrillation (AF) initiated by an atrial premature depolarization of the high right atrium (HRA) (*arrow*) (same patient as in panel A). Note that left atrial (LA) activation precedes low septal right atrial (HBE) and high right atrial (HRA) activation during AV reciprocating tachycardia (RT), suggesting the presence of a left-sided accessory AV connection. A = atrial electrogram, H = His bundle potential. (From Sung RJ, Castellanos A, Mallon SM, et al.: Mechanisms of spontaneous alternation between reciprocating tachycardia and atrial flutter-fibrillation in the Wolff-Parkinson-White syndrome. *Circulation* 56:409, 1977, with permission.)

response when atrial flutter-fibrillation occurs [27,28].

Although the genesis of atrial flutter-fibrillation in patients with preexcitation syndrome is not caused by the presence of an accessory AV connection, rapid ventriculoatrial conduction via the accessory AV connection during the atrial vulnerable phase can trigger an onset of atrial flutter-fibrillation [10,32,33]. During electrophysiologic studies, this may be observed while attempting to terminate AV reciprocating tachycardia or while assessing ventriculoatrial conduction using the technique of ventricular extrastimulation or ventricular overdrive pacing (Figure 9–4). A spontaneously occurring atrial or ventricular premature beat with fast ventriculoatrial conduction through an accessory AV connection can also trigger an onset of atrial flutter-fibrillation (Figures 9–5 and 9–6) [33,34]. Clinically, the frequency

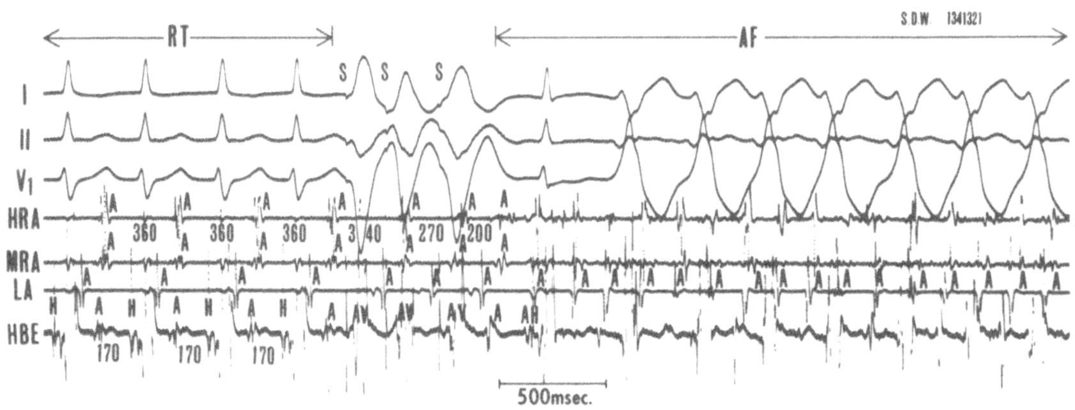

FIGURE 9–4. Conversion of AV reciprocating tachycardia (RT) to atrial flutter-fibrillation (AF) while attempting to terminate reciprocating tachycardia, with ventricular premature stimulation. Note that the sequence of retrograde atrial activation produced by the three successive ventricular premature depolarizations is identical to that recorded during reciprocating tachycardia: left atrial (LA) activities preceding low septal right atrial (in HBE lead), middle right atrial (MRA) and high right atrial (HRA) activation suggestive of ventriculo-atrial conduction via a left-sided accessory AV connection.

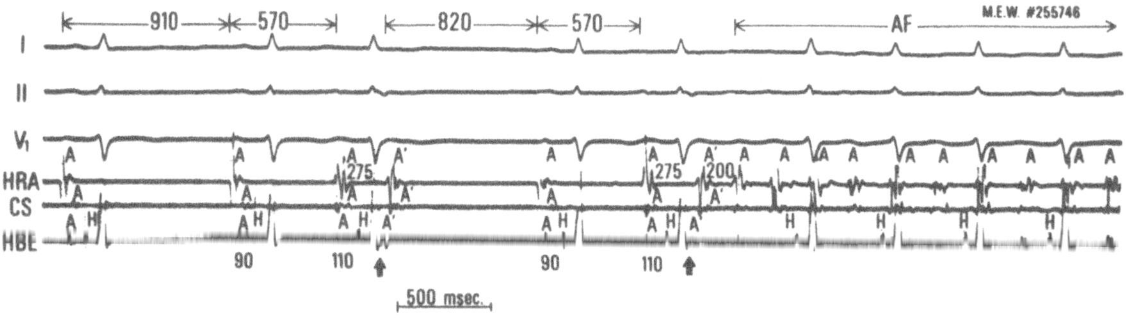

FIGURE 9–5. Atrial premature beat-induced AV reciprocal rhythm and atrial flutter-fibrillation (AF) in a patient with a right-sided septal accessory AV connection. CS = coronary sinus lead; arrows indicate ventriculoatrial activation following atrial premature beats. (From Sung RJ, Gelband H, Castellanos A, et al.: Clinical and electrophysiologic observations in patients with concealed accessory atrioventricular bypass tracts. *Am. J. Cardiol.* 40:839, 1977, with permission.)

with which the onset of atrial flutter-fibrillation is triggered by such a mechanism remains to be determined.

The atrial cycle length during AV reciprocating tachycardia is significantly shorter than that of normal sinus rhythm. Atrial vulnerability is, therefore, expected to be enhanced during AV reciprocating tachycardia especially in adult (i.e., older) patients [25,26]. This may account for the common occurrence of spontaneous conversion of AV reciprocating tachycardia to atrial flutter-fibrillation. Electrophysiologic studies have demonstrated that the abrupt transition from AV reciprocating tachycardia to atrial flutter-fibrillation is usually precipitated by an atrial premature depolarization (Figure 9–3B) [25,35]. The atrial premature depolarization may occur spontaneously during AV recip-

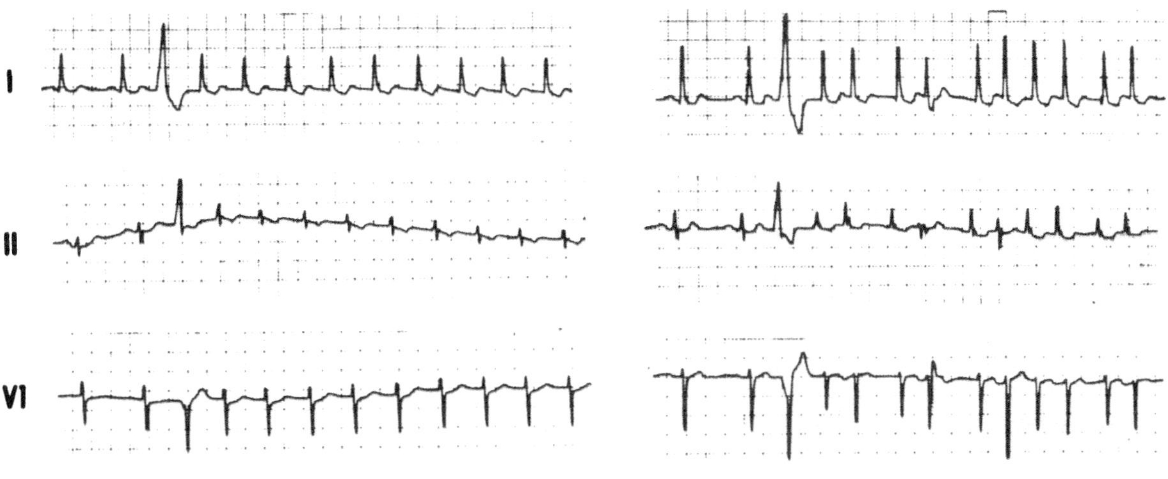

FIGURE 9–6. Initiation of paroxysmal supraventricular tachycardia and atrial fibrillation by spontaneous ventricular premature beats in a patient with concealed Wolff-Parkinson-White syndrome. Left panel: During sinus rhythm at a cycle length of 650 ms, a ventricular premature beat (3rd QRS complex) with a premature coupling interval of 400 ms initiates an onset of supraventricular tachycardia (cycle length 450 ms). Right panel: During sinus rhythm at a cycle length of 700 ms, a ventricular premature beat (3rd QRS complex) with a premature coupling interval of 340 msec precipitates an onset of atrial fibrillation. (From Shen EN and Sung RJ: Initiation of atrial fibrillation by spontaneous ventricular premature beats in concealed Wolff-Parkinson-White syndrome. *Am. Heart J.* 103:911, 1982, with permission.)

rocating tachycardia [36], but may also occur because of (1) the presence of multiple accessory AV connections allowing ventriculoatrial conduction over different conduction pathways during AV reciprocating tachycardia and (2) the occurrence of sinoatrial, AV nodal, or intra-atrial reentry. Additionally, the possibility of mechanical atrial irritation induced by electrode catheter movement should be considered if conversion of AV reciprocating tachycardia to atrial flutter-fibrillation occurs during electrophysiologic studies.

AV RECIPROCATING TACHYCARDIA

The atrium, the two AV conduction pathways (normal and accessory), and the ventricle constitute a reentrant circuit. A premature atrial or ventricular beat can initiate AV reciprocating (circus movement) tachycardia as a result of differences in the electrophysiologic properties of the two AV conduction pathways [37,38]. In most instances, an AV reciprocating tachycardia utilizes the normal AV conduction pathway for anterograde conduction and the accessory AV connection for retrograde conduction — the orthodromic form [38]. The initiation of this form of AV reciprocating tachycardia during programmed atrial stimulation is usually related to anterograde block of an atrial premature beat in the accessory AV connection (Figure 9–7), since the anterograde effective refractory period of the accessory AV connection is usually longer than that of the normal AV conduction pathway. Conversely, the initiation of the orthodromic form of AV reciprocating tachycardia during programmed ventricular stimulation is frequently associated with retrograde block of a ventricular premature beat in the normal AV conduction pathway. This is because the retrograde effective refractory period of the accessory AV connection is usually shorter than that of the normal AV conduction pathway. During AV reciprocating tachycardia of the orthodromic form, the QRS complex is normal unless there is development of functional bundle branch block.

An AV reciprocating tachycardia with a conduction circuit of the reverse direction is uncommon — the antidromic form [39]. During the antidromic form of AV reciprocating tachycardia , the accessory AV connection is used for anterograde conduction and the normal AV

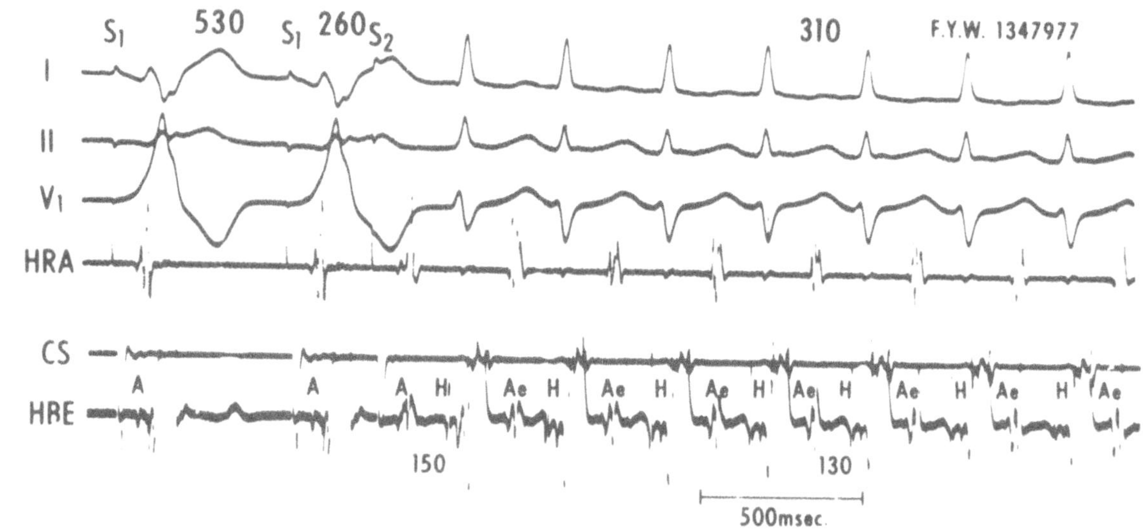

FIGURE 9–7. Initiation of AV reciprocating tachycardia with programmed atrial extrastimulation in the Wolf-Parkinson-White syndrome. ECG leads I, II, and V_1 are simultaneously recorded with high right atrial (HRA), coronary sinus (CS), and His bundle (HBS) electrographic leads. The coronary sinus (CS) is driven at a cycle length (S_1–S_1) of 530 ms. Note ventricular preexcitation with a positive QRS deflection in V_1 during the atrial-paced rhythm (1st and 2nd QRS complexes), suggesting the presence of a left-sided accessory AV connection. An atrial premature beat (S_2) with a premature coupling interval (S_1–S_2) of 260 ms fails to conduct over the accessory AV connection but conducts slowly to the ventricle by way of the normal AV pathway (AV node–His–Purkinje system). The sudden disappearance of the ventricular preexcitation pattern is followed by prolongation of the PR interval, normal QRS complex, and an onset of AV reciprocating tachycardia with a cycle length of 310 ms. During tachycardia, the AV node–His–Purkinje system is used for anterograde conduction, and the left-sided accessory AV connection is used for retrograde conduction (left atrial activation precedes low septal right atrial and high right atrial activation during retrograde atrial activation). A = atrial electrogram; H = His bundle electrogram; A_e = atrial echo.

conduction pathway is used for retrograde conduction. To initiate this form of AV reciprocating tachycardia with programmed atrial stimulation, an atrial premature beat should first fail to conduct over the normal AV conduction pathway as the anterograde effective refractory period of the normal AV conduction pathway is longer than that of the accessory AV connection. Conversely, to initiate the antidromic form of AV reciprocating tachycardia with programmed ventricular stimulation, a ventricular premature beat should first fail to conduct over the accessory AV connection as the retrograde effective refractory period of the normal AV conduction pathway is shorter than that of the accessory AV connection. During the antidromic form of AV reciprocating tachycardia, the QRS complex shows maximal degree of ventricular preexcitation. However, differential diagnoses should include (1) atrial flutter with 1:1 conduction over the accessory AV connection; (2) atrial tachycardia with ventricular preexcitation; (3) ventricular tachycardia; (4) reciprocating tachycardia using an accessory nodoventricular connection for anterograde conduction; (5) AV reciprocating tachycardia involving two accessory AV connections; and (6) AV nodal reentrant tachycardia with "bystander" ventricular excitation over an accessory AV connection [40,41]. Electrophysiologic studies are often required to make a definitive diagnosis.

AV reciprocating tachycardia incorporating two or more accessory AV connections is exceedingly rare [42–44]. The tachycardia (circus movement) uses one accessory AV connection for anterograde conduction and another accessory AV connection for retrograde conduction.

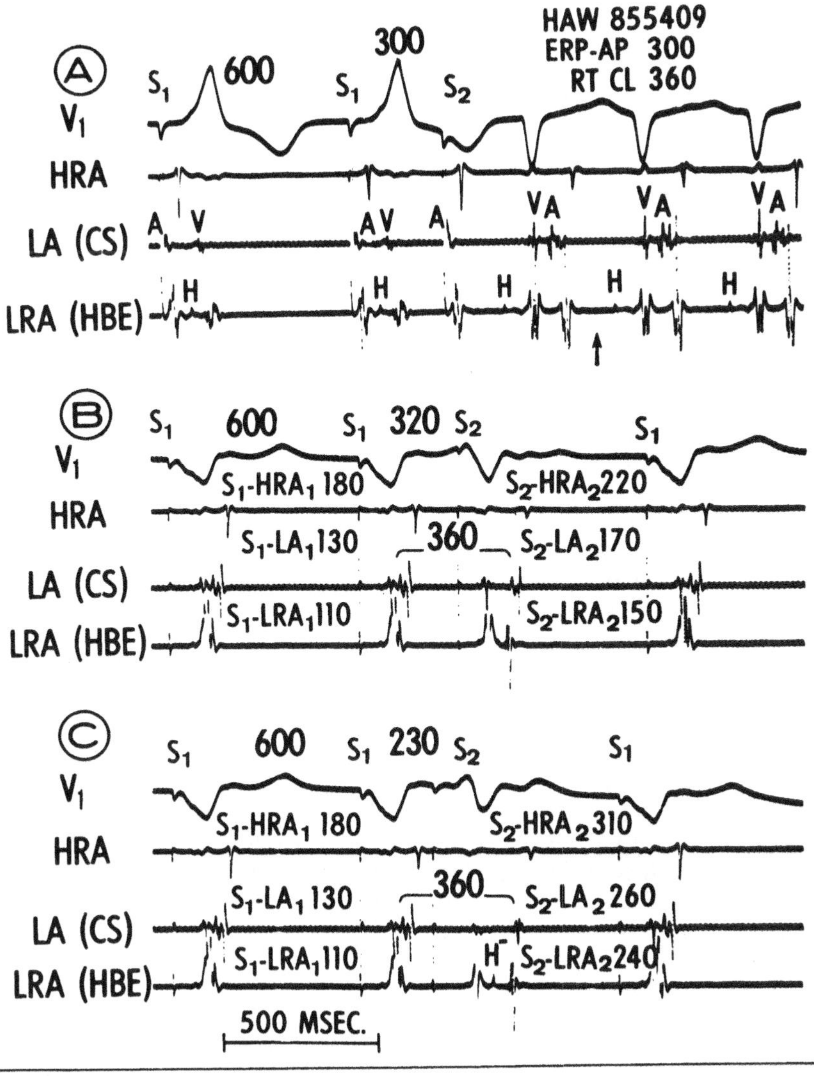

FIGURE 9–8. (A) During left atrial (LA) pacing (S_1-S_1) at a cycle length (CL) of 600 ms, a premature atrial coupling interval (S_1-S_2) of 300 ms results in the disappearance of ventricular preexcitation and initiates reciprocating tachycardia (RT) (*arrow*). Thus, the anterograde effective refractory period (ERP) of the accessory pathway (AP) is 300 ms ($LA_1-LA_2 = S_1-S_2$). The tall R wave in lead V_1 during left atrial pacing and the sequence of atrial activation during reciprocating tachycardia suggest that the accessory pathway is left-sided. (B, C) During right ventricular pacing (S_1-S_1) at a cycle length of 600 ms, there is progressive lengthening of V-A conduction time at all three atrial recording sites (low septal right atrium, LRA; left atrium, LA; and high right atrium, HRA) in response to increasing prematurity of ventricular coupling intervals (S_1-S_2). The low septal right atrium (in His bundle electrographic lead, HBE) is constantly activated 20 and 70 msec before the left atrium and high right atrium, respectively, suggestive of retrograde conduction over the normal pathway. Note LA_1-LA_2 intervals at S_1-S_2 of both 320 and 230 ms are 360 ms, which is beyond the anterograde effective refractory period of the accessory pathway at a comparable cycle length of 600 ms; however, no reciprocating tachycardia is elicited. It is assumed that retrograde concealed conduction of the accessory pathway in response to the ventricular premature beat prevents the transmission of the impulse across the accessory pathway in an anterograde direction. H^- = retrograde His bundle potential. (From Sung RJ, Castellanos A, Mallon SM, et al.: Mode of initiation of reciprocating tachycardia during programmed ventricular stimulation in the Wolff-Parkinson-White syndrome. With reference to various patterns of ventriculoatrial conduction. *Am. J. Cardiol.* 40:24, 1977, with permission.)

The QRS complex also shows maximal preexcitation. Several combinations of reentrant circuits may occur if the normal AV conduction pathway is also involved, and several forms of tachycardia [44] can be initiated in the same patient.

VENTRICULOATRIAL CONDUCTION

In response to increasing prematurity of a ventricular premature beat, retrograde conduction time over the normal AV conduction pathway gradually lengthens, whereas it remains relatively constant over an accessory AV connection [17,45]. Four patterns of ventriculoatrial conduction may be induced during programmed ventricular stimulation and these patterns determine the inducibility of AV reciprocating tachycardia from the venticle [46]: (1) total absence of ventriculoatrial conduction due to retrograde block in both normal and accessory AV conduction pathways — AV reciprocating tachycardia cannot be elicited; (2) persistent retrograde atrial fusion secondary to conduction wave-fronts from both AV conduction pathways with identical retrograde effective refractory periods — AV reciprocating tachycardia cannot be elicited; and (3) predominant or exclusive retrograde atrial activation from the normal AV conduction pathway (Figures 9–8 and 9–9) — rarely, the antidromic form of AV reciprocating tachycardia may be elicited, and (4) predominant or exclusive retrograde atrial activation from the accessory AV conduction pathway — the orthodromic form of AV reciprocating tachycardia may be elicited (Figures 9–10, 9–12).

During programmed ventricular stimulation, the induction of a sustained episode of the orthodromic form of AV reciprocating tachycardia requires (1) an accessory AV connection capable of conduction in the ventriculoatrial direction and having a relatively short effective refractory period compared to that of the AV node–His bundle; (2) minimal retrograde concealed conduction in the normal AV conduction pathway; and (3) the AV node with sufficient conduction delay and a short anterograde effective refractory period. On the other hand, the induction of a sustained episode of the antidromic form of AV reciprocating tachycardia requires (1) the normal AV conduction pathway with a short retrograde effective refractory period; (2) minimal retrograde concealed conduction in the accessory AV connection; and (3) the AV node with sufficient retrograde conduction delay and/or the accessory AV connection with a short anterograde effective refractory period. Retrograde concealed conduction in the accessory AV connection in response to ventricular premature stimulation often precludes anterograde impulse transmission over the accessory AV connection and thereby prevents the initiation of the antidromic form of AV reciprocating tachycardia [46]. (See Figures 9–8 and 9–9.)

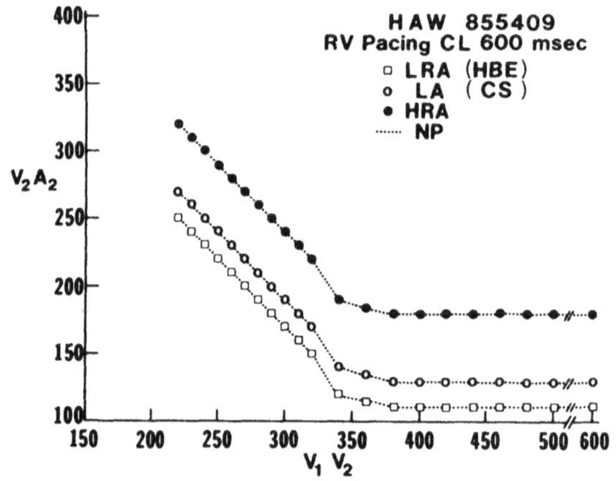

FIGURE 9–9. Same patient as in Figure 9–8. Retrograde conduction time of premature ventricular beats (V_2-A_2) as a function of premature coupling intervals (V_1-V_2) demonstrating exclusive ventriculoatrial conduction through the normal pathway (NP). Note the progressive lengthening of retrograde atrial activation time in three atrial recording sites (high right atrium, HRA; left atrium, LA; low septal right atrium, LRA). CL = cycle length; CS = coronary sinus; HBE = His bundle electrographic lead; RV = right ventricule. (From Sung RJ, Castellanos A, Mallon SM, et al.: Mode of initiation of reciprocating tachycardia during programmed ventricular stimulation in the Wolff-Parkinson-White syndrome. With reference to various patterns of ventriculoatrial conduction. *Am. J. Cardiol.* 40:24, 1977, with permission.)

ACCESSORY AV CONNECTIONS CAPABLE ONLY OF RETROGRADE CONDUCTION (CONCEALED ACCESSORY AV CONNECTION)

The classical electrocardiographic features of ventricular preexcitation (a short PR interval

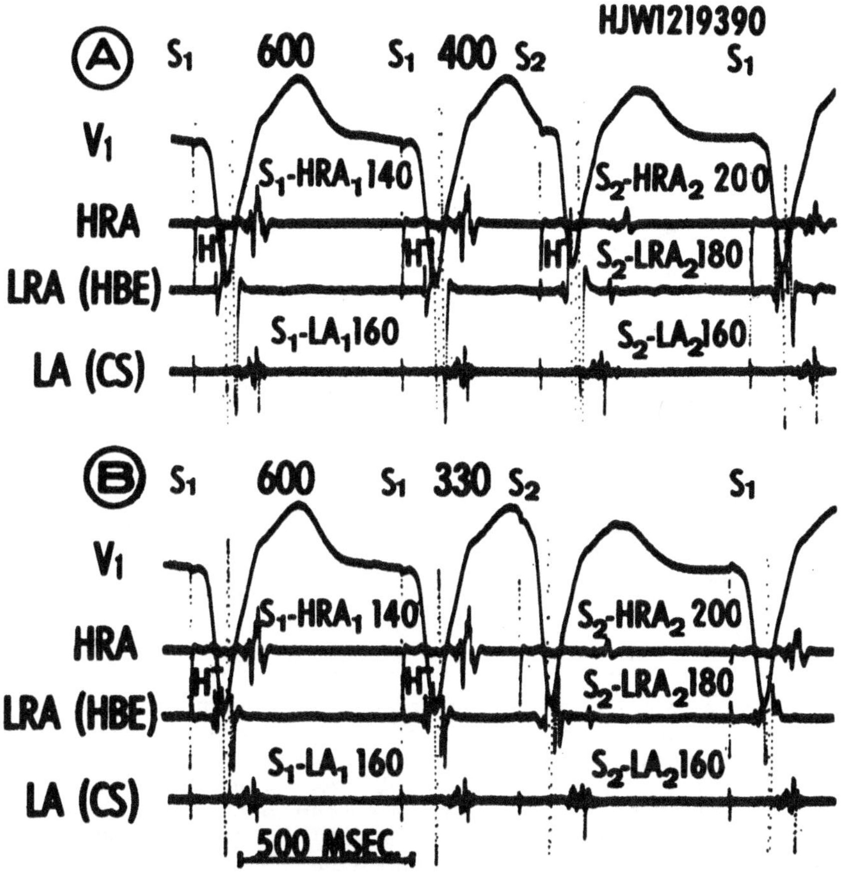

FIGURE 9–10. During right ventricular pacing (S_1-S_1) at a cycle length of 600 ms, high right atrial (HRA) activation precedes left atrial (LA) activation by 20 ms (S_1-HAR_1 = 140 ms, S_1-LA_1 = 160 ms). However, when the premature coupling interval (S_1-S_2) is shortened to 400 ms (A) or less (B), the low septal right atrial (LRA) electrogram (in the His bundle electrographic lead, HBE) becomes discernible. The sequence of atrial activation then reveals that the left atrium was constantly activated 20 and 40 ms, respectively, before the low septal right atrium and the high right atrium, suggestive of a shift in the pattern of ventriculoatrial conduction from retrograde atrial fusion to the one of exclusive retrograde atrial activation through a left-sided accessory pathway. (From Sung RJ, Castellanos A, Mallon SM, et al.: Mode of initiation of reciprocating tachycardia during programmed ventricular stimulation in the Wolff-Parkinson-White syndrome. With reference to various patterns of ventriculoatrial conduction. *Am. J. Cardiol.* 40:24, 1977, with permission.)

and a broad QRS complex with a delta wave) are absent in patients with accessory AV connections capable only of retrograde conduction (anterograde unidirectional block). Such patients are also prone to development of paroxysmal supraventricular tachycardia and atrial flutter-fibrillation and are often referred to as having the concealed WPW syndrome [33,47–49].

During electrophysiologic studies, neither right nor left atrial pacing could produce ventricular preexcitation. However, the sequence of retrograde atrial activation and retrograde AV conduction properties induced by programmed ventricular stimulation are those of accessory AV connections [17,33,45,50]: (1) eccentric atrial activation sequence showing right or left atrial preexcitation; and (2) constant ventriculoatrial conduction time without refractory-dependent delay. Although "impedence mismatch" has been used to explain the development of anterograde unidirectional block in these accessory AV connections [51], the pathophysiology responsible for such develop-

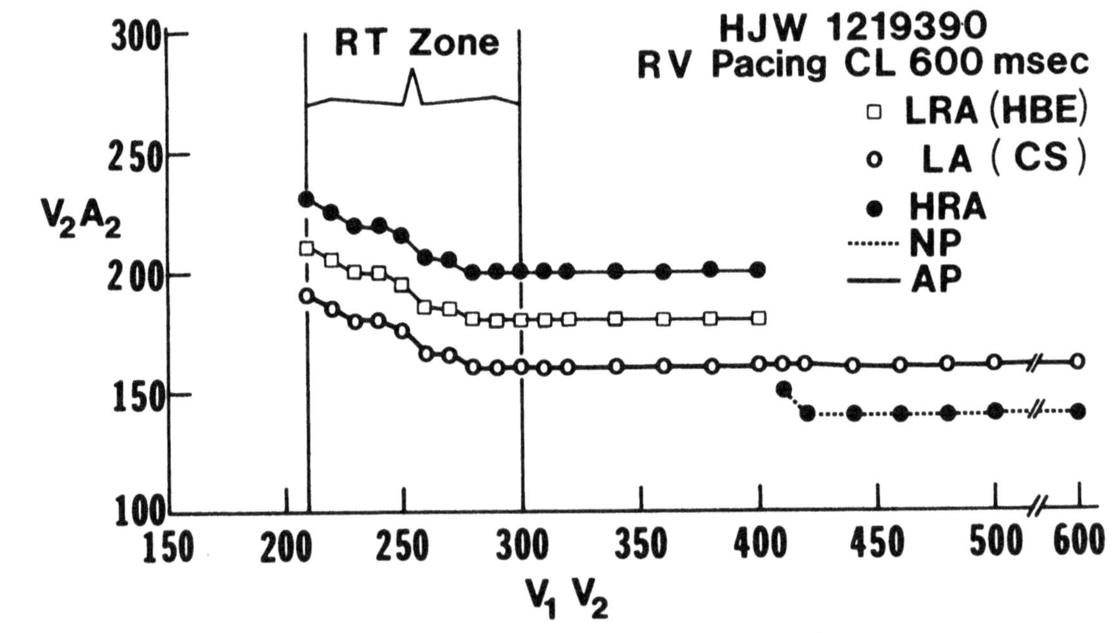

FIGURE 9–11. Same patient as in Figure 9–10. Retrograde conduction time of premature ventricular beats (V_2–A_2) as a function of premature coupling intervals (V_1–V_2), demonstrating a shift of the ventriculoatrial conduction pattern from retrograde atrial fusion to exclusive retrograde atrial activation throught the left-sided accessory pathway (AP). A reciprocating tachycardia (RT) zone is defined between premature coupling intervals (V_1–V_2) of 300 and 210 ms and, in each instance, the onset of reciprocating tachycardia is related to repetitive ventricular responses (see Figure 9–12). (From Sung RJ, Castellanos A, Mallon SM, et al.: Mode of initiation of reciprocating tachycardia during programmed ventricular stimulation in the Wolff-Parkinson-White syndrome. With reference to various patterns of ventriculoatrial conduction. *Am. J. Cardiol.* 40:24, 1977, with permission.)

ment remains unknown. Nevertheless, some of these accessory AV connections actually have extremely long anterograde effective refractory periods. Ventricular preexcitation pattern may thus become overt during sinus bradycardia induced by vagal maneuvers (carotid sinus massage) or during intravenous isoproterenol infusion which may shorten the anterograde effective refractory period of these accessory AV connections [52,53].

The electrophysiologic manifestations of concealed accessory AV connections [33] include: (1) retrograde atrial activation by way of the accessory AV connection resulting in an AV reciprocal rhythm (i.e., nonconducted atrial "echo" beats); (2) perpetuation of AV reciprocal rhythm leading to AV reciprocating tachycardia; and (3) retrograde atrial activation during the atrial vulnerable phase provoking an onset of atrial flutter-fibrillation (See Figures 9–5, 9–13, and 9–14). Because of the presence of anterograde unidirectional block in the accessory AV connection, the AV reciprocating tachycardia is exclusively of the orthodromic form. Furthermore, the AV reciprocating tachycardia can be initiated during sinus rhythm without an atrial or ventricular premature beat or antecedent prolongation of the P-R interval [49,54]. During spontaneous acceleration of the sinus rate, shortening of the sinus cycle length decreases the refractory periods of the atrium and accessory AV connection thereby facilitating retrograde atrial activation. The ease with which AV reciprocation (circus movement) can be initiated explains why it may present clinically as chronic repetitive supraventricular tachycardia (Figure 9–15) [55,56].

Diagnostic clues suggestive of the presence of a concealed accessory AV connection [49] are: (1) presentation as a chronic, repetitive type of supraventricular tachycardia; (2) spontaneous onset of supraventricular tachycardia asso-

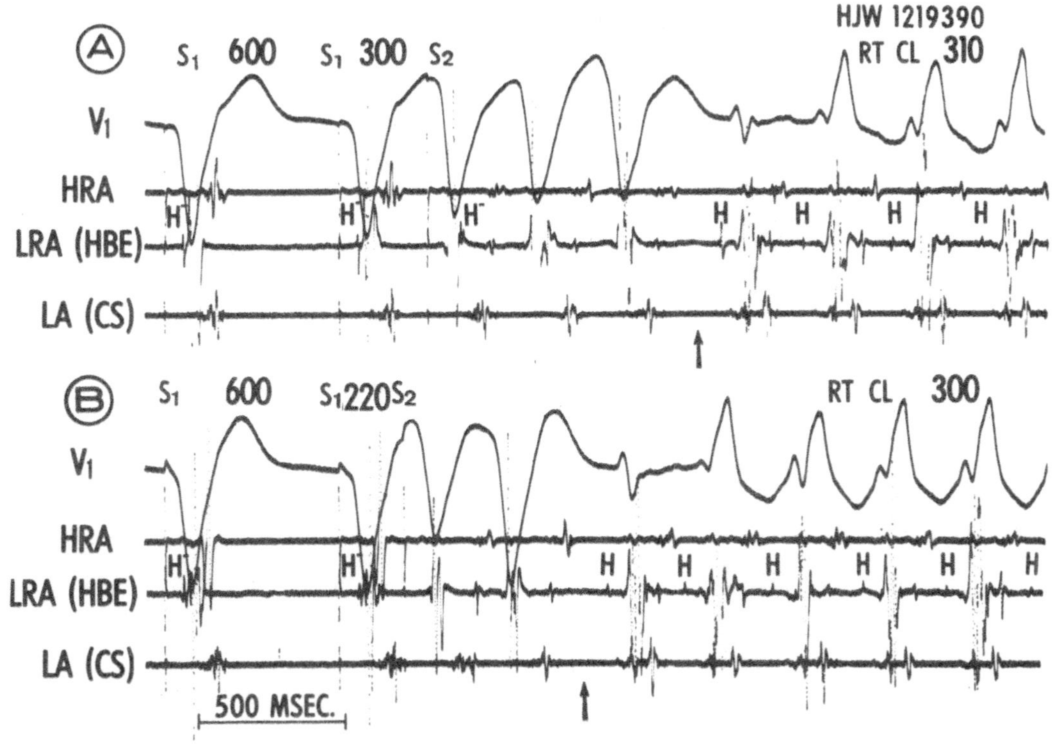

FIGURE 9–12. Same patient as in Figures 9–10 and 9–11. During right ventricular pacing (S_1-S_1) at a cycle length (CL) of 600 ms, repetitive ventricular responses ($V_2V_3V_4$ in A or V_2V_3 in B) at short premature coupling intervals (S_1-S_2) initiate an onset of reciprocating tachycardia (*RT*) (*arrows*). Note persistent retrograde atrial activation from the accessory pathway (AP) during repetitive ventricular responses and the development of a functional complete right bundle branch block pattern during reciprocating tachycardia. It is assumed decremental depolarization of the normal pathway in the retrograde direction induced by repetitive ventricular responses facilitates initiation of reciprocating tachycardia. (From Sung RJ, Castellanos A, Mallons SM, et al.: Mode of initiation of reciprocating tachycardia during programmed ventricular stimulation in the Wolff-Parkinson-White syndrome. With reference to various pattern of ventriculoatrial conduction. *Am. J. Cardiol.* 40: 24, 1977, with permission.)

ciated with an acceleration of the sinus rate; (3) inscription of the retrograde P wave (negative in leads II, III, and aVF) after the QRS complex; (4) initiation of atrial flutter-fibrillation associated with an AV reciprocal rhythm; and (5) slowing of the tachycardia rate associated with development of functional bundle branch block (ipsilateral to the location of the accessory AV connection) (Figure 9–16) [48,49,57].

CONCEALED CONDUCTION IN ACCESSORY AV CONNECTIONS

Concealed conduction occurs when a nonpropagated impulse influences the conduction of a subsequent impulse [58]. In the human heart, this unique electrophysiologic phenomenon has been shown to occur in the atrium, AV node His–Purkinje system [59–61]. Concealed conduction in accessory AV connections has long been suggested [27,28,46] and has recently been systemically demonstrated to occur in both anterograde and retrograde directions using the technique of programmed electrical stimulation in our laboratory (Figures 9–17 and 9–18) [62]. Other investigators have subsequently confirmed these findings [63].

The occurrence of concealed conduction in accessory AV connections in both anterograde and retrograde directions is one of the factors regulating the rate of ventricular response during atrial flutter-fibrillation in the WPW syndrome [27,28]. Further studies should be

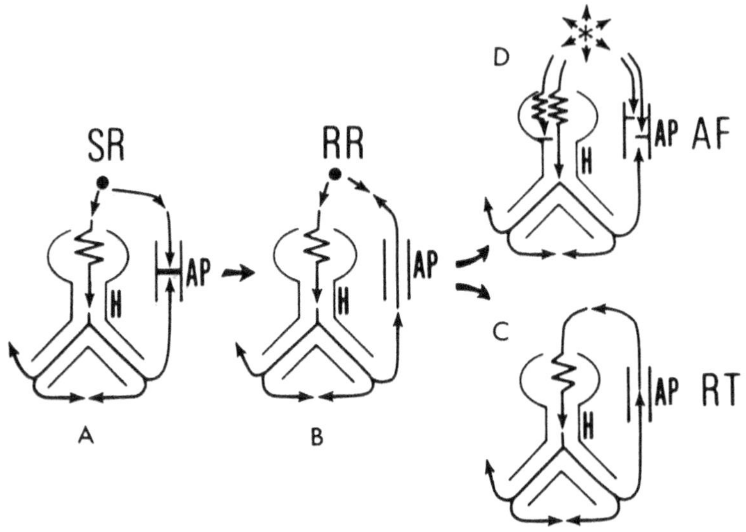

FIGURE 9–13. Schematic representation of the electrophysiologic manifestations of a concealed accessory AV connection. (A) During sinus rhythm (SR), the impulse conducts over the normal AV pathway (AV node–His–Purkinje system) to the ventricle. There is no ventricular preexcitation, because the accessory AV pathway (AP) is capable only of retrograde conduction (anterograde unidirectional block). (B) Retrograde atrial activation by way of the accessory AV pathway (AP) results in an AV reciprocal rhythm (RR). (C) Perpetuation of the AV reciprocal rhythm (RR) leads to AV reciprocating tachycardia (RT). (D) During AV reciprocal rhythm (RR), retrograde atrial activation during the atrial vulnerable phase may provoke an onset of atrial flutter or fibrillation (AF). H = His bundle. (From Sung RJ, Gelband H, Castellanos, A, et al.: Clinical and electrophysiologic observations in patients with concealed accessory atrioventricular bypass tracts. *Am. J. Cardiol.* 40:839, 1977, with permission.)

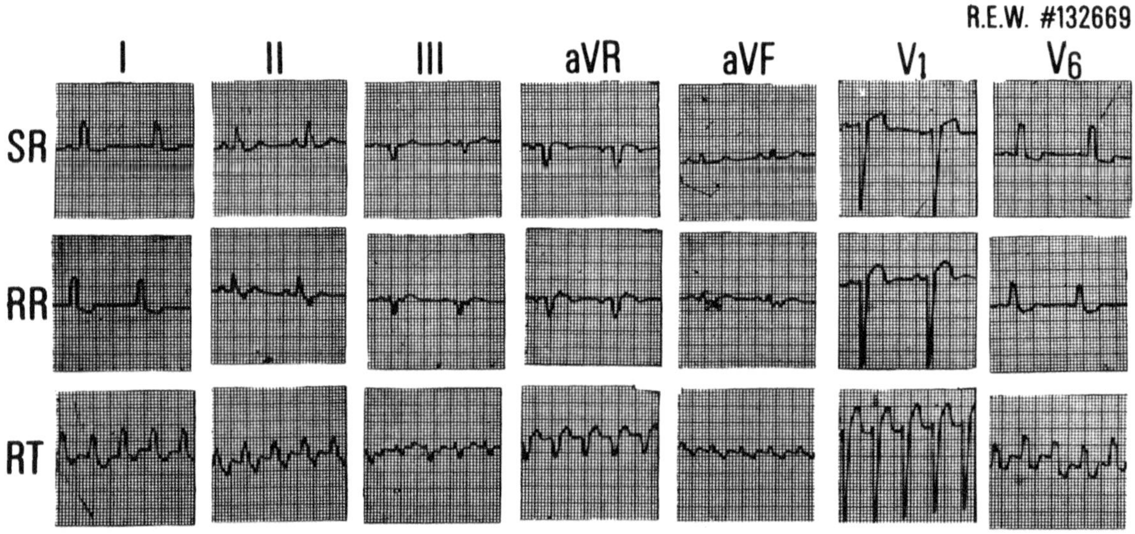

FIGURE 9–14. Sinus rhythm (SR), AV reciprocal rhythm (RR) (i.e., non-conducted atrial "echo" beats), and AV reciprocating tachycardia (RT) in a 71-year-old woman with concealed Wolff-Parkinson-White syndrome. Complete left bundle branch block is present in all three rhythms. The retrograde P wave (negative in leads II, III, and aV_F) has a configuration identical to those seen during AV reciprocal rhythm (RR) and AV reciprocating tachycardia (RT). Note the RP interval is shorter than the PR interval (RP = 0.13 sec vs. PR = 0.16 sec during the AV reciprocal rhythm; RP = 0.13 sec vs. PR = 0.22 sec during AV reciprocating tachycardia. (From Sung RJ, Gelband H, Castellanos A, et al.: Clinical and electrophysiologic observations in patients with concealed accessory atrioventricular bypass tracts. *Am. J. Cardiol.* 40:839, 1977, with permission.)

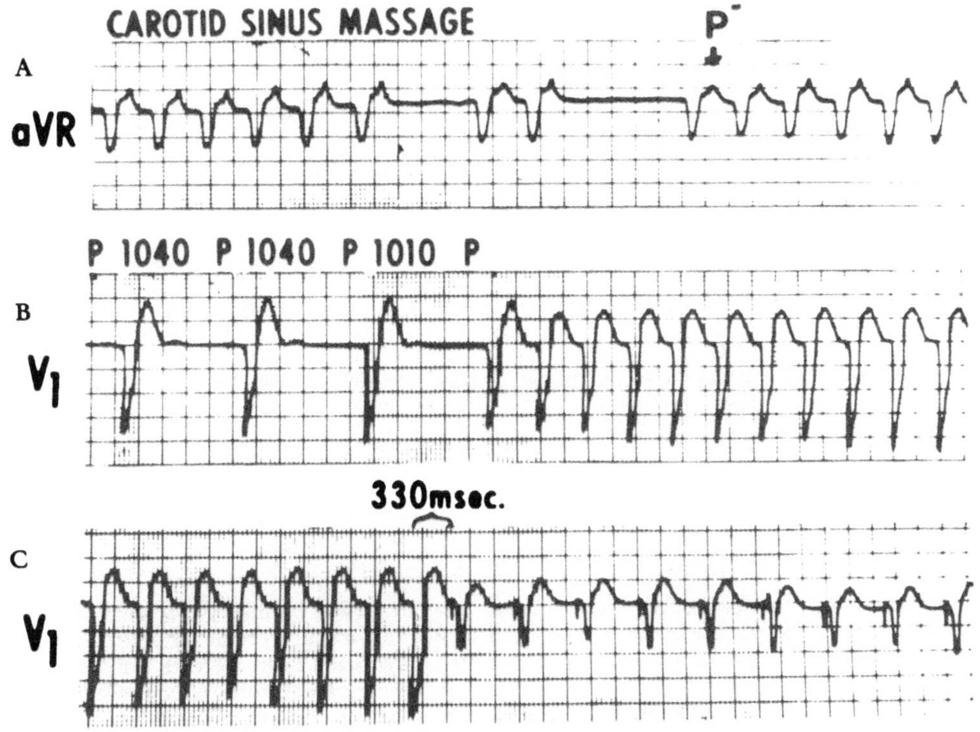

FIGURE 9–15. Chronic repetitive type of supraventricular tachycardia in a 38-year-old man with complete left bundle branch block associated with concealed left-sided accessory pathway. (A) Carotid sinus massage temporarily interrupts the supraventricular tachycardia. Note the retrograde P wave is upright in lead aVR, and the RP interval is shorter than the PR interval during the tachycardia. (B) Spontaneous initiation of the tachycardia after acceleration of the sinus rate (shortening of the sinus cycle length from 1040 to 1010 ms.) (C) The tachycardia is finally controlled by right ventricular pacing at a cycle length of 540 ms. The first pacemaker-captured beat with a ventricular premature coupling interval of 330 ms terminates the tachycardia. (From Sung RJ, Gelband H, Castellanos A, et al.: Clinical and electrophysiologic observations in patients with concealed accessory atrioventricular bypass tracts. *Am. J. Cardiol.* 40:839, 1977, with permission.)

directed toward recording of the electrical activity of accessory AV connections to determine the exact site at which concealed conduction occurs and the effects of antiarrhythmic agents on concealed conduction in accessory AV connections [64].

ACCESSORY AV CONNECTIONS WITH AV NODAL PROPERTIES

Rarely accessory AV connections may exhibit AV node-like properties. The basis for this phenomenon is poorly understood but it may be due to: (1) nonhomogenous physiologic properties of individual myocardial fibers or longitudinal dissociation of the myocardial fibers which make up the accessory AV connection, and (2) presence of cells with functional characteristics of AV nodal cells [7]. Electrophysiologically, refractory-dependent conduction delay (decremental conduction and/or Wenckebach type conduction block) can be demonstrated in accessory AV connections with AV node-like properties.

Clinically, accessory AV connections with AV node-like properties have been mostly described to be located in or close to the atrial septum nearby the AV junction [65–68]. Such accessory AV connections are sometimes called "accessory AV node" because of their proximity to the AV node, and are implicated to be the retrograde limb of the atypical (fast–slow) form of AV junctional reentrant tachycardia [65–68].

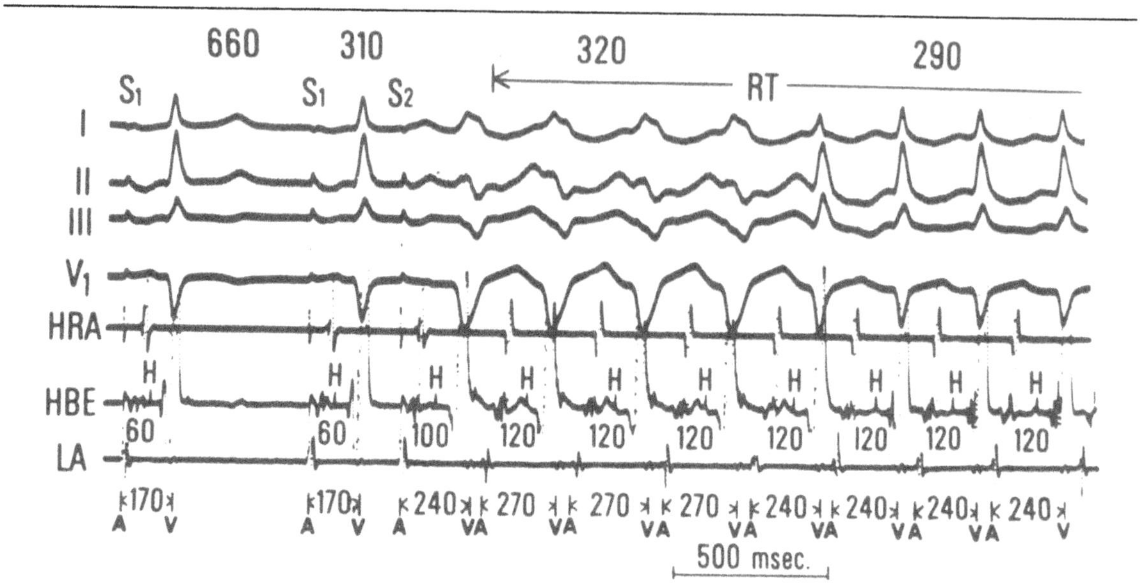

FIGURE 9–16. Slowing of the rate of AV reciprocating tachycardia (RT) during development of functional left bundle branch block in the presence of a concealed accessory AV connection on the left side. During atrial (left atrium) pacing at a cycle length (S_1–S_2) of 660 ms, an atrial premature beat (S_2) with a premature coupling interval (S_1–S_2) of 310 ms initiates an onset of AV reciprocating tachycardia. A concealed accessory AV connection on the left side is used for retrograde conduction during tachycardia. The presence of a concealed accessory AV connection is evidenced by demonstration of retrograde left atrial activation preceding low septal right atrial (HBE) and high right atrial (HRA) activation during tachycardia. The cycle length of tachycardia is 320 ms with 290 ms without the complete left bundle branch block pattern. (From Sung RJ, Gelband H, Castellanos A, et al.: Clinical and electrophysiologic observations in patients with concealed accessory atrioventricular bypass tracts. *Am. J. Cardiol.* 40:839, 1977, with permission.)

Alternative mechanisms responsible for this latter form of AV junctional reentrant tachycardia include: (1) AV nodal reentry using a fast AV nodal pathway for anterograde conduction and a slow AV nodal pathway for retrograde conduction, and (2) AV reciprocation using a fast AV node–His–Purkinje system for anterograde conduction and a slow AV node–nodoventricular connection (with anterograde unidirectional block) for retrograde conduction (Figures 9–19 and 9–20) [56] Electrophysiologic–histologic correlations are ultimately required to clarify the exact anatomic substrate used for retrograde conduction in this atypical (fast–slow) form of AV junctional reentrant tachycardia. Noteworthy is that left-sided lateral (parietal) accessory AV connections with AV node-like properties have recently been described and intravenous verapamil can suppress conduction of such accessory AV connections (Figures 9–21 and 9–22) [69].

EFFECTS OF PHARMACOLOGIC AGENTS ON ACCESSORY AV CONNECTIONS

Various antiarrhythmic agents have been shown to depress conduction and increase refractoriness of accessory AV connections. These agents include quinidine, procainamide, disopyramide, ajmaline, lidocaine, mexiletine, lorcainide, encainide, propafenone [70], and amiodarone [71]. Digitalis and verapamil, particularly the intravenous forms, may decrease the effective refractory periods of accessory AV connections and thereby enhance conduction over accessory AV connections. The effect of digitalis on accessory AV connections probably is mediated by its direct pharmacologic action [72], whereas that of verapamil is secondary to a reflex increase in adrenergic tone resulting from its peripheral vasodilating action [73]. Both intravenous digitalis and verapamil may accelerate the rate of conduction over accessory AV connections during atrial flutter-fibrillation in the

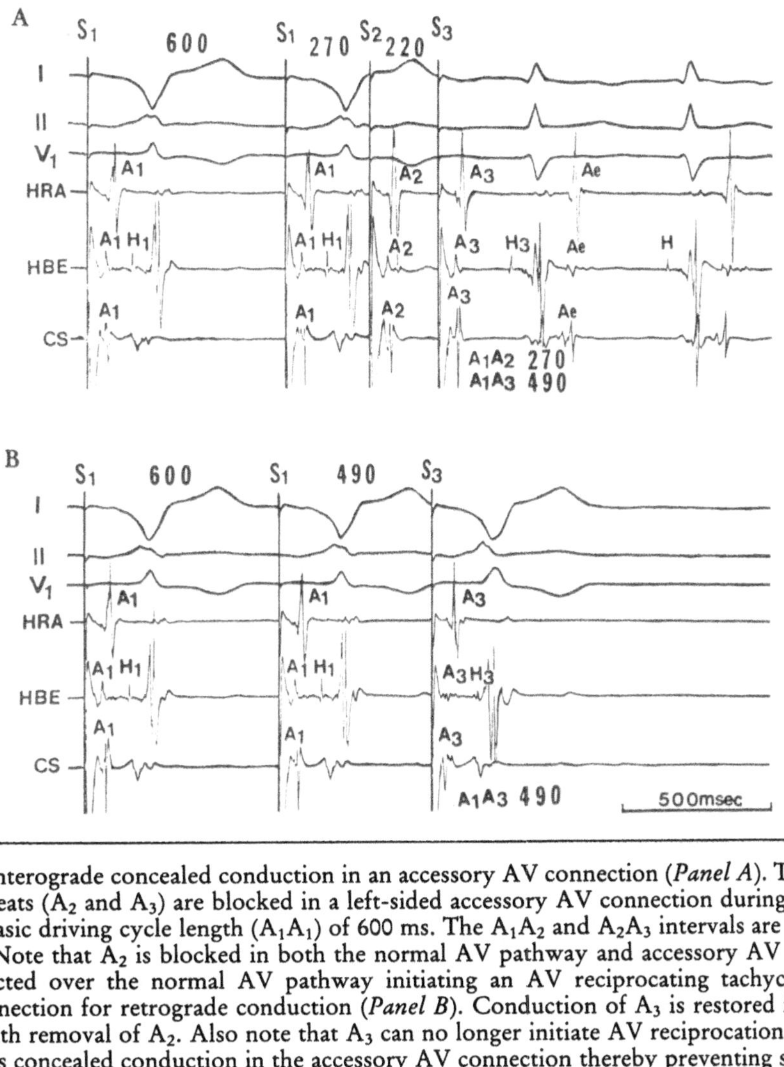

FIGURE 9–17. Anterograde concealed conduction in an accessory AV connection (*Panel A*). Two consecutive atrial premature beats (A_2 and A_3) are blocked in a left-sided accessory AV connection during coronary sinus (CS) pacing at a basic driving cycle length (A_1A_1) of 600 ms. The A_1A_2 and A_2A_3 intervals are 270 ms and 220 ms, respectively. Note that A_2 is blocked in both the normal AV pathway and accessory AV connection and that A_3 is conducted over the normal AV pathway initiating an AV reciprocating tachycardia using the accessory AV connection for retrograde conduction (*Panel B*). Conduction of A_3 is restored in the accessory AV connection with removal of A_2. Also note that A_3 can no longer initiate AV reciprocation. These findings suggest that A_2 has concealed conduction in the accessory AV connection thereby preventing subsequently A_3 conduction in the same conduction pathway in Panel A. (From Svinarich, Tai, Mickelson, et al.: Electrophysiologic demonstration of concealed conduction in anomalous atrioventricular bypass tracts. *J. Am. Coll. Cardiol.* 1985, with permission.)

WPW syndrome (Figure 9–23). If the anterograde effective refractory period of an accessory AV connection is already short, this effect may lead atrial flutter-fibrillation to degenerate into ventricular fibrillation.

Rarely, verapamil may exert depressive action on accessory AV connections and terminate AV reciprocating tachycardia by inducing conduction block in accessory AV connections [69]. This is in contrast to the usual mechanism by which verapamil converts AV reciprocating to normal sinus rhythm [74]. Depending on the functional properties of accessory AV connections, intravenous verapamil may: (1) directly prolong conduction and refractoriness of accessory AV connections with AV node-like properties (See Figures 9–21 and 9–22), and (2) indirectly induce alternating long and short cycle lengths (slow and fast AV nodal conduction) which, in turn, lead to development of the Ashman phenomenon in the accessory AV connection (Figure 9–24).

Changes in autonomic tone can influence the functional electrophysiologic properties of

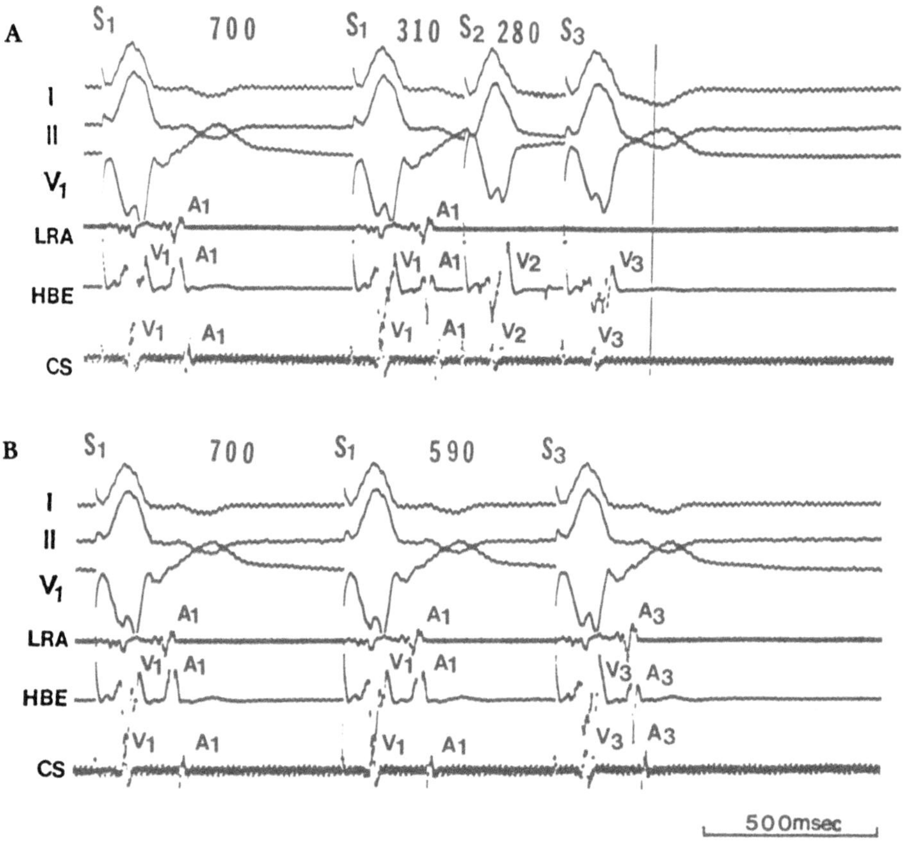

FIGURE 9–18. Retrograde concealed conduction in an accessory Av connection (*Panel A*). V_2 and V_3 are blocked in a right-sided accessory AV connection during right ventricular (RV) pacing at a basic cycle length (V_1V_1) of 700 msec. The V_1V_2 and V_2V_3 intervals are 310 msec and 280 ms, respectively (*Panel B*). Conduction of V_3 is restored in the accessory AV connection with removal of V_2. These findings suggest that V_2 has concealed conduction in the accessory AV connection thereby preventing subsequent V_3 conduction in the same conduction pathway in Panel A. Note atrial preexcitation in which lateral right atrial activation precedes low septal right atrial and left atrial activation during the basic drive. (From Svinarich, Tai, Michelson, et al.: Electrophysiologic demonstration of concealed conduction in anomalous atrioventricular bypass tracts. *J. Am. Coll. Cardiol.* 1985, with permission.)

accessory AV connections [52,53] and affect the rate of ventricular response during atrial flutter-fibrillation. Isoproterenol infusion can significantly shorten the anterograde effective refractory period of the accessory AV connection and thereby increases the rate of conduction over the accessory AV connection during atrial flutter-fibrillation [29,30]. Beta-adrenergic blockade reverses isoproterenol-induced decrease in the effective refractory periods of the atrium, accessory AV connection and the ventricle, and thereby prevents isoproterenol-induced enhanced conduction over the accessory AV connection (Figures 9–25 and 9–26) [75]. Furthermore, beta-adrenergic blockade depresses AV nodal conduction thereby slowing the rate of AV reciprocating tachycardia and may thus reduce atrial vulnerability [25]. Although beta-adrenergic blocking agents are not used for the acute treatment of atrial flutter-fibrillation with ventricular preexcitation associated with the WPW syndrome, chronic treatment with these agents, may be beneficial in patients with WPW syndrome prone to development of atrial flutter-fibrillation [75].

Accessory Nodoventricular and Fasciculoventricular Connections

Accessory nodoventricular and fasciculoventricular connections arise from the AV node and the His bundle or bundle branches, respec-

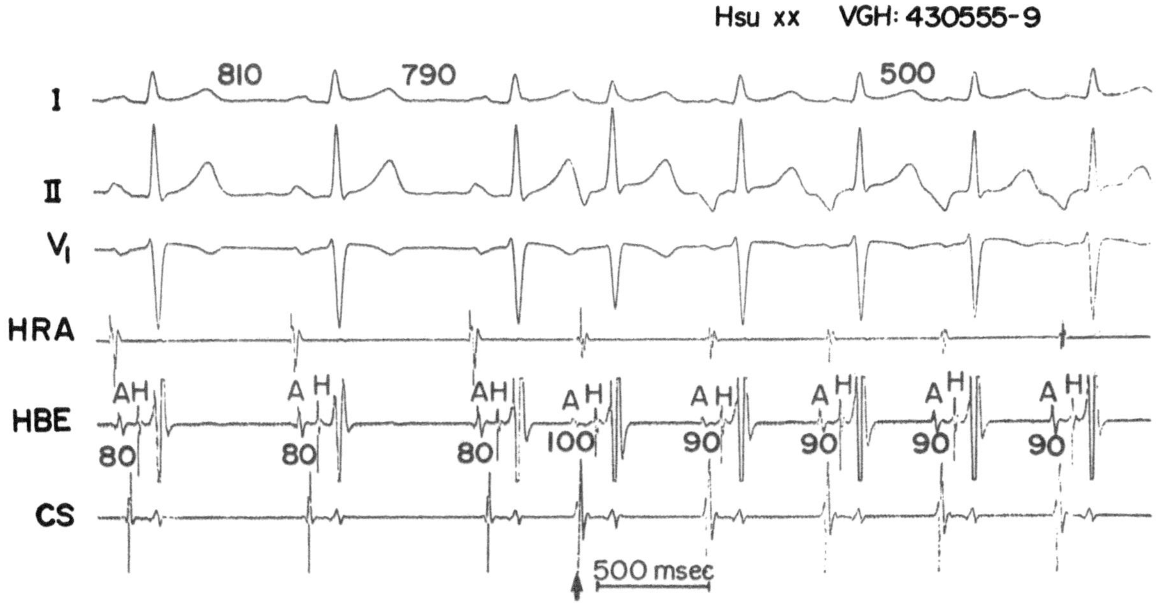

FIGURE 9–19. Spontaneous initiation of the atypical (fast-slow) form of AV junctional reentrant tachycardia during sinus rhythm. Note that shortening of the sinus cycle length from 810 to 790 ms is followed by an onset (arrow) of supraventricular tachycardia. Also note that there is no prolongation of the P-R or A-H interval before the onset of tachycardia and that the retrograde P wave is inscribed far behind the QRS complex with an R-P interval longer than the P-R interval during tachycardia.

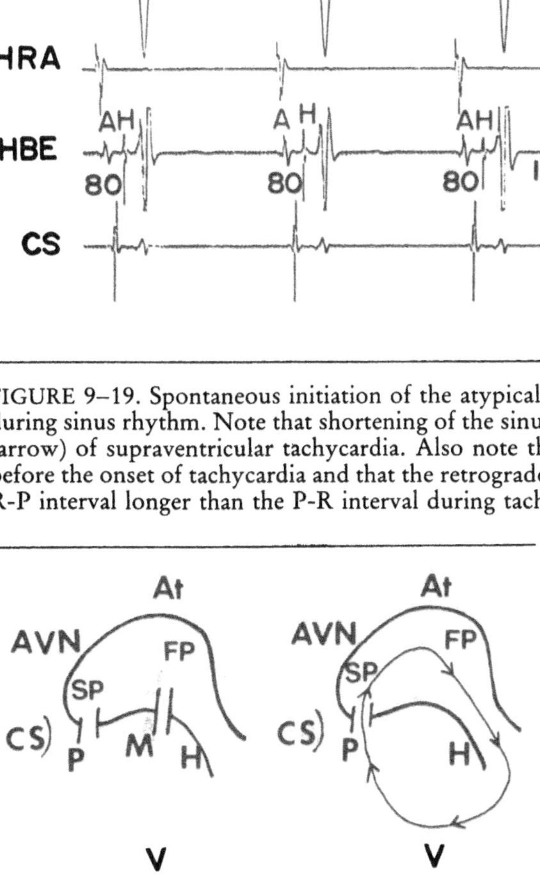

FIGURE 9–20. Schematic representation of the two varieties of nodoventricular connections. Mahaim fiber (M) (*left*) connects the compact (anterior) portion of the atrioventricular node (AVN) to the ventricle and the Paladino fiber (P) connects the transitional cell (posterior) zone of the AVN to the ventricle. [4]. A possible mechanism (*right*) for the fast-slow type of AV junctional reentrant tachycardia involving a concealed nodoventricular connection (capable only of retrograde conduction). The tachycardia uses a fast AVN pathway-His-Purkinje system for anterograde conduction and a slow AVN pathway-nodoventricular connection (Paladino fiber) for retrograde conduction. At = atrium; CS = coronary sinus; FP = fast AVN pathway; SP = slow AVN pathway; H = His bundle; V = ventricle.

tively, and insert into the septum. These accessory connections are often referred to as Mahaim fibers [1,4,76]. The existence of these accessory connections has been confirmed anatomically.

ELECTROCARDIOGRAPHIC FEATURES OF ACCESSORY NODOVENTRICULAR CONNECTIONS

Anatomically, two varieties of accessory nodoventricular connections can be distinguished [4]: one emerging from the transitional cell zone (posterior) and the other from the compact nodal cell zone (anterior) to connect to the septal ventricular myocardium (see Figure 9–20). The former has also been referred to as Paladino fibers [4].

Accessory nodoventricular connections can be associated with either a short or normal PR interval depending on the level of take off relative to the area of AV nodal conduction delay. The QRS complex can be normal or show varying degree of ventricular preexcitation resulting from fusion of impulse propagation by way of the normal AV conduction pathway and the accessory nodoventricular connection. Incremental atrial pacing and pro-

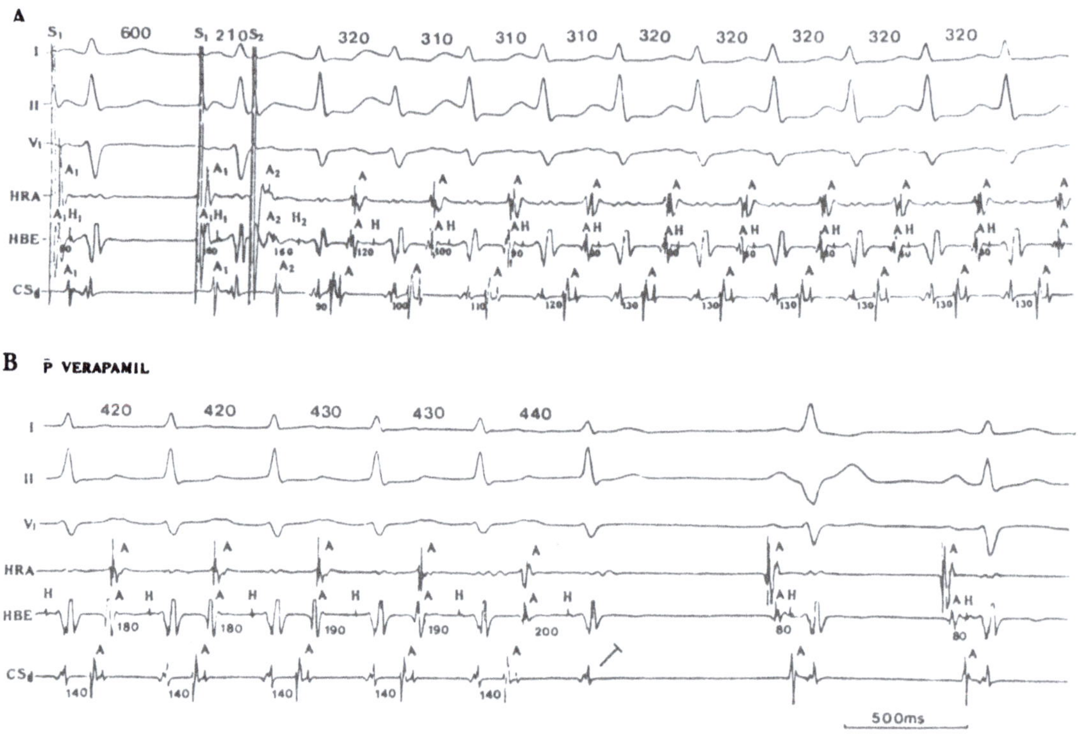

FIGURE 9–21. Termination of AV reciprocating tachycardia by a direct depressive effect of verapamil on the accessory AV connection. (A) AV reciprocating tachycardia is initiated by an atrial premature beat (S_2) with a premature coupling interval (S_1-S_2) of 210 ms during a basic driving cycle length (S_1-S_1) of 600 ms. During the tachycardia, the earliest retrograde atrial activation is recorded at the distal coronary sinus (CSd). Note that ventriculoatrial (VA) conduction time measured from the distal coronary sinus (CSd) progressively prolongs from 90 to 130 ms as AV nodal conduction time (AH interval) gradually shortens from 160 to 80 ms. (B) Verapamil prolongs AV nodal conduction time (AH interval: 180–200 ms) and VA conduction time (110 ms) and terminates AV reciprocating tachycardia by inducing retrograde conduction block in the accessory connection. (From Tai DY, Chang MS, Svinarich JT, et al.: Mechanisms of verapamil-induced conduction block in anomalous atrioventricular bypass tracts. *J. Am. Coll. Cardiol.* 1985, with permission.)

gressive atrial premature stimulation prolong the PR and AH (AV nodal conduction time) intervals and increase the degree of ventricular preexcitation while decreasing the HV interval. The prolongation of the PR interval is lesser than that of the AH interval. Consequently, the His bundle deflection is displaced into the ventricular electrogram and the degree of AV conduction over the nodoventricular connection (ventricular preexcitation) is increased. In all reported cases [18,38,77–81], total ventricular preexcitation observed during reciprocating tachycardia has been of a complete left bundle branch pattern suggesting insertion of the accessory nodoventricular connection into the right ventricle (right ventricular preexcitation). Characteristically, His bundle pacing with the same rate as atrial pacing which induces total ventricular preexcitation will normalize the QRS complex (disappearance of ventricular preexcitation).

RECIPROCATING TACHYCARDIA INVOLVING ACCESSORY NODOVENTRICULAR CONNECTIONS

Sustained paroxysms of reciprocating tachycardia with a QRS morphology resembling complete left bundle branch block pattern can be induced with either programmed atrial or programmed ventricular stimulation in certain

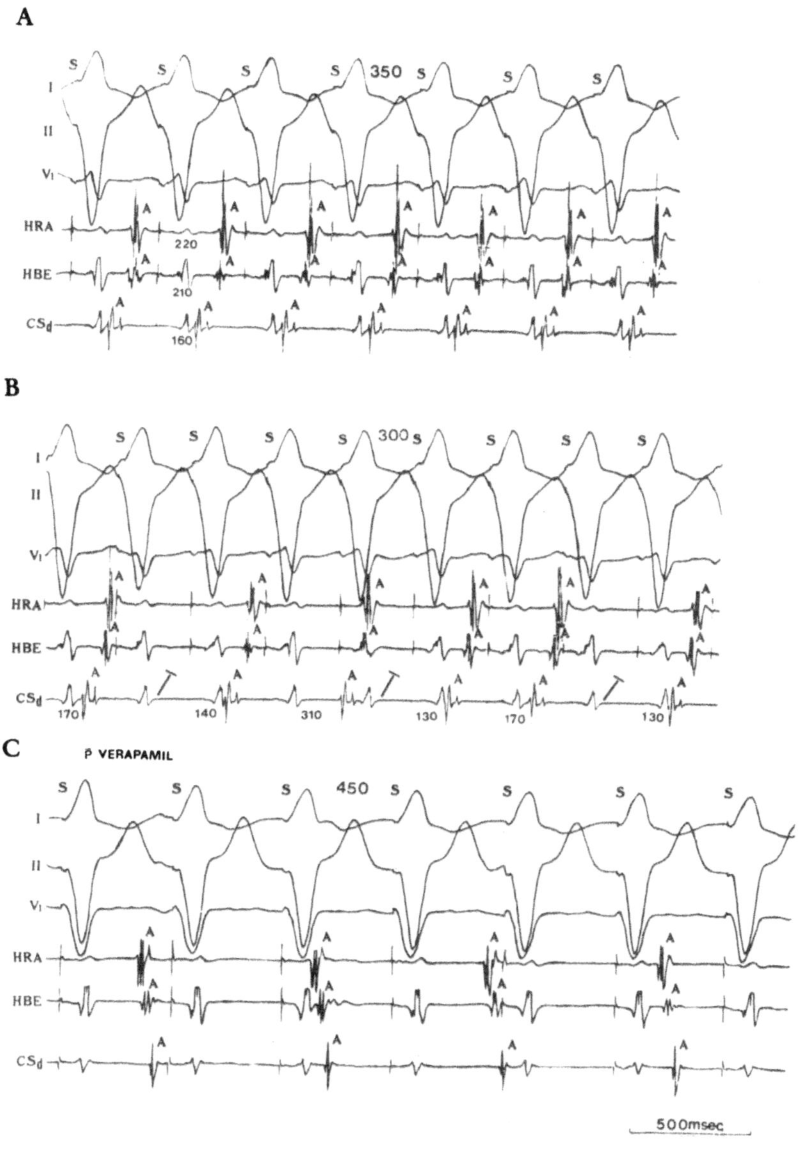

FIGURE 9–22. Effects of intravenous verapamil on ventriculoatrial (VA) conduction during incremental ventricular pacing (same patient as in Figure 9–21). (A) During right ventricular (RV) pacing at a cycle length (SS) of 350 ms, there is a 1:1 VA conduction. The sequence of retrograde atrial activation is identical to that observed during AV reciprocating tachycardia (Figure 9–21). The sequence of retrograde atrial activation is recorded the earliest at the distal coronary sinus (CSd) followed by His bundle (HBE) and high right atrial (HRA) electrographic leads. VA conduction time measured from the distal coronary sinus (CSd) is 160 ms. (B) Right ventricular (RV) pacing at a cycle length (SS) of 300 ms induces a second degree (Wenckebach) VA block in the accessory AV connection. (C) After intravenous infusion of verapamil, complete VA block develops during right ventricular (RV) pacing at a cycle length (SS) of 450 ms. (From Tai DY, Chang MS, Svinarich JT, et al.: Mechanisms of verapamil-induced conduction block in anomalous atrioventricular bypass tracts.* *J. Am. Coll. Cardiol.* 1985, with permission.)

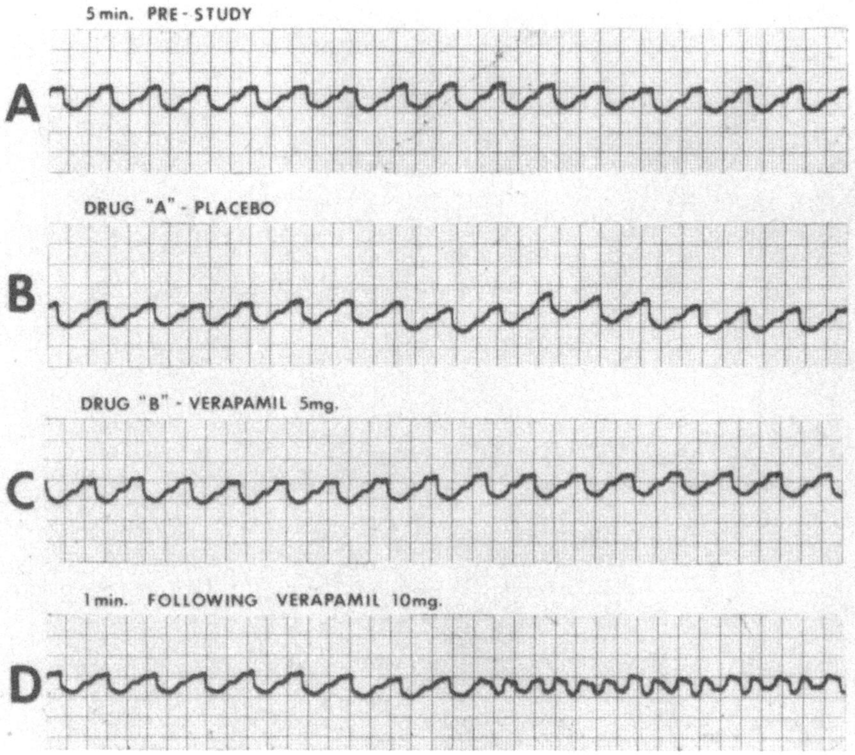

FIGURE 9–23. Acceleration of ventricular responses during atrial flutter in a patient with a left-sided accessory AV conduction. Atrial flutter with 2:1 conduction over the accessory AV connection. (A) Intravenous infusion with either placebo (B) or 5 mg. verapamil (C) exhibits no effect. However, intravenous infusion of 10 mg verapamil (D) accelerates AV conduction from 2:1 to 1:1 conduction over the accessory AV connection.

patients with accessory nodoventricular connections [18,38,77–81]. The most commonly postulated mechanism is a form of reciprocating tachycardia that uses the accessory nodoventricular connection for anterograde conduction to the ventricle and the His–Purkinje system for retrograde conduction to the AV node (Figures 9–27 and 9–28). The atrium is not a necessary link of the reentrant circuit and AV dissociation may occur during reciprocating tachycardia. Alternatively, AV nodal reentry with the nodoventricular connection as a "bystander" for ventricular activation can also produce a similar electrocardiographic pattern [80].

ACCESSORY NODOVENTRICULAR CONNECTIONS, DUAL AV NODAL PATHWAYS, AND THE ATYPICAL (FAST–SLOW) FORM OF AV JUNCTIONAL REENTRANT TACHYCARDIA

In our laboratory, we have observed electrophysiologic findings suggestive of coexistence of accessory nodoventricular connections and dual AV nodal pathways [79,82,83]. These findings are supportive of the presence of two varieties of accessory nodoventricular connections as suggested from anatomic studies [4]. Further the atypical (fast–slow) form of AV junctional reentrant tachycardia may use a concealed accessory nodoventricular connection (capable only of retrograde conduction), which bridges the slow AV nodal pathway and the right ventricular septum, for retrograde conduction (See Figure 9–20) [56].

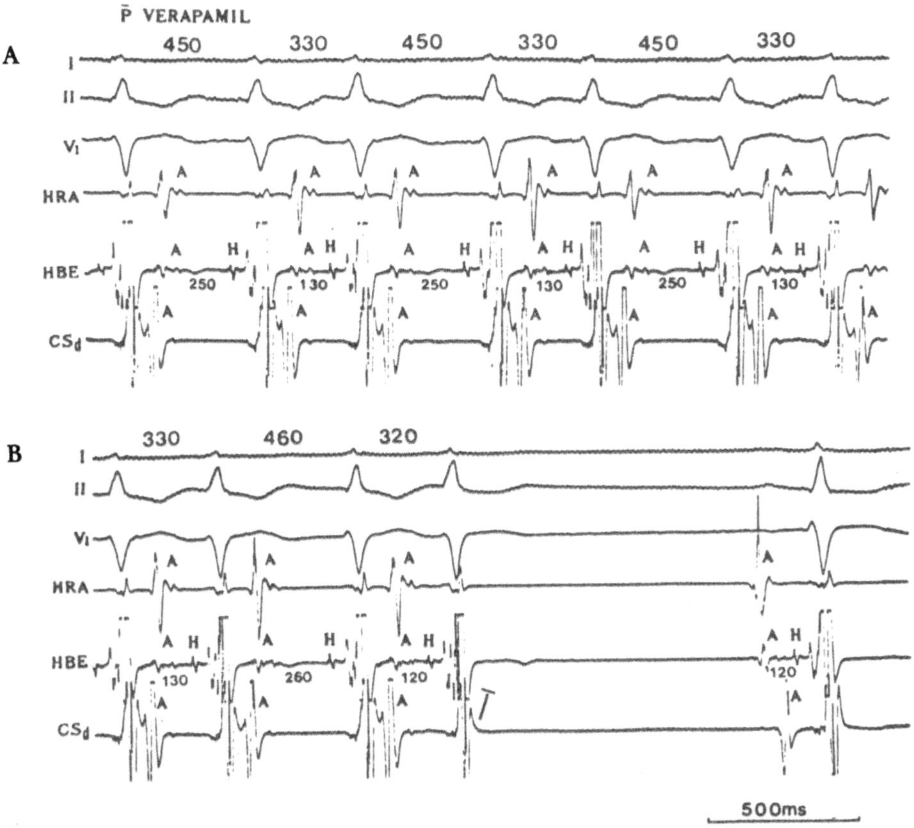

FIGURE 9–24. Termination of AV reciprocating tachycardia by an indirect depressive effect of verapamil on the accessory AV connection. Tracings (A) and (B) are continuous. (A) After intravenous infusion of verapamil, there is development of alternating long and short AV nodal conduction times (AH intervals) of 250 and 130 ms resulting in alternating long and short cycle lengths of 450 and 330 ms during the tachycardia. (B) The tachycardia is terminated by subsequent development of retrograde conduction block in the anomalous AV bypass tract. Note that the development of conduction block in the bypass tract follows a short cycle length of 320 ms (AH interval of 120 ms) which is preceded by a long cycle length of 460 ms (AH interval of 260 ms) consistent with the Ashman phenomenon. (From Tai DY, Chang MS, Svinarich JT, et al.: Mechanisms of verapamil-induced conduction block in anomalous atrioventricular bypass tracts. *J. Am. Coll. Cardiol.* 1985, with permission.)

First of all, patients with accessory nodoventricular connections bridging the fast AV nodal pathway and the right ventricle have the following electrophysiologic characteristics [82]: (1) right ventricular preexcitation is evident during sinus rhythm and becomes more prominent with gradual prolongation of the PR interval with atrial extrastimulation (See Figure 9–29); and (2) during programmed atrial stimulation, a shift from fast to slow AV nodal pathway conduction results in a sudden disappearance of right ventricular preexcitation. Discontinous AV nodal conduction (A_1A_2, A_2H_2 and A_1A_2, H_1H_2) curves may be exposed. In patients with accessory nodoventricular connections bridging the slow AV nodal pathway and the right ventricle have distinctly different electrophysiologic characteristics [82]: (1) right ventricular preexcitation is usually absent during sinus rhythm, and (2) during programmed atrial stimulation, a shift from fast to slow AV nodal pathway conduction results in a sudden

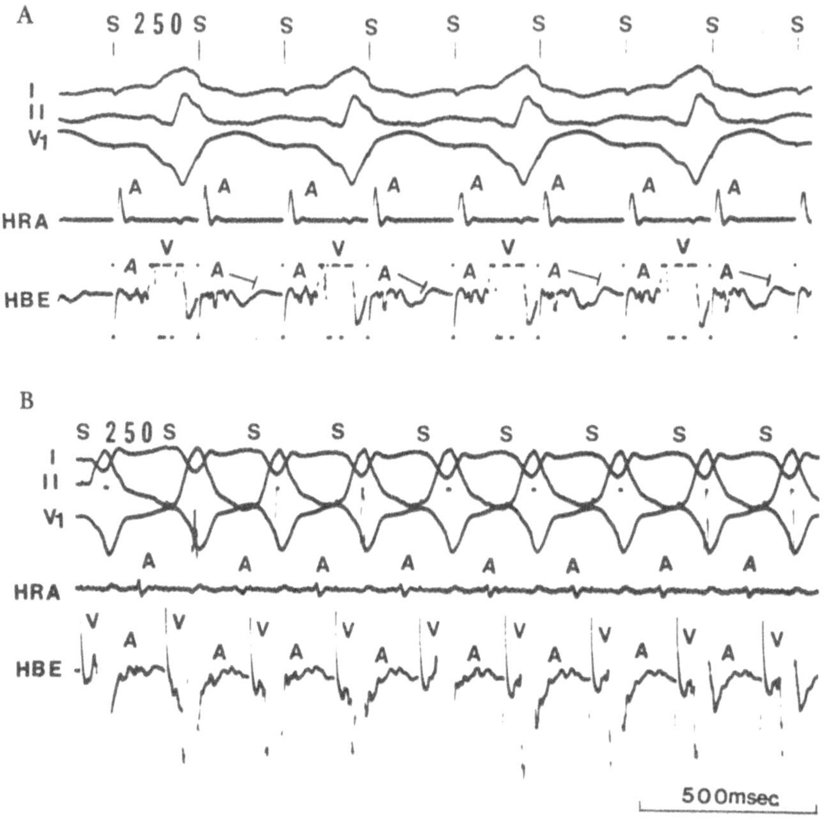

FIGURE 9–25. (A) During high atrial pacing at a cycle length of 250 ms, there is 2:1 AV conduction over a right-sided accessory AV connection. (B) During right ventricular pacing at the same cycle length of 250 ms, there is a 1:1 ventricular caputure. These findings suggest that 2:1 AV conduction is due to 2:1 conduction block in the accessory AV connection at the cycle length of 250 ms. S = electrical stimulus.

appearance of right ventricular preexcitation disrupting AV conduction (A_1A_2, V_1V_2), curves followed by induction of reciprocating tachycardia with a complete left bundle branch block pattern (right ventricular preexcitation) (See Figures 9–27 and 9–28) [79]. The reciprocating tachycardia uses the slow AV nodal pathway–accessory nodoventricular connection for anterograde conduction and the fast AV nodal pathway–His–Purkinje system for retrograde conduction [79].

Second, in patients who manifest both anterograde and retrograde dual AV nodal pathway conduction patterns (discontinuous A_1A_2, A_2H_2; A_1A_2, H_1H_2 and discontinuous V_1V_2, V_2A_2; V_1V_1, A_1A_2 curves), the sequence of retrograde atrial activation abruptly shifts with a change from retrograde fast to retrograde slow AV nodal pathway conduction [83]. During retrograde fast AV nodal pathway conduction, the low septal right atrial activation (recorded from the His bundle electrographic lead) precedes coronary sinus ostial atrial and high right atrial activation. During retrograde slow AV nodal pathway conduction, however, the coronary sinus ostial atrial activation notably precedes the low septal right atrial and high right atrial activation. Thus, the slow AV nodal pathway is probably located inferoposterior to that of the fast AV nodal pathway. These findings seem to correlate with the proposed anatomic classification of accessory nodoventricular connections [4] — one emerging from the transitional cell zone (slow AV nodal pathway) and the other emerging from the compact nodal cell zone (fast AV nodal pathway) to connect to the septal ventricular myocardium.

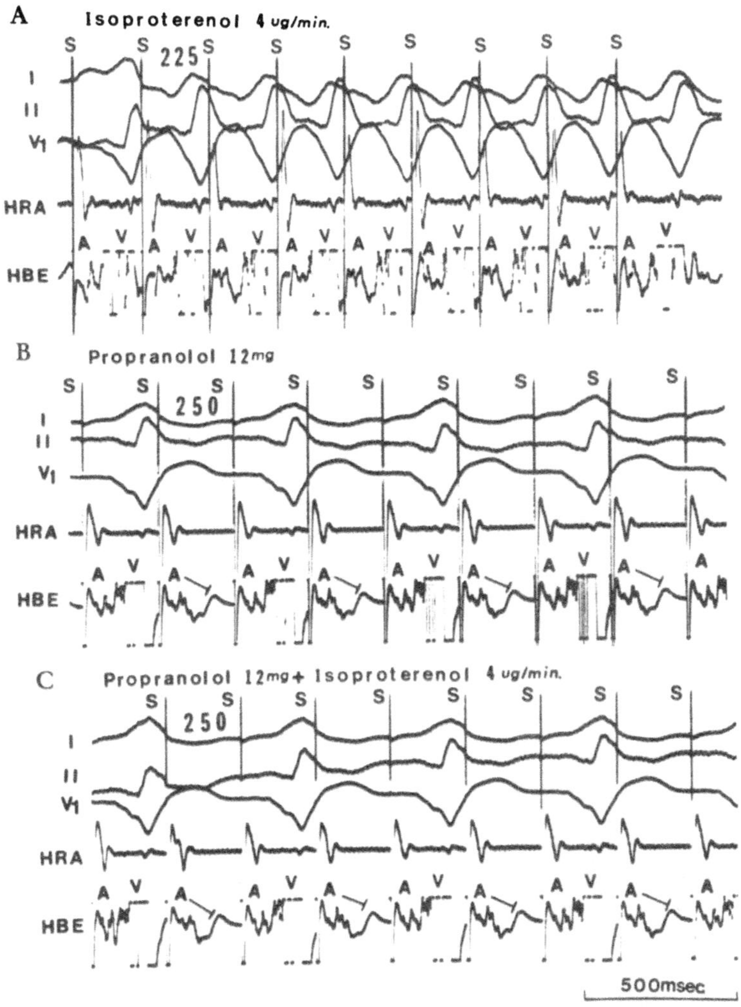

FIGURE 9–26. (A) Isoproterenol infusion at 4 μg/min enhances AV conduction over the accessory AV connection with 1:1 conduction up to a cycle length of 225 ms (same patient as in Figure 9–25). (B) After intravenous infusion of 12 mg propranolol, AV conduction over the accessory is reversed to 2:1. (C) Rechallenge with isoproterenol infusion after propranolol can not accelerate AV conduction over the accessory AV connection.

Although AV nodal (intranodal) reentry remains to be a viable mechanism for the occurrence of the atypical (fast–slow) form of AV junctional reentrant tachycardia [84–88], several investigators favor the involvement of an accessory AV node or accessory AV connection with AV node-like properties as the retrograde limb of the reentrant circuit [65,67,68]. Our observations have, however, led us to suggest that, in some patients, the atypical (fast–slow) form of AV junctional reentrant tachycardia involves a concealed accessory nodoventricular connection (antegrade unidirectional block) bridging the slow AV nodal pathway and the right ventricular septum retrograde conduction (See Figure 9–20) [56]. Participation of such a concealed accessory nodoventricular connection capable only of retrograde conduction is analogous to the situation in which a concealed accessory AV connection is used for retrograde conduction during orthodromic reciprocating tachycardia [33,47–49].

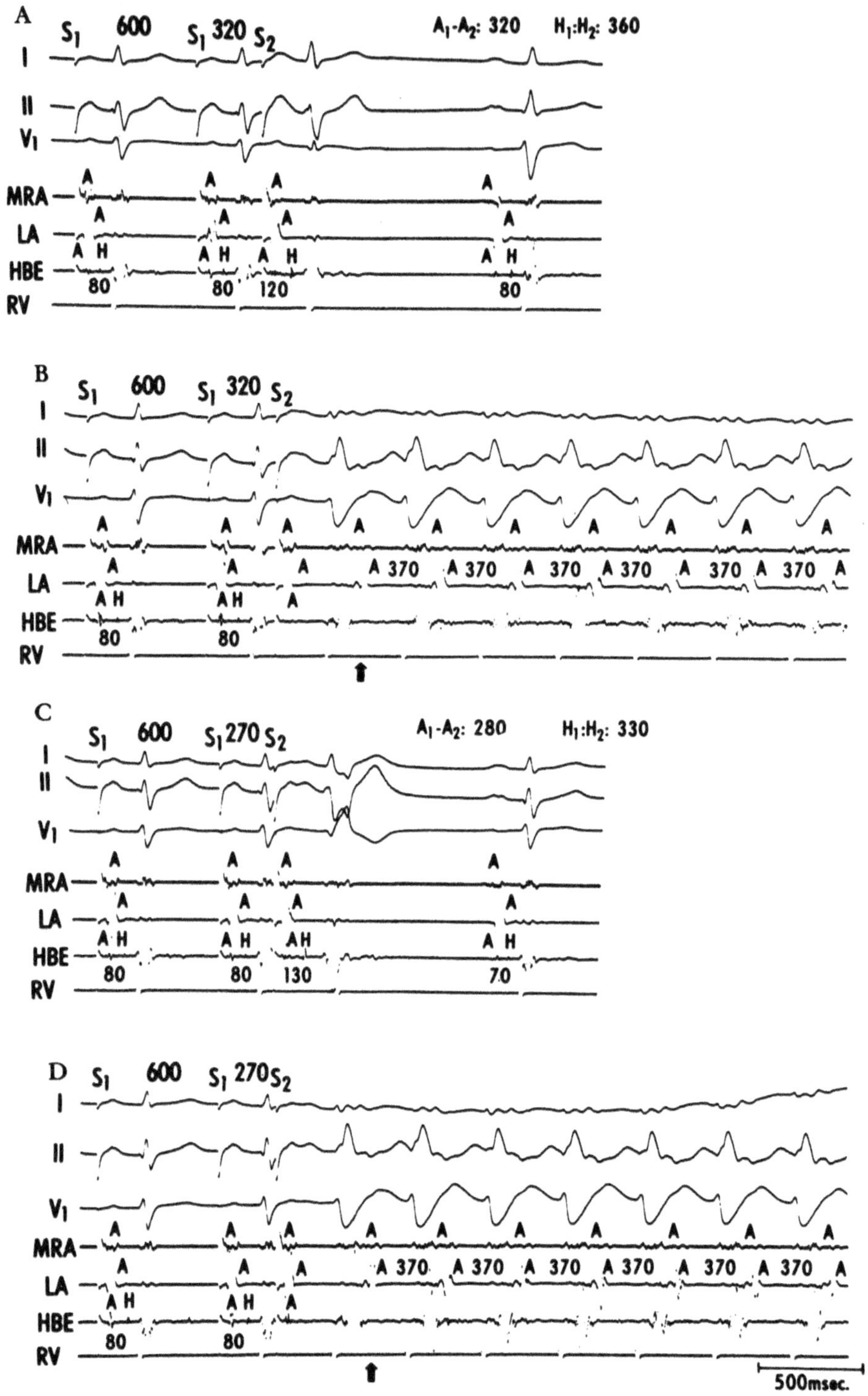

FIGURE 9–27. Atrial premature stimulation with intermittent induction of sustained reciprocating tachycardia in a patient with an accessory nodoventricular connection. The high right atrium (HRA) is driven at a cycle length (S_1S_1) of 600 ms. The atrioventricular (AV) nodal conduction time (AH) lengthens progressively as the atrial premature coupling interval (S_1S_2) gradually shortens. Sustained reciprocating tachycardia could be intermittently induced between premature coupling intervals (S_1S_2) of 320 and 270 ms. (A) An atrial premature beat at a coupling interval (S_1S_2) of 320 ms is conducted to the ventricle with an incomplete right bundle branch block pattern. The corresponding AH, HV intervals are 120 and 50 ms, respectively. (B) An atrial premature beat at the same coupling interval (S_1S_2) of 320 ms conducted to the ventricle with a complete left bundle branch block pattern followed by initiation of a sustained reciprocating trachycardia (*arrow*). Note sudden disappearance

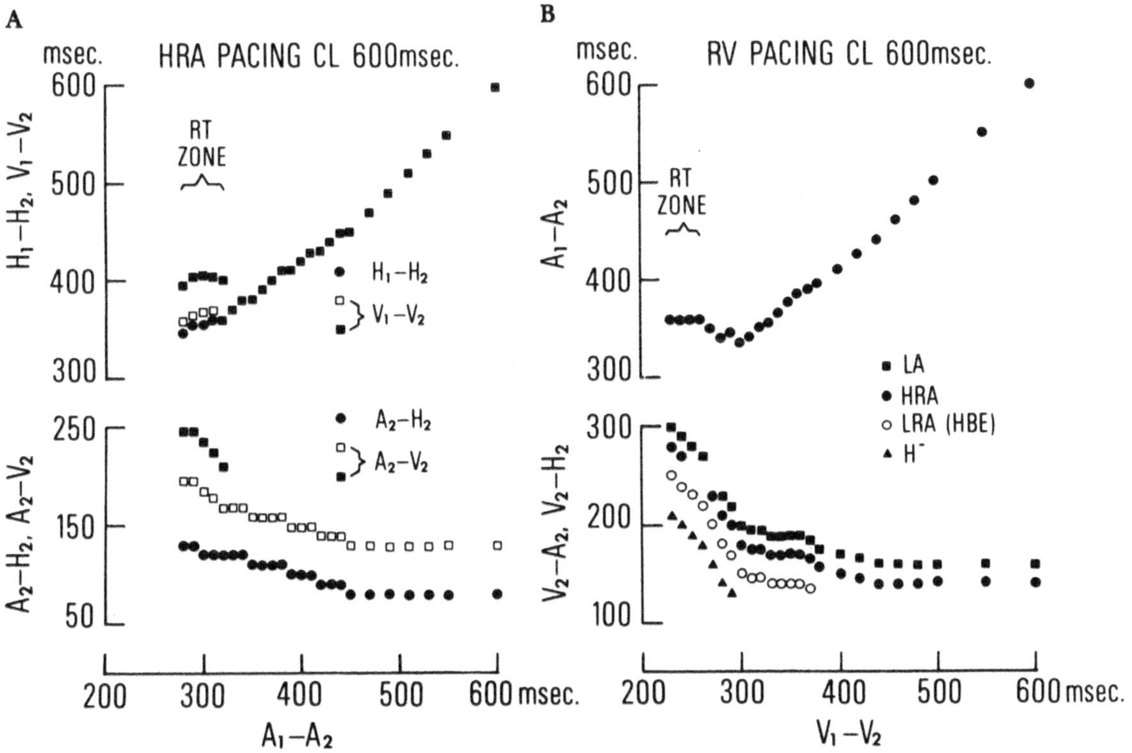

FIGURE 9–28. (A) A_1A_2, H_1H_2 (A_1A_2 V_1V_2) and A_1A_2, A_2H_2 (A_1A_2, A_2V_2) curves during his right atrial (HRA) pacing at a cycle length (CL) of 600 ms (same patient as in Figure 9–27). There is gradual prolongation of atrioventricular (AV) nodal conduction time (A_2H_2) as the atrial premature coupling interval (A_1A_2) progressively shortens, compatible with AV nodal properties. However, between premature coupling intervals (A_1A_2) of 320 and 270 ms, an atrial premature beat (A_2) is conducted to the ventricle with either an incomplete-to-complete right bundle branch block pattern (*open square*) or a complete left bundle block pattern (*closed square*). Of note, when the incomplete-to-complete right bundle block pattern appears, it is always preceded by a His bundle potential with an HV interval of 50–65 ms; when the complete left bundle branch block pattern appears, the His bundle potential suddently disappears and it is followed by initiation of a sustained reciprocating tachycardia (RT) (see Figure 9–27). (B) V_1V_2, V_2A_2 and V_1V_2, A_1A_2 curves during right ventricular (RV) pacing at a CL of 600 ms. Note that the sequence of ventriculoatrial conduction is the low septal right atrium (LRA) first followed by the high right atrium and then the left atrium (LA) compatible with retrograde conduction by way of the AV node–His–Purkinje system. Additionally, the progressive ventriculoatrial conduction delay as the ventricular premature coupling interval (V_1V_2) gradually shortens is in keeping with the retrograde conduction properties of the AV node–His–Purkinje system. Reciprocating tachycardia (RT) could be elicited between ventricular premature coupling intervals of 260 and 230 ms.

of the His bundle potential and prolongation of AV conduction time (A_2V_2) before ventricular activation with a complete left bundle branch block pattern. (C) An atrial premature beat at a coupling interval (S_1S_2) of 270 ms is conducted to the ventricle with a complete right bundle branch block pattern with a superior axis. The corresponding AH and HV intervals are 130 and 65 ms, respectively. (D) An atrial premature beat at the same coupling interval (S_1S_2) of 270 ms is conducted to the ventricle with a complete left bundle branch block pattern, followed by initiation of a sustained reciprocating tachycardia (*arrow*). Also note sudden disappearance of the His bundle potential and prolongation of AV conduction time (A_2V_2) before ventricular activation with a complete left bundle branch block pattern similar to that seen in Panel B. During reciprocating tachycardia (both Panels B and D), the low septal right atrial electrogram cannot be clearly separated from the ventricular electrogram. However, the mid-right atrial (MRA) activation precedes left atrial (LA) activation, and the ventriculoatrial conduction time is constant after initiation of tachycardia. (From Sung RJ, Styperek JL: Electrophysiologic identification of dual atrioventricular nodal pathway conduction in patients with reciprocating tachycardia using anomalous bypass tracts. *Circulation* 60:1464, 1979 with permission.)

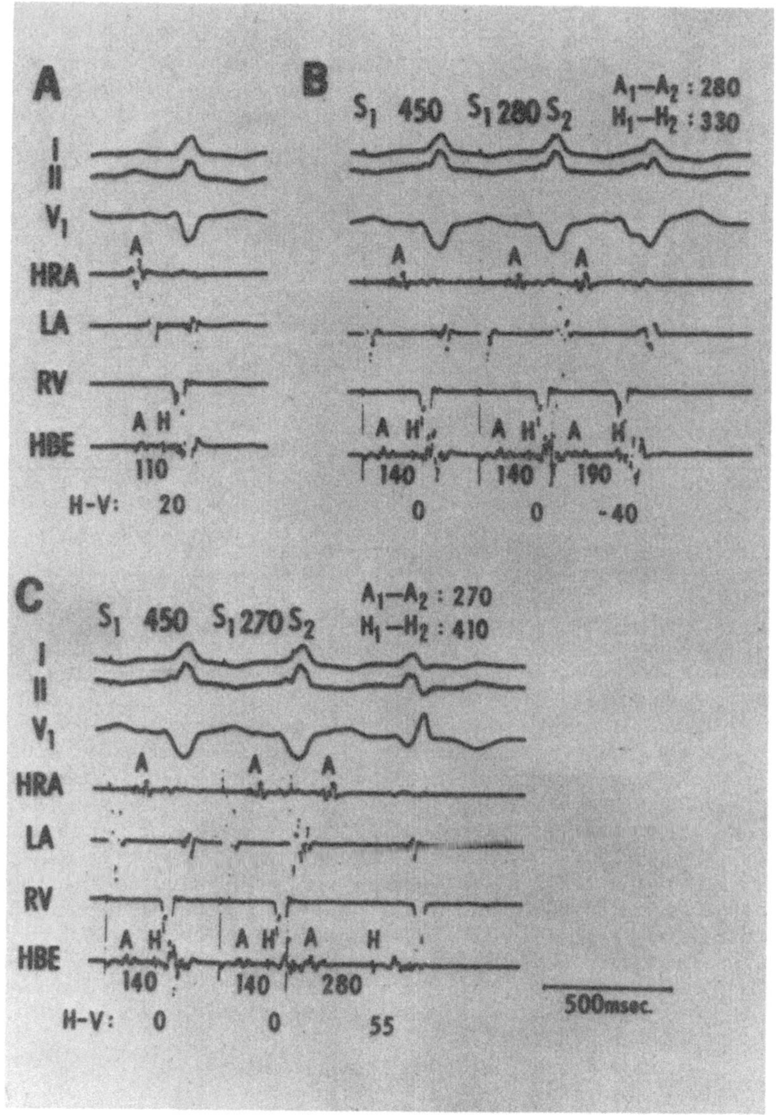

FIGURE 9–29. Effects of atrial premature stimulation on fast AV node–nodoventricular connection. (A) Right ventricular preexcitation is evident during sinus rhythm with an AH interval of 110 ms and a PR interval of 150 ms. (B) During left atrial pacing at a cycle length of 450 ms, the AH interval is increased to 140 ms and the PR interval is increased to 160 ms whereas the HV interval is shortened from 20 to θ ms with more right ventricular preexcitation. An atrial premature stimulation with a premature coupling interval of 280 ms prolongs the AH interval to 190 ms and the PR interval to 180 ms and produces a greater degree of right ventricular preexcitation. Note the HV interval is decreased to −40 ms. (C) Atrial premature stimulation with a premature coupling interval of 270 ms suddenly increased the AH interval to 280 ms (a shift from a fast to a slow AV nodal pathway conduction) and is followed by total disappearance of ventricular preexcitation (the third QRS complex with a right bundle branch block pattern and an HV interval of 55 ms).

ATRIAL FLUTTER-FIBRILLATION AND ACCESSORY NODOVENTRICULAR CONNECTIONS

During atrial flutter or fibrillation anterograde conduction via an accessory nodoventricular connection usually exhibits a complete left bundle branch block pattern (right ventricular preexcitation) [81]. However, if there is a preexisting or functional development of complete right bundle branch block, the QRS complexes may show intermittent complete right and complete left bundle branch block patterns mimicking a status of impending bilateral bundle branch block (Figure 9–30) [79]. Intracardiac recordings should reveal that the QRS complex of a complete right bundle branch block pattern is always preceded by the His bundle potential with an HV interval equal to or longer than the control HV interval. In contrast, the QRS complex of a complete left bundle branch block pattern is either not preceded by the His bundle potential or preceded by the His bundle with an HV interval shorter than the control HV interval.

ACCESSORY FASCICULOVENTRICULAR CONNECTIONS

The PR and AH intervals are normal with isolated accessory fasciculoventricular connections because they arise from the His bundle or bundle branches. The QRS complex may show some degree of ventricular preexcitation (either a right or left bundle branch block pattern) depending on the level of takeoff. In contrast to accessory nodoventricular connections, His bundle pacing is not expected to normalize the QRS complex, and the HV interval is short and fixed. No relations of fasciculoventricular connections to reciprocating tachycardia have been described [81]. Most of the reported cases are combined with other accessory connections mimicking the WPW syndrome [81,89,90].

Atriofascicular Bypass Tracts Intranodal Bypass Tracts and Nodal Malformations

Atriofascicular (or atrio-Hisian) bypass tracts totally bypass the AV node [91, 92], intranodal (atrionodal) bypass tracts (James fibers) partially bypass the AV node [93], and nodal malformations are described as small and immature AV nodes [94,95]. In their presence, the electrocardiogram may show a short or normal PR interval and they may be responsible for some cases of very rapid ventricular response during supraventricular tachyarrhythmias [92,96]. The association of paroxymal supraventricular tachyarrhythmias with a short PR interval and narrow QRS complexes during sinus rhythm is referred to as the Lown-Ganong-Levine syndrome [97,98].

ELECTROPHYSIOLOGIC FINDINGS

Electrophysiologic characteristics of these anatomic varieties are poorly defined and remain debatable. Some cases may have enhanced AV nodal conduction properties [18,99]: (1) AV nodal conduction time (AH interval) in sinus rhythm is less than or equal to 60 ms; (2) 1:1 atrio-His bundle conduction is maintained during atrial pacing at cycle lengths less than 300 ms (200/min); and (3) maximal AH interval prolongation is equal to or less than 100 ms at the shortest cycle length associated with 1:1 atrio-His bundle conduction.

In response to programmed atrial stimulation (incremental atrial pacing and atrial extrastimulation, three types of AV conduction curves have been described to be associated with the Lown-Ganong-Levine syndrome [94,99,100]: (1) a subnormal prolongation of the AH interval suggestive of the presence of an intranodal (atrionodal) bypass tract or a small AV node; (2) no lengthening of the AH interval suggestive of the presence of an atriofascicular (atrio-Hisian) bypass tract; and (3) no lengthening of the AH interval at slow rates and a normal prolongation of the AH interval at fast rates suggestive of the presence of an atriofascicular bypass tract or dual AV nodal pathways.

SUPRAVENTRICULAR TACHYARRHYTHMIAS

Paroxymal supraventricular tachycardia associated with the Lown-Ganong-Levine syndrome has been documented to be either an AV nodal reentrant tachycardia or AV reciprocating tachycardia involving a concealed accessory AV connection for retrograde conduction (Figure 9–31) [98,99,101,102]. The rates of supraventricular tachycardia are significantly higher than those of the same arrhythmia in control patients [99]. Furthermore, the combination of enhanced AV nodal conduction and abbreviated AV nodal refractory periods may result in a very rapid ventricular rate during atrial flutter-

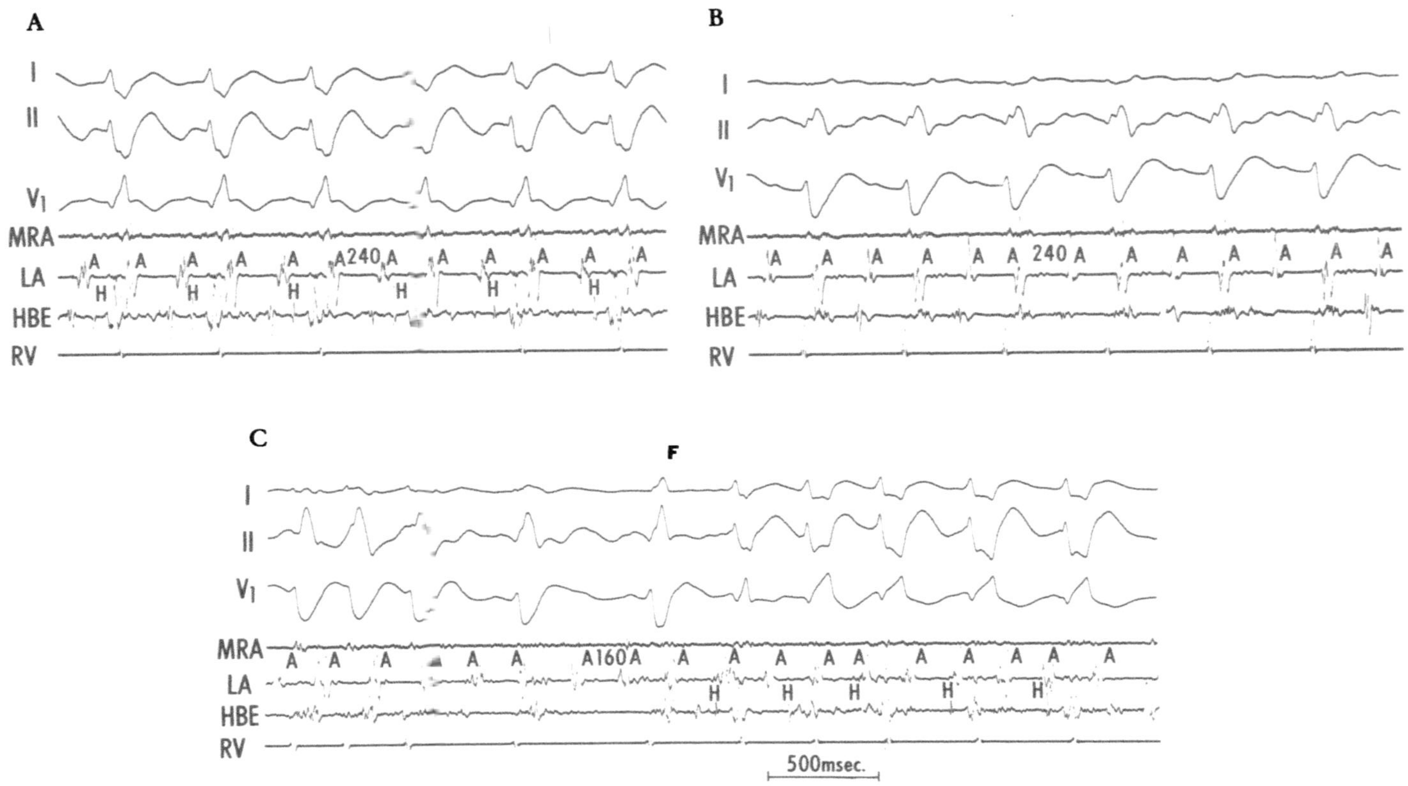

FIGURE 9–30. Intermittent atrioventricular (AV) conduction by way of the fast AV node–His–Purkinje system pathway and the slow AV node–nodoventricular bypass tract pathway during atrial flutter-fibrillation. Panels A and B, atrial flutter (atrial cycle length of 240 ms) manifests 2:1 AV block. Note that the QRS complex of a complete right bundle branch block pattern is always preceded by the His bundle potential with an HV interval of 65 ms (A). In contrast, when the QRS complex shows a complex left bundle branch block pattern, no His bundle activity can be identified (B). Similar phenomena occur during atrial fibrillation with an average atrial cycle length of 160 ms, as shown in Panel C. F = fusion beat. (From Sung RJ, Styperek JL: Electrophysiologic identification of dual atrioventricular nodal pathway conduction in patients with reciprocating tachycardia using anomalous bypass tracts. *Circulation* 60:1664, 1979 with permission.)

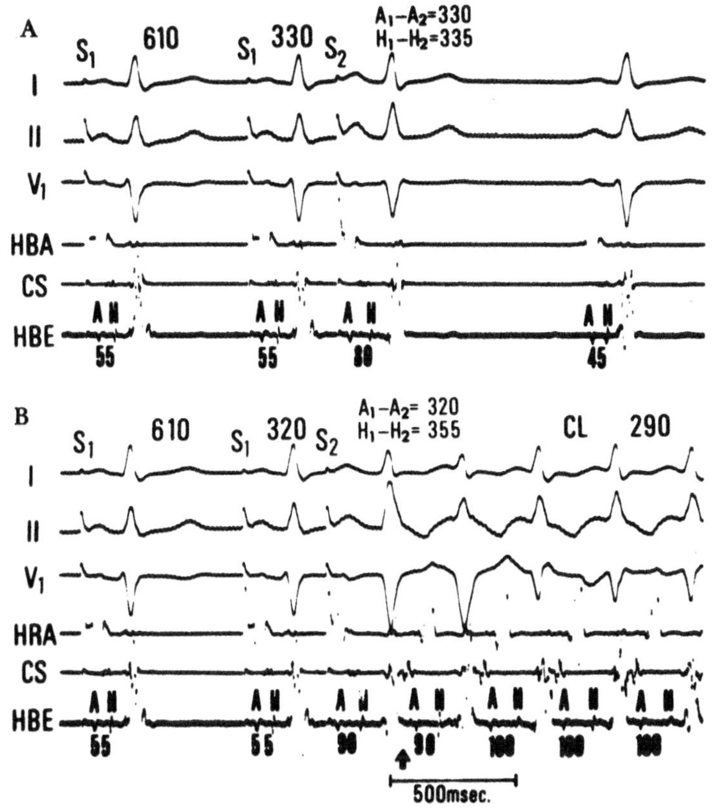

FIGURE 9–31. Induction of AV reciprocating tachycardia involving a concealed left-sided accessory AV connection in a patient with the Lown-Ganong-Levine syndrome. Atrial premature stimulation at cycle length of 610 ms produces subnormal prolongation of AV nodal conduction time (AH interval) — evidence of enhanced AV nodal conduction [18]. The atrial premature coupling interval is 330 ms and the corresponding AH interval is 80 ms. (B) Atrial premature stimulation with a premature coupling interval os 320 ms increases the AH interval to 90 ms and initiates an onset of AV reciprocating tachycardia using a concealed left-sided accessory AV connection for retrograde conduction.

fibrillation similar to that observed in the WPW syndrome [99]. Degeneration of atrial flutter-fibrillation with a fast ventricular response into ventricular fibrillation can also lead to sudden cardiac death [91,92,97,98].

Conclusion

Ventricular preexcitation can be caused by a variety of accessory connections. Most of these accessory connections have been demonstrated anatomically. Some of their electrophysiologic characteristics and functional significance have been elucidated, particularly those of the accessory AV and nodoventricular connections. Further studies on correlation between electrophysiologic findings and morphologic features are still needed for the understanding of certain types of cardiac arrhythmias in relation to the presence of these accessory connections.

References

1. Truex RC, Bishof JK, Hoffman EL: Accessory atrioventricular bundles of the developing human heart. *Anat. Rec.* 135:45, 1958.
2. Lev M: Anatomic basis for atrioventricular block. *Am. J. Med.* 37:742, 1964.
3. Childers R: The AV node: Normal and abnormal physiology. *Prog. Cardiovasc. Dis.* 19:361, 1977.
4. Anderson RH, Becker AE, Brechenmacher C, Davies MJ, Rossi L: Ventricular preexcitation. A proposed nomenclature for its substrates. *Eur. J. Cardiol.* 3:27, 1975.

5. Lev M, Kennamer R, Prinzmetal M, de Mesquita RH: A histopathologic study of the atrioventricular communication in 2 hearts with the Wolff-Parkinson-White syndrome. *Circulation* 24:41, 1961.
6. Lunel AAV: Significance of annulus fibrosis of heart in relation to AV conduction and ventricular activation in case of Wolff-Parkinson-White syndrome. *Br. Heart J.* 34:1263, 1972.
7. Becker AZ, Anderson RH, Durrer D, Wellens HJJ: The anatomic substrates of Wolff-Parkinson-White syndrome — a clinicopathologic correlation in 7 patients. *Circulation* 57:870, 1978.
8. Kent AFS: Reseaches on structure as a function of the mammalian heart. *J. Physiol.* 14:233, 1893.
9. Wellens HJJ, Durrer D: Patterns of ventriculoatrial conduction in the Wolff-Parkinson-White syndrome. *Circulation* 49:22, 1974.
10. Wellens HJJ: The electrophysiologic properties of the accessory pathway in the Wolff-Parkinson-White syndrome. In *The Conduction System of the Heart — Structure, Function and Clinical Implication*. Lea & Febiger, Philadelphia, 1976, pp. 567–587.
11. Moore EN, Spear JE, Boineau JP: Electrophysiological studies on preexcitation in the dog using an electrically simulated atrioventricular bypass pathway. *Circ. Res.* 31:174, 1972.
12. Castellanos A, Chapunoff E, Castillo C, Maytini O, Lemberg L: His bundle electrograms in two cases of Wolff-Parkinson-White syndrome. *Circulation* 41:399, 1970.
13. Gallagher JJ, Pritchett ELC, Sealy WC, Kassell J, Wallace AG: The preexcitation syndrome. *Prog. Cardiovasc. Dis.* 20:285, 1978.
14. Wolff L, Parkinson J, White PD: Bundle-branch block with short P-R interval in healthy young people prone to paroxysmal tachycardia. *Am. Heart J.* 5:685, 1930.
15. Rosenbaum FF, Hecht HH, Wilson FN, Johnston FD: The potential variations of the thorax and the esophagus in anomalous atrioventricular excitation (Wolff-Parkinson-White syndrome). *Am. Heart J.* 29:281, 1945.
16. Boineau JP, Moore EN, Spear JF, Sealy WC: Basis of static and dynamic electrocardiographic variations in Wolff-Parkinson-White syndrome. Anatomic and electrophysiologic observations in right and left ventricular preexcitation. *Am. J. Cardiol.* 32:32, 1973.
17. Svenson RH, Miller HC, Gallagher JJ, Wallace AG: Electrophysiological evaluation of the Wolff-Parkinson-White syndrome. Problems in assessing antegrade and retrograde conduction over the accessory pathway. *Circulation* 52:552, 1975.
18. Gallagher JJ, Sealy WC, Kasell J, Wallace AG: Multiple accessory pathways in patients with the preexcitation syndrome. *Circulation* 54:571, 1976.
19. Mendoza IJ, Castellanos A, Sung RJ: Wolff-Parkinson-White syndrome, Typbe B with tachycardia-dependent (Phase 3) block in the accessory pathway and in left bundle branch block coexisting with rate unrelated right bundle branch block. *Br. Heart J.* 43:481, 1980.
20. Grolleau R, Puech P, Cabasson J, Baissus C, Latour H: Particularitiés de la conduction auriculo-ventriculare dans un syndrome de Wolff-Parkinson-White. *Arch. Mal Coeur* 67:13, 1974.
21. Neuss H, Schlepper M, Spies HF: Double ventricular response to an atrial extrasystole in a patient with WPW syndrome type C. *Eur. J. Cardiol.* 2:175, 1974.
22. Wu D, Denes P, Dhingra R, Pietras RJ, Rosen KM: New manifestations of dual A-V nodal pathways. *Eur. J. Cardiol.* 2:459, 1975.
23. Motte G, Oster G, Coumel PH, Slama R: Tachycardies par rhythme reciproque entre les voies normales et une voie auriculo-hissiene rapide. *Arch. Mal Coeur* 68:673, 1975.
24. Csapo G: Paroxysmal non-reentrant tachycardia due to simultaneous conduction in dual atrioventricular nodal pathways. *Am. J. Cardiol.* 43:1033, 1979.
25. Wyndham CRC, Amat-y-Leon F, Wu D, Denes P, Dhingra R, Simpson R, Rosen K: Effects of cycle length on atrial vulnerability. *Circulation* 55:260, 1977.
26. Sung RJ, Castellanos A, Mallon SM, Bloom MG, Gelband H, Myerburg RJ: Mechanisms of spontaneous alteration between reciprocating tachycardia and atrial flutter-fibrillation in the Wolff-Parkinson-White syndrome. *Circulation* 56:409, 1977.
27. Castellanos A, Jr, Myerburg RJ, Craparo K, Befeler B, Agha AS: Factors regulating ventricular rates during atrial flutter and fibrillation in pre-excitation (Wolff-Parkinson-White) syndrome. *Br. Heart J.* 35:811, 1973.
28. Wellens HJ, Durrer D: Wolff-Parkinson-White syndrome and atrial fibrillation. Relation between refractory period of accessory pathway and ventricular rate during atrial fibrillation. *Am. J. Cardiol.* 34:777, 1974.
29. Wellens HJJ, Brugada P, Roy D, Weiss J, Bar FW: Effect of isoproterenol on the antegrade refractory period of the accessory pathway in patients with the Wolff-Parkinson-White syndrome. *Am. J. Cardiol.* 50:180, 1982.
30. German LD, Gallagher JJ, Broughton A, Giuarnieri T, Trantham JL: Effects of exercise and isoproterenol during atrial fibrillation in patients with Wolff-Parkinson-White syndrome. *Am. J. Cardiol.* 1983; 51:1203, 1983.

31. Klein GJ, Bashore TM, Sellers TD, Pritchett ELC, Smith WM, Gallagher JJ: Ventricular fibrillation in the Wolff-Parkinson-White syndrome. *N. Engl. J. Med.* 301:1080, 1979.
32. Scherf D, Cohen J: Preexcitation syndrome. In *The Atrioventricular Node and Selected Cardiac Arrhythmias.* Grune & Stratton, New York, 1964, pp. 372–447.
33. Sung RJ, Gelband H, Castellanos A, Aranda JM, Myerburg RJ: Clinical and electrophysiologic observations in patients with concealed accessory bypass tracts. *Am. J. Cardiol.* 40:839, 1977.
34. Shen EN, Sung RJ: Initiation of atrial fibrillation by spontaneous ventricular premature beats in concealed Wolff-Parkinson-White syndrome. *Am. Heart J.* 153:911, 1982.
35. Campbell RWF, Smith RA, Gallagher JJ, Pritchett ELC, Wallace AG: Atrial fibrillation in the preexcitation syndrome. *Am. J. Cardiol.* 40:514, 1977.
36. Massing CK, Waldo AL, James TN: Spontaneous atrial premature depolarizations during paroxysmal reentrant tachycardia. *J. Electrocardiol.* 28:263, 1971.
37. Durrer D, Schoo L, Schullenburg RM, Wellens HJJ: The role of premature beats in the initiation and termination of supraventricular tachycardia in the Wolff-Parkinson-White syndrome. *Circulation* 36:644, 1967.
38. Wellens HJJ: Tachycardias related to the preexcitation syndrome. In *Electrical Stimulation of the Heart in the Study and Treatment of Tachycardias.* Ed. by Wellens HJJ Baltimore, University Park Press, 1971, pp. 70–121.
39. Fontaine G, Frank R, Coutte R, Vandel J-P, Grosgogeat Y: Rhythme reciproque antidromique dans un syndrome de Wolff-Parkinson-White de type A. *Ann. Cardiol. Angeiol.* 24:59, 1975.
40. Benditt DG, Pritchett ELC, Gallagher JJ: Spectrum of regular tachycardias with wide QRS complexes in patients with accessory atrioventricular pathways. *Am. J. Cardiol.* 42:828, 1978.
41. Benson DW Jr, Smith WM, Dunnigan A, Sterba R, Gallagher JJ: Mechanisms of regular wide QRS tachycardia in infants and children. *Am. J. Cardiol.* 49:1778, 1982.
42. Denes P, Amat-y-Leon F, Wyndham C, Wu D, Levitsky S, Rosen KM: Electrophysiologic demonstration of bilateral anomalous pathways in a patient with Wolff-Parkinson-White syndrome (Type B preexcitation). *Am. J. Cardiol.* 37:93, 1976.
43. Cinca J, Valle V, Gutiewez L, Figuras J, Ruiz J: Reciprocating tachycardia using bilateral accessory pathways: Electrophysiological and clinical implications. *Circulation* 62:657, 1980.
44. Bardy GH, Packer DL, German LD, Gallagher JJ: Preexcited reciprocating tachycardia in patients with Wolff-Parkinson-White syndrome: Incidence and mechanisms. *Circulation* 70:377, 1984.
45. Wellens HJ, Durrer D: Patterns of ventriculo-atrial conduction in the Wolff-Parkinson-White syndrome. *Circulation* 49:21, 1974.
46. Sung RJ, Castellanos A, Mallon SM, Gelband H, Mendoza I, Myerburg RJ: Mode of initiation of reciprocating tachycardia during programmed ventricular stimulation in the Wolff-Parkinson-White syndrome. With reference to various patterns of ventriculo-atrial conduction. *Am. J. Cardiol.* 40:24, 1977.
47. Slama R, Coumel P, Bouvrain Y: Les syndromes de Wolff-Parkinson-White de type A inapparents ou latents en rhythme sinusal. *Arch. Mal Coeur* 66:639, 1973.
48. Coumel P, Attuel P: Reciprocating tachycardia in overt and latent preexcitation. Influence of functional bundle branch block on the rate of tachycardia . *Eur. J. Cardiol.* 1:423, 1974.
49. Zipes DP, DeJoseph RL, Rothbaum DA: Unusual properties of accessory pathways. *Circulation* 49:1200, 1974.
50. Agha AS, Befeler B, Sung RJ, Castillo CA, Myerburg RJ, Castellanos A: Bipolar catheter electrograms for study of retrograde atrial activation pattern in patients with pre-excitation syndromes. *Br. Heart J.* 38:641, 1976.
51. De las Fuente D, Sasyniuk B, Moe GM: Conduction through a narrow isthmus in isolated canine atrial tissue. A model for the W-P-W syndrome. *Circulation* 44:803, 1971.
52. Przybylski J, Chiale PA, Halpern S, Nau G, Elizari MV, Rosenbaum MB: Unmasking of ventricular pre-excitation by vagal stimulation or isoproterenol administration. *Circulation* 61:1030, 1980.
53. Przybylski J, Chiale PA, Elizari MV, Rosenbaum MB: Physiological properties of accessory pathways. In *Frontiers of Cardiac Electrophysiology.* Ed. by MB Rosenbaum and MV Elizari. Martinus Nijhoff Publishers, Boston, 1983, pp. 702–723.
54. Sung RJ, Castellanos A, Gelband H, Myerburg RJ: Mechanism of reciprocating tachycardia initiated during sinus rhythm in concealed Wolff-Parkinson-White syndrome. *Circulation* 54:338, 1976.
55. Parkinson J, Papp C: Repetitive paroxysmal tachycardia. *Br. Heart J.* 9:241, 1947.
56. Sung RJ: Incessant supraventricular tachycardia. *PACE* 6:1306, 1983.
57. Neuss H, Schlepper M, Thormann J: Analysis of reentry mechanisms in three patients with concealed Wolff-Parkinson-White syndrome. *Circulation* 51:75, 1975.
58. Langendorf R: Concealed A-V conduction: The

effect of blocked impulses on the formation and conduction of subsequent impulses. *Am. Heart J.* 35:542, 1948.
59. Sung RJ, Myerburg RJ, Castellanos A: Electrophysiologic demonstration of concealed conduction in the human atrium. *Circulation* 58:940, 1978.
60. Damato AN, Lau SH, Patton RD, Steiner C Berkowitz WD: A study of atrioventricular conduction in man using premature atrial stimulation and His bundle recordings. *Circulation* 40:61, 1969.
61. Cohen HC, D'Cruz I, Pick A: Concealed intraventricular conduction in the His bundle electrogram. *Circulation* 53:776, 1976.
62. Svinarich JT, Keung EC, Sung RJ: Electrophysiologic demonstration of concealed conduction in anomalous atrioventricular bypass tracts. (Abstract.) *J. Am. Coll. Cardiol.* 3:611, 1984.
63. Klein GJ, Yee R, Sharma: Concealed conduction in accessory atrioventricular pathways: An important determinant of the expression of arrhythmias in the Wolff-Parkinson-White syndrome. (Abstract.) *Clin. Res.* 32:179A, 1984.
64. Svinarich JT, Tai DY, Mickelson J, Keung EC, Sung RJ: Electrophysiologic demonstration of concealed conduction in anomalous atrioventricular bypass tracts. *J. Am. Coll. Cardiol.* 5:898, 1985.
65. Gallagher JJ, Sealy WC: The permanent form of junctional reciprocating tachycardia — further elucidation of the underlying mechanism. *Eur. J. Cardiol.* 8:413, 1978.
66. Denes P, Kehoe R, Rosen KM: Multiple reentrant tachycardias due to retrograde conduction of dual atrioventricular bundles with atrioventricular nodal-like properties. *Am. J. Cardiol.* 44:162, 1979.
67. Epstein ML, Stone FM, Benditt DG: Incessant atrial tachycardia in childhood: Association with rate-dependent conduction in an accessory atrioventricular pathway. *Am. J. Cardiol.* 44:498, 1979.
68. Farre J, Ross P, Weiner I, Bar H, Vanagt EJ, Wellens HJJ: Reciprocal tachycardias using accessory pathway with long conduction times. *Am. J. Cardiol.* 44:1099, 1979.
69. Tai DY, Chang MS, Svinarich JT, Ching BN, Sung RJ: Mechanisms of verapamil-induced conduction block in anomalous atrioventricular bypass tracts. *J. Am. Coll. Cardiol.* 5:311, 1985.
70. Tai DY, Shen EN, Svinarich JT, Michelson J, Dohrmann ML, Sung RJ: Intravenous propafenone — an effective antiarrhythmic agent for tachyarrhythmias associated with Wolff-Parkinson-White syndrome. (Abstract.) *Circulation* 70:II–43, 1984.
71. Rosenbaum MB, Chiale PA, Ryba D, Elizari MV: Control of tachyarrhythmias associated with Wolff-Parkinson-White syndrome by amiodarone hydrochloride. *Am. J. Cardiol.* 34:215, 1974.
72. Sellers TD, Bashore TM, Gallagher JJ: Digitalis in the preexcitation syndrome: Analysis during atrial fibrillation. *Circulation* 52:552, 1975.
73. Gulamhusein S, Ko P, Carruthers G, Klein GJ: Acceleration of the ventricular response during atrial fibrillation in the Wolff-Parkinson-White syndrome after verapamil. *Circulation* 65:348, 1982.
74. Sung RJ, Elser B, McAllister RG, Jr: Intravenous verapamil for termination of re-entrant supraventricular tachycardia: Intracardiac studies correlated with plasma verapamil concentrations. *Ann. Intern. Med.* 93:682, 1978.
75. Svinarich JT, Tai DY, Sung RJ: Is beta-adrenergic blockade contraindicated in Wolff-Parkinson-White patients prone to atrial flutter-fibrillation? (Abstract.) *Circulation* 70:II–251, 1984.
76. Mahaim I, Benatt A: Nouvelles recherches sur les connexions superieures de la branche gauche du faisceau de His-Tawara avec cloison interventriculaire. *Cardiologia* 1:61, 1968.
77. Mark AL, Basta LL: Paroxysmal tachycardia with atrioventricular dissociation in a patient with a variant of pre-excitation syndrome. *J. Electrocardiol.* 7:355, 1974.
78. Tonkin AM, Dugan FA, Svenson RH, Sealy WC, Wallace AG, Gallagher JJ: Coexistence of functional Kent and Mahaim-type tracts in the preexcitation syndrome. Demonstration by catheter techniques and epicardial mapping. *Circulation* 52:193, 1975.
79. Sung RJ, Styperek JL: Electrophysiologic identification of dual atriventricular nodal pathway conduction in patients with reciprocating tachycardia using anomalous bypass tracts. *Circulation* 60:1464, 1979.
80. Ward DE, Carson AJ, Spurrell RAJ: Ventricular preexcitation due to anomalous nodoventricular pathways: Report of 3 patients. *Eur. J. Cardiol.* 9:111, 1979.
81. Gallagher JJ, Smith WM, Kasell JH, Benson DW, Sterba R, Grant AO: Role of Mahaim fibers in cardiac arrhythmias in man. *Circulation* 64:176, 1981.
82. Juma Z, Saksena S, Levy S, Wolff GS, Sung RJ: Electrophysiologic characteristics of nodoventricular bypass tract conduction in patients with dual atrioventricular nodal pathways. (Abstract.) *Circulation* 60 (Suppl III):III–47, 1980.
83. Sung RJ, Waxman H, Juma Z, Saksena S: Sequence of retrograde atrial activation in patients with dual atrioventricular nodal pathways. *Circulation* 64:1059, 1981.
84. Coumel P: Junctional reciprocating tachycardias. The permanent and paroxysmal forms

of AV nodal reciprocating tachycardias. *J. Electrocardiol.* 8:79, 1975.
85. Wu D, Denes P, Amat-y-Leon, Rosen KM: An unusual variety of atrioventricular nodal reentry due to retrograde dual atrioventricular nodal pathways. *Circulation* 56:50, 1977.
86. Sung RJ, Styperek JL, Myerburg RJ, Castellanos A: Initiation of two distinct forms of atrioventricular nodal reentrant tachycardia during programmed ventricular stimulation in man. *Am. J. Cardiol.* 42:404, 1978.
87. Coumel P, Attuel P, Magica J: Junctional reciprocating tachycardia. The permanent form. In *Reentrant Arrhythmias*, Ed. HE Kulbertus. MTP Press, Lancaster 1977, pp. 170–183.
88. Gallagher JJ, Smith WM, Kerr CR: Etiology of long-P-R tachycardia in 33 cases of supraventricular tachycardia. (Abstract.) *Circulation* 64 (Suppl. IV):IV–145, 1981.
89. Lev M, Fox SM, III, Bharati S, Greenfield JC, Jr, Rosen KM, Pick A: Mahaim and James fibers as a basis for a unique variety of ventricular preexcitation. *Am. J. Cardiol.* 36:880, 1975.
90. Neuss H, Thormann J: Functional properties of Mahaim fibers. *Klin. Wochenschr.* 55:1031, 1977.
91. Lev M, Leffler WB, Langendorf R, Pick A: Anatomic findings in a case of ventricular preexcitation (WPW) terminating in complete atrioventricular block. *Circulation* 34:718, 1966.
92. Brechenmacher C, Laham J, Iris L, Gerbeaux A, Lenegre J: Etude histologique des voies anormales de conduction dans un syndrome de Wolff-Parkinson-White et dans un syndrome de Lown-Ganong-Levine. *Arch. Mal Coeur* 67:507, 1974.
93. James TN: Morphology of the human atrioventricular node with remarks pertinent to its electrophysiology. *Am. Heart J.* 62:756, 1961.
94. Caracta AR, Damato AN, Gallagher JJ, Josephson ME, Varghese PJ, Lau SH, Westura EE: Electrophysiologic studies in the syndrome of short P-R interval, normal QRS complex. *Am. J. Cardiol.* 31:245, 1973.
95. Anderson RH, Arnold R, Thapar MK, Jones RS, Hamilton DI: Cardiac specialized tissue in hearts with an apparently single ventricular chamber (Double Inlet Left Ventricle). *Am. J. Cardiol.* 33:95, 1974.
96. Blanc JJ, Fontaliran F, Gerbaux A, Boschat J, Penther P: Atrial flutter with 1–1 atrioventricular conduction: Electrophysiologic and histologic correlations. *Am. Heart J.* 107:1044, 1984.
97. Lown B, Ganong WF, Levine SA: The syndrome of short P-R interval, normal QRS complex and paroxysmal rapid heart action. *Circulation* 5:693, 1952.
98. Castellanos A, Zaman L, Moleiro F, Aranda J, Myerburg RJ: The Lown-Ganong-Levine syndrome. *PACE* 5:715, 1982.
99. Benditt DG, Pritchett ELC, Smith WM, Wallace AG, Gallagher JJ: Characteristics of atrioventricular conduction and the spectrum of arrhythmias in Lown-Ganong-Levine syndrome. *Circulation* 57:454, 1978.
100. Castellanos A, Castillo CA, Agha AS, Tessler M: His bundle electrograms in patients with short P-R intervals, narrow QRS complexes, and paroxysmal tachycardias. *Circulation* 43:667, 1971.
101. Josepheson ME, Kastor JA: Supraventricular tachycardia in Lown-Ganong-Levine syndrome: Atrionodal versus intranodal reentry. *Am. J. Cardiol.* 40:521, 1977.
102. Bauernfeind RA, Ayres BF, Wyndham CC, Rosen KM: Cycle length in atrioventricular nodal reentrant paroxysmal tachycardia with observations on the Lown-Ganong-Levine syndrome. *Am. J. Cardiol.* 45:1148, 1980.

10. ROLE OF NODOVENTRICULAR AND FASCICULOVENTRICULAR CONNECTIONS IN TACHYARRHYTHMIAS

John J. Gallagher

The role of "Mahaim fibers" in the genesis of cardiac arrhythmias in man has been controversial since they were first described [1]. The initial report was limited to fibers connecting the His bundle to the septum but this was soon broadened to include fibers connecting the atrioventricular (AV) node to the septum. Although the existence of these has been confirmed anatomically [2–25], their functional significance has remained controversial [26–80].

In this chapter, electrophysiologic studies in patients with Mahaim fibers will be discussed. Current evidence suggests that some of these fibers do participate in cardiac arrhythmias in man. Furthermore, nonpharmacological forms of therapy are now available for palliation or cure of arrhythmias not controlled by medical therapy.

Terminology

Two main anatomic types of Mahaim fibers have been recognized: nodoventricular (NV) fibers, which arise from the AV node, and fasciculoventricular (FV) fibers which arise from the His bundle and bundle branches [15]. Because the functional consequences are significant, it is useful to consider the two groups separately according to an anatomic and functional classification (Figure 10–1). Anderson [15] has further proposed that two varieties of

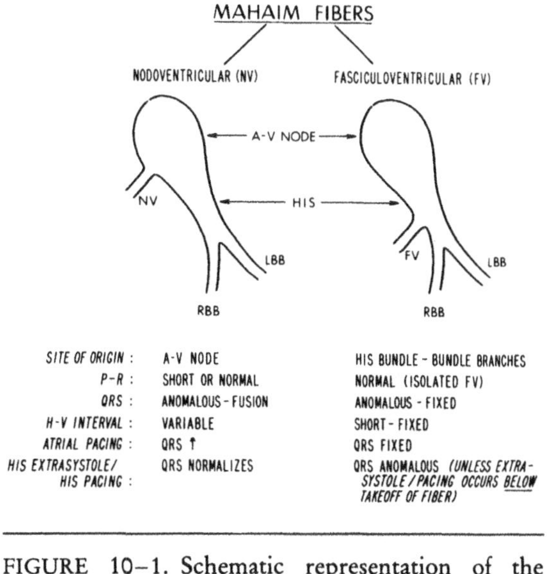

FIGURE 10–1. Schematic representation of the atrioventricular node with two varieties of Mahaim fibers. Nodoventricular (NV) connections arise from the AV node itself, while fasciculoventricular (FV) connections arise from the His bundle or the bundle branches. RBB = right bundle branch; LBB = left bundle branch. Reproduced with permission of the *Am. Heart Assoc.* from Gallagher, JJ et al.: [61].

NV fibers exist: those which arise from the transitional zone of the AV junction and those which arise from the deep, compact nodal portion of the AV junction.

NV fibers, depending on the level of takeoff relative to the area of physiologic AV node delay, can be associated with either a short or normal PR interval. Ventricular activation in this case results from fusion of impulse conduction via the NV fiber and the normal conduction system, resulting in QRS complexes of variable morphology depending upon the degree of anomalous ventricular activation.

FV fibers, arising from the His bundle or bundle branches, result in minor abbreviations of the HV interval and some degree of anomalous QRS morphology. The PR interval however is usually normal in the absence of some other abnormality of AV conduction.

Extrasystoles arising in the His bundle or pacing of the His bundle in the case of NV fibers should normalize the QRS; in the case of FV fibers, the anomalous appearance of the QRS should persist unless the extrasystole arises below the takeoff of the FV fiber, as proposed by Pick and Katz [26] from the study of scalar ECGs.

Nodoventricular Connections

The electrophysiologic findings in a patient felt to have a so-called nodoventricular connection were first reported by Wellens in 1971 [29]. Only a single case report is available that correlates anatomic and electrophysiologic findings in a patient with a nodoventricular connection [78]. All studies have demonstrated certain characteristic features of preexcitation that would be anticipated on the basis of the anatomic connection proposed. Although at the outset the term *nodoventricular* (NV) has been selected to facilitate discussion, it should be emphasized that fibers arising in the AV node may insert into the specialized conduction system (nodofascicular) or ventricular myocardium (nodoventricular). The distinction between these two substrates will be discussed later.

Much of the following commentary is based on detailed electrophysiologic study of 16 patients with NV connections, consisting of 10 males and 6 females aging 4–34 years (mean 20.8 ± 8.6 years). Eight patients had isolated NV fibers; 5 had NV connections, Ebstein's anomaly, and WPW syndrome; 2 had NV connections and WPW syndrome and one had isolated Ebstein's. Two of the WPW patients had their accessory AV pathway divided prior to the study of their NV connection.

STUDIES DURING SINUS RHYTHM/ATRIAL PACING

As anticipated in the schematic presentation in Figure 10–1, the PR interval may be abbreviated but is usually normal (Figure 10–2). Similarly, the surface electrocardiogram during sinus rhythm is almost always normal. In patients with isolated NV connections, the PA interval was prolonged in five patients (four with Ebstein's anomaly, one with isolated atrial septal defect). The AH interval ranged from 40–155 ms (mean 73.7 ± 31.4).

Typically with atrial pacing or premature atrial stimulation (Figure 10–3), the PR interval prolongs and the QRS assumes a left bundle branch block morphology. Intracavitary recordings during pacing demonstrate prolongation of the interval from the atrium to the His deflection (AH) and displacement of the His deflection into the ventricular electrogram. In contrast to accessory AV connections, the PR interval remains normal or prolongs despite the appearance of anomalous conduction. The increment of delay observed with atrial pacing or premature atrial stimulation is rarely greater than 50 ms, indicating a low "safety factor" in intranodal conduction proximal to the takeoff of the connection or within the connection itself. When right atrial pacing is compared to coronary sinus pacing at comparable cycle lengths, the degree of anomalous conduction is invariably greater with right atrial pacing. This latter observation is independent of the AH interval, suggesting that the atrial insertion is functionally related to the right atrium.

In 11 of the 16 patients, it was possible to assess the capacity for antegrade conduction over the NV connection. The minimum cycle length associated with 1:1 AV conduction over the NV connection ranged from 400 to 180 ms (mean 267.3 ms). In only two patients was the minimal cycle length of conduction over the NV connection ≤ to 240 ms. One of these was a 34-year-old woman who developed an increment of only 30 ms during right atrial pacing from cycle length 600 to 200 ms. This suggested origin of the NV connection in the transitional zone of the AV node.

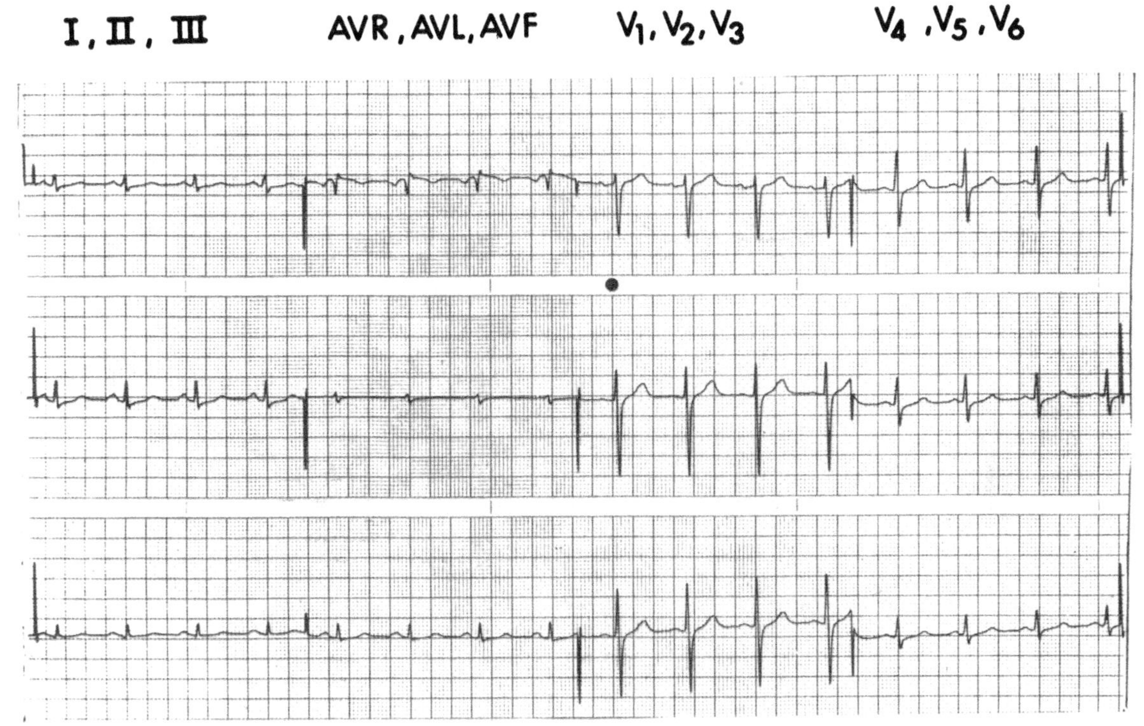

FIGURE 10–2. Normal electrocardiogram recorded in a patient with nodoventricular connection.

(This patient had ventriculoatrial dissociation during reciprocating tachycardia, excluding an accessory AV pathway as the basis of preexcitation.) The other patient, a 4-year-old boy, prolonged AV conduction only by 90 ms during pacing from cycle length 400 to 180 ms. This response may be comparable to the enhanced nodal properties seen in young patients [81]. Administration of isoproterenol has been found to markedly facilitate conduction across a NV connection.

ELECTROCARDIOGRAPHIC MORPHOLOGY OF PREEXCITATION DUE TO A NV CONNECTION

Description of the ECG morphology resulting from preexcitation due to NV connections presents a semantic dilemma. An ECG pattern of left bundle branch block (LBBB) can result whenever the left ventricle is activated after the right ventricle. This can be due to relatively *early* activation of the right ventricle or relatively *late* activation of the left ventricle. Thus preexcitation on the right side or conduction delay/block on the left side of the heart can result in similar ECG patterns. To date, NV connections have appeared to exclusively preexcite the *right* ventricle resulting in left bundle branch block morphology with left axis deviation.

We recently examined our experience with patients presenting with tachycardia associated with left bundle branch block morphology in order to identify ECG clues suggesting the presence of a NV connection [82]. The study group consisted of 13 patients with tachycardia related to a Mahaim fiber, 34 patients with supraventricular tachycardia and aberrant conduction of the left bundle branch block type, 22 patients with ventricular tachycardia, and 18 patients with antidromic tachycardia using a right-sided accessory AV pathway. Six variables present during tachycardia of left bundle branch block morphology were predictive of a Mahaim fiber (Figure 10–4): cycle length between 220 and 450 ms, QRS axis of 0 to −75°, QRS duration 0.15 seconds or less, presence of an R in lead I, rS wave in precordial lead V_1, and a precordial transition from a predominantly negative to a predominantly positive QRS after V_4. All 6

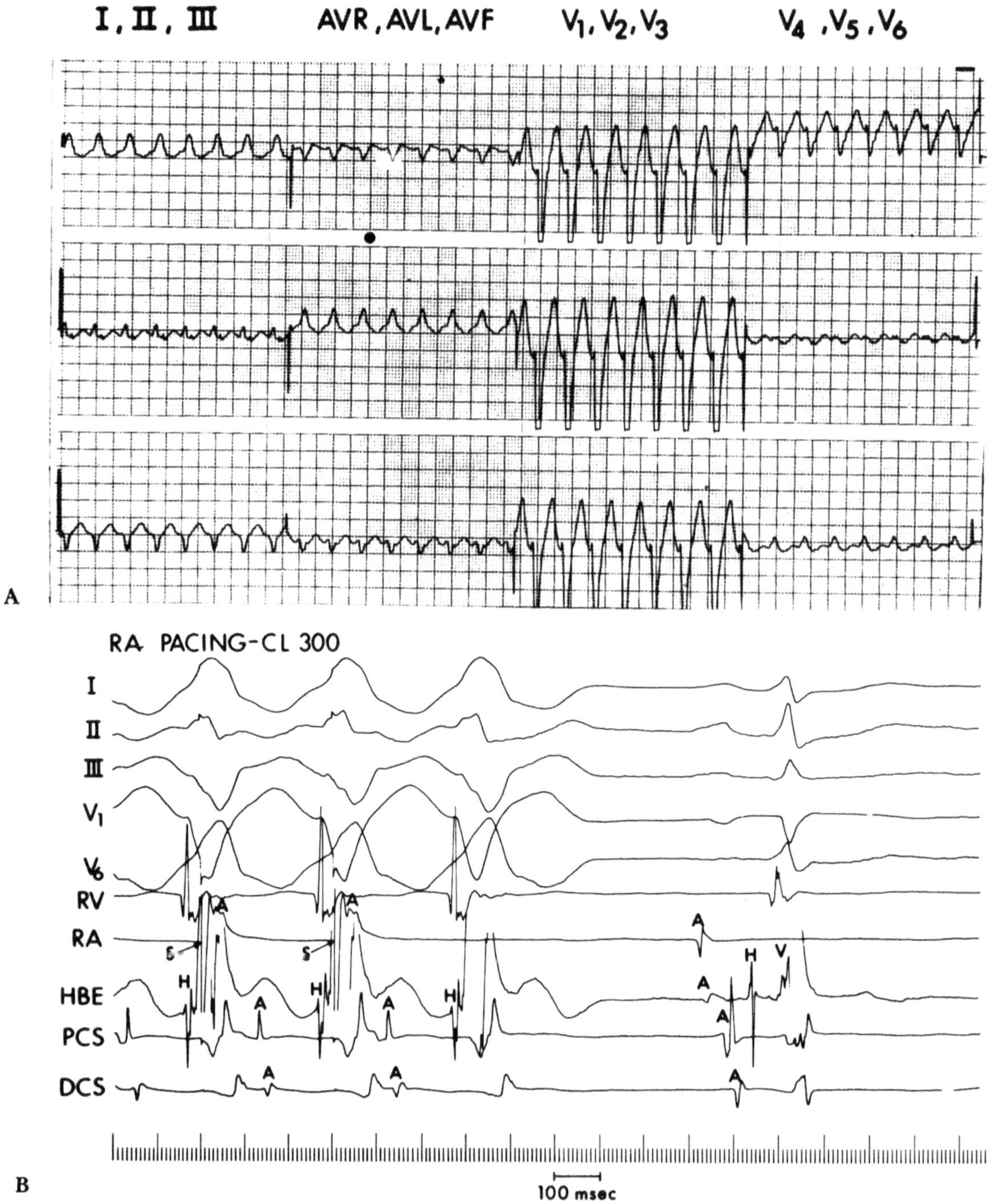

FIGURE 10–3. Recordings from a patient with a nodoventricular connection during atrial pacing. (Panel A) A 12-lead electrocardiogram is shown recorded during atrial pacing which resulted in maximal preexcitation over a nodoventricular fiber. The PR interval is prolonged and a left bundle branch block morphology with left axis deviation is present. (Panel B) Intracavitary recordings during right atrial pacing. Recordings from above down are standard ECG leads I–III, V_1, V_6 and bipolar electrograms recorded from the right ventricular apex (RV), the right atrium (RA), the region of the His bundle (HBE), the proximal coronary sinus (PCS) and the distal coronary sinus (DCS). During pacing at cycle length of 300 ms, the AV interval is prolonged and the His deflection is inscribed after the onset of the QRS complex. With termination of pacing a normally conducted QRS complex is noted, associated with a normal AH and HV interval. A = atrial electrogram; H = His bundle electrogram; V = ventricular electrogram; S = stimulus artifact. Reproduced with permission of Grune and Stratton Publishing Co. from Gallagher et al. [70].

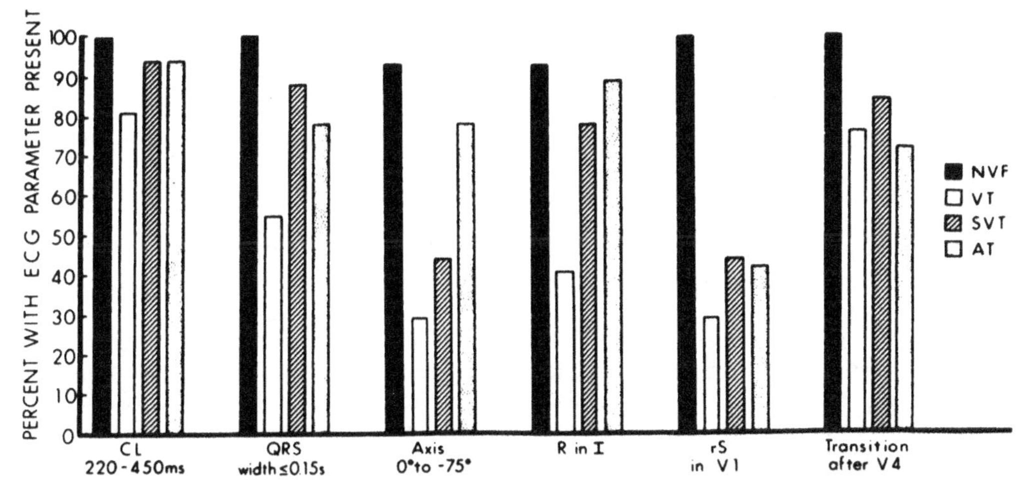

FIGURE 10–4. Relative incidence of six electrocardiographic (ECG) features during tachycardia of left bundle branch block configuration in patients with nodofascicular connection (NVF), ventricular tachycardia (VT), supraventricular tachycardia with aberration (SVT) and antidromic tachycardia (AT). CL = cycle length. (See text for discussion.) Reproduced with permission of Elsevier Science Publishing Company from Bardy et al. [82].

criteria were present in 16 of the 87 patients. No patient with ventricular tachycardia satisfied all of these criteria, whereas 3 of 34 with supraventricular tachycardia, one of 18 with antidromic tachycardia and 12 of 13 with tachycardia using a Mahaim fiber did. Thus the surface ECG recorded during tachycardia can provide clues to the presence of a NV connection although it is not diagnostic. Nevertheless, recognition of the characteristic ECG morphology can direct attention to the possibility of this substrate during a detailed electrophysiologic study.

NORMALIZATION OF PREEXCITATION DUE TO A NV CONNECTION

As noted previously, the QRS complex during sinus rhythm in the presence of a NV connection is generally normal unless there is some other abnormality of AV conduction. Nonetheless, under appropriate autonomic conditions, intermittent preexcitation over a Mahaim connection generally can be observed. Three patients in the study group exhibited almost constant preexcitation over the NV connection but in each case an underlying abnormality could be recognized as the cause: One patient had right bundle branch block due to Ebstein's anomaly, one had right bundle branch block related to previous patch repair of a low atrial septal defect, and one was felt to have a NV connection originating in the transitional zone of the AV node. In cases of intermittent preexcitation, the QRS generally normalized following administration of atropine or isoproterenol (Figure 10–5). Impulse initiation in the His bundle achieved by His bundle pacing (Figure 10–6) or His bundle extrasystoles (Figure 10–7) was observed in the majority of patients and invariably resulted in either a normal (13/16 patients) or right bundle branch block QRS morphology (3/16 patients).

STUDIES DURING VENTRICULAR PACING

Retrograde conduction could be assessed in the absence of an accessory AV pathway in 11 of 16 patients. Retrograde conduction was absent at all paced cycle lengths in 3 patients. In the remaining patients the shortest cycle length with 1:1 ventriculoatrial conduction ranged from 510–250 ms (mean 321.4 ms). The retrograde His deflection preceded the onset of retrograde atrial depolarization which was always initiated in the low interatrial septum with symmetric spread to the lateral right and left atria. Refractory period determinations demonstrated smooth curves.

STUDIES DURING RECIPROCATING TACHYCARDIA

A spontaneous tachycardia with left bundle branch block morphology (cycle length 210–400 ms, mean 306 ± 53.8 ms) was documented in all patients with isolated NV connections. The morphology during tachycardia could be reproduced by overdrive atrial pacing. Left axis deviation (−10° to −75°, mean −38°) was typically present, suggesting that the site of insertion of the connection was related to the posterior-inferior right ventricular septum.

The His deflection *never* preceded QRS complexes with left bundle branch block morphology during tachycardia (Figure 10–8), a situation identical to that observed with overdrive atrial pacing. Ventriculoatrial dissociation was present during tachycardia in 4 patients. In the remainder there was a 1:1 relationship between ventricles and atria which correlated with the presence of retrograde conduction in these patients during ventricular pacing at comparable cycle lengths. The septal sequence of retrograde atrial activation was the same during tachycardia as during ventricular pacing in the absence of an anomalous AV pathway and was indistinguishable from the expected normal sequence of retrograde conduction via the AV node.

Tachycardia induction could be achieved by programmed stimulation from the atrium (Figure 10–9) or the ventricle (Figure 10–10) although in general ventricular stimulation yielded a higher success rate.

Ventriculoatrial dissociation during tachycardia can occur since the atria are not a necessary link, regardless of which mechanism is present [84]. This has been encountered to date in 4/16 patients (Figure 10–11). Reversal of the macroreentry circuit has been observed on two occasions (Figure 10–12), and, curiously, both were patients who exhibited ventriculoatrial dissociation during tachycardia.

During left bundle branch block morphology tachycardia, a retrograde His deflection has been recognized in 11 of the 16 patients. The exact timing of the retrograde His deflection and the implications therein will be addressed in a later section dealing with the site of distal insertion of the NV connection.

MECHANISM OF RECIPROCATING TACHYCARDIA

Two mechanisms have been proposed to explain the manner in which NV (nodoventricular or nodofascicular) connections participate in the genesis of cardiac arrhythmias (Figure 10–13). Whether the connection forms a limb of the reentry circuit [29,61], or merely serves as a "bystander" to reentry confined to the AV node [55,65,83] continues to be controversial.

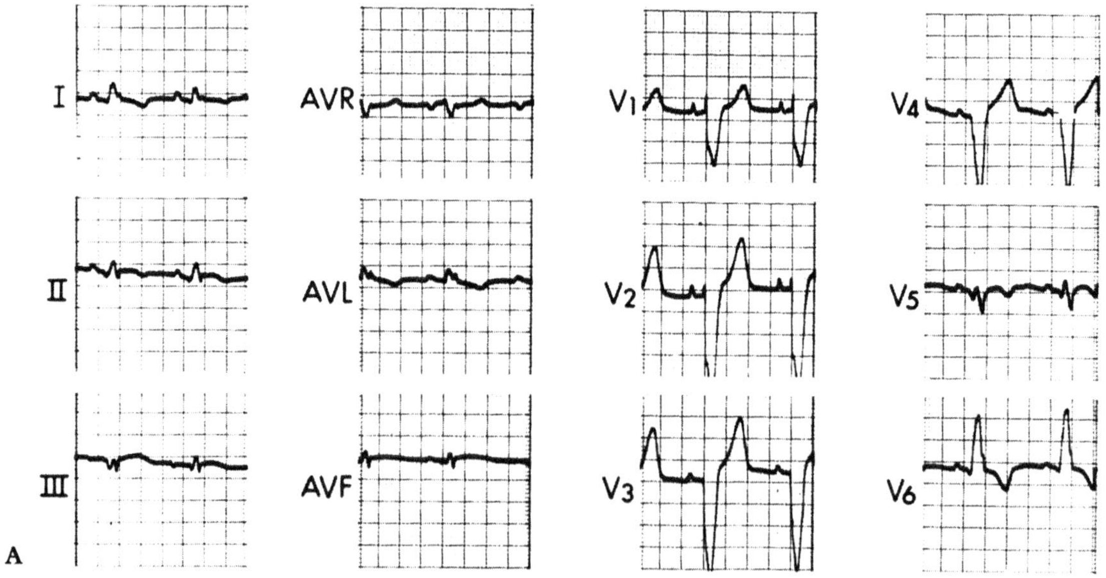

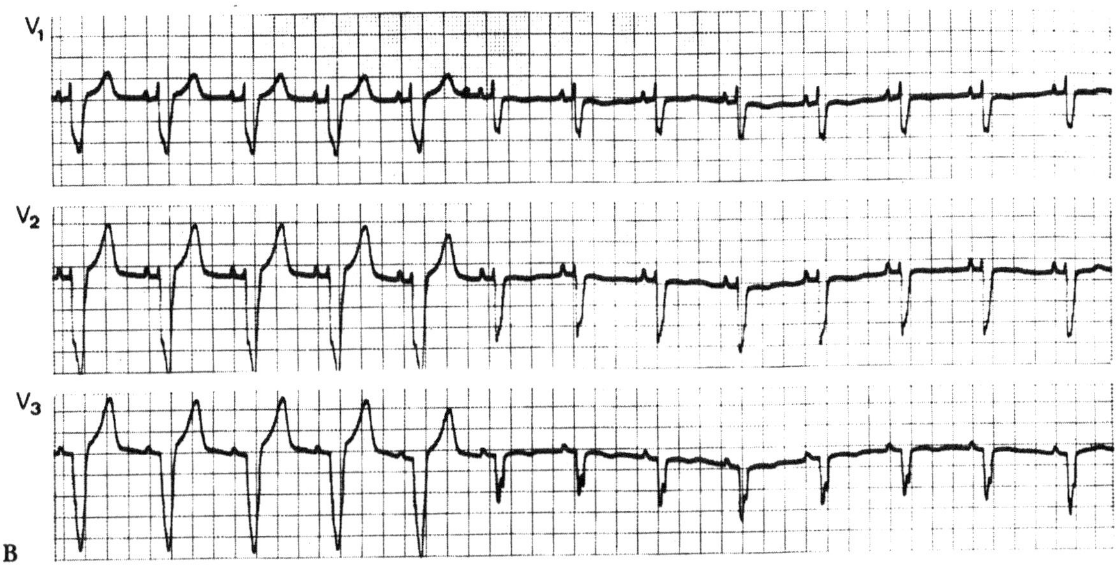

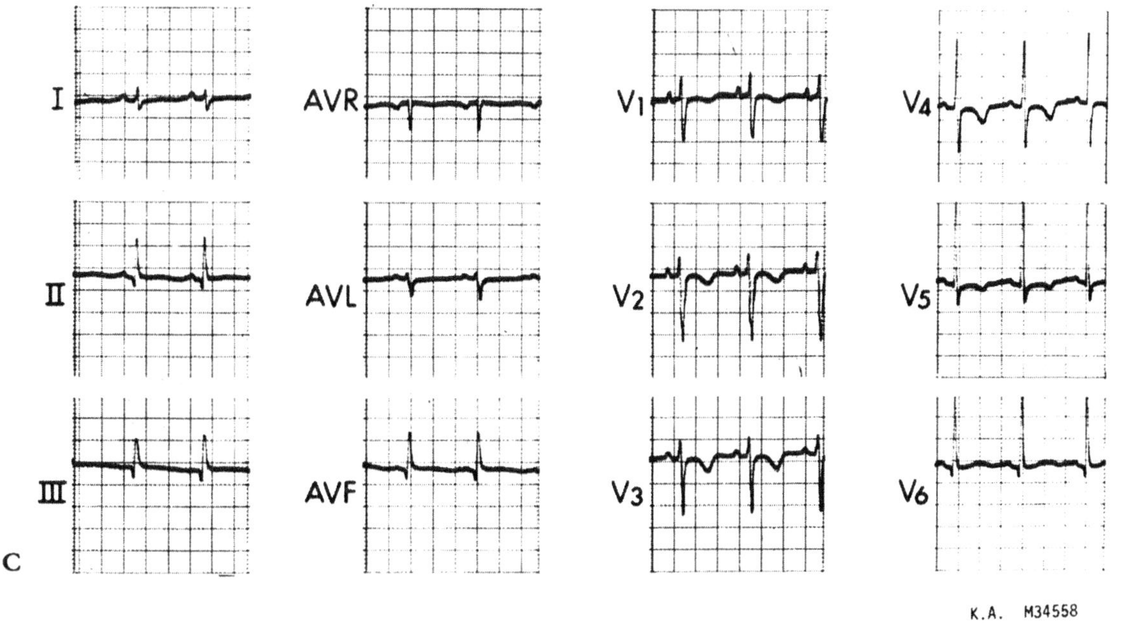

FIGURE 10–5. Normalization of preexcitation due to a nodoventricular connection. (Panel A) 12-lead electrocardiogram recorded during sinus rhythm from a patient with Ebstein's anomaly of the tricuspid valve and a nodoventricular connection. A normal PR interval is present associated with conduction defect of the left bundle branch block type. Q waves are present in the inferior leads related to the coexistence of Ebstein's anomaly. (Panel B) Rhythm strip of electrocardiographic leads V_1–V_3 during the transition to more normal conduction following administration of atropine. (Panel C) Normalization of the QRS complex after administration of atropine. Q waves are still present in the inferior leads due to the associated Ebstein's anomaly. Persistent abnormalities of repolarization are still evident presumably due to "memory" of the pattern of abnormal depolarization as described by Rosenbaum.

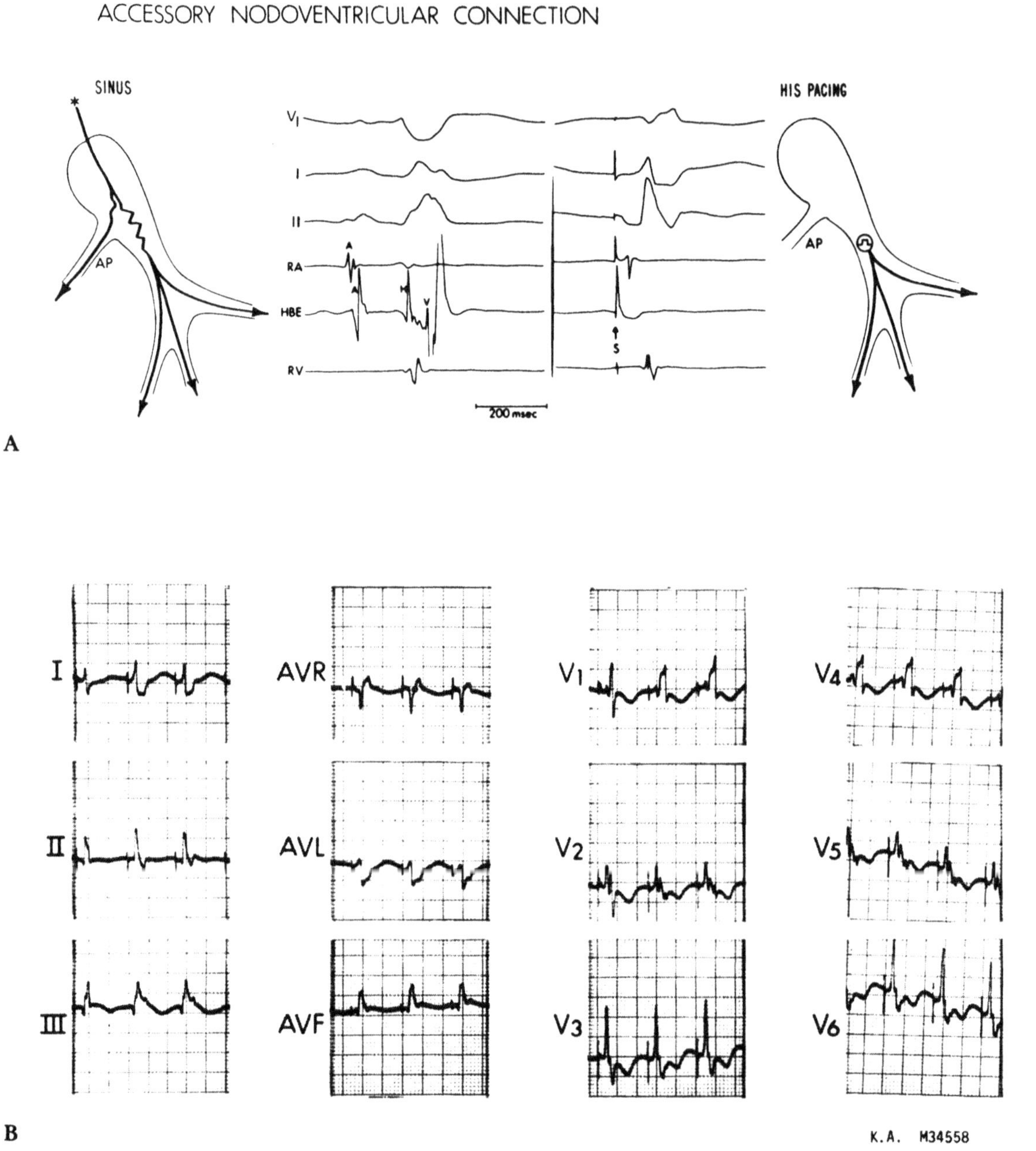

FIGURE 10–6. Normalization of nodoventricular preexcitation by pacing of the His bundle. (Panel A) Intracavitary recordings during sinus rhythm and His bundle pacing in a patient with a nodoventricular fiber. During sinus rhythm the PR interval is normal, the QRS exhibits a pattern of left bundle branch block morphology and the His deflection occurs after the onset of the QRS complex. His bundle pacing results in simultaneous pacing of atria and His bundle. The stimulus – QRS interval is 40 ms and the QRS exhibits a pattern of right bundle branch block due to associated Ebstein's anomaly. (Panel B) 12-lead electrocardiogram (same patient as Panel A) during His bundle pacing.

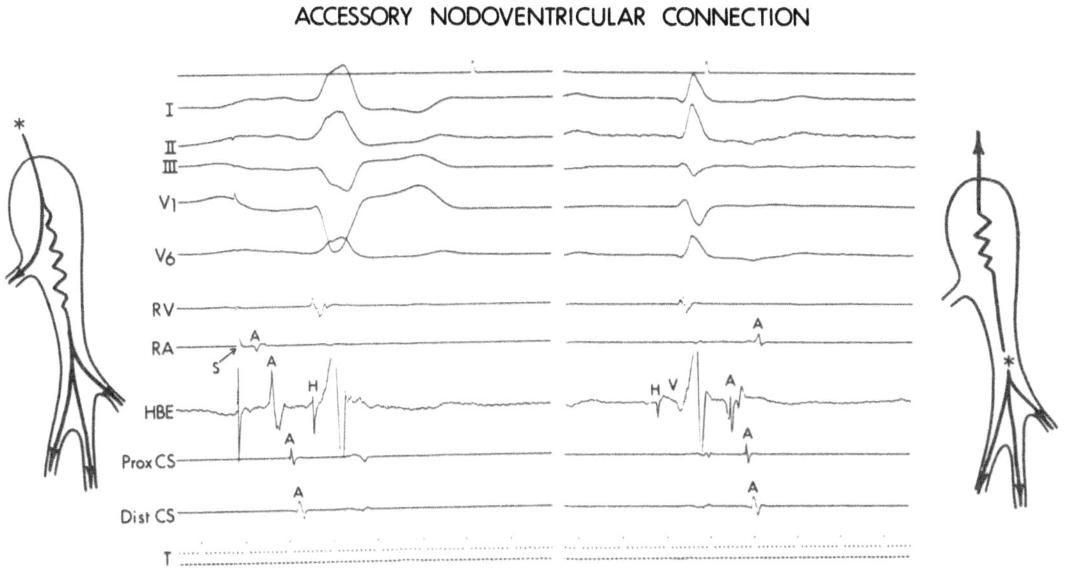

FIGURE 10–7. Normalization of nodoventricular preexcitation by a spontaneous His bundle extrasystole. In the panel to the left, atrial pacing results in a stimulus – QRS of 190 ms associated with a left bundle branch block morphology. The His deflection is inscribed after the onset of the QRS complex. In the panel to the right, a His bundle extrasystole is associated with a normal HV interval, normal QRS complex and retrograde septal spread to the atrium over the AV node. Reproduced with permission of Martinus Nijhoff Publishers from Gallagher et al. [69].

We recently reported [66] a patient with a nodofascicular connection who presented with a narrow QRS tachycardia due to classic reentry confined to the AV node [84]; in addition, two electrophysiologically distinct preexcited tachycardias with left bundle branch block morphology were observed. One of these was due to utilization of the nodofascicular connection as a bystander during reentry confined to the AV node; during this tachycardia, His depolarization preceded depolarization of the right bundle branch. However, during the other preexcited tachycardia, *macro-reentry* utilizing the nodofascicular connection as the antegrade limb of the reentry circuit was strongly suggested by the demonstration that the right bundle branch potential *preceded* the His deflection during tachycardia (Figure 10–14).

BYSTANDER PHENOMENON DURING TACHYCARDIA ASSOCIATED WITH NODOVENTRICULAR CONNECTIONS

The aim of any electrophysiologic study of preexcitation is to define the type and location of the accessory pathway and, more importantly, to document the active participation of the accessory pathway in observed arrhythmias (for obvious therapeutic reasons). The existence of a variety of mechanisms of tachycardia as well as the possibility of multiple accessory pathways can make this differentiation extremely difficult [85]. Not surprisingly, a variety of bystander phenomena involving NV connections was observed in these patients and some representative examples follow.

Figure 10–15 shows electrograms recorded during tachycardias in a 14-year-old girl with Ebstein's anomaly who was proven by pre-

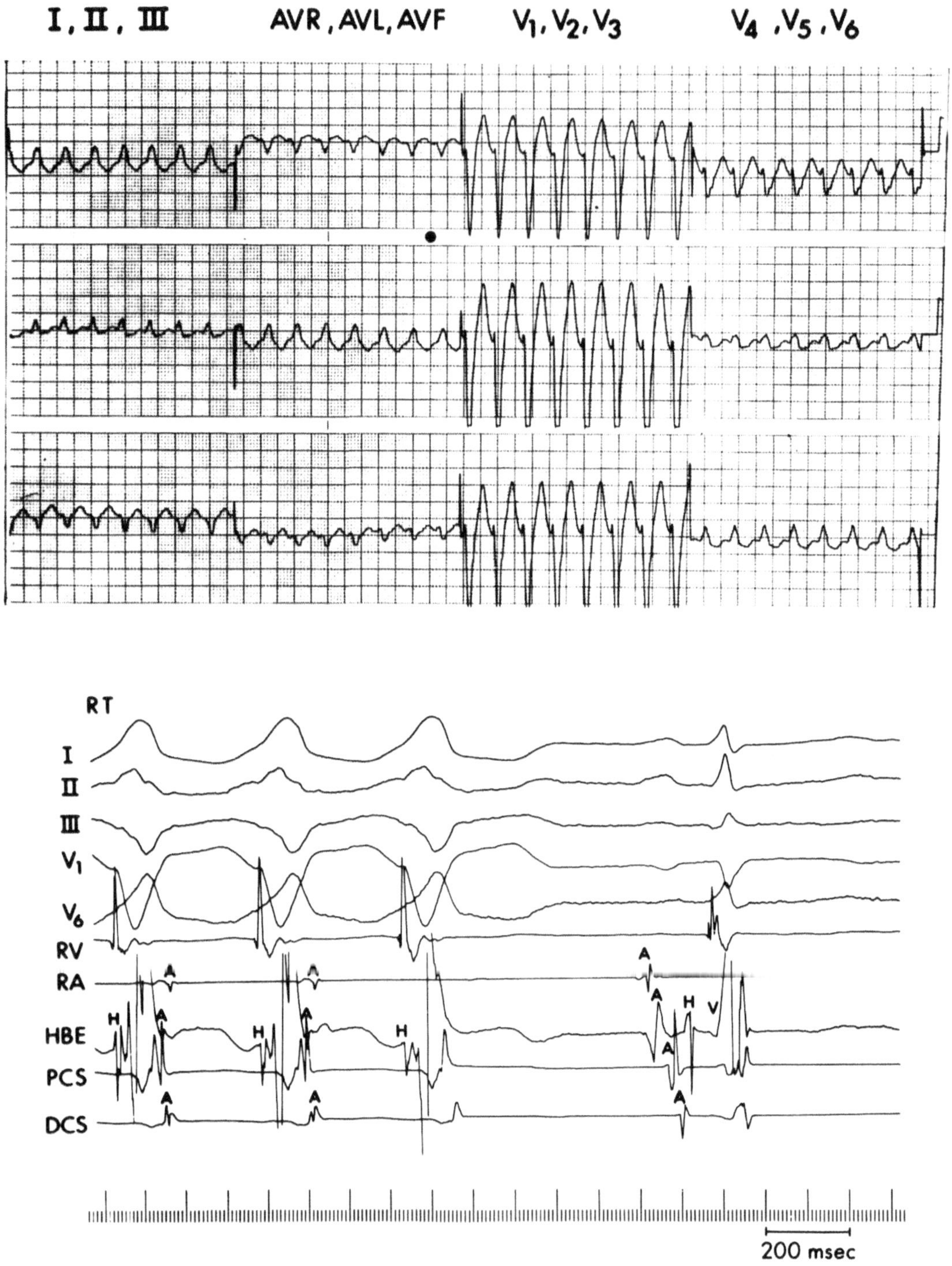

A

B

FIGURE 10–8. Recordings during reciprocating tachycardia in a patient with a nodoventricular connection. (Panel A) 12 lead electrocardiogram recorded during reciprocating tachycardia (same patient as Figure 10–3). Note that left bundle branch block morphology with left axis deviation is present. The electrocardiographic morphology is identical to that produced by atrial pacing as shown previously in Figure 10–3. (Panel B) Intracavitary recordings during reciprocating tachycardia. The His deflection occurs just after the onset of the QRS complex identical to the situation produced by right atrial pacing as shown in Figure 10–3. The tachycardia spontaneously terminates with a ventricular complex followed by a normal sinus complex. Reproduced with permission of Grune and Stratton from Gallagher et al. [70].

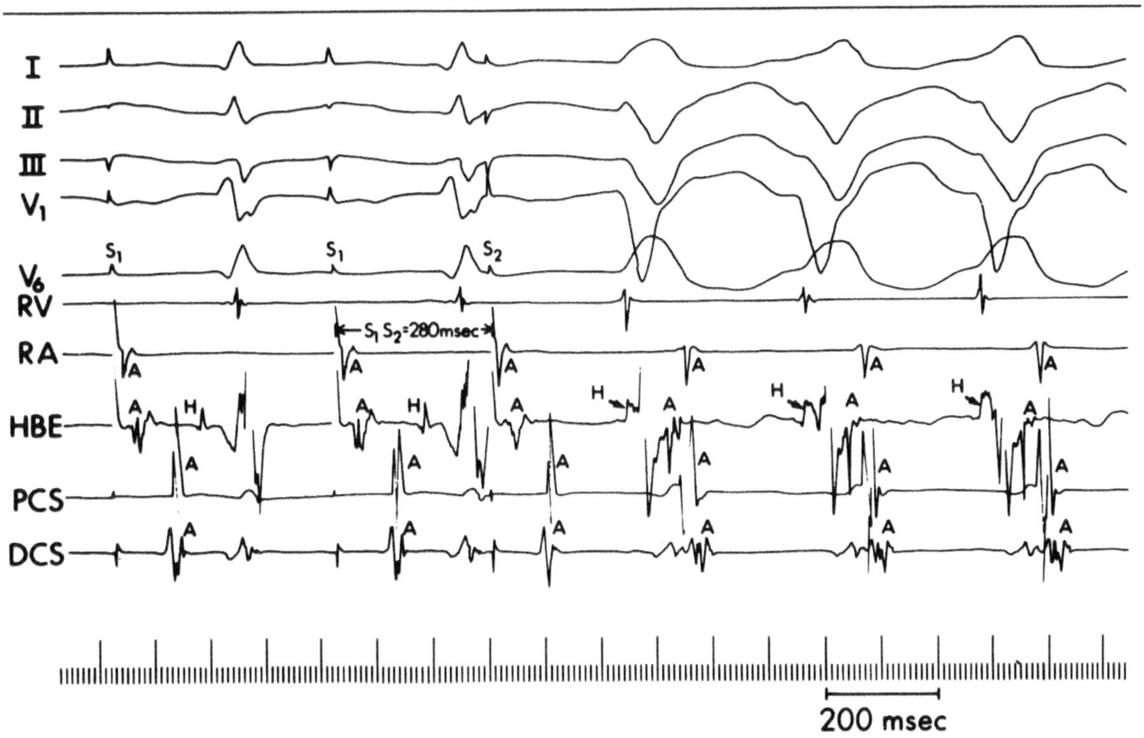

FIGURE 10–9. Tachycardia induction by an atrial premature beat. Recordings of standard ECG leads I–III, V_1, V_6 and selected bipolar recordings are shown during a right atrial refractory period at cycle length 400 ms. The QRS complex during the basic drive beats is normal. A premature stimulus introduced at a coupling interval of 280 ms conducts with 2 long PR and left bundle branch block morphology, resulting in a sustained tachycardia. The retrograde His deflection is barely visible at the onset of the ventricular electrogram.

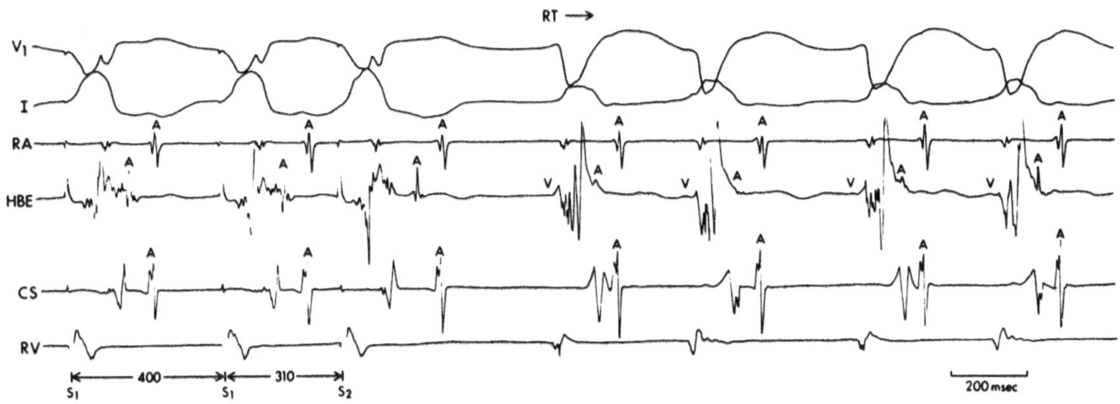

FIGURE 10–10. Tachycardia induction by a ventricular premature beat. Recordings from above down are standard ECG leads V_1 and I, with selected bipolar recordings. During a right ventricular refractory period at a cycle length of 400 ms., a ventricular premature stimulus is introduced at a coupling interval of 310 ms. This resulted in a sustained tachycardia with left bundle branch block morphology identical to that induced by atrial pacing in the same patient. Reproduced with permission of the *Am. Heart Assoc.* from Gallagher et al. [61].

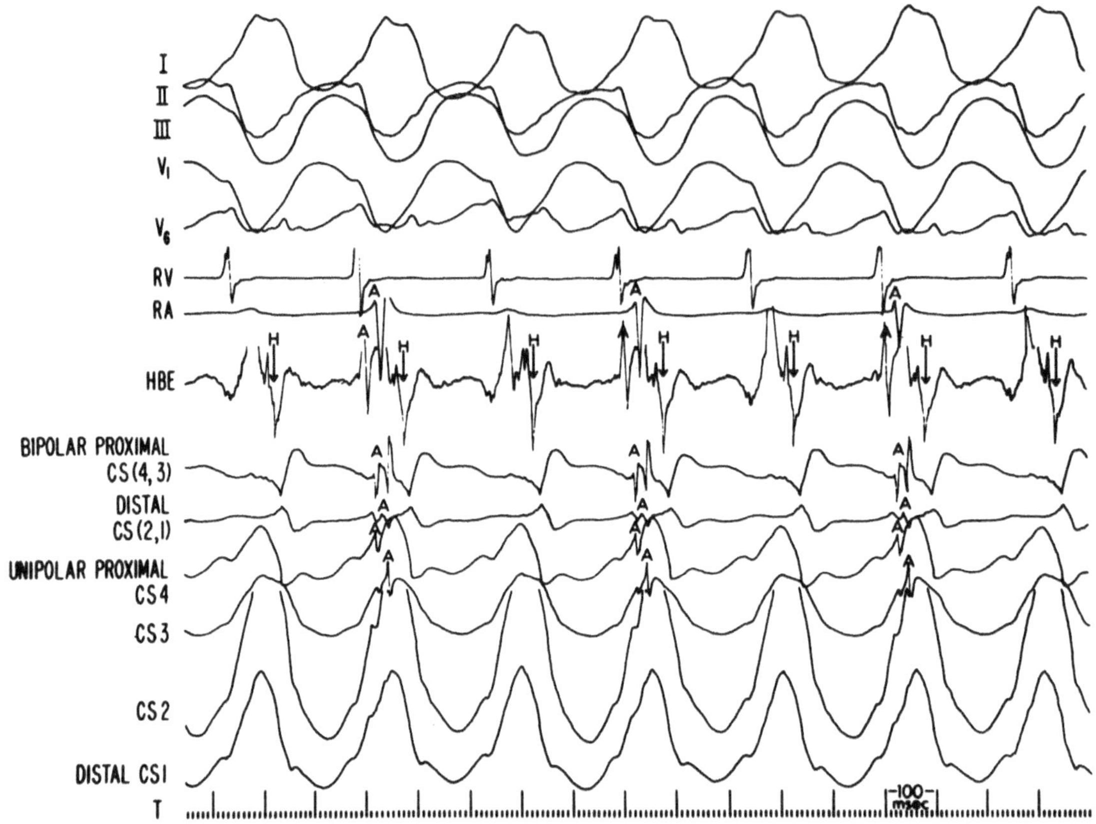

FIGURE 10–11. Recordings during reciprocating tachycardia in a patient with a nodoventricular connection. The tachycardia shows left bundle branch block morphology. A sharp deflection suggestive of a His bundle is inscribed in the ventricular electrogram at a VH interval of 100 ms. 2:1 retrograde conduction is present. Reproduced with permission of the *Am. Heart Assoc.* from Gallagher et al. [61].

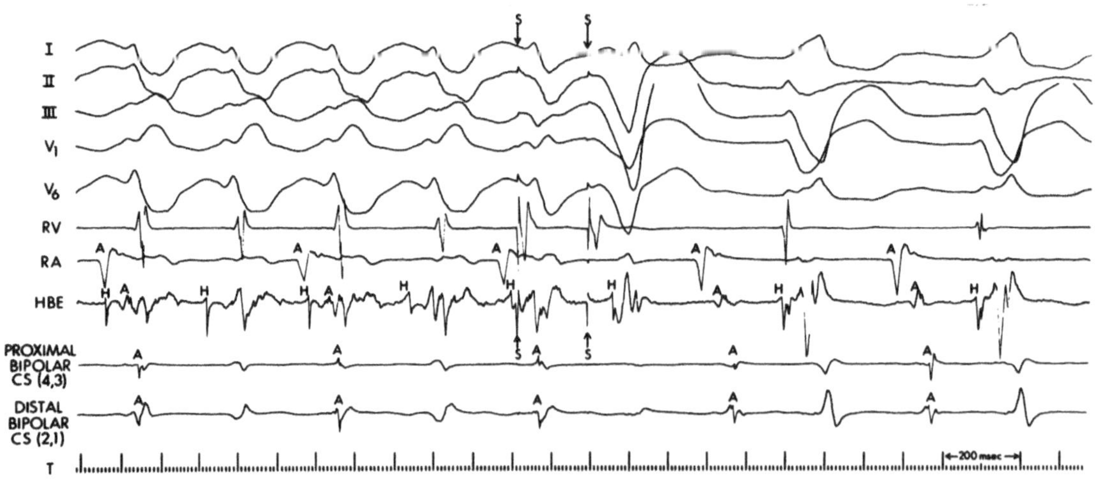

FIGURE 10–12. Reversal of the macro-reentry circuit in a patient with a nodoventricular connection (same patient as Figure 10–11). Tachycardia is initially present with ventriculoatrial dissociation. Each ventricular response is preceded by a His deflection and the surface QRS morphology is that of right bundle branch block. Two successive ventricular premature depolarizations (S) are introduced, resulting in a return to sinus rhythm. The His deflections are not disturbed by the introduction of these ventricular premature depolarizations. With return of sinus rhythm, the left bundle branch block morphology reappears and the His deflection is now inscribed after the onset of the QRS complex. Reproduced with permission of the *Am. Heart Assoc.* from Gallagher et al. [61].

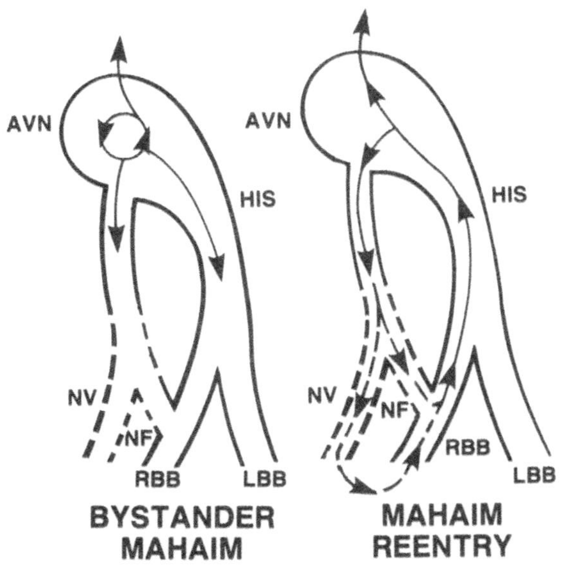

FIGURE 10–13. Schematic representation of possible mechanisms of reciprocating tachycardia in patients with nodoventricular connections. A connection is seen schematically originating from the AV node and inserting either into the right ventricular myocardium (nodoventricular-NV), or the right bundle branch (nodofascicular-NF). In the panel to the left, reentry confined to the AV node is present with "bystander" participation of the connection. In the panel to the right, the anterograde limb of the reentry circuit is provided by the NV-NF connection with the retrograde limb provided by the right bundle branch and His bundle. A portion of the reentry circuit is completed in the AV node. Atrial participation is not necessary with either mechanism.

operative (endocardial) and intraoperative mapping to have both a NV connection and a posterior septal accessory AV pathway. In panel A, tachycardia with a right bundle branch block is present while in panel B tachycardia at an identical cycle length with left bundle branch block morphology is present. The transition from right bundle branch block to left bundle branch block tachycardia was brought about by the introduction of a premature ventricular beat during tachycardia and is shown with intracavitary recordings in Figure 10–16. Initially atrial and ventricular depolarization are simultaneous. The His bundle deflection precedes complexes with right bundle branch block at a normal interval. Following the introduction of a ventricular premature beat there is no change in the cycle length of the tachycardia, the sequence of retrograde atrial activation, HA, and AA intervals. During left bundle branch block morphology, the His bundle deflection is obscured by the ventricular electrogram. This suggests that supraventricular tachycardia due to reentry confined to the AV node was initially present and was converted to reentry confined to the AV node with bystander participation of the NV connection by the premature ventricular depolarization.

Figure 10–17 shows another patient with a proven accessory AV pathway in the right freewall associated with Ebstein's anomaly and a nodoventricular connection. A transition from a narrow QRS supraventricular tachycardia to a left bundle branch block morphology is seen in panel A. In panel B, intracavitary recordings during normal QRS tachycardia show that the low lateral right atrium was activated earliest, consistent with orthodromic reciprocating tachycardia utilizing the AV node-His bundle for the anterograde limb and the right freewall accessory AV pathway as the retrograde limb of the tachycardia circuit. During tachycardia with the "left bundle branch block morphology," the His deflection is inscribed after the beginning of the QRS complex, the retrograde sequence of atrial activation is the same and the cycle length is slightly longer. This sequence was interpreted as demonstrating continued utilization of the right freewall accessory pathway as the retrograde limb of tachycardia with the antegrade limb of tachycardia now provided by the NV connection; it was impossible to establish whether the His deflection was an anterograde deflection (representing fusion) or a retrograde His deflection resulting from activation from the NV connection.

The recordings in Figure 10–18 were obtained from a 21-year-old patient with Ebstein's anomaly and documented accessory AV pathways in the right freewall and in the posterior septal space in addition to a NV connection. Initially, a reciprocating tachycardia with right bundle right block is present at a cycle length of 215 ms. The HV interval is 75 ms. During the first four beats of tachycardia, sinus tachycardia at a cycle length of 360 ms is present and there is VA complete dissociation. Subsequently, there is 1:1 VA association with no change in the cycle length of tachycardia. The earliest retrograde atrial activation is observed in the proximal coronary sinus. This

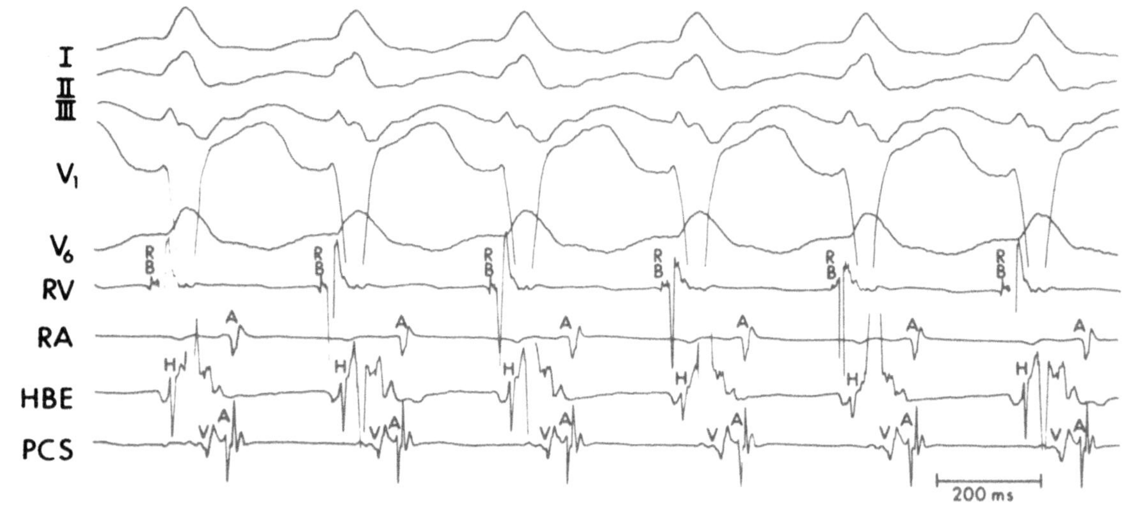

FIGURE 10–14. Preexcited left bundle branch block morphology tachycardia using a nodofascicular connection as a necessary limb of the reentry circuit. Recordings from above down are I–III, V_1, V_6 and selected bipolar recordings. The recording obtained from the proximal right ventricle near the outflow tract demonstrates a sharp deflection arising from the right bundle branch (RB). During this tachycardia, activation of the right bundle potential *precedes* activation of the His deflection, suggesting retrograde depolarization, an observation supportive of marco-reentry. Reproduced with permission of Yorke Publisher from Bardy et al. [66].

sequence was interpreted as representing initial reciprocating tachycardia due to macro-reentry utilizing the AV node-His bundle as the anterograde limb and the NV connection as the retrograde limb with no atrial participation. The appearance of a 1:1 response between ventricle and atrium was felt to represent bystander participation of the septal accessory pathway in the retrograde direction. Although it is conceivable that the retrograde septal sequence merely represents retrograde conduction over the upper portion of the AV node, it is pertinent to note that this sequence was identical to that observed during retrograde conduction over the septal accessory AV pathway later in the same study. A *different* retrograde sequence of atrial activation, initiated in the region of the His bundle, was also observed and interpreted to represent retrograde conduction over the His bundle-AV node.

SITE OF DISTAL INSERTION OF THE NODOVENTRICULAR CONNECTION

In an earlier report [61], findings in 6 patients with reciprocating tachycardia and electrophysiologic evidence of NV connection were presented. A macro-reentrant mechanism of tachycardia in which conduction proceeded anterograde over the NV connection to the right ventricle and retrograde over the His Purkinje system to the AV node was postulated, with reentry being completed within the AV node. During tachycardia, a His deflection well *after* the onset of the QRS complex was observed in 3 patients, with a ventriculo-His (VH) interval comparable to that seen during right ventricular pacing. A total of 16 patients have now been studied. In 3 of these, the unusual finding of 2 distinct and reproducible VH intervals (i.e., a "short VH" interval and a "long VH" interval) during sustained tachycardia was observed [86]. Compared to the VH interval during right ventricular pacing in these patients, the short VH interval was significantly shorter (10–70 ms; mean 26.2 ms) and the long VH interval was significantly longer (95–100 ms; mean 92 ms), thus suggesting that the mechanism of this tachycardia was different from that previously proposed. In these patients the short VH tachycardia exhibited a shorter cycle length than the long VH tachycardia. The two forms of tachycardia converted spontaneously from one to the other or could be converted by means of timed premature ventricular depolarizations

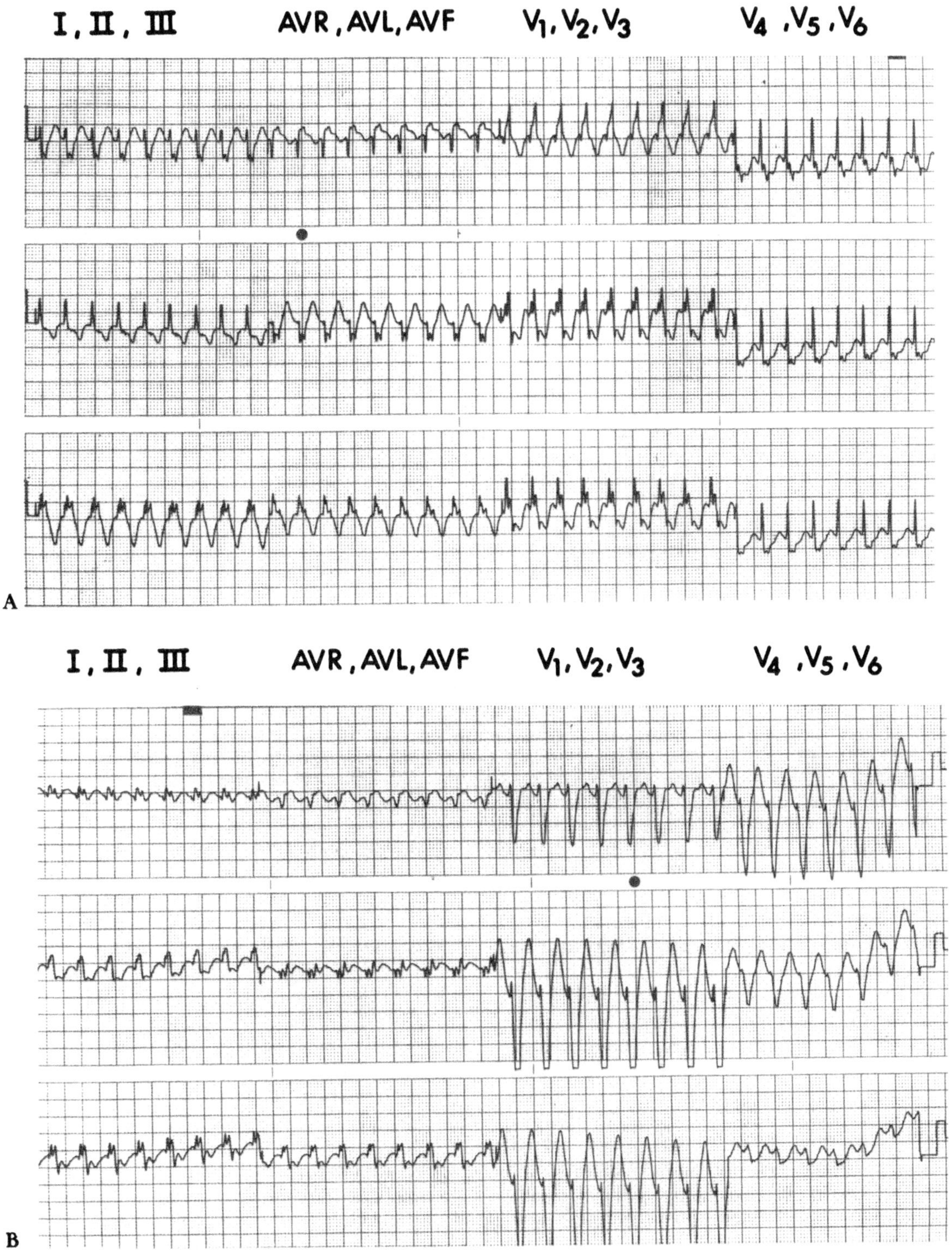

FIGURE 10–15. Bystander participation of a nodoventricular connection in a patient with Ebstein's anomaly and reentry confined to the AV node. (Panel A) Reciprocating tachycardia with right bundle branch block (due to Ebstein's anomaly). (Panel B) Reciprocating tachycardia with left bundle branch block morphology in the same patient. (See text for discussion.) Reproduced with permission of Martinus Nijhoff Publishers from Gallagher et al. [69].

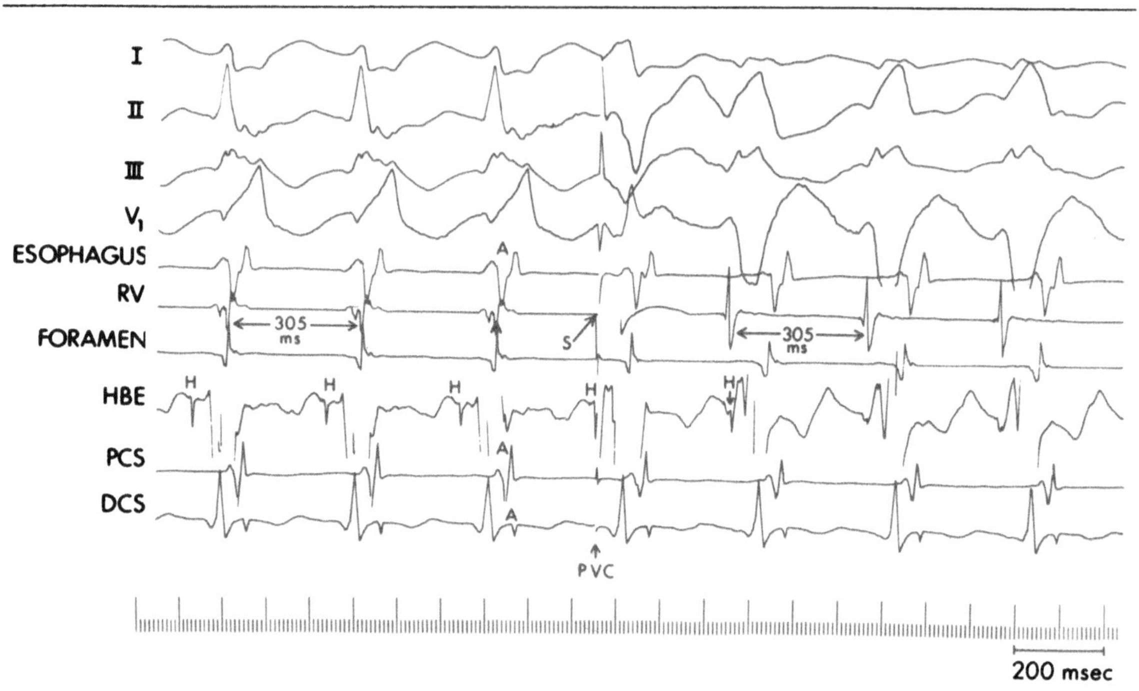

FIGURE 10–16. Bystander participation of a nodoventricular connection in a patient with Ebstein's anomaly and reentry confined to the AV node (same patient as Figure 10–15). Recordings from above down include standard ECG leads I–III, V_1, and bipolar recordings from the esophagus, right ventricle, foramen ovale, region of the His bundle and coronary sinus. Tachycardia is initially present with right bundle branch block at a cycle length of 305 ms; each QRS is preceded by a His deflection at a normal interval. Atrial and ventricular activation are simultaneous, consistent with reentry confined to the AV node. After introduction of a premature ventricular depolarization, left bundle branch block morphology appears with an identical cycle length of 305 ms. Atrial and ventricular activation continues to be near simultaneous. The His deflection is now obscured in the ventricular electrogram. (See text for discussion.) Reproduced with permission of Martinus Nijhoff Publishers from Gallagher et al. [69].

(Figure 10–19). The QRS morphology during both forms of tachycardia was a left bundle branch block morphology. In 2 of the 3 patients, the QRS was identical during both types of tachycardia, while in the third patient periods of alternating QRS axis (−15° and +15°) were seen during the short VH tachycardia. Only a −15° axis was seen during the long VH tachycardia (Figure 10–20). Atrial pacing reproduced the short VH relationship in all patients but never the long VH relationship. The sequence of retrograde atrial activation was identical during both types of tachycardia in each patient.

The observation of two types of VH relationship in these patients has important implications not only for the possible mechanism of reentry involved but also for the location of the NV connection. If the VH relationship is due to equal delay during antegrade conduction from the AV node to the His bundle on the one hand and a NV fiber on the other, then the short VH tachycardia seen could be postulated as being due to reentry confined to the AV node. In this situation, a ventricular insertion into the specialized conduction system of the right ventricle need not be postulated. Long VH tachycardia in this situation could be postulated as either due to reentry confined to the AV node (using another intranodal pathway) or macroreentry with antegrade conduction over the NV connection and retrograde conduction to the AV node over the His bundle (i.e., a second mechanism of tachycardia in the same patient). In the patients studied however, some

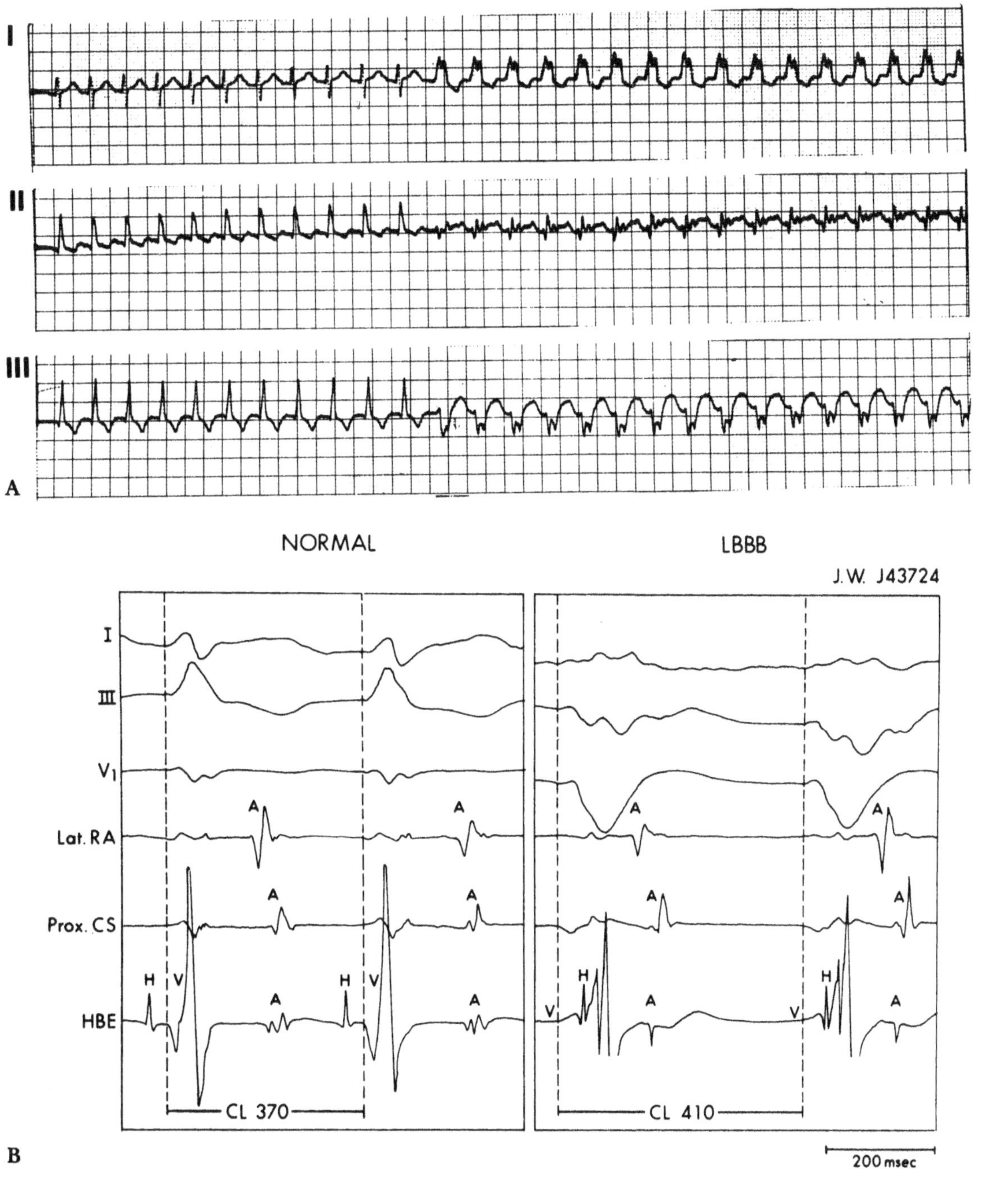

FIGURE 10–17. Bystander participation of a nodoventricular connection in a patient with a right freewall accessory AV pathway. (Panel A) A rhythm strip of standard ECGs I, II, and III are shown during a transition from normal QRS to a left bundle branch block morphology QRS tachycardia. The patient had a right freewall accessory AV pathway in addition to Ebstein's anomaly of the tricuspid valve. (Panel B) Intracavitary recordings before and after the transition shown in Panel A. Recordings from above down are standard ECG leads I, III, V_1, lateral right atrium, proximal coronary sinus and region of the His bundle. In both panels the lateral right atrium is activated earliest during the tachycardia consistent with orthodromic tachycardia utilizing the right freewall pathway in the retrograde direction. During left bundle branch block morphology tachycardia, the His bundle is inscribed in the ventricular electrogram, indicating bystander participation of the nodoventricular connection. Reproduced with permission of the *Am. Heart Assoc.* from Tonkin et al. [37].

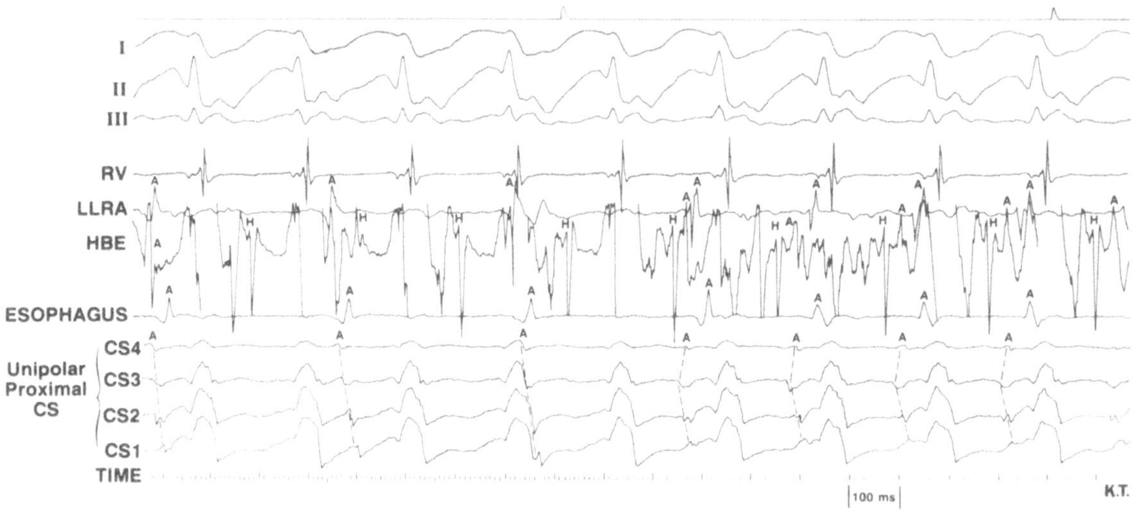

FIGURE 10–18. Bystander participation of a septal accessory AV pathway in the retrograde direction during macro-reentry utilizing a nodoventricular fiber. Recordings from above down are standard ECG leads I, III, and bipolar recordings from the right ventricle (RV), the low lateral right atrium (LLRA), the region of the His bundle (HBE), the esophagus, and unipolar recordings (unipolar proximal CS) recorded from the orifice (CS4) toward the mid-portion (CS1) of the coronary sinus. (See text for discussion.)

observations argued against the short VH relationship being due to equal delays in antegrade conduction:

1. No evidence of fusion was seen during short VH tachycardia. One might have expected during prolonged observation that if the NV connection had in fact been a bystander, some evidence of fusion or block might have been observed. Furthermore a constant tachycardia morphology persisted despite the introduction of atrial and ventricular premature depolarizations. It is impossible, however, to exclude the possibility of repetitive concealed conduction as the cause of constant morphology.
2. No change in QRS morphology or VH interval was observed during either type of tachycardia following the administration of numerous drugs with effects on cardiac conduction, despite a cycle length change in tachycardia. It seems unlikely that equal changes in conduction over the AV node-His bundle *and* the NV connection would have occurred leaving the short VH relationship undisturbed.

An attractive alternative explanation for the short VH relationship is that the Mahaim fiber inserts into the specialized conduction system of the right ventricle and thus is more properly termed a *nodofascicular* tract. In this situation, exclusive antegrade conduction could occur via the Mahaim fiber to the right bundle branch with subsequent equal conduction delay retrograde to the His deflection and antegrade to the ventricle being responsible for the short VH relationship. The long VH relationship could result from functional block in the right bundle branch with retrograde conduction to the His bundle now occurring via ventricular myocardium to the left bundle branch (i.e., concealed right bundle branch block). In this case, both short VH and long VH tachycardia would be due to a macro-reentrant circuit. A number of observations favor this latter hypothesis:

1. Long VH tachycardias were accompanied by longer VA intervals and tachycardia cycle lengths than observed during short VH tachycardias.
2. The VH intervals observed during right ventricular pacing were intermediate to those seen in Short VH and Long VH tachycardias.
3. Catheter ablation of the AV node – proximal His bundle in one patient abolished further episodes of tachycardia yet left intact antegrade conduction over the Mahaim fiber with a persistent short VH relationship [69].

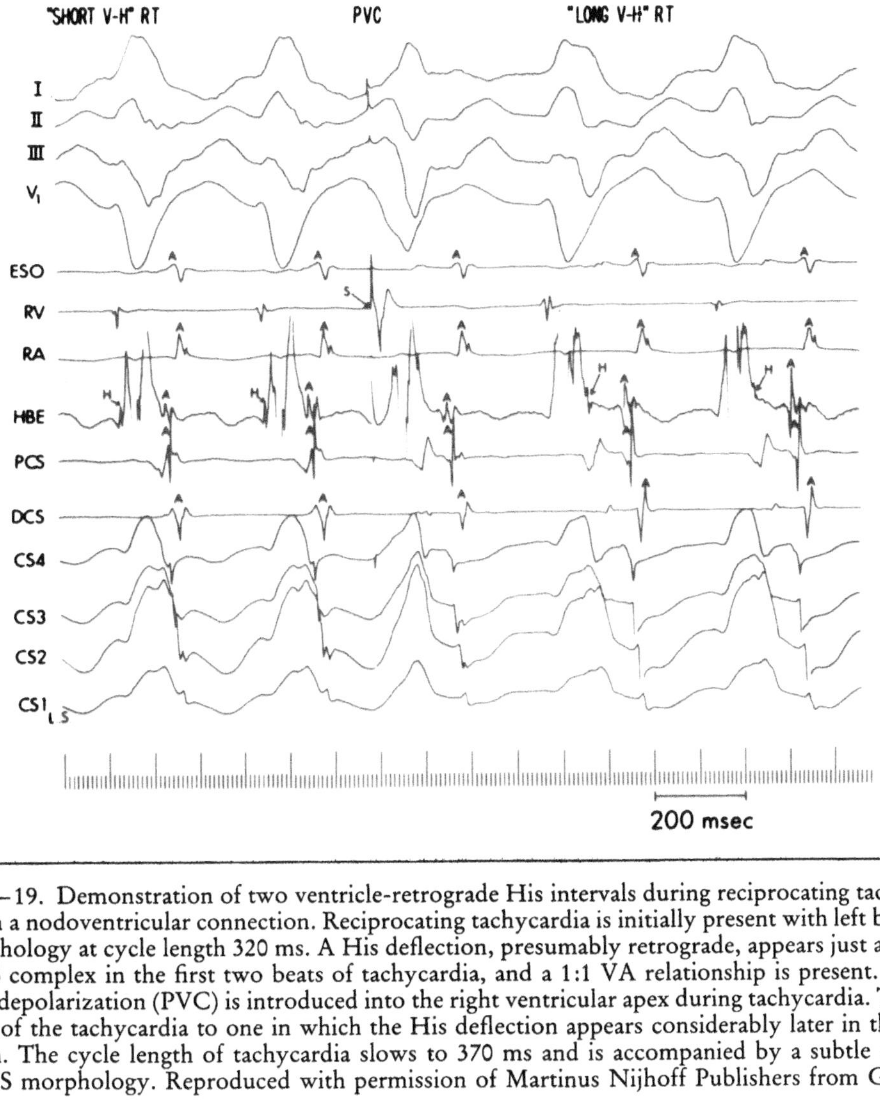

FIGURE 10–19. Demonstration of two ventricle-retrograde His intervals during reciprocating tachycardia in a patient with a nodoventricular connection. Reciprocating tachycardia is initially present with left bundle branch block morphology at cycle length 320 ms. A His deflection, presumably retrograde, appears just after the onset of the QRS complex in the first two beats of tachycardia, and a 1:1 VA relationship is present. A premature ventricular depolarization (PVC) is introduced into the right ventricular apex during tachycardia. This results in conversion of the tachycardia to one in which the His deflection appears considerably later in the ventricular electrogram. The cycle length of tachycardia slows to 370 ms and is accompanied by a subtle change in the surface QRS morphology. Reproduced with permission of Martinus Nijhoff Publishers from Gallagher et al [69].

4. Termination of reciprocating tachycardia was temporally related to trauma to the NV connection in two instances and to the right bundle branch in another instance, both being required portions of the postulated macroreentry circuit.
6. Ventriculoatrial dissociation was observed in 4 of the 14 patients studied. Although ventriculoatrial dissociation has been reported during reentry confined to the AV node, it still presents an unusual finding.

In the final analysis it is difficult to be certain concerning the mechanism of the reentry and the distal insertion site of these connections. The evidence to date however suggests that the accessory connection may arise within the AV node and insert into the specialized conducting tissues of the right ventricle. Alternatively, multiple NV connections might be postulated [64].

VENTRICULAR RESPONSE DURING ATRIAL FIBRILLATION

The ability of the NV connection to conduct during atrial fibrillation could be observed in the absence of additional anomalies of AV conduction in 11 of 16 patients. The shortest RR between 2 consecutive beats conducted over the Mahaim fiber ranged from 204–305 ms

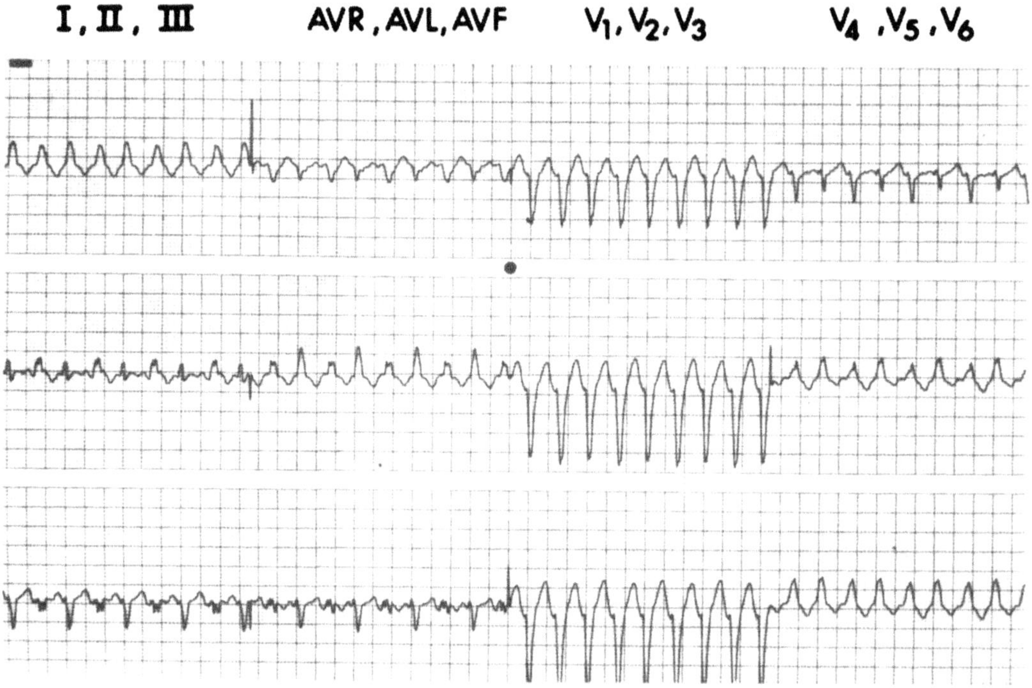

FIGURE 10–20. Alterations in axis during reciprocating tachycardia in a patient with a nodoventricular connection. (See text for discussion.)

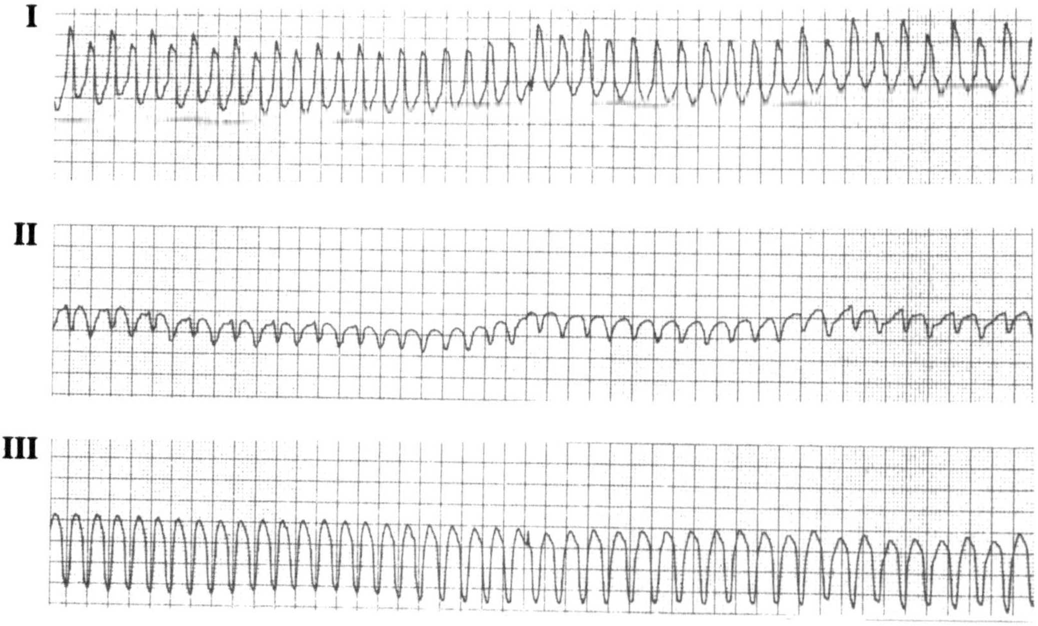

FIGURE 10–21. Ventricular response during atrial flutter in a patient with a nodoventricular connection presumably arising in the transitional zone of the AV node. All QRS complexes are conducted via the nodoventricular connection and the shortest RR interval is 200 ms. The same patient suffered from reciprocating tachycardia with an identical QRS morphology during which there was ventriculoatrial dissociation.

(mean 262.4 ms). The average ventricular response ranged from 282–518 ms (mean 374.1 ms). In general therefore, conduction over the AV node – NV connection complex was only moderate except in 2 patients who exhibited extremely short RR intervals during atrial fibrillation. In one of these (Figure 10–21), ventriculoatrial dissociation was observed during macro-reentry utilizing the NV connection, excluding an accessory AV pathway. These observations are most consistent with probable origin of the NV connection in the transitional cell zone of the AV node in these cases.

Problems still remain in distinguishing NV fiber from accessory AV connections which exhibit decremental properties [87,88]. Previous studies have shown that decremental properties during retrograde conduction over accessory AV pathways can be observed during programmed stimulation. One might therefore reasonably question whether NV connections may in fact represent accessory AV pathways operating with decremental properties in the antegrade direction [88–90]. In four of the cases described in this report, this possibility appears excluded by the observation that ventriculoatrial dissociation was noted during macro-reentry tachycardia. Furthermore, the QRS morphology due to nodoventricular fibers appears to differ significantly from that associated with accessory AV pathways located in the right anterior septal/paraseptal region [85].

TREATMENT

Fifteen of the 16 patients described required therapy. The response to medical therapy alone could be observed in 9 patients and consisted of verapamil plus digoxin (2 patients), verapamil alone (1 patient), verapamil plus a type I agent (1 patient), a type I agent alone (4 patients), and a type I agent combined with propranolol (1 patient). One patient had a radiofrequency atrial pacemaker inplanted and one underwent catheter ablation of the AV node–His bundle. The remaining 4 patients underwent surgery. Of these, one encountered heartblock during replacement of the tricuspid valve related to Ebstein's anomaly and had no further tachycardias. The remaining 3 were taken to surgery because of associated accessory AV pathways. In each of these 3 patients, dissection of the posterior septal pathway [91] simultaneously abolished further conduction in the NV connection with *preservation* of normal conduction in the AV node–His bundle. None of these patients suffered further tachycardia.

Catheter ablation of the AV node–His bundle [69] was undertaken in one patient who failed treatment with multiple antiarrhythmic agents in addition to use of a radiofrequency pacemaker. The previously described technique of catheter ablation of the His bundle [92] was utilized (same patient as Figure 10–8). Delivery of a direct current shock through a catheter recording a His potential, resulted in appearance of a maximally preexcited left bundle branch block morphology QRS complex (Figure 10–22). Intracavitary recordings following ablation demonstrated a deflection arising in specialized conduction tissue (? distal His bundle versus right bundle branch potential) when the catheter was slightly advanced into the ventricle. The interval from the onset of ventricular depolarization to this deflection was 0 to −5 ms. Retrograde conduction was absent. A prophylactic permanent pacemaker was implanted. Subsequent attempts to reinduce tachycardia were unsuccessful and the patient has remained free of tachycardia on no medication for over 2 years in follow-up.

INTRAOPERATIVE STUDY OF NODOVENTRICULAR CONNECTIONS

I have had the opportunity of mapping the ventricular sequence of activation during exclusive conduction over the Mahaim fiber in three patients to date (Figure 10–23). In each case, there was not evidence of early activation of the base of the right ventricle, excluding an accessory AV pathway. Earliest activation was noted after the onset of the QRS over a large portion of the anterior right ventricle. Direct recordings of the His bundle verified that His bundle depolarization was occurring after the onset of the QRS complex.

SURGICAL INTERRUPTION OF NODOVENTRICULAR CONNECTION

As mentioned earlier, four patients underwent surgical dissection of coexisting posterior septal accessory AV pathways [91]. In one of these, tricuspid valve replacement was indicated because of severe tricuspid regurgitation associated with Ebstein's anomaly. Complete heart block in both the antegrade and retrograde direction resulted from suturing of the prosthetic tricuspid valve and there were no further observed arrhythmias. In the remaining three patients however, it was of interest that there was *no postoperative evidence of conduction over the NV connection following*

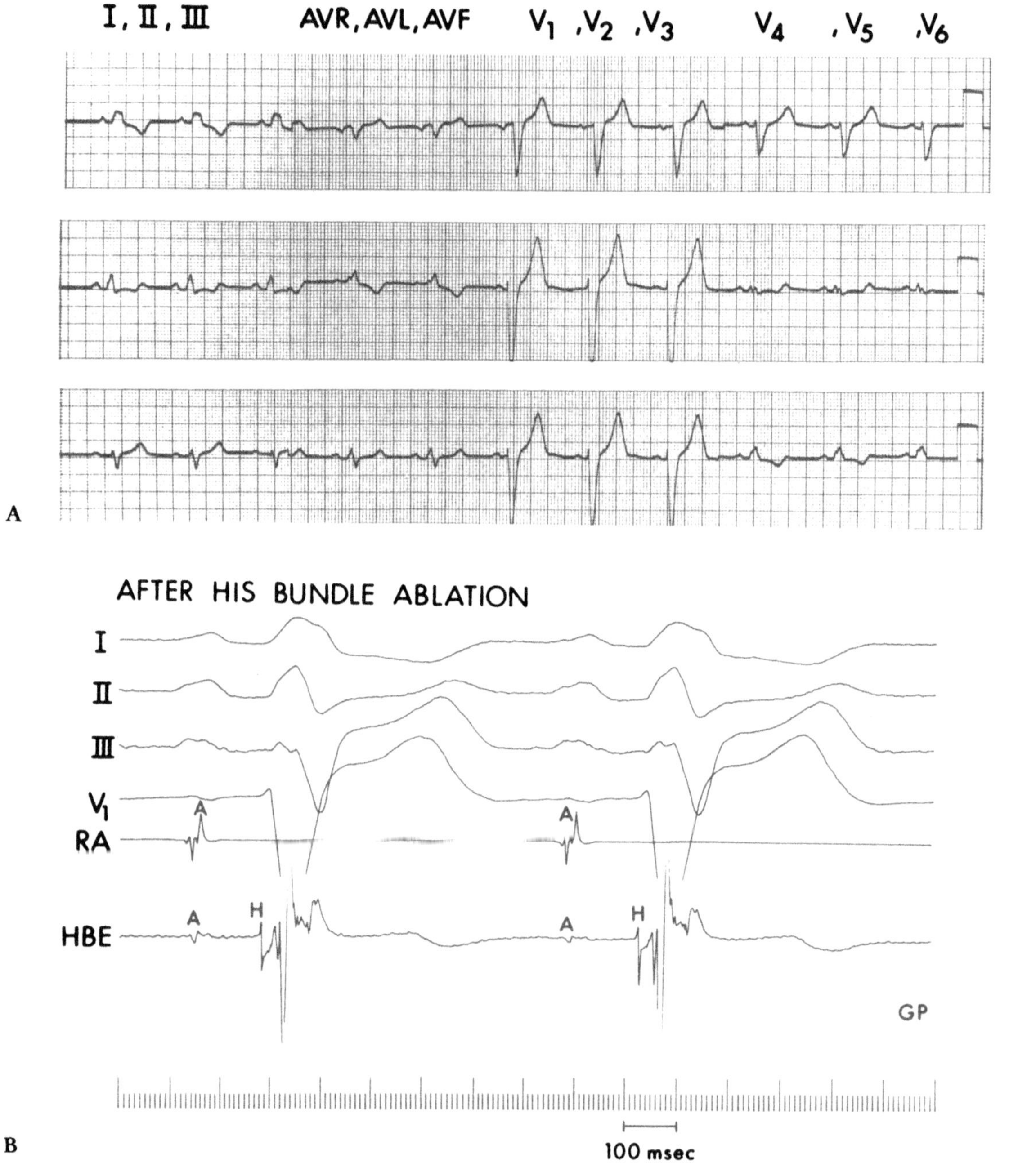

FIGURE 10–22. Recordings obtained after ablation of the His bundle in a patient with a nodoventricular connection. (Panel A) During sinus rhythm there is a persistent left bundle branch block morphology. The PR interval is 0.18 seconds. The QRS morphology is identical to that observed previously during reciprocating tachycardia (Figure 10–3) and during right atrial pacing (Figure 10–8). (Panel B) Intracavitary recordings following His bundle ablation. The His bundle catheter was advanced slightly distal to the position used to record the electrograms shown in Figure 10–3. As a result the size of the atrial electrogram is smaller. A deflection which may represent either distal His bundle or right bundle branch is noted at the onset of the QRS complex and is identical in timing to that demonstrated during reciprocating tachycardia in Figure 10–8. Reproduced with permission by Martinus Nijhoff Publishers from Gallagher et al. [69].

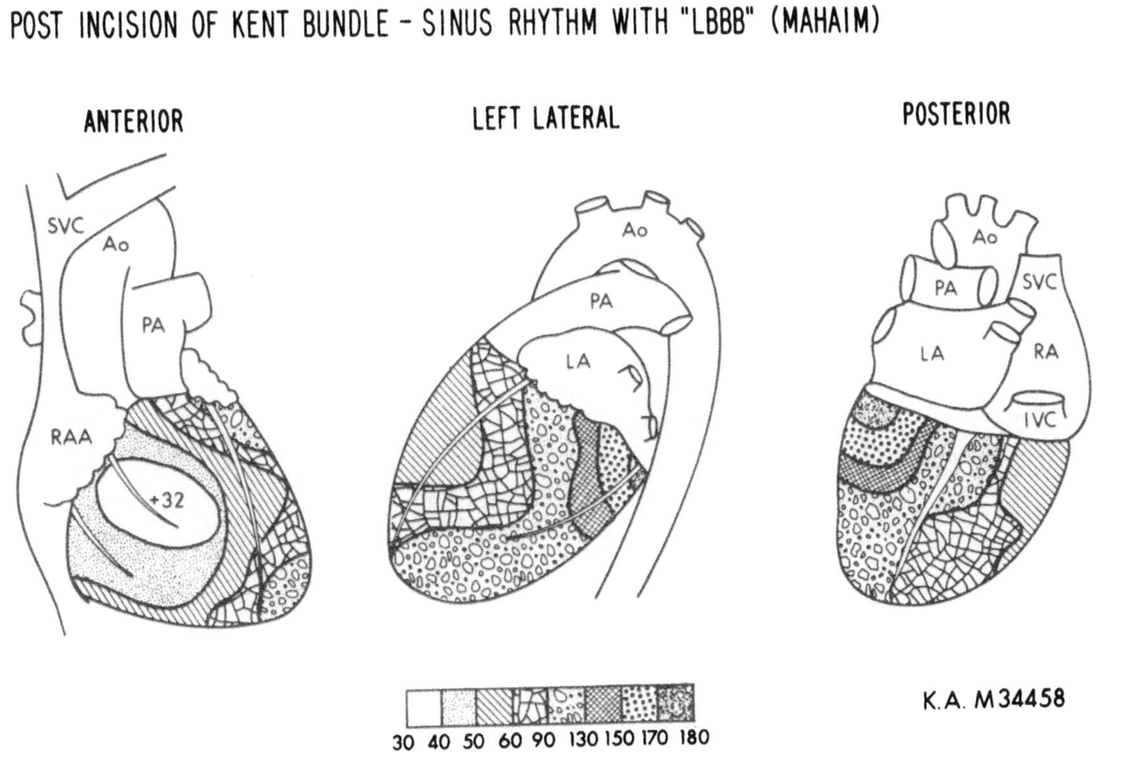

FIGURE 10–23. Epicardial map of the sequence of ventricular activation in a patient with a nodoventricular connection. The epicardial map shown was obtained in a patient with Ebstein's anomaly of the tricuspid valve after successful surgical interruption of a posterior septal accessory pathway. A long PR and left bundle branch block was present and it was verified that the His deflection was occurring after the onset of the QRS. The epicardial map demonstrates earliest breakthrough on the anterior right ventricle 32 ms after the onset of the QRS complex. A late area of activation separates this early area from all basal portions of the ventricles. A larger-than-normal area of epicardial breakthrough is noted and may be related to the thin wall of the right ventricle in this patient with associated Ebstein's anomaly. Reproduced with premission of the *Am. Heart Assoc.*

posterior septal space dissections. A representative example follows. The patient was an 18-year-old male with Ebstein's anomaly of the tricuspid valve with typical associated accessory AV pathways of the posterior septal and right freewall type. In addition, he was found to have a NV connection which participated in reciprocating tachycardia (Figure 10–24). Intraoperatively, the usual dissection for right freewall and posterior septal accessory pathways was carried out, with extension of the posterior septal dissection up to the posterior margin of the right fibrous trigone. Postoperatively (Figure 10–25) intermittent Wenckebach in the AV node was observed, without any further evidence of conduction over the NV connection. Conduction normalized with atropine or with exercise. Despite atrial pacing and programmed stimulation of atrium and ventricle, no further tachycardias could be induced. These observations suggested that both accessory AV pathways and the NV connection had been successfully divided. The same observation has been made in two additional cases. Despite the apparent intimate relationship of the NV connection with the AV node–His bundle [93], it thus appears possible to interrupt the ventricular insertion of the NV connection without producing heart block.

Fasciculoventricular Connections

Fasciculoventricular (FV) connections arise from the His bundle and bundle branches; the PR interval might therefore be expected to be

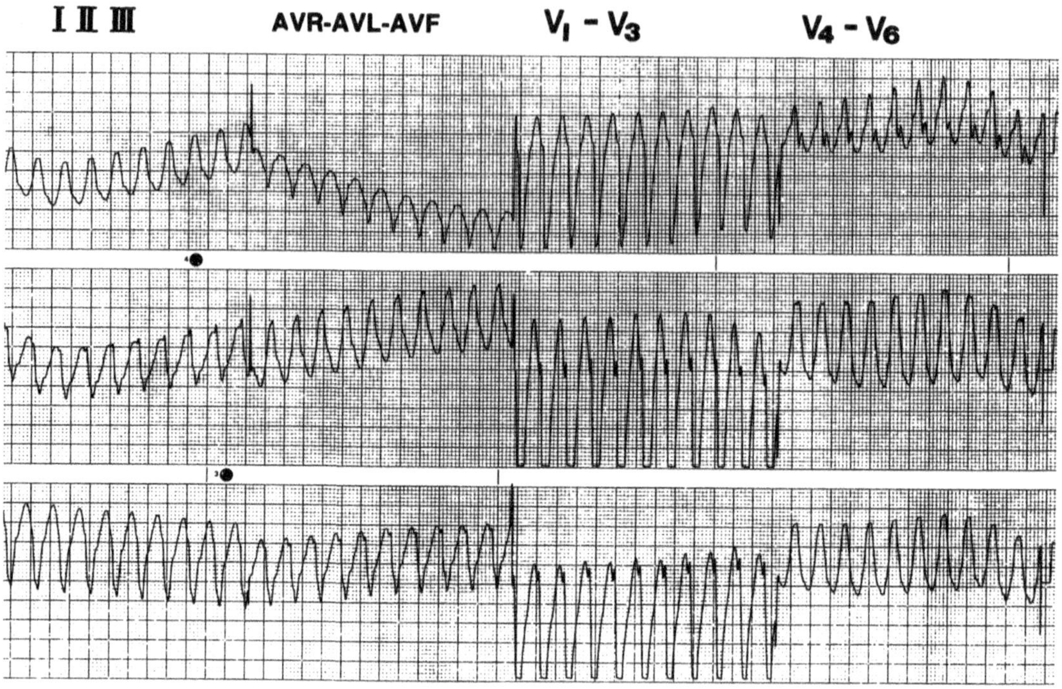

FIGURE 10–24. Reciprocating tachycardia in a patient with a nodoventricular connection. The QRS morphology exhibits the typical pattern associated with a nodoventricular fiber. (See text for discussion.)

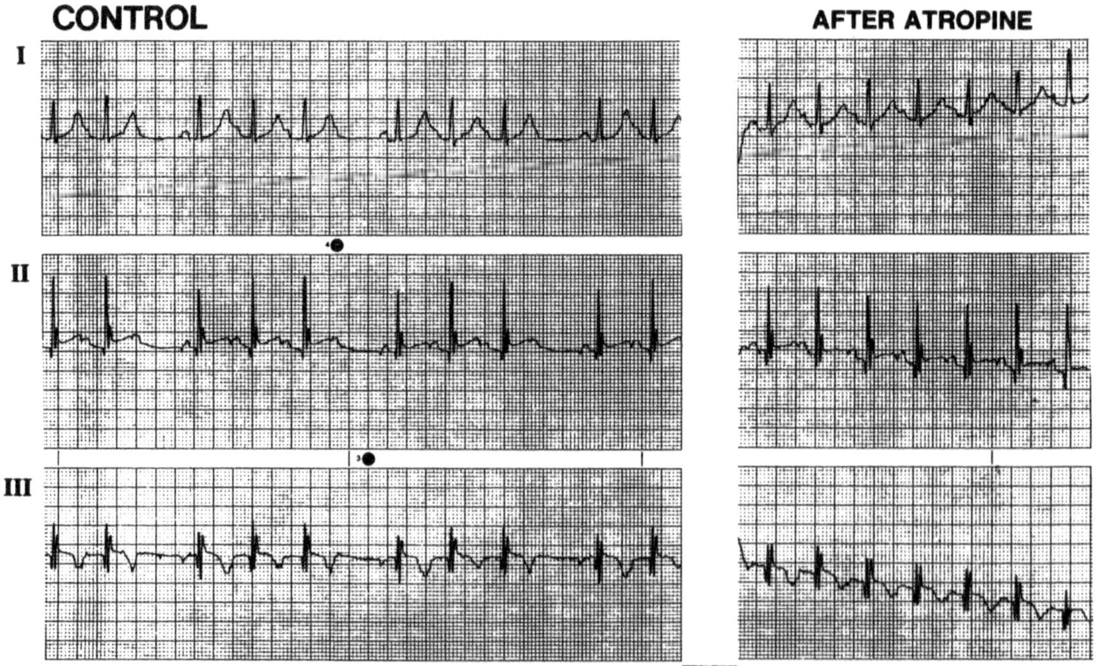

FIGURE 10–25. Postoperative electrocardiograms before and after administration of atropine in a patient with apparent surgical interruption of a nodoventricular connection (same patient as Figure 10–24). In the panel to the left, a rhythm strip shows spontaneous Wenckebach periods while in the panel to the right, administration of atropine resulted in normalization of conduction. Q waves are evident in the inferior leads and there is terminal delay in the QRS due to right bundle branch block, both related to the presence of Ebstein's anomaly.

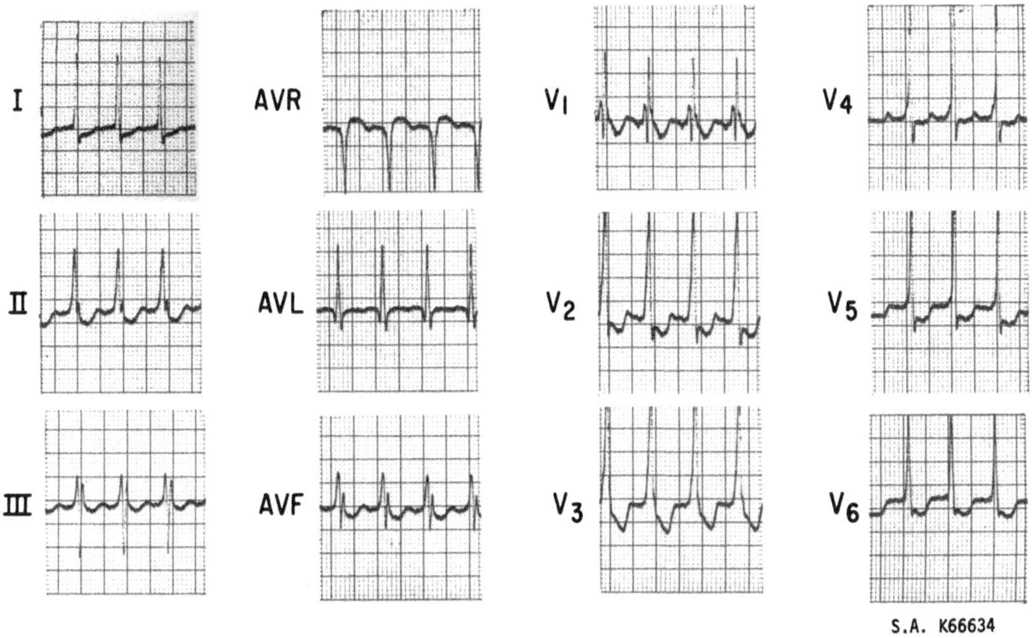

FIGURE 10–26. Atrial flutter in a patient with fasciculoventricular connection. This 12-lead electrocardiogram was recorded during an episode of atrial flutter with 2:1 block. The ventricular complexes exhibit slurring of the initial forces which is most evident in the precordial leads. A pattern of incomplete right bundle branch block is evident.

normal unless another anomaly of AV conduction is present. The QRS complex associated with FV connections may be anomalous depending on the origin of the connection, but variable fusion is not expected and the QRS morphology should be reasonably constant.

Eleven patients with FV connections have been studied consisting of males and 2 females ranging in age from 8 to 61 years (mean 31.7 years). Associated anomalies were present in all 11 patients and consisted of: enhanced conduction in the AV node (4 patients); a syndrome of sinus node dysfunction, familial tendency to complete heart block and cardiomyopathy (3 patients); WPW syndrome (3 patients); and rheumatic heart disease, sick sinus syndrome, and enhanced conduction in the AV node (1 patient). The patients with WPW syndrome had their accessory AV pathways surgically divided before being studied. In the remaining cases, patients were selected for study because of rapid ventricular responses during atrial flutter-fibrillation due to enhanced conduction in the AV node.

STUDIES DURING SINUS RHYTHM/ ATRIAL PACING

During sinus rhythm the PR interval was abbreviated in the majority of patients because of associated enhanced conduction in the AV node. The QRS complex was slightly prolonged (0.10–0.12 seconds, mean 0.11 seconds) with slurring of the initial forces suggesting a small delta wave. The QRS complex exhibited a pattern of incomplete right bundle branch block in eight patients and incomplete left bundle branch block in three patients.

A representative example is shown in Figure 10–26 recorded in a 61-year-old woman presenting with atrial flutter 2:1 AV conduction, and a FV fiber. A pattern of incomplete right bundle branch block is evident. Intracavitary recordings during sinus rhythm in the same patient (Figure 10–27) demonstrated abbreviation of the AH interval (30 ms) as well as the HV interval (25 ms). The AH interval was abbreviated in the majority of patients because of the presence of enhanced conduction in the AV node. The HV interval ranged from 15–30 msec (mean 23 ms).

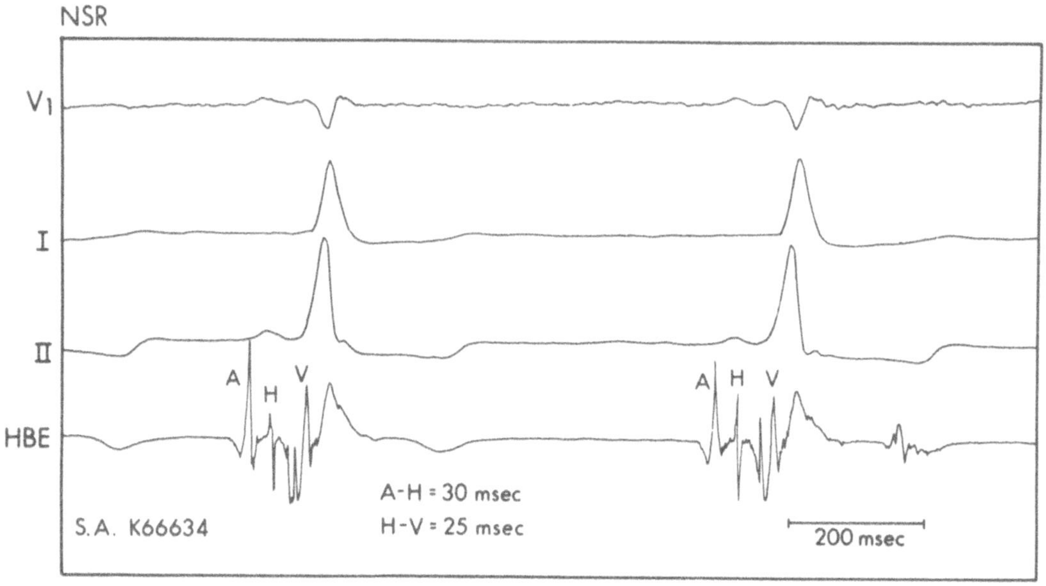

FIGURE 10–27. Intracavitary recordings in a patient with enhanced conduction in the AV node and a fasciculoventricular fiber. Note that the AH interval is 30 ms and the HV interval is 25 ms. Reproduced with permission of the *Am. Heart Assoc.* from Gallagher et al. [39].

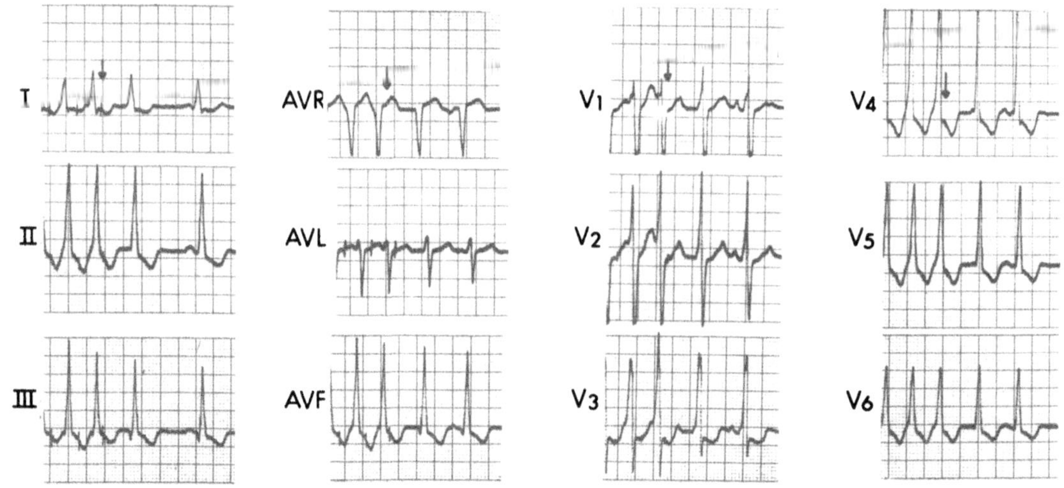

FIGURE 10–28. Refractory period determination in a patient with enhanced conduction in the AV node and a fasciculoventricular fiber. In each strip of the ECG, the last two drive beats of an atrial refractory period at cycle length 300 ms with introduction of a premature atrial depolarization at a coupling interval of 240 ms is shown (*arrow*). Note that in the drive beat, the PR interval is abbreviated and there is slurring of the initial forces, most evident in the precordial leads. Introduction of the premature beat results in prolongation of the PR interval but the QRS morphology remains unchanged.

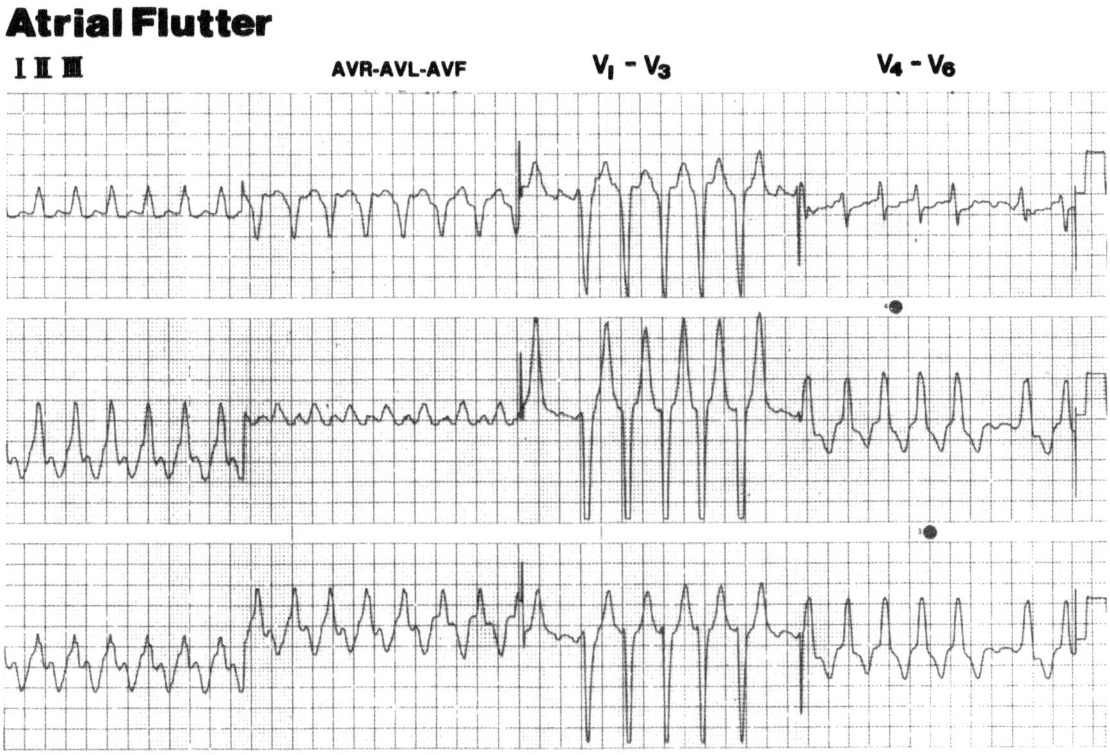

FIGURE 10–29. Atrial flutter in a patient with enhanced conduction in the AV node and a fasciculoventricular fiber. The QRS complexes are anomalous due to the presence of fasciculoventricular fiber. The HV interval recorded during this tachycardia was 10 ms.

No fusion was observed during sinus rhythm or with atrial pacing from the right atrium or the coronary sinus. Programmed stimulation of the atrium invariably resulted in prolongation of the AH interval; the HV interval remained constant, associated with a constant degree of preexcitation (Figure 10–28).

THE EFFECT OF IMPULSE FORMATION IN THE REGION OF THE HIS BUNDLE

His bundle extrasystoles and/or His bundle pacing demonstrated the same abbreviated HV intervals observed during sinus rhythm. The surface delta wave was unchanged with these extrasystoles (Figure 10–28). Although it is possible to observe complete normalization of the QRS complex with impulse formation *below* the takeoff of the FV connection, we did not observe this in our study group.

STUDIES DURING VENTRICULAR PACING

Ventriculoatrial conduction during ventricular pacing appeared to spread retrograde over the His bundle followed by a normal sequence of retrograde atrial activation. Enhanced conduction in the retrograde direction was almost invariably present in the same patients who had shown enhanced conduction in the AV node in the antegrade direction.

STUDIES DURING OBSERVED ARRHYTHMIAS

No observed arrhythmia in our study group could be causally related to the presence of the FV connection. Most patients exhibited a rapid ventricular response during atrial fibrillation because of the associated anomaly of enhanced conduction in the AV node. During atrial fibrillation, the QRS complexes were predominantly preexcited and fusion beats were not observed. It thus appears that the presence of the FV connection was coincidental. Bharati [20] has reported a patient with ventricular tachycardia associated with a left bundle branch block morphology. Pathological examination of the heart revealed an abnormally septated His bundle. It appears conceivable that a

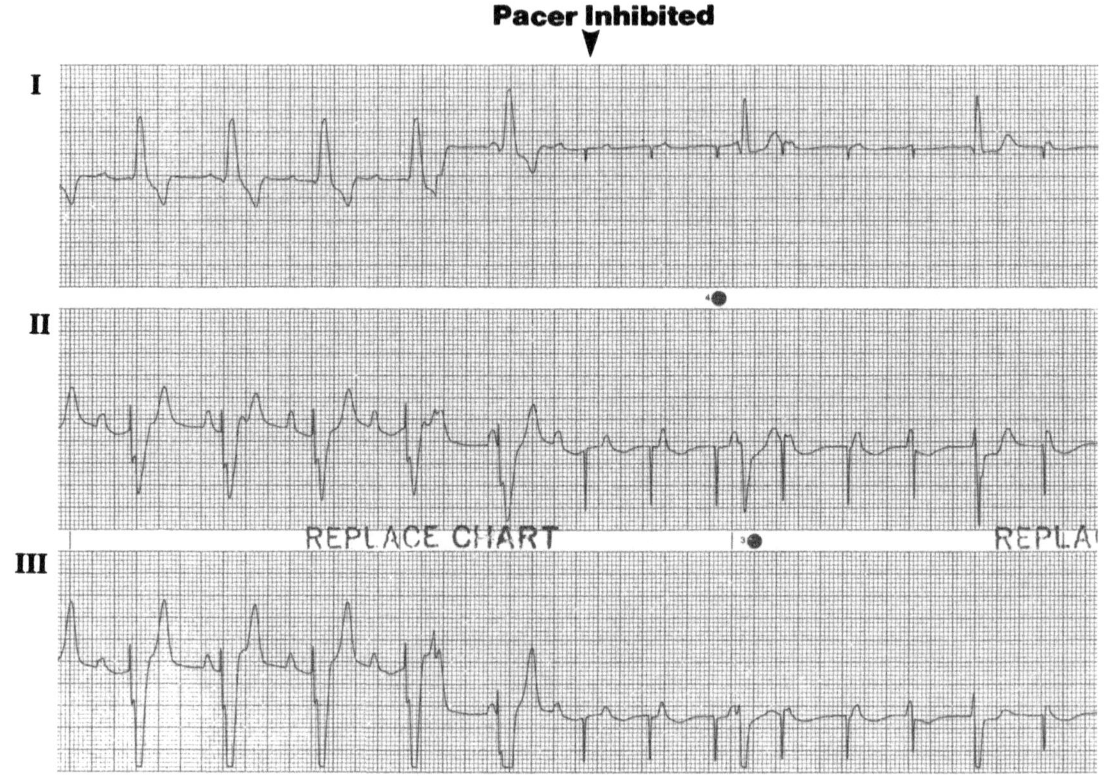

FIGURE 10–30. Escape rhythm following catheter ablation of the AV node–His bundle (same patient as Figure 10–29). A ventricular demand pacemaker captures the ventricle and complete heart block is evident. The pacemaker is then inhibited by chest wall stimulation resulting in the appearance of an escape rhythm with left anterior hemiblock. (See text for discussion.)

reentry mechanism might be sustained in some cases of FV connections, resulting in a pattern of ventricular tachycardia although we did not observe this.

TREATMENT

Some patients require treatment because of the abnormally rapid response during atrial fibrillation due to associated enhanced conduction in the AV node. These in general responded to a type I drug alone or in combination with propranolol. One patient underwent cryosurgery of the AV node–His bundle as an adjunctive procedure to replacement of a rheumatic mitral valve. The final patient proved refractory to medical management and underwent catheter ablation of the AV node–His bundle (Figure 10–29). Following inhibition of the ventricular demand pacemaker, an escape rhythm with left anterior hemiblock was observed, presumably due to an escape rhythm arising *below* the takeoff of the FV connection (Figure 10–30).

INTRAOPERATIVE STUDIES

A single patient underwent intraoperative mapping because of the need to replace a rheumatic mitral valve with severe regurgitation (same patient as Figures 10–26 and 10–27). Epicardial mapping at the time of surgery (Figure 10–31) failed to demonstrate any early activation at the base of the ventricles, excluding an accessory AV pathway. Instead, earliest activation occurred well after the onset of the QRS complex over the lower anterior and posterior interventricular septum.

Conclusion

The presence of Mahaim fibers appear to be ubiquitous during histological examination of the conduction system in man. Some of these connections appear functional. Nodoventricular (NV) connections can mimic the presence of left bundle branch block and can participate in sustained reciprocating tachycardia. The

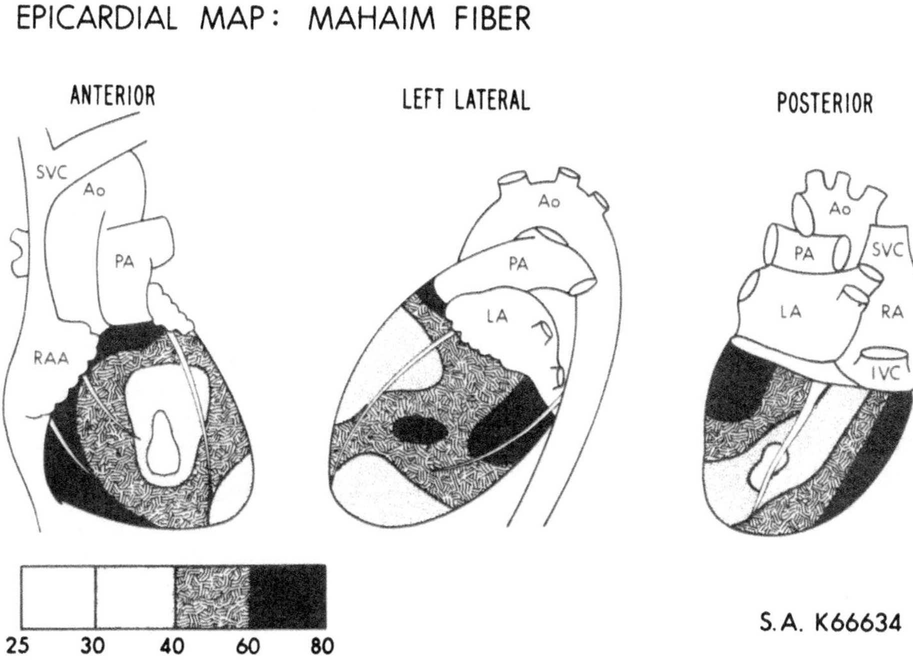

FIGURE 10–31. Ventricular activation due to a fasciculoventricular connection. Earliest activation is noted in normal breakthrough areas over the lower anterior right ventricle and over the posterior interventricular septum where activation of 25 ms. is noted. There is no early activation of the base of the ventricles. The right ventricle is slightly delayed relative to the left ventricle accounting for the pattern of incomplete right bundle branch block observed in this patient (same patient as Figure 10–26). Reproduced with permission from the *Am. Heart Assoc.* from Gallagher et al [39].

resulting tachycardia can mimic ventricular tachycardia because of the absence of a His deflection before the QRS complexes and in some instances because of ventriculoatrial dissociation. Fasciculoventricular (FV) connections can mimic intraventricular conduction defects but to date we have found no direct relationship between FV connections and arrhythmias.

Acknowledgment

The author gratefully acknowledges Mrs. Judy Ballard for her preparation of the manuscript and coordination of patient care. Also acknowledged is the collaboration of my many former colleagues at Duke University Medical Center; the members of the Electrophysiology Group of the Sanger Clinic: Drs. Robert H. Svenson, Samuel H. Zimmern, John M. Fedor, Will C. Sealy, and Jay G. Selle, and colleagues of the Sanger Clinic.

References

1. Mahaim I, Benatt A: Nouvelles recherches sur les connexions superieures de la branche gauche du faisceau de His–Tawara avec cloison interventriculaire. Cardiologia 1:61, 1938.
2. Mahaim I, Winston MR: Recherches d'anatomie comparee et de pathologie experimentale sur les connexions hautes de faisceau de His–Tawara. Cardiologia 5:189–260, 1941.
3. Mahaim I: Kent's fibers and the A–V paraspecific conduction through the upper connections of the bundle of His–Tawara. *Am. Heart J.* 33:651, 1947.
4. Lev M, Lerner R: The theory of Kent. A histologic study of the normal atrioventricular communications of the human heart. Circulation 12:176, 1955.
5. Lev M, Gibson S, Miller RA: Ebstein's disease with Wolff-Parkinson-White syndrome. *Am. Heart J.* 49:724, 1955.
6. Truex RC, Bishop JK, Hoffman EL: (1958) Accessory atrioventricular muscle bundles of the developing human heart. Anat Rec 131:45, 1958.

7. James TN: Morphology of the human atrioventricular node with remarks pertinent to its electrophysiology. *Am. Heart J.* 62:756, 1961.
8. Lev M, Sodi-Pollares D, Friedland C: A histopathologic study of the atrioventricular communications in a case of WPW with incomplete left bundle branch block. *Am. Heart J.* 66:399, 1963.
9. Lev M, Leffler WB, Langendorf R, Pick A: Anatomic findings in a case of ventricular preexcitation (WPW) terminating in complete atrioventricular block. Circulation 34:718, 1966.
10. Lunel AAV: Significance of annulus fibrosis of heart in relation to AV conduction and ventricular activation in cases of Wolff-Parkinson-White syndrome. *Br. Heart J.* 34:1283, 1972.
11. Okada R, Mizutani T, Mochizuki S: A morphologic study of a case of idiopathic cardiomyopathy which showed the electrocardiographic features of WPW syndrome. Heart 6:630, 1974.
12. James TN, Marilley RJ Jr, Marriott HJL: De subitaneis mortibus. XI. Young girl with palpitations. *Circulation* 51:743, 1975.
13. Bharati S, Lev M: The course of the conduction system in single ventricle with inverted (L–) loop and inverted (L–) transposition. *Circulation* 51:723, 1975.
14. Lev M, Fox SM, Bharati S, Greenfield JC Jr, Rosen KM, Pick A: Mahaim and James fibers as a basis for a unique variety of ventricular preexcitiation. *Am. J. Cardiol.* 36:880, 1975.
15. Anderson RH, Becker AE, Brechenmacher C, Davies MJ, Rossi L: Ventricular preexcitation. A proposed nomenclature for its substrates. *Eur. J. Cardiol.* 3:27, 1975.
16. Brechenmacher C, Courtadon M, Jourde M, Yermia JC, Cheyneo J, Voogtlin R: Syndrome de Wolff-Parkinson-White par association de fibres atrio-hissiennes et de fibres de Mahaim. *Arch. Mal. Coeur.* 69:1275, 1976.
17. Becker AE, Anderson RH: Morphology of the human atrioventricular junctional area. *In:* The Conduction System of the Heart. Edited by HJJ Wellens, KI Lie, MJ Janse. Leiden, HE Stenfert Kroese BV, 1976, pp. 263–286.
18. Anderson RH, Wenick AC, Losekoot TG, Becker AE: Congenitally complete heart block. Development aspects. *Circulation* 56:90, 1977.
19. Becker AE, Anderson RH, Durrer D, Wellens HJJ: The anatomic substrates of Wolff-Parkinson-White syndrome. *Circulation* 57:870, 1978.
20. Bharati S, Bauernfiend R, Scheinman M, Massie B, Cheitlin M, Denes P, Wu P, Lev M, Rosen KM: Congenital abnormalities of the conduction system in two patients with tachyarrhythmias. *Circulation* 59:593, 1979.
21. Brechenmacher C: *In:* Les troubles du rhytme cardiaque, Le Group de Rythmologie de la Societé Francaise de Cardiologie. Roussel, Paris, 1979, pp. 13–19.
22. Bharati S, Lev M: The conduction system in hypoplasia of the aortic tract complex. *Circulation* 59:1324, 1979.
23. Thiene G, Pennelli N, Rossi L: Cardiac conduction system abnormalities as a possible cause of sudden death in young athletes. Hum Pathol Aug 14:704, 1983.
24. Rossi L, Thiene G: Arrhythmologic pathology of sudden cardiac death. Casa Editrice Ambrosiana, Milano, 1983.
25. Marino TA, Kane BM: Cardiac atrioventricular junctional tissues in hearts from infants who died suddenly. *JACC* 5:1178, 1985.
26. Pick A, Katz LN: Disturbance of impulse formation and conduction in the preexcitation syndrome: their bearing on its mechanism. *Am. J. Med.* 19:759, 1955.
27. Massumi RA: His bundle recordings in bilateral bundle branch block combined with WPW syndrome: Antegrade type II (Mobitz) block and 1:1 retrograde conduction through the anomalous bundle. *Circulation* 42:287, 1970.
28. Coumel P, Waynberger M, Slama R, Bouvrain Y: Interest de l'enregistrement des potentiels hisienes au cours du syndrome de Wolff-Parkinson-White. A propos de six observations. *Acta. Cardiol.* 26:188, 1971.
29. Wellens HJJ: Eectrical Stimulation of the Heart in the Study and Treatment of Tachycardias. University Park Press, Baltimore, Maryland, 1971, p. 97.
30. Moore EN: Electrophysiological studies on preexcitation in dog using an electronically simulated atrioventricular bypass pathway. *Circ. Res.* 31:174, 1972.
31. Coumel P, Wayneberger M, Fabiato A, Slama R, Aigueperse A, Bouvrain Y: Wolff-Parkinson-White syndrome: problems in evaluation of multiple accessory pathways and surgical therapy. *Circulation* 45:1216, 1972.
32. Marco J, Salvador M, Couderc JJ, Dardenne P: Syndrome de Wolff-Parkinson-White avec PR normal: preexcitation du type Mahaim, association probable d' un faisceau de Kent. Etude du potentiel hisien. Rev Med Toulouse 8:229, 1972.
33. Stefanov G: Paroxysmal tachycardia in the probable presence of Mahaim's fibers. *Vutr Boles* 12:124, 1973.
34. Stefanov G: Three electrocardiographic variants of paroxysmal tachycardia with the probable presence of Mahaim fibers. *Vutr Boles* 13:42, 1974.
35. Mark AL, Basta LL: (1974) Paroxysmal tachycardia with atrioventricular dissociation in a patient with a variant of preexcitation syndrome. J. Electrocardiol 7:355, 1974.
36. Castellano A, Agha AS, Befeller B, Myerburg

RJ: Double accessory pathways in Wolff-Parkinson-White syndrome. *Circulation* 51:1020, 1975.
37. Tonkin AM, Dugan FA, Svenson RH, Sealy WC Wallace AG, Gallagher JJ: Coexistence of functional Kent and Mahaim-type tracts in the preexcitation syndrome. Demonstration by catheter techniques and epicardial mapping. *Circulation* 52:193, 1975.
38. Touboul P, Huerta F, Arnaud P, Porte J, Delahaye JP: Etude electrophysiologique de deux cas de preexcitation ventriculaire compatibles avec la presence de fibres de Mahaim. *Arch. Mal. Coeur.* 68:841, 1975.
39. Gallagher JJ, Sealy WC, Kasell J, Wallace AG: Multiple accessory pathways in patients with the preexcitation syndrome. *Circulation* 54:571, 1976.
40. Okumura M, Koike Y, Hattori M, Tsuzuke J, Tanahashi Y: A case of preexcitation syndrome due to possible Mahaim-fiber conduction. *Respir. Circ.* 24:891, 1976.
41. Castellanos A, Sung RJ, Castillo CA, Agha AS, Befeler B, Myerburg RJ: His bundle recordings in diagnosis of impulse formation in Kent and Mahaim tracts. *Br. Heart J.* 38:1173, 1976.
42. Touboul P, Gressard A, Vexler RM, Chatelain MT: Unusual re-entrant tachycardias associated with accessory pathways. *In:* Reentrant Arrhythmias. Edited by HE Kulbertus, MTP Press Ltd., Lancaster, 1977, pp. 132–143.
43. Donzeau JP, Constans R, Bernadet P, Bounhoore JP, Calazel P: Nodal tachycardia with atrioventricular dissociation probably connected with Mahaim's bundle undetectable in sinus rhythm. *Ann Cardiol Angeiol* 26:413, 1977.
44. Neuss H Thormann J: Functional properties of Mahaim fibers. *Klin. Wochenschr* 55:1031, 1977.
45. Gomes JA, Haft JI: His bundle electrocardiography in the Wolff-Parkinson-White syndrome. Evidence for combination of James and Mahaim conduction. *Cardiologia* 62:355, 1977.
46. Ikram H: Direct demonstration of pure infranodal preexcitation (Mahaim conduction) by A-V nodal and His bundle electrography. *Angiology* 28:376, 1977.
47. Probst P, Pachinger U, Steinbach R, Kaindl F: Preexcitation of the ventricle associated with total intra His bundle block. *Am. Heart J.* 94:96, 1977.
48. Motte G, Guillevin L, Dessouter P, Fruchaud J: (1978) Nodo-ventricular accessory pathway unmasked by a block in the trunk of the bundle of His. *Arch. Mal. Coeur.* 71:227, 1978.
49. Touboul P, Vexler RM, Chatelain MT: Re-entry via Mahaim fibres as a possible basis for tachycardia. *Br. Heart J.* 40:806, 1978.
50. Boroumand K, Armstrong PW: Preservation of preexcitation despite acute myocardial infarction complicated by complete heart block. *Can. Med. Assoc. J.* 119:139, 1978.
51. Matsuguchi H, Takeshita A, Makino N, Tanaka S, Nakagaki U, Kuroiwa A, Nakamura M.: Mahaim conduction producing left axis deviation and normal QRS. *Br. Heart J.* 40:902, 1978.
52. Rossi L, Thiene G, Knippel M: A case of surgically corrected Wolff-Parkinson-White syndrome. Clinical and histological data. *Br. Heart J.* 40:581, 1978.
53. Benditt DG, Pritchett ELC, Gallagher JJ: Spectrum of regular tachycardias with wide QRS complexes in patients with accessory atrioventricular pathways. *Am. J. Cardiol.* 42:828, 1978.
54. Long-Tai Fu, Iunama H, Watanabe T, Koyama S: Functional accessory pathway in ventricular preexcitation without short P-R. VIII World Congress of Cardiology Abstracts II:31, 1978.
55. Ward DE, Camm AJ, Spurrell RAJ: Ventricular preexcitation due to anomalous nodoventricular pathways: report of 3 patients. *Eur. J. Cardiol.* 9:111, 1979.
56. Motte G, Slama R: Les Tachycardies Ventriculaires. Edited by Laboratories Servier, Edi Conseil, Paris, 1979, p. 20.
57. Gallagher JJ, Pritchett ELC, Sealy WC, Kasell J, Wallace AG: The preexcitation syndromes. *Prog. Cardiovasc. Dis.* 20:285, 1978.
58. Josephson ME, Seides SF: Clinical Cardiac Electrophysiology. Lea and Febiger, Philadelphia, pp. 240, 1979.
59. Sung RJ, Styperek JL: Electrophysiologic identification of dual atrioventricular nodal pathway conduction in patients with reciprocating tachycardia using anomalous bypass tracts. *Circulation* 60:1464, 1979.
60. Pick A: Complex ECG patterns of Wolff-Parkinson-White syndrome. *In:* Cardiac Arrhythmias. Edited by OS Narula, Williams and Wilkins, Baltimore, 1979, p. 565.
61. Gallagher JJ, Smith WM, Kasell J, Benson DW, Sterba R, Grant AO: Role of Mahaim fibers in cardiac arrhythmias in man. *Circulation* 64:176, 1981.
62. Lerman BB, Waxman HL, Proclemer A, Josephson ME: Supraventricular tachycardia associated with nodventricular and concealed atrioventricular bypass tracts. *Am. Heart J.* 104:1097, 1982.
63. Reiter MJ, Smith WM, Gallagher JJ: Clinical spectrum of ventricular tachycardia with left bundle branch morphology. *Am. J. Cardiol.* 51:113, 1983.
64. Benditt DG, Epstein ML, Benson DW Jr: Dual accessory nodoventricular pathways: Role in paroxysmal wide QRS reciprocating tachycardia. *PACE* 6:577, 1983.
65. Morady F, Scheinman MM, Gonzalez R, Hess D: His-ventricular dissociation in a patient with

reciprocating tachycardia and a nodoventricular bypass tract. *Circulation* 64:839, 1981.
66. Bardy GH, German LD, Packer DL, Coltorti F, Gallagher JJ: Mechanism of tachycardia using a nodofascicular Mahaim fiber. *Am. J. Cardiol.* 54:1140, 1984.
67. Bhandari A, Morady F, Shan EN, Schwartz AB, Botvinick E, Scheinman MM: Catheter-induced His bundle ablation in a patient with reentrant tachycardia associated with a nodoventricular tract. *J. Am. Coll. Cardiol.* 4:611, 1984.
68. Zaman L, Garcia N, Luceri RM, Castellanos A, Myerburg RJ: Ectopic left atrial rhythm that produces QRS changes in absence of Wolff-Parkinson-White syndrome. *Circulation* 68:704, 1983.
69. Gallagher JJ, German LD, Broughton A, Guarnieri T, Trantham JL: Variants of the preexcitation syndromes. *In:* Frontiers of Cardiac Electrophysiology. Ed. by MB Rosenbaum and MV Elizari, Martinus Nijhoff, The Hague, 1983, pp. 724–772.
70. Gallagher JJ: Variants of preexcitation: Update 1984. *In:* Cardiac Electrophysiology and Arrhythmias. Grune and Stratton, 1984, pp. 419–433.
71. Matsuguchi H, Takeshita A, Makino N, et al: Mahaim conduction producing left axis deviation and normal QRS. *Br. Heart J.* 40:902, 1978.
72. Montely JM, Hanania G, Barrillon A, et al.: Fibres de Mahaim nodoventriculaires. Deux cas mis en evidence a l'exploration electrophysiologique. *Arch. Mal. Coeur.* 75:801, 1982.
73. Rakovec P, Cijan A: Lown-Ganong-Levine syndrome associated with Mahaim nodoventricular fibres. *Texas Heart Inst. J.* 10:289, 1983.
74. Garcia Civera R, Ferrero Cabedo JA, Sanjuan M[illegible] D, et al.: Diagnostico electrofisiologico y significado clinico de la preexcitation pro fibras fasciculoventriculares, *Rev. Lat. Cardiol.* 4:133, 1983.
75. Reiter MJ, Smith WM, Gallagher JJ: Clinical spectrum of ventricular tachycardia with left bundle branch morphology. *Am. J. Cardiol.* 51:113, 1983.
76. Rakovec P, Kranjec I, Fettich JJ, Pohar B, Fidler V: Multiple accessory pathways: a combined electrophysiological and radionuclide study. *PACE* 8:60, 1985.
77. Anderson RH, Becker AE, Brechenmacher C, Davies MJ, Rossi L: Ventricular preexcitation, a proposed nomenclature for its substrates. *Eur. J. Cardio.* 3:27, 1975.
78. Motte G, Brenchenmacher C, Davy JM, Belhassen B: Association de fibers nodoventriculaires et atrioventriculaires a l'origine de tachycardies reciproques. *Arch. Mal. Coeur.* 73:737, 1980.
79. Rossi L: Histopatologia del sindrome de Wolff-Parkinson-White. *Rev. Lat. Cardiol.* 4:99, 1983.
80. Rossi L: A histological survey of preexcitation and related arrhythmias. 5:816, 1975.
81. Pahlajani DB, Miller RA, Serrato M: Patterns of atrioventricular conduction in children, *Am. Heart J.* 90:165, 1975.
82. Bardy GH, Fedor JM, German LD, Packer DL, Gallagher JJ: Surface electrocardiographic clues suggesting presence of a nodofascicular Mahaim fiber *J. Am. Coll. Cardiol.* 3:1161, 1984.
83. Smith WM, Broughton A, Reiter M, Benson DW, Grant AO, Gallagher JJ: Bystander accessory pathway during AV node reentrant tachycardia. *PACE* 6:537, 1983.
84. Kerr CR, Benson DW, Gallagher JJ: Role of specialized conducting fibers in the genesis of "AV nodal" reentry tachycardia. *PACE* 6:171, 1983.
85. Bardy GH, Packer DL, German LD, Gallagher JJ: Preexcited reciprocating tachycardia in patients with Wolff-Parkinson-White syndrome: incidence and mechanisms. *Circulation* 70:377–391, 1984.
86. Trantham JL, Broughton A, Guarnieri T, German LD, Gallagher JJ: (1982) Two distinct V-H intervals in tachycardia associated with nodoventricular Mahaim fibers (Abstract.) *Circulation* 66:II–269, 1982.
87. Klein GJ, Prystowsky EN, Pritchett ELC, Davis D, Gallagher JJ: Atypical patterns of retrograde conduction over accessory atrioventricular pathways in the Wolff-Parkinson-White syndrome. *Circulation* 60:1477, 1979.
88. Gillette PC, Garson A Cooley DA, McNamara DG: Prolonged and decremental antegrade conduction properties in right anterior accessory connections. Wide QRS antidromic tachycardia of left bundle branch block pattern without Wolff-Parkinson-White configuration in sinus rhythm. *Am. Heart J.* 103:66, 1982.
89. Wellens HJJ, Durrer D: Combined conduction disturbances in two AV pathways in patients wtih Wolff-Parkinson-White syndrome. *Eur. J. Cardiol.* 1:23, 1973.
90. Moene R, Roos J: (1973) Transient Wolff-Parkinson-White syndrome and neonatal reciprocating tachycardia. *Circulation* 48:443, 1973.
91. Sealy WC, Mikat EM: Anatomical problems with identification and interruption of posterior septal Kent bundles. *Ann. Thorac. Surg.* 36:584, 1983.
92. Gallagher JJ, Svenson RH, Kasell JH, German LD, Bardy GH, Broughton A, Critelli G: Catheter technique for closed chest ablation of the atrioventricular conduction system. *N. Engl. J. Med.* 306:194, 1982.
93. Davies MJ, Anderson RH, Becker AE: The conduction system of the heart. Butterworths, Boston, 1983.

11. THE PERMANENT FORM OF JUNCTIONAL RECIPROCATING TACHYCARDIA

Giuseppe Critelli
John J. Gallagher
Gaetano Thiene
Lino Rossi

In 1967, Coumel et al. [1] described a fascinating tachycardia with a normal QRS occurring predominantly in infants and children. Due to the incessant nature of this tachycardia the arrhythmia was named "permanent junctional reciprocating tachycardia" (PJRT). Although the clinical characteristics and electrocardiographic findings of PJRT have been confirmed following the original reports of the French authors, controversy has persisted for many years concerning the pathophysiologic substrate of this arrhythmia [2–9]. Recent data strongly suggest that PJRT represents a "variant" form of the preexcitation syndromes [10–17].

Clinical Characteristics

PJRT is rarely detected at birth [5], but is often discovered during the first year of life [18] or at least by the age of 10 years [19]. However, in some cases PJRT may not be recognized until adulthood [12]. Published cases have suggested a male predominance. PJRT is not definitely associated with other congenital heart disease but moderate or severe cardiac dysfunction and/or congestive failure is often present. In affected individuals the tachycardia is characteristically incessant with heart rates ranging between 130 and 240 beats/min, and is usually unresponsive to pharmacologic treatment.

Electrocardiographic Features

The standard ECG during tachycardia (Figure 11–1, top) shows a 1:1 atrioventricular (AV) relationship with a retrograde P wave (P′) negative in leads II, III, and aVF. A peculiarity of the arrhythmia is the timing of the P′ wave, which occurs closer to the succeeding QRS complex than the preceding one ("long R–P" tachycardia), resulting in an R-P′/P′-R ratio greater than 1.0.

Spontaneous restoration of sinus rhythm is frequently observed but the tachycardia generally starts again after a few sinus beats (Figure 11–1, bottom). During sinus rhythm, the PR interval is normal and there is no evidence of a delta wave or prolonged QRS.

The onset of tachycardia is most commonly due to acceleration of the sinus rate without PR prolongation [1,18,20]. However, as in other reentrant tachycardias [20–22], spontaneous onset may occur with a variety of initiating

The authors wish to gratefully acknowledge Ms. Judy Ballard of the Sanger Clinic for preparing this manuscript.

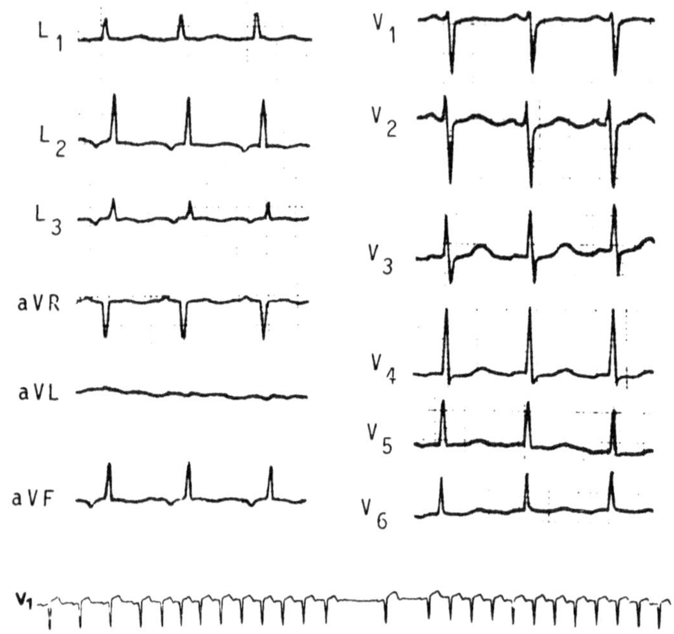

FIGURE 11–1. (*Top*) Standard electrocardiogram obtained from a patient with PJRT. Negative P waves in Leads II, III, aVF are present; the R-P′ interval is greater than P′-R interval. (*Bottom*) ECG strip showing the almost incessant nature of the tachycardia: When spontaneous restoration of sinus rhythm occurs, tachycardia starts again after two sinus beats.

mechanisms: (1) atrial premature beats with lengthening of the PR interval; (2) critical shortening of the PP interval; (3) junctional escape beats; (4) premature ventricular beats (Figure 11–2)

Electrophysiologic Substrate: Current Hypotheses

In order to explain the electrocardiographic peculiarities of PJRT — namely, the absence of preexcitation during sinus rhythm and the long R-P′ interval during tachycardia — the following possible mechanisms have been hypothesized: (1) unusual ("fast–slow") intranodal reentry [2–4]; (2) reentry utilizing a concealed accessory pathway with a long conduction time [5–10]; (3) an accessory AV node [5,10]; and (4) retrogradely conducting nodoventricular connection (with decremental conduction) in series with a "bystander" atriofascicular tract (resulting in two distinct sequences of atrial activation). The controversial state of current views concerning the underlying mechanisms of PJRT is due in part to the rarity of this tachyarrhythmia, the paucity of histological data in cases of PJRT, and the possibility that more than one mechanism is operative in patients with tachycardia of similar ECG features.

A number of recent observations provide strong support for the hypothesis that an accessory AV pathway with "decremental" properties is the substrate for the clinical arrhythmia known as PJRT. These observations have been derived from electrophysiologic investigation of patients with PJRT, studies performed following ablation of *either* the AV node–His bundle *or* the accessory pathway, and from postmortem histopathological findings in a patient with PJRT [10–17].

Electrophysiologic Investigation of PJRT

Certain characteristic findings are typically demonstrated during electrophysiologic study of patients with PJRT:

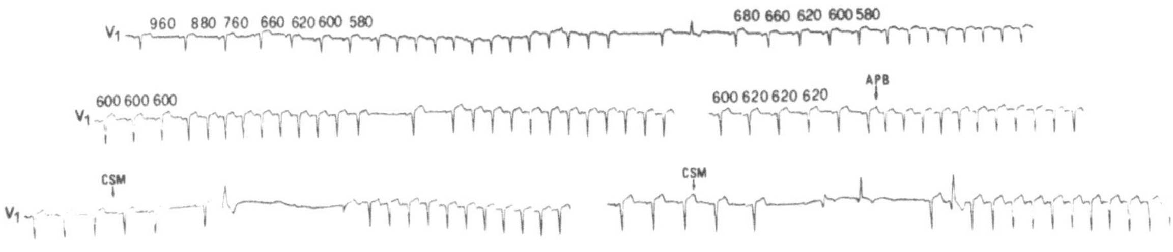

FIGURE 11–2. ECG strips showing several initiating mechanisms in PJRT: (a) critical shortening of the PP cycle (*top*); (b) no modification of the PP cycle and PR interval (*middle left*); (c) atrial premature beat (APB) (*middle right*); (d) junctional (*bottom left*) and ventricular (*bottom right*) escape beat elicited with carotid sinus massage (CSM). RR intervals indicated in milliseconds.

1. A long ventriculoatrial (VA) conduction time is evident during tachycardia and is responsive to changes in autonomic tone.
2. The earliest retrograde atrial activation is recorded just inside the orifice of the coronary sinus.
3. Premature stimulation of the ventricle during tachycardia at a time when the His bundle is refractory typically shortens the ensuing atrial cycle length (i.e., "preexcites" the atria) without a change in atrial activation sequence (Figure 11–3), a demonstration in support of existence of an accessory pathway [23,24]. Earlier premature stimulation of the ventricle can terminate the tachycardia without conduction to the atria (due to block in the pathway) (Figure 11–4).
4. With appropriate maneuvers during ventricular stimulation, two distinct sequences of atrial activation [25–27] are found: one initiated near the coronary sinus orifice and presumably due to conduction over the accessory pathway; the other initiated in the atrial septum near the His bundle, presumably due to conduction of the normal AV node (Figure 11–5).

Caution must be exercised in the interpretation of retrograde atrial activation sequences. A study of the sequence of *normal* retrograde atrial activation [25] has shown that the earliest site of retrograde atrial activation can be located in the orifice of the coronary sinus (one-third of cases), the atrial septum near the His bundle (one-third of cases) or near-simultaneous in both of these areas (one-third of cases). What distinguishes PJRT is that *two* distinct sequences can be recorded in the same patient. Studies of rabbit AV node in vitro [28] have demonstrated the possibility of two exit points from the AV node, but we have never observed *two* distinct sequences by *catheter* technique in the *absence* of an accessory pathway.

The above findings in concert suggest that the retrograde limb of the tachycardia circuit is an accessory pathway with decremental properties coursing from ventricle to atrium near the coronary sinus orifice. The existence of such an accessory pathway is further supported by the results of ablation procedures. Ablation of the AV node–His bundle results in complete heart block but persistence of retrograde conduction, while dissection of the posterior septum near the coronary sinus abolishes tachycardia while preserving conduction in the normal conduction system [5,16].

One point deserves further emphasis. The phenomenon of "retrograde preexcitation of the atria" shown in Figure 11–3 is a pivotal demonstration which helps exclude further consideration of an alternative diagnosis: the unusual ("fast-slow") variety of intranodal reentry. It has been stressed that the accessory pathway exhibits decremental properties; indeed, early premature ventricular stimulation results in block in the accessory pathway as shown in Figure 11–4. One might expect therefore that a critically timed premature stimulation of the ventricle would engage the retrograde limb and paradoxically *delay* the ensuing atrial response because of conduction delay in the accessory pathway. This has in fact been demonstrated now in three consecutive cases where it was looked for (Figure 11–6). A further implication

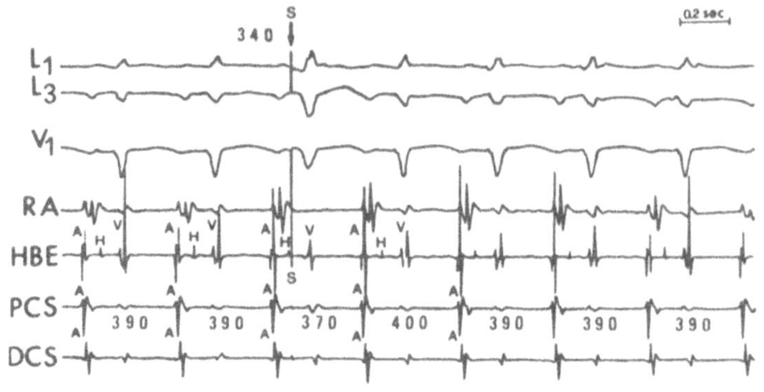

FIGURE 11–3. Endocardial mapping of right atrium and coronary sinus during tachycardia. A long VA interval (390 ms) is evident; the earliest retrograde electrogram is recorded near the coronary sinus orifice. A premature ventricular depolarizaiton(s) (*arrow*) introduced when the His bundle is refractory results in shortening of the AA interval (370 ms) without disturbing the sequence of atrial activation. RA: right atrium electrogram; HBE: His bundle electrogram; PCS: proximal coronary sinus electrogram; DCS: distal coronary sinus electrogram.

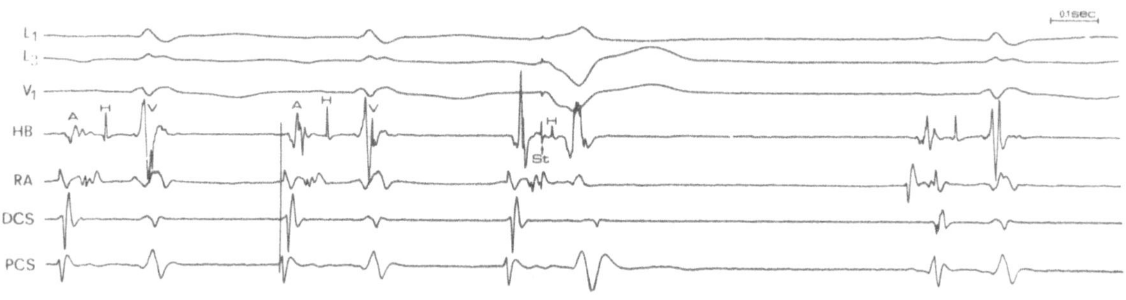

FIGURE 11–4. Termination of tachycardia by premature ventricular stimulation (st) without conduction to the atria. With resumption of sinus rhythm the AH intervals are normal. Abbreviations as in Figure 11–3.

follows: Compensatory delays in the retrograde limb might *conceal* retrograde preexcitation, obscuring the true diagnosis. To avoid this problem, we recommend very detailed scanning of the ventricle with tiny increments in coupling interval. Administration of isoproterenol minimizes the possibility of retrograde block/delay in the accessory pathway and should be used when equivocal results are obtained.

Observations After His Bundle Ablation

Interruption of the AV node–His bundle provides a *direct* demonstration of the presence of an accessory pathway in patients with PJRT. Anterograde conduction over an accessory pathway with decremental properties was noted for the first time in two patients after catheter ablation of the AV node–His bundle [29,30] and retrospectively in another patient who underwent surgical ablation of the AV node–His bundle [5]. After the procedure, there was no evidence of anterograde conduction of the AV node–His bundle. Conduction to the ventricles now occurred over the accessory pathway resulting in an anomalous QRS complex (Figure 11–7). No spontaneous tachycardia was observed nor could any be induced by atrial or ventricular pacing.

Decremental *anterograde* conduction in the

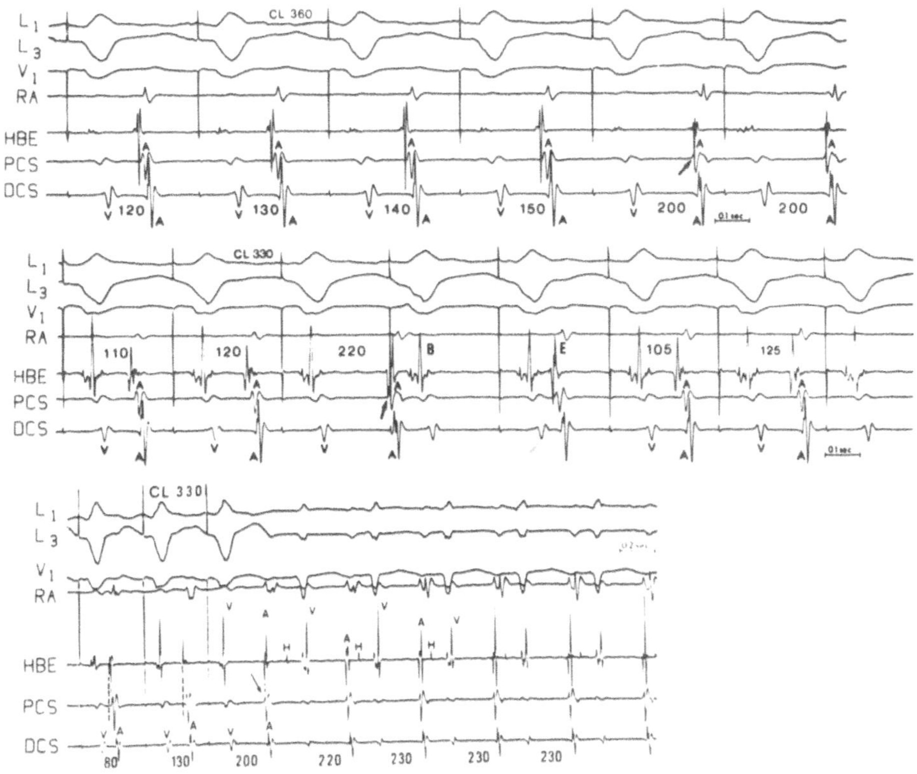

FIGURE 11–5. Endocardial mapping of the right atrium and coronary sinus during ventricular pacing. At a cycle length (CL) of 360 ms (*top*) the earliest retrograde atrial activation is recorded on the His bundle electrogram; a gradual lengthening of the VA interval is evident. After the fifth QRS complex, a sudden increase of the VA interval simultaneous with a change (earliest electrogram in proximal coronary sinus) in the sequence of atrial activation (*arrow*) occurs. Pacing at a CL of 330 ms (*middle*) results in a similar pattern, followed by retrograde block (B) and an atrial escape beat (E). The retrograde conduction then resumes with the same atrial activation sequence and VA behavior as seen before the block. In the *lower panel*, tachycardia induction is shown. It occurs when a sudden increase of VA conduction simultaneous with a change in the retrograde activation sequence (*arrow*) is achieved. Abbreviations as in Figure 11–3.

accessory pathway was manifested by transient spontaneous Wenckebach phenomenon in all patients (Figure 11–7). In addition, complete AV block with junctional escape rhythm was observed spontaneously and during carotid sinus massage in one patient (Figure 11–8). Stable 1:1 AV conduction over the accessory pathway was noted in all patients with a long PR interval (340,320, and 280 ms, respectively) and a QRS configuration suggesting posterior septal preexcitation (initial forces negative in leads II, III, aVF and positive in leads I, aVL and V_1–V_6) (Figure 11–9). Of interest was the disappearance of the pattern of myocardial infarction which had been evident before His bundle ablation in one patient (Figure 11–10).

The decremental properties of *retrograde* conduction over the accessory pathway were confirmed after His bundle ablation in all three patients. Figure 11–11 shows the pattern of retrograde conduction in one of these. During ventricular pacing, the retrograde sequence of atrial activation was now always initiated in the coronary sinus orifice.

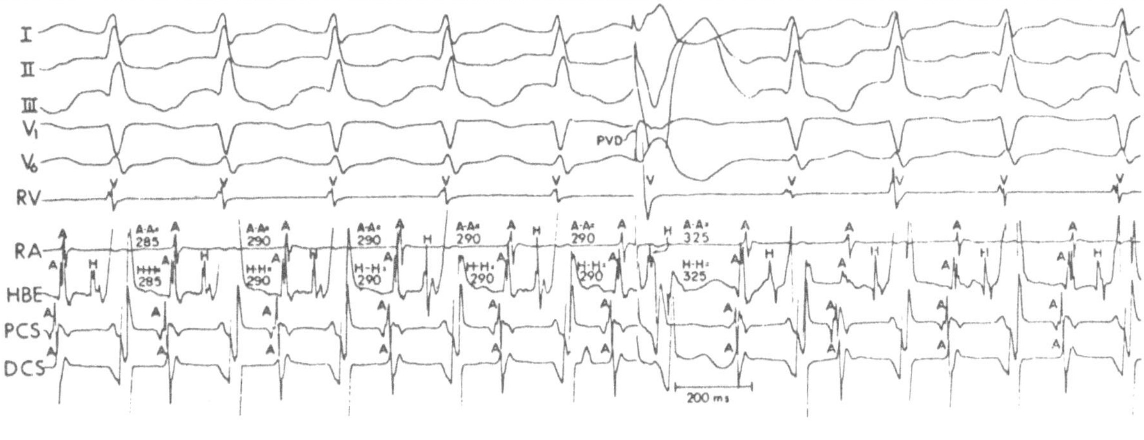

FIGURE 11–6. "Paradoxic" preexcitation by ventricular stimulation in PJRT. Tracings from above down are standard ECG leads I–III, V_1, V_6 and bipolar electrograms from the right ventricle (RV), His bundle region (HBE), proximal coronary sinus (PCS) and distal coronary sinus (DCS). Tachycardia is present with a cycle length of 290 ms. A premature ventricular depolarization (PVD) is introduced without disturbing the His deflection. The PVD conducts retrogradely with the same sequence as in tachycardia (earliest in proximal CS), but is delayed, prolonging the atrial cycle length to 325 ms.

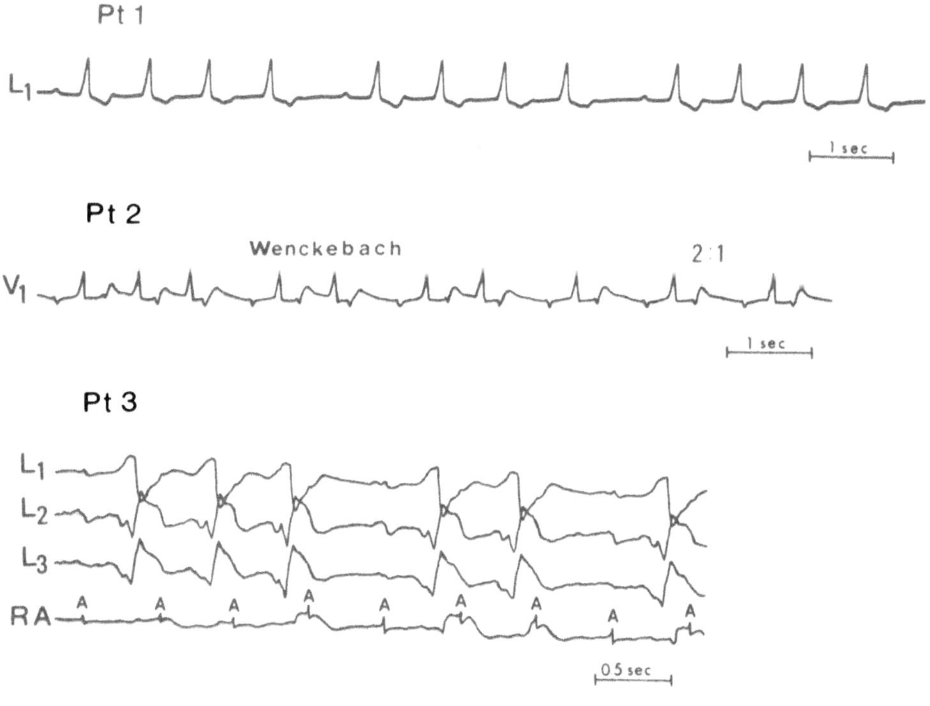

FIGURE 11–7. Electrocardiographic recordings obtained after His bundle ablation from three patients with PJRT. Sinus rhythm with a long PR interval and Wenckebach type block is present in all patients. In patient 2, 2:1 AV block is also evident. The QRS configuration is consistent with posterior septal preexcitation (see also Figure 11–8). Abbreviations as in Figure 11–3.

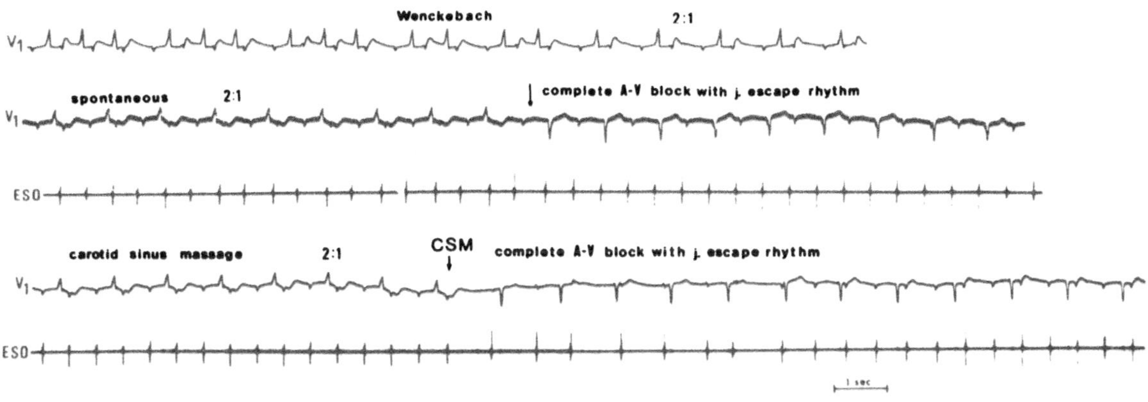

FIGURE 11–8. Surface electrocardiogram (V_1) and atrial electrogram recorded by esophagus five days after His bundle ablation. A long PR interval with spontaneous Wenckebach-type and 2:1 AV block are present. Complete AV block with junctional escape rhythm is also observed spontaneously and during carotid sinus massage (CSM).

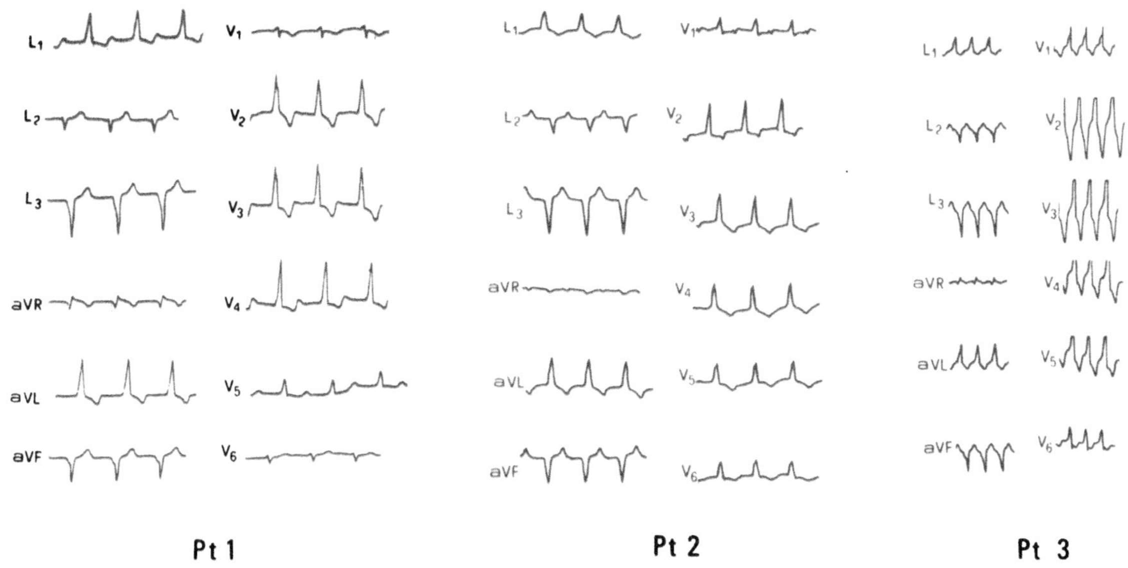

FIGURE 11–9. Standard electrocardiograms recorded 2 to 3 weeks after His bundle ablation in three patients (the same shown in Figure 11–6) with PJRT. Stable sinus rhythm (with sinus tachycardia in patient 3) is present. The PR interval measures 340, 320, and 280 ms, respectively. The QRS configuration suggests posteroseptal preexcitation. (See text for further details.)

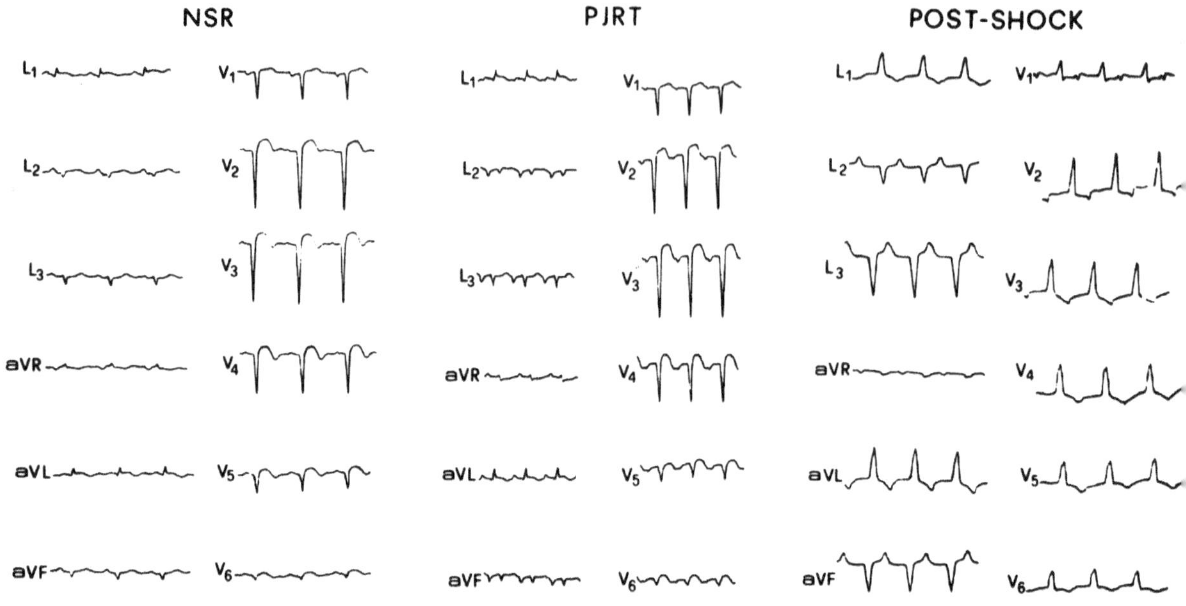

FIGURE 11–10. Standard electrocardiograms obtained before and after His bundle ablation in a patient with PJRT and a previous myocardial infarction. Before the shock a pattern of anterior myocardial infarction during tachycardia (PJRT) is evident. After His bundle ablation, sinus rhythm with a long (280 ms) PR interval and QRS morphology consistent with posterior septal preexcitation is present. Note the disappearance of the myocardial infarction pattern after His bundle ablation.

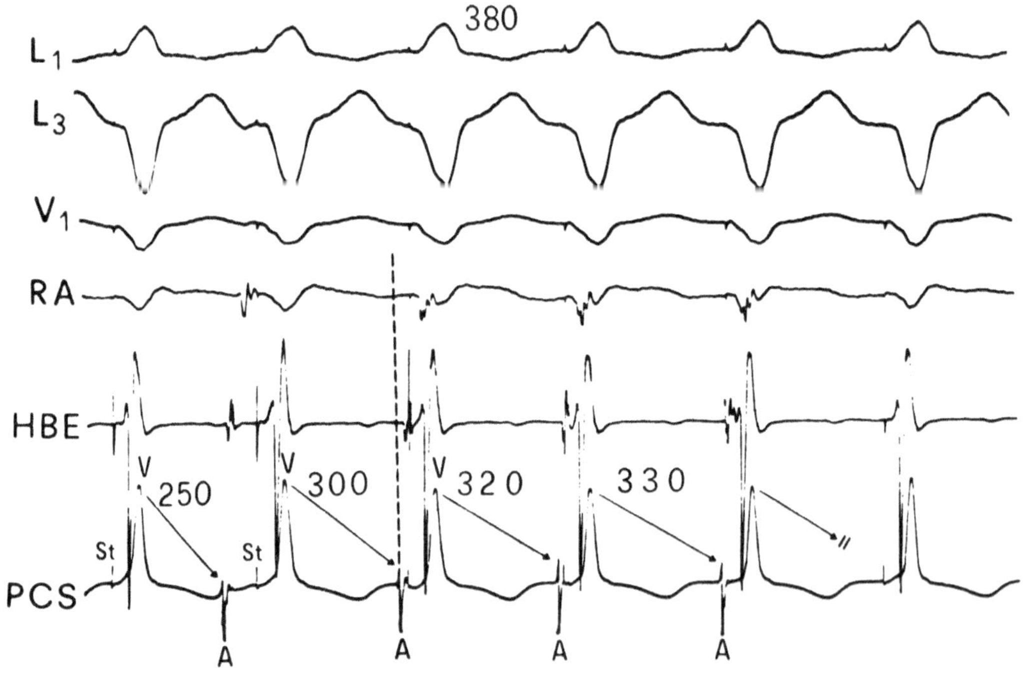

FIGURE 11–11. The pattern of VA conduction after His bundle ablation. Ventricular pacing (St) at a CL of 380 ms results in a long VA interval with retrograde Wenckebach phenomenon; the earliest atrial electrogram is recorded in the proximal coronary sinus. Abbreviations as in Figure 11–3.

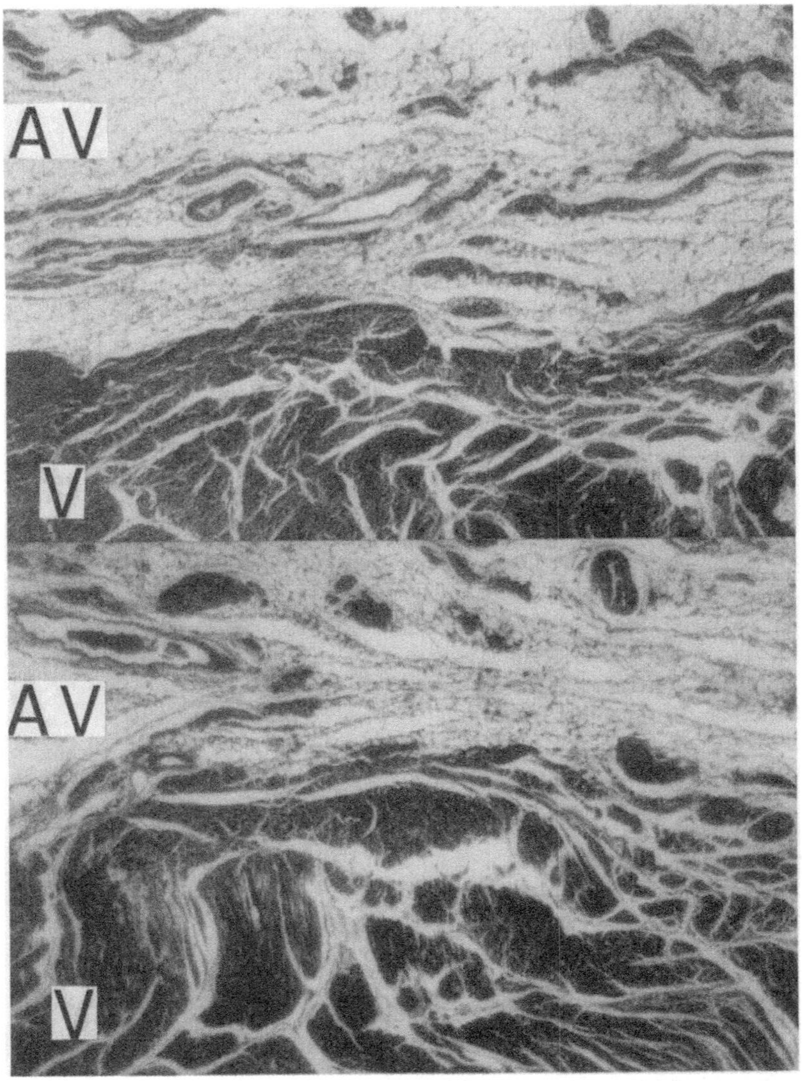

FIGURE 11–12. Photomicrographs taken from serial sections of the right atrioventricular junction (*top*) and the level of the ventricular end of the accessory pathway (*bottom*) in a patient with PJRT who suddenly died five months after closed chest ablation of the His bundle. (*Top*) Note atrial fascicles passing from the right atrium across the fat of the atrioventricular (AV) sulcus to join the ventricle (V) through gaps in the AV anulus. (*Bottom*) The anastomosing AV accessory fibers change direction and show sclerotic replacement (Hematoxylin-eosin stain; original magnification × 19).

Histologic Observations

Postmortem documentation of the accessory pathway was achieved in one patient who developed a ventricular aneurysm as a result of previous myocardial infarction and died suddenly 5 months after His bundle ablation [12].

Extensive coronary artery disease and myocardial infarction with aneurysm formation was present. Histologic examination of the posterior AV sulcus was revealing. A group of tiny atrial fibromuscular bundles were seen to descend into and to criss-cross the fat of the AV sulcus, approaching and intermingling with fascicles belonging to the uppermost ventricular muscle through narrow clefts of rudimentary fenestrated AV anulus, immediately behind the central fibrous body (Figure 11–12, top).

The accessory pathway originated from the lower rim of the coronary sinus. No specialized tissue was observed in the accessory pathway. The accessory pathway exhibited spotty interstitial fibrosis where individual fibers inserted on the ventricular myocardium through the narrow fissures of the AV anulus. Because the general orientation of the anastomosing fascicles was perpendicular to the cut, the AV contiguity was barely evident on individual sections. At the ventricular end of the connection, some ventricular bundles bent so sharply as to present parallel to the plane of section, whereas more laterally, a patch of pronounced sclerosis disrupted the myocardium (Figure 11–12, bottom).

On further serial sections, histological lesions induced at the AV junction by catheter ablation were analyzed. The AV node (Figure 11–13) exhibited severe fibrotic scarring (with numerous newly formed capillaries) of its outer layer, with complete interruption of the atrial–AV nodal connection. The upper and penetrating His bundle was replaced by fibrosis; the overlying endocardium on the right side was markedly thickened. The bifurcating His bundle was slightly lipomatous but well preserved (Figure 11–14). The roots of both bundle branches, separated from each other by a fibrous spur, were normal. The details of the AV node–His bundle histology resulting from catheter ablation [28,29] are reported in detail elsewhere [13].

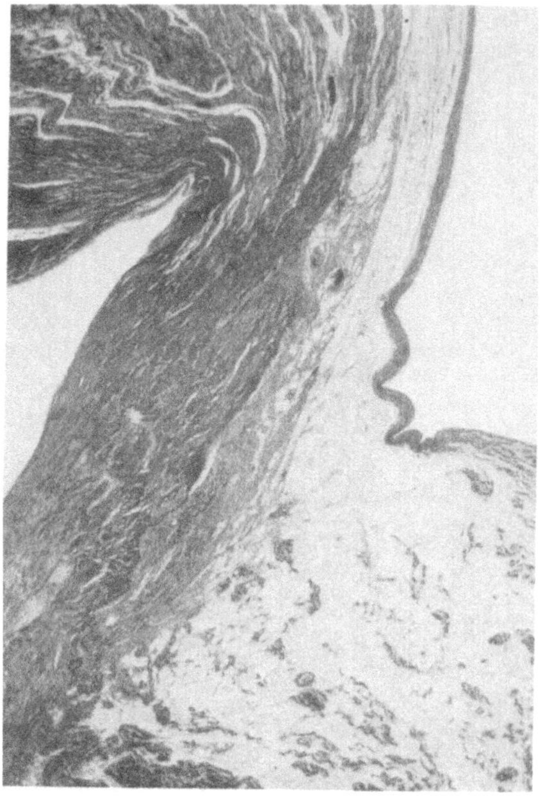

FIGURE 11–13. Same case as in Figure 11–12. Serial sections of atrioventricular junctional tissue. Severe fibrosis of AV node (*arrow*) and nearby AV node. (Trichromic Heidenhain's (azan) stain; original magnification × 15.)

A Unified Hypothesis about the Structural – Functional Substrate

On the basis of the above findings, it is possible to define the anatomic and electrophysiologic substrate of PJRT.

1. *A ventriculoatrial accessory pathway with decremental properties provides the retrograde limb of the reentry circuit (Figure 11–15).*

It is conceivable that a nodoventricular connection provides the retrograde limb of the reentry circuit in PJRT. In this case, "retrograde preexcitation" of the atrium during tachycardia could only be explained by postulating longitudinal dissociation within the AV node, with two separate exit points from the AV node required to explain the observed sequences of atrial activation. The findings obtained from the pa-

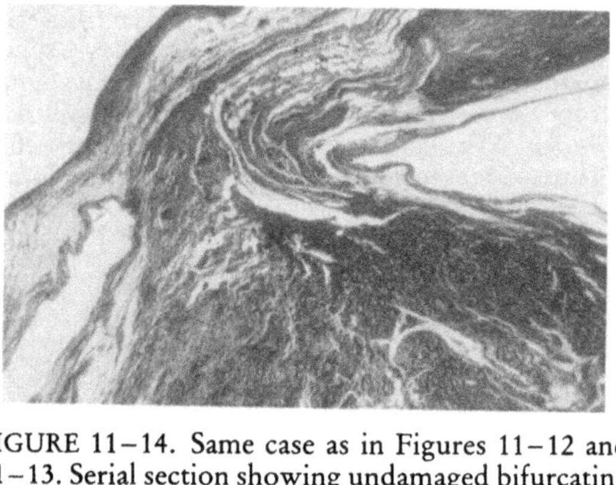

FIGURE 11–14. Same case as in Figures 11–12 and 11–13. Serial section showing undamaged bifurcating His bundle (*arrow*) astride and crest of ventricular septum. (Trichromic Heidenhain's (azan) stain; original magnification × 15.)

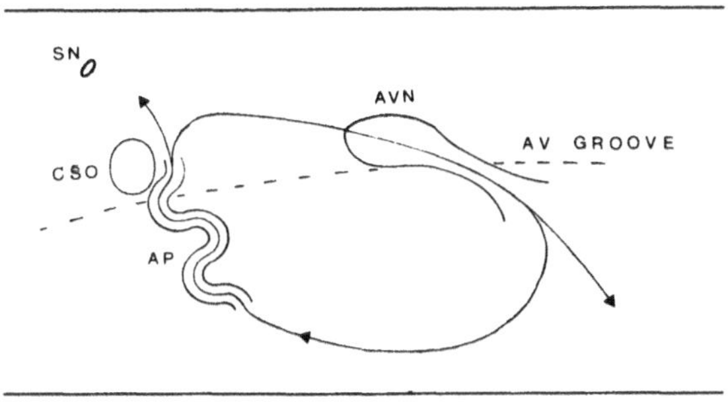

FIGURE 11–15. Schematic representation of the AV junctional region illustrating the reentry circuit in PJRT. The relation of the accessory pathway (AP) to the coronary sinus orifice (CSO) is shown. The tortuosity of AP is also defined. SN: sinus node; AVN: atrioventricular node.

tient in whom postmortem examination was performed are against this theoretical possibility. Indeed, the lesions observed in the AV region showed severe fibrosis of the AV node with complete interruption of the approaches to the AV node and penetrating His bundle, making the persistence of a hypothetical nodoventricular fiber unlikely.

2. *The accessory pathway is located in the posterior pyramidal space.*

The posterior septal location of the accessory pathway in PJRT is suggested by the location of the atrial and ventricular insertions: (1) earliest atrial activity recorded during retrograde conduction over the accessory pathway is situated just inside the orifice of the coronary sinus; (2) the ECG obtained after His bundle ablation shows sinus rhythm with an anomalous QRS configuration, consistent with a ventricular insertion in the posteroseptal region; (3) surgical dissection of the posterior pyramidal space in patients with PJRT [6,10,17,31] results in interruption of the accessory pathway while preserving conduction in the AV node–His bundle and; (4) the single case with histological demonstration of an accessory pathway showed a posterior septal location.

3. *The accessory pathway can conduct in the anterograde direction in the absence of conduction over the AV node–His bundle (Figure 11–16).*

Despite the widely held belief that the accessory pathway in patients with PJRT can conduct only in the retrograde direction, conduction in the anterograde direction over the accessory pathway (with a long PR interval) was noted after ablation of the AV node–His bundle in each of the three patients in whom this intervention was undertaken. These observations prompt consideration about the lack of preexcitation during sinus rhythm (see later section).

4. *Decremental properties of the accessory pathway may be explained by anatomic considerations.*

Spach [32] emphasized the important influence that geometric features can have on the propagation of depolarization in normal and abnormal cardiac muscle. As mentioned above, the accessory pathway was characterized by pronounced tortuosity of the fibers bridging the AV sulcus. Theoretically one would expect substantial disorders in axial resistivity to be present along the course of a fiber that pursued such a sinuous path. As a result of changing cross-sectional area, such a fiber might predictably exhibit slow conduction similar to that of a normally functioning AV node. The structural and geometric asymmetry of the accessory pathway, as found in our patient, may be critical to decremental conduction. Although this case is not necessarily representative of all patients with PJRT, one can speculate that directional distortion and partial fibrotic thinning of the accessory pathway may have a significant bearing on impairment in impulse propagation along the accessory pathway itself.

It seems reasonable therefore to modify some currently accepted concepts in PJRT.

1. *Impedance mismatch is not responsible for the lack of preexcitation in sinus rhythm.*

The absence of preexcitation during sinus rhythm, although attributed in some cases to fibrosis of the accessory pathway and/or neurolesions [33–35], has generally suggested that the accessory pathway is unable to conduct in the anterograde direction because of the presence of "impedance mismatch" [36]. This phenomenon has been demonstrated experimentally in a narrow isthmus of muscle joining a broad sheet of atrial myocardium with a three-dimensional mass of ventricular muscle. Thus the limited wave front in the accessory pathway might be insufficient to bring the larger volume of ventricular cells to threshold during *anterograde* conduction but would be sufficient to bring the atrium to threshold

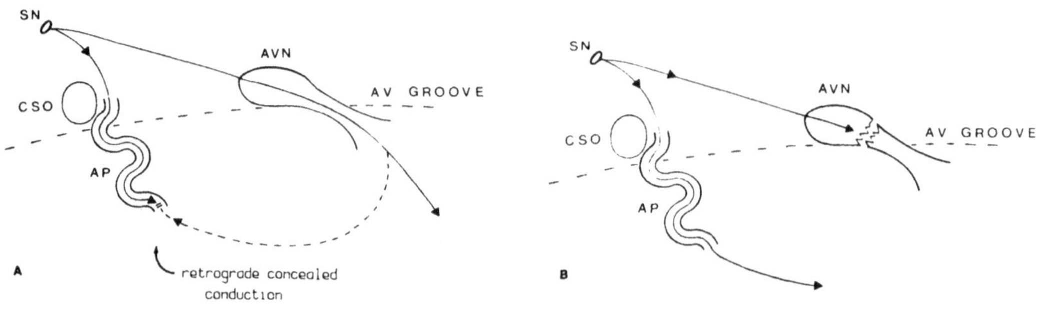

FIGURE 11–16. Schematic representation of the AV junctional region showing the pathway of anterograde conduction in PJRT before and after His bundle ablation. (Panel A) Proposed hypothesis to explain the absence of preexcitation during sinus rhythm in PJRT. (Panel B) In the absence of conduction over the normal conduction system the activation of ventricles occurs through the accessory pathway (AP) with decremental properties. (See text for details.)

during *retrograde* conduction. If this were true, we should have observed complete AV block after His bundle ablation instead of anomalous 1:1 AV conduction. On the contrary [12], we believe that competitive concealed retrograde conduction from the normal conduction system to the ventricular insertion of the accessory pathway must be invoked to explain the absence of preexcitation during sinus rhythm (Figure 11–16, Panel A). With *removal* of this influence by His bundle ablation, the accessory pathway is capable of manifesting anterograde conduction (Figure 11–16, Panel B). This interpretation is also supported by observations in a patient in whom it was necessary to deliver two shocks to the His bundle (Figure 11–17). The first shock only resulted in reversible damage of the His bundle followed by reappearance of the tachyarrhythmia. Initially, anterograde conduction was present over the accessory pathway. At the end of a Wenckebach cycle in the accessory pathway, conduction over the AV node His bundle (with right bundle branch block due to the shock) suddenly appeared. It is reasonable to believe that in that moment, conduction over the normal pathway (which was previously inhibited due to concealed retrograde penetration by the impulse coming from the accessory pathway) was now possible because block in the accessory pathway prevented retrograde concealed conduction into the normal pathway. Once ventricular activation occurred by the normal conduction system, an analogous mechanism — namely, retrograde concealed conduction from the normal to the anomalous pathway — prevented activation of the ventricles by the accessory pathway. After the second shock, irreversible damage was induced below the His bundle (Figure 11–18). Concealed conduction into the accessory pathway no longer occurred and stable ventricular activation over the accessory pathway was now present.

2. *Critical shortening of the PP cycle is not the only initiating mechanism.*

Initiation of tachycardia in PJRT is commonly associated with acceleration of the sinus rate without PR prolongation [1,18,20]. On the contrary, as shown in Figure 11–2, several mechanisms other than critical shortening of the PP cycle can be responsible for tachycardia initiation.

3. *Fast–slow intranodal reentry should not be invoked as the underlying mechanism.*

In the few cases in which a "fast–slow" atypical variety of intranodal reentry was invoked as the explanation for "long R–P reciprocating tachycardia" [2,4,37], an accessory pathway utilized in the retrograde direction by the tachycardia was not excluded. Indeed a discontinuous curve is not peculiar to dual intranodal pathways, since the same pattern is usually observed in the presence of an accessory pathway with retrograde decremental properties (Figure 11–5). Thus the behavior of VA conduction cannot be used to distinguish whether retrograde conduc-

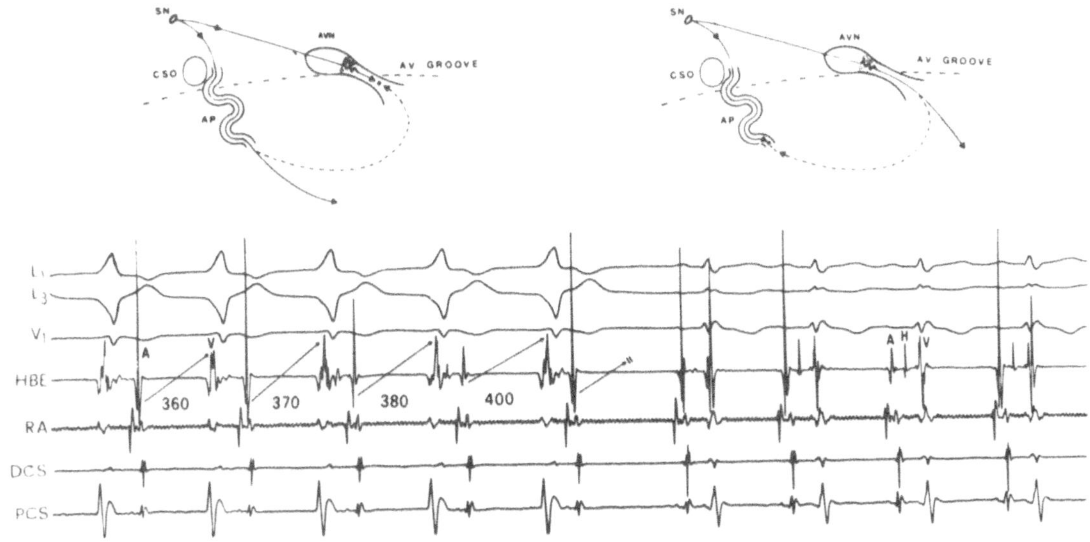

FIGURE 11–17. Surface electrocardiograms and His bundle electrogram (HB) obtained from a patient with PJRT after the first attempt of interrupting the His bundle by catheter technique. (*Left*) Sinus rhythm with Wenckebach-type block over the accessory pathway (AP) is present in the first five beats; the conduction over the normal conduction system is inhibited because of retrograde concealed penetration by the impulse coming from the accessory pathway. The His bundle deflection results from anterograde conduction over the normal conduction system, which is interrupted below the His bundle. (*Right*) At the end of the Wenckebach phenomenon, conduction over the normal conduction system resumes with normal AH and HV intervals (and right bundle branch block as a consequence of the shock). (See text for details.)

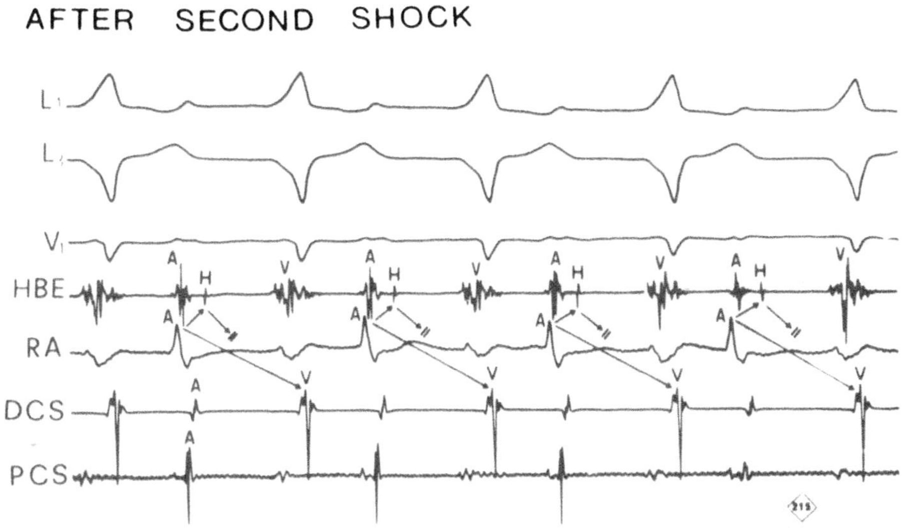

FIGURE 11–18. Same patient as in Figure 11–17. Surface electrocardiograms and His bundle electrogram obtained after the second shock. Stable 1:1 conduction with a long PR interval occurs over the accessory pathway. (See text for details.)

tion occurs over an accessory pathway with atypical properties or through the AV node. Multiple atrial electrograms must also be recorded to define the pathway of retrograde conduction [26]. As noted above, compensatory delays in retrograde accessory pathway conduction may preclude demonstration of atrial preexcitation during ventricular stimulation during tachycardia. Only one observation in this situation can support the diagnosis of intranodal reentry while excluding PJRT: persistence of tachycardia despite AV block [38–40].

New Trends in the Treatment of PJRT

Since tachycardia in patients with PJRT is often refractory to pharmacologic therapy, alternative treatment methods have often been necessary. Coumel [41] has utilized AV sequential pacing as a possible treatment modality although in our own experience, it is difficult to prevent tachycardia initiation by this method during changing autonomic conditions. The presence of an accessory pathway with decremental properties as the substrate of arrhythmia however provides two further potential therapeutic possibilities: ablation of the normal *or* the accessory pathway. AV node-His bundle ablation can be accomplished by the closed chest catheter technique as was performed in two of our patients. Because of the latent capability of the AP to conduct in the anterograde direction, pacemaker dependence will not necessarily occur; nonetheless pacemaker implantation in this situation is recommended. The decremental properties of the accessory pathway will prevent a rapid ventricular response in the event of atrial flutter-fibrillation. Alternatively, surgical dissection of the posterior septal pathway has been reported [10,17,31] in cases of PJRT, leaving the AV node–His bundle intact. This possibility has also been recently realized by a catheter technique [14,42].

Catheter Ablation of the Accessory Pathway

Intentional closed chest ablation of the accessory pathway by delivery of a direct current shock at the coronary sinus was performed in a patient who had previously undergone unsuccessful ablation of the AV node–His bundle. The patient was a 37-year-old woman with a previous history of PJRT for 15 years. The ECG (Figure 11–19, top) showed a persistent 1:1 AV relationship with RP' longer than P'R interval. A previous electrophysiologic study documented that an accessory AV pathway with a long conduction time comprised the retrograde limb of the reentry circuit; the atrial end of this anomalous pathway was located near the coronary sinus orifice.

One year previously, a 280-joule shock delivered to the region of the His bundle by the closed chest technique had resulted in sinus rhythm with first degree block and a QRS configuration consistent with posterior septal preexcitation (Figure 11–19, bottom). A permanent demand (VVI) pacemaker had been implanted and no further episodes of reciprocating tachycardia occurred. Nonetheless, one year later, intermittent conduction over the AV node was documented and shortly therafter the typical pattern of PJRT recurred. The patient was readmitted for possible closed chest ablation of the accessory pathway.

The procedure was performed in June 1983 in an operating room with a cardiovascular team on standby. A #6 French quadripolar catheter was placed in the coronary sinus. Two #6 French bipolar catheters were positioned in the region of the His bundle and in the right ventricular apex respectively, and an esophageal lead was introduced into the distal esophagus. Tachycardia was initially present. During positioning of the His bundle catheter, the tachycardia terminated and once again first degree block with maximal preexcitation over the accessory pathway was evident. No evidence of conduction over the AV node His bundle could be detected, presumably due to transient catheter trauma. Right ventricular pacing at a cycle length of 480 ms. demonstrated 1:1 retrograde conduction. Coronary sinus mapping showed earliest activity by unipolar recording to be 1–2 cm inside the orifice of the coronary sinus (Figure 11–20) identical to the pattern previously observed during tachycardia. The electrode exhibiting the earliest activity (VA interval = 276 ms) was connected to the cathodal side of a standard defibrillator while the anodal output was connected to a plate placed over the left precordium. The patient was sedated with Pentobarbital and a 120-joule shock was deli-

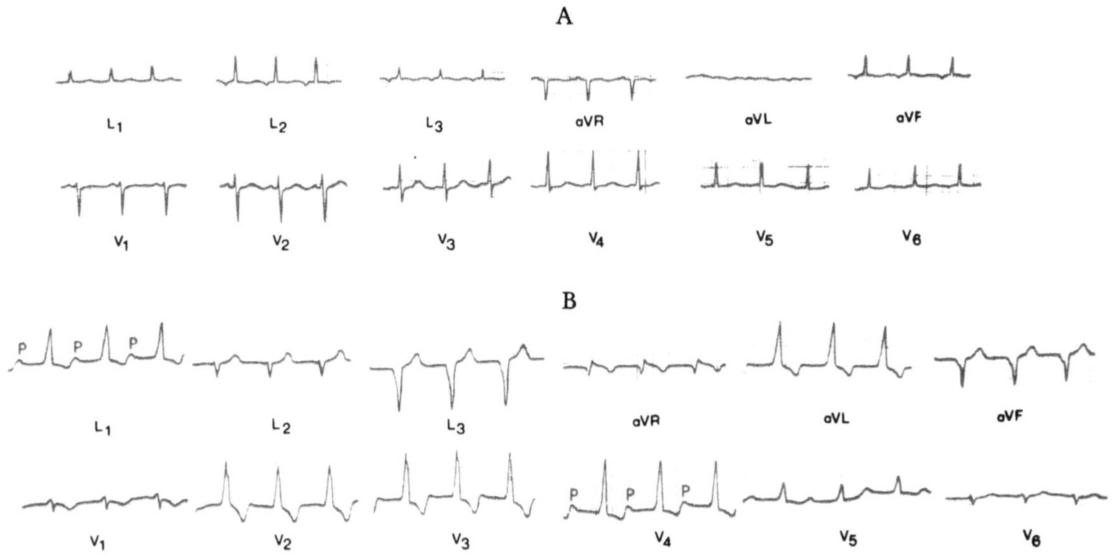

FIGURE 11–19. Standard electrocardiogram obtained from a patient with PJRT before (A) and after (B) His bundle ablation. The typical pattern of PJRT is evident before the procedure. After His bundle ablation 1:1 conduction (with a long PR interval) over the accessory pathway is present.

vered. An additional shock of 120 joules was also delivered to a closely adjacent electrode (VA interval = 284 ms) which had also recorded early activity prior to the first shock. VA dissociation was immediately evident. Complete AV block appeared on discontinuation of temporary pacing and inhibition of the permanent pacemaker. This suggested that the accessory pathway was no longer conducting in either the anterograde or retrograde direction and the His bundle was still blocked. Ten minutes later, conduction resumed over the AV node His bundle but retrograde conduction was still absent. Tachycardia could not be elicited by either atrial or ventricular pacing even with the administration of isoproterenol, and no further conduction over the accessory pathway was observed.

The patient tolerated the procedure well and the subsequent hospital course was unremarkable. Sinus rhythm with incomplete right bundle branch block (noted after His bundle ablation one year before) persisted. Figure 11–21 shows the standard ECG before and after the procedure.

One week later, a repeat electrophysiologic study showed no retrograde conduction with ventricular pacing at cycle length 540 ms; transesophageal atrial pacing resulted in second degree AV block, without tachycardia induction (Figure 11–22). During the follow-up (31 months) the patient has remained free of tachycardia on no medication.

The successful ablation of the accessory pathway was also demonstrated by the different response of AV conduction to intravenous ajmaline injection as compared to that observed before the shock (Figure 11–23, top). Before the shock, administration of ajmaline blocked conduction in the normal conduction system, unmasking stable anterograde conduction over the accessory pathway; this pattern was observed for 50 minutes until conduction over the AV node His bundle reappeared. Probably because of the residual damage due to the shock delivered to the His bundle one year before, ajmaline induced complete block in the normal conduction system thus disclosing anterograde conduction over the accessory pathway. After ablation of the accessory pathway by delivery of shocks to the coronary sinus (Figure 11–23, bottom), injection of ajmaline resulted in complete AV block without evidence of conduction either over the accessory pathway or the normal

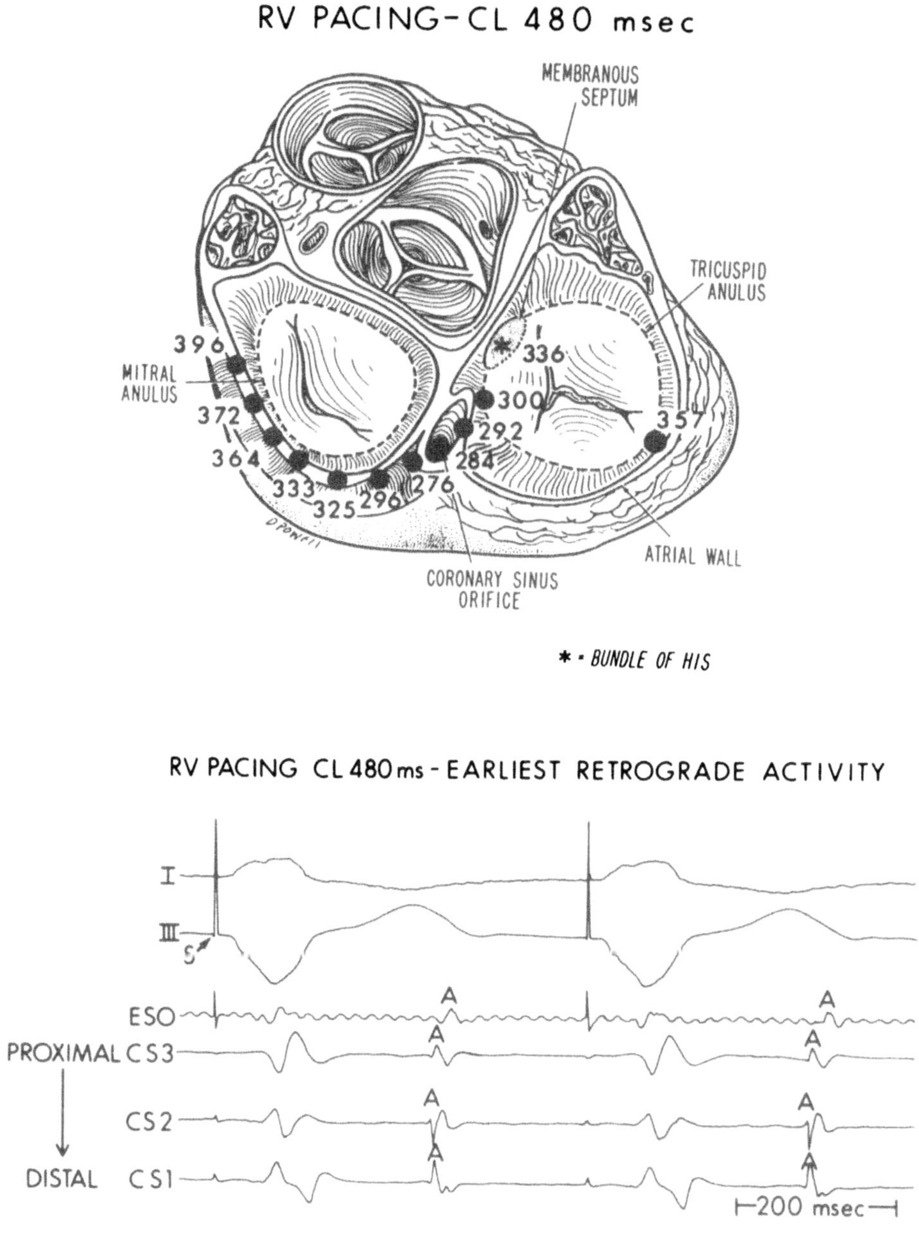

FIGURE 11–20. Same patient as in Figure 11–19. Retrograde atrial activation during right ventricular pacing. (*Top*) Schematic cross section of the heart at the level of the AV groove showing the VA intervals recorded from eleven sites of the coronary sinus. (*Bottom*) Selected recordings from the earliest areas of retrograde activation, occurring 1–1.5 cm. inside the coronary sinus orifice. (See text for further explanation.)

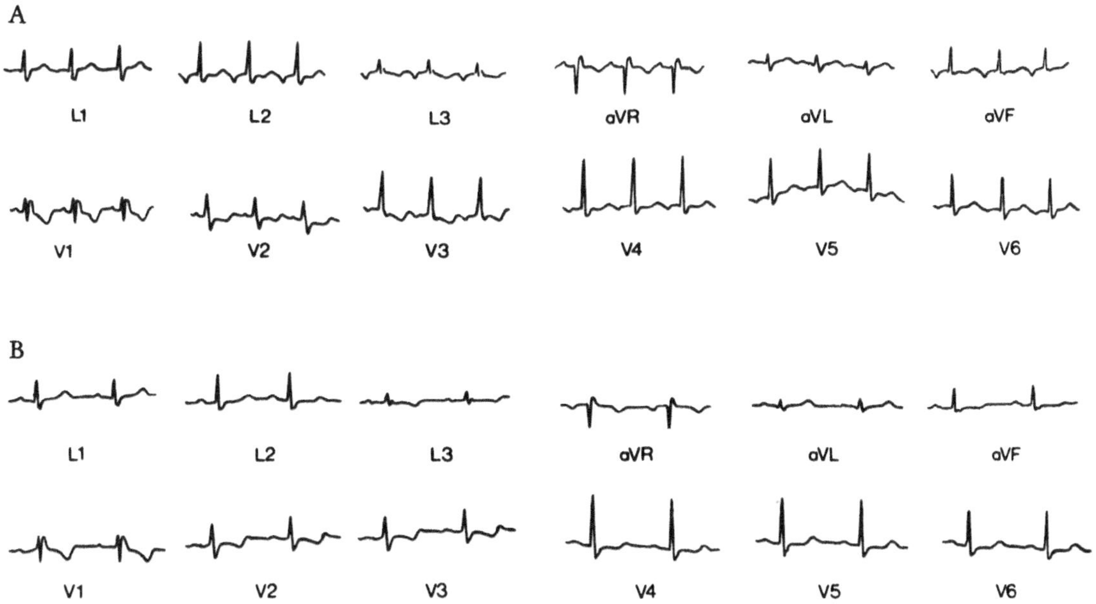

FIGURE 11–21. Same patient as in Figures 11–19 and 11–20. Standard electrocardiogram recorded before (A) and after (B) interruption of the accessory pathway by delivery of shocks in coronary sinus. Stable sinus rhythm is evident after the procedure. Right bundle branch block is present in both tracings, as a consequence of previously attempted interruption of the His bundle.

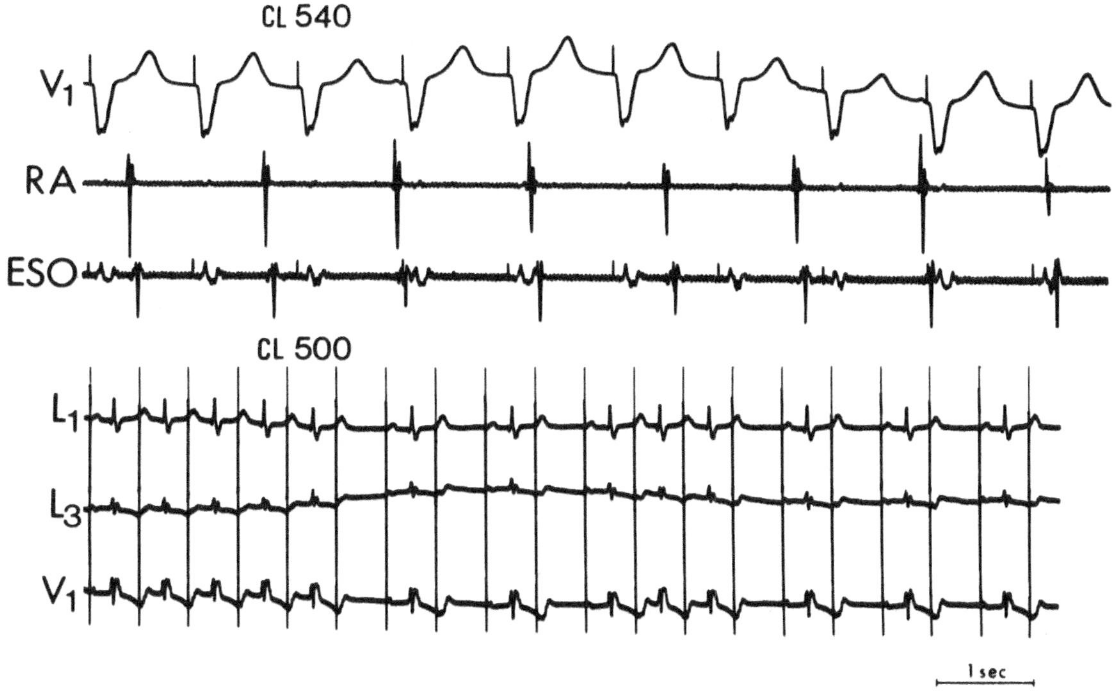

FIGURE 11–22. Same patient as in Figures 11–19 to 11–21. Evaluation of retrograde and anterograde conduction following ablation of the AP. (*Top*) Ventriculoatrial dissociation is evident during ventricular pacing. (*Bottom*) Wenckebach-type and 2:1 AV block occurs during transesophageal atrial pacing.

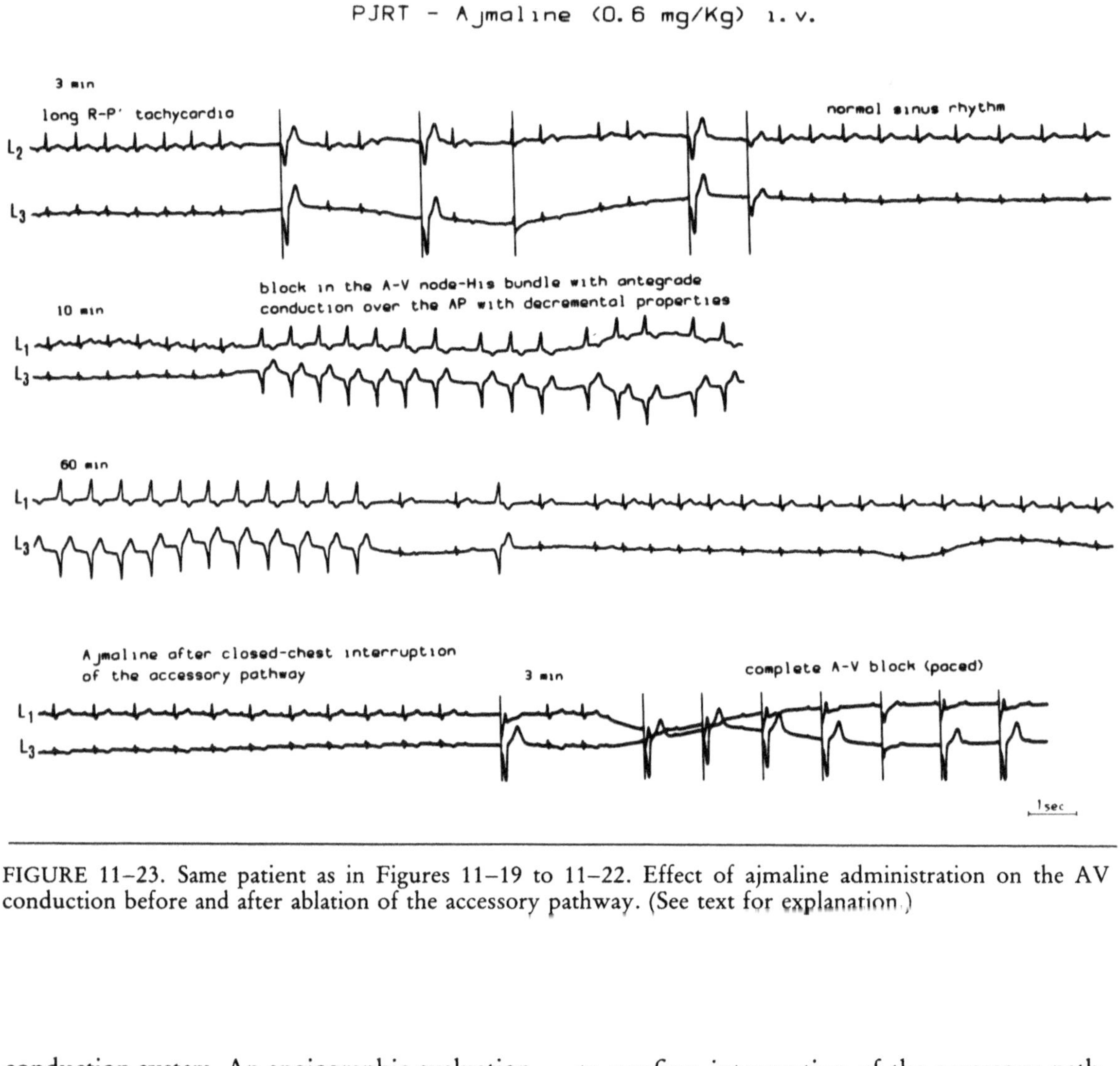

FIGURE 11–23. Same patient as in Figures 11–19 to 11–22. Effect of ajmaline administration on the AV conduction before and after ablation of the accessory pathway. (See text for explanation.)

conduction system. An angiographic evaluation performed seven months after the procedure showed that the coronary sinus was intact (Figure 11–24); no evidence of mitral valve regurgitation was observed (Figure 11–25).

In our patient, closed chest ablation of the accessory pathway was undertaken because of reappearance of conduction in the normal conduction system following attempted His bundle ablation and because of the proximity of the anomalous pathway to the orifice of the coronary sinus. As a precaution, the procedure was performed in an operating room with a cardiovascular team in attendance. No untoward effect however was noted and pacing studies performed during the follow-up have continued to confirm interruption of the accessory pathway. To our knowledge this is the first report of sustained ablation of the accessory pathway in PJRT deliberately induced by the closed chest technique. After initial unsatisfactory results [42–44], successful interruption of posterior septal accessory pathways in some patients with typical WPW syndrome have been recently achieved [45].

Our preliminary results suggest potential application of the closed chest ablation technique for treatment of PJRT. Optimal catheter design, mode of discharge, and effective but safe energy levels need to be defined before this technique can be advocated more widely.

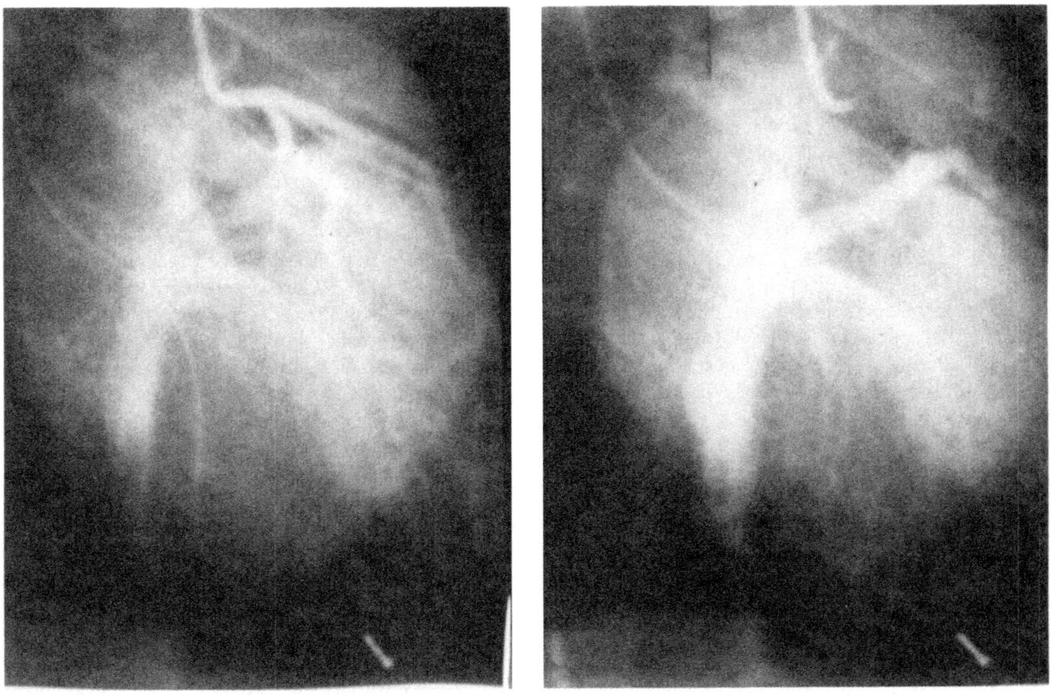

FIGURE 11–24. Same patient as in Figures 11–19 to 11–23. Angiography of the coronary sinus, performed seven months after ablation of the accessory pathway, showing a patent coronary sinus without damage.

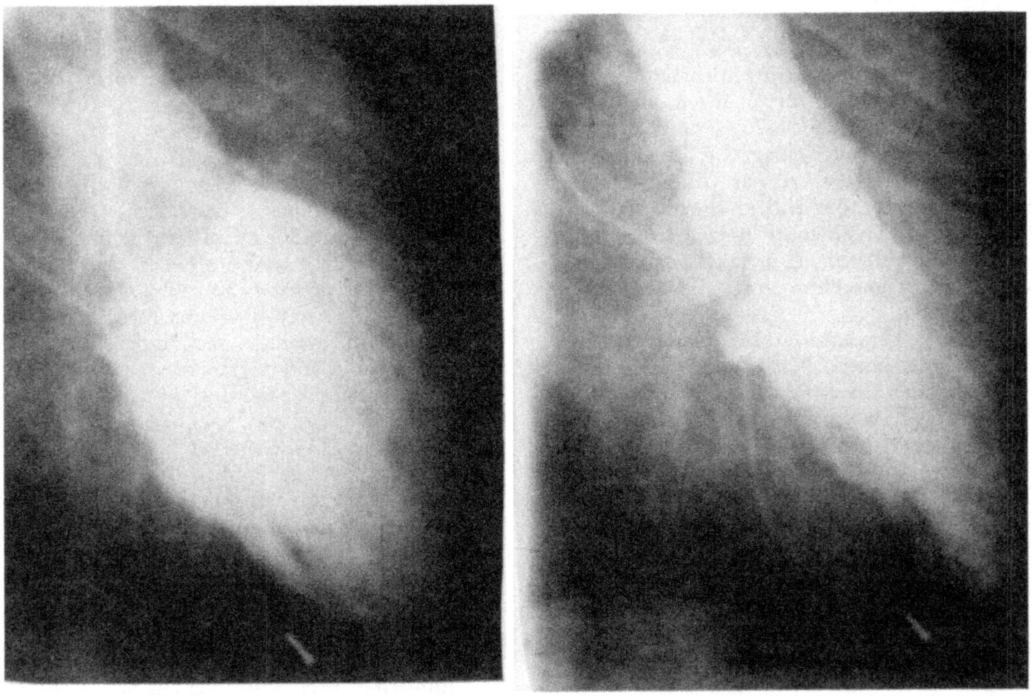

FIGURE 11–25. Same patient as in Figures 11–19 to 11–24. No evidence of mitral valve regurgitation is present seven months after the shock in coronary sinus.

References

1. Coumel P, Cabrol C, Fabiato A, Gourgon R, Salma R: Tachycardie permanente par rythme reciproque. *Arch. Mal Coeur* 60:1830, 1967.
2. Strasberg B, Swiryn S, Bauernfeind R, Palileo E, Scagliott D, Duffy CE, Rosen KM: Retrograde dual atrioventricular nodal pathways. *Am. J. Cardiol.* 48:639, 1981.
3. Gallagher JJ, Smith WM, Kerr CR, German LD, Sterba R, Sealy WC: Etiology of long RP tachycardia in 33 cases of supravenricular tachycardia. (Abstract.) *Circulation* 64:IV–145, 1981.
4. Wu D, Denes P, Amat-y-Leon F, Wyndam CRC, Dhingra R, Rosen KM: An unusual variety of atrioventricular nodal reentry due to retrograde dual atrioventricular nodal pathways. *Circulation* 56:50, 1977.
5. Gallagher JJ, Sealy WC: The permanent form of junctional reciprocating tachycardia. Further elucidation of the underlying mechanism. *Eur. J. Cardiol.* 8:413, 1978.
6. Gallagher JJ, Sealy WC, Kasell J, Klein GJ, Pritchett ELC, Davis D: The permanent form of junctional reciprocating tachycardia: evidence for an accessory ventriculoatrial pathway as the underlying substrate. *PACE* 2:A21, 1979.
7. Epstein ML, Stone FM, Benditt DG: Incessant atrial tachycardia in childhood: association with rate-dependent conduction in accessory atrioventricular pathway. *Am. J. Cardiol.* 44:498, 1979.
8. Brugada P, Vanagt EJ, Bar FW, Wellens HJJ: Incessant reciprocating atrioventricular tachycardia. Factors playing a role in the mechanism of the arrhythmia. *PACE* 3:670, 1980.
9. Brugada P, Bar FW, Vanagt EJ, Friedman PL, Wellens HJJ: Observations on patients showing AV junctional echoes with a shorter P-R than R-P interval. Distinction between intranodal reentry or reentry using an accessory pathway with a long conduction time. *Am. J. Cardiol.* 48:611, 1981.
10. Gallagher JJ, German LD, Broughton A, Guarnieri T, Trantham JL: Variants of the preexcitation syndromes. In: Rosenbaum MB, Elizari MV Frontiers of Cardiac Electrophysiology. (eds.) The Hague: Martinus Nijhoff Publishers 724–772, 1983.
11. Critelli G, Perticone F, Coltorti F, Monda V, Gallagher JJ: Antegrade slow bypass conduction after closed-chest ablation of the His bundle in permanent junctional reciprocating tachycardia. *Circulation* 67:687, 1983.
12. Critelli G, Gallagher JJ, Monda V, Coltorti F, Scherillo M, Rossi L: Anatomic and electrophysiologic substrate of the permanent form of junctional reciprocating tachycardia. *J. Am. Coll. Cardiol.* 4:601, 1984.
13. Critelli G, Gallagher JJ, Thiene G, Perticone F, Monda V, Rossi L: Histological observations after closed-chest ablation of the atrioventricular conduction system. *JAMA* 252:2604, 1984.
14. Critelli G, Gallagher JJ, Thiene G, Perticone F, Coltorti F, Rossi L: Electrophysiologic and histopathologic correlations in a case of permanent form of reciprocating tachycardia. *Eur. Heart J.* 6, 130, 1985
15. Gallagher JJ: Variants of preexcitation — update 1984. In: Cardiac Electrophysiology and Arrhythmias. Eds. Zipes DP and Jalife J. Grune and Stratton, New York, 1985, pp. 419–433.
16. Guarnieri T, Sealy WC, German LD: Utilization of an accessory pathway as the anterograde limb during the permanent form of junctional reciprocating tachycardia. *Am. J. Cardiol.* 53:365, 1984.
17. Guarnieri T, Sealy WC, Kasell JH: The nonpharmacologic management of the permanent form of junctional reciprocating tachycardia. *Circulation* 69:269 1984.
18. Lucet V, Do-Ngoc D, Tounmieux MC, Fidelle J, Coumel Ph: Permanent junctional reentrant tachycardia in children: long-term follow-up and treatment. In "Recent Advances in Cardiac Arrhythmias." S Levy, R Gerard (eds.) John Libbey, London, 1983, p. 278.
19. Smith RT, Gillette PC, Garson A, Massumi A, McVey P: Evidence that some "AV node reentry" involves two anatomically separated pathways. (Abstract.) *J. Am. Coll. Cardiol.* 3:483, 1984.
20. Coumel P, Fidelle J, Cloup M, Toumieux ML, Attuel P: Les tachycardies reciproques a evolution prolongee chez l'enfant. *Arch. Mal Coeur* 67:23, 1974.
21. Krikler DM, Curry P, Attuel P, Coumel P: "Incessant" tachycardias in Wolff-Parkinson-White syndrome. I: Initiation without antecedent extrastimulus or PR lengthening, with reference to reciprocation after shortening of cycle length. *Br. Heart J.* 38:885, 1976.
22. Coumel P, Attuel P, Slama R, Curry P, Krikler DM: "Incessant" tachycardias in Wolff-Parkinson-White syndrome II: Role of atypical cycle length dependence and nodal–His escape beats in initiation of reciprocating tachycardias. *Br. Heart J.* 38:897, 1976
23. Coumel P, Attuel P, Motte G, Slama R, Bouvrain Y: Les tachycardies jonctionelles paroxystiques. Evaluation du point de jonction inferieur du circuit de reentree. Demembrement des "rythmes" reciproques intra-nodaux. *Arch. Mal Coeur* 68:1255, 1975.
24. Sellers TD, Gallagher JJ, Cope GD, Tonkin AM, Wallace AG: Retrograde atrial preexcitation following premature ventricular beats during reciprocating tachycardia. *Eur. J. Cardiol.* 4:283, 1976.

25. Gallagher JJ, Pritchett ELC, Benditt DA, Tonkin AM, Campbell RWF, Dugan FA, Bashore TM, Tower A, Wallace AG: New catheter techniques for analysis of the sequence of retrograde atrial activation. *Eur. J. Cardiol.* 6:1, 1977.
26. Svenson RH, Miller RH, Gallagher JJ, Wallace WG: Electrophysiologic evaluation of the Wolff-Parkinson-White syndrome. Problems in assessing anterograde and retrograde conduction over the accessory pathway. *Circulation* 52:552, 1975.
27. Wellens HJJ, Durrer D: Patterns of ventriculo-atrial conduction in the Wolff-Parkinson-White syndrome. *Circulation* 49:22, 1974.
28. Janse MJ, Van Capelle FJL, Anderson RH, Touboul P, Billette J: Electrophysiology and structure of the atrioventricular node of the isolated rabbit heart. In *The Conduction System of the Heart*, MJJ Wellens, KI Lie, and MJ Janse (eds.) Lea and Febiger, Philadelphia, 1976, pp. 296–315.
29. Gallagher JJ, Svenson RH, Kasell J, German LD, Bardy GH, Broughton A, Critelli G: Catheter technique for closed-chest ablation of the atrioventricular conduction system: a therapeutic alternative for the treatment of refractory supraventricular tachycardia. *N. Engl. J. Med.* 306:194, 1982.
30. Scheinman M, Morady F, Hess D, Gonzales R: Catheter induced ablation of the atrioventricular junction to control refractory supraventricular arrhythmias. *JAMA* 243:851, 1982.
31. Sealy WC, Gallagher JJ: The surgical approach to the septal area of the heart based on experiences with 45 patients with Kent bundles. *J. Thorac. Cardiovasc. Surg.* 79:542, 1980.
32. Spach MS: The electrical representation of cardiac muscle based on discontinuities of atrial resistivity at a microscopic and macroscopic level. A basis for saltatory propagation in cardiac muscle. In *Normal and Abnormal Conduction in the Heart* de Carvalho AP, Hoffman BF, Liebermann M (eds.). Biophysics, Physiology, Pharmacology and Ultrastructure. Mount Kisco, New York. Futura Publishing Company, 1982, pp. 145–153.
33. Klein GJ, Hackel DB, Gallagher JJ: Anatomic substrate of impaired antegrade conduction over an accessory pathway in the Wolff-Parkinson-White syndrome. *Circulation* 61:1249, 1980.
34. Prystowsky EN, Heger JJ, Jackman WM, Naccarelli GV, Zipes DP: Post-myocardial infarction incessant supraventricular tachycardia due to concealed accessory pathway. *Am. Heart J.* 103:426, 1982.
35. Rossi L: The pathologic basis of cardiac arrhythmias. *Cardiol. Clin.* 1:13, 1983.
36. De La Fuente D, Sasyniuk B, Moe GK: Conduction through a narrow isthmus in isolated canine atrial tissue. A model of the WPW syndrome. *Circulation* 44:803, 1971.
37. Wolff GS, Sung RJ, Pickoff A, Garcia OL, Werblim R, P Ferrer PL, Tamer D, Gelband H: The fast-slow form of atrioventricular nodal reentrant tachycardia in children, *Am. J. Cardiol.* 43:1181, 1979.
38. Wellens HJJ, Wesdorp JC, Diiren DR, Lie KI: Second degree block during reciprocal atrioventricular nodal tachycardia. *Circulation* 53:595, 1976.
39. Josephson ME and Kastor JA: Paroxysmal supraventricular tachycardia. Is the atrium a necessary link? *Circulation* 54:430, 1976.
40. Bauernfeind RA, Wu D, Denes P, Rosen GM: Retrograde block during dual pathway atrioventricular nodal reentrant paroxysmal tachycardia. *Am. J. Cardiol.* 42:499, 1978.
41. Coumel P: Different modes of pacemaking in the long-term management of paroxysmal tachycardia in Symposium on Cardiac Arrhythmias, E Sandoe. E Jlensted-Jenson, and KH Olesen (eds.). AB Astra, Sweden, 1970, pp. 783–806.
42. Critelli G, Monda V, Perticone F, Coltorti F, Scherillo M, Condorelli M: Interruzione a torace chiuso dei fasci anomali di conduzione. Impiego in un caso di tachicardia incessante guidato da un modello sperimentale. *G. Ital. Cardiolx.* 16:181, 1984.
43. Fisher JD, Brodman R, Kim SG, Motos JA: Wolff-Parkinson-White syndrome: nonsurgical Kent bundle ablation via the coronary sinus. *PACE* 6A:18, 1983.
44. Weber H, Schmitz L: Catheter technique for closed-chest ablation of an accessoary atrioventricular pathway. *N. Engl. J. Med.* 308:653, 1983.
45. Morady F, Scheinman MM: Transvenous catheter ablation of a posterior septal accessory pathway in a patient with the Wolff-Parkinson-White syndrome. *N. Engl.* J. Med. 310:705, 1984.

12. AV NODE BYPASS TRACTS AND ENHANCED AV CONDUCTION: RELATION TO VENTRICULAR PREEXCITATION

David G. Benditt
David Dunbar
Adrian Almquist
Shanda Pool-Schneider

The preexcitation syndromes comprise a diverse group of conduction disturbances in which the common thread is the ability of atrial impulses to activate all or part of the ventricular myocardium earlier than would have been expected had AV conduction been restricted to the normal cardiac conduction system [1–4]. Despite earlier doubts [5–7], it is now generally agreed that most forms of ventricular preexcitation are best accounted for by the presence of functioning accessory conduction tissue bypassing all or portions of the specialized cardiac conduction system. [1–4,8,9]. However, controversy continues to surround the subset of preexcitation syndromes in which the principal conduction disturbance appears to be a "short-circuiting" of the primary physiologic function of the AV node, namely, the slowing of conduction of supraventricular impulses between the atria and His bundle.

At the present time, it is uncertain whether disturbances of AV node capacity to induce appropriate degrees of AV conduction slowing in the antegrade direction are the result of accessory conduction tissue bypassing all or part of the AV node [10–15], structural or functional disturbances within the node itself [16,17], or possibly of heterogeneous origin with multiple, but variable, contributing elements resulting in a common electrophysiologic picture. The purposes of this chapter are; (1) to review the potential anatomic, electrophysiologic, and neural substrates which may contribute to the apparent "bypass" of AV node conduction slowing; (2) to delineate the electrocardiographic and clinical electrophysiologic features of the syndrome; and (3) to assess the significance of subnormal AV nodal conduction delay in the context of susceptibility to and treatment of supraventricular and ventricular tachyarrhythmias. Electrophysiologic observations on the

This work was supported in part by a grant-in-aid HL 29460 (DGB) and a NRSA grant HL 07047 (DD) from the National Institutes of Health, Bethesda, Maryland, and was completed during Dr. Benditt's tenure as an Established Investigator of the American Heart Association, Dallas, Texas. Dr. Almquist is supported by a fellowship grant of the North American Society of Pacing and Electrophysiology (NASPE).
The authors would like to express their appreciation to Wendy Markuson and Barry L.S. Detloff for assistance in preparation of the manuscript.

characteristics of ventriculoatrial conduction in a similar setting is presented in the following chapter.

Pathogenesis: Potential Factors Contributing to Subnormal Conduction Slowing Within the AV Node

STRUCTURAL DETERMINANTS OF AV NODE CONDUCTION

Disturbances of both AV node structure and development have been implicated, at least theoretically, as potential causes of "subnormal" AV node conduction slowing. Most important among these are (1) accessory conduction tissue bypassing part or all of the AV node, and (2) developmental disturbances altering AV node size and/or histologic makeup.

AV Nodal Bypass Tracts. The presence of accessory conduction tissue bypassing part or all of the AV node is commonly invoked to explain instances in which AV nodal conduction slowing appears to be subnormal. Two types of AV nodal bypasses are pertinent in this context (Figure 12–1): (1) bypass tracts circumventing the AV node completely and connecting the atria to the penetrating bundle of the specialized cardiac conduction system (His bundle) [12–15], and (2) bypass tracts which divert the atrial impulse wavefront to enter the AV node beyond the zone which is most critical for producing conduction delay [10,13,18]. In either case, the functional capacity of the AV node to slow atrial impulses would be attenuated, yet infranodal ventricular activation would remain normal (in the absence of either other forms of ventricular preexcitation or underlying cardiac conduction system disease).

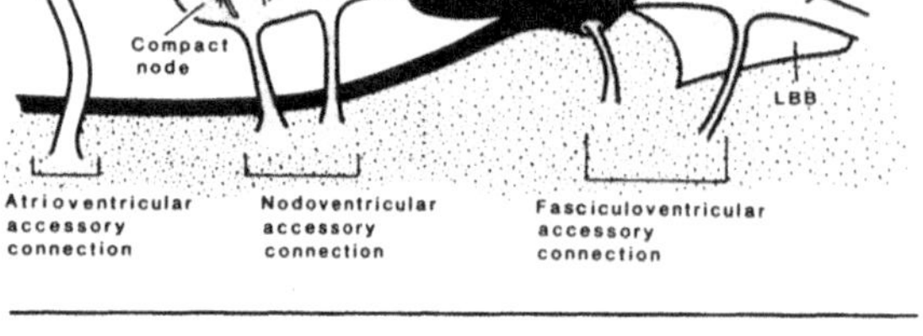

FIGURE 12–1. Schematic depicting the known types of accessory connections (after Anderson et al. [13]). Atrionodal and atriofascicular bypass tracts are the most pertinent in the context of this chapter. RBB = right bundle branch, LBB = left bundle branch.

ATRIOFASCICULAR TRACTS. It is now accepted that excitable tissue bypassing the AV node and inserting into the His bundle (atriofascicular bypass tracts [13]) may occur in man, but they appear to be extremely rare. James [10] schematically illustrated the possibility of such connections (his Figure 11), but provided no histologic demonstration. On the other hand, Brechenmacher described such tracts in 2 patients [12,14]. In each case the fibers originated in the interatrial septum and bypasssed the right lateral surface of the AV node. In the first reported case, a patient with a short PR interval on surface ECG, the bypass tract joined the His bundle at a point where it was beginning to enter the central fibrous body of the heart. In the second instance, a patient with a normal PR interval presumably on the basis of associated infranodal conduction system disease, the bypass tract penetrated the specialized cardiac conduction system at a point near its site of branching. In both patients the tracts were described as being comprised of cells similar in morphology to those of the His bundle, but differing from the His bundle in that they run "approximately perpendicular to it." In all, Brechenmacher observed such tracts in only 2 of 687 (0.3%) hearts submitted to detailed histologic examination of the cardiac conduction system [14]. To our knowledge, in only 1 other instance has a bypass tract connecting the atrial septum to the penetrating portion or the AV bundle been described in association with ventricular preexcitation, and in that instance the coexistence of apparently functioning nodoventricular connections resulted in an anomalous QRS complex suggesting Wolff-Parkinson-White (WPW) syndrome [19]. On other occassions such tracts have been noted, but in the absence of evidence supporting their functional capacity [20].

The frequency with which atriofascicular bypass tracts of the type described by Brechenmacher occur in the human heart [14], appears to be too uncommon to explain most instances of apparently subnormal AV nodal conduction delay (although it must be noted that the precise frequency with which the latter occurs among the general population is unknown). Further, although histologic confirmation is essential, electrophysiologic evidence in the vast majority of patients with either short PR intervals or other findings indicative of accelerated AV nodal conduction, do not support the concept of accessory conduction tissue connecting the atria directly to the His bundle (see below).

ATRIONODAL (INTRANODAL) TRACTS. In contrast to the rarity of atriofascicular tracts, atrial fibers skirting portions of the AV node and entering the compact node at a more distal point (atrionodal tracts), are ubiquitous in the adult human. James [10] described the latter tracts as containing "numerous Purkinje fibers ... but also ordinary-appearing myocardial fibers." However, while he indicated that they may permit atrial impulses to "circumvent the AV node," he pointed out that their presence alone did not imply participation in AV conduction.

The functional significance of atrionodal connections has been a particularly controversial issue. Antagonists indicate that such connections are found too frequently in man to be accepted as the histologic substrate for AV nodal bypass in the selected group of patients who manifest subnormal AV node conduction slowing. In addition, it has been pointed out that there is considerable variation in the manner in which the compact node is approached by transitional fibers, suggesting that atrionodal connections of the type described by James may reflect normal variation of the approaches to the node [18,21]. Based on the latter argument, it has been suggested that if these fibers are to be termed bypass tracts at all, they should be considered to be intranodal [13]. On the other hand, the concept of atrionodal tracts is theoretically consistent with electrophysiologic findings in the majority of patients in whom subnormal AV node conduction delay has been demonstrated (see below). Further, functional atrionodal connections provide a plausible basis for both the phenomenon of "dual AV node conduction" [22–24], and the development of reciprocating tachycardia within the AV node [25].

Given the difficulty of obtaining functional-morphologic correlations in human studies, it seems unlikely that the role of so-called atrionodal tracts (or intranodal bypass tracts [13]) will be clarified in the foreseeable future. However, it is of interest that apparently similar tracts have been shown to permit atrial impulses to bypass the AV node in the rabbit. However, in the latter studies, bypass tract function was only demonstrable after normal AV node conduction had been impaired by acetylcholine administration, and the atria stimulated from a site anterior to the junction of the right atrium with the inferior vena cava [26].

AV NODAL SIZE AND DEVELOPMENT. Although it has been suggested that an anatomically smaller than normal AV node may result in diminished AV nodal conduction slowing [11], a comparative study designed to evaluate the impact of AV node size on physiologic function has not been undertaken. Furthermore, the functional importance of differences in AV node size cannot be assessed readily in vivo in humans. Consequently, at the present time we can only obtain a rough approximation of the effect of dimension on nodal conduction properties by comparing PR intervals, normalized for heart rate, in a variety of species [17]. For example, in the mouse, adult human, and elephant, the range of usual PR interval duration is respectively, 0.02–0.04 sec, 0.14–0.20 sec, and 0.28–0.41 sec [27]. Normalizing PR intervals for baseline differences in cardiac frequency, and assuming a linear relation between cardiac frequency and PR duration [16], the resulting normalized mean PR interval ratios (at a cardiac frequency of 1 Hz, 60 beats/minute) in these three species would be, 0.02:1:3.3. Presumably, if AV node size were a critical factor in effecting PR interval duration, one would anticipate that the relationship among AV node dimensions in these species would parallel this ratio. Unfortunately, precise measurements of AV node size are not readily available However, the calculated PR interval ratios are smaller than are the respective interspecies relationships among heart weight, body weight, or body surface area. Thus, as animal size becomes larger, the influence of the presumably parallel increase in AV node size on slowing of AV conduction is diminished. This conclusion is consistent with observations on heart rate during atrial fibrillation in various species reported by Meijler et al. [28,29]. Consequently, overall dimensions of the AV node are not likely a critical factor in determining its conduction characteristics.

The possibility exists that developmental differences in cell size [30] or number, "slow channel" versus "fast channel" responsiveness, or resistance of intercellular connections within the specialized AV conduction system may contribute to age-related differences in AV nodal conduction responses [31–32]. For example, in calf cardiac Purkinje fibers, which have been shown to be smaller than adult bovine Purkinje fibers [33], action potential durations are often equal to those of ventricular myocardium. By contrast, in the adult cardiac Purkinje fiber, action potential durations are usually longer than those recorded from myocardial cells [30]. Whether analogous size–function relationships apply within AV nodal tissue has not been assessed directly. However, comparative electrophysiologic studies of AV conduction in newborn and older animals suggest that similar relationships may hold. For instance Preston et al. [34] demonstrated in a variety of young nonprimate mammals that refractoriness of the AV conduction system was actually less than that of ventricular muscle, the reverse of the case in the adult. Additionally, young animals appeared to be susceptible to repetitive ventricular responses and even ventricular fibrillation as a result of unimpeded conduction of premature atrial impulses to a presumably incompletely recovered myocardium. However, the latter observations may not apply directly to man. The findings of Janse et al. [35] in isolated fetal heart suggest that unlike in other mammals, the human AV conduction system is capable of protecting the ventricles "in the same manner as does this system in the adult" from a very early stage of development.

The development of AV nodal architecture with age may also play a role in determining electrophysiologic response. In the fetus and neonate, the AV node has been characterized as a relatively large and irregular structure [36] which, in conjunction with the central fibrous body of the heart, continues to undergo morphologic change in the postnatal period. Ultimately, the normally developed adult AV node is more circumscribed than the fetal node, but differs in being comprised of profusely anastomosing fibers [10]. The latter circumstance may lead to the possibility of multiple circuitous conduction routes with complex electrotonic interactions and slow wavefront propagation [37–40]. Conceivably, postnatal failure of development of this complex nodal structure, may diminish AV nodal capacity to slow AV conduction appropriately. Conversely, it is possible that the complex structure of a normally developed node could be "simplified" by acquired disease states, thereby explaining the apparent de novo occurrence of diminished AV nodal conduction delay in older patients, or patients with degenerative or infiltrative conduction system disease such as has been suggested in both Fabry's disease [41] and Pompe's disease [42]. Finally, the possibility remains that an abnormality restricted to the number or electrophysiologic characteristics of the subset of AV nodal cells thought to be critical for decremental conduction slowing (i.e., N zone cells [43]), may account for apparently subnormal AV node physiologic delav.

OTHER ELECTROPHYSIOLOGIC DETERMINANTS OF AV NODE CONDUCTION

Apart from the presence of accessory conduction tissue having electrophysiologic characteristics which differ from AV nodal cells and the possibility that altered nodal structure may affect intranodal electrotonic interactions, conduction delay within the AV node may be influenced by other electrophysiologic factors, including: (1) direction and timing of the atrial wavefront arriving at the AV node, (2) intercellular and membrane resistances of nodal cells, and (3) cellular responsiveness to locally released and circulating neurohumoral mediators.

Nodal inputs. The manner in which the AV node is activated by arrival of the atrial excitation wavefront may influence AV conduction time of atrial impulses. For example, under normal conditions the AV node in both the adult dog [44] and the rabbit [43] exhibits dual atrial inputs; a posterior input from the crista terminalis, and an anterior input from the interatrial septum (Figure 12–2). Simultaneous stimulation of both inputs, presumably as a result of summation of wavefronts, has been shown experimentally to both improve chances of AV conduction [45] and diminish AV conduction time [43] of premature atrial beats. Potentially a similar phenomenon could in part explain the reduced AH interval increment and the more rapid 1:1 AV conduction rates achievable in humans during coronary sinus pacing versus high right atrial stimulation [46–48], thereby providing a basis for subnormal AV conduction slowing. Alternatively, it has been

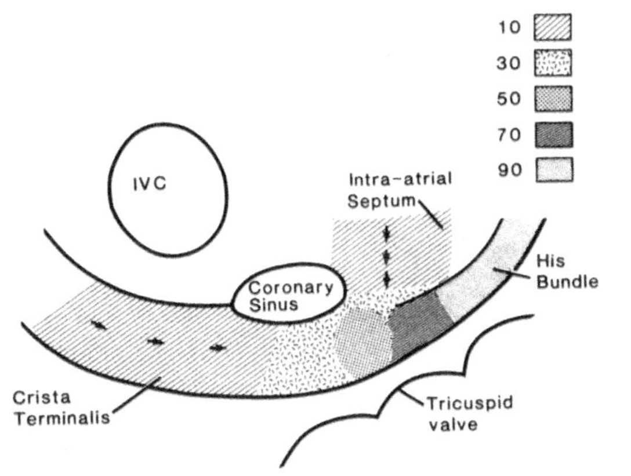

FIGURE 12–2. Illustration of the AV nodal area of the rabbit heart depicting the sequence of normal antegrade activation (after Janse et al. [38]). There is a dual input to the AV node; a posterior input activates the AV node from the crista terminalis, and an anterior input activates the node from the region of the inter-atrial septum. Background patterns indicate the approximate temporal sequence of AV node and His bundle activation (see Key, ms).

proposed that in certain as yet undefined instances eccentric activation of the AV node may accentuate AV conduction over ubiquitous atrionodal ("intranodal" [13]) fibers, thereby resulting in partial bypass of usual AV node delay [7,10,49]. Although the latter possibility has yet to be demonstrated in man, it remains a potential explanation for the findings of Sano et al. in the rabbit [26], in which apparent AV node bypass was observed during pacing-induced eccentric atrial activation.

Intercellular and Nonjunctional Membrane Resistances of Nodal Cells. The velocity with which electrical impulses progress along a series of excitable cells depends in large part upon the spread of local currents induced by already depolarized tissues. Although the mechanisms are not yet clearly worked out [50], the ability of depolarized cells in the normal AV node to influence tissues farther downstream (i.e., space constant) is diminished by virtue of the combined effects of slow-rising transmembrane action potential upstrokes, and relatively high intercellular resistances to current flow [37,40] in association with relatively lower resistances of nonjunctional membranes [51]. Agents which accentuate these electrophysiologic features of the AV node (e.g., acetylcholine, cardiac glycosides [40,51,52]) would be expected to slow AV conduction, whereas the converse would be expected to occur in the presence of factors reversing these characteristics (e.g., angiotensin II [53]).

At present the possible contribution of these cellular electrophysiologic factors to clinical syndromes associated with subnormal AV node physiologic delay is beyond the resolution of electrophysiologic study in man. However, their potential role merits consideration since it may have therapeutic implications.

Cellular Responsiveness to Neurohumoral Mediators. Developmental differences in responsiveness of cardiac tissues to neurohumoral mediators are characteristic of the mammalian heart [54]. For example, acetylcholine (1×10^{-9}M) increases automaticity in Purkinje fibers of the newborn dog, a finding which differs markedly from the slowing observed in Purkinje fibers from adult animals [55]. In addition, automaticity in neonatal tissues appears to be more sensitive to catecholamine stimulation than is the case for tissues from the adult animal [56]. Whether analogous developmental differential sensitivities to locally released or circulating neurohumors may account for differences in AV nodal conduction properties in animals or man is unknown.

Influence of Sympathetic and Parasympathetic Innervation. Apart from tissue sensitivity to, and the nature of the response elicited by sympathetic and parasympathetic neural mediators, AV node conduction characteristics may be influenced by the extent of nodal innervation and the balance between the influences of the two major limbs of the autonomic nervous system. In mammals, development of cardiac sympathetic innervation continues into the postnatal period [57], whereas in most tissues studied, parasympathetic neural input appears to be complete at birth [58]. Variation in the extent of this developmental process would be expected to be especially critical in regions as dependent on neural control as the AV node.

In both animals [59,60] and humans [17,61], the effects of sympathetic and parasympathetic innervation on AV node conduction properties appears to be more or less equally balanced in the resting state. In dogs, absence of electrical stimulation of either vagal or sympathetic neural inputs to the AV node was associated with a PR interval which was unchanged from the resting innervated state [59]. Similarly, we have recently observed that AV node response to both incremental atrial pacing and atrial extrastimulus testing did not differ significantly in awake chronically instrumented control dogs, and dogs having undergone orthotopic cardiac transplantation [60]. In humans with normal AV node conduction properties, recent studies indicate that the minimum paced cycle length with sustained 1:1 AV conduction remained essentially unchanged from baseline values following pharmacologic autonomic blockade with atropine and propranolol [17,61] (Figure 12–3). AV node functional refractory periods tended to behave similarly.

The possibility that neural factors may play a role in clinical syndromes of subnormal AV node physiologic conduction delay recently has been demonstrated [17]. In contrast to findings in normal subjects, pharmacologic autonomic blockade prolonged the minimum cycle length at which 1:1 AV conduction was maintained (i.e., moved the point at which AV Wenkebach block occurred to a slower heart rate) and resulted in a similar directional change for AV node functional refractoriness (Figure 12–3). These observations suggested that patients with subnormal AV node conduction slowing exhibited predominance of sympathetic neural input to the node. However, it should be pointed out that autonomic blockade did not normalize AV node conduction properties in these patients; both minimum cycle length with 1:1 AV conduction and AV node functional refractory periods remained significantly shorter than those in the control subjects [17].

Electrocardiographic and Clinical Electrophysiologic Features

ELECTROCARDIOGRAPHIC FINDINGS

The capacity of the AV node to induce physiologic conduction delay cannot be adequately assessed by examination of the surface electrocardiogram alone. For instance, the presence of a short PR interval in adult patients (i.e., a PR interval less than or equal to 120 ms) may result for a number of reasons [62], of which diminished AV node conduction time is only one.

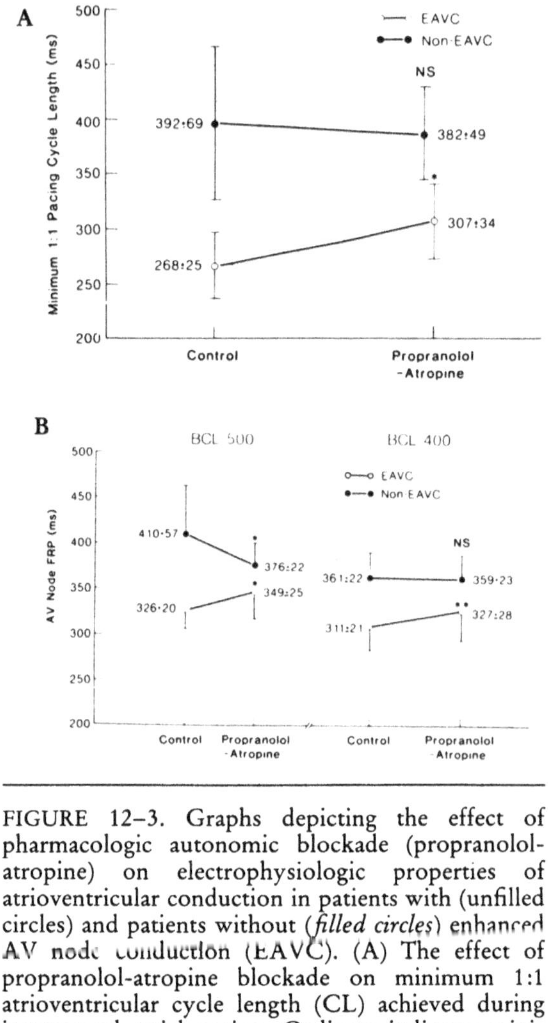

FIGURE 12–3. Graphs depicting the effect of pharmacologic autonomic blockade (propranolol-atropine) on electrophysiologic properties of atrioventricular conduction in patients with (unfilled circles) and patients without (*filled circles*) enhanced AV node conduction (EAVC). (A) The effect of propranolol-atropine blockade on minimum 1:1 atrioventricular cycle length (CL) achieved during incremental atrial pacing. Ordinate indicates minimum 1:1 CL in milliseconds (ms), and the abscissa indicates the patient groups and test conditions. Findings in EAVC patients are depicted by the unfilled circles and those in non-EAVC patients by filled circles. *$p < .01$, control vs. propranolol-atropine. (B) The effect of propranolol-atropine blockade on atrioventricular nodal functional refractory period (AV FRP) measurements at basic pacing cycle lengths (BCLs) of 500 and 400 msec. An FRP is indicated in milliseconds (ms) on the ordinate and the test conditions are noted on the abscissa. Unfilled circles represent findings in EAVC patients, and filled circles those in non-EAVC patients. Data are mean ± SD, *$p < .05$, **$p = .07$, control vs. propranolol-atropine. (Reprinted by permission of the *Am. Heart Assoc.* from Benditt DG, Klein GJ, Kriett JM, Dunnigan A, Benson DW Jr.: Enhanced atrioventricular nodal conduction in man: electrophysiologic effect of pharmacologic autonomic blockade. *Circulation* 69:1088, 1984.)

TABLE 12–1.

	Normal PR		Normal PR		Short PR
	Normal AV Conduction	P	EAVC	P	
RT CL (ms)	349 ± 58	<0.05	288 ± 44	NS	272 ± 58
A Fib					
Shortest RR (ms)	353 ± 59	<0.01	256 ± 36	NS	254 ± 42
Mean RR (ms)	463 ± 78	<0.05	359 ± 36	NS	372 ± 89
At ERP (600) (ms)	353 ± 59	NS	210 ± 41	NS	224 ± 39
AVN ERP (600) (ms)	303 ± 50	NS	275 ± 24	NS	256 ± 33
AVN FRP (600) (ms)	412 ± 51	<0.05	349 ± 33	NS	357 ± 32
At ERP (400) (ms)	227 ± 36	<0.05	192 ± 28	NS	208 ± 40
AVN ERP (400) (ms)	280 ± 19	<0.05	246 ± 25	NS	255 ± 37
AVN FRP (400) (ms)	372 ± 41	<0.01	320 ± 41	NS	317 ± 41

Abbreviations: A Fib = atrial fibrillation; At = atrial; AVN = AV node; ERP = effective refractory period; FRP = functional refractory period; RT = reciprocating tachycardia; CL = cycle length.

Alternatively, a normal PR interval does not preclude AV conduction being sustained to very rapid heart rates with minimal prolongation of AV nodal conduction time (as assessed by rate-related increment of AH interval measurement) over baseline value. By way of example, Table 12–1 summarizes electrophysiologic findings from this laboratory in 3 groups of patients recently studied for evaluation of recurrent supraventricular tachycardias. Group 1 comprised 18 patients (age, 42+/−13 years, mean +/−SD) with normal PR intervals, baseline AH intervals greater than 60 ms, and normal AV conduction responses during incremental right atrial pacing. Group 2 consisted of 9 patients (age, 38+/−19 years) with baseline AH intervals less than or equal to 60 ms, and sustained 1:1 AV conduction to heart rates greater than 200/minute (i.e., cycle lengths less than 300 ms). Group 3 included 12 adult patients (age, 30+/−17 years) with short PR intervals. In brief, AV node functional refractory periods (measured at 2 basic pacing cycle lengths, 600 and 400 ms), cycle lengths during reciprocating tachycardia, and both mean and shortest RR intervals during atrial fibrillation were significantly shorter in both Group 2 and Group 3 patients compared to Group 1. Furthermore, there was no statistically significant difference between results in Group 2 and Group 3 patients.

Heart rate response during supraventricular tachyarrhythmias also may lead to a misinterpretation of AV nodal conduction properties. For example, the development of excessively rapid ventricular responses during certain supraventricular tachycardias (Figures 12–4, 12–5), in particular atrial flutter, atrial fibrillation, and reciprocating tachycardia utilizing an accessory AV connection, have been associated with subnormal conduction slowing within the AV node [16]. However, this relation does not hold in the case of reciprocating tachycardia due to reentry within the AV node [16,63]. Thus tachycardia rate cannot necessarily be considered a reliable indicator of underlying AV nodal conduction properties.

ELECTROPHYSIOLOGIC STUDIES IN MAN

Normal variation of AV node response. It is widely accepted that the PR interval on the surface electrocardiogram (an imprecise correlate of AV nodal conduction time) encompasses a broad unimodal range of values [64], with no obvious demarcation between values in adult patients exhibiting conventionally defined short PR intervals (i.e., less than or equal to 120 ms), and the remainder of the population. Recently, it has become apparent that clinical electrophysiologic characteristics of AV node conduction behave similarly. For example. Figure 12–6 illustrates the spectrum of AH interval versus atrial pacing cycle length responses in 33 patients undergoing electrophysiologic study for evaluation of recurrent supraventricular tachycardias [16]. Patients with evidence of accessory AV connections capable of conduction in the antegrade direction were excluded from the

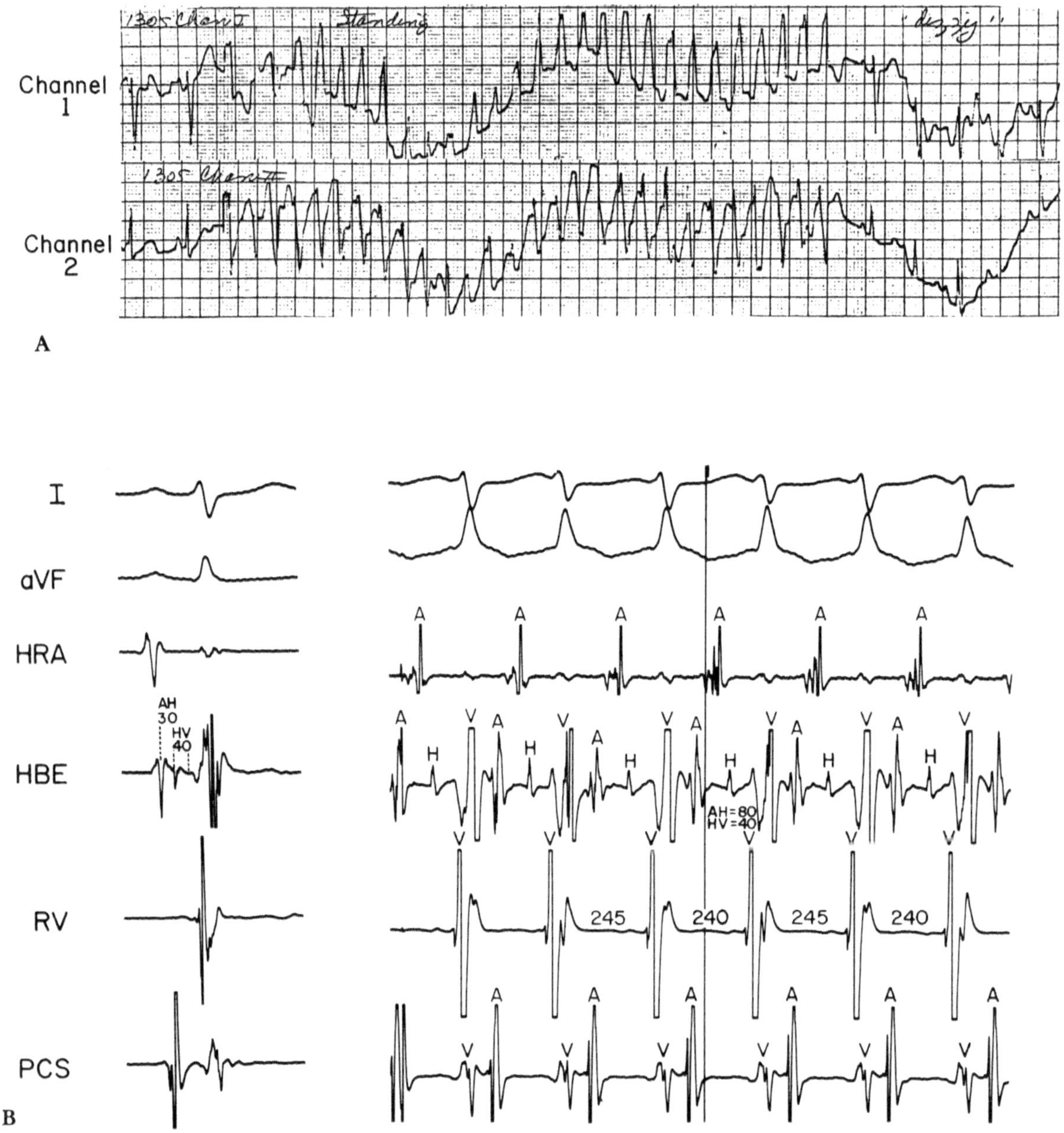

FIGURE 12–4. Electrocardiographic and intracardiac recordings during paroxysmal reciprocating tachycardia in a 15-year-old female with enhanced AV node conduction (EAVC) and a concealed posterior septal accessory AV connection. (A) Electrocardiographic recording obtained during a period of ambulatory monitoring, illustrating spontaneous paroxysmal tachycardia associated with symptoms of dizziness. (B) Electrocardiographic and intracardiac recording obtained during clinical electrophysiologic study. Traces from top to bottom are ECG leads I, and aVF, and intracardiac recordings from the high right atrium (HRA), His bundle region (HBE), right ventricle (RV), and proximal coronary sinus (PCS). At left, a brief recording during sinus rhythm illustrates the short AH and normal HV intervals. At right reciprocating tachycardia with a cycle length of 240–245 ms and an AH interval of 80 ms is illustrated.

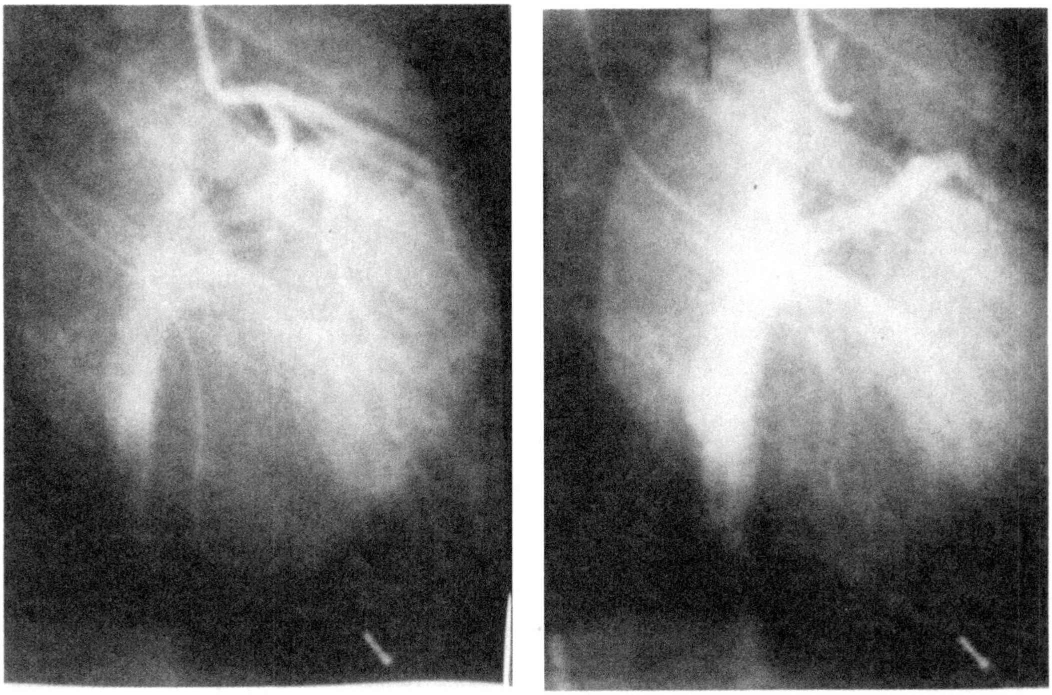

FIGURE 11–24. Same patient as in Figures 11–19 to 11–23. Angiography of the coronary sinus, performed seven months after ablation of the accessory pathway, showing a patent coronary sinus without damage.

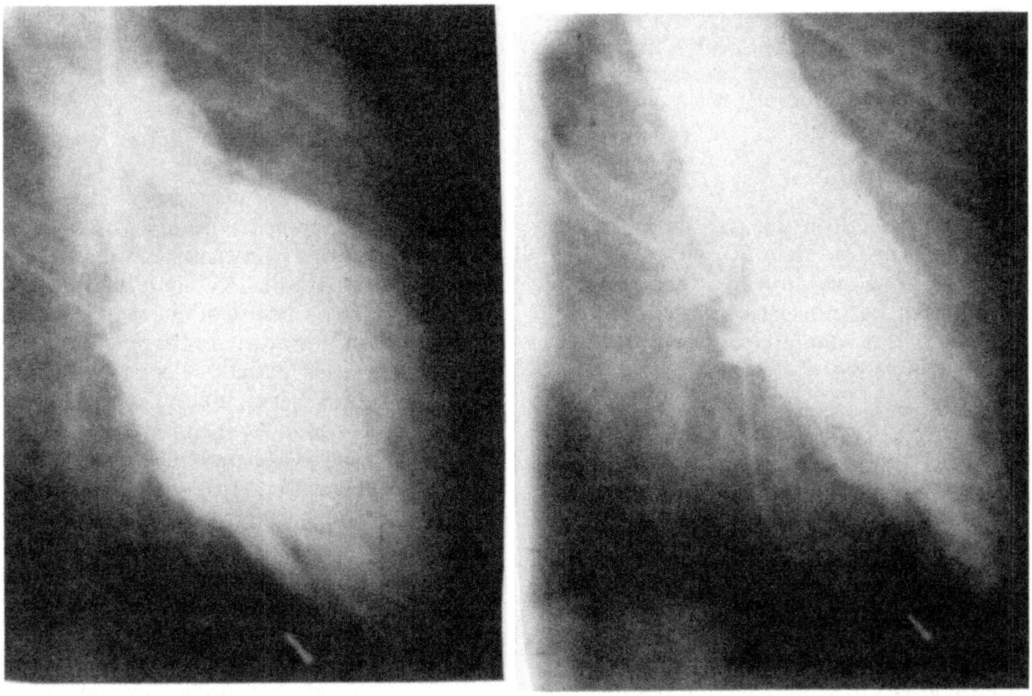

FIGURE 11–25. Same patient as in Figures 11–19 to 11–24. No evidence of mitral valve regurgitation is present seven months after the shock in coronary sinus.

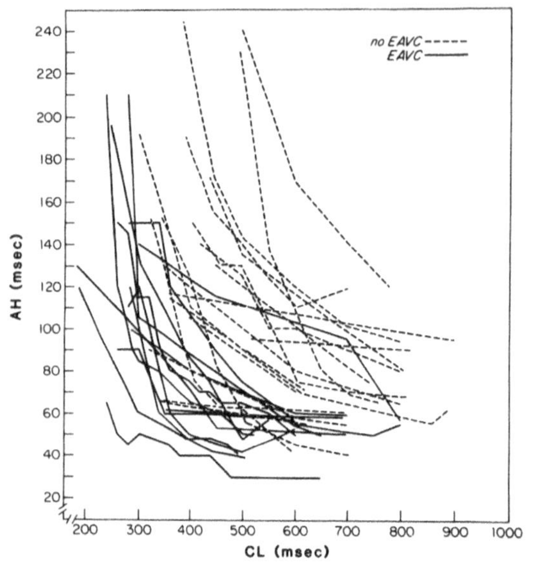

FIGURE 12–6. Graph illustrating the spectrum of atrioventricular (AV) conduction properties in 33 patients in whom atrial pacing cycle length was progressively reduced until the shortest pacing cycle length with 1:1 AV conduction was achieved. EAVC = enhanced AV conduction. (Reproduced with permission of the *Am. Heart Assoc.*, from Benditt DG, Epstein ML, Arentzen CE, Kriett JN and Klein GJ: Enhanced atrioventricular conduction in patients without preexcitation syndrome: relation to heart rate in paroxysmal reciprocating tachycardia. *Circulation* 65:1474, 1982.)

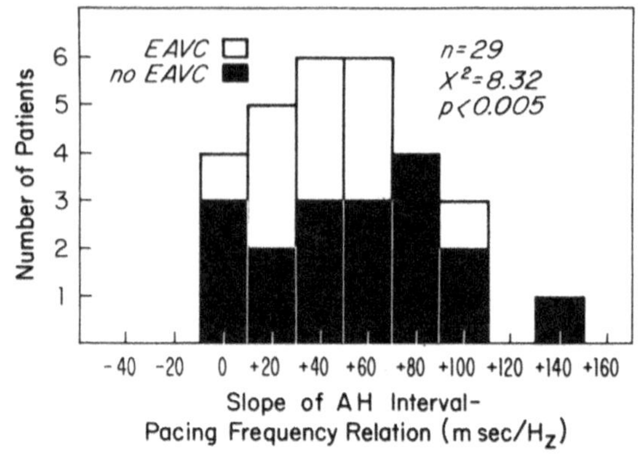

FIGURE 12–7. Graph depicting the unimodal frequency distribution of the slope of the AH interval-pacing frequency relation in 29 patients in whom the AH interval was clearly measurable at 3 or more pacing cycle lengths. EAVC = enhanced atrioventricular conduction. Normality of this distribution was assessed by chi-square test for goodness of fit. (Reproduced with permission of the *Am. Heart Assoc.*, from Benditt DG, Epstein ML, Arentzen CE, Kriett JN and Klein GJ: Enhanced atrioventricular conduction in patients without preexcitation syndrome: relation to heart rate in paroxysmal reciprocating tachycardia. *Circulation* 65:1474, 1982.)

bundle maintained during right atrial pacing at cycle lengths less than 300 ms;

3. AH interval prolongation less than or equal to 100 ms at the shortest cycle length associated with 1:1 conduction compared to sinus rhythm valve.

Subsequently, the definition of EAVC was broadened by altering the last criterion to include patients in whom the maximum increment of the AH interval remained less than or equal to 100 ms, between the value in sinus rhythm and that at pacing cycle length 300 ms (200 beats/minute) [67]. This revision expanded the number of potential EAVC patients and may have muddied the waters by permitting inclusion of individuals in whom substantial degrees of AV node conduction delay become manifest at pacing cycle lengths less than 300 ms. Nonetheless, the revised definition has supplanted the original [3,4,9].

Although in recent years EAVC has provided a useful framework within which one can compare findings in patients exhibiting approximately comparable AV conduction characteristics, a large body of literature evaluating subnormal AV node conduction responses is based on *similar* patient selection criteria. For example, Holmes et al. [68,69] utilized the terms *enhanced AV node conduction* [68] and *accelerated AV node conduction* [69] based upon the single criterion that 1:1 AV conduction was sustained at rates in excess of 200 beats/minute. A similar single criterion was employed by Frank et al. [70] in characterizing the attenuated nodal response. Consequently, care must be taken in evaluating published reports detailing electrophysiologic characteristics in patients with subnormal AV node conduction properties, even if termed EAVC.

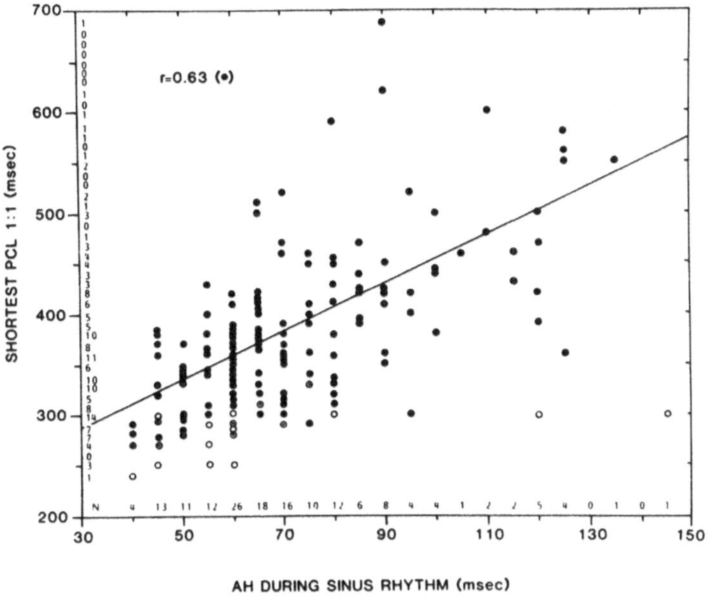

FIGURE 12–8. Graph illustrating shortest right atrial pacing cycle length maintaining 1:1 atrioventricular nodal conduction (shortest PCL 1:1) plotted as a function of AH interval measured during sinus rhythm. The frequency distributions for the two variables are listed along the ordinate and abscissa, respectively. Linear regression analysis incorporated only patients in whom the shortest PCL 1:1 was determined definitively (filled circles, $n = 141$). Unfilled circles represent patients in whom incremental atrial pacing was terminated before the onset of atrioventricular nodal block. Actual values for the shortest PCL 1:1 in those patients are the same or less than value plotted. Target symbols represent superimposed filled and unfilled circles. Note the wide range of shortest PCL 1:1 for each value of AH interval. (Reproduced with permission of the *Am. Heart Assoc.* from Jackman WM, Prystowsky EN, Naccarelli GV, Fineberg NS, Rahilly GT, Heger JJ, Zipes DP: Reevaluation of enhanced atrioventricular nodal conduction: Evidence to suggest a continuum of normal atrioventricular nodal physiology. *Circulation* 67:441, 1983.)

Spectrum of subnormal AV node conduction responses. Published electrophysiologic findings in patients exhibiting markedly diminished AV conduction delay suggest that at least a segment of functioning delay-producing AV nodal tissue is utilized during antegrade conduction in the vast majority of instances. Specifically, at least some degree of AH interval prolongation usually is observed during either incremental right atrial pacing or following insertion of progressively more premature atrial extrastimuli (Figure 12–9) [11,16,67,71–77]. Further, the capacity for concealed conduction to occur within the AV node in the antegrade direction, although probably diminished given the fact that extremely short RR intervals are often conducted [16], is nonetheless present [66]. Finally, for the most part AV conduction in this setting has been shown to respond in a directionally appropriate manner (i.e., by further slowing) following administration of cardiac glycosides, propranolol, verapamil, and adenosine triphosphate (ATP) [70,76–80].

CONDUCTION CURVES. Although the PR interval is not a precise predictor of AV node conduction characteristics (see above), patients with short PR intervals often exhibit subnormal AV node conduction slowing [11,67,81]. By way of example, Caracta et al. [11] noted that most patients with short PR intervals exhibited abbreviated AH values during sinus rhythm (i.e., <60 ms), and that the magnitude of AH

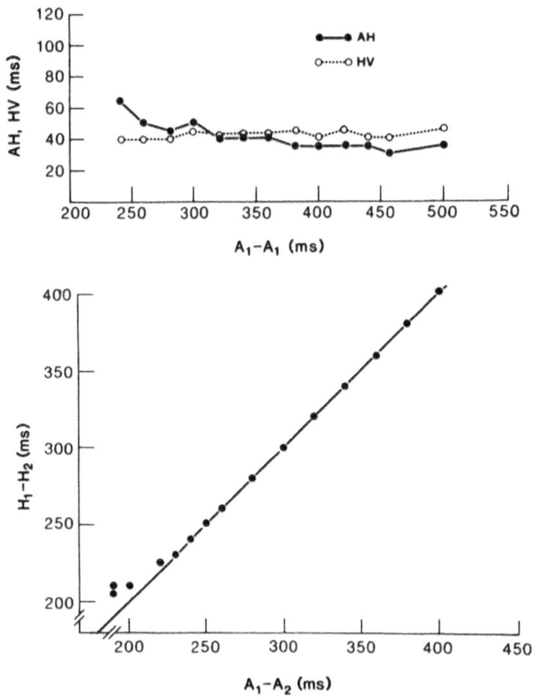

FIGURE 12–9. Graphs illustrating electrophysiologic characteristics of atrioventricular conduction in a 15-year-old female with reciprocating tachycardia and EAVC (same patient as in Figure 12–4). (*Top Panel*) Effect of decreasing atrial pacing cycle length (abscissa, A_1–A_1, ms) on AH (*filled circles*) and HV (*unfilled circles*) intervals (ordinate). Although the AH interval remained relatively flat, over most of the pacing cycle length range, measurable AH prolongation occurred at cycle lengths less than 320 ms. (*Bottom Panel*) Effect of decreasing atrial extrastimulus coupling interval (abscissa A_1–A_2, ms) on H_1–H_2 interval. For the most part, the H_1–H_2 interval followed the line of identity, with minimal AV conduction slowing being observed at A_1–A_2 coupling intervals less than 240 ms.

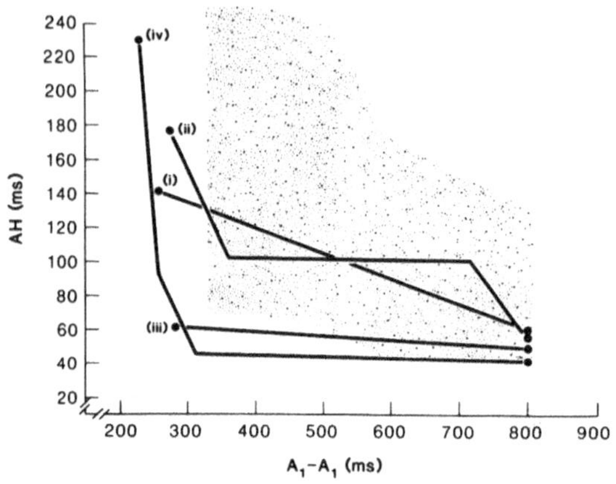

FIGURE 12–10. Graphs illustrating the four types of AV node conduction patterns observed in patients with "subnormal" AV node conduction delay. Atrial pacing cycle length (A_1–A_2, ms) is plotted on the abscissa, and the AH interval (ms) is plotted on the ordinate. The approximate range of "normal" AV node responses is (*shaded area*) is derived from the findings of Benditt et al. [16]. See text for details.

interval change during incremental atrial pacing (range 50 to 100 ms) was less in patients with short PR intervals than in control subjects (mean value approximately 120 ms). Of note, the criteria subsequently used to define enhanced AV node conduction (EAVC [66,67] were based largely on these initial observations. Nonetheless, while EAVC criteria are fulfilled in approximately 60 percent of patients with short PR intervals referred for electrophysiologic evaluation of tachyarrhythmias, almost 30 percent of tachyarrhythmia patients with normal PR intervals also exhibit this phenomenon [67].

Apart from the observation that the magnitude of the AH change with increasing heart rate is often subnormal in patients with short PR intervals, the manner in which the AH interval changes has drawn considerable attention. Caracta et al. [11] noted three relatively distinctive patterns: (1) a monotonic increase in AH interval, similar to but less marked than that observed in control subjects; (2) an initial AH interval prolongation, interrupted by a plateau zone of variable duration, followed by further AH increase; the total AH interval increment being less than in control subjects; and (3) an essentially flat AH interval response during atrial pacing at incrementally increased rates. In general, these patterns (Figure 12–10) have been corroborated by other investigators, although a fourth pattern has been observed as well: that is, an initially relatively flat AH versus cycle length relation, which only begins to exhibit marked AH prolongation at cycle lengths less than 300 ms [67,70,72,73].

Whether each of the AV conduction patterns described above can be attributed to a specific structural or functional substrate within the AV

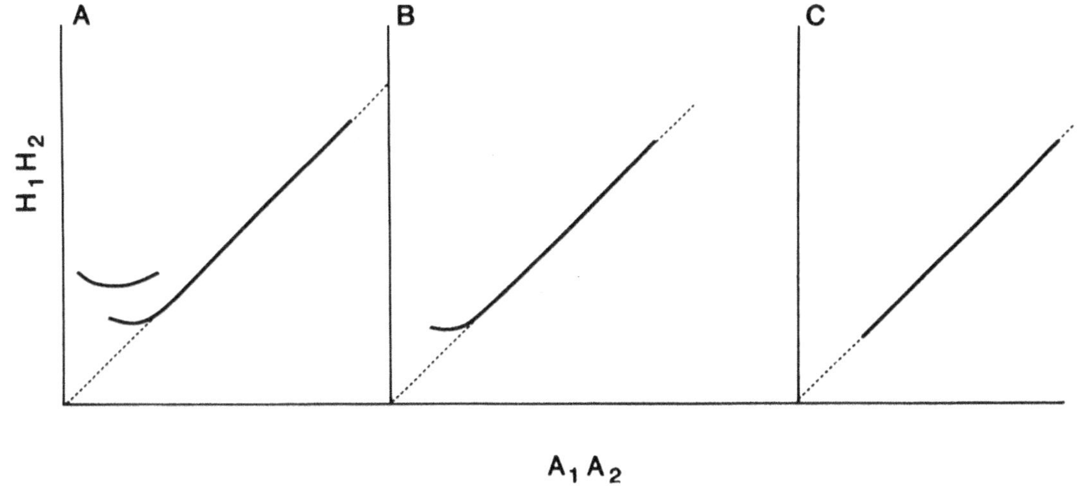

FIGURE 12–11. Graphs depicting the patterns of AV nodal response during atrial extrastimulus testing in patients with "subnormal" AV node conduction delay. The coupling interval of the atrial premature beat is indicated on the abscissa and the resulting H_1–H_2 interval is plotted on the ordinate. The hatched line indicates the line of identity (i.e., H_1–H_2 = A_1–A_2). (A) Discontinuous curves suggesting presence of "dual AV nodal pathways." (B) AV conduction slowing of premature atrial impulses occurs only at very short A_1–A_2 coupling intervals. (C) Throughout the range of coupling intervals of atrial premature beats conducted to the His bundle, there is no evidence of AV nodal conduction slowing (i.e., H_1H_2 = A_1–A_2 at all coupling intervals greater than the atrial effective refractory period).

junction remains conjectural. However, there has been some thought provoking speculation in this regard [70,77]. The first pattern (Figure, 12–10, type i) suggests that excitable tissue exhibiting decremental conduction properties is utilized for conduction in the antegrade direction over a wide range of cycle lengths, but that the ability of this tissue to induce conduction slowing is less than normal. Such a situation might be compatible with a small AV node [11], partial AV node bypass via an atrionodal (intranodal [13]) tract [10], or altered cellular electrophysiologic properties within the node (see above). The type ii response (Figure 12–10), in which a plateau occurs between the cycle length zones exhibiting decremental conduction, may be attributed to presence of several conduction routes, at least one of which bypasses the zone of decremental conduction within the AV node. Over the cycle length range that the bypass predominates, it manifests a fixed conduction time. Subsequently bypass conduction blocks at shorter cycle lengths and decremental conduction, more typical of AV nodal tissue, becomes evident again. The type iii (Figure 12–10) or flat AH response is relatively rare and is suggestive of a true atriofascicular bypass tract [14,15]. The latter argument would be strongly supported by a similarly flat response during atrial extrastimulus testing (Figures 12–11 and 12–12). The fourth conduction pattern (Figure 12–10, type iv) suggests that at relatively long cycle lengths AV conduction bypasses tissues usually exhibiting decremental conduction. At shorter cycle lengths the factor(s) resulting in apparent bypass of AV conduction delay vanish (e.g., development of block within an atrionodal bypass tract), thereby unmasking slower conduction through normal AV nodal tissues. An unanswered question in several of these hypotheses is the absence of marked conduction curve discontinuities between the plateau and the decrement segments of the curves.

REFRACTORY PERIODS. Atrial and AV node responses to atrial extrastimuli have been compared in patients with short PR intervals, EAVC patients, and control subjects. In comparison to combined findings in the former two patient groups (see above, Table 12–1), control subjects tend to manifest similar atrial refrac-

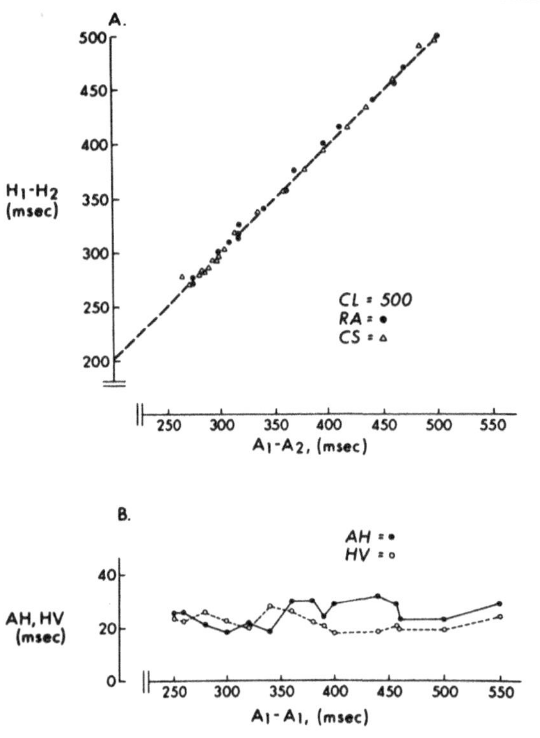

FIGURE 12–12. Graphs illustrating electrophysiologic characteristics of AV node conduction in a patient with a short PR interval and probable atriofasicular bypass tract. (Reproduced with the permission of the *Am. Heart Assoc.* from Benditt DG, Pritchett ELC, Smith WM, Wallace AG, Gallagher JJ: Characteristics of atrioventricular conduction and the spectrum of arrhythmias in Lown-Ganong-Levine syndrome. *Circulation* 57:454–465, 1978.) (A) AV node response (H_1–H_2, ordinate) during atrial (both right atrial and coronary sinus) extrastimulus testing at progressively shorter coupling intervals (A_1–A_2, abscissa) reveals no deviation from the line of identity (hatched line). (B) AV node (AH interval, ordinate) and infra-nodal (HV interval, abscissa) response during right atrial pacing at progressively faster rates (i.e., progressively shorter cycle lengths, A_1–A_2, abscissa). Both AH and HV intervals remain relatively constant throughout the range of pacing cycle lengths tested.

toriness, but longer AV node effective and functional refractory periods [67,72].

The possibility that the attenuated AV nodal response in EAVC patients (with or without a short PR interval) may be due to conduction over the fast pathway in the setting of so-called dual AV nodal pathway physiology [22–24, Figure 12–11A] is often raised and remains an intriguing question. Benditt et al. [67] noted discontinuous curves in 3/12 (25%) patients with short PR intervals and recurrent tachyarrhythmias. In similar subsets of patients, Frank et al. [70] observed discontinuous refractory period curves in 4/29 (14%) patients, while Ward et al. [76] reported this finding in 10/21 (48%) individuals. Conceivably, the true incidence of this phenomenon may be higher, but usually one is only able to discern those instances in which the effective refractory period of the fast pathway is longer than that of the slow pathway. Nonetheless, Ward et al. [76] pointed out that while the fast pathway exhibited electrophysiologic features which could account for the phenomenon of subnormal AV node conduction delay, refractoriness of the slow pathway was also markedly shorter in patients with short PR intervals than in normals. Thus, if one accepts the concept of "dual AV nodal pathways" in this setting, it seems that both limbs of intranodal conduction exhibit subnormal conduction delay. Given this additional abnormality in the so-called slow pathway, it seems unlikely that either EAVC or short PR intervals are solely the result of a normal AV node in which, for unknown reasons, conduction in the antegrade direction occurs over the fast segment of "dual AV nodal pathways."

In patients with EAVC, measurement of AV node effective refractory periods frequently is limited by atrial refractoriness; however, the pattern of the nodal response during atrial extrastimulus testing can be ascertained (i.e., the A_1A_2, H_1H_2 relation) and may give some insight into the nature of the conducting tissues. Frank et al. [70] noted that prolongation of the H_1H_2 interval in the terminal portion (i.e., at the shortest coupling intervals) of the extrastimulus response suggested the presence of tissue exhibiting decremental conduction properties (Figures 12–9 and 12–11B) in 19/29 (66%) patients with short PR intervals. In 7/29 (24%) patients in the latter study, but in only 1/12 (8%) of the patients described by Benditt et al. [67], the AV node response (i.e., the H_1H_2 interval) to atrial extrastimuli did not deviate from the line of identity (Figures 12–11C and 12–12). The latter response would seem to be most consistent with an atriofascicular bypass tract, although an intranodal fast pathway with a short effective refractory period is a plausible alternative explanation.

In summary, subnormal AV node conduction delay may manifest as any of a variety of AV nodal electrophysiologic responses during incremental atrial pacing or atrial extrastimulus testing. Consequently, the basis for this phenomenon is likely diverse, and at present it is best viewed as an electrophysiologic syndrome [81], the clinical significance of which must be assessed on an individual basis.

Clinical Implications

The relationship between subnormal AV node conduction slowing and the relatively frequent occurrence of rapid heart beating has long been a curiousity. In 1938, Clerc, Robert-Levy, and Cristesco [82] reported electrocardiographic and clinical findings in 21 patients with short PR intervals, and noted the strong association of this electrocardiographic finding with complaints of palpitations (approximately 50% of their patients, and almost 80% if one excludes those patients with other significant heart disease such as rheumatic valvular conditions, heart failure, or hypertension). Subsequently, Lown, Ganong, and Levine [83] reported a 12% incidence of rapid heart beating following retrospective analysis of symptoms among individuals in whom a short PR interval was detected (23/200 in patients with short PR intervals versus 1/200 in patients with normal PR intervals). Presumably, the true frequency of tachyarrhythmias in patients with short PR intervals lies somewhere in between the findings in these two reports.

Why patients with diminished conduction slowing capacity within the AV junction (i.e., EAVC patients, and the majority of patients with short PR intervals) tend to have a high incidence of symptomatic tachyarrhythmias is still uncertain. However, recent electrophysiologic and electropharmacologic studies have improved our appreciation of the spectrum of arrhythmias observed, and the impact that AV node conduction characteristics have on tachycardia rate and response to therapeutic interventions in this subset of patients.

SPECTRUM OF TACHYARRHYTHMIAS OBSERVED

In most cases where tachycardias have been reported in association with short PR intervals or EAVC, the arrhythmias have been paroxysmal supraventricular tachycardias. Nonetheless, ventricular tachyarrhythmias have been observed in a few instances (Figure 12–13). In a report of historical importance, Lown, Ganong, and Levine [83] noted that 12/23 patients with short PR intervals (i.e., less than or equal to .12 seconds) had "paroxysmal auricular tachycardia." Ten of the latter 12 patients had either atrial flutter or fibrillation, and it was among the patients with atrial fibrillation that the 2 deaths in the series occurred. However, in a number of these patients more than one kind of rapid heart action was noted, while in others the nature of the dysrhythmia(s) was not delineated. More recently, Benditt et al. [67] noted that while regular narrow QRS reciprocating tachycardias were the most frequent rhythm disturbance among 12 patients with short PR intervals (6/12, 50%), both primary atrial tachycardias (atrial flutter or fibrillation 3/12, 25%) and severe ventricular arrhythmias (4/12, 33%) were surprisingly common.

In an effort to better understand the apparent relation between subnormal AV node conduction delay and occurrence of reciprocating tachycardia, a number of attempts have been made to examine the nature of reentrant supraventricular tachyarrhythmias in both patients with short PR intervals and patients with EAVC. Unfortunately, many of these studies are deficient in that it is unclear whether the possible participation of accessory connections capable of conduction in only the retrograde direction (i.e., concealed accessory connections) was assessed appropriately. Among studies in which such connections were looked for, Benditt et al. [67] found their participation in symptomatic tachyarrhythmias in 2/7 (29%) patients with short PR intervals and paroxysmal reciprocating tachycardia, while Ward et al. [84] reported involvement of concealed connections in 9/12 (75%) tachycardias in 11 similar patients. Analogous results have been obtained in EAVC patients without short PR intervals)e.g., 50% [6/12 patients] incidence of concealed accessory connections [67]). In the remaining patients in each of these studies, paroxysmal reciprocating tachycardias were found to be due to reentry within the AV node.

As noted previously, it has been proposed that short PR intervals and/or EAVC represent so-called fast-pathway conduction in patients with "dual AV nodal conduction pathways." This theory suggests that the presumed presence of dual-pathways leads to a greater than expected

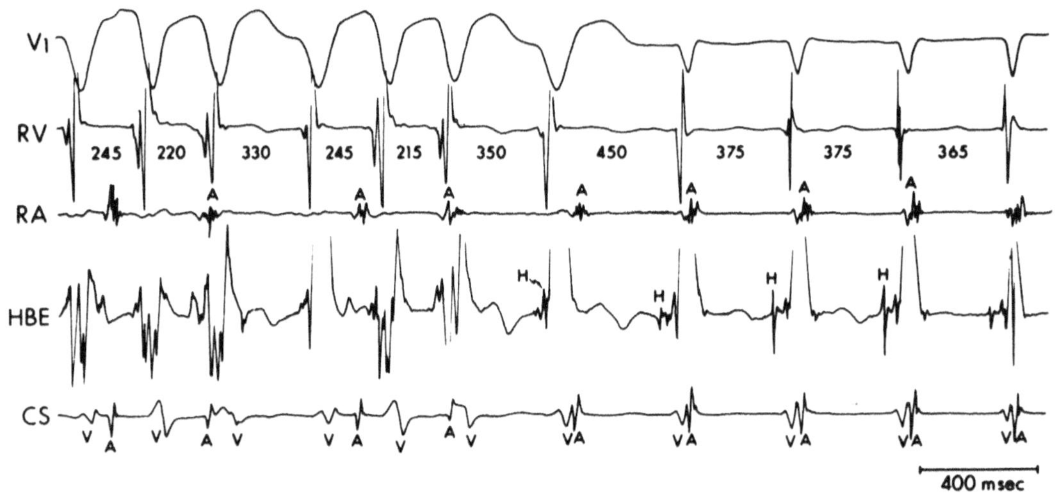

FIGURE 12–13. Electrocardiogram and intracardiac electrograms from a patient with a short PR interval and repetitive tachyarrhythmias. From top to bottom, traces and ECG lead V_1, and electrograms from the right ventricle (RV), right atrium (RA), His bundle region (HBE) and coronary sinus (CS). At left paroxysmal ventricular tachycardia was documented, with subsequent spontaneous orthodromic reciprocating tachycardia at the right. (Reproduced with the permission of the *Am. Heart Assoc.* from Benditt DG, Pritchett ELC, Smith WM, Wallace AG, Gallagher JJ: Characteristics of atrioventricular conduction and the spectrum of arrhythmias in Lown-Ganong-Levine syndrome. *Circulation* 57:454–465, 1978.)

propensity for development of reciprocating tachycardia due to reentry within the AV node [85]. However, as noted above, the role of the fast-pathway in EAVC is far from clear. Further, the relative frequency with which concealed accessory connections participate in paroxysmal reciprocating tachycardia in patients with short PR intervals and/or EAVC appears to be approximately the same as in the general population of patients with episodic supraventricular tachycardias [2,9]. Therefore, while it may be true that the incidence of symptomatic tachyarrhythmias is higher in patients with short PR intervals or EAVC than in normals, the view that this is due to "increased incidence of sustained AV nodal reentrant tachycardias in patients with short PR intervals" [81] does not appear to be well substantiated. Indeed, there is reason to hypothesize that the incidence of reentry within the AV node should be less in patients with subnormal AV node conduction slowing than in patients with normal AV conduction characteristics, since in the former instances it would seem to be more difficult to achieve sufficient AV conduction slowing in the antegrade (AV) direction. In our own reported series of 35 patients with reciprocating tachycardia [16], reentry within the AV node occurred in 16/23 (70%) of patients with normal AV conduction, versus 6/12 (50%) in EAVC patients.

The relationship between the presence of diminished AV conduction delay and the propensity for development of symptomatic atrial flutter or fibrillation remains poorly understood. However, this association may be largely coincidental. Given the potential, in this setting, for occurrence of very rapid (and therefore presumably hemodynamically disturbing) heart rates during these particular arrhythmias [16], their occurrence would be expected to result in clinically significant symptoms. In addition, a connection has been made between excessively rapid ventricular response during supraventricular tachyarrhythmias and the development of ventricular fibrillation [61,86,87]. Alternatively, there is growing evidence that otherwise apparently healthy individuals, presenting initially with primary atrial tachycardias, may have a high incidence of subtle underlying cardiomyopathy [88,89]. Conceivably, the latter association in conjunction with a rapid ventricular rate may increase the likelihood of symptom development or perhaps the chance of initiation of potentially lethal arrhythmias.

IMPACT OF AV NODE CONDUCTION CHARACTERISTICS ON TACHYCARDIA RATE

The relationship between subnormal AV node conduction delay and heart rates during supraventricular tachyarrhythmias has been a source of controversy. Initially, Gallagher et al. [66] pointed out that the coexistence of EAVC in patients with accessory AV conduction pathways was associated with more rapid heart rates during both reciprocating tachycardia and atrial fibrillation than were observed in the absence of EAVC. Further, the difference in heart rates was entirely attributable to shorter AH intervals during tachycardia in EAVC patients. The findings of Gallagher et al. [66] were later extended to patients with short PR intervals and paroxysmal tachycardias (i.e., Lown-Ganong-Levine syndrome), in whom Benditt et al. [67] reported a relatively high incidence of EAVC (58% overall, 75% among patients with reciprocating tachycardia). In the latter report, reciprocating tachycardias due to both reentry within the AV node and reentry using a concealed accessory connection had shorter cycle lengths (faster heart rates) than did the same tachycardias in control patients with normal PR intervals. Similarly, patients with short PR intervals manifested more rapid ventricular responses (both mean and shortest RR intervals) during atrial fibrillation than did control subjects.

Recently, Bauernfeind et al. [63] were unable to substantiate a statistically significant association between either short PR or AH intervals and development of faster than expected tachycardia heart rates (of whom 14/65 patients had short PR and/or AH intervals) with dual AV nodal pathways and reciprocating tachycardia due to reentry within the AV node, despite an apparently weak relationship between AH intervals less than 60 ms and a tendency to shorter tachycardia cycle lengths (see Figure 12–3, Panel B in reference 63). Not surprisingly, these authors indicated that tachycardia cycle length correlated most strongly with the AH interval of the slow pathway (i.e., the AH interval measured just to the left of the discontinuity in the A_1–A_2, H_1–H_2 relation) (Figure 12–14).

In part, differences between the findings in patients with tachycardia due to reentry within

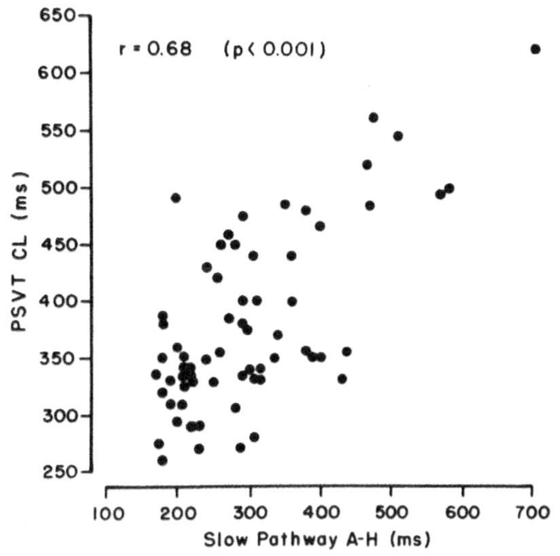

FIGURE 12–14. Relation between the slow pathway AH interval (abscissa) and the cycle length of A–V nodal reentrant paroxysmal tachycardia (PSVT CL, ordinate). (Reproduced with permission of Technical Publishing, Inc. from Bauernfeind et al.: Cycle length in atrioventricular nodal reentrant paroxysmal tachycardia with observations on the Lown-Ganong-Levine syndrome. *Am. J. Cardiol.* 45:1148–1153, 1980.)

the AV node reported by Baurenfeind et al. [63], and those reported earlier by Benditt et al. [67], may have been a function of the basis upon which AV node conduction was assessed. In the former study [63] AV conduction was characterized by static PR or AH values, whereas the definition of EAVC as applied in the latter study [67] necessitates a more dynamic characterization of AV nodal properties. Nonetheless, in an attempt to resolve the apparent discrepancy between these reports we reexamined the relation between EAVC and tachycardia rates in a larger series of patients with reciprocating tachycardias [16]. Again, EAVC patients tended to exhibit more rapid heart rates during reciprocating tachycardia than did individuals with normal AV node conduction delay (Figure 12–15, left panel); however, the differences in tachycardia rates primarily resulted from significantly faster rates in EAVC patients with reciprocating tachycardia due to reentry using concealed accessory connections (Figure 12–15, middle panel). On the other hand, while tachycardia rates tended to be somewhat faster (i.e., shorter cycle lengths) in EAVC patients with

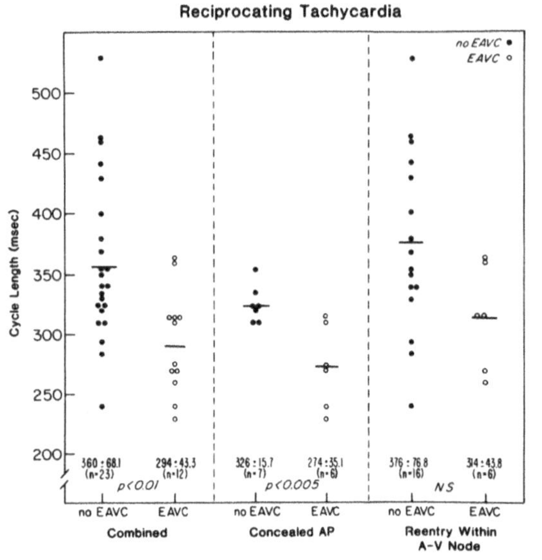

FIGURE 12–15. Comparison of reciprocating tachycardia (RT) cycle lengths in patients with and without enhanced atrioventricular conduction (EAVC). (*Left*) Comparison of RT cycle lengths in all patients independent of RT mechanism, demonstrating the tendency toward shorter RT cycle lengths in patients with EAVC. (*Middle*) Comparison of RT cycle lengths in patients with RT due to reentry via concealed accessory AV pathways (AP), illustrating the preponderance of shorter RT cycle lengths in patients with EAVC than in those without EAVC. (*Right*) RT cycle lengths in patient swith RT due to reenty iwthin the AV node. There is no statistically significant difference between RT cycle lengths in patients with and without EAVC. (Reproduced with permission of the *Am. Heart Assoc.* from Benditt DG, Epstein ML, Arentzen CE, Kriett JM, Klein GJ: Enhanced atioventricular conduction in patients without preexcitation syndrome: Relation to heart rate in paroxysmal reciprocating tachycardia. *Circulation* 65:1474–1479, 1982.)

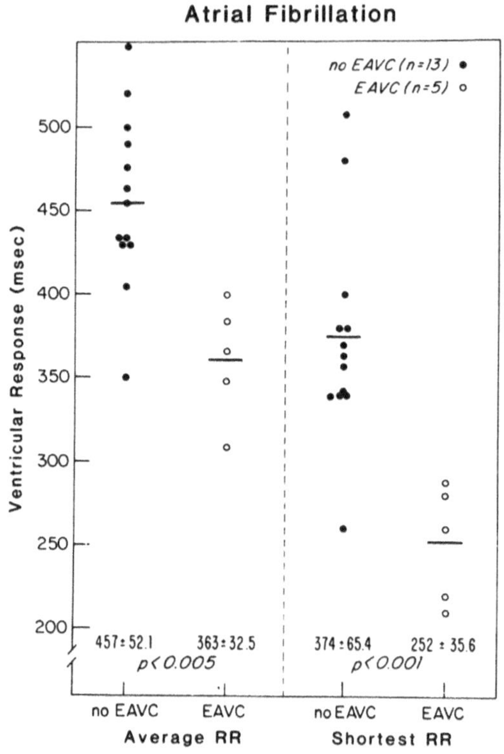

FIGURE 12–16. Graph illustrating that both the average RR interval (*left*) and shortest RR intervals (*right*) during pacing-induced atrial fibrillation were shorter in patients with enhanced atrioventricular conduction (EAVC) than in patients without EAVC. (Reproduced with permission of the *Am. Heart Assoc.* from Benditt DG, Epstein ML, Arentzen CE, Kriett JM, Klein GJ: Enhanced atioventricular conduction in patients without preexcitation syndrome: Relation to heart rate in paroxysmal reciprocating tachycardia. *Circulation* 65:1474–1479, 1982.)

reentry within the AV node than in non-EAVC patients, the difference was not statistically significant (Figure 12–15, right panel). The relationship between EAVC and more rapid ventricular responses during atrial fibrillation was confirmed (Figure 12–16) [16].

The relationship between AV node conduction characteristics and heart rate during reciprocating tachycardias due to reentry using an accessory connection or reentry within the AV node is consistent with our understanding of the role played by the AV node in these arrhythmias. In reciprocating tachycardia utilizing an accessory connection, the entire AV node usually comprises a portion of the antegrade limb of the reentry pathway while the accessory connection is contained within the retrograde limb. Thus, in this setting the aspects of AV node conduction assessed by atrial pacing and extrastimulus studies would be expected to be precisely those which determine the characteristics of AV conduction during the tachyarrhythmia. Conversely, during reciprocating tachycardia due to reentry within the AV node the segment of the AV node which determines tachycardia rate is not so clearly evaluated by these same techniques, and consequently absence of a strong correlation between AV node conduction properties and tachycardia characteristics is not entirely surprising.

THERAPEUTIC IMPLICATIONS

The treatment of paroxysmal supraventricular tachycardias, including both reciprocating tachycardias and primary atrial tachyarrhythmias such as atrial fibrillation [88], relies heavily on drug effects on AV nodal conduction properties. Consequently, it is understandable that altered AV node responsiveness to commonly used pharmacologic agents (e.g., cardiac glycosides, beta-adrenergic blockers, calcium channel blockers) may be associated with diminished effectiveness of standard medical treatment.

Cardiac glycosides. A prospective study correlating the magnitude of the electrophysiologic effects of cardiac glycosides on AV node conduction and refractoriness with underlying AV node conduction properties has yet to be carried out. However, in a study comprising eight patients with enhanced AV nodal conduction and medically refractory reciprocating tachycardias utilizing concealed accessory AV connections, Holmes et al. [68] reported that digitalis produced "little or no slowing of anterograde conduction and little or no prolongation of anterograde AV nodal refractory periods." These finding are consistent with our own observations; namely, that EAVC is associated with either diminished capacity within the AV node for enlisting additional parasympathetic neural influence or with a level of background sympathetic tone capable of effectively diminishing efficacy of vagomimetic agents [17]. Thus, since the predominant electrophysiologic effects of cardiac glycosides on the AV node are believed to be the result of glycoside-mediated accentuation of parasympathetic tone, both the report by Holmes et al. [68] and theoretical considerations suggest that cardiac glycosides may be of limited value for either treatment or prophylaxis of supraventricular tachycardias in patients exhibiting subnormal AV node physiologic conduction delay.

Beta-adrenergic blocking drugs. Recently we compared acute electrophysiologic effects of high dose propranolol (0.2 mg/kg i.v.) on AV node conduction and refractoriness in 10 patients with EAVC and 12 non-EAVC control subjects. In EAVC patients, propranolol decreased the maximum atrial paced rate with sustained 1:1 AV conduction from a mean of 224 beats/minute to 179 beats/minute (a 20% change). In non-EAVC subjects, the maximum atrial paced rate with 1:1 AV conduction was reduced from 153 beats/minute to 134 beats/minute (a 12% change). Findings were comparable for AV node functional refractory periods (AVNFRP). At basic pacing cycle length 500 ms, propranolol increased AVNFRP by 7% in EAVC patients, and by 6% in non-EAVC subjects. Therefore, our findings suggest the beta-adrenergic blockade appears to be at least as effective in EAVC patients as in patients with normal AV nodal conduction slowing. Whether this apparent similarity of electrophysiologic effect translates into comparable therapeutic effectiveness remains to be evaluated. Of note, however, 5/8 patients in the study reported by Holmes et al. [68], had been treated with propranolol unsuccessfully. On the other hand, the latter patients had also been concomitantly exposed to a variety of other drug regimens, and neither the doses of propranolol nor the doses of the other agents were specified. At the present time, we conclude that beta-adrenergic blocking drugs are likely to provide a useful addition to antiarrhythmic treatment in the setting of apparently subnormal AV node conduction slowing.

Calcium channel blocking drugs. Of the various calcium channel blocking drugs, the electrophysiologic effects of verapamil have been most extensively evaluated in patients with diminished AV node conduction delay (i.e., short PR interval, EAVC). However, the findings have been somewhat variable. For example, Seipel et al. [77] examined AV node conduction and refractoriness in eight patients with short PR intervals prior to and following the administration of intravenous verapamil (0.1 mg/kg), and compared the results with observations reported separately in 10 control subjects with normal PR intervals [90]. Although detailed electrophysiologic results were not presented, verapamil was reported to have little or no effect on AV nodal conduction characteristics in the patients with short PR intervals [77]. Further, any effects that were observed were said to be markedly less impressive in patients with short PR intervals compared to control subjects. On the other hand, in a similar group of patients, Moro and Cosio [80] reported that verapamil significantly prolonged AH intervals during sinus rhythm (although the effect on sinus cycle length is unclear), and both AV node effective and functional refractory periods. The latter findings are supported by the observations of Disertori et al. [75] and tend to parallel our own experience following verapamil administration in patients with EAVC.

In summary, it appears that the acute electrophysiologic effects of intravenously administered verapamil on AV conduction may be less prominent in patients with subnormal AV node conduction delay than in normal subjects. Consistent with these findings are the observations by Ward and Camm [84] that verapamil was entirely ineffective or only marginally effective in treating supraventricular tachycardias in 6/9 patients with short PR intervals. Consequently, given the fact that oral verapamil is often less effective than the parenterally administered compound for treating paroxysmal supraventricular tachycardias, the usefulness of verapamil and other calcium channel blockers for long-term tachycardia prophylaxis may be reduced in the setting of diminished AV nodal conduction delay.

Other antiarrhythmic drugs. It would not be surprising if direct acting antiarrhythmic compounds with predominantly sodium-channel (fast channel) blocking action tended to exert a more prominent negative dromotropic effect on AV conduction in patients with subnormal AV conduction slowing than in normal subjects. This suggestion is based on the supposition that, in the former instance, AV conduction appears to be both less dependent on calcium-channel dependent tissues, and by virtue of diminished parasympathetic influence, less susceptible to the often present vagolytic side-effects of certain type 1 antiarrhythmic drugs (especially quinidine and disopyramide). Clearly, an assessment of the relationship between baseline electrophysiologic properties of AV node conduction and the action of various antiarrhythmic compounds is warranted.

Other therapeutic modalities. In those instances when subnormal AV node conduction delay is associated with drug refractory supraventicular tachycardias, alternative therapeutic techniques must be considered. Obviously, surgical ablation of an accessory AV connection with sparing of the AV node–His bundle is now a widely accepted and highly successful procedure. However, in many patients the principal rhythm disturbances are primary atrial tachycardias [88] with a rapid ventricular response due to diminished physiologic delay within the AV node, or tachycardias in which the AV node alone or the AV node along with physically closely associated nodoventricular or fasciculoventricular connections participate [2,25]. In the latter instances, appropriate modification of AV node conduction by surgical techniques such as placement of discrete cryolesions or laser lesions in the vicinity of the AV node may become a reality (see Cox et al., this volume). However, at the present time ablation of the AV node–His bundle axis may be indicated. For example, in 3/6 patients presenting with EAVC alone and either atrial flutter with 1:1 AV conduction, or ventricular fibrillation due to an excessively rapid ventricular response during atrial fibrillation, Gallagher et al. [91] found pharmacologic therapy to be inadequate and therefore undertook ablation of the cardiac conduction system. At the present time, transection of the AV node–His bundle can be achieved with a high degree of reliability, and with relatively little risk by electrode catheter technique [92,93.]

Conclusion

In humans, AV node conduction properties comprise a wide spectrum with no clearcut boundaries dividing normal from abnormal; whether the abnormality in question be inappropriately slow AV conduction or excessively rapid AV conduction (i.e., short PR, EAVC). Nonetheless we now recognize that diminished AV nodal capacity for inducing physiologic conduction delay is associated with the potential for development of excessively rapid heart rates among patients with certain forms of supraventricular tachycardia, and that effectiveness of pharmacologic intervention depends in part on the manner in which AV nodal conduction is disturbed. Consequently, despite the fact that the diagnostic criteria are arbitrary, and regardless of whether the substrate of the conduction disturbance differs from patient to patient, there appears to be merit in our attempting to identify individuals at risk of excessively rapid heart rates.

Ultimately, the ability to evaluate interactions among the developmental, anatomic, electrophysiologic, and neural influences determining AV nodal conduction properties in individual patients, may have practical therapeutic implications.

References

1. Ohnell RF: Preexcitation, a cardiac abnormality *Acta Med. Scand.* (Supp) 152:1, 1944.
2. Gallagher JJ, Pritchett ELC, Sealy WC, Kasell J, Wallace AG: The preexcitation syndromes. *Prog. Cardiovasc. Dis.* 20:285, 1978.
3. Durrer D, Schuilenberg RM, Wellens HJJ: Preexcitation revisited *Am. J. Cardiol.* 25:690, 1970.
4. Prystowsky EN, Miles WM, Heger JJ, Zipes DP: Preexcitation syndromes. Mechanisms and management *Med. Clin. N.A.* 68:831, 1984.
5. James TN: The Wolff-Parkinson-White syndrome: Evolving concepts of its pathogenesis. *Prog. Cardiovasc. Dis.* 13:159, 1970.
6. James TN: Heuristic thoughts on the Wolff-Parkinson-White syndrome. In *Advances in Electrocardiography* (Vol. 2) Schlant RC, Hurst JW (eds.), New York, Grune and Stratton, 1976, pp. 199–217.
7. Sherf L: The atrial conduction system: clinical implications. *Am. J. Cardiol.* 37:814, 1976.
8. Gallagher JJ, Sealy WC Wallace AG, Kasell J: Correlation between catheter electrophysiologic studies and findings on mapping ventricular excitation in the WPW syndrome. In *The Conduction System of the Heart.* Wellens HJJ Lie KI, Janse MJ, (eds.) The Netherlands, Martinus Nijhoff, 1976, pp. 588–612.
9. Fisher JD: Role of electrophysiologic testing in the diagnosis and treatment of patients with known and suspected bradycardias and tachycardias. *Prog. Cardiovasc: Dis.* 24:25, 1981.
10. James TN: Morphology of the human atrioventricular node, with remarks pertinent to its electrophysiology. *Am. Heart J.* 6:756, 1961.
11. Caracta AR, Damato AN, Gallagher JJ, Josephson ME, Varghese PH, Lau SH Westura EE: Electrophysiologic studies in the syndrome of short interval, normal QRS complex. *Am. J. Cardiol.* 31:245, 1973.
12. Brechenmacher C, Laham J, Iris L, Gerbaux A, Lenegre J: Etude histologique des voies anormales de conduction dans un syndrome de Wolff-Parkinson-White et dans un syndrome de Lown-Ganong-Levine. *Arch. Mal Coeur* 67:507, 1974.
13. Anderson RH, Becker AE, Brechenmacher C, Davies MJ, Rossi L: Ventricular preexcitation. A proposed nomenclature for its substrates. *Cardiology* 3:27, 1975.
14. Brechenmacher C: Atrio-His bundle tracts. *Br. Heart J.* 37:853, 1975.
15. Brechenmacher C, Courtadon M, Jourde M, Yermia JC, Cheynel J, Voegtlin R: Syndrome de Wolff-Parkinson-White par association de fibres atrio-hissienes et de fibres de Mahaim: Confrontation entre l'electrophysiologie et l'histologie. *Arch. Mal Coeur* 69:1275, 1976.
16. Benditt DG, Epstein ML, Arentzen CE, Kriett JM, Klein GJ: Enhanced atrioventricular conduction in patients without preexcitation syndrome: Relation to heart rate in paroxysmal reciprocating tachycardia. *Circulation* 65:1474, 1982.
17. Benditt DG, Klein GJ, Kriett JM, Dunnigan A, Benson DW Jr: Enhanced atrioventricular nodal conduction in man: electrophysiologic effect of pharmacologic autonomic blockade. *Circulation* 69:1088, 1984.
18. Anderson RH, Becker AE, Brechenmacher C, Davies MJ, Rossi L: The human atrioventricular junctional area. A morphological study of the node and bundle. *Eur. J. Cardiol.* 3:11, 1975.
19. Lev M, Leffler WB, Langendorf R, Pick A: Anatomic findings in a case of ventricular preexcitation (WPW) terminating in complete atrioventricular block. *Circulation* 34:718, 1966.
20. Rossi L: Histopathologic features of cardiac arrhythmias. Casa Editrice Ambrosiana, Milan, 1969.
21. Becker AE, Anderson RH: Morphology of the human atrioventricular junctional area. In *The Conduction System of the Heart.* Wellens HJJ, Lie KI, Janse MJ (eds.). The Netherlands, Martinus Nijhoff, 1976, pp. 263–286.
22. Moe GK, Preston JB, Burlington H: Physiologic evidence for a dual AV transmission system. *Circ. Res.* 4:357, 1956.
23. Mendez C, Moe GK: Demonstration of a dual AV nodal conduction system in the isolated rabbit heart. *Circ. Res.* 19:378, 1966.
24. Rosen KM, Mehta A, Miller RA: Demonstration of dual atrioventricular nodal pathways in man. *Am. J. Cardiol.* 33:291, 1974.
25. Kerr CR, Benson DW Jr, Gallagher JJ: Role of specialized conducting fibers in the genesis of "AV nodal" reentry tachycardia. *PACE* 6:171, 1983.
26. Sano T, Suzuki F, Tsuchihashi H: Function of potential bypass tracts for atrioventricular conduction. *Circulation* 41:413, 1970.
27. King RL, Jenks JL, White PD: The electrocardiogram of a beluga whale. *Circulation* 8:387, 1953.
28. Meijler F, Van der Tweel I, Herbschleb JN, Heethaar RM, Borst C: Lessons from comparative studies of atrial fibrillation in dog, human, and horse. In *Cardiac Electrophysiology and Arrhythmias* Zipes DP, Jalife J (eds.). Orlando,

Grune and Stratton, 1985, pp. 489–493.
29. Meijler FL: Atrioventricular conduction versus heart size from mouse to whale (editorial). *J. Am. Coll. Cardiol.* 5:363, 1985.
30. Moore EN: Atrioventricular transmission in newborn calves. *Ann. N.Y. Acad. Sci.* 127:113, 1965.
31. Abella J, Trixeira OHP, Misra KP, Hastreiter AR: Changes of atrioventricular conduction with age in infants and children. *Am. J. Cardiol.* 30:876, 1972.
32. DuBrow IW, Fisher EA, Amat-Y-Leon F, Denes P, Wu D, Rosen K, Hastreiter AR: Comparison of cardiac refractory periods in children and adults. *Circulation* 51:485, 1975.
33. Truex RC, Copenhaver WM: Histology of the moderator band in man and other animals with special reference to the conduction system. *Am. J. Cardiol.* 80:173–202, 1947.
34. Preston JB, McFadden S, Moe GK: Atrioventricular transmission in young mammals. *Am. J. Physiol.* 197:236–240, 1959.
35. Janse MJ, Anderson RH, Capelle FJL, Durrer D: A combined electrophysiological and anatomical study of the human fetal heart. *Am. Heart J.* 91: 556, 1976.
36. James TN: Normal and abnormal variations in anatomy of the atrioventricular node and His bundle and their relevance to the pathogenesis of reentrant tachycardias and parasystolic rhythms. In *Cardiac Electrophysiology and Arrhythmias.* Zipes DP, Jalife J (eds.). Orlando, Grune and Stratton, 1985, pp. 301–310.
37. Lieberman M, Kootsey JM, Johnson EA, Sawanobori T: Slow conduction in cardiac muscle. *Biophys. J.* 13:37, 1973.
38. Van Capelle FJL, Janse MJ: Influence of geometry on the shape of the propagated action potential. In *Conduction System of the Heart.* Wellens HJJ, Lie KI, Janse MJ (eds.). The Netherlands, Martinus Nijhoff 1976, 316–335.
39. Mendez C, Moe GK: Atrioventricular transmission. In *Electrical Phenomena in the Heart.* DeMello WC (ed.). New York, Academic Press, 1972, pp. 263–391.
40. De Mello WC: Passive electrical properties of the atrio-ventricular node. *Pflugers Arch.* 371:135, 1977.
41. Mehta J, Tuna N, Moller JH, Desnick RJ: Electrocardiographic and vectorcardiographic abnormalities in Fabry's disease. *Am. Heart J.* 93:699, 1977.
42. Gillette PC, Nihill MR, Singer DB: Electrophysiological mechanism of the short PR interval in Pompe disease. *Am. J. Dis. Child.* 128:622, 1974.
43. Janse MJ, Van Capelle FJL, Anderson RH, Touboul P, Billette J: Electrophysiology and structure of the atrioventricular node of the isolated rabbit heart. In *The Conduction System of the Heart.* Wellens HJJ, Lie KI, Janse MJ (eds.). The Netherlands, Martinus Nijhoff, 1976 pp. 296–315.
44. Spach MS, Lieberman M, Scott JG, Barr RC, Johnson EA, Kootsey JM: Excitation sequences of the atrial septum and the AV node in isolated hearts of the dog and rabbit. *Circ. Res.* 29:156, 1971.
45. Zipes DP, Mendez C, Moe GK: Evidence for summation and voltage dependency in rabbit atrioventricular nodal fibers. *Circ. Res.* 32:170, 1973.
46. Batsford WP, Akhtar M, Caracta AR, Josephson ME, Seides SF, Damato AN: Effect of atrial stimulation site on the electrophysiological properties of the atrioventricular node in man. *Circulation* 50:283, 1974.
47. Aranda J, Castellanos A, Moleiro F, Befeler B: Effects of the pacing site on AH conduction and refractoriness in patients with short PR intervals. *Circulation* 53:33, 1976.
48. Childers R: The AV node: Normal and abnormal physiology. *Prog. Cardiovasc. Dis.* 19:361, 1977.
49. Sherf L, James TN: A new look at some old questions in clinical electrocardiography. *Henry Ford Hosp. Med. Bull.* 14:265, 1966.
50. Mendez C: Characteristics of impulse propagation in the mammalian atioventricular node. In *Normal and Abnormal Conduction in the Heart.* Paes de Carvalho A, Hoffman BF Lieberman M (eds.). Mount Kisco NY, Futura, 1982, pp. 363–376.
51. De Mello WC: Intercellular communication in heart. In *Intercellular Communication.* De Mello WC (ed.). New York, Plenum 1977, pp. 87–125.
52. De Mello WC: Intercellular communication in cardiac muscle: Physiological and pathological implications. In *Cardiac Electrophysiology and Arrhythmias.* Zipes DP, Jalife J (eds.). Orlando Grune and Stratton, 1985, pp. 65–72.
53. Hermsmeyer K: Angiotensin II increases electrical coupling in mammalian ventricular myocardium. *Circ. Res.* 47:524, 1980.
54. Rosen MR, Robinson RB, Danilo P Jr: Developmental changes in cardiac-autonomic interactions. In *Cardiac Electrophysiology and Arrhythmias.* Zipes DP, Jalife J (eds.). Orlando, Grune and Stratton, 1984, pp. 159–164.
55. Danilo P Jr, Rosen MR, Hordof AJ: Effects of acetylcholine on the ventricular specialized conduction system of neonatal and adult dog. *Circ. Res.* 43:777, 1978.
56. Rosen MR, Hordof AJ, Ilvento JP, Danilo P, Jr: Effects of adrenergic amines on electrophysiological properties and automatic neonatal and adult canine Purkinje fibers. Evidence for alpha and beta adrenergic actions. *Circ. Res.* 40:390, 1977.
57. Friedman WF, Pool PE, Jacobowitz D, Seagren S, Braunwald E: Sympathetic innervation of the

developing rabbit heart: biochemical and histochemical comparison of fetal, neonatal, and adult myocardium. *Circ. Res.* 23:25, 1968.
58. Schifferli PY, Caldeyro-Barcia R: Effects of atropine and beta-adrenergic drugs on the heart rate of the human fetus. In *Fetal Pharmacology.* Boreus LO (ed.). New York, Raven Press, 1973, pp. 259–268.
59. Levy MN, Zieske H: Autonomic control of cardiac pacemaker activity and atrioventricular transmission. *J. Appl. Physiol.* 27:465, 1969.
60. Qi A, Tuna IC, Gornick C, Ring WS, Bolman RM, Benditt DG: Potentiation of cardiac electrophysiologic effects of verapamil following autonomic blockade or cardiac transplantation. (Abstract.) *Clin. Res.* 33:218A, 1985.
61. Prystowsky EN, Jackman WM, Rinkenberger RL, Heger JJ, Zipes DP: Effect of autonomic blockade on ventricular refractoriness and atrioventricular nodal conduction in humans. Evidence supporting a direct cholinergic action on ventricular muscle refractoriness. *Circ. Res.* 49:511 1981.
62. Castellanos A, Zaman L, Moleiro F, Aranda JM, Myerburg RJ: The Lown-Ganong-Levine syndrome. *PACE* 5:715, 1982.
63. Bauernfeind RA, Ayres BF, Wyndham CC, Dhingra RC, Swiryn SP, Strasberg B, Rosen KM: Cycle length in atrioventricular nodal reentrant paroxysmal tachycardia, observations on the Lown-Ganong-Levine syndrome. *Am. J. Cardiol.* 45:1148, 1980.
64. Lepeshkin E: Modern Electrocardiography. Volume I. The P-Q-R-S-T-U Complex. Baltimore, Williams and Wilkins, 1951, p. 237.
65. Jackman WM, Prystowsky EN, Naccarelli GV, Fineberg NS, Rahilly GT, Heger JJ, Zipes DP: Reevaluation of enhanced atrioventricular nodal conduction: Evidence to suggest a continuum of normal atrioventricular nodal physiology. *Circulation* 67:441, 1983.
66. Gallagher JJ, Sealy WC, Kasell J, Wallace AG: Multiple accessory pathways in patients with the pre-excitation syndrome. *Circulation* 54:571, 1976.
67. Benditt DG, Pritchett ELC, Smith WM, Wallace AG, Gallagher JJ: Characteristics of atrioventricular conduction and the spectrum of arrhythmias in Lown-Ganong-Levine syndrome. *Circulation* 57:454, 1978.
68. Holmes DR Jr, Hartzler GO, Maloney JD: Concealed retrograde bypass tracts and enhanced atrioventricular conduction. An unusual subset patients with refractory paroxysmal supraventricular tachycardia. *Am. J. Cardiol.* 45:1053, 1980.
69. Holmes DR Jr, Hartzler GO, Meredith J: The clinical and electrophysiologic characteristics of patients with accelerated atrioventricular nodal conduction. *Mayo Clin. Proc.* 57:339, 1982.
70. Frank R, Phan-Thuc H, Blanc P, Allali I, Goutte R, Vedel J, Fontaine G, Grosgogeat Y: La reponse nodale attenuee. *Arch. Mal Coeur* 73: 1007, 1980.
71. Bissett JK, Thompson AJ, deSoyza N, Murphy ML: Atrioventricular conduction in patients with short PR intervals and normal QRS complex. *Br. Heart J.* 35:123, 1973.
72. Bissett JK, deSoyza N, Kane JJ, Murphy ML: Altered refractory periods in patients with short PR intervals and normal QRS complex. *Am. J. Cardiol.* 35:487, 1975.
73. Iannone LA: Electrophysiology of atrial pacing in patients with short PR interval, normal QRS complex. *Am. Heart J.* 89:74, 1975.
74. Moleiro F, Mendoza IJ, Medina-Ravell V, Castellanos A, Myerburg RJ: One to one atrioventricular conduction during atrial pacing at rates of 300/minute in absence of Wolff-Parkinson-White syndrome. *Am. J. Cardiol.* 48:789, 1981.
75. Disertori M, Vergara G, Cozzi F, Inama G, Furlanello F: Il fenomeno della conduzione A-V accelerta. Studio elettrofisiologico con un farmaco calcioantagonista "selettivo" (Verapamil). *G. Ital. Cardiol.* II:447, 1981.
76. Ward DE, Bexton R, Camm AJ: Characteristics of atrio-His conduction in the short PR interval, normal QRS complex syndrome. Evidence for enhanced slow pathway conduction. *Eur. Heart J.* 4:882, 1983.
77. Seipel L, Breithardt G, Both A: Atrioventricular (AV) and ventriculoatrial (VA) conduction pattern in patients with short PR interval and normal QRS complex. In *Cardiac Pacing. Diagnostic and Therapeutic Tools.* Luderlitz B (ed.). Berlin, Springer-Verlag, 1976, pp. 152–163.
78. Wu D, Denes P, Dhingra R, Khan A, Rosen KM: The effects of propranolol on induction of AV nodal reentrant paroxysmal tachycardia. *Circulation* 50:665, 1974.
79. Wu D, Wyndham CC, Amat-Y-Leon F, Denes P, Dhingra RC, Rosen KM: The effects of ouabain on induction of atrioventricular reentrant paroxysmal supraventricular tachycardia. *Circulation* 52:201 1975.
80. Moro C, Cosio FG: Electrophysiologic study of patients with short PR interval and normal QRS complex. *Eur. J. Cardiol.* II:81, 1980.
81. Wiener I: Syndromes of Lown-Ganong-Levine and enhanced atrioventricular nodal conduction. *Am. J. Cardiol.* 52:637, 1983.
82. Clerc A, Robert-Levy, Cristesco C: A propos du raccourcissement permanent de l'espace P-R de l'electrocardiogramme sans deformation du complexe ventriculaire. *Arch. Mal Coeur* 31:569, 1938.
83. Lown B, Ganong WF, Levine SA: The syndrome of short PR interval, normal QRS complex and

paroxysmal rapid heart action. *Circulation* 5: 693, 1952.
84. Ward DE, Camm J: Mechanisms of junctional tachycardias in the Lown-Ganong-Levine syndrome. *Am. Heart J.* 105:169, 1983.
85. Josephson ME, Kastor JA: Supraventricular tachycardia in the Lown-Ganong-Levine syndrome: atrionodal versus intranodal reentry. *Am. J. Cardiol.* 40:521, 1977.
86. Castellanos A, Vagueiro MC, Befeler B, Myerburg RJ: Syndrome of short PR, narrow QRS and repetitive supraventricular tachyarrhythmias: the possible occurrence of the R-on-T phenomenon and the limits of syndrome. *Eur. J. Cardiol.* 2:337, 1975.
87. Myerburg RJ, Sung RJ, Castellanos A: Ventricular tachycardia and ventricular fibrillation in patients with short P-R intervals and narrow QRS complexes. *PACE* 2:568, 1979.
88. Benditt DG, Benson DW Jr, Dunnigan A, Gornick CC, Anderson RW: Atrial flutter, atrial fibrillation, and other primary atrial tachycardias. *Med. Clin. N.A.* 68:895, 1984.
89. Dunnigan A, Pierpont ME, Smith SA, Breningstall G, Benditt DG, Benson DW, Jr: Cardiac and skeletal myopathy associated with cardiac dysrhythmias. *Am. J. Cardiol.* 53:731, 1984.
90. Seipel L, Both A, Loggen F: Die atrioventrikulare Erregungsleitung beim Lown-Ganong-Levine-Syndrome. *Z. Kardiol.* 64:20, 1975.
91. Gallagher JJ, German LD, Broughton A, Guarnieri T, Trantham JL: Variants of the preexcitation syndrome. In *Frontiers of Cardiac Electrophysiology*. Rosenbaum MB, Elizari MV (eds.). Boston, Martinus Nijhoff 1983, pp. 724–772.
92. Scheinman MM, Morady F, Hess DS, Gonzales P: Catheter-induced ablation of the atrioventricular junction to control refractory suppraventricular arrhythmias. *JAMA* 278:851, 1982.
93. Scheinman MM, Evans-Bell T and the Executive Committee of the Percutaneous Cardiac Mapping and Ablation Registry: Catheter ablation of the atrioventricular junction: a report of the percutaneous mapping and ablation registry. *Circulation* 70:1024, 1984.

13. ENHANCED AV CONDUCTION: CHARACTERISTICS OF RETROGRADE CONDUCTION

Anne Hamilton Dougherty
Gerald V. Naccarelli

Enhanced atrioventricular conduction (EAVC) is an electrophysiologic descriptor applied to one extreme in the clinical spectrum of atrioventricular (AV) nodal conduction properties [1]. Although EAVC has been variously defined (see Benditt et al. this volume), it is used in this chapter to indicate the presence of 1:1 AV conduction at cycle lengths of 300 ms or less.

EAVC achieves clinical significance only when associated with arrhythmias. A rapidly conducting AV node increases susceptibility to very rapid tachycardia rates during certain supraventricular tachyarrhythmias and consequently hemodynamic compromise may occur. Supraventricular tachyarrhythmias which have been described in patients with EAVC include atrial fibrillation and flutter, ectopic atrial tachycardia, intraatrial and sinus node reentrant tachycardia, reciprocating tachycardia (RT) due to reentry within the AV node, and RT associated with accessory AV connections [2–5]. It is the purpose of this discussion to explore the electrophysiologic characteristics of ventriculoatrial (VA) conduction in EAVC patients without accessory AV connections.

Benditt, D.G. and Benson, D.W., Cardiac Preexcitation Syndromes.

Characteristics of retrograde AV nodal conduction

As a preface to the decription of retrograde conduction in EAVC patients, it is useful to review what is know about retrograde (VA) conduction. Schuilenburg [6] has demonstrated that, among patients with normal antegrade AV node conduction, 68% were capable of retrograde atrial activation via the AV node during ventricular pacing. With increasing degrees of antegrade AV nodal dysfunction, the fraction capable of retrograde conduction was diminishingly small. Akhtar et al. [7] determined that antegrade AV conduction could be maintained at faster pacing rates than retrograde VA conduction in most patients (72%), whereas retrograde conduction was "better than" antegrade in only 12%. On the other hand, retrograde VA conduction intervals are typically shorter than AV conduction intervals [8].

The anatomic pathway which maintains VA conduction in patients without accessory AV connections remains a source of speculation. In many individuals, VA conduction intervals prolong very little in response to incremental ventricular pacing and block occurs abruptly. This "all-or-none" phenomenon, which resembles that seen in accessory AV connections more closely than it does the behavior of the antegrade AV nodal system [9], has led to the suggestion that the VA conduction system is anatomically separate from the AV node, formed by either an extranodal AV connection in close proximity to the node or by the atriofascicular bypass tracts described by Brechenmacher [10–12]. Compelling evidence against this hypothesis includes the fact that during RT due to reentry within the AV node, the atrium can be shown not to be a necessary part of the reentrant circuit [5,13,14], suggesting that VA conduction occurs within the AV node.

The observed differences in electrophysiologic characteristics of antegrade and retrograde conduction via the AV node are consistant with the theory of summation [15,16,17,18]. Whereas the wavefront of activation arrives at the upper portion of the AV node in a broad, heterogenous fashion in the antegrade direction, the retrograde input is funneled through the penetrating bundle of the specialized cardiac conduction system in a synchronized wavefront, potentially facilitating conduction by summation of input. Another factor which may influence conduction properties in the same tissue is the direction in which interfaces (e.g., the atrial muscle-transitional cell interface) are approached. This effect has been demonstrated in the isthmus preparation described by de la Fuente et al. [19].

Characteristics of retrograde conduction in EAVC

We have studied retrograde conduction in 21 EAVC patients without accessory AV connections. VA conduction was demonstrated in 17/21 (81%) EAVC patients compared to 64% in a control group of patients with normal AV node conduction characteristics in the antegrade direction. Furthermore, 1:1 VA conduction was maintained at significantly faster pacing rates in EAVC patients compared to controls, correlating well with the rates to which 1:1 antegrade AV conduction could be maintained (see Figure 13–1) [20]. Similar conclusions were reached by Bauernfeind et al. [21], who found that among all patients with "dual AV nodal physiology," those with shorter AH intervals were more likely to have retrograde VA conduction and more likely to have clinical RT.

Among EAVC patients in whom VA conduction was present, 1:1 AV conduction could be maintained at faster pacing rates than 1:1 VA conduction. Retrograde conduction was "better than" antegrade in 2/21 (9.5%) and equal to antegrade conduction in another 2/21 (9.5%). In control patients with normal AV node function, results were similar to those reported by Akhtar et al. [7]; antegrade conduction was "better" in 10/14 (71%) and "worse" in 4/14 (29%).

VA conduction time curves determined during incremental ventricular pacing in 15 EAVC patients without accessory AV connections are shown in Figure 13–2. Although several curves terminate with Wenckebach periodicity, 9/15 remain quite flat (maximum increase in VA interval from sinus cycle length to minimal paced cycle length maintaining 1:1 VA conduction ≤20 msec). The absence of progressive prolongation in VA intervals with increasing pacing rates in these 10 patients is similar to that observed in patients with accessory AV connections [9] (Figure 13–3). The site of retrograde block was clearly identified in 7 patients, and in all instances block occurred above the level of the His bundle. "Dual AV nodal physiology" in the antegrade direction was observed in eight patients and dual AV nodal physiology in the retrograde direction in 4. Two of the 21 patients were observed to have discontinuous curves in both the antegrade and retrograde directions.

Detailed sequences of retrograde atrial septal activation have not been specifically studied in EAVC patients. In unselected patients with symptomatic RT due to reentry within the AV node, however, atrial activation is first observed in the low septal right atrium near the orifice of the coronary sinus or in the vicinity of the His bundle [13].

Dual AV nodal physiology in EAVC

Dual AV nodal physiology has been frequently observed in patients with and without EAVC, and reentry within the AV node is a common mechanism of paroxsymal supraventricular tachycardia in these patients [4–5]. As in patients without EAVC, the slower AV nodal pathway usually forms the antegrade limb and the fast nodal pathway the retrograde limb of the circuit in EAVC patients. Because of similarities in their electrophysiologic properties, it is commonly assumed that the retrograde "fast" pathway traversed during tachycardia is anatomically the same as the antegrade fast pathway observed during sinus or atrial-paced rhythms; however, this concept remains unproven and will be discussed later.

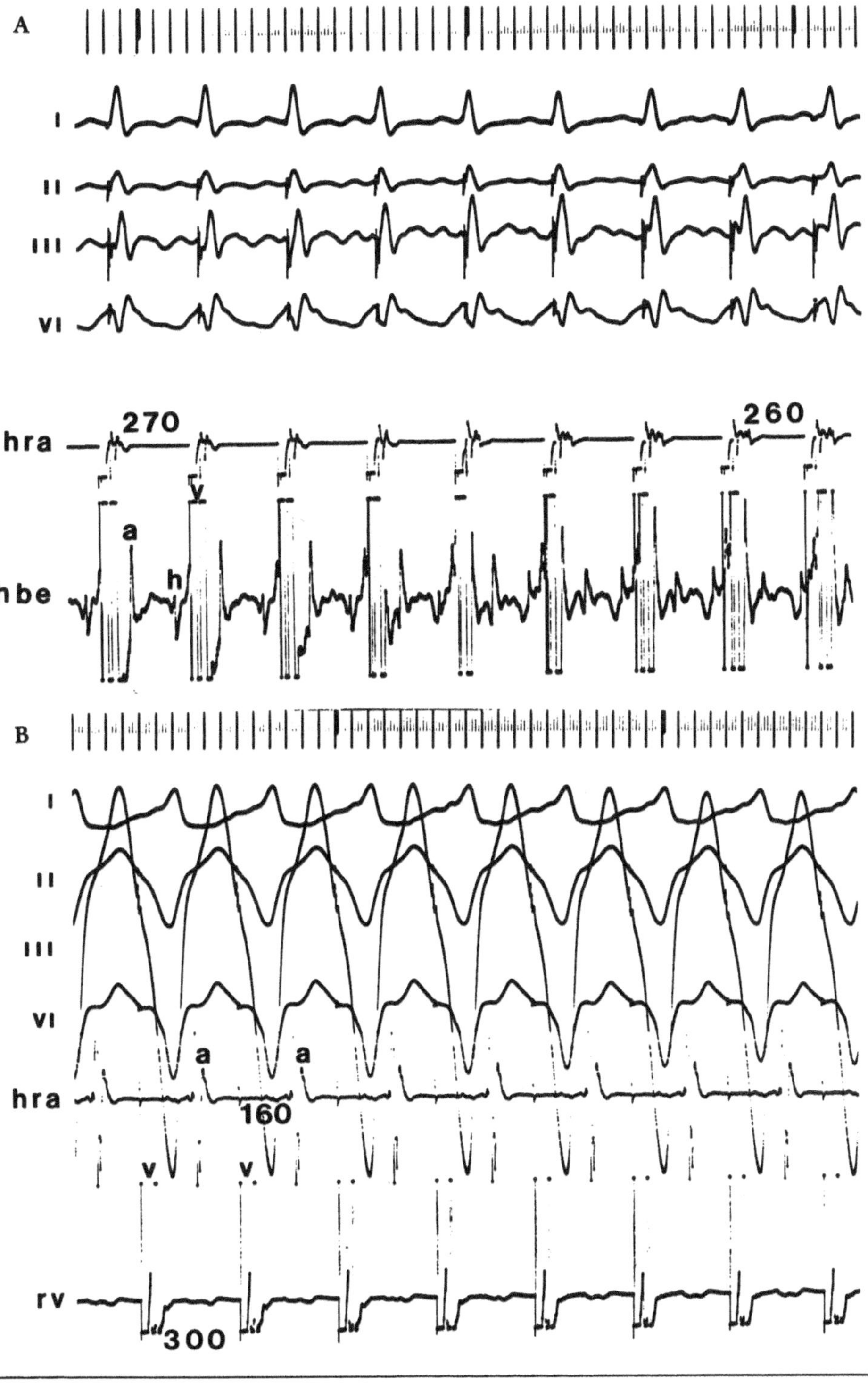

FIGURE 13–1. Rapid antegrade and retrograde AV nodal conduction in an EAVC patient with paroxysmal atrial fibrillation. (A) demonstrates 1:1 AV conduction during incremental atrial pacing at cycle lengths up to 270 msec. At this rate, the AH interval is minimally prolonged (120 msec). (B) shows incremental ventricular pacing in the same patient showing maintenance of 1:1 VA conduction at a cycle length of 300 ms.

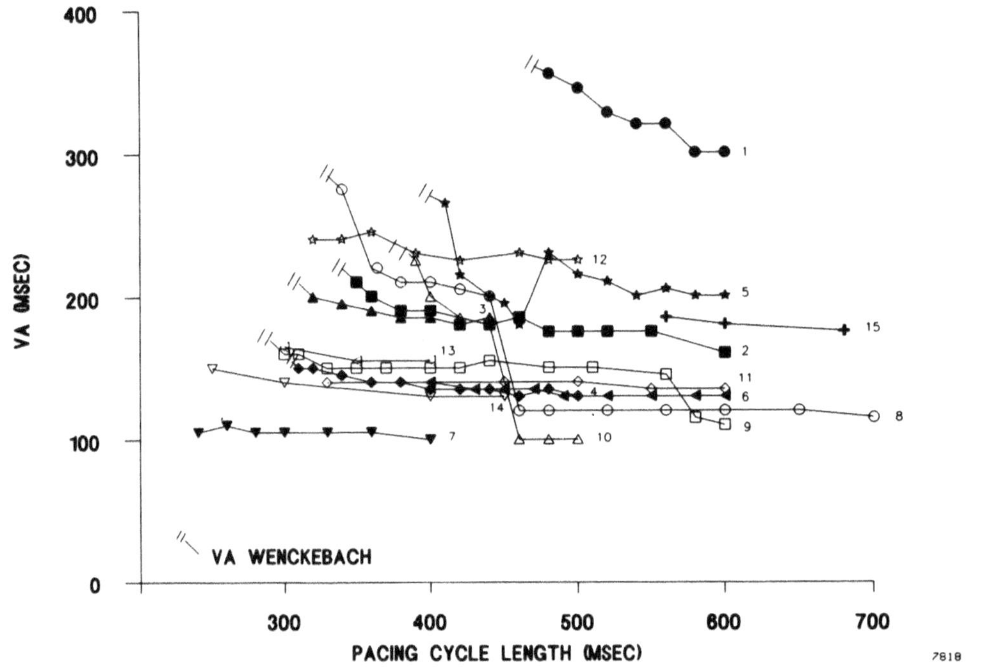

FIGURE 13–2. VA conduction intervals during incremental ventricular pacing in 15 patients without accessory AV connections capable of 1:1 antegrade AV conduction at atrial pacing cycle lengths ≤300 ms. Patients numbered 5, 8, 10, and 12 showed evidence of "dual AV nodal physiology" in the retrograde direction during either incremental ventricular pacing or extrastimulus technique.

The tachycardia rate in AV nodal reentry is not significantly faster than that in similar patients without EAVC because the cycle length is determined primarily by the conduction velocity of the slower antegrade pathway, which becomes the rate-limiting limb [22–23]. EAVC patients, however, may be susceptible to frequent sustained tachycardias if both antegrade and retrograde limbs are fast [21].

In contrast, when RT utilizes an accessory AV connection in patients with EAVC, the tachycardia rate is significantly faster [23–24] than in non-EAVC patients. Orthodromic RT traversing the enhanced AV node antegrade and the accessory AV connection retrograde may be particularly rapid, characteristically over 200 bpm. In this case, the tachycardia cycle length is determined predominantly by the characteristics of the accessory connection, which may be slower than the antegrade limb. Theoretically, orthodromic RT may be less frequently inducible or sustainable in EAVC than in non-EAVC patients if the critical antegrade AV nodal delay necessary to initiate tachycardia is not present [24].

An unusual form of AV nodal RT associated with dual AV nodal physiology in the retrograde direction has been described by Wu et al. in patients without EAVC [25]. As opposed to the more common slow-fast RT, the unusual form traverses a fast AV nodal pathway in the antegrade direction and a slow AV nodal pathway in the retrograde direction. Strasberg et al. [26] have demonstrated dual AV nodal physiology in the retrograde direction in 3.5% of their patients. Both slow-fast and fast-slow AV nodal RT could be induced in this group. A noteworthy finding was that several patients (23%) were capable of 1:1 AV conduction at rates of 200 bpm or more, including one patient with a documented history of spontaneous sustained fast-slow RT. These patients may present with an incessant tachycardia, which has been described in young patients [27–28].

Evidence has been presented to suggest that, specifically in the presence of dual AV nodal

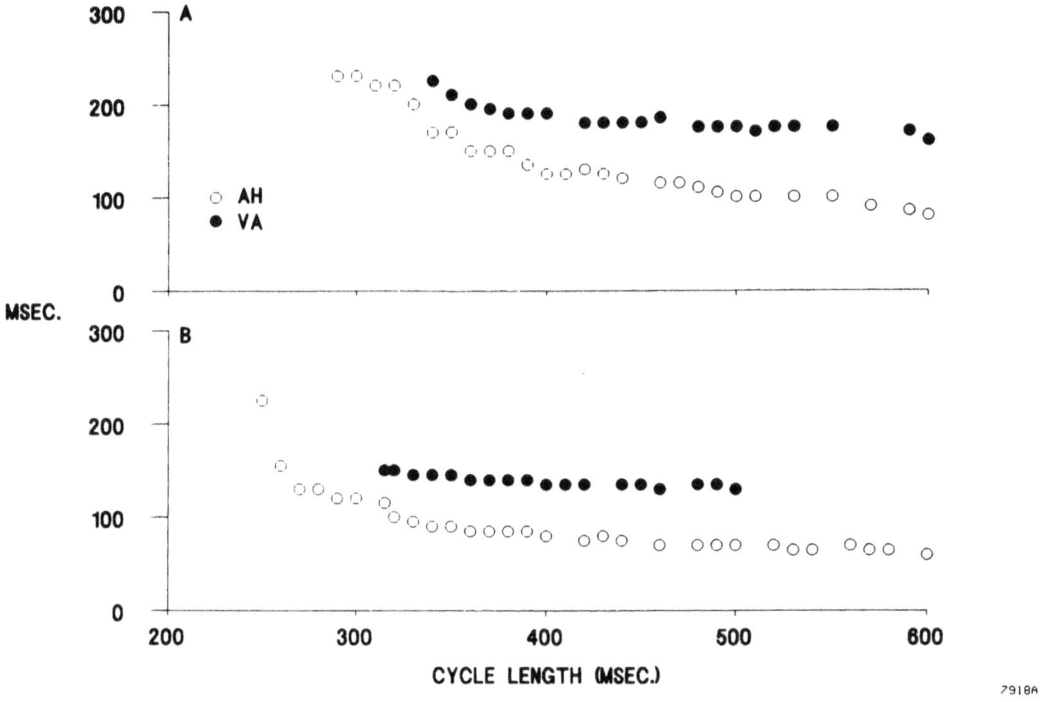

FIGURE 13–3. Antegrade and retrograde conduction intervals in two patients with incremental atrial (O = AH interval) and ventricular (● = VA interval) pacing. (A) Patient with AV node-like retrograde conduction. Antegrade 1:1 AV conduction is maintained to a cycle length of 290 ms, although progressive AH prolongation occurs. Gradual prolongation of VA conduction time with ventricular pacing is also observed. (B) Patient with accessory AV connection-like retrograde conduction. Minimal prolongation of VA conduction intervals occurs with incremental ventricular pacing.

physiology in the retrograde direction, two anatomically separate retrograde pathways are involved. Sung et al. showed varying atrial activation sequences, depending on whether the fast or slow pathway was traversed [29]. Earliest activation was observed in the low septal right atrium near the His bundle when the fast pathway was utilized and in the region of the proximal coronary sinus with slow pathway conduction. Similar conclusions were reached by Smith et al. [30] who were able to ablate conduction by either antegrade or retrograde pathway alone by catheter technique without affecting function in the other pathway in patients with dual AV nodal physiology in the retrograde direction. Furthermore, Gomes et al. were able to demonstrate a differential effect of procainimide on the antegrade and retrograde fast pathways, enhancing the former and depressing the latter in the same patients [31]. This discrepancy led the authors to conclude that the fast pathway in the antegrade direction is not necessarily the same as the fast pathway in the retrograde direction.

Modulators of Retrograde AV Nodal Conduction (Ventriculoatrial Conduction)

Our data suggests that retrograde AV nodal conduction in normal and EAVC patients is modulated by the autonomic nervous system in a balanced fashion (Figure 13–4). This effect appears to be concordant in magnitude and direction to the effect on antegrade conduction in a given patient [20]. Furthermore, following autonomic blockade with atropine and propranolol, intrinsic retrograde AV nodal conduction closely parallels intrinsic antegrade conduction.

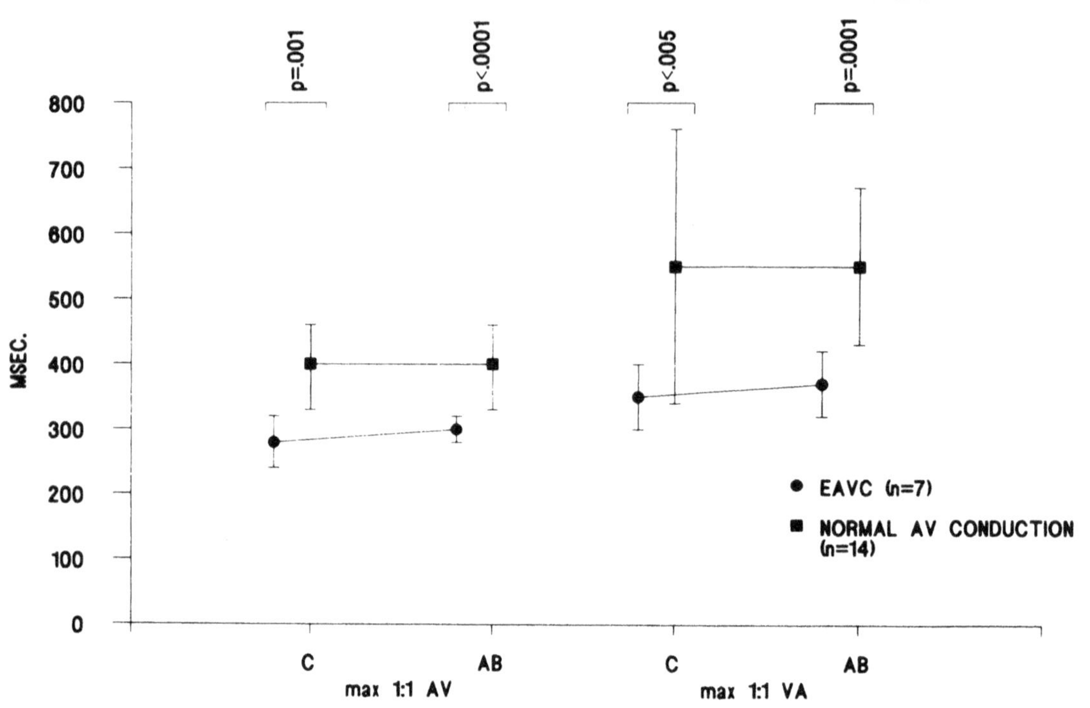

FIGURE 13–4. Effect of autonomic blockade (AB) with atropine and propranolol in patients with normal AV node conduction and EAVC. No significant mean change in either antegrade or retrograde conduction was observed in either group, suggesting a balanced sympathetic and parasympathetic effect. 1:1 VA conduction is maintained to a significantly faster rate in EAVC patients in both control (C) and AB states.

Although we were unable to demonstrate a significant mean change in either antegrade or retrograde conduction following autonomic blockade, Benditt et al. [32] did show a small, but significant lengthening of the minimum paced cycle length maintaining 1:1 antegrade AV conduction in EAVC patients, but not in other patients. This suggests a predominant sympathetic influence on antegrade conduction. Nonetheless, antegrade conduction did not normalize in the EAVC group, leading the authors to conclude (as we have) that there was a significant intrinsic difference between the two groups, independent of autonomic effects.

The effects of digitalis and antiarrhythmic drugs on retrograde conduction have not been demonstrated specifically in patients with EAVC, and can only be inferred from studies on unselected patients with RT within the AV node and on pacemaker patients with undesired VA conduction. Gomes et al. [11] noted that ouabain slowed or blocked retrograde conduction only in those patients who had in the control study demonstrated longer H-Ae (His to atrial echo) intervals and a progressive increase in VA conduction time during incremental ventricular pacing, analogous to the Wenckebach periodicity commonly observed during conduction in the antegrade direction. Retrograde pathways with short H-Ae intervals and flat VA interval curves (resembling accessory AV connection curves) were unaffected by ouabain.

Calcium channel blockade with intravenous verapamil produces prolongation of retrograde VA conduction intervals in most patients and occasionally produces VA block [33–36]. Hamer et al. [36] have demonstrated that the extent of this effect can, in fact, be predicted from the characteristics of retrograde conduction in the control state. As in the ouabain-sensitive group described by Gomes et al. [11], those patients exhibiting progressive delay in VA conduction intervals during incremental ventricular pacing were most susceptible to verapamil-induced conduction delay and block. Those with fixed VA conduction with pacing (flat curves), however, showed neither conduction delay nor block after verapamil.

Antiarrhythmic drugs which act primarily by blocking the sodium channel appear to have more potent effects on retrograde conduction. The results are similar to those observed in Purkinje fibers and accessory AV connections. Uniform slowing of VA conduction and occasional VA block have been demonstrated with procainamide, quinidine, ajmaline, and flecainide [31,35,37,38]. The latter may be the most potent, producing VA block in 10/14 patients in one series [35].

The variability in functional characteristics of VA conduction and its response to pharmacologic interventions suggests that there may be many types of functional or anatomic pathways within the AV node, with individual properties governing direction of conduction, sensitivity to autonomic manipulation, and sodium and calcium channel dependence. Although perhaps functionally insulated from one another, the tracts need not necessarily be anatomically separate. The relative density of each type of pathway in a given patient as well as the absolute volume of AV nodal tissue may then determine the functional characteristics of antegrade and retrograde conduction in that individual. It appears that there is far more variability in the retrograde conduction system than in the antegrade.

Clinical Significance of Retrograde Conduction Characteristics

Whether RT is due to reentry within the AV node or utilizes an accessory AV connection, the relationship between conduction and refractoriness of the antegrade and retrograde pathways determines the probability of initiating and sustaining tachycardia by governing the width of the echo zone. If the conduction time of the reentry circuit is longer than the effective refractory periods of any of its parts, RT can be established and maintained. However, when one limb is capable of very rapid conduction, as is the antegrade limb in EAVC patients, a critical delay must occur in the other limb in order to permit initiation of and sustaining RT. Since EAVC patients tend also to have more rapid retrograde conduction, RT may actually be less likely to occur, unless the refractory periods of both limbs are also short. In this instance, however, extremely rapid tachycardia rates are possible. A high rate of symptoms with very rapid rates may, in fact, account for disproportionate selection of these patients for electrophysiologic study.

Antiarrhythmic agents which slow retrograde conduction without total blockade may actually widen the echo zone and increase the frequency of spontaneous, albeit slower, tachycardia. Retrograde conduction may be particularly difficult to block in EAVC patients with an underdeveloped AV node and rapid retrograde conduction. Therefore, antiarrhythmic agents used to attack retrograde conduction should be selected for a high probability of total VA blockade or used in combination with agents which depress antegrade conduction or prolong refractoriness. Nonpharmacologic ablative techniques may be necessary to block retrograde conduction in selected patients unresponsive to drug therapy.

Summary

VA conduction is a common finding in EAVC patients. Compared to patients with normal AV node conduction in the antegrade direction, 1:1 retrograde conduction can be maintained at faster pacing rates in this group. Although VA conduction curves in some EAVC patients exhibit Wenckebach periodicity similar to that seen in antegrade AV node conduction, many others show a flat all-or-none response similar to that observed in accessory AV connection tissue. The anatomic structure(s) responsible for retrograde conduction have not been clearly demonstrated, although it is probably the AV node in most patients.

Modulation of retrograde conduction by the autonomic nervous system is balanced in EAVC patients, as it is in normal patients. Following pharmacologic autonomic blockade, changes are concordant in magnitude and direction in individual patients to the effects on antegrade AV node conduction. Although not specifically tested in a large group of EAVC patients, it is presumed from studies on other patients that sodium channel blocking agents have more potent inhibitory effects on retrograde conduction than do either ouabain or calcium channel blocking agents. Furthermore, the response to antiarrhythmic drugs may be dependent upon the baseline characteristics of the retrograde conduction system.

The characteristics of the VA conduction system are clinically important in EAVC patients with RT involving reentry within the AV node, as well as in those with RT associated with accessory AV connections. In those patients with rapid retrograde conduction, pharmacologic blockade of the retrograde limb may be particularly difficult. Further elucidation of the anatomy and physiology of the VA conduction system in these patients may lead to more effective antiarrhythmic therapy.

References

1. Jackman WM, Prystowsky EN, Naccarelli GV, Fineberg NS, Rahilly GT, Heger JJ, Zipes DP: Reevaluation of enhanced atrioventricular nodal conduction: evidence to suggest a continuum of normal atrioventricular nodal physiology. *Circulation* 67:441, 1983.
2. Lown B, Ganong WF, Levine SA. The syndrome of short PR interval, normal QRS complex and paroxysmal rapid heart action. *Circulation* 5:693, 1952.
3. Benditt DG, Pritchett ELC, Smith WM, Wallace AG, Gallagher JJ. Characteristics of atrioventricular conduction and the spectrum of arrhythmias in Lown-Ganong-Levine syndrome. *Circulation* 57:454, 1978.
4. Castellanos A, Castillo CA, Agha AS, Tessler M. His bundle electrograms in patients with short PR intervals, narrow QRS complexes, and paroxysmal tachycardias. *Circulation* 43:667, 1971.
5. Josephson ME, Kastor JA. Supraventricular tachycardia in Lown-Ganong-Levine syndrome: atrionodal versus intranodal reentry. *Am. J. Cardiol.* 40:521, 1977.
6. Schuilenburg RM: Patterns of V–A conduction in the human heart in the presence of normal and abnormal A–V conduction. In *The conduction system of the heart: structure, function and clinical implications*, Wellens HJJ, Lie KI, Janse MJ. (eds.). Philadelphia, 1976, Lea and Febiger, p. 485.
7. Akhtar M, Damato AN, Batsford WP, Ruskin JN, Ogunkelu JB: A comparative analysis of antegrade and retrograde conduction patterns in man. *Circulation* 52:766, 1975.
8. Narula OS: Retrograde pre-excitation: comparison of antegrade and retrograde conduction intervals in man. *Circulation* 50:1129, 1974.
9. Svenson RH, Miller HC, Gallagher JJ, Wallace AG: Electrophysiological evaluation of the Wolff-Parkinson-White syndrome: problems in assessing antegrade and retrograde conduction over the accessory pathway. *Circulation* 52:552, 1975.
10. Brechenmacher C: Atrio-His bundle tracts. *Br. Heart J.* 37:853, 1975.
11. Gomes JAC, Dhatt MS, Rubenson DS, Damato AN: Electrophysiologic evidence for selective retrograde utilization of a specialized conducting system in atrioventricular nodal reentrant tachycardia. *Am. J. Cardiol.* 43:687, 1979.
12. Gomes JAC, Dhatt MS, Damato AN, Akhtar M, Holder CA: Incidence, determinants and significance of fixed retrograde conduction in the region of the atrioventricular node. *Am. J. Cardiol.* 44:1089, 1979.
13. Kerr CR, Benson DW, Gallagher JJ: Role of specialized conducting fibers in the genesis of "AV nodal" re-entry tachycardia. *PACE* 6:171, 1983.
14. Ko PT, Naccarelli GV, Gulamhusein S, Prystowsky EN, Zipes DP, Klein GJ: Atrioventricular dissociation during paroxysmal junctional tachycardia. *PACE* 4:670, 1981.
15. Cranefield PF, Hoffman BF: Conduction of the cardiac impulse. II. summation and inhibition. *Circ. Res.* 28:220, 1971.
16. Janse MJ: Influence of the direction of the atrial wave front on A–V nodal transmission in isolated hearts of rabbits. *Circ. Res.* 25:439, 1969.
17. Zipes DP, Mendez C, Moe GK: Evidence for summation and voltage dependency in rabbit atrioventricular nodal fibers. *Circ. Res.* 32:170, 1973.
18. Wu D: Dual atrioventricular nodal pathways: a reappraisal. *PACE* 5:72, 1982.
19. De la Fuente D, Sasynink B, Moe GK: Conduction through a narrow isthmus in isolated canine atrial tissue: a model of the W-P-W syndrome. *Circulation* 44:803, 1971.
20. Dougherty AH, Naccarelli GV, Rinkenberger RL: Ventriculoatrial and atrioventricular conduction during autonomic blockade. (Abstract.) *Circulation* 70:II-375, 1984.
21. Bauernfiend, RA, Swiryn S, Strasberg B, Palileo E, Wyndham C, Duffy CE, Rosen KM: Analysis of anterograde and retrograde fast pathway properties in patients with dual atrioventricular nodal pathways: observations regarding the pathophysiology of the Lown-Ganong-Levine syndrome. *Am. J. Cardiol.* 49:283, 1982.
22. Bauernfiend RA, Ayres BF, Wyndham CC, Dhingra RC, Swiryn SP, Strasberg B, Rosen KM: Cycle length in atrioventricular nodal reentrant paroxysmal tachycardia with observations

on the Lown-Ganong-Levine Syndrome. *Am. J. Cardiol.* 45:1148, 1980.
23. Benditt DG, Epstein ML Arentzen CE, Kriett JM, Klein GJ: Enhanced atrioventricular conduction in patients without preexcitation syndrome: relation to heart rate in paroxysmal reciprocating tachycardia. *Circulation* 65:1474, 1982.
24. Gallagher JJ, Sealy WC, Kasell J, Wallace AG: Multiple accessory pathways in patients with the pre-excitation syndrome. *Circulation* 54:571, 1976.
25. Wu D, Denes P, Amat-y-Leon F, Wyndham CRC, Dhingra R, Rosen KM: An unususal variety of atrioventricular nodal re-entry due to retrograde dual atrioventricular nodal pathways.*Circulation* 56:50, 1977.
26. Strasberg B, Swiryn S, Bauernfeind R, Palileo E, Scagliotti D, Duffy CE, Rosen KM: Retrograde dual atrioventricular nodal pathways. *Am. J. Cardiol.* 48:639, 1981.
27. Coumel P: Junctional reciprocating tachycardias. The permanent and paroxsymal forms of A-V nodal reciprocating tachycardias. *J. Electrocardiol.* 8:79, 1975.
28. Wolff GS, Sung RJ, Pickoff A, Garcia OL, Werblin R, Ferrer PL, Tamer D, Gelband H: The fast-slow form of atrioventricular nodal reentrant tachycardia in children. *Am. J. Cardiol.* 43:1181, 1979.
29. Sung RJ, Waxman HL: Physiologic shift of retrograde atrioventricular nodal output mimicking retrograde accessory pathway conduction (Abstract.) *Circulation* 60:II–191, 1979.
30. Smith RT, Gillette PC, Garson A, Massumi A, MeVey P: Evidence that some "AV node reentry" involves two anatomically separate pathways. (Abstract.) *J. Am. Coll. Cardiol.* 3:483, 1984.
31. Gomes JAC, Kang PS, Kelen G, Khan R, El-Sherif N: Simultaneous anterograde fast-slow atrioventricular nodal pathway conduction after procainamide. *Am. J. Cardiol.* 46:677, 1980.
32. Benditt DG, Klein GJ, Kriett JM, Dunnigan A, Benson DW: Enhanced atrioventricular nodal conduction in man: electrophysiologic effects of pharmacologic autonomic blockade. *Circulation* 69:1088, 1984.
33. Klein GJ, Gulamhusein S, Prystowsky EN, Carruthers SG, Donner AP, Ko PT: Comparison of the electrophysiologic effects of intraveneous and oral verapamil in patients with paroxsymal supraventricular tachycardia. *Am. J. Cardiol.* 49:117, 1982.
34. Shenasa M, Denker S, Mahmud R, Lehmann M, Murthy VS, Akhtar M: Effect of verapamil on retrograde atrioventricular nodal conduction in the human heart. *J. Am. Coll. Cardiol.* 2:545, 1983.
35. Morley CA, Perrins EJ, Dixey J, Sutton R: The pharmacological blockade of retrograde atrioventricular conduction in paced patients. (Abstract.) *PACE* 6:312, 1983.
36. Hamer A, Peter T, Mandel W: Atrioventricular node reentry: intravenous verapamil as a method of defining multiple electrophysiologic types. *Am. Heart J.* 105:629, 1983.
37. Bauernfeind RA, Wyndham CR, Dhingra RC, Swiryn SP, Palileo E, Strasberg B, Rosen KM: Serial electrophysiologic testing of multiple drugs in patients with atrioventricular nodal reentrant paroxsymal tachycardia. *Circulation* 62:1341, 1980.
38. Shenasa M, Gilbert CJ, Schmidt DH, Akhtar M: Procainamide and retrograde atrioventricular nodal conduction in man. *Circulation* 65:355, 1982.

14. PREEXCITATION SYNDROMES ASSOCIATED WITH CONGENITAL HEART DISEASE

Co-burn J. Porter
David R. Holmes, Jr.

Although preexcitation is a congenital heart defect, the focus of this chapter will be on the congenital heart abnormalities associated with preexcitation. The simultaneous occurrence of preexcitation syndromes with tachyarrhythmias and certain types of congenital heart disease — for example, Ebstein's malformation — is not unexpected, considering the developmental abnormalities and anatomic substrates involved. Each separate problem may affect the clinical presentation and the management of the other. Because structural anomalies and hemodynamic abnormalities result in dilatation and fibrosis, causing atrial and ventricular ectopy, episodes of tachycardia may be frequent and poorly tolerated. Conversely, frequent episodic or prolonged tachycardia (or both) may result in further deterioration of hemodynamics, in subendocardial ischemia, and in the development of additional structural abnormalities with further fibrosis and chamber dilatation. In addition to these interrelationships, treatment may be affected by the simultaneous occurrence of tachycardia and structural or hemodynamic abnormalities. For example, the use of beta-adrenergic blockers, while helpful in treating many patients with preexcitation syndromes and supraventricular tachycardia, may aggravate or be contraindicated in patients with congenital heart disease and ventricular dysfunction.

The two problems of preexcitation syndrome and congenital heart disease entail evaluation of the anatomic-pathophysiologic substrates involved with each. This chapter evaluates the combined problems and addresses the factors that influence clinical management, including medical and surgical therapy of the most common congenital heart disease associated with preexcitation syndrome, Ebstein's anomaly. Once the philosophy in managing patients with Ebstein's anomaly and preexcitation syndrome is understood, these same principles of management can be applied to other patients with congenital heart disease and preexcitation syndrome.

Definitions and Anatomy

The term *preexcitation* was first used by Öhnell in 1944 [1]. Initially, it was defined as a condition in which all or part of the ventricular myocardium is activated by an atrial impulse earlier than if that atrial impulse had traveled through the normal specialized conduction tissues alone to activate the ventricle [2]. The concept explains the electrocardiographic findings seen in patients with the Wolff-Parkinson-White (WPW) syndrome, in which the PR interval generally is short, reflecting the lack of usual delayed conduction through the

Benditt, D.G. and Benson, D.W., Cardiac Preexcitation Syndromes.

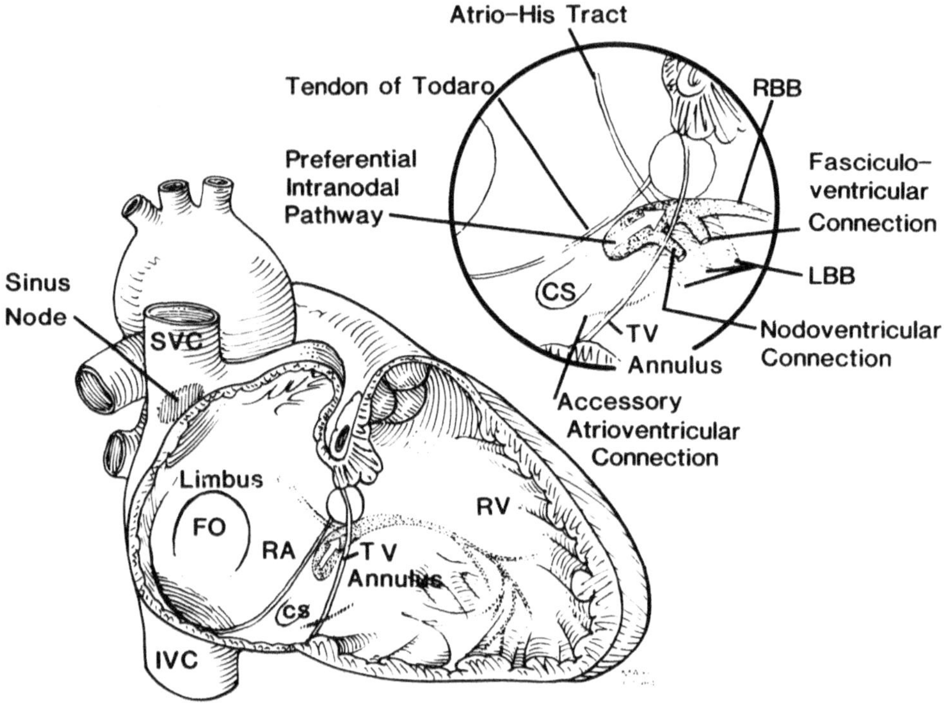

FIGURE 14–1. Drawing showing possible anatomic substrates causing preexcitation syndromes. *CS* = coronary sinus; *FO* = foramen ovale; *IVC* = inferior vena cava; *LBB* = left bundle branch; *RA* = right atrium; *RBB* = right bundle branch; *RV* = right ventricle; *SVC* = superior vena cava; and *TV* = tricuspid valve. See text. (By permission of Mayo Foundation.)

atrioventricular node and the broadened QRS complex with a delta wave representing varied degrees of fusion between the normal QRS complex and the premature ventricular activation. Since then, the concept of preexcitation has been broadened to include anatomic pathways that allow impulses to travel retrogradely from the ventricle to the atrium without traversing the specialized conduction tissue [3]. In this latter type, the surface electrocardiogram is normal, but similar arrhythmias may be seen as in patients with preexcitation. For this presentation both categories will be included.

Anatomic substrates that can explain the preexcitation syndromes have been proposed and documented histologically, electrophysiologically, and both (Figure 14–1). The classification of accessory pathways proposed by the European Study Group for Preexcitation will be used: the term *connection* describes anomalous conduction pathways that insert into ventricular muscle and the term *tract* describes anomalous conduction pathways that insert into specialized conduction tissue [4]. Accessory atrioventricular (AV) muscle connections, formerly known as Kent bundles, originate from and insert into working myocardium and may be free-wall or septal in location.

Controversy has existed concerning AV nodal bypass tracts with direct connections from the atrium to the His bundle (atriofascicular bypass tracts) or from the atrium to the lower AV noda via intranodal bypass tracts [5–8]. Preexcitation may also be the result of accessory nodoventricular or fasciculoventricular connections (Mahaim fibers). Accessory nodoventricular connections originate from the AV node and insert into either the ventricular myocardium or possibly the specialized cardiac conduction system, whereas accessory fasciculoventricular connections connect the specialized cardiac conduction system to the ventricular myocardium.

Developmental Aspects

In early cardiac development, the embryonic heart tube folds on itself and divides into four separate chambers with four separate valves. During this process, the AV junction undergoes a transformation whereby the atrial musculature is separated and insulated from that of the ventricles by the fibrofatty tissue that becomes the tricuspid and mitral valve anuli [9]. During this time, defects in the formation of the AV junction can occur, resulting in a congenital heart defect that also may arrest the development of a mature fibrous (insulated) AV anulus and cause retention of accessory AV muscle connections. In addition, there are specific differences in the formation of the mitral and tricuspid anuli that make the tricuspid anulus more likely to retain an embryonic AV communication. The left-sided mitral anulus is composed of a firm band of collagen, whereas the right-sided tricuspid anulus forms a much thinner ring with many interruptions [9]. In the sites void of collagen tissue, fibrofatty tissues of the atrioventricular sulcus separate the atrial from the ventricular myocardium. Occasionally, in normal hearts, remnants of the specialized tissue of the embryonic AV ring can be found in the atrial aspect of the AV junction. Although these remnants are not direct connections responsible for preexcitation, they illustrate the variability in cardiac development. These remnants are more commonly found on the right and may be the connections described by Kent.

Another important area to consider during embryogenesis in the relationship to preexcitation syndromes is the central fibrous body. In normal hearts, the nodal bundle axis is completely encased in collagen, where it penetrates onto the crest of the ventricular septum [9]. However, during development in some hearts, there is poor formation of the central fibrous body with less complete envelopment of the bundle and the potential for atrial fibers to contact the nodal bundle axis more peripherally. There may even be contacts between the nodal bundle axis and the ventricular myocardium, resulting in nodoventricular or fasciculoventricular connections.

In Ebstein's anomaly, right-sided accessory AV muscle connections are frequently found. During normal embryogenesis, the AV valve leaflets and tensor apparatus are formed by delamination of the inner layers of the inlet zone of the ventricles [10]. In Ebstein's anomaly, the insertions of the inferior and septal leaflets are displaced to the junction of the inlet and trabecular part of the ventricle, suggesting improper delamination. The anterior leaflet is formed from tissue that initially separated the inlet and trabecular zones. The AV junction is juxtaposed to the inlet zone, such that abnormal delamination and displacement of the junction of the inlet and trabecular septum could arrest the development of the right-sided AV anulus, resulting in remnants of AV connections. When Ebstein's anomaly of the left AV valve is associated with situs solitus and AV discordance, there may be an accessory AV connection on the left side, which demonstrates the developmental association of the accessory connection being ipsilateral to the abnormal valve.

Congential Heart Defects Associated with Preexcitation

The incidence of the WPW syndrome in the general population is not known precisely but has been reported to be between 0.1% and 0.2% [11]. To determine the incidence of concealed AV pathways or other variations of preexcitation is a more difficult task because these patients come to the attention of a physician only if they are symptomatic from tachyarrhythmia. However, fairly accurate studies have searched for preexcitation in populations with congenital heart disease because most of these patients have serial electrocardiograms obtained during their evaluation. The incidence of WPW syndrome in patients with congenital heart disease has been reported to be between 0.27% and 0.86% [12–14]. Conversely, in large series of pediatric patients with WPW syndrome, between 32% and 46% of patients have associated congenital heart disease [12,15]. The most frequent congenital heart defect is Ebstein's anomaly of the tricuspid valve, the incidence varying between 10% and 29%.

Although Ebstein's anomaly is the congenital heart defect reported most often with preexcitation syndromes, a variety of associated congenital heart defects have been reported. In the early 1940s, several European authors reported the association of congenital heart disease and the WPW syndrome [16–18]. In 1946, in the American literature, Bodlander [19] and Moore and Dimond [20] reported patients with coarctation of the aorta and WPW syndrome. Since that time, the WPW syndrome and tachycardia have been found in association with: (1) ventricular septal defect [21–23], (2) *d*-transposition of the great arteries [24,25], (3) atrial septal defect [26,27], (4) tetralogy of Fallot [28], (5) corrected transposition (or atrioventricular discordance) [23,29,30], (6) atrioventricular canal defect [23], (7) univentricular heart [23], (8) tricuspid atresia [31], (9) complex congenital aortic stenosis [32], (10) isolated mirror-image dextrocardia [33], and (11) Marfan's syndrome with mitral insufficiency and atrial septal defect [34]. However, the incidences of these and other congenital heart defects in patients with the WPW syndrome are low in comparison to the incidence of Ebstein's anomaly. Conversely, the incidence of WPW syndrome in patients with Ebstein's anomaly is also high, varying from 4% to 26% [35–37].

In 1955, Lev et al. [38] were the first to report a case of the WPW syndrome and Ebstein's anomaly in which they found postmortem evidence of accessory AV conduction tissue between the right atrium and the right ventricle. They analyzed the entire conduction system and AV rings and found a large AV communication in the parietal wall of the right ventricle and a small, high communication between the right bundle branch and the ventricle. They postulated that either abnormality could give rise to the electrocardiographic pattern of ventricular preexcitation. In 1971, Rosenberg et al. [22] studied postmortem specimens in two cases of WPW syndrome, one of a ventricular septal defect, and the other of Ebstein's anomaly. These authors found anatomic evidence of accessory atrioventricular connections from the right atrium to the right ventricle in both cases. Thus, from these detailed studies, evidence was accumulated supporting a morphologic basis for the electrocardiographic pattern of the WPW syndrome in patients with congenital heart disease.

Clinical Presentation of Patients with Congential Heart Disease and Preexcitation

Patients with congenital heart disease and preexcitation syndrome may be at a higher risk to develop symptoms than are patients with either condition alone. First, as a result of the congenital heart defect, such patients frequently have dilated chambers caused by volume or pressure overload, which provide a substrate for atrial or ventricular extrasystoles. These extrasystoles in turn may initiate reentrant tachycardia. Second, when tachycardia occurs, it is more likely to produce a low output state or significant cyanosis from a right-to-left shunt. Finally, tachycardia may result in more severe symptoms at a lower heart rate in patients with abnormal hemodynamics from underlying congenital heart disease than in patients without congenital heart disease.

Ebstein's Anomaly

CLINICAL FEATURES

Ebstein's anomaly is characterized by abnormal attachments of the tricuspid valve which vary from minor abnormalities that produce little or no clinical symptoms to major defects that are incompatible with life. Usually, there is displacement of the septal and posterior (inferior) leaflets of the tricuspid valve, with maximal displacement at the commissure between the leaflets [10]. The two leaflets are usually dysplastic, with the septal leaflet showing more dysplasia. The anterior leaflet is not displaced but is abnormally large and has fibrous strands running through it. This leaflet is abnormally attached posteroinferiorly to the ledge between the inlet and the trabecular portions of the right ventricle. The right atrium is usually dilated, and the right AV junction is enlarged. Because of the displaced tricuspid valve, the right ventricle is divided into two parts: the inlet portion ("atrialized" ventricle) and the trabecular and outlet portions (functional ventricle). Frequently, there is a true atrial septal defect, and many patients have a patent foramen ovale. Associated pulmonary stenosis or atresia may be found less commonly. Because of obstruction to blood flow from the right atrium to the right ventricle and into the pulmonary artery and the frequent atrial septal communication, right-to-left shunts are present, resulting in clinical cyanosis.

Ebstein's anomaly appears to involve both sexes equally and can be manifested at any age (range, 1 day to 80 years in a series from the Mayo Clinic) [37]. The defect is diagnosed frequently at the time of physical examination, when the clinician hears the typical multiplicity of heart sounds and murmurs.

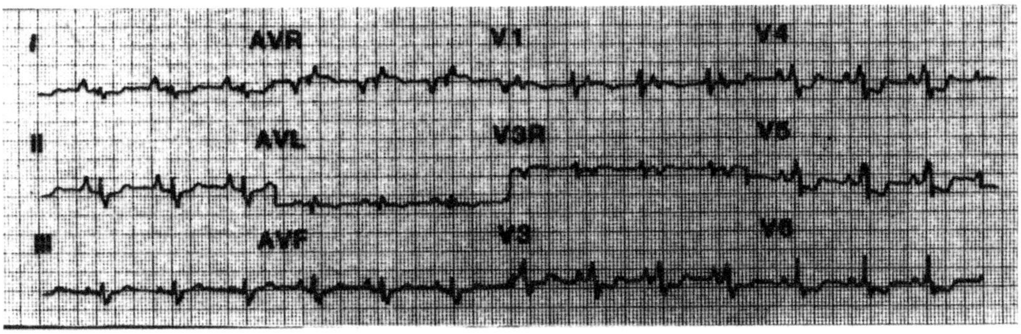

FIGURE 14–2. Electrocardiogram of 13-year-old girl with Ebstein's anomaly and no preexcitation shows a normal PR interval, evidence of right atrial enlargement, and right bundle-branch block.

The electrocardiogram is usually abnormal and helps in confirming the clinical diagnosis (Figure 14–2). Although sinus rhythm is usually present, AV dissociation or atrial fibrillation can be found in few patients. In any large series, one-third to one-half the patients have prolonged PR interval [35], and one-fourth to three-fourths of patients meet criteria for right atrial enlargement [35,37]. Most patients have right bundle-branch block, either complete or incomplete.

From 4% to 26% of patients with Ebstein's anomaly [35–37] have the WPW syndrome. Several resting or exercise electrocardiograms or 24-hour ambulatory electrocardiograms may have to be examined to find the characteristic electrocardiographic pattern (Figure 14–3). Occasionally, the pattern is transient or intermittent [12,39,40]. The absence of anterograde preexcitation neither indicates that the accessory connection is no longer present nor that the patient is no longer susceptible to tachycardia. Also, apparent patterns of the WPW syndrome may be some other form preexcitation, which may have to be evaluated during an electrophysiologic study. Patients with a normal PR interval and a delta wave with left-axis deviation and Ebstein's anomaly should be suspected of having an accessory nodoventricular connection [41].

However, if there is enhanced AV node conduction [3] and an accessory nodoventricular connection, there could appear to be a typical WPW pattern. Finally, patients with Ebstein's anomaly who have undergone division of an accessory AV connection may have an accessory nodoventricular preexcitation pattern later [42].

ELECTROPHYSIOLOGIC ASSESSMENT

The electrophysiologic assessment of patients with WPW syndrome undergoing evaluation at the Mayo Clinic has been previously described [43]. Briefly, this is summarized as follows. The electrophysiologic evaluation is carried out after cardioactive medications have been discontinued for at least 48 hours. Depending on the age and cooperation of the patient, either premedications are not used or meperidine (2 mg/kg), chlorpromazine (1 mg/kg), and promethazine (1 mg/kg) are used. Quadripolar electrode catheters are positioned in the high right atrium, at the right ventricular apex, and in the coronary sinus for recording and stimulation; a tripolar catheter is positioned against the ventricular septum near the tricuspid annulus for recording the His bundle potentials. Difficulty may be encountered during positioning of the catheter because of the dilated right atrium and enlarged anulus of the right AV valve in addition to the abnormal tricuspid valve. If the position of the catheter is difficult to determine by fluoroscopy, the electrograms may be helpful, or in the case of the ventricular catheter, ventricular pacing can be used to document satisfactory position. Simultaneous intracardiac electrograms filtered at 30 and 500 Hz and multiple surface electrocardiograms are displayed on an oscilloscope and recorded on photographic paper at 100 to 200 mm/sec. Incremental pacing and programmed stimulation are performed with a programmable stimulator.

Twenty-three patients with Ebstein's anomaly of the tricuspid valve underwent electrophysiology testing at the Mayo Clinic between 1974 and 1984. All patients were evaluated because of recurrent symptomatic tachycardia or as a part

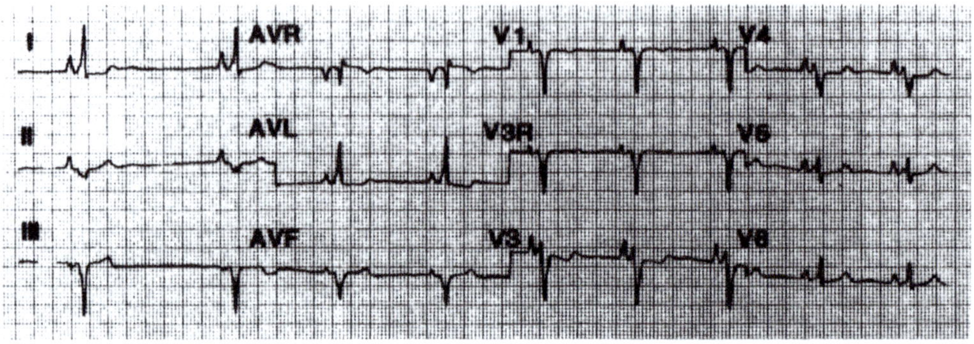

FIGURE 14–3. Electrocardiogram of 13-year-old girl with Ebstein's anomaly and preexcitation shows evidence of right atrial enlargement and Wolff-Parkinson-White syndrome (type B with delta waves in leads, I, AVL, and V4–6).

of their preoperative assessment before valvuloplasty or tricuspid valve replacement. Of the 23 patients, 12 had both Ebstein's anomaly and preexcitation and underwent valve surgery with ablation of accessory AV connections. Six of the patients were males and 6 were females, with ages ranging from 13 to 35 years (mean, 21). Eleven of the 12 patients had a history of medically treated tachycardia before the electrophysiology study, and 1 had evidence of anterograde preexcitation without a history of tachycardia. The latter patient had an electrophysiology study to determine the location of the accessory AV connection prior to valve surgery since it has previously been recommended that patients with preexcitation undergoing surgery for congenital heart disease should have accessory pathway ablation even in the absence of previously documented tachycardia [28,52]. Two additional patients underwent surgery early in our experience and did not have a preoperative electrophysiology study.

The other large series of patients with Ebstein's anomaly and preexcitation undergoing surgical ablation of an accessory pathway was reported by Smith et al. [44] from Duke University Medical Center. Of their 15 patients, 9 were females and 6 males, with ages averaging 27 years (range, 10 to 45), and all 15 underwent surgery between 1969 and December 1980. Where appropriate, comparisons will be made between our 12 patients and their 15 patients.

Basic Intervals. In 10/12 patients with preoperative electrophysiology study, the average PA interval was 37 msec (range, 15 to 63) and the average AH interval was 86 msec (range, 70 to 120); 5 of the 10 patients had enhanced AV nodal conduction and 1 patient had dual AV nodal physiology. In the series reported by Smith et al. [44], the average PA interval was 44 msec (range, 18 to 80) and the average AH interval was 80 msec (range, 45 to 140).

Accessory AV Connections. Preoperative electrophysiology study in 10 patients disclosed a right free-wall pathway in 6 patients and a septal pathway in 5 patients. However, at surgery 2 of the 5 presumed septal pathways were found to be free-wall. Therefore, in the 12 patients undergoing surgery, 10 accessory pathways were right free-wall and 3 were septal; 1 patient had both a right free-wall and a septal pathway. In the series reported by Smith et al. [44], 11 patients had a free-wall pathway, 7 had a septal pathway, and 4 had both; and 1 patient with a presumed right posterior septal pathway was found to have a right posterior free-wall pathway at surgery. In 2 other patients, right anterolateral pathways that were found by endocardial mapping were ultimately localized to a right posterolateral position at surgery. In patients with Ebstein's anomaly discordances between the preoperative endocardial map and the intraoperative epicardial map are common and may be due to right atrial enlargement and tricuspid valve displacement.

Mechanisms of Tachycardia. During preoperative electrophysiology testing, six patients were found to have one mechanism and four patients to have two mechanisms for their arrhythmia. Orthodromic reciprocating tachycardia was found in seven patients: four who had reentrant tachycardia only and three who also had atrial flutter/fibrillation. In these latter seven patients, the mean heart rate during tachycardia was 180 beats/min (range, 150 to 220). During the study, one patient had reciprocating tachycardia due to reentry within the AV node, one had both intraatrial reentry tachycardia and atrial flutter/fibrillation, and one had only atrial flutter. No patient had antidromic reciprocating tachycardia or evidence of an accessory nodoventricular or fasciculoventricular connection. No patient had induction of ventricular tachycardia. All patients in the series of Smith et al. [44] had evidence of orthodromic reciprocating tachycardia; one also was suspected of having antidromic reciprocating tachycardia, three were believed to have an additional accessory nodoventricular or fasciculoventricular pathway, and one had inducible ventricular tachycardia.

Difficulties in Electrophysiologic Evaluation. Patients with multiple accessory AV connections provide a challenge to the electrophys iologist when determining the site of the pathway and its participation in the tachycardia circuit. It is well known that patients with WPW syndrome can have multiple accessory atrioventricular connections, some of which are "manifest" (anterograde conduction) and others "concealed" (retrograde conduction), and only one or both or none of the pathways may participate in a reciprocating tachycardia. Figure 14–4 is an example of a posterior paraseptal accessory AV connection that conducts anterogradely, resulting in the WPW pattern on surface electrocardiogram, but this pathway does not participate in the patient's spontaneously occurring orthodromic reciprocating tachycardia. A second pathway that is right anterior and conducts only retrogradely is the participant in the patient's reentrant tachycardia. A more complex situation occurs when the patient has an accessory AV pathway and a concomitant accessory nodoventricular connection.

Tonkin et al. [45] described a patient with Ebstein's anomaly and WPW syndrome in whom ventricular preexcitation was due to conduction over both a right posterior accessory atrioventricular pathway and an accessory nodoventricular connection. The patient had two distinct types of tachycardia: one involving anterograde conduction over the AV node and retrograde via the accessory AV pathway and the other characterized by a slower rate and a left bundle-branch block pattern (related to anterograde conduction over the accessory nodoventricular connection) that was consistent with reciprocating tachycardia due to reentry within the AV node. Similarly, others [46] have reported the association of multiple accessory connections and/or tracts. These findings stress the importance of a detailed electrophysiologic catheterization to elucidate the mechanisms of tachycardia and the location of the accessory pathway(s) prior to undertaking any intracardiac repair and accessory pathway ablation.

During the electrophysiologic catheterization, it is important to (1) inspect carefully the surface electrocardiogram obtained at rest, (2) perform atrial stimulation at increasing rates and multiple sites, (3) analyze atrial excitation during reentrant tachycardia, and (4) perform ventricular stimulation with atrial recordings to evaluate the location and properties of the different pathways [47]. Antidromic reciprocating tachycardia occurs rarely but has been noted in patients with Ebstein's anomaly [44,48]. In addition, accessory connections occasionally are not involved during tachycardia, and the reentry circuit is localized within the AV node [44,49]. Finally, in patients with Ebstein's anomaly and a history of tachycardia, either atrial flutter or fibrillation may be the primary rhythm disturbance, with evidence of an accessory AV pathway.

Surgical Treatment

INDICATIONS FOR SURGICAL TREATMENT OF ACCESSORY AV PATHWAYS

Recently, more emphasis has been placed on the surgical management of accessory AV pathways, especially in patients with congenital heart disease. Three major reasons for this shift include: (1) the high incidence of atrial fibrillation in patients with the WPW syndrome and the associated risk of sudden death from ventricular fibrillation, (2) uncontrollable reciprocating tachycardia resulting in low output and sometimes death during the immediate postoperative period in patients undergoing intracardiac repair of a congenital heart defect, and

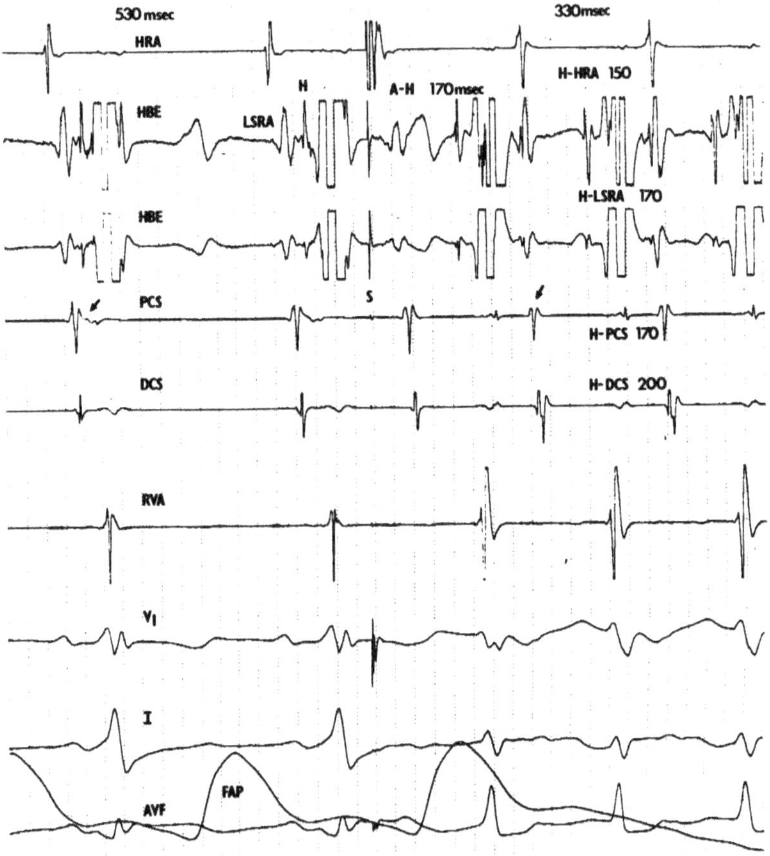

FIGURE 14–4. Intracardiac electrograms and surface electrocardiograms of 10-year-old boy with two separate accessory atrioventricular connections. Posterior paraseptal pathway conducts only anterograde, and right anterior pathway conducts only retrograde. During sinus rhythm (left side of tracing), there is preexcitation with early activation of the posterior left ventricle, seen in the proximal coronary sinus electrogram (*arrow* on the left). A premature atrial stimulus (S) at 260 ms blocks in the anterograde pathway, resulting in a narrow QRS complex, but travels through the atrioventricular node slowly (AH interval 170 ms) to activate the ventricle and return to the atrium via the right anterior pathway. An episode of orthodromic reciprocating tachycardia is started (right side of tracing). During tachycardia, the left atrium (seen on the proximal coronary sinus electrogram, *right arrow*) is activated later (H-PCS 170 ms) than the right atrium (seen in HRA electrogram, H-HRA 150 ms), indicating ventriculoatrial conduction via the right anterior pathway. (HRA = high right atrium; HBE = His bundle electrogram; PCS = proximal coronary sinus; DCS = distal coronary sinus; RVA = right ventricular apex; V, I, AVF = surface electrocardiographic leads; FAP = femoral artery pressure curve).

(3) for those patients having intracardiac repair, the convenience of undergoing only one thoracotomy and eliminating the necessity of long-term antiarrhythmic therapy. These issues will be addressed in more detail.

Atrial fibrillation is found in one-fourth to one-third of adults with WPW syndrome [3]. Atrial fibrillation by itself is not a problem unless conduction via the accessory pathway results in excessively rapid ventricular response resulting in ventricular tachycardia or development of ventricular fibrillation. Klein et al. [50] examined the risk of ventricular fibrillation during electrophysiologic testing in two groups of patients with WPW syndrome, one having a history of spontaneous ventricular fibrillation and the other without such a history. The authors hypothesized that ventricular fibrillation occurred during atrial fibrillation presumably due to rapid conduction over the accessory pathway. They noted that patients with spontaneous ventricular fibrillation had a higher prevalence of both reciprocating tachycardia and atrial fibrillation and multiple accessory pathways. The shortest preexcitation RR interval during atrial fibrillation was less in the group with spontaneous ventricular fibrillation, as was the average RR interval. The importance of these findings has not been determined on the pediatric age group since atrial flutter and fibrillation have only rarely been reported in the very young patient with WPW syndrome [51].

Although infrequent, refractory reciprocating tachycardia resulting in low cardiac output and even death can occur in the WPW syndrome after intracardiac repair of a congenital heart defect [28,52]. This emphasizes the necessity of performing detailed preoperative electrophysiologic investigations to localize any accessory atrioventricular connection(s) and of combining intracardiac repair of a congenital heart defect with division or ablation of an accessory pathway. Kugler et al. [52] reported the results of atrial septal defect closure and tricuspid valve commissurotomy in a teenage girl with Ebstein's anomaly. In the postoperative period, severe tricuspid insufficiency and recurrent reciprocating tachycardia resulted in low cardiac output and profuse chest drainage. Consequently, the patient underwent a second intracardiac surgical procedure four weeks after the first in order to replace the tricuspid valve and divide the accessory pathway.

The case reported by Kugler et al. [52] illustrates an additional point. It is preferable to perform one thoracotomy, repair the congenital heart defect, and divide the accessory connection, and thereby eliminate the need for antiarrhythmic medication or the possibility of developing atrial fibrillation resulting in ventricular fibrillation. Patients who have undergone cardiopulmonary bypass and especially those with repaired congenital heart defects are likely to experience atrial arrhythmias, including atrial flutter/fibrillation. If an accessory AV pathway with a short refractory period is still intact when atrial flutter/fibrillation occurs, the patient is at risk of sudden cardiac arrest.

EARLY SURGICAL EXPERIENCE WITH PREEXCITATION

Credit for the early work in epicardial mapping during surgery of patients with WPW syndrome must be given to Durrer and Roos [53]. In January 1967, they reported their work involving epicardial mapping of a patient with an atrial septal defect and type B WPW syndrome. They determined that the early activation of the ventricles was due to an accessory pathway between the right atrium and the closely adjacent right ventricular surface. In November 1967, Burchell et al. [54] described an early attempt at destroying a right accessory AV pathway in a patient during repair of an atrial septal defect. After careful epicardial mapping of the right ventricle and localization of the pathway, a solution of 1% procaine was injected into the right ventricular myocardium, resulting in disappearance of the preexcitation pattern. After this, a 1-cm long incision was made on the inside of the right atrium, close to and parallel to the atrioventricular ring. Just after the chest was closed, the electrocardiogram showed a return of the preexcited complexes. However, this case indicated the feasibility of a surgical approach.

INDICATIONS FOR SURGERY IN EBSTEIN'S ANOMALY

In 1982, Danielson and Fuster [55] reported the results of surgery in 42 consecutive patients with Ebstein's anomaly who underwent operation at the Mayo Clinic between April 1972 and January 1982. The ages ranged from 11 months to 52 years (median, 17 years). The hemoglobin level ranged between 10.8 and 23.4 g/dl (mean, 16.4), cardiothoracic ratio between 0.49 and 0.96 (mean, 0.67), and arterial oxygen saturation between 65% and 98% (mean, 89.6%). Three hospital deaths occurred (7.1%), one of whom was of an infant with an associated hypoplastic right ventricular outflow tract. There were no late deaths. Before this report, intracardiac repair for Ebstein's anomaly had almost ceased being performed at all because of complications, such as heart block, and the high mortality. However, that report documented not only improved survival but also improvement in NYHA functional class and reduction in cardiothoracic ratio. Although the indications for surgery evolved over the 10-year period, the authors stated that indications for surgical intervention were still incompletely defined. They believed that most patients in functional classes I and II should be managed medically. Factors that prompted earlier surgery included: (1) moderate-to-severe cyanosis, (2) paradoxic emboli, (3) right ventricular outflow tract obstruction, (4) progression to classes III and IV, (5) progressive increase in heart size (relative indication), and (6) accessory AV pathway resulting in refractory or life-threatening arrhythmia. Operation should be undertaken if the overall functional status warrants surgical intervention, not just because atrial, junctional, or ventricular arrhythmias are poorly controlled.

Of our 12 patients who had both Ebstein's anomaly and preexcitation and underwent intracardiac repair with ablation of the accessory AV pathway, 9 had a tricuspid valve anuloplasty and 3 required tricuspid valve replacement (Dr. Gordon K. Danielson performed the intracardiac repair in these patients). All 9 patients had abolition of anterograde conduction over the accessory AV pathway, and all were symptomatically improved. Of the 15 patients reported by Smith et al. [44], 7 had tricuspid valve replacement and 8 had no surgery on the tricuspid valve. Anterograde conduction over the accessory AV pathway was abolished in 14 of the 15 patients.

IMPORTANT CONSIDERATIONS FOR SURGICAL TREATMENT

The importance of a preoperative electrophysiologic catheterization in patients with Ebstein's anomaly cannot be overemphasized. There are various reasons for this. First, in spite of the presence of anterograde preexcitation during sinus rhythm, associated tachycardia may not be due to the usual form of AV reentry, but may be caused by atrial flutter/fibrillation, other atrial tachycardia or reentry within the AV node, or ventricular tachycardia. The significance of this may become more apparent during the postoperative period, when, in spite of the absence of a delta wave, the patient may have a tachyarrhythmia requiring immediate intervention [56]. Second, although most patients with Ebstein's anomaly and accessory AV pathways have right free-wall pathways, a small percentage of patients have septal pathways that require more extensive yet cautious surgery in the septal region to eliminate the accessory pathway and preserve normal conduction through the AV node and His-Purkinje system [57,58]. The extensiveness of the surgery should be known in advance. Third, multiple accessory AV pathways are found in a small but significant number of patients with Ebstein's malformation, which can result in confusion intraoperatively or postoperatively [59]. A preoperative electrophysiologic catheterization may identify two separate accessory AV pathways, and after abolition of the first pathway, the second one may become active and manifest itself as a participant in a reciprocating tachycardia. In other cases, two pathways may be identified by preoperative electrophysiology study, but during the operative procedure, the second pathway is not active, perhaps as a result of anesthetic medications. The preoperative map is most helpful in this unusual situation. Lastly, some pathways conduct only in the retrograde direction, and therefore, their presence might not be known without electrophysiologic study.

The issue of right free-wall versus septal accessory connections in patients with Ebstein's anomaly is important (Figure 14–5). As mentioned, septal pathways require extensive but cautious tissue dissection. However, the im-

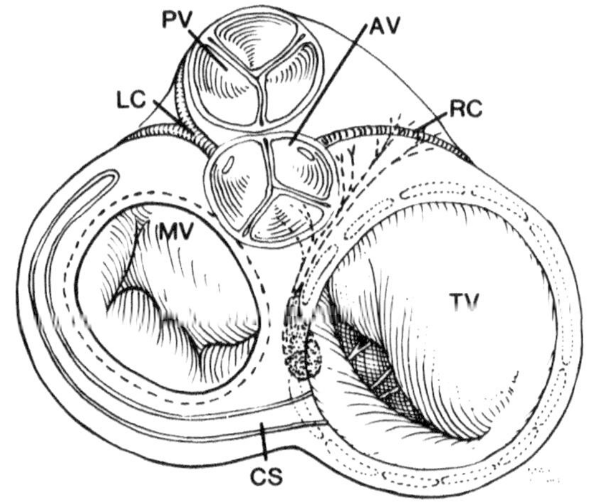

FIGURE 14–5. Diagram of cross section of heart with Ebstein's anomaly, through a plane to include atrioventricular valve rings and the semilunar valves. Tricuspid valve anulus and anterior leaflet are enlarged. Septal and posterior leaflets are dysplastic, small, and displaced. Tricuspid anulus is thinner than mitral anulus and has sites that are void of collagen tissue, making it easier to retain atrioventricular connections. Posterior paraseptal accessory atrioventricular connections can be very near the atrioventricular node and His bundle structures. *AV* = aortic valve; *CS* = coronary sinus; *LC* = left main coronary artery; *MV* = mitral valve; *PV* = pulmonary valve; *RC* = right coronary artery; and *TV* = tricuspid valve. (By permission of Mayo Foundation.)

portance of complete evaluation of free-wall pathways must be emphasized also. The extensive work by Sealy et al. [58] in developing the surgical technique for abolition of accessory AV pathways has revealed the following important facts. In general, right free-wall accessory pathways can be either adjacent to the anulus fibrosus or far out in the coronary sulcus fat, away from the anulus. In patients with Ebstein's anomaly, there is even more variation in the right free-wall pathways. Because of the overlap of the right ventricle on the external surface of the right atrium, there can be an unusually wide accessory atrioventricular connection or the usual endocardial incision through the atrium may not be successful in dividing the pathway. In the approach to right free-wall pathways, one assumes that they can be located adjacent to the anulus fibrosus or underneath the epicardium. Thus the fat in the coronary sulcus must be separated from the atrium as well as the ventricle, and the endocardial incision should be made above the anulus, completely dividing the right atrium from the anulus.

However, the posterior septal region has been the source of most difficulties for surgeons. Septal pathways can be located at sites that start at the insertion of the atrial septum into the right fibrous trigone and extend posteriorly to the crux. Because of this, the surgical technique requires an endocardial incision from just anterior to the coronary sinus ostium but posterior to the atrial septum toward the crux and for 1 cm onto the free wall. This leads into a triangular space, the floor of which is the ventricular septum and the posterior-superior process of the left ventricle. The fat in this space is separated from the septum, with care being taken to avoid the atrioventricular nodal artery. Because of the distortion of anatomy in Ebstein's anomaly, this area may be more difficult to incise and dissect.

During operation on the tricuspid valve in patients with Ebstein's anomaly, experienced surgical assessment must be used to decide between repair of the tricuspid valve and valve replacement [55]. If repair of the tricuspid valve is performed, we prefer to place ventricular plication sutures so as to avoid the posterior descending coronary artery and obvious large branches of the right coronary artery [55]. It is preferable to avoid suture placement in the septum in order to prevent heart block. If the valve is so dysplastic that it must be replaced, a bioprosthetic valve is preferred. Again, to avoid producing heart block, the suture line is carried on the atrial side of the coronary sinus and the atrioventricular node.

Preexcitation Associated with Mitral Value Prolapse Syndrome

Mitral valve prolapse is a very common cardiac abnormality [60,61]. Whether it is congenital or acquired remains to be determined. However, an association of mitral valve prolapse and preexcitation has been recognized [3,62]. Although ventricular arrhythmias are suspected and detected in many patients with mitral valve prolapse and palpitations, a few patients have sustained reciprocating tachycardia as the mechanism of their arrhythmias. Gallagher et al. [3] and Josephson et al. [62] have described patients with mitral valve prolapse and accessory AV pathways that conduct bidirectionally or only in the retrograde direction.

Conclusion

In patients with congenital heart disease, especially Ebstein's anomaly of the tricuspid valve; and a history of tachycardia, the mechanism of tachycardia should be documented to determine if it is related to an accessory AV pathway. This is particularly true in patients who are candidates for intracardiac repair because the goal in patients with symptomatic reciprocating tachycardia and accessory AV pathway should be not only correcting or palliating the congenital heart defect but also abolishing the anatomic pathophysiologic substrate for tachycardia.

References

1. Öhnell RF: Pre-excitation: a cardiac abnormality; patho-physiological, patho-anatomical and clinical studies of an excitatory spread phenomenon bearing upon the problem of the WPW (Wolff-Parkinson and White) electrocardiogram and paroxysmal tachycardia. *Acta Med. Scand.* [Suppl] 152:1, 1944.
2. Durrer D: Electrical aspects of human cardiac activity: a clinical-physiological approach to excitation and stimulation. *Cardiovasc. Res.* 2:1, 1968.
3. Gallagher JJ, Pritchett ELC, Sealy WC, Kasell J, Wallace AG: The preexcitation syndromes. *Prog. Cardiovasc. Dis.* 20:285, 1978.
4. Anderson RH, Becker AE, Brechenmacher C,

Davies MJ, Rossi L: Ventricular preexcitation: a proposed nomenclature for its substrates. *Eur. J. Cardiol.* 3:27, 1975.
5. Lev M, Leffler WB, Langendorf R, Pick A: Anatomic findings in a case of ventricular preexcitation (WPW) terminating in complete atrioventricular block. *Circulation* 34:718, 1966.
6. James TN: Morphology of the human atrioventricular node, with remarks pertinent to its electrophysiology. *Am. Heart J.* 62:756, 1961.
7. Denes P, Wu D, Dhingra RC, Chuquimia R, Rosen KM: Demonstration of dual A-V nodal pathways in patients with paroxysmal supraventricular tachycardia. *Circulation* 48:549, 1973.
8. Josephson ME, Kastor JA: Supraventricular tachycardia in Lown-Ganong-Levine syndrome: atrionodal versus intranodal reentry. *Am. J. Cardiol.* 40:521, 1977.
9. Davies MJ, Anderson RH, Becker AE: The Conduction System of the Heart. London, Butterworth, 1983, pp. 181–202.
10. Anderson KR, Zuberbuhler JR, Anderson RH, Becker AE, Lie JT: Morphologic spectrum of Ebstein's anomaly of the heart: a review. *Mayo Clin. Proc.* 54:174, 1979.
11. Katz LN, Pick A: Cited by Schiebler GL, Adams P Jr, Anderson RC[12]
12. Schiebler GL, Adams P Jr, Anderson RC: The Wolff-Parkinson-White syndrome in infants and children: a review and a report of 28 cases. *Pediatrics* 24:585, 1959.
13. Metianu C, de Balsac RH: Les troubles congénitaux de la conduction et du rythme. In *Traité des Cardiopathies Congénitales*, Donzelot E, D'Allaines F (eds.). Paris, Masson, 1954, p. 1025.
14. Hecht HH (moderator): Anomalous atrioventricular excitation: panel discussion. *Ann. N.Y. Acad. Sci.* 65:826, 1957.
15. Giardina ACV, Ehlers KH, Engle MA: Wolff-Parkinson-White syndrome in infants and children: a long-term follow-up study. *Br. Heart J.* 34:839, 1972.
16. Pohlmann F: Beitrag zur Frage der verkürzten Vorhof-Kammerleitung. *Ztschr. Klin. Med.* 140:1, 1941.
17. Kiss P von: "Paladino-Kent-Bündel" beim Kinde. *Arch. Kinderheilkd.* 122:29, 1941.
18. Nádrai A: Die Elektrokardiographie im Säuglings–und Kindesalter. *Ergeb. Inn. Med. Kinderheilkd.* 60:688, 1941.
19. Bodlander JW: The Wolff-Parkinson-White syndrome in association with congenital heart disease: coarctation of the aorta; report of a case. *Am. Heart J.* 31:785, 1946.
20. Moore RM, Dimond G: Case of coarctation of aorta (adult type) with Wolff-Parkinson-White syndrome. *J. Indiana Med. Assoc.* 39:352, 1946.
21. Segers M, Sanabria T, Lequime J, Denolin H: Le syndrome de Wolff-Parkinson-White: mise en evidence d'une connexion A-V septale directe. *Acta Cardiol.* 2:21, 1947.
22. Rosenberg HS, Klima T, McNamara DG, Leachman RD: Atrioventricular communication in the Wolff-Parkinson-White syndrome. *Am. J. Clin. Pathol.* 56:79, 1971.
23. Gillette PC, Garson A Jr, Kugler JD: Wolff-Parkinson-White syndrome in children: electrophysiologic and pharmacologic characteristics. *Circulation* 60:1487, 1979.
24. Hejtmancik MR, Herrmann GR: The electrocardiographic syndrome of short P–R interval and broad QRS complexes: a clinical study of 80 cases. *Am. Heart J.* 54:708, 1957.
25. El-Said G, Rosenberg HS, Mullins CE, Hallman GL, Cooley DA, McNamara DG: Dysrhythmias after Mustard's operation for transposition of the great arteries. *Am. J. Cardiol.* 30:526, 1972.
26. Neutze J, Kerr AR, Whitlock RML: Epicardial mapping in a variant of type A Wolff-Parkinson-White syndrome. *Circulation* 48:662, 1973.
27. Gomi H, Karasu K, Nishimaru I, Iikawa T, Kazama S: Case of surgery on Wolff-Parkinson-White syndrome. *Kyobu. Geka.* 27:129, 1974.
28. Mantakas ME, McCue CM, Miller WW: Natural history of Wolff-Parkinson-White syndrome discovered in infancy. *Am. J. Cardiol.* 41:1097, 1978.
29. Symons JC, Shinebourne EA, Joseph MC, Lincoln C, Ho Y, Anderson RH: Criss-cross heart with congenitally corrected transposition: report of a case with d-transposed aorta and ventricular preexcitation. *Eur. J. Cardiol.* 5:493, 1977.
30. Benson DW Jr, Gallagher JJ, Oldham HN, Sealy WC, Sterba R, Spach MS: Corrected transposition with severe intracardiac deformities with Wolff-Parkinson-White syndrome in a child: electrophysiologic investigation and surgical correction. *Circulation* 61:1256, 1980.
31. Dick M II, Behrendt DM, Byrum CJ, Sealy WC, Stern AM, Hees P, Rosenthal A: Tricuspid atresia and the Wolff-Parkinson-White syndrome: evaluation methodology and successful surgical treatment of the combined disorders. *Am. Heart J.* 101:496, 1981.
32. Vanetti A, Donzeau-Gouge GP, Frank R, Fourati M, Evans J, Ismail MB, Daumet P: Surgical treatment for a complicated congenital aortic stenosis: the association of a three-level obstruction of the left ventricular outflow tract with mitral incompetence, coarctation of the aorta, and the Wolff-Parkinson-White syndrome. *J. Thorac. Cardiovasc. Surg.* 77:230, 1979.
33. Wellens HJJ, Gorgels AP: Mirror image dextrocardia and the Wolff-Parkinson-White syndrome. *Chest* 76:91, 1979.
34. Hiejima K, Tsuchiya S, Sakamoto Y, Shiina S: Two cases of Marfan's syndrome associated re-

spectively with subacute bacterial endocarditis and the Wolff-Parkinson-White syndrome. *Jpn. Heart J.* 9:208, 1968.

35. Schiebler GL, Adams P Jr, Anderson RC, Amplatz K, Lester RG: Clinical study of twenty-three cases of Ebstein's anomaly of the tricuspid valve. *Circulation* 19:165, 1959.
36. Soulié P, Heulin A, Pauly-Laubry C, Degeorges M: Maladie d'Ebstein etude clinique et évolution (a propos de 40 observations dont 9 chirurgicales). *Arch. Mal Coeur* 63:615, 1970.
37. Giuliani ER, Fuster V, Brandenburg RO, Mair DD: Ebstein's anomaly: the clinical features and natural history of Ebstein's anomaly of the tricuspid valve. *Mayo Clin. Proc.* 54:163, 1979.
38. Lev M, Gibson S, Miller RA: Ebstein's disease with Wolff-Parkinson-White syndrome: report of a case with a histopathologic study of possible conduction pathways. *Am. Heart J.* 49:724, 1955.
39. Friedman S, Wells CRE, Amiri S: The transient nature of Wolff-Parkinson-White anomaly in childhood. *J. Pediatr.* 74:296, 1969.
40. Klein GJ, Gulamhusein SS: Intermittent preexcitation in the Wolff-Parkinson-White syndrome. *Am. J. Cardiol.* 52:292, 1983.
41. Follath F, Hallidie-Smith KA: Unusual electrocardiographic changes in Ebstein's anomaly. *Br. Heart J.* 34:513, 1972.
42. Gallagher JJ, Smith WM, Kasell JH, Benson DW Jr, Sterba R, Grant AO: Role of Mahaim fibers in cardiac arrhythmias in man. *Circulation* 64:176, 1981.
43. Holmes DR Jr, Osborn MJ, Gersh B, Maloney JD, Danielson GK: The Wolff-Parkinson-White syndrome: a surgical approach. *Mayo Clin. Proc.* 57:345, 1982.
44. Smith WM, Gallagher JJ, Kerr CR, Sealy WC, Kasell JH, Benson DW Jr, Reiter MJ, Sterba R, Grant AO: The electrophysiologic basis and management of symptomatic recurrent tachycardia in patients with Ebstein's anomaly of the tricuspid valve. *Am. J. Cardiol.* 49:1223, 1982.
45. Tonkin AM, Dugan FA, Svenson RH, Sealy WC, Wallace AG, Gallagher JJ: Coexistence of functional Kent and Mahaim-type tracts in the pre-excitation syndrome: demonstration by catheter techniques and epicardial mapping. *Circulation* 52:193, 1975.
46. Castellanos A, Agha AS, Befeler B, Myerburg RJ: Double accessory pathways in Wolff-Parkinson-White syndrome. *Circulation* 51:1020, 1975.
47. Edvardsson N, Blomström P, Olsson SB: Identification of multiple pathways in the Wolff-Parkinson-White syndrome: diagnostic problems and therapeutic implications. *Cardiology* 71:20, 1984.
48. Inoue H, Matsuo H, Takayanagi K, Ishimitsu T, Murao S: Antidromic reciprocating tachycardia via a slow Kent bundle in Ebstein's anomaly. *Am. Heart J.* 106:147, 1983.
49. Smith WM, Broughton A, Reiter MJ, Benson DW Jr, Grant AO, Gallagher JJ: Bystander accessory pathway during AV node re-entrant tachycardia. *PACE* 6:537, 1983.
50. Klein GJ, Bashore TM, Sellers TD, Pritchett ELC, Smith WM, Gallagher JJ: Ventricular fibrillation in the Wolff-Parkinson-White syndrome. *N. Engl. J. Med.* 301:1080, 1979.
51. Mehta AV, Pickoff AS, Raptoulis A, Wolff GS, Garcia OL, Tamer DF, Ferrer PL, Gelband H: Atrial flutter and atrial fibrillation associated with Wolff-Parkinson-White syndrome in childhood. *Pediatr. Cardiol.* 1:197, 1980.
52. Kugler JD, Gillette PC, Duff DF, Cooley DA, McNamara DG: Elective mapping and surgical division of the bundle of Kent in a patient with Ebstein's anomaly who required tricuspid valve replacement. *Am. J. Cardiol.* 41:602, 1978.
53. Durrer D, Roos JP: Epicardial excitation of the ventricles in a patient with Wolff-Parkinson-White syndrome (type B). *Circulation* 35:15, 1967.
54. Burchell HB, Frye RL, Anderson MW, McGoon DC: Atrioventricular and ventriculoatrial excitation in Wolff-Parkinson-White syndrome (type B): temporary ablation at surgery. *Circulation* 36:663, 1967.
55. Danielson GK, Fuster V: Surgical repair of Ebstein's anomaly. *Ann. Surg.* 196:499, 1982.
56. Westaby S, Karp RB, Kirklin JW, Waldo AL, Blackstone EH: Surgical treatment in Ebstein's malformation. *Ann. Thorac. Surg.* 34:388, 1982.
57. Sealy WC, Gallagher JJ, Pritchett ELC, Wallace AG: Surgical treatment of tachyarrhythmias in patients with both an Ebstein anomaly and a Kent bundle. *J. Thorac. Cardiovasc. Surg.* 75:847, 1978.
58. Sealy WC, Gallagher JJ, Pritchett ELC: The surgical anatomy of Kent bundles based on electrophysiological mapping and surgical exploration. *J. Thorac. Cardiovasc. Surg.* 76:804, 1978.
59. Iwa T, Magara T, Watanabe Y, Kawasuji M, Misaki T: Interruption of multiple accessory conduction pathways in the Wolff-Parkinson-White syndrome. *Ann. Thorac. Surg.* 30:313, 1980.
60. Devereux RB, Perloff JK, Reichek N, Josephson ME: Mitral valve prolapse. *Circulation* 54:3, 1976.
61. Procacci PM, Savran SV, Schreiter SL, Bryson AL: Prevalence of clinical mitral-valve prolapse in 1169 young women. *N. Engl. J. Med.* 294:1086, 1976.
62. Josephson Me, Horowitz LN, Kastor JA: Paroxysmal supraventricular tachycardia in patients with mitral valve prolapse. *Circulation* 57:111, 1978.

IV.
ELECTROPHYSIOLOGIC EVALUATION

15. INITIAL EVALUATION OF PATIENTS WITH THE WOLFF-PARKINSON-WHITE SYNDROME

George J. Klein
Arjun D. Sharma
Simon Milstein

The classic electrocardiographic Wolff-Parkinson-White (WPW) pattern has been estimated to occur in 1 to 3 per 1,000 individuals [1]. Strictly speaking, only patients with a manifest delta wave and rapid-heart-beating should be considered as having WPW syndrome [2] but it is now known that many patients with the underlying substrate for this syndrome — namely, the accessory atrioventricular pathway — have "concealed" accessory pathways and have normal PR intervals and QRS morphology as the pathways conduct only in the retrograde direction [3,4]. The spectrum of WPW patients includes those with a purely benign "cosmetic" delta wave, those with troublesome but not life-threatening paroxysmal tachycardia, and those with a potentially life-threatening arrhythmia (most often atrial fibrillation with a rapid ventricular response that could lead to ventricular fibrillation) [5]. The evaluation of the patient with WPW syndrome depends a great deal on the clinical presentation. The main challenge to the physician is to find the relatively infrequent WPW patient who is at risk for a potentially lethal arrhythmia and to distinguish this patient from those that can be reassured or treated in a more methodical fashion with empirical drug trials.

This work was supported by a grant from the Heart and Stroke Foundation of Ontario, Toronto, Ontario, Canada. The authors wish to thank Suzanme Stewart for preparing the manuscript.

The Asymptomatic Patient

It is now widely believed that sudden death in the WPW syndrome occurs as a result of atrial fibrillation with a rapid ventricular response over the accessory pathway ultimately leading to ventricular fibrillation [5]. Although most patients who experience ventricular fibrillation have a previous history of both reciprocating tachycardia and atrial fibrillation, unfortunately, ventricular fibrillation can be the initial manifestation of this syndrome, even in the previously asymptomatic patient. Patients with a short anterograde refractory period of the accessory pathway (less than 270 ms) are capable of a rapid ventricular response in the event of atrial fibrillation [6]. Conversely, patients with a long anterograde refractory period of the accessory pathway would not be expected to be at risk for sudden death provided that other serious concomitant cardiac disease is absent.

The initial evaluation of the asymptomatic patient should include a complete history, a thorough clinical examination, and those noninvasive investigations necessary to establish the presence or absence of associated cardiac anomalies [7]. In patients with preexcitation the location of the accessory pathway can be approximated by electrocardiographic criteria [8] or by observation of earliest ventricular activation by echocardiography [9] or myocardial imaging [10]. The latter is initially only of academic importance since the location of the accessory pathway does not predict its electrophysiologic properties. The crucial element in the initial evaluation of the patient is to derive an approximation of the anterograde effective refractory period [ERP] of the accessory pathway. In the adult patient, the important distinction to be made is that between the patients with a "long" ERP (greater than 270 msec) versus a "short" ERP (less than 270 msec). Fortunately, several noninvasive techniques are of value.

SERIAL ELECTROCARDIOGRAMS AND AMBULATORY ELECTROCARDIOGRAPHY

Sudden and unexpected loss of the delta wave (normalization of the QRS complex) has long been observed in the WPW syndrome [11,12] (Figures 15–1 and 15–2). Loss of the delta wave in this fasion can be related to a critically rapid (or slow) heart rate although, most often, loss of the delta wave occurs in a sporadic fashion [13,14]. Intuitively, one would expect that such loss of the delta would indicate "precarious" conduction over the accessory pathway or, at least, an accessory pathway with a long anterograde refractory period. This was indeed found to be the case when patients with intermittent loss of the delta wave were evaluated by invasive electrophysiologic studies [13]. Patients showing intermittent preexcitation invariably had a long ERP of the accessory pathway and relatively slow ventricular rates during atrial fibrillation. Examination of serial electrocardiograms and ambulatory monitoring records may reveal this phenomenon in up to 50% or more of patients and can accurately categorize them into a low risk subgroup [13,15].

Several notes of caution must be made in identifying the phenomenon of QRS normalization. First, the delta wave should be reasonably obvious and QRS normalization should be accompanied by prolongation of the PR interval and, usually, repolarization changes. One should be very hesitant in diagnosing this phenomenon (i.e., QRS normalization) when the delta wave is subtle or when the QRS normalizes gradually without prolongation of the PR interval. In the latter instance, one may merely be observing acceleration of normal AV nodal conduction due to sympathetic influences with a resultant greater contribution of the normal AV conduction system to ventricular activation. Second, the normalized QRS should be preceded by a P wave since normalized QRSs without a preceding P wave may represent His bundle extrasystoles or junctional escape complexes that would not be expected to be preexcited even if the accessory pathway had a short ERP (Figure 15–3). Finally, normalization of a QRS immediately after a ventricular extrasystole should be interpreted with caution (Figure 15–4). In the latter example, concealed retrograde conduction into the accessory pathway following a ventricular complex may result in failure of the subsequent atrial complex to conduct with preexcitation even if the accessory pathway usually exhibited a short ERP [16].

EXERCISE TESTING

Exercise testing in the WPW syndrome is of limited value in assessment of arrhythmias since paroxysmal tachycardias are rarely provoked during exercise testing [13,17,18,19]. Furthermore, abnormal repolarization as a result of preexcitation greatly limits the usefulness of treadmill testing in diagnosing myocardial ischemia in WPW patients. However, the acceleration of the heart rate with exercise may result in sudden loss of the delta wave, a finding which identifies the patient with a long ERP of the accessory pathway [13,17,20] (see Figures 15–5, 15–6). To interpret this finding properly, it is critical that there be abrupt loss ("Mobitz II") of an obvious delta wave as viewed on multiple ECG leads during the exercise test. Since the PR interval may shorten with exercise, a gradual diminution of preexcitation during exercise not accompanied by PR prolongation cannot be considered to represent loss of preexcitation. Multiple leads should be examined since preexcitation may appear to be lost in some leads (probably due to "opposite" PR segment changes) while clearly still present in other leads [13].

USE OF ANTIARRHYTHMIC AGENTS IN PREDICTING THE ERP OF THE ACCESSORY PATHWAY

The use of an antiarrhythmic agent, administered as a bolus to predict the anterograde ERP

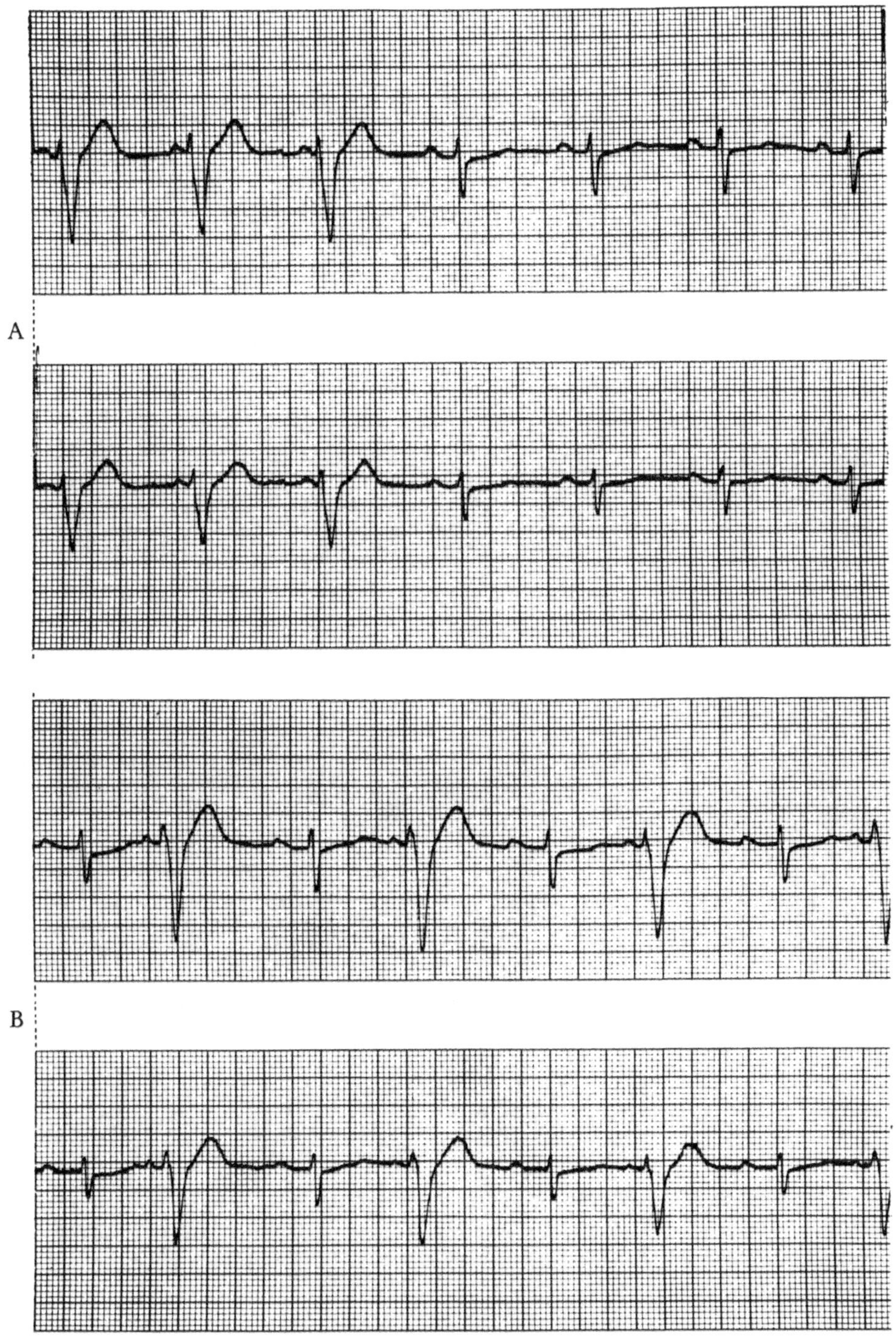

FIGURE 15–1. Intermittent loss of the delta wave on ambulatory monitor. (A) The 2-channel ambulatory electrocardiogram shows sudden loss of the delta wave on the fourth complex with prolongation of the PR interval, normalization of the QRS and change in the repolarization pattern. There is no appreciable change in the heart rate. (B) The 2-channel ambulatory record also shows instances of 2:1 ("Mobitz II") block over the accessory pathway with alternating preexcitation.

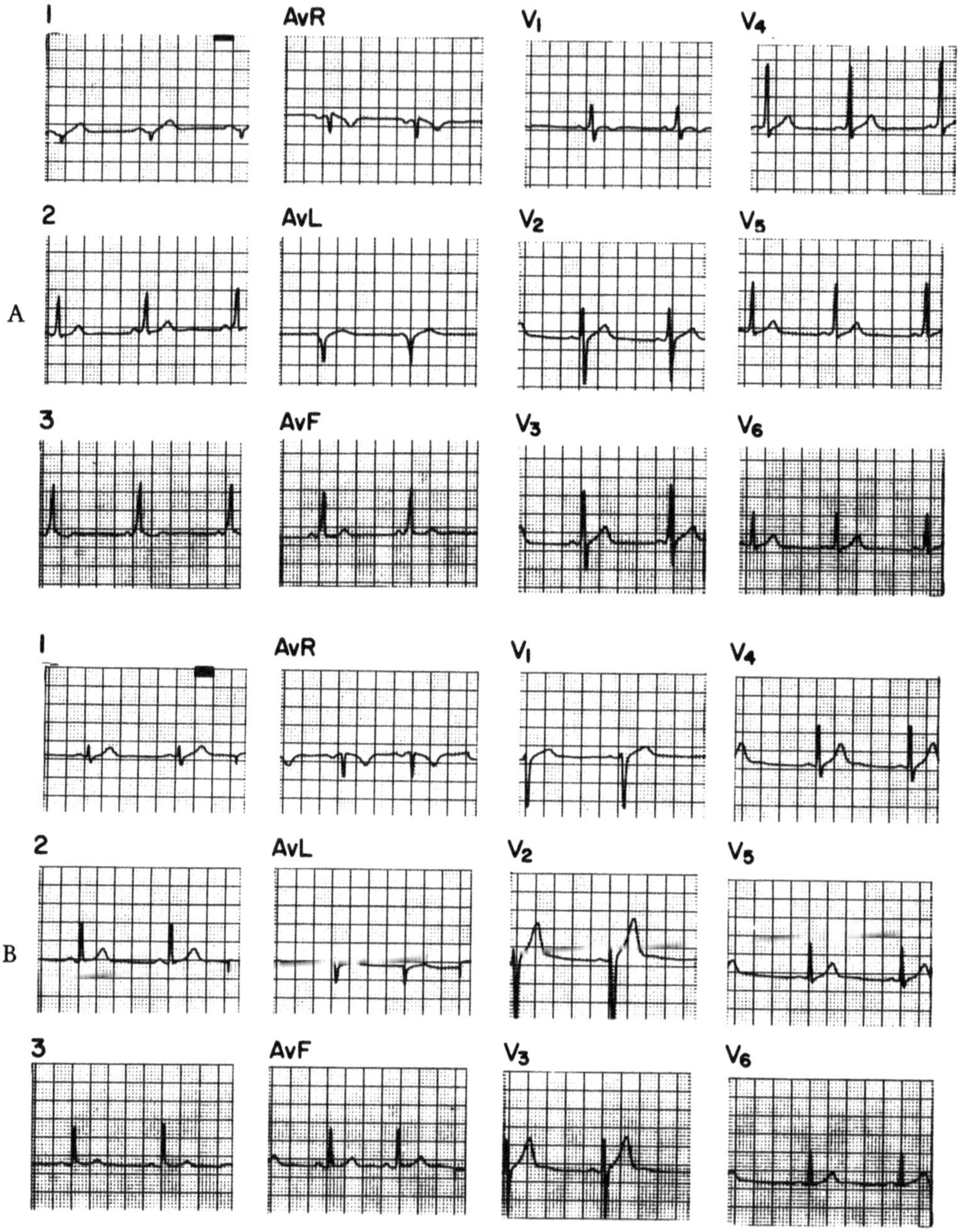

FIGURE 15–2. Intermittent preexcitation. (A) shows a 12-lead electrocardiogram recorded at the initial assessment showing preexcitation. (B) is an electrocardiogram recorded during a follow-up visit on the same patient and is entirely normal.

FIGURE 15–3. Normalization with a junctional escape rhythm. (A) shows a 12-lead electrocardiogram with obvious preexcitation. (B) is the electrocardiogram recorded on the same patient during a vasovagal episode occurring with insertion of an intravenous. *P* waves are not apparent and a junctional escape rhythm is observed. The QRS complex is normalized. In this example, normalization is merely the result of activation of the ventricle via a junctional rhythm that does not have an opportunity to reach the accessory pathway. The refractory period of the accessory pathway in this patient was short.

A

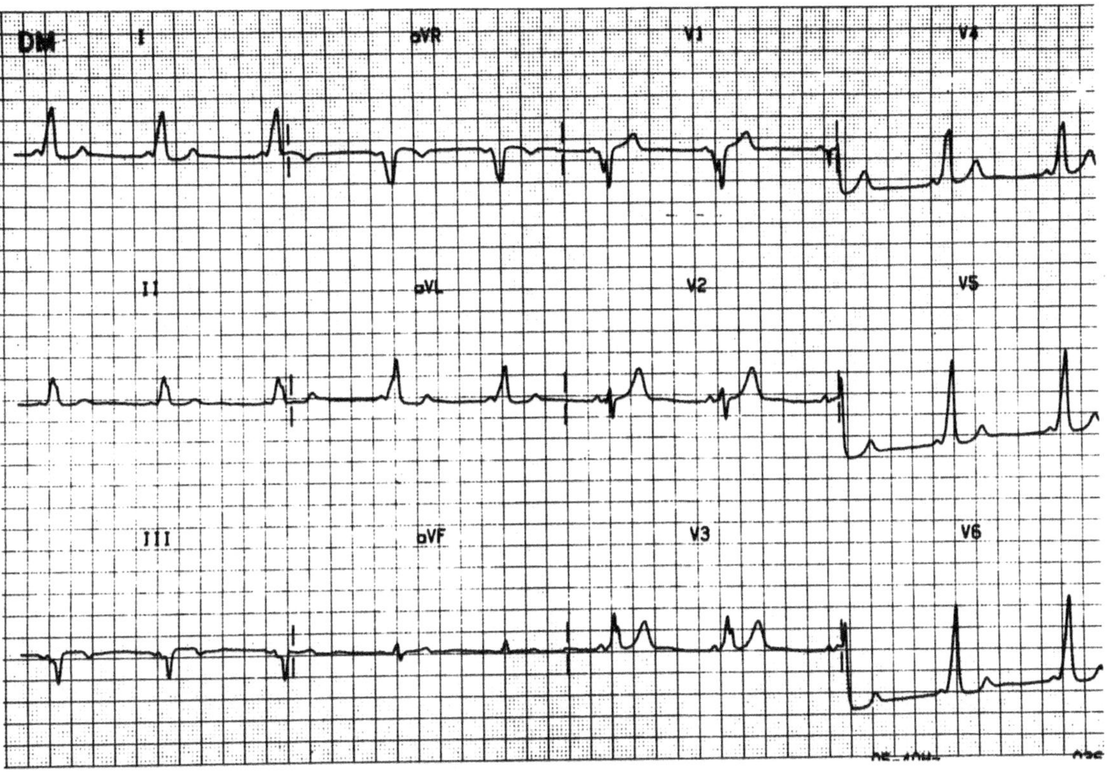
DM
I
aVR
V1
V4
II
aVL
V2
V5
III
aVF
V3
V6

B

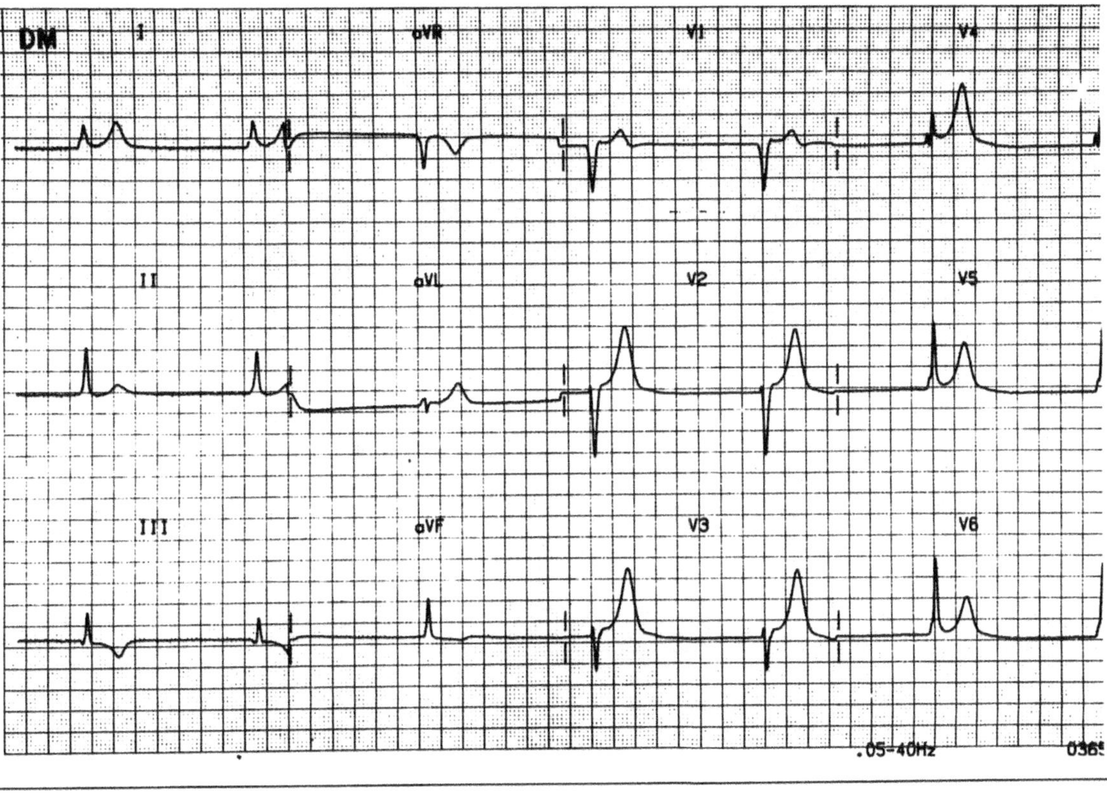
DM
I
aVR
V1
V4
II
aVL
V2
V5
III
aVF
V3
V6
.05-40Hz

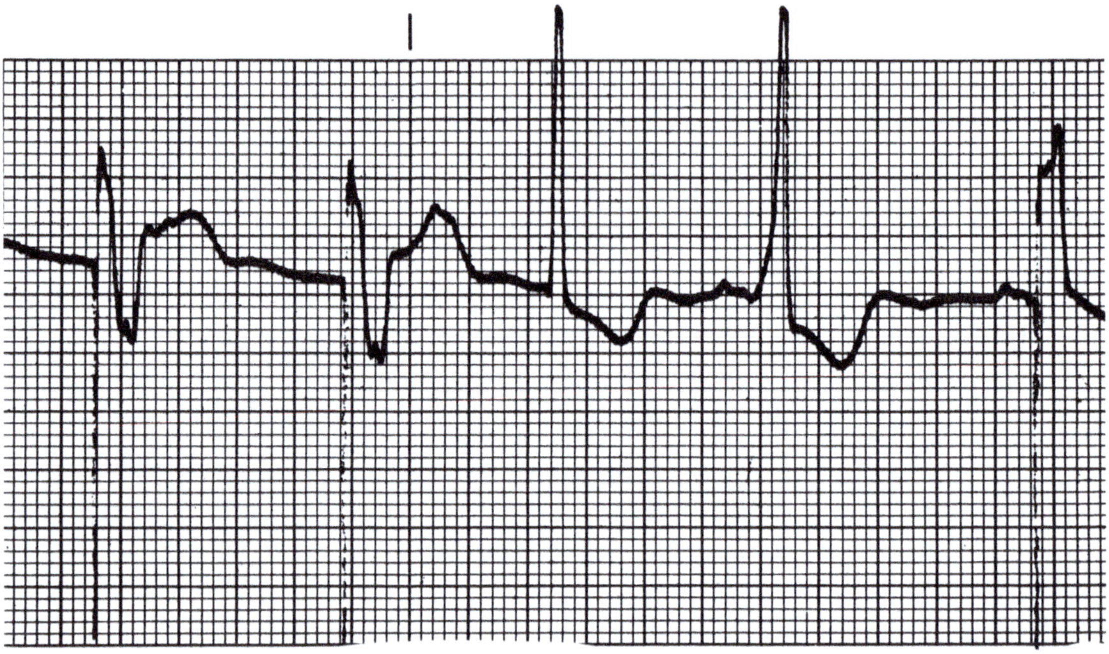

FIGURE 15–4. Loss of preexcitation after ventricular stimulation. In this patient, a sinus capture beat is observed immediately after a ventricular paced complex. The PR interval is prolonged and the QRS complex is normalized. In the cycle following immediately, preexcitation is evident. In this example, normalization of the QRS can be entirely explained by concealed retrograde conduction into the accessory pathway by the preceding ventricular complex and need not indicate an accessory pathway with a long refractory period.

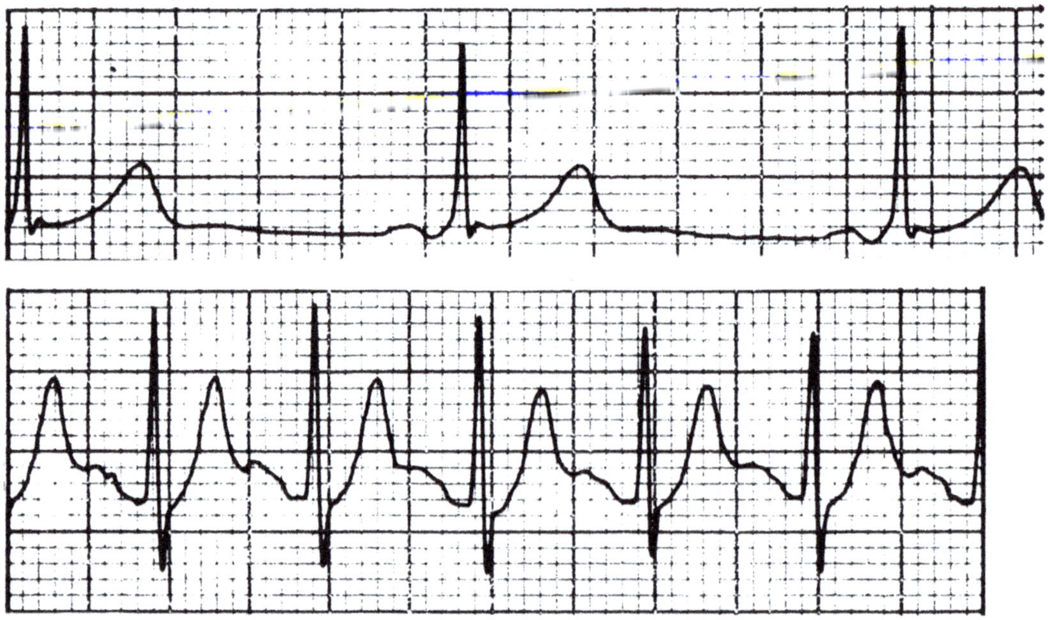

B

FIGURE 15–5. Loss of preexcitation with exercise. (A) shows a preexcited QRS in the basal state. With exercise, (B), the heart rate accelerates and preexcitation is abruptly lost.

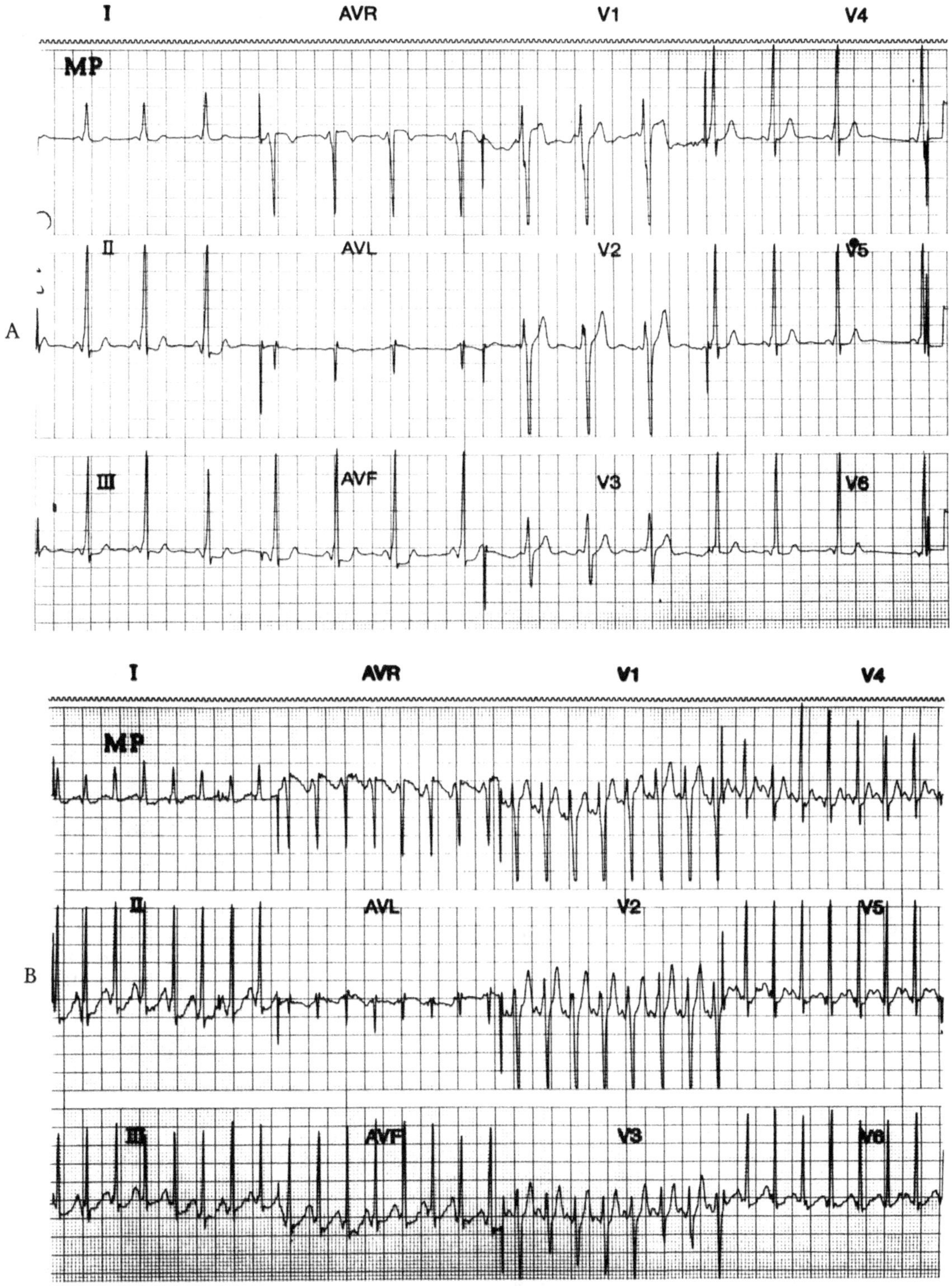

FIGURE 15–6. Legend on page 312.

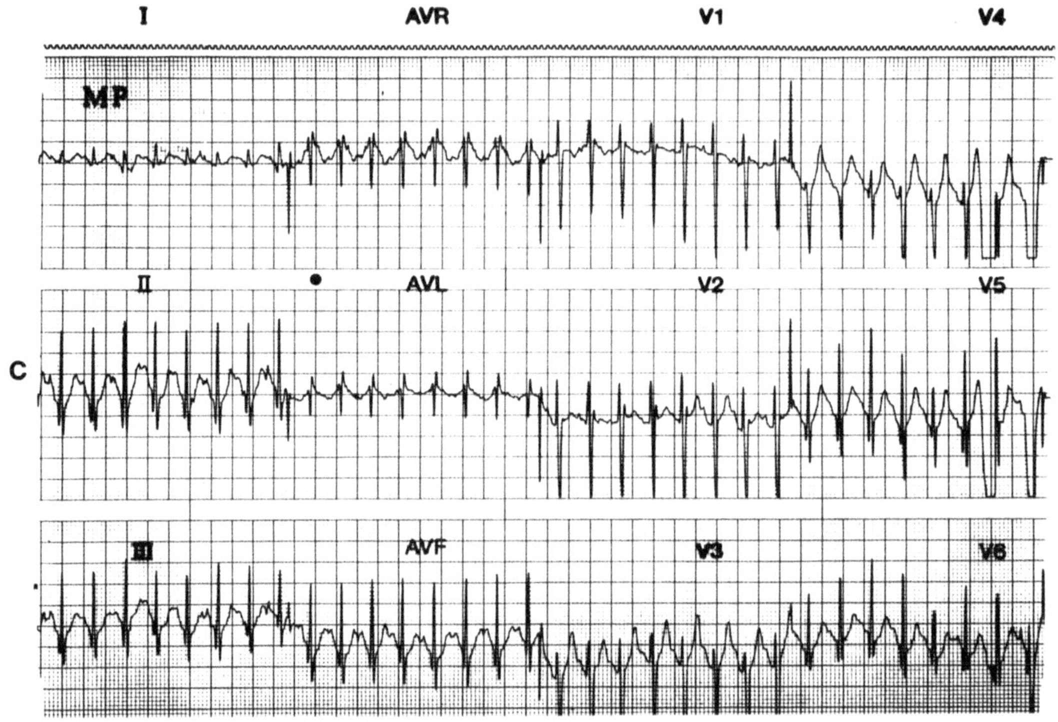

FIGURE 15–6. Loss of preexcitation with exercise. (AS) shows the electrocardiogram at rest with an obvious delta wave. During stress (B), the delta wave persists but is abruptly lost at maximum stress (C). Delta waves are best seen in the inferior leads.

of the accessory pathway is based on Wellen's [21] observation. He noted that the magnitude of the increase in the refractory period after intravenous injection of a class I antiarrhythmic agent (procainamide, quinidine, ajmaline) is related to the initial ERP of the accessory pathway, being relatively small if the effective refractory period is less than 270 and relatively great if the refractory period is greater than this. In other words, these antiarrhythmic agents are most effective when the control (i.e., no drug) ERP of the accessory pathway is relatively long. This observation prompted Wellens to propose the "ajmaline test" [22] in which 50 mg of ajmaline are given intravenously over 3 minutes. In most patients, this results in disappearance of the delta wave if the refractory period is greater than 270 msec. Wellens also proposed that procainamide can be used in the same way [23] and showed that procainamide given in a dosage of 10 mg/kg over 5 minutes results in loss of the delta wave in most patients in whom the anterograde refractory period is greater than 270 msec. Both of these tests were associated, however, with a small number of false positives in which disappearance of the delta wave occurred in patients with a short ERP of the accessory pathway. We have found that the class I agent disopyramide, 2 mg/kg given over 2 minutes, can be used in the same way with similar results [24] (Figure 15–7), observing loss of the delta wave in 86% of a population of patients found to have a shortest RR interval between preexcited beats in atrial fibrillation greater than 290 msec. In the latter study, the use of the disopyramide test and "Mobitz II" loss of the delta wave during treadmill testing allowed identification of 92% of the patients with a long refractory period of the accessory pathway with a specificity of 89% and a predictive value of 75%. Infrequent false positives with the disopyramide test (2 of 49 patients) were observed as a result of disappearance of the delta wave due to a combination of intraatrial conduction delay and prolongation of accessory pathway conduction time (but no refractoriness) after disopyramide.

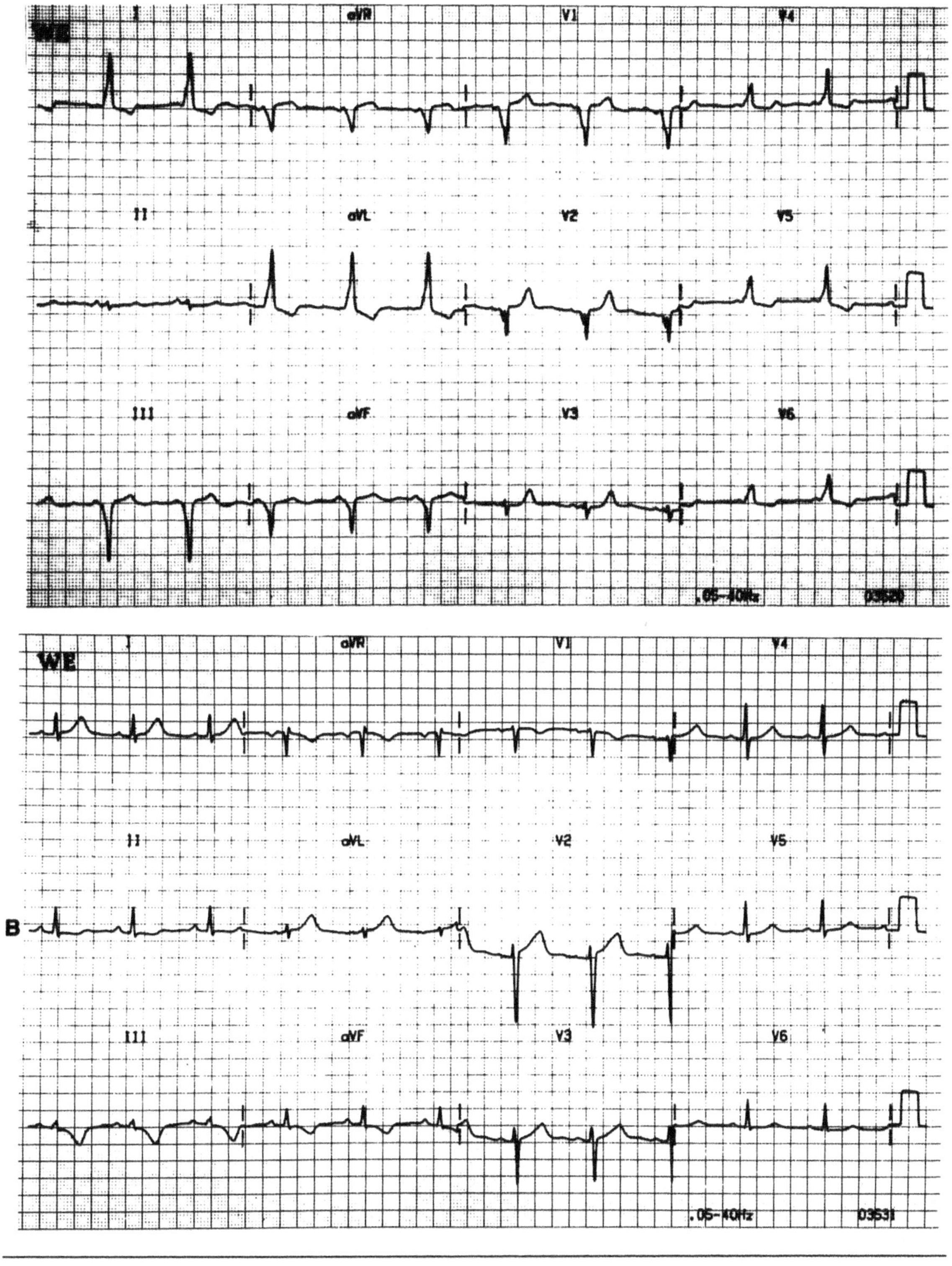

FIGURE 15–7. Loss of preexcitation after disopyramide. (A) shows a 12-lead electrocardiogram with obvious preexcitation. (B) is the electrocardiogram of the same patient 2 minutes after disopyramide, 2 mg/kg. The delta wave disappeared abruptly and the QRS is now entirely normal. This patient had no preexcited QRS complexes during induced atrial fibrillation in the absence of medication.

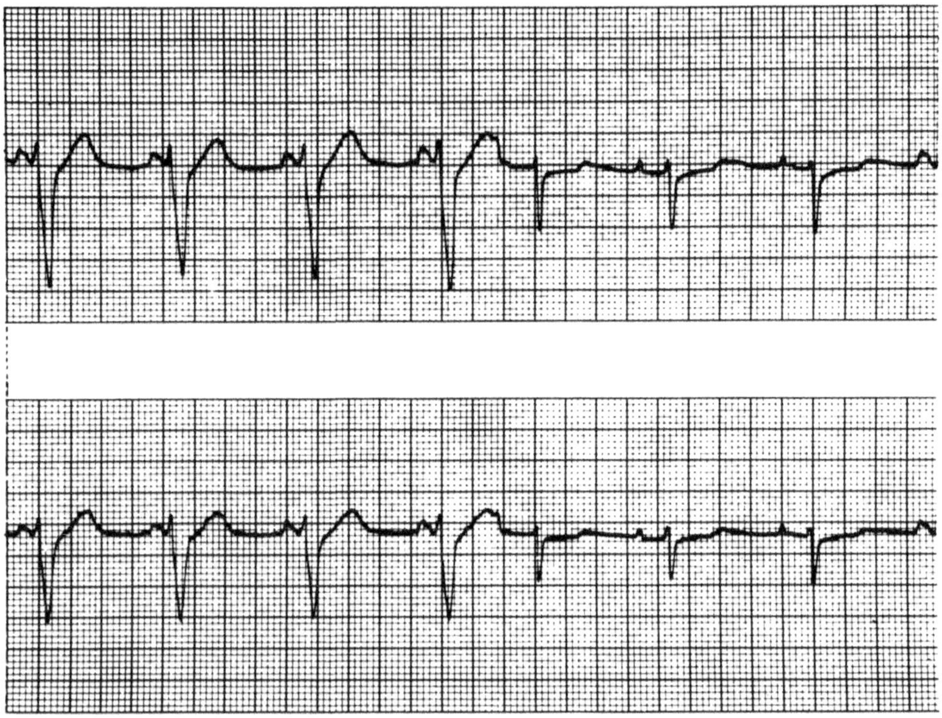

FIGURE 15–8. Ambulatory monitoring in a patient assessed for WPW syndrome. In this 2-channel recording, a spontaneous atrial extrasystole occurs after the fourth complex and conducts with a normalized QRS complex. From the record, it is clear that the ERP of the accessory pathway in this patient is at least 400 ms.

ESOPHAGEAL PACING

Esophageal pacing is a minimally invasive procedure that can provide a direct measurement of the refractory period of the accessory pathway and can be used for the induction of atrial fibrillation. This technique can certainly be a valuable maneuver when other noninvasive tests are equivocal and is discussed elsewhere in this book.

Patients Presenting with Recurrent Reciprocating Tachycardia

When a patient with WPW syndrome presents only with a history of recurrent paroxysmal tachycardia, the decision must be made whether to treat the patient empirically or proceed with invasive electrophysiologic studies. However, it is well known that some antiarrhythmic agents, notably verapamil [25] and digitalis [5], can accelerate the ventricular response during atrial fibrillation and it is also known that patients who present initially with reciprocating tachycardia may later develop atrial fibrillation. It is thus important that the clinician be reasonably confident that the ERP of the accessory pathway is "relatively long" (greater than 270 msec for all practical purposes). If this information can be obtained by the noninvasive tests enumerated above, the clinician may reasonably proceed with empirical drug trials. Ambulatory monitoring may be especially helpful in this respect if one is fortunate enough to observe normalization of the QRS with premature atrial depolarizations (Figure 15–8) and thus obtain a "natural" estimate of the ERP of the accessory pathway. It is our belief that invasive electrophysiologic studies are indicated in those WPW patients where one cannot determine the status of the anterograde refractory period of the accessory pathway. Although the severity of clinical symptoms such as chest pain or presyncope may incline the clinician towards the performance of electrophysiologic studies, the severity of symptoms does not necessarily predict a rapid ventricular response in the event of atrial fibrillation. For example, we have recently observed [26] that patients with a history of syncope during tachycardia do not have a more malignant electrophysiologic profile or an increased incidence of rapid ventricular responses during atrial fibrillation than their counterparts without this symptom.

The Patient with Documented Atrial Fibrillation

If atrial fibrillation has been documented electrocardiographically, the clinician has the most important piece of information to determine whether or not to proceed with further invasive studies. The demonstration of a rapid ventricular response during atrial fibrillation (shortest RR interval between preexcited beats less than 250 msec) clearly identifies patients with a potential for degeneration of this arrhythmia to ventricular fibrillation [5] and such patients should proceed with electrophysiologic studies with a view to establishing drug efficacy or as a prelude to surgical correction.

Initial Management of the Patient Presenting with Tachycardia

By far, the most common arrhythmias in patients with the WPW syndrome are orthodromic reciprocating tachycardia ("PAT," "RT," circus movement tachycardia) and atrial fibrillation.

PRESENTATION WITH RECIPROCATING TACHYCARDIA

Patients presenting acutely with regular, supraventricular tachycardia are most likely to have atrioventricular reentry utilizing a manifest or concealed accessory pathway as the retrograde limb of the circuit [7]. Atrioventricular nodal reentry, ectopic atrial tachycardia and atrial flutter with 2:1 AV block occur less frequently in patients with WPW syndrome. Factors favouring a diagnosis of atrioventricular reentry include:

1. Age of presentation under 21 years [7].
2. Tachycardia rate greater than 200/minute in the adult patient.
3. Bundle branch block aberration, especially if a rate change is observed after normalization of the QRS [3].
4. Identification of a retrograde P wave, where the RP interval is less than the PR interval [7].
5. Presence of a previous ECG showing the WPW pattern during sinus rhythm.
6. Electrical alternans of the QRS during tachycardia [27].
7. Alternation of long with short cycle lengths during tachycardia [28] (Figure 15–9). Although the latter can occur with AV nodal reentry, in our experience, it is usually seen with atrioventricular reentry utilizing an accessory AV pathway.

From a therapeutic standpoint, initial therapy does not depend critically on determining the mechanism of tachycardia. The following provides a standard approach to terminating reciprocating tachycardia:

1. One should try vagal stimulation techniques [29], utilizing carotid sinus massage alone, or in conjunction with edrophonium (Tensilon), 5–10 mg IV, or phenylephrine, .5–1 mg IV. Atrial flutter or ectopic atrial tachycardia will usually become apparent at this stage by observation of continuing tachycardia in the face of transient AV block. Reciprocating tachycardia will slow slightly and terminate or continue.
2. The initial drug of choice if vagotonic maneuvers fail is 5–10 mg verapamil intravenously. The great majority of reciprocating tachycardias involving the AV node as part of the circuit will terminate within 5–10 minutes after this drug. Verapamil should be administered slowly to avoid inducing hypotension due to peripheral vascular dilatation and should be used cautiously in patients taking beta-adrenergic blocking drugs, using more conservative doses of 2.5 to 5 mg intravenously. Although many authors advise against the use of the verapamil in this setting, we have not observed adverse effects when verapamil is added to beta-adrenergic blockers in younger patients without organic heart disease who are likely to have normal sinus node function [30].
3. Alternative drug regimens may be aimed at the AV nodal limb of the reentrant circuit (i.e., propranolol 5–10 mg IV) or the retro-

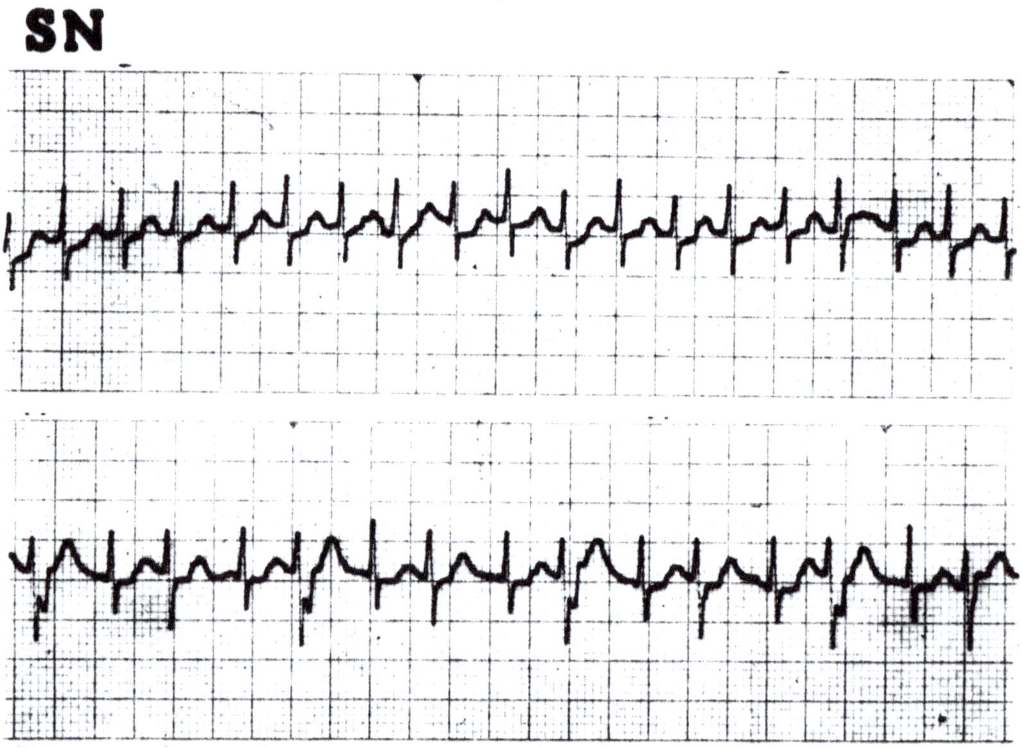

FIGURE 15–9. Cycle length alternans. In this patient with WPW syndrome, both regular SVT (*top panel*) and SVT with cycle length alternans (*bottom panel*) can be observed.

grade limb, be it an accessory pathway or a "fast" retrograde AV nodal pathway (i.e., disopyramide 2 mg/kg IV or procainamide 5–10 mg/kg IV).

4. Pacing techniques (burst pacing or atrial extrastimuli) can terminate reentrant tachycardia and pacing can be achieved by a trasvenous catheter or with an esophageal electrode. These techniques are discussed more fully elsewhere in this volume.
5. Synchronized transthoracic shock can be used if the above fail or if severe hemodynamic decompensation occurs at any stage. Note, however, that termination of tachycardia may not fully reverse hypotension induced by rapid infusion of verapamil (see above).

A note of caution is warranted if intravenous digitalis or verapamil is used. The latter may result in acceleration of the ventricular response in atrial fibrillation in WPW [5,25]. Consequently, patients should be closely observed with the physician ready to proceed with transthoracic cardioversion/defibrillation should reciprocating tachycardia degenerate into atrial fibrillation. After termination of the acute episode, further investigation should proceed as outlined previously.

PRESENTATION WITH ATRIAL FIBRILLATION

Atrial fibrillation with predominantly preexcited QRS complexes may be a life-threatening arrhythmia (Figure 15–10) with average ventricular rates up to 300 per minute or greater. Surprisingly, these rates may be reasonably well tolerated for some time in patients without heart disease and, if so, intravenous medication can be tried. Medications that prolong the antegrade refractory period of the accessory pathway, such as disopyramide 2 mg/kg IV or procainamide 5–10 mg/kg IV, may slow the ventricular response and even terminate the arrhythmia. However, the patient should be carefully watched with resort to transthoracic shock in the event of hemodynamic decompensation. Intravenous administration of either

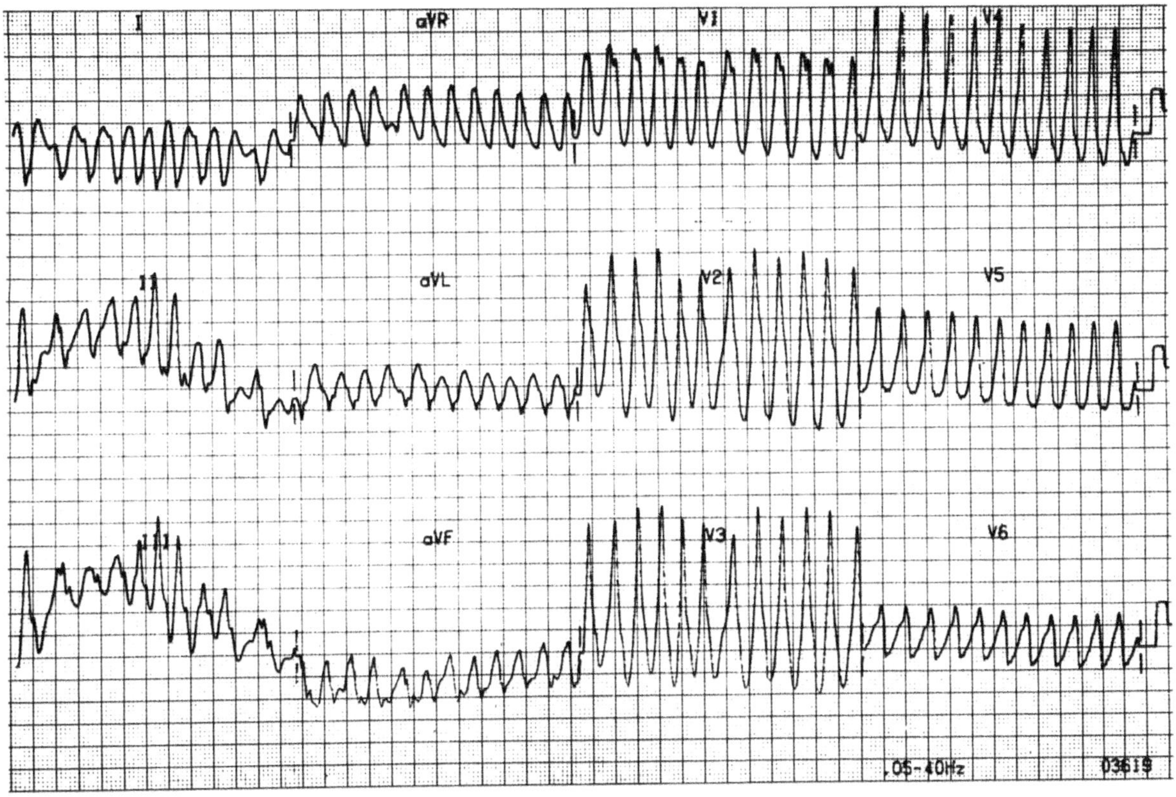

FIGURE 15–10. Atrial fibrillation in WPW syndrome. In this patient with a left lateral accessory pathway, the average ventricular response is greater than 250 per minute. Sinus rhythm was restored after disopyramide, 2 mg/kg.

digitalis or verapamil is *contraindicated* in this setting as they may be associated with acceleration of the ventricular response leading to ventricular fibrillation [5,25,31].

After termination of the episode, management should include electrophysiologic testing to verify drug efficacy or as a prelude to surgical correction [32]. However, if an impressive slowing of rate with reversion to sinus rhythm was observed with the use of procainamide or disopyramide, it would be reasonable for the patient to have an empirical trial with these medications orally. On oral therapy, an attempt should be made to replicate the plasma levels of the drug achieved with the beneficial intravenous injection.

Conclusion

The initial problem of the clinician in dealing with a patient with the WPW syndrome, regardless of the presentation, is to derive some estimate of the anterograde refractory period of the accessory pathway with a view to identifying those patients with potentially malignant ventricular responses in the event of atrial fibrillation. The noninvasive methods described are very useful in deciding in which WPW syndrome patients electrophysiologic testing is advised and which patients can be left untreated or treated empirically. Although ventricular fibrillation in the WPW syndrome is uncommon, it is certainly a tragedy to miss such a patient considering the relative ease and efficacy of modern management once the problem is identified.

References

1. Chung KY, Walsh TJ, Massie E: Wolff-Parkinson-White syndrome. *Am. Heart J.* 69:116, 1965.

2. Wolff L, White PD: Syndrome of short P-R interval with abnormal QRS complexes and paroxysmal tachycardia. *Arch. Intern. Med.* 82:446, 1948.
3. Coumel P, Attuel P: Reciprocating tachycardia in overt and latent preexcitation: Influence of bundle branch block on the rate of the tachycardia. *Eur. J. Cardiol.* 1:423, 1974.
4. Pritchett ELC, Gallagher JJ, Sealy WC, Gallagher JJ: Supraventricular tachycardia dependent upon accessory pathways in the absence of ventricular preexcitation. *Am. J. Med.* 64:214, 1978.
5. Klein GJ, Bashore TM, Sellers TD, Pritchett ELC, Smith WM, Gallagher JJ: Ventricular fibrillation in the Wolff-Parkinson-White syndrome. *N. Engl. J. Med.* 301:1080, 1979.
6. Wellens HJJ, Durrer D: Wolff-Parkinson-White syndrome and atrial fibrillation. Relation between refractory period of the accessory pathway and ventricular rate during atrial fibrillation. *Am. J. Cardiol.* 34:777, 1974.
7. Wellens HJJ, Farre J, Bar FWHM: The Wolff-Parkinson-White syndrome. In *Cardiac Arrhythmias*, WJ Mandel (eds.), JB Lippincott, Philadelphia, 1980 pp. 342–365.
8. Prystowsky EN, Miles WM, Heger JJ, Zipes DP: Preexcitation syndromes. Mechanisms and management. *Med. Clin. N. A.* 68:831, 1984.
9. Hishida H, Sotobata I, Koike Y, Okumura M, Mizuno Y. Echocardiographic patterns of ventricular contraction in the Wolff-Parkinson-White syndrome. *Circulation* 54:567, 1976.
10. Chan WWC, Kalff V, Dick M, Rabinovitch MA, Jenkins J, Thrall JH, Pitt B: Topography of preemptying ventricular segments in patients with Wolff-Parkinson-White syndrome using scintigraphic phase mapping and esophageal pacing. *Circulation* 67:1139, 1983.
11. Ohnell RF: Preexcitation: A cardiac abnormality. *Acta Med. Scand.* (Suppl) 152:1, 1944.
12. Hamburger WW: Bundle branch block: Four cases of intraventricular block showing some interesting and unusual clinical features. *Med. Clin. N. A.* 13:343, 1929.
13. Klein GJ, Gulamhusein SS: Intermittent preexcitation in the Wolff-Parkinson-White syndrome. *Am. J. Cardiol.* 52:292, 1983.
14. Hindman MC, Last JH, Rosen KM: Wolff-Parkinson-White syndrome observed by portable monitoring. *Ann. Intern. Med.* 79:654, 1973.
15. Wellens HJJ, Bar FW, Farre J, Ross D, Vanagt EJ: Sudden death in the Wolff-Parkinson-White syndrome. In *Sudden Death*, HE Kulbertus, HJJ Wellens (eds.). Martinus Nijhoff, Boston, 1980, pp. 392–399.
16. Klein GJ, Yee R, Sharma AD: Concealed conduction in accessory atrioventricular pathways: An important determinant of the expression of arrhythmias in patients with Wolff-Parkinson-White syndrome. *Circulation* 70:402, 1984.
17. Strasberg B, Ashley WW, Wyndham CRC, Bauernfeind RA, Swiryn SP, Dhingra RC, Rosen KM: Treadmill exercise testing in the Wolff-Parkinson-White syndrome. *Am. J. Cardiol.* 45:742, 1980.
18. Force T, Graboys TB: Exercise testing and ambulatory monitoring in patients with preexcitation syndrome. *Arch. Intern. Med.* 141:88, 1981.
19. Sherf L, Neufeld HN: The Pre-excitation Syndrome: Facts and Theories, Yorke Medical Books, New York, 1978, pp. 117–142.
20. Lévy S, Broustet JP, Clementy J, Circoulon B, Bricaud H, Gerard R: Value of noninvasive techniques in the Wolff-Parkinson-White syndrome with particular reference to exercise testing. In *Cardiac Arrhythmias*, S Lévy, MM Scheinman (eds.). Futura Publishing Company, New York, 1984, pp. 301–312.
21. Wellens HJJ, Bar FW, Dassen WRM, Brugada P, Vanagt EJ, Farre J: Effect of drugs in the Wolff-Parkinson-White syndrome. *Am. J. Cardiol.* 46:665, 1980.
22. Wellens HJJ, Bar FW, Gorgels AP: Use of ajmaline in identifying patients with the Wolff-Parkinson-White syndrome and a short refractory period of their accessory pathway. *Am. J. Cardiol.* 45:63, 1980.
23. Wellens HJJ, Braat S, Brugada P, Gorgels APM, Bar FW: Use of procainamide in patients with the Wolff-Parkinson-White syndrome to disclose a short refractory period of the accessory pathway. *Am. J. Cardiol.* 50:1087, 1982.
24. Sharma AD, Klein GJ, Yee R, Milstein S: Noninvasive assessment of accessory pathway conduction in the Wolff-Parkinson-White syndrome. (Abstract.) *Clin. Invest. Med.* (Suppl X) X:43, 1984.
25. Gulamhusein S, Ko P, Carruthers SG, Klein GJ: Acceleration of the ventricular response during atrial fibrillation in the Wolff-Parkinson-White syndrome after verapamil. *Circulation* 65:348, 1982.
26. Yee R, Klein GJ: Syncope in the Wolff-Parkinson-White syndrome: Incidence and electrophysiologic correlates. *PACE* 7:381, 1984.
27. Green M, Heddle B, Dassen W, Wehr M, Abdollah H, Brugada P, Wellens HJJ: Value of QRS alternation in determining the site of origin of narrow QRS supraventricular tachycardia. *Circulation* 68:368, 1983.
28. Ross DL, Dassen WRM, Vanagt EJ, Brugada P, Bar FWHM, Wellens HJJ: Cycle length alternation in circus movement tachycardia using an atrioventricular accessory pathway. *Circulation* 65:862, 1982.
29. Waxman MB, Wald RW, Sharma AD, Hverta F,

Cameron DA: Vagal techniques for termination of paroxysmal supraventricular tachycardia. *Am. J. Cardiol.* 46:655, 1980.

30. Yee R, Gulamhusein SS, Klein GJ: Combined verapamil and propranolol for supraventricular tachycardia. *Am. J. Cardiol.* 53:757, 1984.

31. Gulamhusein S, Ko P, Klein GJ: Ventricular fibrillation following verapamil in the Wolff-Parkinson-White syndrome. *Am. Heart J.* 106:145, 1983.

32. Klein GJ, Guiraudon GM: Surgical therapy of cardiac arrhythmias. *Cardiol. Clin.* 1:323, 1983.

16. TRANSESOPHAGEAL RECORDING AND PACING TECHNIQUES FOR EVALUATION OF PATIENTS WITH PREEXCITATION

David C. Chung
Charles R. Kerr

Preexcitation of the ventricle may be associated with (1) one or more accessory (anomalous) atrioventricular (AV) pathways, (2) an atriofascicular bypass tract, (3) an intranodal bypass tract, or (4) a nodoventricular or fasciculoventricular connection. However, ventricular preexcitation in association with an accessory AV pathway seen in the so-called Wolff-Parkinson-White (WPW) syndrome [1–5] is the most common. Victims of this syndrome frequently have disabling and occasionally life-threatening arrhythmias [6–12]. The term *preexcitation syndrome* is used in this chapter to mean the WPW syndrome unless otherwise stated.

Conduction of impulses across an accessory AV pathway in the antegrade direction is usually more rapid than across the AV node, resulting in fusion of ventricular activation during sinus rhythm and accounting for the delta wave of ventricular preexcitation superimposed on the QRS complex of normal ventricular excitation.

This project is supported in part by grants from the British Columbia Heart Foundation and the Medical Research Council of Canada.

This syndrome affects patients of all ages [7]. According to most studies the incidence of WPW syndrome varies between 0.12 and 0.2% in the general population [13–16]: between 54 and 70% of the affected patients are men [17–19], and 60 to 70% of the cases are found in healthy individuals without organic heart disease [2,8,19,20].

Depending on the series, the incidence of paroxysmal tachycardias among patients who have the WPW syndrome varies between 40 and 80% [6,7,19–21]. The most frequent arrhythmia is orthodromic reciprocating (reentrant) tachycardia, with antegrade conduction via the AV node and His bundle–Purkinje system and retrograde conduction via the accessory pathway as shown in Figure 16–1B [9]. In rare occasions, tachycardia utilizing a reentrant circuit in the reverse direction as shown in Figure 16–1C (antidromic reciprocating tachycardia) can also occur [22,23]. A variant of this syndrome, in which the accessory pathway is capable of conduction *only in the retrograde direction* (concealed pathways), has been recognized recently [24–27]. These pathways are capable of perpetuating an orthodromic reciprocating tachycardia, but preexcitation is not seen during sinus rhythm.

Whereas paroxysmal reciprocating tachycardia may be a frequent and disabling tachycardia

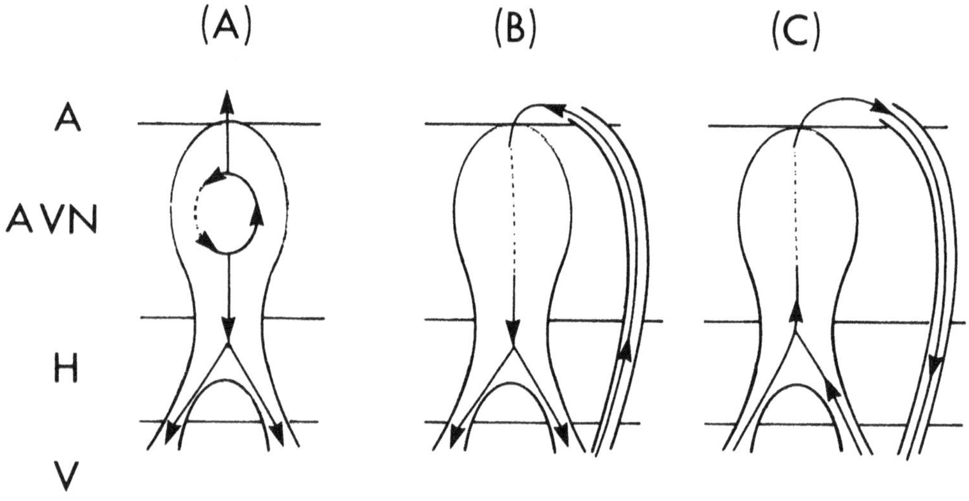

FIGURE 16–1. Mechanisms of reciprocating supraventricular tachycardia: (A) reentry within the AV node, (B) orthodromic atrioventricular reentry utilizing an accessory AV pathway, and (C) antidromic atrioventricular reentry utilizing an accessory AV pathway.

seen in patients with preexcitation, atrial fibrillation, or flutter may be life-threatening. These two arrhythmias account for nearly a quarter of all tachycardias seen in these patients [10], but atrial flutter alone is extremely rare. If the accessory pathway has a short antegrade effective refractory period, atrial fibrillation or flutter may result in rapid ventricular response that can deteriorate into ventricular fibrillation [11,28,29]. This potential risk may be compounded further by the administration of digitalis [30–32] or verapamil [33–35]. These two drugs are commonly prescribed for the treatment of paroxysmal supraventricular tachyarrhythmias and may shorten refractoriness of the accessory pathway, accelerate the ventricular response during atrial fibrillation, and facilitate the progression to ventricular fibrillation.

The clinical importance of identifying patients who have the WPW syndrome or its variant, of determining the behavior of the ventricles during atrial fibrillation or flutter, and of following the effects of therapy is self-evident. In the past, endocardial recording and pacing was the only method available for this purpose. More recently, transesophageal recording and pacing has become a valuable noninvasive means of diagnosing the mechanisms of supraventricular tachycardia and of assessing the efficacy of therapeutic agents.

History of Esophageal Recording and Pacing

Due to the proximity between the esophagus and the posterior aspect of the heart, the possibility of using an esophageal electrode for recording cardiac electrograms has captivated the imagination of physicians since the turn of the century. The first successful attempt was accredited to Cremer [36], but his report, dated back to 1906, attracted little attention owing to the size of the electrode he used. It measured 10 cm long and 1.5 cm in diameter, and his subject was a professional sword swallower. As a result, the method failed to become popular but was revived by Lieberson and Liberson [37] after a hiatus of nearly 30 years. At about the same time, Brown [38,39] studied the anatomic position of the esophageal electrode in relation to the left atrium and systematically analysed the relationship between the atrial and ventricular deflections of transesophageal electrograms obtained during sinus rhythm and during atrial arrhythmias, ventricular extrasystoles, and bundle branch block. He published his wealth of experience on the subject in 1936, providing the groundwork for much of our current understanding of this subject. Since then, there have been a series of reports advocating the use of transesophageal recording of electrograms in the diagnosis of tachyarrhythmias [40–45]. In 1979 the technique of transesophageal recording was developed further by Jenkins et al. [46], who introduced a swallowable electrode encased in a gelatin capsule. They used this pill electrode for long-term monitoring and found the recordings suitable for computer assisted analysis. In that same year, Benditt and his coworkers [47] introduced the ventricle-to-atrium activation interval recorded by endocardial leads during reciprocating supraventricular tachycardia as a means of differentiating reentry utilizing an accessory AV pathway from reentry within the AV node. In the following year, Gallagher et al. [48] reported similar discriminant value of the ventricle-to-atrium activation interval obtained from transesophageal recordings.

Besides these milestones in the transesophageal recording of the cardiac electrogram, there has been equal enthusiasm in pacing the heart via the esophagus. In 1952 Zoll [49] attempted transesophageal ventricular pacing in dogs, and in 1957 Shafiroff and Linder [50] applied this technique in man. In 1966 McNally [51] used an electrode in the esophagus to defibrillate the atria and noted that this technique required lower energy than conventional methods. Subsequently in 1969 Burack and Furman [52] reported successful tranesophageal ventricular pacing in a patient for 60 hours, and in 1971 Lubell [53] reported similar success in 3 of 5 patients who had complete AV block and slow ventricular rhythm. Stopczyk and his colleagues [54] used transesophageal atrial pacing in a patient with sinus node dysfunction and for the determination of AV nodal refractory period in 1972, and Montoyo [55] employed rapid atrial pacing via an esophageal lead to terminate reciprocating supraventricular tachycardia in 1973. The feasibility of this last technique was confirmed in 1982 by Gallagher and his associates [56], who also used the same procedure to induce reciprocating supraventricular tachycardia in susceptible patients. Similarly, Kerr et al. [57] used the transesophageal technique to induce atrial fibrillation or flutter and to terminate atrial flutter. In addition to these studies there have been sporadic applications of transesophageal cardiac pacing in resuscitation [58–60], and Andersen and Pless have shown that both atrial and ventricular pacing could be achieved reliably by using esophageal balloon leads [61].

Despite concerns about the possibility of electrical burns at the site of the stimulating electrodes, such complication has been reported following transesophageal cardiac pacing. The patient in the report of Burack and Furman [52] died after 60 hours of continuous pacing. At autopsy, no coagulative necrosis was observed in the esophagus; the esophageal mucosa was normal except for two small areas of pressure necrosis at the site of the electrode. Similarly no erythema, erosions, or ulceration was observed in another patient reported by Shaw and his colleagues [58] at esophagoscopy done after 30 minutes of transesophageal pacing. The absence of any complications is also confirmed by our own experience of approximately 150 cases of transesophageal pacing.

Origin of the Atrial Component of the Transesophageal Electrogram

As it descends in the posterior mediastinum, the lower half of the esophagus emerges from behind the carina of the trachea to run directly against the posterior surface of the heart and in front of the descending aorta before it disappears into the abdominal cavity through the diaphragmatic hiatus (Figures 16–2 and 16–3). The posterior aspect of the heart is formed to a large extent by the free wall of the left atrium superiorly with only a small contribution from the base of the left ventricle inferiorly. In situ, the left atrium extends between the body of the fifth thoracic vertebra and the T8–9 intervertebral disc; it is separated from the esophagus only by the pericardium. The distance between an electrode placed in the esophagus at this level and the wall of the left atrium is no more than 0.5 to 1 cm [41]. The close proximity between the esophageal electrode and the posterior left atrial wall has been confirmed recently by left atrial cineangiography [62]. It is little wonder that the atrial component of the electrogram recorded at this level of the esophagus has been attributed to left atrial depolarization [62–64].

However, this interpretation based on anatomic relationships was questioned by Prystowsky et al. [65]. In their attempt to localize the origin of the atrial component of the transesophageal electrogram in man, these authors followed the sequence of retrograde atrial activation in 16 patients. Eleven of these patients had reentrant tachycardia involving ret-

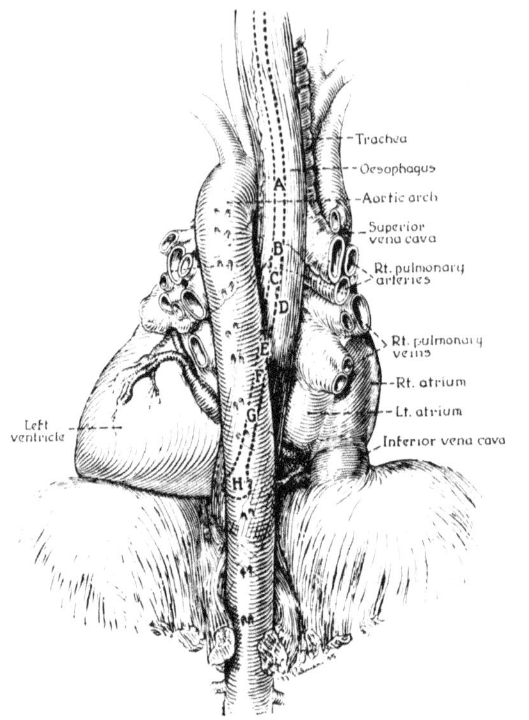

FIGURE 16–2. A diagram illustrating the anatomic relationship between the distal esophagus and the posterior surface of the heart: This portion of the esophagus lies largely in apposition to the posterior free wall of the left atrium [38]. For the purpose of transesophageal recording and pacing, the electrode is placed at a level between E and G. (Reproduced with the permission of the publisher.)

rograde conduction across an accessory pathway; 1 of the 16 had reentry in the AV node; the other 4 had retrograde conduction during ventricular pacing. They compared the ventricle-to-atrium activation interval recorded in the transesophageal electrogram to that obtained by endocardial mapping with catheter electrodes exploring the right atrium, the atrial septum, and the left atrium via the coronary sinus. Their results showed that in 5 out of 7 patients with left lateral accessory pathways, the ventricle-to-atrium activation interval measured from transesophageal electrograms was significantly longer than the ventricle-to-left-atrium activation interval measured by intracardiac mapping. In fact, the ventricle-to-atrium activation interval recorded by the transesophageal electrogram correlated best with ventricle-to-septal activation in all 16 patients. They suggested that the atrial component of electrograms recorded in the distal esophagus probably reflects posterior paraseptal atrial and not left atrial depolarization.

In support of their findings these authors referred to cross-sections obtained at this level of the thorax by computer assisted tomography, showing the proximity between the esophagus and the atrial septum [66]. This anatomic relationship is also confirmed by the drawings of Brown (Figure 16–3C) [38]. Nevertheless, similar retrograde activation intervals ascertained from transesophageal electrograms and those obtained by endocardial mapping can only be regarded as indirect evidence that the atrial component of electrograms recorded in the distal esophagus reflects atrial septal depolarization. The origin of the atrial complex seen on transesophageal electrograms remains unsettled. Despite this controversy, however, there is empiric evidence that the time from ventricular to atrial activation obtained from transesophageal electrograms can be used to identify patients who utilize an accessory pathway during paroxysmal reciprocating supraventricular tachycardia (see the next section in this chapter).

Diagnostic Functions of Esophageal Recording and Pacing

TO IDENTIFY THE USE OF AN ACCESSORY PATHWAY IN RECIPROCATING SUPRAVENTRICULAR TACHYCARDIA

Reentry using an accessory pathway and reentry confined within the AV node are two of the most common mechanisms of paroxysmal reciprocating supraventricular tachycardia [67,68]. However, in the absence of overt preexcitation during sinus rhythm, the participation of an accessory pathway in the arrhythmia may be overlooked. In the past, the mechanism of a reciprocating supraventricular tachycardia has been attributed to AV nodal reentry if ventricular preexcitation was not observed during sinus rhythm. Recent improvement in diagnostic techniques has shown however that a high percentage of patients with recurrent tachycardias have accessory pathways capable of only retrograde conduction (concealed pathways). This is particularly true in cases that are refractory to drug therapy. Because of the potential for surgical ablation of the accessory AV path-

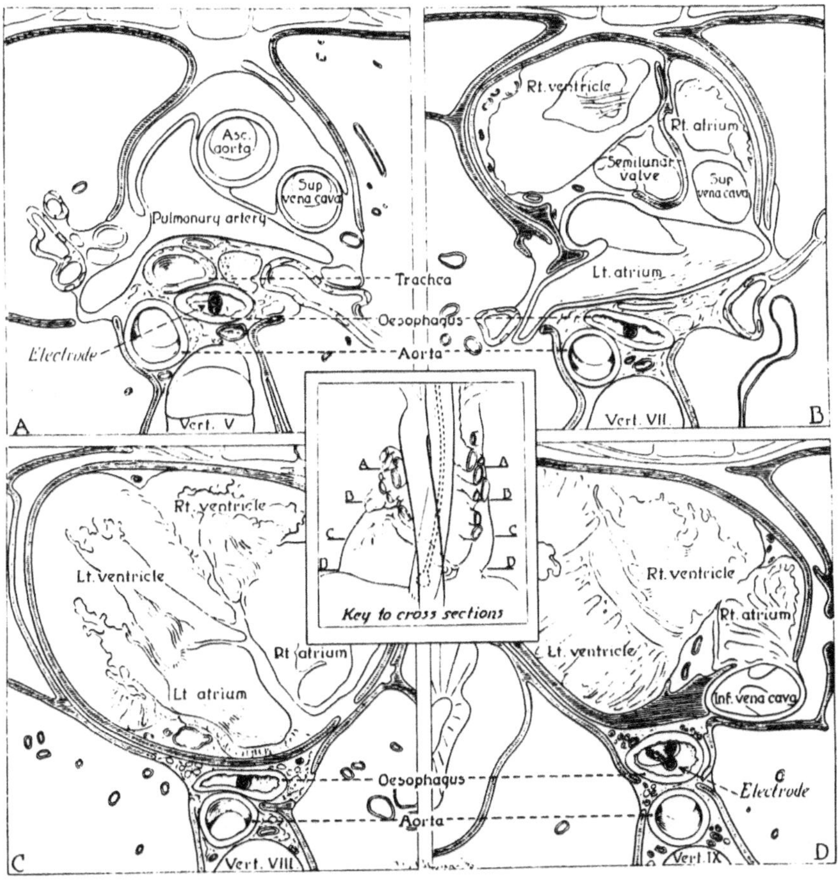

FIGURE 16–3. Cross-sections of the mediastinum illustrating the relationship between the distal esophagus and the heart: In (C) the esophagus is shown lying against the posterior free wall of the left atrium. At this level it is also in close proximity to the atrial septum [38]. (Reproduced with the permission of the publisher.)

way, the differentiation between these two mechanisms is extremely important.

In reentry confined to the AV node (Figure 16–1A), the retrograde limb of the reentry circuit is characterized by rapid conduction in the majority of cases (slow-fast form) — that is, the impulse rapidly returns to the upper part of the AV node and the atrium. Consequently, the atria and ventricles, both being activated as offshoots of the reentry circuit, are excited at approximately the same time. In contrast, during tachycardia utilizing an accessory pathway (Figure 16–1B) the impulse must sequentially traverse the AV node, His-Purkinje system, ventricle, accessory pathway, and atrium — thus creating a delay between the earliest ventricular and atrial activation (the ventricle-to-atrium activation or VA interval).

The time relationship between the QRS complex and the retrograde P wave (the VA interval on the surface electrocardiogram) during tachycardia has been exploited previously by the astute electrocardiographer to determine the underlying mechanism of the tachycardia. In a correlation of electrocardiographic and intracardiac electrophysiologic observations in 79 patients with paroxysmal supraventricular tachycardia, Wu and his associates [69] found that reciprocating tachycardia involving a concealed accessory pathway was characterized by a P wave following the QRS complex during tachycardia whereas AV nodal reentrant tachycardia was characterized by the absence of visible P wave in most instances because of its synchronous occurrence with the QRS complex. The importance of these electrocardiographic signs has been confirmed also by others [70]. Unfortunately, identification of the P wave on the surface electrocardiogram during tachycardia may be difficult because of its superposition on the ST–T wave.

In 1979 Benditt et al. [47] reported results of a retrospective analysis of data obtained during intracardiac electrophysiologic studies in 65 patients with the preexcitation syndrome and in 15 patients with AV nodal reentrant tachycardia. They showed that both the time from ventricular depolarization to the earliest atrial deflection (VA-min) and the time from ventricular activation to depolarization of the high right atrium (VA-hra) were significantly longer in patients who had reciprocating tachycardia involving an accessory pathway than in those who had AV nodal reentrant tachycardia. They suggested that a VA-min of 61 ms or less and a VA-hra of 95 ms or less during an episode of tachycardia excluded the participation of an accessory pathway in reciprocating tachycardia.

In the following year, Gallagher and his associates [48] compared the application of the VA intervals during tachycardia obtained from transesophageal recordings to those obtained with multielectrode intracardiac recordings. In their study of 28 patients, ages 2 to 65 years, reciprocating supraventricular tachycardia either occurred spontaneously or was induced by atrial pacing. During tachycardia, electrograms in the distal esophagus were mapped (from the most distal point where an atrial component could be recorded and at 1-cm intervals cephalad until the atrial complex was no longer recordable), and the shortest VA interval recorded by the esophageal lead (VA-eso) was compared to the intracardiac VA-min. They found that the latter was shorter than the former; but both were useful in differentiating reentry involving an accessory pathway from reentry in the AV node. All 16 patients in the study who had reciprocating tachycardia involving an accessory pathway had a VA-eso longer than 70 ms, although 1 of 12 patients who had AV nodal reentrant tachycardia also had a VA-eso longer than 70 msec. These authors proposed that the long VA-eso interval found in this patient was due either to his having a slow conducting segment interposed

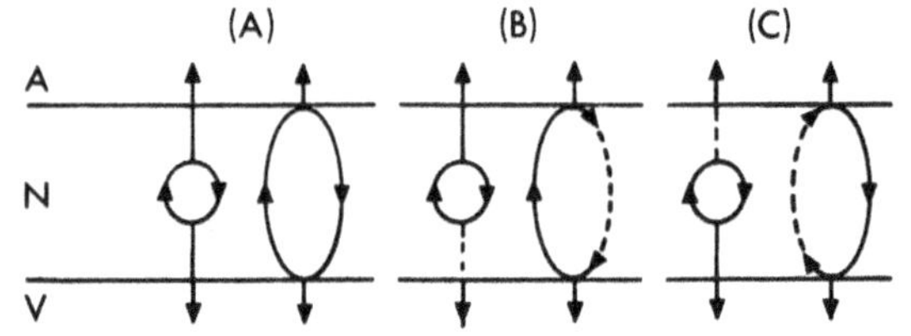

FIGURE 16–4. Possible circuits of reentry within the AV node: The pathways of slow conduction are represented by broken lines. In (A) and (B) atrial activation follows ventricular excitation in rapid sequence, and the ventricle-to-atrium activation interval (VA-eso) recorded by the esophageal lead is short. In (C) retrograde conduction involves slow pathways and the VA-eso may be longer than 70 ms. (Adapted from Gallagher et al. [48].)

between the reentrant circuit and the retrograde common pathway or to his using the slowly conducting AV pathway as the retrograde limb of the reentrant circuit (the "fast-slow" type of reentry) as shown in Figure 16–4C — thus accounting for his long VA-eso during reciprocating tachycardia.

In a subsequent study, Benson et al. [71] applied this technique to 14 infants between 1 and 84 days in age, all of whom had episodes of supraventricular tachycardia and three of whom had electrocardiographic features of ventricular preexcitation involving an accessory AV pathway. In contrast to the study described above [48], they recorded the electrogram only at the level of largest atrial deflections instead of mapping atrial activities in the distal esophagus. They found that the VA-eso was longer than 70 ms in all their infants and attributed this to involvement of accessory AV pathways in perpetuating the supraventricular tachycardia. Therefore a VA-eso of greater than 70 ms during tachycardia appears to be a generally reliable indicator of the participation of an accessory pathway in paroxysmal supraventricular tachycardia, whereas a VA-eso less than 70 ms is indicative of reentry confined to the AV node (Figures 16–5 and 16–6).

TO DETERMINE THE VENTRICULAR RESPONSE DURING ATRIAL FIBRILLATION

In conjunction with transesophageal recording, transesophageal atrial pacing plays an important role in diagnosis of arrhythmias. First of all, it is

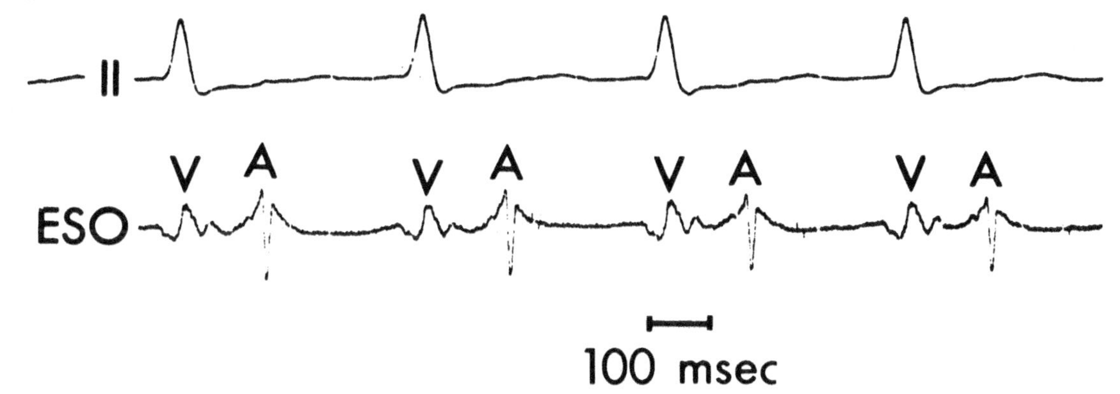

FIGURE 16–5. The ventricle-to-atrium activation interval (VA-eso) in a patient who has reciprocating supraventricular tachycardia involving an accessory pathway: This interval is obtained from the transesophageal cardiac electrogram (ESO). It measures from the beginning of the V wave to the most rapid intrinsic deflection of the A wave and is 160 ms in this instance. A VA-eso longer than 70 ms during reciprocating supraventricular tachycardia is a reliable indicator of the participation of an accessory pathway in the tachycardia.

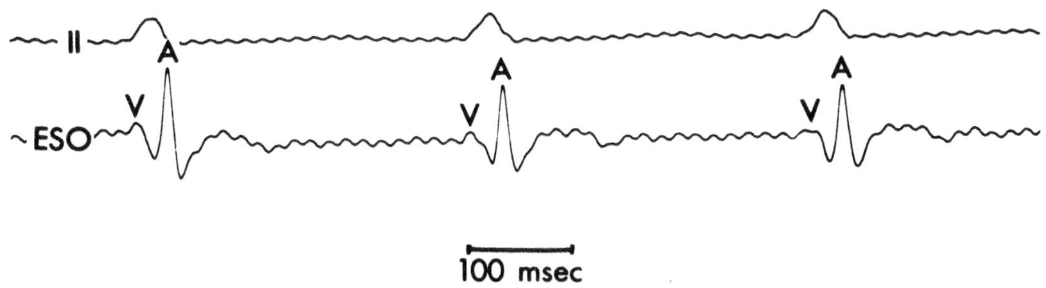

FIGURE 16–6. The ventricle-to-atrium activation interval (VA-eso) in a patient who has reciprocating supraventricular tachycardia involving reentry within the AV node: This interval is obtained from the transesophageal cardiac electrogram (ESO). The A wave follows the V wave in rapid sequence during AV nodal reentrant tachycardia. A comparison of the electrogram recorded during tachycardia to that obtained during sinus rhythm will facilitate the identification of these two components. The VA-eso is 35 ms in this instance (see also Figure 16–4). A VA-eso of less than 70 ms is a reliable indicator that the mechanism of the reciprocating supraventricular tachycardia is reentry within the AV node.

often necessary to induce reciprocating tachycardia by rapid transesophageal atrial pacing (Figure 16–7) in order to measure the VA-eso interval (see "Putting transesophageal recording and pacing into practice" later in this Chapter). Second, atrial fibrillation or flutter should be induced in these patients in order to assess the ventricular response.

For almost 40 years, ventricular preexcitation involving an accessory AV pathway found in patients without organic heart disease was assumed to be a benign electrocardiographic anomaly with excellent prognosis. Nevertheless, cases of ventricular fibrillation and sudden death among these apparently healthy patients have been reported in both the cardiology literature and actuarial studies [11,28,29,72]. In more recent reports, a direct link between ven-

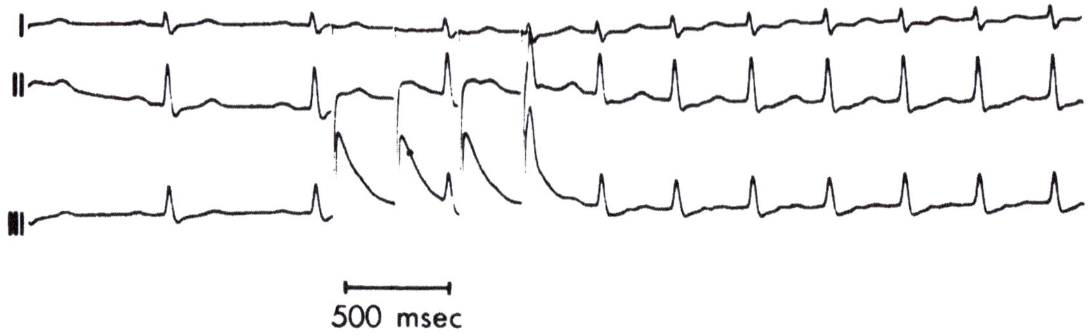

FIGURE 16–7. Induction of reciprocating supraventricular tachycardia involving an accessory AV pathway by rapid transesophageal atrial pacing: Sinus rhythm (cycle length = 710 ms) on the left hand side of this figure is converted to reciprocating supraventricular tachycardia (cycle length = 350 ms) by a four-beat burst of atrial pacing at a cycle length of 300 ms.

tricular rate recorded during atrial fibrillation and the risk of development of ventricular fibrillation has been established [28,29,73–76].

During atrial fibrillation, whether antegrade conduction is sustained by the AV node or the accessory pathway is determined by the conduction properties and refractoriness of these two pathways [74]. According to Wellens and Durrer [73], many factors affecting both the AV node and the accessory pathway as well as those affecting the ventricle can determine the rate of ventricular response during atrial fibrillation in these patients. Whereas the ventricular refractory period is the final determinant of this rate, the refractory periods of the AV node and the accessory pathway, the conduction properties of these two structures, and the presence of concealed conduction in the AV node and the accessory pathway all may affect the ventricular rate.

Castellanos et al. [75] found that in three patients in whom the antegrade effective refractory period of the accessory pathway was longer than that of the AV node, the ventricular rate was less than 210/min during atrial fibrillation or flutter; but in 3 others in whom the antegrade effective refractory period of the pathway was less than 220 ms, the ventricular rate could exceed 300/min. The majority of supraventricular impulses reached the ventricles via the normal AV nodal pathway in the first group and via the accessory pathway in the latter group of patients. The importance of the antegrade effective refractory period as a major determinant of ventricular rate during atrial fibrillation in patients who have the preexcitation syndrome was upheld by Wellens and Durrer [73]. They found that the shorter the antegrade effective refractory period of the accessory pathway, the faster the ventricular rate (as indicated by a short averaged RR interval) during atrial fibrillation. In the same study, these authors also observed that the shortest RR interval during atrial fibrillation in these patients was directly related to the antegrade effective refractory period of the pathway. However, this last observation has not been confirmed by that of others [29].

Klein et al. [29] compared two groups of patients with WPW syndrome: a control group without history of ventricular fibrillation and a second group with a history of ventricular fibrillation without other identifiable causes. They found that the second group of patients could be identified by these clinical features: a history of both atrial fibrillation and reciprocating tachycardia and the presence of more than one accessory AV pathway. Furthermore, these groups differed electrophysiologically by several parameters. The antegrade effective refractory periods of the accessory pathways in all the patients with a history of ventricular fibrillation were less than 350 ms; the ventricular rate of these patients during atrial fibrillation was faster than that of the control group — the averaged RR interval being 269 ± 62 and 340 ± 80 ms (mean ± S.D.) respectively; and their shortest RR interval between preexcited beats was shorter than that of the control group — 180 ± 29 and 240 ± 63 ms (mean ± S.D.), respectively. Among the electrophysiologic factors, the shortest RR interval between preexcited beats during atrial fibrillation was found by Klein and his colleagues to be the most useful indicator of patients at risk of having ventricular fibrillation. All the patients in the ventricular fibrillation group had shortest RR interval of 250 ms or less.

These observations have raised the possibility that the measurement of the shortest RR interval between preexcitated beats during induced atrial fibrillation may be a means of identifying patients who are at risk of developing ventricular fibrillation. Although the determination of the antegrade effective refractory period of the accessory pathway has similar predictive value, its measurement is not always possible because it is frequently shorter than the functional refractory period of atrial muscle. The use of the shortest RR interval between preexcitated beats during atrial fibrillation is both simple and reliable. Several authors have stressed the importance of inducing atrial fibrillation to evaluate the vulnerability to a rapid ventricular response [29,76,77].

Although similar data on the prognostic value of the shortest RR interval between preexcited beats during atrial flutter are not available, Castellanos et al. [75] did find an inverse relationship between the antegrade effective refractory period of the accessory pathway and the rate of ventricular response during atrial flutter. Therefore, it would not be unreasonable to assume that rapid conduction across the accessory pathway during atrial flutter that results in 1:1 ventricular response carries similar prognostic importance. The report of a patient who initially presented with atrial flutter associated with 1:1 ventricular response and subsequently developed atrial fibrillation followed by ventricular fibrillation [29] would seem to confirm this impression.

Whereas atrial fibrillation was induced by intracardiac pacing in earlier reports, Kerr et al. [57] demonstrated that atrial fibrillation or flutter could be reliably induced by transesophageal atrial pacing at cycle lengths between 60 and 200 ms. These authors were successful in inducing atrial flutter or fibrillation in 22 of 23 patients: fibrillation alone in 11, flutter alone in 6, and both fibrillation and flutter in 5. In the other patient, induction of fibrillation or flutter proved difficult, even by intracardiac pacing techniques. They suggested that the intentional induction of atrial fibrillation or flutter by transesophageal pacing may be used to study the behavior of the ventricles in patients who have ventricular preexcitation. This technique was applied successfully by Critelli and his colleagues [77] to follow the progress of treatment with amiodarone in 5 patients; they were successful in inducing atrial fibrillation in all 5 patients on more than one occasion by pacing at cycle lengths between 60 and 120 ms. Before amiodarone therapy the shortest RR intervals between preexcited beats of these 5 patients were between 190 and 210 ms (the mean being 198 ms). After amiodarone therapy, no ventricular preexcitation was observed in 2 patients and the shortest RR interval between preexcitated beats varied from 240 to 370 ms (the mean being 300 ms).

It has been suggested that there are other noninvasive methods to exclude accessory AV pathways with a short antegrade effective refractory period [78]. These include intermittent preexcitation during sinus rhythm [79], disappearance of preexcitation during exercise stress test [80], and development of antegrade block in the accessory pathway after intravenous administration of ajmaline [81] or procainamide [78]. However, like the effective refractory period of atrial or ventricular myocardium, that of the accessory pathway can decrease and its conduction capacity can increase during rapid atrial depolarization [76, 77]. None of these three methods have taken this factor into account and failures of these methods to exclude a rapid ventricular response during atrial fibrillation can be found in the report of Critelli et al. [77]. Pacing induced atrial fibrillation or flutter may be the most reliable means of assessing the potential for rapid ventricular response in patients with WPW syndrome.

Therapeutic Functions of Esophageal Recording and Pacing

Besides the diagnostic application of transesophageal pacing mentioned above, this technique can also be used to terminate all types of reciprocating supraventricular tachycardia, including that associated with an accessory AV pathway, irrespective of whether this pathway

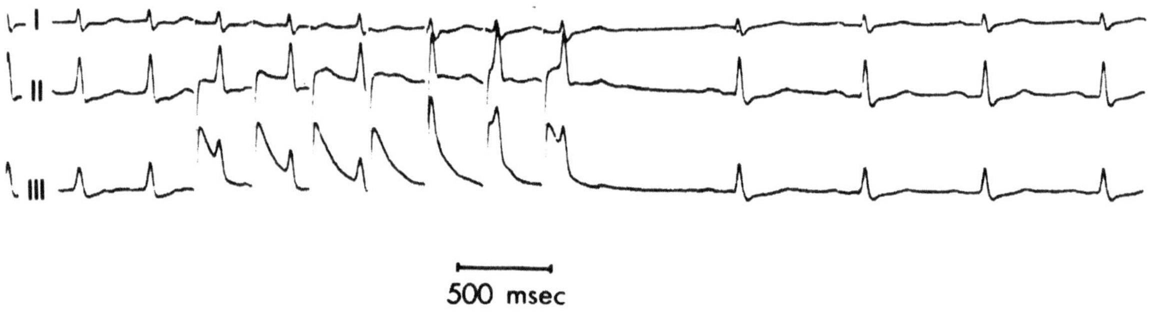

FIGURE 16–8. Termination of reciprocating supraventricular tachycardia involving an accessory AV pathway by rapid transesophageal atrial pacing: Reciprocating supraventricular tachycardia (cycle length = 360 ms) on the left hand side of this figure is converted to sinus rhythm (cycle length = 640 ms) by a seven-best burst of atrial pacing at a cycle length of 300 ms.

causes preexcitation or is concealed (Figure 16–8). Although this technique was first described in 1973 [55], its use had not increased until Gallagher et al. improved the reliability of atrial capture [56]. These authors found that a bipolar electrode with an interpolar distance of 29 mm was optimum for this purpose. The electrode was positioned in the esophagus at a level where the atrial component of the *unipolar* electrogram obtained with the proximal pole exhibited the greatest amplitude and the most rapid deflections. They showed that consistant atrial capture could be achieved in 26 of 39 patients if the pulse width was 1.0 ms and the mean pulse amplitude 21 ± 5 mA, in 33 of 39 patients if the pulse width was 2.0 ms and the mean pulse amplitude 18 ± 5 mA, and in 39 of 39 patients if the pulse width was 9.9 ms and the mean pulse amplitude 11 ± 5 mA. They also observed that, by using a stimulus with a pulse width between 7.0 to 9.9 ms and a mean pulse amplitude of 15 mA, it was possible to induce supraventricular tachycardia in 35 of 38 patients by pacing at a cycle length between 240 and 400 ms. In the other 3 patients, supraventricuar tachycardia was inducible only by direct ventricular pacing. (Thirty-three of the patients had reentrant tachycardia involving accessory pathways and 5 had reciprocating tachycardia associated with AV nodal reentry.) After supraventricular tachycardia was induced in these 38 patients, it was possible to terminate the arrhythmia one or more times in 33. In the other 5 patients the outcome was variable: the induced tachycardia was converted to atrial fibrillation which reverted to sinus rhythm spontaneously in 4; supraventricular tachycardia could not be terminated by transesophageal pacing in the other and drug therapy was required.

Subsequently, the reliability of inducing and terminating supraventricuar tachycardia in infants was tested by Benson et al. [71]. They used bipolar electrodes with an interpolar distance of 15 or 22 mm placed in the esophagus at a level where the atrial component of the *bipolar* electrogram was largest. The pulse width was 9.9 ms and the pulse amplitude between 10 to 20 mA. For the induction of tachycardia during sinus rhythm, they utilized one of the following protocols: (1) pacing the heart at incremental rates until the development of second degree heart block, (2) applying premature stimuli during normal sinus rhythm, or (3) applying extrastimuli at the end of a pacing drive of 350 or 400 ms cycle length. For termination of supraventricular tachycardia, they used burst pacing (a train of 2 to 8 stimuli) at a cycle length that was between 10 and 80 ms shorter than the cycle length of the tachycardia. They found that this technique was successful in 12 out of 12 infants.

In addition to the use of transesophageal pacing to terminate supraventricular tachycardia, Kerr et al. [57] reported that it was possible to use this technique to terminate atrial flutter (Figure 16–9). Using a bipolar electrode with an interpolar distance of 29 mm, a pulse width of 7.0 to 9.9 ms, a pulse amplitude just sufficient to capture the atria, and a cycle length between 10

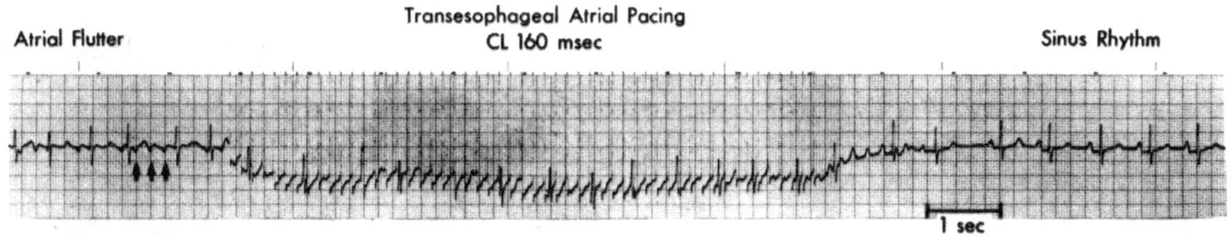

FIGURE 16–9. Termination of atrial flutter by rapid transesophageal atrial pacing: Atrial flutter on the left hand side of this figure is converted to sinus rhythm by a burst of atrial pacing. This technique is applicable to both induced and spontaneous atrial flutter.

and 60 ms shorter than the atrial flutter cycle lengths, they were successful in converting atrial flutter to sinus rhythm in 8 of 10 patients. In 7 of these patients, conversion was immediate; on one occasion, the transition was preceded by a brief period of junctional rhythm. In the other two patients who had flutter waves of extremely short cycle lengths (160 and 170 ms) termination of atrial flutter by transesophageal pacing was not successful. These authors attributed these two failures to the shorter cycle length of the flutter waves. Since this report, similar successes in the termination of induced or spontaneous atrial flutter by transesophageal atrial pacing have been reported by others [82–84]. Therefore transesophageal atrial pacing can be used both to induce atrial fibrillation or flutter in order to assess the ventricular response and to terminate atrial flutter in patients in whom this rhythm is induced. Subsequently, we have expanded our experience to the termination of spontaneous atrial flutter and have been successful in 20 of 24 patients presenting with this arrhythmia.

Technical Considerations in the Use of Esophageal Recording and Pacing

The successful application of esophageal recording and pacing in diagnosis and therapy depends on the use of appropriate equipment to record high-quality electrograms from the distal esophagus and to pace and capture the atria reliably. Therefore, a discussion on the choice of electrodes, pulse generators, and amplifiers and recorders is necessary.

THE ESOPHAGEAL ELECTRODE

Many designs of the esophageal electrode for either recording or pacing have been proposed. For the purpose of recording and pacing in the same sitting, as is required in an electrophysiology study, the use of a bipolar electrode is imperative. A bipolar electrode [85–87], together with proper filter settings of the amplifier [88] (see "The Amplifier and Recorder" in this chapter), will not only eliminate baseline drift and give transesophageal electrograms of the best quality but also assure consistant pacing and capturing. Thin, flexible catheter electrodes embedded in silicone rubber will also improve acceptance by the patient. Many authors used commercially available catheter electrodes designed for permanent transvenous pacing for this purpose. Originally Gallagher and his colleagues used the Medtronic 6904 endocardial lead with an interpolar distance of 16 mm for recording in adult patients [48]. Subsequently they found the Medtronic 6992 bipolar transvenous pacing electrode with an interpolar distance of 29 mm more suitable for pacing [56]. Critelli and his coworkers also successfully used the same Medtronic 6992 electrode for both recording and pacing [77]. Benson et al. [71], on the other hand, used the Medtronic 6902 electrode with an interpolar distance of 15 mm and the Medtronic 6904-A lead with an interpolar distance of 22 mm for recording and pacing in their infants. They reported equally satisfactory results with both. In our own laboratory we routinely use the Medtronic 6992 bipolar endocardial pacing electrode for both pacing and recording (Figure 16–10B).

THE PULSE GENERATOR

During endocardial pacing, little decrease in threshold is achieved by increasing the pulse width beyond 2 ms. During atrial pacing via the esophagus using the Medtronic 6992 electrode, Gallagher et al. [56] showed that pulse amplitude fell progressively when pulse width was increased in steps to 9.9 ms (Figure 16–11).

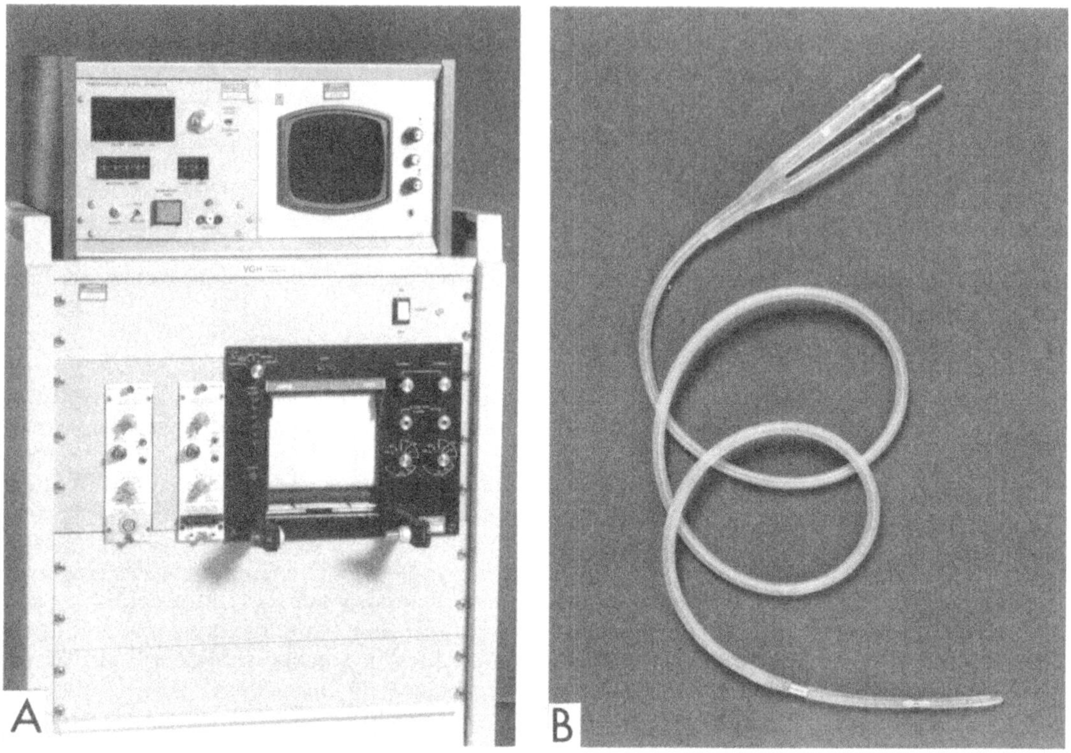

FIGURE 16-10. Transesophageal recording and pacing equipment: (A) the pulse generator, amplifiers, oscilloscope, and chart recorder and (B) the Medtronic 6992 pacing electrode.

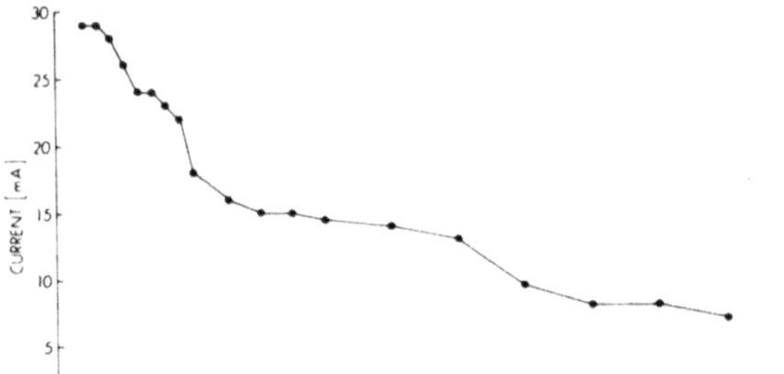

FIGURE 16-11. A representative strength-duration curve of transesophageal atrial pacing: The threshold current required to capture the atria falls progressively as the pulse width is increased to 10 ms [56]. (Reproduced with the permission of the authors and publisher.)

Similarly, the number of patients successfully paced also increased with a stepwise increase in pulse width. When the pulse width was between 8.0 and 9.9 ms, consistent atrial capture was achieved in all their patients. In a separate study, Benson and his associates [89] used a bipolar electrode with an interpolar distance of 15 or 22 mm in infants and an electrode with interpolar distance of 22 or 28 mm for adults. They found that these differences in interpolar distance had little effect on the pacing threshold. Furthermore, they reported that increasing the pulse width to 15 or 20 ms caused an insignificant fall in the pacing threshold obtained with a pulse width of 10 ms. The need of using a pulse width of about 10 ms has been repeatedly emphasized by Gallagher and Benson [56,89]. The long pulse width improves the reliability of capture and eliminates the necessity of a high current output, which is the major source of discomfort to the patient.

Most portable pulse generators used in endocardial pacing are capable of generating a square-wave pulse of no more than 2 ms in width and no more than 20 mA in output. For the purpose of transesophageal pacing, a variable pulse generator capable of generating a pulse up to 10 ms (9.9 ms) in width and up to 20 mA in amplitude is required. It should be capable of pacing at variable cycle lengths ranging between 50 and 1000 ms. The ability to discharge an extrastimulus at variable coupling intervals following a basic pacing drive is also a desirable feature but not absolutely necessary. We routinely set the pulse width at its maximum (i.e., 9.9 ms) and increase the output in steps until consistant capture of the atria is attained.

THE AMPLIFIER AND RECORDER

In order to record high-quality transesophageal electrograms for analysis, a bipolar electrode is necessary and proper filtering of the signals is equally important. While Gallagher et al. [48] used filter settings of 50 and 1000 Hz for their bipolar recordings, Benson and his group [71] used settings of 0.5 and 40 Hz obtained with standard ECG monitoring equipment. In our own laboratory, we filter our signals between 15 and 1000 Hz and find these settings satisfactory. The lower filter setting can be adjusted to minimize baseline drift and optimize the quality of the recording. The output from the amplifier should be directed to both an oscilloscope and a chart recorder.

With respect to the recorder, one with variable paper speeds is necessary. A paper speed of 100 mm/s is recommended for the measurement of VA-eso and shortest RR intervals. Time marks that are accurate to 10 ms and incorporated directly onto the record will improve the accuracy of these measurements. We use a two-channel recorder in our laboratory: one channel for the transesophageal recording and the other for lead II electrocardiogram. The pulse generator, amplifiers, oscilloscope, and recorder can be mounted on a cart to form an integral unit as shown in Figure 16–10A.

PUTTING TRANSESOPHAGEAL RECORDING AND PACING INTO PRACTICE

In earlier sections, the theoretical and empirical bases for the use of transesophageal recording and pacing as a diagnostic and therapeutic tool in patients who have ventricular preexcitation in association with accessory AV pathways have been outlined; the technical specifications of instruments required for this purpose have also been delineated. In order to reap the full benefit of this technique, it must be done properly. In this section, the conduct of the procedure is recapitulated for the benefit of those who are not familiar with the technique.

Being minimally invasive in nature, transesophageal recording and pacing can be done as an outpatient procedure. However, the technique does carry certain potential risks: they include pacing of the ventricles or phrenic nerve, pacing the brachial plexus in small infants, tracheal irritation, and the precipitation of a tachycardia that requires electrical cardioversion. Other discomfort is usually mild. Most patients will complain of a tingling or burning sensation in the precordial region during pacing and, although not usually necessary, the administration of diazepam with or without meperidine may be required. The procedure should be performed in the postabsorptive state as placement of the lead may cause gagging and vomiting. In all cases a freely running intravenous infusion should be established before the procedure, and the patient should be monitored continuously by ECG. The procedure itself can be done in an electrophysiology laboratory, in the emergency department, or at the patient's bedside; *but equipment for resuscitation should be immediately available.*

In our laboratory, the electrode is well-lubricated with lidocaine jelly and introduced into the distal esophagus through the nares with the patient lying supine. The proper position of the electrode can be confirmed by either (1) monitoring the bipolar esophageal electrogram as the electrode courses its way down the esophagus and the site of minimum pacing threshold is approximately at the level at which the atrial component of the electrogram shows the largest and fastest deflection [71,89], or (2) using the graph relating the ideal depth of insertion to the height of the patient proposed by Benson et al. (Figure 16–12) [89]. The second method is more expedient, particularly in an emergency.

If the patient is in sinus rhythm, induction of supraventricular tachycardia and atrial fibrillation or flutter is necessary before recording is made for the determination of the VA-eso and the shortest RR interval between preexcited beats, respectively. Reciprocating supraventric-

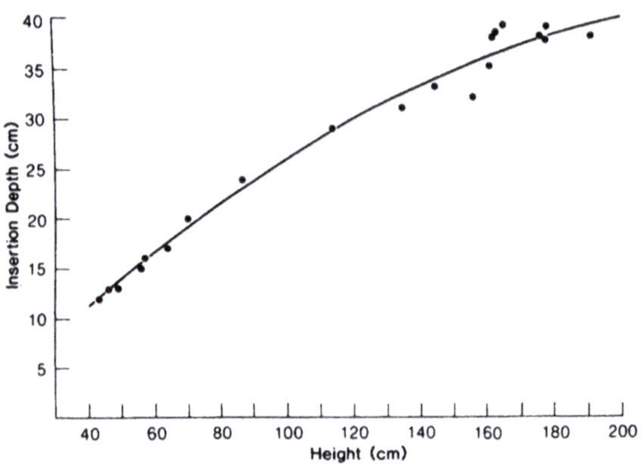

FIGURE 16–12. A graph relating the optimum depth of insertion of the esophageal electrode (measured from the nares) to the height of the patient: At the optimum depth of insertion the atrial pacing threshold is minimum [89]. (Reproduced with the permission of the authors and publisher.)

ular tachycardia can be induced by the introduction of extrastimuli or by bursts of rapid atrial pacing, and atrial fibrillation or flutter can be induced by rapid atrial pacing.

Pacing should commence at a relatively slow rate and observations should be made to rule out ventricular pacing, tracheal irritation, and phrenic nerve or brachial plexus stimulation. If any one of these adverse side effects is present, adjustment in the position of the electrode is indicated. We routinely commence pacing using a pulse width of 9.9 ms, a pulse amplitude of 12 mA, and a cycle length approximately 10% shorter than that of the patient's spontaneous sinus rate. A graded increase in the pulse amplitude may be required to achieve reliable atrial capture, and a stepwise decrease in cycle length may be necessary to provoke the desired tachycardia. In general capture is seen with a pulse amplitude of less than 15 mA and induction of supraventricular tachycardia is successful at pacing cycle length between 400 and 240 ms. In order to achieve atrial fibrillation or atrial flutter, pacing at cycle lengths between 80 and 60 ms may be necessary.

If transesophageal atrial pacing is used to terminate supraventricular tachycardia or atrial flutter, the presence of atrial capture may be difficult to observe. The absence of ventricular pacing should first be assured by pacing at a cycle length slightly shorter than the ventricular cycle length. We arbitrarily choose a pulse amplitude of 12 to 15 mA and commence pacing at a cycle length approximately 10% shorter than the atrial cycle length previously determined by esophageal recording. The presence of atrial capture is assumed if there is perturbation of the ventricular cycle on the surface recording or by termination of the arrhythmia. Initially, short bursts of pacing that last 2 to 10 beats are introduced. If termination is not achieved, progressively faster rates, longer bursts, and stronger pulse currents are used. Termination of atrial flutter may require pacing cycle lengths as short as 60–80 ms and bursts of up to 30 sec.

Summary

In the management of patients who are suspected to have the preexcitation syndrome, it is necessary to confirm the mechanism of the reciprocating supraventricular tachycardia and to identify the subgroup that is at risk of sudden death due to ventricular fibrillation. The noninvasive technique of transesophageal recording and pacing can be applied successfully to achieve these aims. A ventricle-to-atrium activation interval (VA-eso) of 70 ms or longer recorded on the transesophageal electrogram during reciprocating supraventricular tachycardia is a reliable indicator that the mechanism of the tachycardia involves atrioventricular reentry utilizing an accessory pathway. A shortest RR interval between preexcited beats of 250 ms or less recorded during atrial fibrillation or flutter would suggest that the patient is at risk of having a fast ventricular response that can degenerate into ventricular fibrillation. This shortest RR interval can also be used to monitor the effect of drugs on antegrade conduction in the accessory pathway during these atrial arrhythmias. If the patient is in sinus rhythm before these recordings are made, reciprocating tachycardia and atrial fibrillation or flutter can be induced by programmed atrial pacing via the esophageal electrode. In addition, transesophageal atrial pacing can be used to terminate reciprocating supraventicular tachycardia or atrial flutter. However, endocardial recording and pacing is still required for localization of the accessory pathway, particularly in preparation for the surgical interruption of the pathway.

References

1. Wolff L, Parkinson J, White PD: Bundle branch block with short P-R interval in healthy young people prone to paroxysmal tachycardia. *Am. Heart J.* 5:685, 1930.
2. Wolff L: Anomalous atrioventricular excitation (Wolff-Parkinson-White syndrome). *Circulation* 19:14, 1959.
3. Wolff L: The WPW syndrome. *Am. Heart J.* 63:284, 1962.
4. Zipes DP, Rothbaum DA, DeJoseph RL: Pre-excitation syndrome. *Cardiovasc. Clin.* 6:209, 1974.
5. Gallagher JJ, Pritchett ELC, Sealy WC, Kasell J, Wallace AG: The preexcitation syndromes. *Prog. Cardiovasc. Dis.* 20:285, 1978.
6. Wolff L and White PD: Syndrome of short P-R interval with abnormal QRS complexes and paroxysmal tachycardia. *Arch. Intern. Med.* 28:446, 1948.
7. Wolff L: Syndrome of short P-R interval with abnormal QRS complexes and paroxysmal tachycardia (WPW syndrome). *Circulation* 10:282, 1954.
8. Chung KY, Walsh TJ, Massie E: Wolff-Parkinson-White syndrome. *Am. Heart J.* 69:116, 1965.
9. Newman BJ, Donoso E, Friedberg CK: Arrhythmias in the Wolff-Parkinson-White syndrome. *Prog. Cardiovasc. Dis.* 9:147, 1966.
10. Chung EK: Wolff-Parkinson-White Syndrome — Current Views. *Am. J. Med.* 62:252, 1977.
11. Kaplan MA and Cohen KL: Ventricular Fibrillation in the Wolff-Parkinson-White syndrome. *Am. J. Cardiol.* 24:259, 1969.
12. Campbell RWF, Smith RA, Gallagher JJ, Pritchett ELC, Wallace AG: Atrial fibrillation in the preexcitation syndrome. *Am. J. Cardiol.* 40:514, 1977.
13. Graybiel A, McFarland RA, Gates DC, Webster FA: Analysis of the electrocardiograms obtained from 1,000 young health aviators. *Am. Heart J.* 27:524, 1944.
14. Manning GW: Electrocardiography in the selection of Royal Canadian Air Force aircrew. *Circulation* 10:401, 1954.
15. Packard JM, Graettinger JS, Graybiel A: Analysis of the electrocardiograms obtained from 1,000 young healthy aviators: ten year follow-up. *Circulation* 10:384, 1954.
16. Averill KH, Fosmoe RJ, Lamb LE: Electrocardiographic findings in 67,375 asymptomatic subjects: IV. Wolff-Parkinson-White syndrome. *Am. J. Cardiol.* 6:108, 1960.
17. Wolff L. and White PD: The cardinal aspects of paroxysmal rapid heart action. *N. Engl. J. Med.* 226:640, 1942.
18. Öhnell RF: Pre-excitation, a cardiac abnormality. PA Norstedt and Loner: Stockholm, 1944.
19. Willus FA and Carryer HM: Electrocardiograms displaying short P-R intervals with prolonged QRS complexes: An analysis of sixty-five cases. *Proc. Staff Meet., Mayo Clin.* 21:438, 1946.
20. Hejtmancik MT and Herrman GR: The electrocardiographic syndrome of short P-R interval and broad QRS complexes: A clinical study of 80 cases. *Am. Heart J.* 54:708, 1957.
21. Hecht HH, Kennamer R, Prinzmetal M, Rosenbaum FF, Sodi-Pallares D, Wolff L, Brooks C, Pick A, Rijlant P, Robb JS: Anomalous atrioventricular excitation. Panel discussion, *Ann. N.Y. Acad. Sci.* 65:826, 1956.
22. Wellens HJJ, Schuilenburg RM, Durrer D: Electrical stimulation of the heart in patients with Wolff-Parkinson-White syndrome, type A. *Circulation* 43:99, 1971.
23. Fontaine G, Frank R, Coutte R, et al.: Rhythme reciproque antidromique dans un syndrome de Wolff-Parkinson-White de type A. *Ann. Cardiol. Angeiol.* (Paris), 59:59, 1975.
24. Zipes DP, DeJoseph RL, Rothbaum DA: Unusual properties of accessory pathways. *Circulation* 49:1200, 1974.
25. Neuss H, Schlepper M, Thormann J: Analysis of reentry mechanisms in three patients with concealed Wolff-Parkinson-White syndrome. *Circulation* 51:75, 1975.
26. Tonkin AM, Gallagher JJ, Svenson RH, Wallace AG, Sealy WC: Antegrade block in accessory pathways with retrograde conduction in reciprocating tachycardia. *Eur. J. Cardiol.* 3:143, 1975.
27. Sung RJ, Castellanos A, Gelband H, Myerburg RJ: Mechanism of reciprocating tachycardia during sinus rhythm in concealed Wolff-Parkinson-White syndrome. *Circulation* 54:338, 1976.
28. Dreifus LS, Haiat R, Watanabe Y, Arriaga J, Reitman N: Ventricular fibrillation: A possible mechanism of sudden death in patients with Wolff-Parkinson-White syndrome. *Circulation* 43:520, 1971.
29. Klein GJ, Bashore TM, Sellers TD, Pritchett ELC, Smith WM, Gallagher JJ: Ventricular fibrillation in the Wolff-Parkinson-White syndrome. *N. Engl. J. Med.* 301:1080, 1979.
30. Wellens HJ and Durrer D: Effect of digitalis on atrioventricular conduction and circus-movement tachycardias in patients with Wolff-Parkinson-White syndrome. *Circulation* 47:1229, 1973.
31. Sellers TD, Bashore, TM, Gallagher JJ: Digitalis in the pre-excitation syndrome: Analysis during atrial fibrillation. *Circulation* 56:260, 1977.
32. Byrum CJ, Wahl RA, Behrendt DM, Dick M: Ventricular fibrillation associated with use of digitalis in a newborn infant with Wolff-Parkinson-White syndrome. *J. Pediatr.* 101:400, 1982.

33. Neuss H and Schlepper M: Influence of various antiarrhythmic drugs (aprindine, ajmaline, verapamil, oxprenolol, orciprenaline) on the functional properties of accessory AV pathways. *Acta Cardiol.* 18 (suppl):279, 1974.
34. Petri H, Kafka W, Hall D, Rudolph W: Potential acceleration of the ventricular rate in WPW with atrial fibrillation after verapamil. *Circulation* 62 (suppl III):III–262, 1980.
35. Gulamhusein S, Ko P, Carruthers SG, Klein GJ: Acceleration of the ventricular response during atrial fibrillation in the Wolff-Parkinson-White syndrome after verapamil. *Circulation* 65:348, 1982.
36. Cremer M: Ueber die direkte ableitung der aktionsstrome der menschlichen herzens vom oesophagus und ueber das elektrokardiogramm des foetus. *Munchen Med. Wchnschr.*, 53:811, 1906.
37. Lieberson A and Liberson F: An internal electrocardiographic lead. *Proc. Soc. Exp. Biol. Med.* 31:441, 1934.
38. Brown WH: A study of the esophageal lead in clinical electrocardiography: Part I. The application of the esophageal lead to the human subject with observations on the Ta-wave, extrasystoles and bundle-branch block. *Am. Heart J.* 12:1, 1936.
39. Brown WH: A study of the esophageal lead in clinical electrocardiography: Part II. An electrocardiographic study of auricular disorders in the human subject by means of the esophageal lead. *Am. Heart J.* 12:307, 1936.
40. Butterworth S and Poindexter CA: The esophageal electrocardiogram in arrhythmias and tachycardias. *Am. Heart J.* 32:681, 1946.
41. Kistin AD, Brill WD, Robb GP: Normal esophageal and gastric electrocardiograms: Description, statistical analysis and bearing on theories of "eletrocardiographic position." *Circulation* 2:578, 1950.
42. Enselberg CD: The esophageal electrocardiogram in the study of atrial activity and cardiac arrhythmias. *Am. Heart J.* 41:382, 1951.
43. Oblath R and Karpman H: The normal esophageal lead electrocardiogram. *Am. Heart J.* 41:369, 1951.
44. Kistin AD and Bruce JC: Simultaneous esophageal and standard electrocardiographic leads for the study of cardiac arrhythmias. *Am. Heart J.* 53:65, 1957.
45. Rubin IL, Jagendorf B, Goldberg AL: The esophageal lead in the diagnosis of tachycardias with aberrant ventricular conduction. *Am. Heart J.* 57:19, 1959.
46. Jenkins JM, Wu D, Arzbaecher RC: Computer diagnosis of supraventricular and ventricular arrhythmias: A new esophageal technique. *Circulation* 60:977, 1979.
47. Benditt DG, Pritchett ELC, Smith WM, Gallagher JJ: Ventriculoatrial intervals: Diagnostic use in paroxysmal supraventricular tachycardia. *Ann. Intern. Med.* 91:161, 1979.
48. Gallagher JJ, Smith WM, Kasell J, Smith WM, Grant AO, Benson DW, Jr: Use of the esophageal lead in the diagnosis of mechanisms of reciprocating supraventricular tachycardia. *PACE* 3:440, 1980.
49. Zoll PM: Resuscitation of the heart in ventricular standstill by external electrical stimulation. *N. Engl. J. Med.* 247:768, 1952.
50. Shafiroff BFP and Linder J: Effects of external electrical pacemaker stimuli on the human heart. *J. Thorac. Cardiovasc. Surg.* 33:544, 1957.
51. McNally EM, Meyer EC, Langendorf R: Elective countershock in unanesthetized patients with use of an esophageal electrode. *Circulation* 33:124, 1966.
52. Burack B and Furman S: Transesophageal cardiac pacing. *Am. J. Cardiol.* 23:469, 1969.
53. Lubell DL: Cardiac pacing from the esophagus. *Am. J. Cardiol.* 27:641, 1971.
54. Stopczyk MJ, Zochowski RJ, Sadowski Z: P wave triggered permanent atrial pacing in a case of transient sinus arrest. *Br. Heart J.* 34:318. 1972.
55. Montoyo JV, Angel J, Valle V, Gausi C: Cardioversion of tachycardias by transesophageal atrial pacing. *Am. J. Cardiol.* 32:85, 1973.
56. Gallagher JJ, Smith WM, Kerr CR, Kasell J, Cook L, Reiter M, Sterba R, Harte M: Esophageal pacing: A diagnostic and therapeutic tool. *Circulation* 65:336, 1982.
57. Kerr CR, Gallagher JJ, Smith WM, Sterba R, German LD, Cook L, Kasell JH: The induction of atrial flutter and fibrillation and the termination of atrial flutter by esophageal pacing. *PACE* 6:60, 1983.
58. Shaw RJ, Berman LH, Hinton JM: Successful emergency transoesophageal cardiac pacing with subsequent endoscopy. *Br. Med. J.* 284:309, 1982.
59. Touborg P, Andersen HR, Pless P: Low-current bedside emergency atrial and ventricular cardiac pacing from the oesophagus. *Lancet* 1:166, 1982.
60. Cooper DN: Temporary cardiac pacing via the oesophagus. *Postgrad. Med. J.* 58:45, 1982.
61. Andersen HR and Pless P: Trans-esophageal pacing. *PACE* 6:674, 1983.
62. Binkley PF, Bush CA, Kolibash AJ, Magorien RD, Hamlin RL, Leier CV: The anatomic relationship of the esophageal lead to the left atrium. *PACE* 5:853, 1982.
63. Massumi RA, Sarin RK, Tawakkol AA, Rios JC, Jackson H: Time sequence of right and left atrial depolarization as a guide to the origin of the P waves. *Am. J. Cardiol.* 24:28, 1969.
64. Puech P: The P wave: Correlation of surface and

intra-atrial electrograms. *Cardiovasc. Clin.* 6:43, 1974.
65. Prystowsky EN, Pritchett ELC and Gallagher JJ: Origin of the atrial electrogram recorded from the esophagus. *Circulation* 61:1017, 1980.
66. Ledley RS, Huang HK, Mazziotta JC: Cross-sectional Anatomy — An Atlas for Computerized Tomography. Williams & Wilkins: Baltimore, 1977.
67. Josephson ME and Seides SF: *Clinical Cardiac Electrophysiology Techniques and Interpretations.* Lea & Febiger: Philadelphia, 1979.
68. Bär FW, Brugada P, Dassen WRM, Wellens HJJ: Differential diagnosis of tachycardia with narrow QRS complex (shorter than 0.12 second). *Am. J. Cardiol.* 54:555, 1984.
69. Wu D, Denes P, Amat-Y-Leon F, Dhingra R, Wydham CRC, Bauernfeind R, Latif P, Rosen KM: Clinical electrocardiographic and electrophysiologic observations in patients with paroxysmal supraventricular tachycardia. *Am. J. Cardiol.* 41:1045, 1978.
70. Josephson ME: Paroxysmal supraventricular tachycardia: An electrophysiologic approach. *Am. J. Cardiol.* 41:1123, 1978.
71. Benson DW, Jr, Dunnigan A, Benditt DG, Pritzker MR, Thompson TR: Transesophageal study of infant supraventricular tachycardia: Electrophysiologic characteristics. *Am. J. Cardiol.* 52:1002, 1983.
72. Smith RF: The Wolff-Parkinson-White syndrome as an aviation risk. *Circulation* 29:672, 1964.
73. Wellens HJ and Durrer D: Wolff-Parkinson-White syndrome and atrial fibrillation: Relation between refractory period of accessory pathway and ventricular rate during atrial fibrillation. *Am. J. Cardiol.* 34:777, 1974.
74. Castellanos A, Jr, Castillo CA, Agha AS, Befeler B, Myerburg RJ: Functional properties of accessory AV pathways during premature atrial stimulation. *Br. Heart J.* 35:578, 1973.
75. Castellanos A, Jr, Myerburg RJ, Craparo K, Befeler B, Agha AS: Factors regulating ventricular rates during atrial flutter and fibrillation in pre-excitation (Wolff-Parkinson-White) syndrome. *Br. Heart J.* 35:811, 1973.
76. Tonkin AM, Miller HC, Svenson RH, Wallace AG, Gallagher JJ: Refractory periods of the accessory pathway in the Wolff-Parkinson-White syndrome. *Circulation* 52:563, 1975.
77. Critelli G, Grassi G, Perticone F, Coltorti F, Monda V, Condorelli M: Transesophageal pacing for prognostic evaluation of preexcitation syndrome and assessment of protective therapy. *Am. J. Cardiol.* 51:513, 1983.
78. Wellens HJJ and Brugada P: Value of programmed stimulation of the heart in patients with Wolff-Parkinson-White syndrome. In *Tachycardias: Mechanisms, Diagnosis, Treatment.* ME Josephson and HJJ Wellens (eds.). Lea & Febiger: Philadelphia, 1984.
79. Wellens HJJ, Bar FW, Farre J, Ross D, Vanagt EJ: Sudden death in the Wolff-Parkinson-White syndrome. In *Sudden Death.* HE Kulbertus and HJJ Wellens (eds.). Martinus Nijhoff: Boston, 1980.
80. Lévy S, Broustet JP, Clementy J, Guern B, Vircoulon B, Guern P, Bricaud H: Syndrome de Wolff-Parkinson-White: Correlations entre l'exploration electrophysiologique et l'effet de l'epreuve d'effort sur l'aspect electrocardiographique de preexcitation. *Arch. Mal Coeur* 72:634, 1979.
81. Wellens HJJ, Bar FW, Gorgels AP, Vanagt EJ: Use of ajmaline in patients with the Wolff-Parkinson-White syndrome to discover short refractory period of the accessory pathway. *Am. J. Cardiol.* 45:130, 1980.
82. Benson DW, Jr, Dunnigan A, Benditt DG, Pritzker HR: Transesophageal conversion of atrial flutter in infants, children and young adults. (Abstract.) *Circulation* 66:II–316, 1982.
83. Dunnigan A, Benson DW, Jr, Benditt DG: Atrial flutter in infancy: Diagnosis, clinical features, and treatment, *Pediatrics* 75:725, 1985.
84. Disertori M, Inama G, Vergara G, Guarnerio M, Furlanello F: Impiego della stimolazione atriale transesofagea nel trattamento del flutter atriale. *G. Ital. Cardiol.* 14:153, 1984.
85. Brody DA, Harris TR, Romans WE: A simple method for obtaining esophageal electrocardiograms of good diagnostic quality. *Am. Heart J.* 50:923, 1955.
86. Brody DA and Copeland GD: The principles of esophageal electrocardiography. *Am. Heart J.* 57:3, 1959.
87. Copeland GD, Tullis IF, Brody DA: Clinical evaluation of a new esophageal electrode, with particular reference to the bipolar esophageal electrocardiogram: Part I. Normal sinus mechanism. *Am. Heart J.* 57:862, 1959.
88. Barold SS: Filtered bipolar esophageal electrocardiography. *Am. Heart J.* 83:431, 1972.
89. Benson DW, Jr, Sanford M, Dunnigan A, Benditt DG: Transesophageal atrial pacing threshold: Role of interelectrode spacing, pulse width and catheter insertion depth. *Am. J. Cardiol.* 53:63, 1984.

17. THE ROLE OF INVASIVE ELECTROPHYSIOLOGIC STUDIES IN PREEXCITATION SYNDROMES

Lawrence D. German, Marcel R. Gilbert, and Jackie H. Kasell

Invasive electrophysiologic studies have made important contributions toward our understanding of the preexcitation syndrome. Among these have been the elucidation of both the physiologic basis for preexcitation [1–17] and the mechanisms of the various associated arrhythmias [18–46]. Demonstration of accessory pathway participation in arrhythmia has made certain forms of therapy possible [1,47–52]. For example, the effects of specific antiarrhythmic drugs on accessory pathway function can be assessed in individual patients [53–56]. Furthermore, potential adverse drug effects can be studied, and patients who are potentially at risk for lethal arrhythmias can be identified [29,31,41,52,54].

An additional contribution of the electrophysiologic study has been identification of patients with accessory pathways functioning in the retrograde direction only (i.e., "concealed" accessory pathway), and therefore without ECG evidence of preexcitation [3,23,28,30,57–59]. The management of these patients may be improved by a correct diagnosis.

Invasive studies make possible the use of antitachycardia pacemakers to treat reciprocating tachycardia. The electrophysiologic study is essential to determine the potential effectiveness of a particular pacing device prior to implantation [52]. Lastly, the possibility of ablation of accessory pathways has been explored and shown to be an important form of therapy in the future [1,11,47–49,61]. The ablation of accessory atrioventricular (AV) pathways with elimination of both the arrhythmias and the ECG abnormality is one of the most dramatic examples of surgical correction of a congenital heart defect.

Indications for Invasive Studies (Table 17–1)

TABLE 17–1. Indications for invasive studies in the preexcitation syndromes

A. Diagnosis
   1. Establish accessory pathway presence
   2. Establish accessory pathway participation
   3. Exclude presence of coexisting forms of PSVT
   4. Assess the risk of atrial fibrillation
B. Therapy
   1. Following unsuccessful attempts at empiric therapy of PSVT
   2. Prior to surgery
   3. Prior to antitachycardia pacemaker implantation
   4. Prior to catheter ablation
   5. To assess adequacy of treatment for atrial fibrillation

DIAGNOSIS

The use of electrophysiologic studies in patients with preexcitation syndrome has been the subject of numerous reviews [8,9,11,36,43,62–66]. One of the most fundamental indications for performing invasive electrophysiologic studies is to establish an accurate diagnosis. A precise diagnosis forms the basis for all future management of the patient and may have significant prognostic implications. The diagnosis of preexcitation may be evident if anomalous QRS morphology (i.e., overt delta wave) is seen on the surface ECG, although other conditions result in mimickry of a delta wave [67]. The presence of preexcitation does not insure that tachycardia is due to circus movement utilizing the accessory pathway. The observed tachycardia may be the result of another mechanism, such as reentry within the AV node with "bystander" participation of the accessory pathway [20,22,68–70]. Furthermore, the absence of preexcitation on a given surface ECG tracing does not exclude the presence of a surgically or medically remediable accessory pathway [3,23,28,30,57–60]. In most populations of patients with paroxysmal superventricular tachycardia (PSVT) without preexcitation, a significant number are found to have tachycardia that utilizes an accessory AV pathway that does not result in preexcitation.

A number of distinct forms of supraventricular tachycardia have been identified by means of invasive electrophysiologic studies. These include reentry within the AV node, intraatrial reentry, atrial flutter, and ectopic atrial tachycardia, all of which may occur coincidentally in patients with preexcitation syndrome and simulate reciprocating tachycardia utilizing an accessory pathway. In addition to these tachycardias, Figure 17–1 illustrates four entities which may provide the substrate for tachyarrhythmias in the preexcitation syndrome. Although clues to the specific mechanism present in any given patient may be present on the surface ECG, invasive electrophysiologic studies are often required to establish the diagnosis.

The most common form of preexcitation is that associated with accessory AV pathways which are the basis for the Wolff-Parkinson-White (WPW) Syndrome. Preexcitation may also occur from the presence of accessory nodoventricular or nodofascicular fibers (Mahaim fibers) that also support reentrant tachycardia [7,10,32,71]. In this group, as well as some patients with accessory AV pathway, tachycardia may be associated with a wide QRS, thereby mimicking ventricular tachycardia [34]. In addition, a distinct group of patients may be found to have an unusual accessory AV pathway in the posterior septal region displaying decremental conduction properties. These patients often have virtually incessant AV reciprocating tachycardia and are said to have the "permanent form of junctional reciprocating tachycardia" (PJRT) [33,45,50,72,73]. Finally, a variety of patients with short PR intervals and "enhanced AV nodal conduction" may be identified [37,38,74–76]. These patients may have the Lown-Ganong-Levine syndrome [77] consisting of a short PR interval, normal QRS, and rapid heart beating; the latter is most often due to reentry within the AV node or reentry utilizing a concealed accessory AV pathway. Often, patients with enhanced AV node conduction (defined as an AH interval of less than 60 ms, 1:1 conduction at pacing cycle lengths less than 300 ms, and failure of the AH interval to prolong by over 100 ms at the point where Wenckebach block occurs) [76] simply represent one end of the spectrum of normal conduction. The possibility that enhanced AV conduction and/or short PR interval may be due to the presence of an atriofascicular (atrio-Hisian) bypass tract (Brechenmacher) or intranodal bypass tracts (James) has not been confirmed. Enhanced AV node conduction is discussed in the chapter by Benditt et al. in this volume.

The role of the electrophysiologic study in patients with known preexcitation is not only to document the presence of specific arrhythmias, but to demonstrate that the clinically relevent arrhythmia actually uses the accessory pathway. Thus, patients with clear ECG evidence of preexciation may have reentry within the AV node as the clinical arrhythmia, with the accessory pathway playing no causal role in tachycardia. The implications for therapy are clear, and efforts directed at the accessory pathway such as surgery, catheter ablation, or specific drugs may be to no avail.

THERAPY

The necessity for differentiating between the various forms of PSVT in the absence of preexcitation during sinus rhythm may be questioned. In these patients, the differential diagnosis is primarily between reentry within the AV

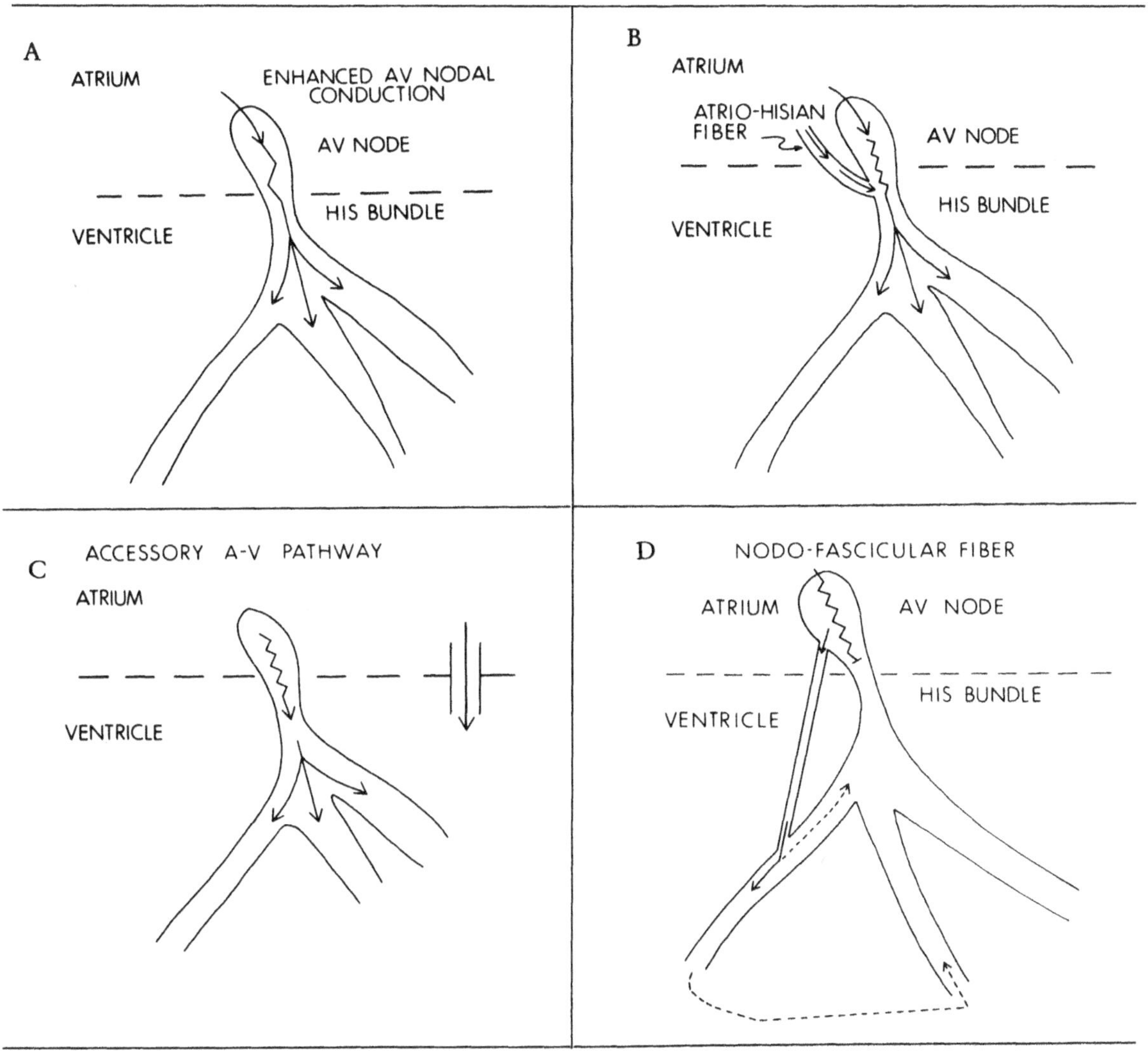

FIGURE 17–1. Mechanisms of Preexcitation. (A) Enhanced AV nodal conduction. No anatomically abnormal accessory pathways are present, but conduction occurs through the AV node without the normal amount of delay, resulting in a short PR interval and unusually rapid ventricular rates during atrial fibrillation. (B) Atriofascicular (Atrio-Hisian) fiber. An accessory pathway is present from the atrium to the Bundle of His, bypassing the AV node and resulting in similar electrocardiographic findings as enhanced AV nodal conduction. The PR interval may be short, and rapid conduction from atrium to ventricle may be present. The QRS complex would be expected to be normal, as with enhanced AV nodal conduction. (C) An accessory AV pathway. An accessory pathway connecting atrium and ventricle forms the basis for the WPW syndrome. The accessory pathway may function in both antegrade and retrograde directions or in only one or the other. Conduction in the antegrade direction via the accessory pathway results in a preexcited (anomalous) QRS complex. Reciprocating tachycardia using the accessory pathway occurs in either the orthodromic or antidromic forms. In the former, conduction proceeds down the normal conduction pathways and in retrograde direction up the accessory pathway, whereas during antidromic tachycardia, conduction proceeds down the accessory pathway and in the ventriculoatrial direction up the normal conduction pathway. An accessory AV pathway with decremental properties is found in the "PJRT" variant. (D) A nodofascicular or nodoventricular connection. An accessory pathway may connect the lower parts of the AV node with either one of the conduction fascicles or the ventricular myocardium itself. The QRS complex may be mildly preexcited during sinus rhythm but with atrial pacing, and resultant delay in the AV node, more conduction occurs across the accessory pathway resulting in a preexcited QRS complex. Reciprocating tachycardia usually occurs with a preexcited QRS complex due to conduction proceeding down the accessory pathway and returning up the normal conduction system into the AV node. Reciprocating tachycardia does not involve the atrium, as opposed to the case with an accessory atrioventricular pathway.

node, and reciprocating tachycardia using a concealed accessory AV pathway, and invasive studies are not always required to make the distinction. Measurement of the VA interval during tachycardia using an esophageal electrode may be diagnostic [78]. Furthermore, if esophageal recordings can be made during tachycardia in which the QRS complexes exhibit both bundle branch block as well as normal morphologies, a more definite statement about arrhythmia mechanism and accessory pathway location can be made [79].

Pharmacologic therapy. In most patients with PSVT, an initial attempt at empiric therapy is justified, and the same drugs may be expected to be effective in patients with reciprocating tachycardias due either to reentry within the AV node or utilizing an accessory pathway. It may not be necessary to pursue invasive electrophysiologic studies prior to initial attempts at therapy in these patients. However, serial electrophysiologic studies have been shown to be an effective method of choosing antiarrhythmic drug regimens in patients with PSVT [56], and are indicated when initial attempts at empiric therapy have failed, or when tachycardia is associated with severe symptoms. The demonstration that PSVT involves reentry using an accessory AV pathway, or a nodoventricular pathway, may prompt use of a combination of antiarrhythmic agents that act on both the normal conduction system, and the accessory pathway. Certain antiarrhythmic agents (e.g., digitalis) may be contraindicated in some forms of the preexcitation syndrome and useful in others [80,81]. Drugs such as beta-blockers and calcium antagonists may also have useful applications in some patients. Alternatively, drugs such as quinidine or procainamide, that are generally effective in slowing accessory pathway conduction, may be ineffective in some patients and even aggravate reciprocating tachycardia in others.

Nonpharmacologic therapy. When nonpharmacologic treatment modalities are being considered, including surgical or electrode catheter ablation of the accessory pathway, invasive studies are required. The most common alternative to drug therapy in patients with the preexcitation syndrome is surgical division of an accessory AV pathway. Invasive studies are required prior to considering surgery to demonstrate participation of the accessory pathway in the clinically documented arrhythmia, to provide preoperative localization of the accessory pathway, and to detect the presence of multiple pathways [44,82–86]. Confirmation of pathway location is important prior to surgery in order to provide the patient with an estimate of the potential risk of damaging the normal conduction system, resulting in heart block. The surgical approach may also depend on pathway location, making this information necessary prior to the time of operation. Surgical manipulation or anesthetic drugs may also result in failure of the accessory pathway to function at the time of intraoperative mapping, making prior knowledge of pathway location critical.

The development of antitachycardia pacing devices has provided an additional alternative for treating some patients with PSVT due to preexcitation syndromes. The feasibility of these devices in any given patient depends on several characteristics of the tachycardia being treated and the propensity of the patient to develop atrial fibrillation. Characteristics of tachycardia that bear on the ability of antitachycardia pacing devices to interrupt the reentrant circuit include the rate of the arrhythmia, and the location of the accessory pathway. Careful testing of the proposed method of tachycardia termination prior to implantation is necessary and can only be performed during invasive testing. Such testing should consider the possible complicating influences of posture, exercise, and concomitant drug therapy.

Invasive studies are indicated when catheter ablation techniques are being considered. Catheter ablation of the AV junction has been shown to be successful in creating complete heart block, and therefore will be effective in preventing reciprocating tachycardia in patients with single accessory pathways. This technique is an indirect method of treating these patients, at best, and does nothing to affect conduction over the accessory pathway. Selection of patients for catheter ablation of the AV junction is critical, and the technique should be reserved for patients in whom a rapid ventricular response during atrial fibrillation is not considered a problem, and in whom direct division of the accessory pathway(s) is not possible. A possible exception to this is the role of catheter ablation of the AV junction in patients with nodofascicular (nodoventricular) fibers. In these patients, ablation of the AV junction may eliminate tachycardia, with AV conduction being preserved over the accessory connection, and obviating patient dependence on a pacemaker [48,87].

Only limited success has been achieved to this point with direct catheter ablation of accessory pathways (see Scheinman, this volume). The long-term consequences of electric shocks near coronary arteries within the AV groove are not known, and these techniques must still be considered highly investigational. Nevertheless, continued research into nonoperative techniques for ablating accessory pathways can be expected, and invasive studies are clearly required for their success.

ASSESSING THE RISK OF SUDDEN DEATH

Although sudden death due to ventricular fibrillation occurs in only a minority of patients with the preexcitation syndrome, the risk is unpredictable on the basis of the ECG alone. Invasive studies may be indicated in symptomatic patients with preexcitation to assess the risk of atrial fibrillation with a rapid ventricular response leading to ventricular fibrillation [29,31,41,53,54,88]. The use of electrophysiologic testing to induce atrial fibrillation in a controlled setting, prior to and following infusion of isoproterenol to accentuate conduction over the accessory pathway, may provide an estimation of the risk for rapid conduction during atrial fibrillation [55]. The use of isoproterenol during these studies may be particularly important in patients planning vigorous physical activity, those engaged in potentially dangerous sports, or those employed in "public risk" occupations (e.g., airline pilots). Any patient with preexcitation who has experienced syncope or presyncope due to atrial fibrillation should be promptly and thoroughly evaluated. Empiric therapy in these patients is justified only until specific therapy (i.e., therapy whose effectiveness is documented by electrophysiologic testing) can be instituted.

Techniques of Electrophysiologic Study

THE DIAGNOSTIC STUDY FOR PSVT

The electrophysiologic catheter study performed in the patient with preexcitation syndrome has certain features that should be performed routinely. Variations on the general technique described here may be employed (e.g., intraarterial pressure recording), depending on personal preference. At a minimum the diagnostic study in patients suspected of the preexcitation syndrome involves the placement of four transvenous electrode catheters. In our laboratory, we routinely use an esophageal lead placed transnasally. The esophageal electrode is positioned at the beginning of the study prior to other catheter insertion to permit atrial recording and pacing should arrhythmias be induced during transvenous catheter manipulation.

The first catheter placed is the coronary sinus catheter, whose purpose is to record left atrial activity near the mitral anulus. This catheter may be placed via either the left subclavian or median basilic vein. The subclavian vein approach provides maximum stability during the study and is convenient if the catheter is to be left in place following the study. Catheter position in the coronary sinus is confirmed fluoroscopically and by recording typical electrograms that show both atrial and ventricular activation.

Three catheters are then placed via the right femoral vein. Catheters may be placed in the left femoral vein if necessary, but advancement to the heart and catheter manipulation may be more difficult from this site, especially with the His bundle catheter. These catheters are placed to permit electrogram recordings from the apex of the right ventricle, the His bundle region, and the right atrium respectively. A specialized catheter is preferred for mapping the tricuspid anulus. This mapping catheter has closely spaced (5 mm) bipolar pair of electrodes at its tip, and alumen through which a curved stylet is inserted. The stylet incorporates a position indicator at its hub to show the orientation of the curve in the heart. Following the mapping procedures this catheter will be exchanged for a quadripolar catheter positioned in the atrial appendage or the high lateral atrial position.

Mapping the mitral anulus is performed by carefully moving the coronary sinus catheter under fluoroscopic control. Alternatively, use of a hexapolar, octapolar, or decapolar electrode catheters within the coronary sinus may eliminate the need to move the catheter during the study. Mapping the right atrium is carried out by moving the bipolar atrial mapping catheter to selected sites within the right atrium. The His bundle catheter and the ventricular catheter remain fixed during the study in order to provide relatively stable reference points, although it must be remembered that there may be considerable motion of the His bundle recording catheter with cardiac contraction, pacing, and during tachycardia.

The catheter placement described above is necessary in the diagnostic evaluation of patients for preexcitation syndrome, since eccentric retrograde activation over an accessory pathway may be missed, simulating conduction over the normal conduction system, if both coronary sinus and right atrial mapping is not performed. Even when preexcitation is known, such as in patients with obvious delta waves on the surface ECG, the multiple catheter recordings are necessary to exclude the presence of multiple pathways. Antegrade accessory pathway function may also be missed if pacing near the atrial insertion of the pathway is not performed.

ELECTROCARDIOGRAPHIC AND INTRACARDIAC ELECTROGRAM RECORDINGS

Data are recorded on three types of recorders during the electrophysiologic study: (1) the standard 12 lead ECG recorder, (2) a chart recorder capable of high frequency response, rapid paper speeds, and multichannel recordings, and (3) magnetic FM tape. Standard 12 lead ECG recordings, obtained periodically throughout the procedure, are essential to document arrhythmias induced during the study for comparison with spontaneously occurring arrhythmias and for analysis of QRS morphology. However, in our laboratory, the bulk of the recordings obtained during an electrophysiologic study will be recorded on chart paper at a speed of 200–250 mm/sec. These rapid speeds allow accurate measurement of intervals and separation of the various intracardiac electrograms. A time marker channel should be present on the paper with 10 ms and 100 ms divisions. Lastly, the use of continuous magnetic FM tape recordings during the study permits later playback of any potentially critical events occurring when the chart paper was not running. The data from the study may be saved on magnetic FM tape for further analysis at a later date, or the tape may be erased and reused once data analysis is complete.

Of great importance to the data acquisition system is the filtering and amplification of the signals from the patients. Both bipolar and unipolar recordings are routinely made during the electrophysiologic study. Unipolar recordings are referenced to the left leg electrode and filtered between 0.15 and 1000 Hz. Bipolar electrograms are filtered from 50 to 1000 Hz, and surface ECG leads are filtered from 0.5 to 30 Hz. The 0.5 Hz frequency limit is chosen to prevent baseline drift of the ECG leads during the study. Amplification of the signals varies depending on recording site. A 1 mv calibration signal should be recorded on the paper at the beginning of the study for each channel, and subsequent changes in gain setting recorded, or new calibrations made.

The number of channels recorded during the study may vary, but for a complete study in patients suspected of preexcitation, a minimum of 16 channels is recommended (Figure 17–2). Five channels are allocated to surface ECG leads (I,II,III,VI, and V6), one channel to electrograms from the right ventricle, His bundle, and right atrium, and six channels to the coronary sinus electrograms (proximal and distal bipolar, and four unipolar recordings). Left ventricular recordings may also be obtained in some instances.

In addition to the recording devices described above, an oscilloscope capable of storing the displaying data at rapid sweep speeds is used for on-line timing of intracardiac electrograms. A digital timer may also be incorporated into the recording circuits to continuously display cycle lengths or other intervals.

PACING PROCEDURES

A predetermined study protocol is followed during catheter studies for preexcitation, with modifications in the order of the protocol being made to accommodate unexpected findings, or the occurrence of spontaneous arrhythmias. Adherence to a predefined protocol assures that there will be a logical, thorough progression of the study with efficient use of time, that important observations will be made during the study permitting further observations to be made to clarify unexpected findings, and that all important data will be collected. The electrophysiologic study should be a scientific exercise with each component having a clearly understood purpose. Certain basic electrophysiologic techniques such as pacing at progressively more rapid rates and refractory period determinations are always performed from several sites during these studies. Other special techniques designed

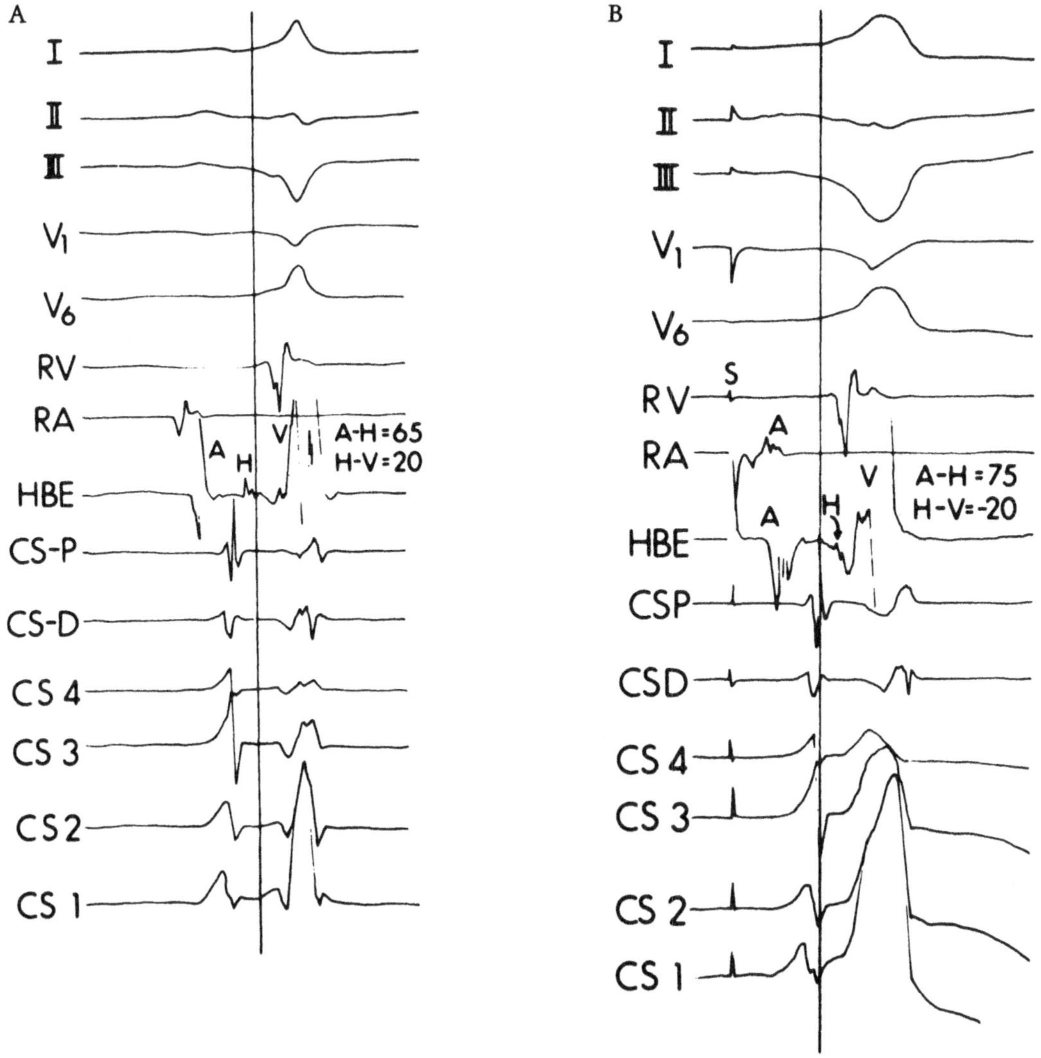

FIGURE 17–2. (A) Basic intervals recorded at the beginning of an electrophysiologic study in a patient with WPW syndrome showing the routine array of surface ECG leads and intracardiac electrograms. Note the short HV interval due to the presence of baseline preexcitation. Abbreviations RV = right ventricle, RA = right atrium, HBE = His bundle electrogram, CS = coronary sinus. The coronary sinus leads are displayed as proximal and distal bipolar and proximal (4) to distal (1) unipolar recordings. (B) Right atrial pacing in the same patient as in Panel A showing a more preexcited QRS complex with displacement of the His bundle electrogram into the QRS resulting in a negative HV interval. Abbreviations: same as in Panel A.

for evaluation of preexcitation syndromes are also required and are discussed briefly below.

Atrial mapping Mapping of the sequence of retrograde atrial activation is performed both during right ventricular pacing and reciprocating tachycardia. During ventricular pacing, relatively rapid rates are used to produce a small amount of physiologic delay in conduction over the AV node, thus accentuating the retrograde activation over the accessory pathway(s). Mapping is accomplished by carefully moving the mapping catheter to preselected sites around the atrioventricular ring. During the mapping procedure, the electrograms from the right atrial catheter, the His bundle catheter, and the coronary sinus catheter are displayed on the oscilloscope at a rapid sweep speed to allow comparison of the relative timing of the atrial events (Figure 17–3).

Following mapping of the right atrium, mapping of the left atrium is performed by sequential pull-backs of the coronary sinus catheter until a cavity potential is recorded on the most proximal pole. This indicates that the catheter has been withdrawn to the orifice of the coronary sinus.

Differential atrial pacing. The purpose of differential atrial pacing is to assess varying degrees of preexcitation while pacing at a constant cycle length from different sites in the atria

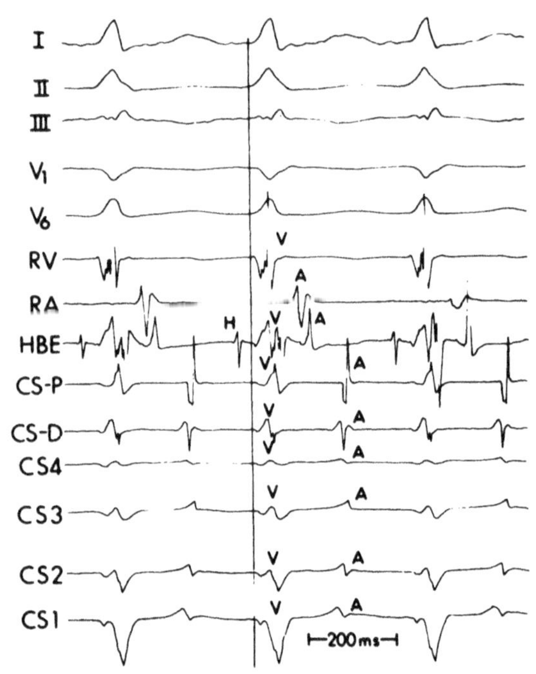

FIGURE 17–3. Orthodromic reciprocating tachycardia in a patient with WPW syndrome. Note the normal HV interval preceding the onset of the QRS (vertical line). Retrograde atrial activation occurs earliest in the right atrium followed by the His bundle atrial electrogram, with the coronary sinus activating late. Abbreviations: same as Figure 17–2.

[89] (Figure 17–4). QRS morphology, and the interval from stimulus to delta wave is assessed at each pacing site based on standard ECG recording. The use of differential pacing is discussed in more detail in the section on interpretation of the electrophysiologic study.

Premature ventricular stimulation during reciprocating tachycardia. An important observation to be made during PSVT is the effect of premature ventricular stimuli that occur during the time that the His bundle is refractory. The ability of such a premature stimulus to affect the atrium proves the existence of an accessory pathway (Figure 17–5).

Premature right ventricular stimuli may fail to preexcite the atrium in patients with left lateral accessory pathways. In such patients, atrial preexcitation may be demonstrated using double premature stimuli, with the first placed just prior to the His bundle electrogram, and the second placed just before the following His deflection. Alternatively, in patients with left-sided pathways, if sustained tachycardia with left bundle branch block can be induced, premature stimuli from the right ventricle will often preexcite the left atrium. Left ventricular stimulation should be considered when right ventricular stimulation fails to induce atrial preexcitation during tachycardia.

Bundle branch block during reciprocating tachycardia. An important observation to be made during the study is the effect of spontaneous development of bundle branch block during reciprocating tachycardia. The presence of bundle branch block ipsilateral to a freewall accessory pathway will result in prolongation of the VA interval by more than 35 ms [40] (Figure 17–6). Failure to prolong the VA interval by at least this amount with bundle branch block (right and left) suggests a septal pathway.

Bundle branch block usually develops on initiation of tachycardia, especially following ventricular burst pacing, and is often transient, converting to a normal QRS morphology within a few beats. When bundle branch block is sustained, an appropriately placed PVC will often result in normalization of the QRS. When transient bundle branch block during tachycardia cannot be induced despite repeated efforts, the administration of a type I antiarrhythmic agent, such as procainamide, may facilitate its occurrence.

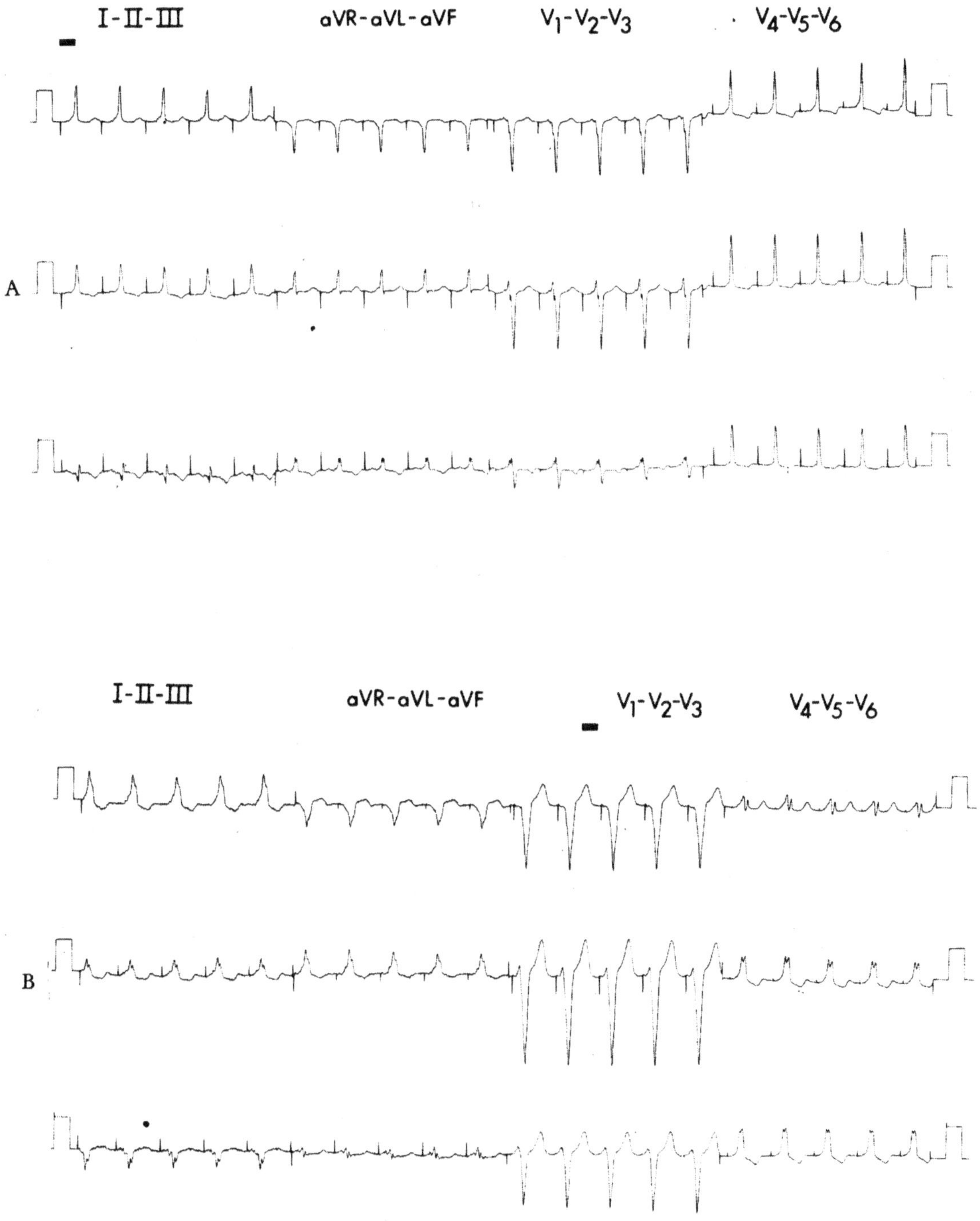

FIGURE 17–4. Differential atrial pacing in a patient with a right-sided accessory pathway. (A) Pacing from the distal coronary sinus results in a minimally preexcited QRS complex. (B) Pacing at the same cycle length from the right atrial appendage results in maximally preexcited QRS complex.

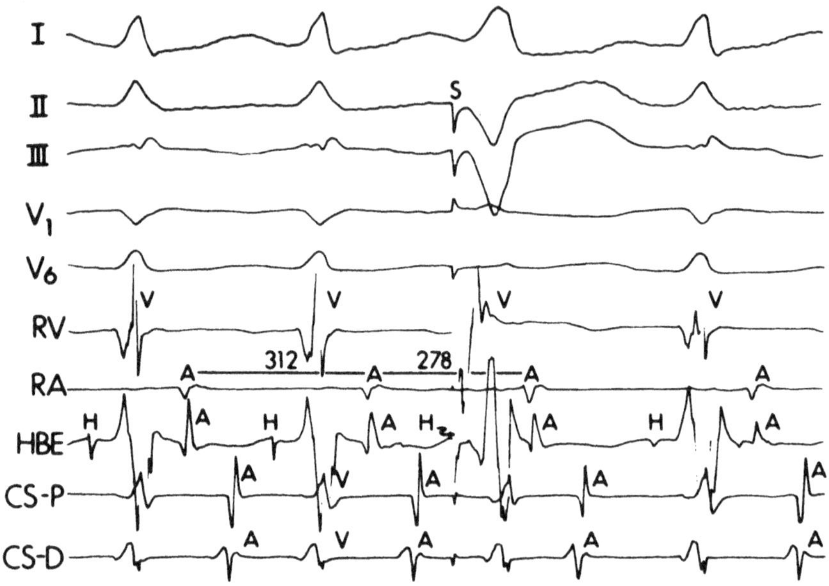

FIGURE 17–5. Premature ventricular stimulation during orthodromic reciprocating tachycardia in a patient with WPW syndrome. The premature stimulus (S) is timed to occur during the refractory period of the His bundle, thereby precluding the possibility of retrograde conduction up the normal conduction system. The premature stimulus results in the atrial electrograms occurring earlier than expected, although the retrograde atrial activation sequence is unchanged, proving the presence of an accessory atrioventricular pathway.

His bundle pacing. Normalization of the QRS morphology with His bundle pacing or by His bundle extrasystoles in a patient with preexcitation demonstrates the dependence of the anomalous QRS on fusion over pathways (normal and accessory) and precludes the presence of a fasciculoventricular fiber.

SERIAL STUDIES

It is often necessary to perform serial tests of arrhythmia induction over several days following the original study. This may be easily accomplished by leaving the coronary sinus catheter in situ at the end of the study or by use of an esophageal electrode, if esophageal pacing reliably induced the arrhythmia during the original study. The ability to reinduce arrhythmias repeatedly permits evaluation of drug efficacy and greatly aids selection of an effective antiarrhythmic regimen.

When evaluation of a pacing device for control of reciprocating tachycardia is desired, the use of a temporary catheter is also of great help. External simulators that mimic the operation of the implanted device may be connected to the temporary catheter and their efficacy observed over several days prior to implantation of the permanent device. Likewise, use of a patient activated device can be tested to insure that the patient will be able to detect the terminate tachycardia reliably.

If pacing the right atrial appendage is desired instead of the coronary sinus, the coronary sinus catheter is removed at the end of the original study and replaced with a temporary atrial "J" pacing lead.

EVALUATION DURING INDUCED ATRIAL FIBRILLATION

When the principal goal of the evaluation of a patient with preexcitation is to determine the potential for excessively rapid ventricular rates during atrial fibrillation, a complete diagnostic catheter study may be unnecessary. To perform this evaluation, we recommend induction of atrial fibrillation in the control state and during infusion of isoproterenol [55]. In our experience, isoproterenol administration during atrial

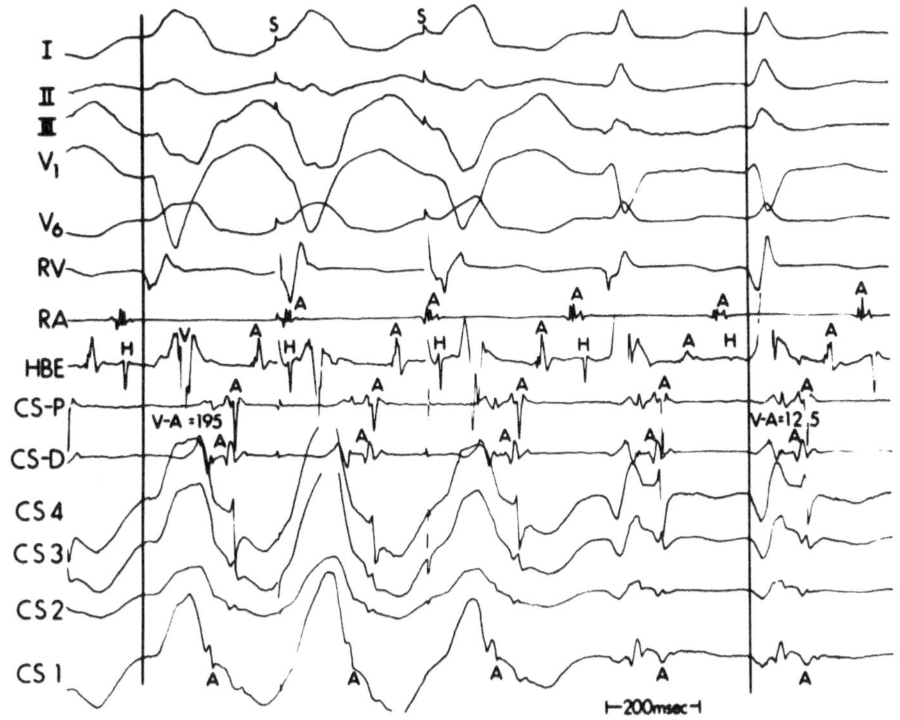

FIGURE 17–6. Conversion of left bundle branch block to normal QRS orthodromic reciprocating tachycardia. Introduction of two critically times PVSs during left bundle morphology reciprocating tachycardia results in normalization of the QRS complex while the tachycardia continues. The VA intervals shorten by 70 ms consistent with the presence of a left-sided accessory pathway. Note the early activation of the coronary sinus (CS-1) consistent with retrograde function of a left-sided accessory pathway during tachycardia.

fibrillation gives the best estimate of the patient's potential for rapid conduction over the accessory pathway. Exercise may also be performed but has not proven to be a valuable means of assessing risk for atrial fibrillation in patients with preexcitation [90]. Observations in patients with documented ventricular fibrillation resulting from rapid conduction during atrial fibrillation have suggested that the risk for lethal ventricular tachyarrhythmias is greatest in patients in whom the shortest RR interval between preexcited beats in atrial fibrillation is below 250 ms [91]. Correlation between the refractory period of the accessory pathway and ventricular rate during atrial fibrillation has been shown, and rapid ventricular rates during atrial fibrillation commonly occur when the accessory pathway effective refractory period is less than 220 ms [92,29].

Patients at risk for rapid ventricular rates during atrial fibrillation should be treated prophylactically with agents shown to decrease accessory pathway conduction, such as quinidine or procainamide, even when otherwise asymptomatic. Documentation of a beneficial effect should be made by repeat testing on stable serum drug concentrations. When patients present following a symptomatic episode of rapid atrial fibrillation, a decision regarding future therapy must be made, and the role of surgery should be considered.

Complications of Invasive Studies (Table 17–2)

ARRHYTHMIAS

Atrial fibrillation. The most troublesome arrhythmia encountered during most invasive studies in patients with preexcitation syndromes

TABLE 17–2. Complications of invasive studies

A. Arrhythmias
   1. Atrial fibrillation
   2. Reciprocating tachycardia
   3. Ventricular tachycardia/fibrillation

B. Mechanical
   1. Cardiac tamponade
   2. Catheter-induced block of accessory pathway
   3. Hematoma from arterial or venous puncture
   4. False aneurysm (femoral artery)
   5. Femoral arteriovenous fistula

C. Infection

D. Embolism

E. Myocardial ischemia

F. Hypotension, low cardiac output during rapid pacing

is sustained atrial fibrillation. This may result from catheter manipulation in the right atrium, frequently the atrial appendage, or may develop during pacing, refractory period determinations, or from rapid reciprocating tachycardia. In many patients, atrial fibrillation may be transient and terminate spontaneously. Unfortunately, many patients undergoing invasive studies have easily induced and sustained atrial fibrillation as a major clinical manifestation of their cardiac problems, and in these patients, multiple long episodes of atrial fibrillation can be anticipated during the study.

The unscheduled appearance of atrial fibrillation that fails to spontaneously terminate presents two problems. First, the study cannot proceed without restoration of sinus rhythm. Atrial fibrillation precludes any further useful observations regarding accessory pathway location, and unless that arrhythmia has developed fortuitously at the end of the study, no satisfactory alternative is available except cardioversion. The administration of drugs to slow or terminate atrial fibrillation will affect electrophysiologic results for the remainder of the study and may make induction of reciprocating tachycardia more difficult, thus preventing other important observations from being made.

The second problem that arises as a result of the development of atrial fibrillation in patients with extremely rapid antegrade conduction is that of hemodynamic deterioration, or even ventricular fibrillation. In these situations, cardioversion is necessary. It is unusual to experience sufficiently severe hypotension as to preclude prior administration of a short-acting anesthetic agent. Even when the ventricular response during atrial fibrillation is quite rapid, blood pressure is usually supported adequately with the patient in the supine position to obtain both surface ECG tracings to examine delta wave morphology, and chart paper recordings to measure shortest and average RR intervals.

Rarely, it will be impossible to maintain sinus rhythm or reciprocating tachycardia long enough to make any useful observations without the development of atrial fibrillation intervening. In these situations, the gradual administration of procainamide intravenously may be helpful in preventing atrial fibrillation or may cause it to terminate spontaneously. It may then be possible to proceed with the study; however, findings must be interpreted carefully in view of the presence of the drug.

Reciprocating tachycardia. Reciprocating tachycardia is rarely a problem during the invasive study of patients with preexcitation syndromes, except for those instances when it cannot be induced. The arrhythmia may be quite rapid in some patients, but is usually well enough tolerated to permit mapping or other observations to be made without having to terminate the tachycardia. When patient discomfort or hypotension makes brief episodes of tachycardia necessary, the arrhythmia can almost always be interrupted easily by atrial or ventricular burst pacing or by critically timed atrial or ventricular extrastimuli. In some patients, reciprocating tachycardia is refractory to termination by any pacing modality involving one chamber. In these cases, simultaneous pacing of the ventricle and atrium will usually permit tachycardia termination. It should be remembered that pacing as close to the pathway location as possible will be most likely to be effective in terminating the tachycardia.

Ventricular tachcyardia/ventricular fibrillation. Patients with preexcitation syndromes are not immune from the development of serious ventricular arrhythmias, either due to the presence of predisposing cardiac disease, or due to rapid ventricular rates during tachycardia. Apparently healthy, normal young adults may develop ventricular fibrillation during pacing or extrastimulus refractory period determinations. Sustained ventricular tachycardia may be managed by pacing techniques, if possible, or by cardioversion, but ventricular fibrillation requires defibrillation.

CATHETER RELATED COMPLICATIONS
Serious complications of invasive electrophysiologic studies may result from catheter manipulation. In addition to provoking arrhythmias, as mentioned above, the danger of cardiac perforation exists. Whereas arrhythmias during electrophysiologic studies are often anticipated and are seldom life-threatening, hemodynamic complications, notably cardiac tamponade, is potentially life-threatening if not recognized and treated quickly.

The heart is vulnerable to catheter perforation in the right ventricle, right atrium, and coronary sinus during routine electrophysiologic studies. Any of these structures may be thin walled and easily penetrated by the relatively stiff electrode catheters. Perforation of the right ventricle by pacing catheters may not be immediately apparent. Heparin administration may aggravate the risk of bleeding.

The occurrence of cardiac perforation during the study may be manifested by chest pain, especially when it has pleuritic qualities, and hypotension. Although hypotension and bradycardia may be the result of hypervagatonia and respond to saline administration and reassurance, the presence of prolonged hypotension associated with chest pain should always raise the question of tamponade. The diagnosis of tamponade may be made on physical examination and emergency pericardiocentesis performed if severe hypotension is present. Often, saline administration and dopamine infusion can stabilize the patient until the presence of pericardial fluid can be documented echocardiographically.

Cardiac perforation can be prevented if catheter manipulation is performed carefully. The patient is especially vulnerable to catheter trauma during cardioversion. Catheters that have warmed to body temperature are seldom likely to perforate during cardioversion if they have been placed correctly. The mapping catheters used in the right atrium, however, include a stiff stylet that must be removed before cardioversion is performed.

Catheter trauma to the accessory pathway may also occur during the study. This may render the accessory pathway nonfunctional temporarily, thus effectively preventing any further observations at that time [93]. The time course of recovery of pathway function after such an incident is unpredictable.

ARTERIAL PUNCTURE
Inadvertent arterial puncture may occur during insertion of the femoral vein catheters or the subclavian catheter. This is not usually a serious complication if recognized prior to insertion of the introducer. False aneurysm formation is possible following arterial puncture. If a catheter is introduced through the femoral artery into the vein, the potential for creating a chronic arteriovenous fistula exists.

COEXISTING CARDIAC CONDITIONS
The presence of coexisting cardiac conditions must always be kept in mind when performing invasive studies. The most frequent coexisting abnormality encountered is coronary artery disease. In these patients, there may be a higher propensity for developing ventricular tachycardia during ventricular pacing, and atrial fibrillation or reciprocating tachycardia may not be well tolerated. In addition, ischemia may develop during rapid atrial pacing. Patients with obstructive hypertrophic cardiomyopathy and valvular aortic stenosis are also at risk for hemodynamic complications during the electrophysiologic study and may not tolerate rapid heart rates.

Interpretation of the Electrophysiologic Study

The electrophysiologic study of patients suspected of preexcitation should be a carefully thought out exercise whose purpose is to martial data to support or refute the presence of an accessory pathway. The data acquired during the study should therefore be considered in terms of the evidence it provides toward this purpose. A complete electrophysiologic study provides evidence to: (1) substantiate the presence of an accessory pathway, (2) determine the location of the accessory pathway, and (3) assess participation of the accessory pathway in the tachycardia. In addition, data regarding the functional characteristics of the accessory pathway, potential arrhythmias supported by the accessory pathway, the effect of drugs on the accessory pathway, and the ability of pacing techniques to terminate arrhythmias must be gathered (Table 17–3).

TABLE 17–3. Important observations during electrophysiologic study of the preexcitation syndromes

1. Presence of an accessory pathway
2. Location of the accessory pathway
3. Participation of the accessory pathway in the patient's tachycardias
4. Functional characteristics of the accessory pathway
5. The effect of drugs/exercise on the accessory pathway
6. Arrhythmias observed
7. The effect of pacing on the observed arrhythmias

PRESENCE OF AN ACCESSORY PATHWAY

The presence of an accessory pathway may be inferred from the observation of a preexcited QRS morphology on the surface ECG, although the absence of a typical delta wave does not exclude the presence of an accessory pathway. When delta waves are not clearly present on the surface ECG, the presence of ventricular preexcitation may be suggested by demonstrating a short HV interval on intracavitary recordings. With greater degrees of preexcitation, the His deflection is progressively displaced into the surface QRS until a negative HV interval is produced (Figure 17–2). This phenomenon may be produced during the electrophysiologic study by atrial pacing at progressively more rapid rates. As conduction slows across the normal AV node with increasing heart rate, ventricular activation occurs to a greater extent over the accessory pathway and preexcitation becomes more evident. As the His deflection is displaced into the QRS, the interval from the atrial electrogram to the delta wave remains constant, reflecting relatively nondecremental conduction over the accessory pathway.

AV nodal bypass tracts (atriofascicular or intranodal) are rarely found. In these patients, a short AH interval may be present, and atrial pacing at progressively more rapid rates may result in no appreciable lengthening of the AH interval. A "jump" in AV conduction time may occur if refractoriness in the accessory pathway is encountered before refractoriness of the AV node. The absence of decremental conduction prior to the "jump," in addition to the short AH interval, distinguishes these patients from those with dual AV nodal physiology.

Nodoventricular (nodofascicular) bypass tracts are usually associated with some degree of decremental conduction due to the presence of AV nodal tissue proximal to the fiber's ventricular insertion. As conduction occurs preferentially over the nodoventricular fiber at faster pacing rates, the QRS assumes a preexcited morphology, usually resembling left bundle branch block. Reciprocating tachycardia utilizing a nodoventricular bypass tract is typically preexcited, with a QRS morphology resembling left bundle branch block with a leftward QRS frontal axis.

Evidence that an anomalous QRS represents fusion over an accessory AV pathway may be obtained through the observation that the QRS normalizes during orthodromic reciprocating tachycardia, with spontaneously His bundle extrasystoles, or with His bundle pacing.

Evidence for the retrograde function of an accessory AV pathway is obtained by observation of eccentric sequence of atrial activation during ventricular pacing or during reciprocating tachycardia. In addition, the absence of decremental conduction during ventricular pacing or refractory period determination favors the existence of an accessory pathway functioning in the retrograde direction (Figure 17–7). Some accessory pathways, however, may exhibit decremental properties [94,17], including those found in the PJRT variant. Nodoventricular fibers may also appear to display retrograde decremental conduction due to their insertion into the AV node.

Lastly, the ability of premature ventricular stimuli inserted during reciprocating tachycardia and timed to occur when the His bundle is refractory (and therefore incapable of retrograde conduction over the AV node-His bundle axis) to advance activation of the atria, provides strong evidence for the presence of a functioning accessory AV pathway.

Multiple accessory pathways are present in a small percentage of patients with preexcitation syndrome [44,83–87]. The presence of multiple pathways has been associated with Ebstein's anomaly [95] and with a history of ventricular fibrillation [92]. The occurrence of antidromic reciprocating tachycardia should also alert one to the possible presence of multiple accessory pathways [24]. A frequent finding, especially in patients with Ebstein's anomaly, is the combination of a nodoventricular fiber, with a right-sided or posterior septal accessory AV pathway.

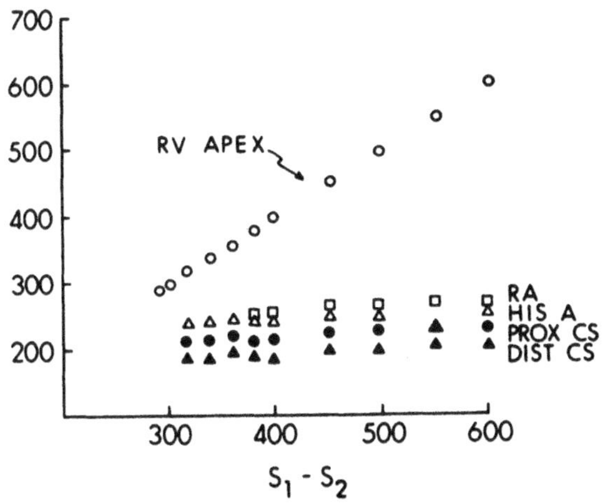

FIGURE 17–7. A retrograde (ventricular) refractory period determination in a patient with an accessory AV pathway located on the left side. Retrograde atrial activation occurs earliest in the distal coronary sinus followed by the proximal coronary sinus, medial RA (HBE) and right atrium. As the premature coupling intervals (S1–S2) abscissa, in the RV apex are decreased (*open circles*) there is no decrement in VA conduction, (ms) ordmate, as would be expected if conduction were occurring over the normal conduction system. Failure of conduction in the retrograde direction over the accessory pathway occurs just prior to loss of capture in the right ventricle. Flat retrograde conduction curves such as this are typical of accessory pathways. Axes are both in milliseconds.

The presence of multiple pathways may be suspected during electrophysiologic study through the observation of one or more of the following phenomena:

1. More than one preexcited QRS morphology, either spontaneously, during differential atrial pacing, or during atrial fibrillation. Rhythm strips of the various ECG leads during atrial fibrillation may help to identify different QRS morphologies.
2. Antidromic reciprocating tachycardia with an eccentric retrograde activation sequence. The presence of one pathway is demonstrated by the preexcited QRS, and the presence of another is proved by the anomalous retrograde activation.
3. Orthodromic reciprocating tachycardia (normal QRS) with varying retrograde activation sequences. The normal conduction system is being used for the antegrade limb of the circuit, and the different retrograde activation sequences prove the presence of multiple accessory pathways.
4. The occurrence of orthodromic or antidromic reciprocating tachycardia at different cycle lengths. This implies the presence of at least two different reentrant circuits, of different size, although changes in conduction through the AV node alone may account for such changes in some patients. The presence of dual AV nodal physiology may also account for this finding.
5. Spontaneous or premature beat-induced conversion from a preexcited QRS to a normal QRS (or vice versa) during reciprocating tachycardia. This demonstrates the bystander function of an accessory pathway not involved in the reentrant circuit. AV nodal reentry must be excluded as the mechanism for the arrhythmia.

When multiple pathways are suspected, their participation in the observed arrhythmias must be demonstrated through other maneuvers such as critically timed extrastimuli during tachycardia when portions of the reentrant circuit are refractory [24,85].

LOCATION OF THE ACCESSORY PATHWAY

The location of the accessory pathway is an important concern when surgical or pacing techniques are considered for therapy. Estimation of pathway location can often be made by a trained observer from evaluation of the delta wave on the surface ECG. However, the precision of such an estimation relies on the presence of maximal preexcitation, is only applicable to pathways which conduct in the antegrade direction, and is confounded if more than one accessory pathway is present. Differential atrial pacing also provides a good estimation of pathway location since the shortest stimulus to delta interval observed will correspond to the pacing site closest to the atrial insertion of the pathway (Figure 17–4). An interval between pacing stimulus and delta wave onset of 0.08 seconds or less is often found at the site nearest the atrial insertion of the accessory pathway, although this value may be longer when it is not possible to position the pacing catheter directly at the atrial insertion of the accessory pathway. The relative value compared to measurements obtained from a variety of sites is of use.

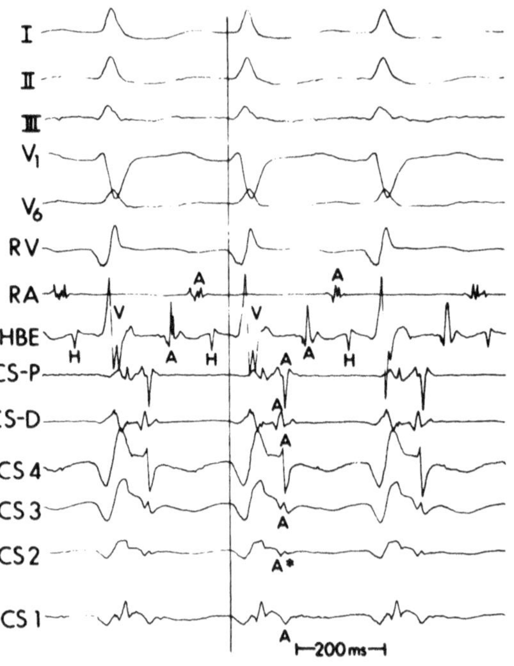

FIGURE 17–8. Coronary sinus mapping during reciprocating tachycardia in a patient with a left-sided accessory pathway. The coronary sinus catheter has been positioned over the accessory pathway so that earliest atrial activation occurs in coronary sinus pole 2 (*). Activation distal (CS-1), and proximal in the coronary sinus (CS-3, CS-4, CS-P) as well as in the medial and lateral right atrium occurs later.

Data from retrograde pathway function may also be helpful in localization. The earliest site of atrial activation during ventricular pacing or reciprocating tachycardia corresponds to the site of the pathway (Figure 17–8). The ventriculoatrial conduction time following critical timed right ventricular extrasystoles has also been proposed as a method of separating septal from free wall accessory pathways [96].

Changes in tachycardia cycle length or VA intervals with the development of bundle branch block also provide strong evidence that the pathway is located ipsilateral to the site of bundle branch block [40,23] (Figure 17–6).

PARTICIPATION OF THE ACCESSORY PATHWAY IN TACHYCARDIA

Patients with accessory pathways may also suffer from forms of tachycardia that do not actually use the accessory pathway. In these patients, the accessory pathway is said to be a bystander. The electrophysiologic study must demonstrate actual dependance of the tachycardia on the accessory pathway. This is done by demonstrating the effect on the tachycardia of bundle branch block and the effect of premature stimuli from the ventricle or atrium, as mentioned above. By carefully observing the effect of premature stimuli during tachycardia, the various limbs of the reentrant circuit can be identified, or participation of certain regions of the heart in the reentrant circuit can be excluded. These maneuvers are particularly helpful in patients with nodoventricular fibers, in whom reciprocating tachycardia may involve either or both bundle branches in the retrograde direction, and in antidromic tachycardias where participation of the normal conduction system may be involved, as opposed to a second accessory pathway functioning in the retrograde direction. In patients with tachycardias associated with a wide QRS complex, the differentiation between antidromic tachycardia and AV nodal reentry with bystander participation of an accessory pathway is critical, if surgery or other nonmedical forms of therapy are being considered.

FUNCTIONAL PROPERTIES OF THE ACCESSORY PATHWAY

It is necessary to know the functional characteristics of the accessory pathway for characterization of the risk from atrial fibrillation, and evaluation of the potential effectiveness of medical management. The refractory period of the accessory pathway has been used as one indicator of the ability of the pathway to support rapid conduction during atrial fibrillation and has been shown to correlate with ventricular response during atrial fibrillation. Likewise, accessory pathways with very short refractory periods are less likely to respond significantly to conventional antiarrhythmic agents.

EFFECTS OF DRUGS AND EXERCISE ON ACCESSORY PATHWAY FUNCTION

We have found that the use of isoproterenol during electrophysiologic testing gives a good assessment of the potential for rapid ventricular rates during atrial fibrillation. Exercise has not been found to be a reliable method for assessing arrhythmias due to preexcitation syndromes, but an assessment of the effects of exercise may be desirable in young, active patients. The effects of other drugs on accessory pathway function may also be important to evaluate, including beta-blockers, calcium antagonists, or digitalis, if therapy with these agents is contemplated. The effects of certain type I antiarrhythmic agents may be more complex. Drugs such as procainamide may slow conduction over the accessory pathway and provide protection against atrial fibrillation, while at the same time making reciprocating tachycardia more inducible and occasionally incessant.

ARRHYTHMIAS OBSERVED

The various arrhythmias observed during the study should be clearly reported, along with the mode of induction, cycle length (rate), mechanism, and mode of termination. Attempts should be made to induce atrial fibrillation and reciprocating tachycardia in every patient. The presence of antidromic tachycardia should be specifically mentioned, since this may be confused later for ventricular tachycardia and may often imply the presence of multiple pathways. When atrial fibrillation is recorded, the average and shortest RR intervals and percentage of preexcited beats are reported.

EFFECTS OF PACING

The effects of various pacing modalities should be studied, so that an assessment of their potential role in treating reciprocating tachycardia can be made. The ease with which tachycardia can be interrupted from different pacing sites should be studied, and the potential for the induction of atrial fibrillation by the pacing methods found to be effective in terminating tachycardia should be examined. In addition to the potential for the induction of complicating arrhythmias such as atrial fibrillation and the ability to terminate the tachycardia from the coronary sinus and the right atrial appendage, the effectiveness of different modalities of pacing, either bursts, or critically timed extrastimuli should be tested.

Conclusion

Invasive electrophysiologic studies are essential in establishing diagnosis, documenting tachycardia mechanism, and guiding therapy in symptomatic patients in whom the preexcitation syndrome is suspected. Although initial empiric therapy may be justified in mildly symptomatic patients, invasive studies provide efficient evaluation of antiarrhythmic therapy and may permit an objective assessment of life-threatening risk from arrhythmia in patients with preexcitation syndrome.

Many patients with PSVT will be found to have a variant of the preexcitation syndrome, often with a surgically correctable accessory pathway. Thus invasive studies may reveal important therapeutic options that would otherwise not be considered. When surgery is considered for patients with the preexcitation syndrome, a thorough electrophysiologic study performed by experienced personnel is essential.

References

1. Jackman WM, Friday KJ, Scherlag BJ, Dehning MM, Schechter E, Reynolds DW, Olson EG, Berbari EJ, Harrison LA, Lazzara R: Direct endocardial recording from an accessory atrioventricular pathway: localization of the site of block, effect of antiarrhythmic drugs, and attempt at non-surgical ablation. *Circulation* 68:906, 1983.
2. Prystowsky EN, Browne KF, Zipes DP: Intracardiac recording by catheter electrode of accessory pathway depolarization. *J. Am. Coll. Cardiol.* 1:468, 1983.
3. Klein GJ, Hackel DB, Gallagher JJ: Anatomic substrate of impaired antegrade conduction over an accessory atrioventricular pathway in the Wolff-Parkinson-White syndrome. *Circulation* 61:1249, 1980.
4. Rosenberg HS, Klima T, McNamara DG, Leachman RD: Atrioventricular communication in the Wolff-Parkinson-White syndrome. *Am. J. Clin. Pathol.* 56:79, 1971.
5. Boineau JP, Moore EN, Spear JF, Sealy WC: Basis of static and dynamic electrocardiographic variations in Wolff-Parkinson-White syndrome. *Am. J. Cardiol.* 32:32, 1973.
6. Untereker WJ, Litwak RS, Mindich BP, Wiemann G, Goldberg S, Gorlin R, Kupersmith J: Superficial accessory pathway in the Wolff-Parkinson-White syndrome — electrophysiological, surgical and histologic demonstration. *J. Electrocardiol.* 13:393, 1980.
7. Castellanos A, Sung RJ, Castillo CA, Agha AS, Befler B, Myerburg RJ: His bundle recordings in diagnosis of impulse formation in Kent and Mahaim tracts. *Br. Heart J.* 38:1173, 1976.
8. Wellens HJJ: Contribution of cardiac pacing to our understanding of the Wolff-Parkinson-White syndrome. *Br. Heart J.* 37:231, 1975.
9. Svenson RH, Miller HS, Gallagher JJ, Wallace AG: Electrophysiological evaluation of the

Wolff-Parkinson-White syndrome. Problems in assessing antegrade and retrograde conduction over the accessory pathway. *Circulation* 52:552, 1975.
10. Tonkin AM, Dugan FA, Svenson RH, Sealy WC, Wallace AG, Gallagher JJ: Coexistence of functional Kent and Mahaim-type tracts in the preexcitation syndrome. Demonstration by catheter techniques and epicardial mapping. *Circulation* 52:193, 1975.
11. Gallagher JJ, Gilbert M, Svenson RH, Sealy SC, Kasell J and Wallace AG: Wolff-Parkinson-White syndrome. The problem, evaluation, and surgical correction. *Circulation* 51:767, 1975.
12. Castellanos A, Jr, Chapunoff E, Castillo CA, Maytin O, Lemburg L: His bundle electrograms in two cases of Wolff-Parkinson-White (preexcitation) syndrome. *Circulation* 41:399, 1975.
13. Touboul P, Tessier Y, Magrina J, Clement C, Delahaye JP: His bundle recording and electrical stimulation of the atria in patients with Wolff-Parkinson-White syndrome type A. *Br. Heart J.* 34:623, 1972.
14. Durrer D, Roos JP: Epicardial excitation of the ventricles in a patient with Wolff-Parkinson-White syndrome (type B). *Circulation* 35:15, 1967.
15. Burchell HB, Frye RL, Anderson MW, McGoon DC: Atrioventricular and ventriculoatrial excitation in Wolff-Parkinson-White syndrome (type B). *Circulation* 36:663, 1967.
16. Boineau JP, Moore EN: Evidence for propagation of activation across an accessory atrioventricular connection in types A and B preexcitation. *Circulation* 41:375, 1970.
17. Wellens HJJ, Durrer D: Patterns of ventriculo-atrial conduction in the Wolff-Parkinson-White syndrome. *Circulation* 49:22, 1974.
18. Lister JW, Worthington FX, Gentsch TO, Svenson JA, Nathan DA, Grosselin AJ: Preexcitation and tachycardias in the Wolff-Parkinson-White syndrome, type B. *Circulation* 45:1081, 1972.
19. Durrer D, Schoo L, Schuilenburg RM, Wellens HJJ: The role of premature beats in the termination of supraventricular tachycardia in the Wolff-Parkinson-White syndrome. *Circulation* 36:644, 1967.
20. Adams JR, Hess D, Scheinman MM: Mechanism of spontaneous tachycardia termination in a patient with the Wolff-Parkinson-White syndrome and dual atrioventricular nodal pathways. *PACE* 4:367, 1981.
21. Castillo CA, Castellanos A, Jr: His bundle recordings in patients with Wolff-Parkinson-White syndrome. *Circulation* 42:271, 1970.
22. Rosen KM: AV nodal reentrance. An unexpected mechanism of paroxysmal tachycardia in a patient with preexcitation. *Circulation* 47:1267, 1973.
23. Coumel P, Attuel P: Reciprocating tachycardia in overt and latent preexcitation. *Eur. J. Cardiol.* 1:423, 1974.
24. Bardy GH, Packer DL, German LD, Gallagher JJ: Preexcited reciprocating tachycardia in patients with Wolff-Parkinson-White syndrome: incidence and mechanisms. *Circulation* 70:377, 1984.
25. Roelandt J, Van der Hawwaert LG: Atrial reciprocating rhythm and reciprocating tachycardias in the Wolff-Parkinson-White syndrome. *Circulation* 38:64, 1968.
26. Sung RJ, Castellanos A, Gelband H, Myerburg RJ: Mechanism of reciprocating tachycardia initiated during sinus rhythm in concealed Wolff-Parkinson-White syndrome. *Circulation* 54:338, 1976.
27. Wellens HJJ, Durrer D: The role of an accessory atrioventricular pathway in reciprocating tachycardia. Observations in patients with and without the Wolff-Parkinson-White syndrome. *Circulation* 52:58, 1975.
28. Gillette P: Concealed anomalous cardiac conduction pathways: A frequent cause of supraventricular tachycardia. *Am. J. Cardiol.* 40:848, 1977.
29. Wellens HJJ, Durrer D: Wolff-Parkinson-White syndrome and atrial fibrillation. Relation between refractory period of accessory pathway and ventricular rate during atrial fibrillation. *Am. J. Cardiol.* 34:777, 1974.
30. Tonkin AM, Gallagher JJ, Svenson RH, Wallace AG, Sealy WC: Anterograde block in accessory pathways with retrograde conduction in reciprocating tachycardia. *Eur. J. Cardiol.* 3:143, 1975.
31. Campbell RWF, Smith, RA, Gallagher JJ, Pritchett ELC, Wallace AG: Atrial fibrillation in the preexcitation syndrome. *Am. J. Cardiol.* 40:514, 1977.
32. Gallagher JJ, Smith WM, Kasell JH, Benson DW, Jr, Sterba R, Grant AO: Role of Mahaim fibers in cardiac arrhythmias in man. *Circulation* 64:176, 1981.
33. Gallagher JJ, Sealy WC: The permanent form of junctional reciprocating tachycardia: further elucidation of the underlying mechanism. *Eur. J. Cardiol.* 8:413, 1978.
34. Benditt DG, Pritchett ELC, Gallagher JJ: Spectrum of regular tachycardias with wide QRS complexes in patients with accessory atrioventricular pathways. *Am. J. Cardiol.* 42:828, 1978.
35. Akhtar M, Shenasa M, Schmidt DH: Role of retrograde His Purkinje block in the initiation of supraventricular tachycardia by ventricular premature stimulation in the Wolff-Parkinson-White syndrome. *J. Clin. Invest.* 67:1047, 1981.
36. Sung RJ, Castellanos A: Supraventricular tachycardia: Mechanisms and treatment. *Cardiovasc. Clin.* 11:27, 1980.

37. Benditt DG, Pritchett ELC, Smith WM, Wallace AG, Gallagher JJ: Characteristics of atrioventricular conduction and the spectrum of arrhythmias in Lown-Ganong-Levine syndrome. *Circulation* 57:454, 1978.
38. Josephson ME, Kastor JA: Supraventricular tachycardia in Lown-Ganong-Levine syndrome: atrionodal versus intranodal reentry. *Am. J. Cardiol.* 40:521, 1977.
39. Garson A, Jr, Gillette PC: Electrophysiologic studies of supraventricular tachycardia in children. I. Clinical – electrophysiologic correlations. *Am. Heart J.* 102:233, 1981.
40. Pritchett ELC, Tonkin AM, Dugan FA, Wallace AG, Gallagher JJ: Ventriculoatrial conduction time during reciprocating tachycardia with intermittent bundle branch block in Wolff-Parkinson-White syndrome. *Br. Heart J.* 38:1058, 1976.
41. Cosio FG, Benson DW, Jr, Anderson RW, Hession WT, Pritzker MR, Kriett JM, Benditt DG: Onset of atrial fibrillation during antidromic tachycardia: Association with sudden cardiac arrest and ventricular fibrillation in a patient with Wolff-Parkinson-White syndrome. *Am. J. Cardiol.* 50:353, 1982.
42. Golitsyn SP, Sokolov SF, Mazur NA: The importance of electrophysiological studies of atrioventricular conduction for diagnosis of some forms of paroxysmal supraventricular tachycardia. *Adv. Cardiol.* 28:140, 1981.
43. Ezri MD: Electrophysiologic testing in the diagnosis and management of cardiac arrhythmias. *Chest* 84:481, 1983.
44. Portillo B, Portillo-Leon N, Zaman L, Castellanos A: Quintuple pathways participating in three distinct types of atrioventricular reciprocating tachycardia in a patient with Wolff-Parkinson-White syndrome. *Am. J. Cardiol.* 50:347, 1982.
45. Critelli G, Gallagher JJ, Monda V, Coltorti F, Scherillo M, Rossi L: Anatomic and electrophysiologic substrate of the permanent form of junctional reciprocating tachycardia. *J. Am. Coll. Cardiol.* 4:601, 1984.
46. Sung RJ, Styperek JL: Electrophysiologic identification of dual atrioventricular nodal pathway conduction in patients with reciprocating tachycardia using anomalous bypass tracts. *Circulation* 60:1464, 1979.
47. Gallagher JJ, Sealy WC, Kasell J: Intraoperative mapping studies in the Wolff-Parkinson-White syndrome. *PACE* 2:523, 1979.
48. Bhandari A, Morady F, Shen EN, Schwertz AB, Botvinick E, Scheinman MM: Catheter-induced His bundle ablation in a patient with reentrant tachycardia associated with a nodoventricular tract. *J. Am. Coll. Cardiol.* 4:611, 1984.
49. Fisher JD, Brodman R, Kim SG, Matos JA, Brodman LE, Wallerson D, Waspe LE: Attempted non-surgical electrical ablation of accessory pathways via the coronary sinus in the Wolff-Parkinson-White syndrome. *J. Am. Coll. Cardiol.* 4:685, 1984.
50. Guarnieri T, Sealy WC, Kasell JH, German LD, Gallagher JJ: The nonpharmacologic management of the permanent form of junctional reciprocating tachycardia. *Circulation* 69:269, 1984.
51. Spurrell RAJ, Nathan AW, Bexton RS, Hellestrand KJ, Nappholz T, Camm AJ: Implantable automatic scanning pacemaker for termination of supraventricular tachycardia. *Am. J. Cardiol.* 49:753, 1982.
52. German LD, Strauss HC: Electrical termination of tachyarrhythmias by discrete pulses. *PACE* 7:514, 1984.
53. Morady F, Sledge C, Shen E, Sung RJ, Gonzales R, Scheinman MM: Electrophysiologic testing in the management of patients with Wolff-Parkinson-White syndrome and atrial fibrillation. *Am. J. Cardiol.* 51:1623, 1983.
54. Bauernfeind RA, Swiryn SP, Strasberg B, Palileo E, Scagliotti D, Rosen KM: Electrophysiologic drug testing in prophylaxis of sporadic paroxysmal atrial fibrillation: technique, application and efficacy in severely symptomatic preexcitation patients. *Am. Heart. J.* 103:941, 1982.
55. German LD, Gallagher JJ, Broughton A, Guarnieri T, Trantham JL: Effects of exercise and isoproterenol during atrial fibrillation in patients with Wolff-Parkinson-White syndrome. *Am. J. Cardiol.* 51:1203, 1983.
56. Wu D, Amat-Y-Leon F, Simpson RJ Jr, Latif P, Wyndham CRC, Denes P, Rosen KM: Electrophysiological studies with multiple drugs in patients with atrioventricular reentrant tachycardias utilizing an extranodal pathway. *Circulation* 56:727, 1977.
57. Krikler D: Concealed preexcitation. (Editorial.) *J. Electrocardiol.* 11:209, 1978.
58. Zipes DP, DeJoseph RL, Rothbaum DA: Unusual properties of accessory pathways. *Circulation* 49:1200, 1974.
59. Sung RJ, Gelband H, Castellanos A, Aranda JM, Myersburg RJ: Clinical and electrophysiologic observations in patients with concealed accessory atrioventricular bypass tract. *Am. J. Cardiol.* 40:839, 1977.
60. Klein GJ, Yee R, Sharma AD: Concealed conduction in accessory atrioventricular pathways: an important determinant of the expression of arrhythmias in patients with Wolff-Parkinson-White syndrome. *Circulation* 70:402, 1984.
61. Bardy GH, Poole JE, Coltorti F, Ivey TD, Block TA, Trobaugh GB, Greene HL: Catheter ablation of a concealed accessory pathway. *Am. J. Cardiol.* 54:1366, 1984.
62. Wiener I: Current applications of clinical electrophysiologic study in the diagnosis and treat-

ment of cardiac arrhythmias. *Am. J. Cardiol.* 49:1287, 1982.
63. Michelson EL, Dreifus LS: Present status of clinical electrophysiologic studies: Introduction — What studies are necessary. *PACE* 7:421, 1984.
64. Hart R, Peters R, Rubinstein M, Desai J, O'Young J, Thomas A, Scheinman MM: A review of instrumentation and therapeutic techniques in the diagnosis and management of supraventricular tachycardia. *Med. Instrum.* 12:268, 1978.
65. Fisher JD: Role of electrophysiologic testing in the diagnosis and treatment of patients with known and suspected bradycardias and tachycardias. *Prog. Cardiovasc. Dis.* 24:25, 1981.
66. Breithardt G, Borggrefe M: Induced arrhythmias in clinical decision making. *Eur. Heart J.* 5 (Suppl B):35, 1984.
67. Zaman L, Garcia N, Luceri RM, Castellanos A, Myerburg RJ: Ectopic left atrial rhythm that produces QRS changes in absence of Wolff-Parkinson-White syndrome. *Circulation* 68:701, 1983.
68. Smith WM, Broughton A, Reiter MJ, Benson DW, Jr, Grant AO, Gallagher JJ: Bystander accessory pathway during AV node reentrant tachycardia. *PACE* 6:537, 1983.
69. Mandel WJ, Laks MM, and Obayashi K: Atrioventricular nodal reentry in the Wolff-Parkinson-White syndrome. *Chest* 68:321, 1975.
70. Neuss H, Schlepper M: Unusual reentry mechanisms in patients with Wolff-Parkinson-White syndrome. *Br. Heart J.* 36:880, 1974.
71. Bardy GH, Fedor JM, German LD, Packer DL, Gallagher JJ: Surface electrocardiographic clues suggesting the presence of a nodofascicular Mahaim fiber. *J. Am. Coll. Cardiol.* 3:1161, 1984.
72. Guarnieri T, Sealy WC, German LD, Gallagher JJ: Utilization of an accessory pathway as the anterograde limb during the permanent form of junctional reciprocating tachycardia. *Am. J. Cardiol.* 53:365, 1984.
73. Coumel P, Cabrol C, Fabiato A, Gourgon R, Slama R: Tachycardie permanente par rhythme reciproque. *Arch. Mal Coeur.* 60:1830, 1967.
74. Moro C, Cosio FG: Electrophysiologic study of patients with short P-R interval and normal QRS complex. *Eur. J. Cardiol.* 11:81, 1980.
75. Mandel WJ, Danzig R, Hoyakawa H: Lown-Ganong-Levine syndrome. A study using His bundle electrograms. *Circulation* 44:696, 1973.
76. Caracta AR, Damato AN, Gallagher JJ, Josephson ME, Varghese PJ, Lou SH, Westura EE: Electrophysiological studies in the syndrome of short P-R interval, normal QRS complex. *Am. J. Cardiol.* 31:245, 1973.
77. Lown B, Ganong WF, Levine SA: The syndrome of short P-R interval, normal QRS complex, and paroxysmal rapid heart action. *Circulation* 5:693, 1952.
78. Benditt DG, Pritchett ELC, Smith WM, Gallagher JJ: Ventriculoatrial intervals: Diagnostic use in paroxysmal supraventricular tachycardia. *Ann. Intern. Med.* 91:161, 1979.
79. Broughton A, Gallagher JJ, German LD, Guarnieri T, Trantham JL: Differentiation of septal from free wall accessory pathway location: observations during bundle branch block in reciprocating tachycardia in the presence of type I antiarrhythmic drugs. *Am. J. Cardiol.* 52:751, 1983.
80. Sellers TD, Jr, Bashore TM, Gallagher JJ: Digitalis in the preexcitation syndrome. Analysis during atrial fibrillation. *Circulation* 56:260, 1977.
81. Wellens HJJ, Durrer D: Effect of digitalis on atrioventricular conduction and circus movement tachycardias in patients with Wolff-Parkinson-White syndrome. *Circulation* 47:1229, 1973.
82. Edvardsson N, Blomstrom P, Olsson SB: Identification of multiple pathways in the Wolff-Parkinson-White syndrome. *Cardiology* 71:20, 1984.
83. Denes P, Amat-Y-Leon F, Wyndham C, Wu D, Levitsky S, Rosen KM: Electrophysiologic demonstration of bilateral anomalous pathways in a patient with Wolff-Parkinson-White syndrome (Type B preexcitation). *Am. J. Cardiol.* 37:93, 1976.
84. Gallagher JJ, Sealy WC, Kasell J, Wallace AG: Multiple accessory pathways in patients with the preexcitation syndrome. *Circulation* 54:571, 1976.
85. Coumel P, Waynberger M, Fabiato A, Slama R, Aiqueperse J, Bouvrain G: Wolff-Parkinson-White syndrome. Problems in evaluation of multiple accessory pathways and surgical therapy. *Circulation* 45:1216, 1972.
86. Castellanos A, Agha AS, Befeler B, Myerburg RJ: Double accessory pathways in Wolff-Parkinson-White syndrome. *Circulation* 51:1020, 1975.
87. Ellenbogen KA, O'Callaghan WG, Colavita PG, Packer DL, Gilbert MR, German LD: Catheter His ablation for recurrent supraventricular tachycardia in two patients with nodoventricular fibers. *Am. J. Cardiol.* (In press.)
88. Sung RJ, Castellanos A, Mallon SM, Bloom MG, Gelband H, Myerburg RJ: Mechanisms of spontaneous alternation between reciprocating tachycardia and atrial flutter – fibrillation in the Wolff-Parkinson-White syndrome. *Circulation* 56:409, 1977.
89. Denes P, Wyndham CR, Amat-Y-Leon F, Wu D, Dhingra RC, Miller RH, Rosen KM: Atrial pacing at multiple sites in the Wolff-Parkinson-White syndrome. *Br. Heart J.* 39:506, 1977.
90. Strasberg B, Ashley WW, Wyndham CRC,

Bavernfeind RA, Swiryn SP, Dhingra RC, Rosen KM: Treadmill exercise testing in the Wolff-Parkinson-White syndrome. *Am. J. Cardiol.* 45:742, 1980.
91. Klein GJ, Bashore TM, Sellers TD, Pritchett ELC, Smith WM, Gallagher JJ: Ventricular fibrillation in the Wolff-Parkinson-White syndrome. *N. Engl. J. Med.* 301:1080, 1979.
92. Castellanos A, Jr, Myerburg RJ, Craparo K, Befeler B, Agha AS: Factors regulating ventricular rates during atrial flutter and fibrillation in preexcitation (Wolff-Parkinson-White) syndrome. *Br. Heart J.* 35:811, 1973.
93. Novick TL, Pritchett ELC, Campbell RWF, Rogers GC, Wallace AC, Gallagher JJ: Temporary, catheter-induced block in accessory pathways. *Circulation* 58:932, 1978.
94. Klein GJ, Prystowsky EN, Pritchett ELC, Davis D, Gallagher JJ: Atypical patterns of retrograde conduction over accessory atrioventricular pathways in the Wolff-Parkinson-White syndrome. *Circulation* 60:1477, 1979.
95. Smith WM, Gallagher JJ, Kerr CR, Sealy WC, Kasell JH, Benson DW, Jr, Reiter MJ, Sterba R, Grant AO: The electrophysiologic basis and management of symptomatic recurrent tachycardia in patients with Ebstein's anomaly of the tricuspid valve. *Am. J. Cardiol.* 49:1223, 1982.
96. Weiss J. Brugada P, Roy D, Bar FWHM, Wellens HJJ: Localization of the accessory pathway in the Wolff-Parkinson-White syndrome from the ventriculo-atrial conduction time of right ventricular apical extrasystoles. *PACE* 6:260, 1983.

18. EVALUATION OF PEDIATRIC PATIENTS WITH PREEXCITATION SYNDROMES

John D. Kugler

In this chapter, the following areas are addressed: (1) history and physical examination (signs and symptoms), (2) noninvasive testing, (3) invasive testing and, (4) indications for evaluation. Emphasis on the evaluation of the pediatric patients with one of the preexcitation syndromes is directed toward age as well as the presence of specific symptoms, both important factors when considering whether noninvasive and/or invasive testing is needed. At the outset of the chapter, the discussion of the presentation of pediatric patients includes general features followed by details of signs and symptoms relative to the age of the child. Together, the history and physical examination are paramount in the evaluation of the pediatric patient because the extent of evaluation virtually always depends on the specific signs and symptoms. Next, the chapter includes discussion of the available noninvasive tests with findings, advantages, and limitations of each relative to the pediatric patient. Invasive testing discussion includes similar but more detailed analysis of invasive electrophysiology studies, and lastly, attention is given to indications for evaluation, that is, to the problems of clinicians when they are confronted with a neonate or infant or older child/adolescent who has the preexcitation syndrome. When is evaluation indicated? If evaluation is indicated, are noninvasive and/or invasive testing necessary?

Evaluation by History and Physical Examination

Before discussing each pediatric age group separately, general comments are indicated regarding history and physical examination.

HISTORY

Symptoms may differ among patients with preexcitation syndromes in different age groups due to variations in the hemodynamic effects of arrhythmias or to the capacity of the child to express discomfort. For example, low cardiac output may cause decreased coronary blood flow, expressed as angina in the adolescent or manifested in the infant by sudden paleness, lethargy, outbursts of unexplained irritability, crying, or diaphoresis.

It is important to investigate associated activity and body position (supine, sitting, walking, exercise) preceding and during symptoms. The same arrhythmia causing lethargy and angina in the supine or sitting patient may cause syncope or sudden death (the latter resulting from progressive coronary insufficiency which causes eventual ventricular fibrillation) in the upright or vasodilated patient. Vasodilation may be produced by: exercise or any activity associated with high cardiac output, alcohol consumption, hot bath or jacuzzi, hot weather or environment, dehydration, vasodilating drugs. Onset of rapid tachycardia during any of these circumstances may result in profound symptoms [1,2]. History of antiarrhythmic medications is an important consideration in the evaluation of young patients with preexcitation. In some individuals, specific antiarrhythmia drugs may aggravate tachycardia. Additionally, there has been concern regarding the possibility that digitalis and verapamil may result in syncope and/or sudden death secondary to increased rate of atrial impulses conducted via the accessory atrioventricular (AV) connection during atrial flutter-fibrillation [3–10].

Other arrhythmias, not directly associated with ventricular preexcitation, may be found in patients of any age who have preexcitation syndromes. These arrhythmias may include ventricular tachycardia, ventricular fibrillation and long QT interval-associated *torsade de pointe*. The latter may be related to iatrogenic/drug causes in these patients (type 1 drugs, hypokalemia, etc.) [11–12]. Underlying structural heart disease or other system diseases are important historic data because symptoms may be related to these problems rather than arrhythmias associated with preexcitation syndrome. On the other hand, it is possible in such patients that symptoms related to preexcitation arrhythmias are exacerbated because of other underlying disease.

A critical historic observation in any patient with one of the preexcitation syndromes relates to whether or not syncope or cardiac arrest has occurred. The occurrence of a seizure requires a detailed history of preseizure activity, onset, seizure and postseizure activity. It is not uncommon in the young patient for syncope to present as a "seizure" [13]. Only detailed history of the witnessed event reveals a pale, glassy-eyed child who suddenly becomes unconscious, begins noisy, erratic breathing, or becomes apneic followed by tonic (±clonic) movements. If the life-threatening arrhythmia spontaneously resolves or changes to enable more effective cardiac output, the patient may recover immediately or manifest postictal symptoms (when cerebral hypoxia has in fact caused a seizure). If the arrhythmia continues, cardiopulmonary resuscitation is required for the patient to survive. If preexcitation syndrome is known or discovered in a young patient with syncope, the initial assumption should be that the episode is related to a life-threatening arrhythmia. This assumption is based upon the observation that syncope or cardiac arrest occur in young patients with preexcitation syndromes, and these potentially catastrophic symptoms may be the initial manifestation of one of the preexcitation syndromes [1,3].

Family history also is important in evaluating the pediatric patient. Positive family history especially is helpful when a patient also has underlying congenital or other structural heart disease, sudden death, or other unexplained cardiac death. There have been rare reports of an autosomal dominant heritance of Wolff-Parkinson-White (WPW) syndrome [14–16]. Gallagher et al. reported an asymptomatic patient with a family history of sudden cardiac arrest in whom preexcitation syndrome was found and in whom prophylactic division of the accessory AV connection was carried out [16]. Also, there is a positive family history of paroxysmal tachycardia in approximately 3% of infants who have the WPW syndrome, but in most patients, family history is negative [17].

The *physical examination* should be focused on detecting associated/underlying structural abnormalities and to assess hemodynamic effects of tachycardia if present (e.g., severity of congestive heart failure). Approximately 15–30% of infants with preexcitation syndrome also have congenital heart disease [18–25]. Ebstein's anomaly is the congenital heart defect most widely known to be associated with WPW syndrome [26,27]. Approximately 15–25% of patients who have Ebstein's anomaly also have accessory AV connections, whereas, others have preexcitation due to nodofasicular and fasiculoventricular connections [28]. Other congenital heart defects that have been reported with associated preexcitation include corrected transposition of the great arteries (probably because of increased incidence of Ebstein's malformation of left-sided AV valve) [29,30], tricuspid atresia [31], ventricular septal defect [32], endocardial cushion defect [33], arrhythmogenic right ventricular dysplasia [34], left ventricular fibroelastosis [35], complete transposition of the great arteries (see Figure 18–4), mitral valve prolapse [36–38], and hypertrophic cardiomyopathy [39] (see Chapter 14 by Porter and Holmes).

Age-Related Signs and Symptoms

Specific signs and symptoms, historic, and physical data relative to age of the pediatric patient are essential to determine the significance of the problem, and thus determine the extent of evaluation. Initially, the infant (< 1 yr of age) is discussed followed by the young and older child (1–3; 4–12 years) and lastly the adolescent (13–20 years).

INFANTS

The symptomatic newborn or older infant who has the preexcitation syndrome most often presents with a normal QRS tachycardia (250–350 bpm) with or without signs and symptoms of congestive heart failure [17–25]. Following conversion of the tachycardia, preexcitation is noted during sinus rhythm (Figure 18–1). Occasionally, the fetus with tachycardia develops heart failure in utero (nonimmune hydrops fetalis) [40]. However, tachycardia may not be present when the hydrops is detected. After birth, the cause of the hydrops may be inferred from ECG evidence of preexcitation or documentation of tachycardia. Similarly, when an infant with congenital heart disease presents with signs and symptoms of congestive heart failure and ECG evidence of preexcitation syndrome is present, it is not immediately known whether or not the neonate has frequent/long episodes of tachycardia contributing to the congestive heart failure. Further evaluation usually reveals whether the underlying heart disease or tachycardia or both contribute to the signs and symptoms. However, in a recent interinstitutional study of 321 infants (≤4 months old) who had WPW syndrome, the presence of congenital heart disease did not influence whether or not low cardiac output was found at initial presentation (53% of total vs. 53% of 49 infants who had congenital heart disease) [17].

It is believed that the duration and rate of tachycardia determine the severity of congestive heart failure; thus, at the usual rates of 280–300 bpm, signs and symptoms of congestive heart failure are noted within 12–24 hours. At slower tachycardia rates, problems are not noted as early and the presentation of infants with "chronic" tachycardia often is insidious, encompassing weeks or months [41–43]. Repetitive, incessant, or continuous tachycardia is more common in infants with other mechanisms of tachycardia (e.g., automatic atrial or chronic junctional reciprocating) but it can be found in infants with an accessory AV connection [41]. This incessant tachycardia can cause chronic left ventricular dysfunction and infants who have this combination present with failure to thrive and chronic congestive heart failure (see Chapter 11 by Critelli et al.).

It is uncommon for infants who have preexcitation syndrome to present with only signs of intermittent, infrequent tachycardia. Occasionally the parent notices "palpitations" or a heart rate "too fast to count" if the baby is held tightly during tachycardia. These episodes may be accompanied by unexplained irritability, crying, paleness, or diaphoresis. The most common type of presentation in infants who have congenital or other underlying heart disease occurs during initial evaluation for murmur, cyanosis, congestive heart failure etc. As part of the evaluation, an ECG is obtained showing preexcitation syndrome.

Syncope is uncommon in infants who have the preexcitation syndrome. None of the 321 infants in the interinstitutional WPW syndrome study presented with a syncopal episode [17]. In this interinstitutional study, 12 patients had documented atrial flutter, fibrillation, or both and only one had documented ventricular fibrillation from atrial flutter-fibrillation. Although none of these 12 died, three of the 321 patients died suddenly in infancy. Although the cause of sudden death is uncertain, a definite possibility includes ventricular tachycardia/fibrillation preceded by atrial fibrillation and a rapid ventricular rate due to rapid conduction via the accessory AV connection. Interpretation of death in the three infants is difficult since each was taking maintenance digitalis. Gillette et al. [5] and later Jedeikin et al. [10] showed that acute administration of digitalis shortens the antegrade effective refractory period of accessory AV connections in some pediatric patients (5/8; 9/21, respectively). Atrial flutter-fibrillation producing ventricular fibrillation has been documented in a neonate who had WPW syndrome and who was being treated with digitalis to control reciprocating tachycardia [7].

Another possible cause of sudden cardiac death in infants with preexcitation syndrome may relate to rapid rates during tachycardia. With very high tachycardia rates (350 bpm) it is possible that coronary ischemia, perhaps exacerbated by the presence of undetected congestive heart failure, also could result in ventricular tachycardia/fibrillation [44]. It must also be considered that apparently normal infants die of noncardiac causes. This usually relates to the dilemma surrounding the cause of Sudden Infant Death syndrome (SIDS) — most likely a multifactorial problem [45,46].

Although the incidence of infant sudden death in the interinstitutional WPW syndrome study is low, nevertheless three unexplained sudden deaths occurred and it can be argued that one sudden death in any group of children who have preexcitation syndrome is too many. It is also possible that the true incidence of life-threatening arrhythmias related to the preexcitation syndrome producing syncope and/or sudden death is underestimated in this age group. Reasons include the possibilities that (1) intermittent syncopal episodes may go undetected, especially if self-terminated within seconds, (2) infants are virtually always in supine or near-supine body position and thereby cerebral perfusion, although greatly diminished, is maintained during a life-threatening tachyarrhythmia and, (3) "seizures", near-miss SIDS, SIDS, or other catastrophic events may not be considered as manifestations of preexcitation syndrome. Thus ECG/cardiac evaluation is never obtained [44–46].

YOUNG AND OLDER CHILD

The young child (age 1–3) with preexcitation syndrome displays signs and symptoms similar to the infant, but is less likely to develop congestive heart failure. Other differences in presentation include: (1) with rapid tachycardia and accompanying acute low cardiac output, syncope may occur more readily due to upright posture in the ambulatory child, (2) the older child's longer neck facilitates the recognition of palpitations.

It is not entirely clear why congestive heart failure is less common in children than infants but possible explanations include slower heart rate, shorter duration of tachycardia before recognition, and better ventricular function in children than in infants. The tachycardia rate is slower in the older child probably because they have slower conducting tissue in all areas of the reentry circuit but especially through the AV node. Unless an incessant type of tachycardia occurs, the duration of rapid tachycardia in the older child usually is much less than in infants because the older child is noted earlier to have the tachycardia.

In the older child — usually at least 4–5 years of age — who is able to verbally express and describe symptoms of "racing heart, chest pain, dizziness, light headedness, blacking out, fainting," it becomes easier to determine whether or not symptomatic arrhythmia has occurred. Moreover, it is again emphasized that if a young pediatric patient has near-syncope or syncope, until proven contrary, the cause should be assumed related to tachycardia when ECG evidence of preexcitation is found.

ADOLESCENT

The most common sign/symptom at presentation in this age group is palpitations. Palpitations frequently are accompanied by "light headedness or dizziness." Occasionally more severe complaints of typical angina are elicited. Any of these symptoms may be exacerbated when the adolescent is active, e.g., any exercise activity.

A difficult problem arises when an adolescent with preexcitation syndrome experiences near-syncope and/or syncope. Vasovagal syncope is common in normal adolescents [47,48]. However, as in the younger pediatric patient, the adolescent who has the preexcitation syndrome and syncope is considered to have an arrhythmia-related life-threatening problem until absolutely proven otherwise. Supporting this view, at this age the incidence of atrial flutter-fibrillation in patients who also have the preexcitation syndrome appears much higher than in any other pediatric age group (see Chapter 2 by Dunnigan). When atrial flutter-fibrillation begins, the signs and symptoms change if reciprocating tachycardia also is or has been experienced. If the refractory period of the accessory AV connection is long then the detected heart rate during atrial flutter-fibrillation, may be slower and more irregular with virtually no other sign/symptom. If the accessory AV connection antegrade refractory period is short and atrial flutter-fibrillation occurs, a fast irregular rate results and the patient may have symptoms of cerebral/myocardial vascular insufficiency producing dizziness, near-syncope/syncope, angina, or cardiac arrest [3,49,50].

The reason why adolescents with preexcitation syndromes have a higher incidence of atrial flutter-fibrillation is unclear. The explanation is probably related to the unexpected finding by Gillette and associates when they studied the antegrade refractory period of the accessory AV connection in pediatric patients [5]. These investigators found that as a group pediatric patients (median age 8 years) had a longer mean antegrade refractory period of the accessory AV

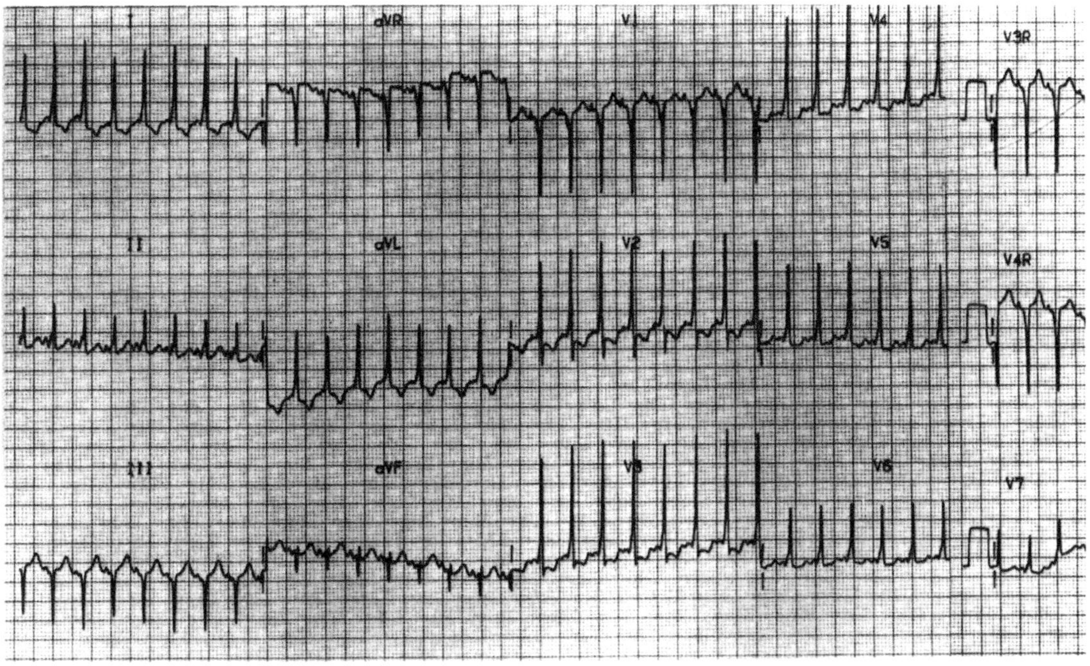

FIGURE 18–1. 15-lead ECG from a 4-month-old girl who presented with normal QRS tachycardia. Short PR interval with prominent delta wave demonstrates preexcitation syndrome, most likely Wolff-Parkinson-White Syndrome. (In the first 12 leads, the three ECG channels, top to bottom, are recorded simultaneously and continuously.)

connection than reported by Tonkin et al. for adults [51]. Gillette et al. speculated that the two age groups were probably each selected because of presentation differences that relate to age. The pediatric patients undergoing evaluation most commonly presented with tachycardia with a normal QRS and the adults undergoing evaluation often presented with atrial flutter-fibrillation. Thus pediatric patients with short antegrade refractory period accessory AV connections most often present later in adolescence or adulthood when atrial flutter-fibrillation is more common.

Noninvasive and Mimimally Invasive Evaluation

The available noninvasive and minimally invasive (e.g., transesophageal testing) tests are discussed in this section of the chapter. Pertinent to the pediatric patient who has preexcitation syndrome, the expected, elicited information of each test are discussed with inclusion of advantages and limitations. Although some discussion of indications of each test is unavoidable, the major emphasis on indications appears at the end of the chapter.

ELECTROCARDIOGRAM

The diagnosis of preexcitation syndromes are usually made by surface ECG (see also Chapter 4). In the presence of increasing technology including intracardiac catheter evaluation, the simple, inexpensive standard 12 or 15 (V_3R, V_4R and V_7 added), lead ECG remains a useful noninvasive test (Figures 18–1 and 18–2). In patients with accessory AV connections, prediction of the ventricular preexcitation site during sinus rhythm was demonstrated by Tonkin et al. and Gallagher et al. [52,53]. They determined that predictable delta wave axes were associated with certain sites of accessory AV connections. Although the important limitation of overlap was found, this study improved the value of the ECG compared to that of the earlier scheme of Rosenbaum et al. [54].

In patients with accessory AV connections, tachycardia is usually associated with a normal QRS (orthodromic reciprocating tachycardia).

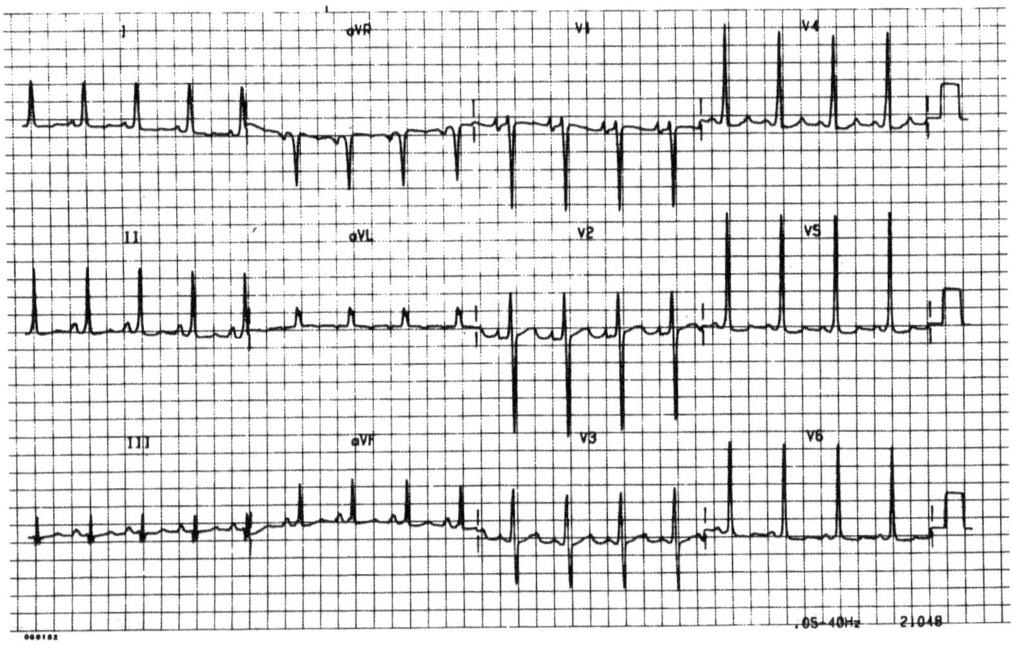

FIGURE 18–2. 12-lead ECG from a 14 year old boy who also had preexcited beats during reciprocating tachycardia. During electrophysiology study (see Figure 18–30), the preexcited beats were found to result from antegrade conduction through a fasciculoventricular connection. (The three ECG channels, top to bottom, are recorded simultaneously and continuously.)

Several ECG features are characteristic of orthodromic reciprocating tachycardia [55–59]. Although in infants and young children visible *p* waves are infrequent, use of double standard facilitates identification as shown in Figure 18–3. If identifiable, the frontal *p* wave axis may aid in localizing the site of accessory AV connection (Figure 18–3). Also, with higher speed recordings and distinct visible onset of p waves the ventriculoatrial interval (conduction time) is measurable (see Chapter 16 by Chung and Kerr). The frontal plane *p* wave axis during tachycardia is most helpful when it ranges from (−)120° to (−)180°. Thus negative *p* waves are found in all leads except AVR, III, and occasionally AVF and the greatest amplitude negative *p* waves exist in Leads I and AVL. This pattern would indicate that retrograde atrial activation proceeds left to right and the site of accessory AV connection therefore is left. When any other *p* wave axis is found, the specificity decreases because right-sided and septal accessory AV connection retrograde *p* waves are similarly superior in orientation.

Measurement of the RR interval during tachycardia also aids in determining whether or not conduction in the retrograde direction via accessory AV connection is present in the tachycardia circuit. Green et al. studied 163 regular tachycardias with a normal QRS in 161 adults to determine whether or not RR interval alternans or amplitude of the QRS was predictive of tachycardia that involved retrograde conduction via accessory AV connection [59]. These investigators found 33 of 36 tachycardias with RR interval alternans were circus movement tachycardias utilizing accessory AV connections. Although this finding appears helpful in adults, it has not been studied in the pediatric age group.

When wide QRS tachycardia occurs, it is important to note the QRS morphology/axis and associated tachycardia cycle length [60–63]. This is helpful for the following reasons. First, a regular pattern of left bundle branch morphology and left axis deviation during tachycardia in a patient who has preexcitation strongly suggests the possibility of a nodoventricular accessory

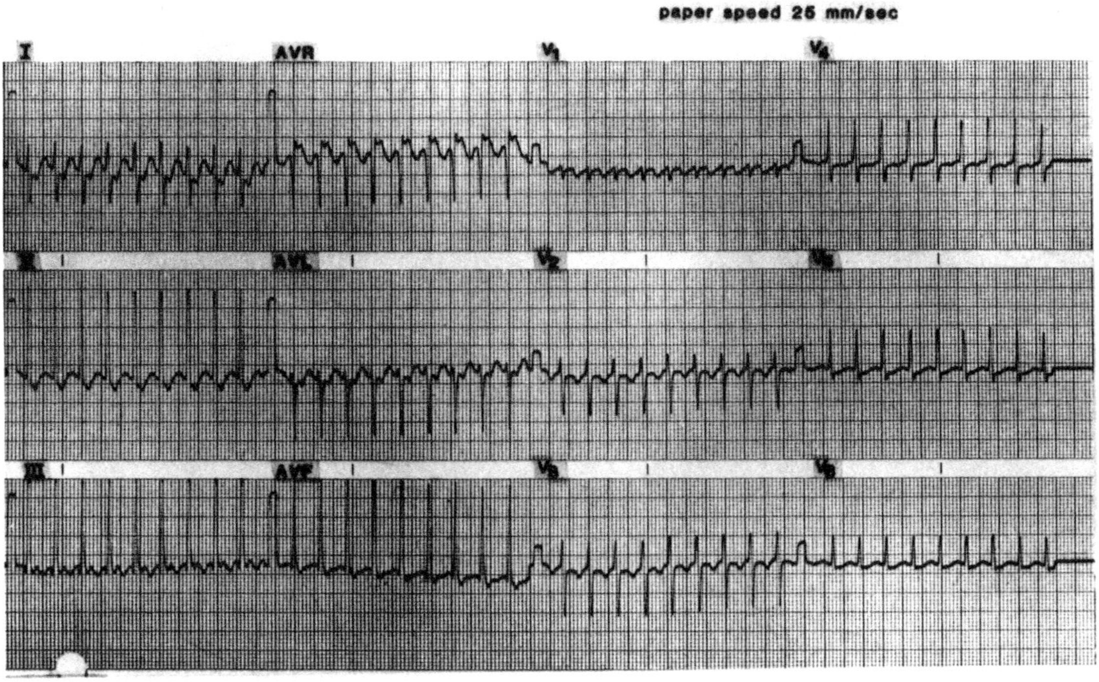

FIGURE 18–3. 12-lead ECG from a 7-year-old boy during tachycardia (SVT) at rate of 214 bpm. The limb leads are recorded at twice standard amplitude to better visualize *p* waves. Note the *p* wave axis is near (−) 180 degrees suggesting atrial activation starting within the left atrium. A lateral left-sided accessory AV connection with only retrograde conducting properties was found during subsequent electrophysiology study. (The three ECG channels, top to bottom, are recorded simultaneously and continuously.)

connection [62,64]. Second, the association of bundle branch block during orthodromic reciprocating tachycardia with prolongation of tachycardia and cycle length suggests that the reentry circuit involves conduction through that bundle branch system and implies the presence of an ipsilateral accessory AV connection to that side [60]. For example, if the QRS changes from an incomplete right bundle branch block to complete left bundle branch block and the tachycardia rate slows from 250 to 200 bpm, the patient most likely has a left-sided accessory AV connection. Third, if wide-QRS complexes similar to the resting preexcited beats occur (especially with irregular intervals) atrial flutter-fibrillation most likely is present [60,61]. Reciprocating tachycardia may convert to atrial-flutter fibrillation and vice versa [65]. Fourth, in contrast to the usual orthodromic (antegrade AVN/His-Purkinje, retrograde accessory AV connection) normal-QRS tachycardia in patients with WPW syndrome, occasional antidromic (antegrade accessory AV connection, retrograde His-Purkinje/AV node) tachycardia may occur, producing wide-QRS tachycardia [60,61,66]. By noting the QRS morphology the site of anomalous ventricular activation can be estimated. Fifth, functional (rate-dependent) bundle branch block may result from circus movement reciprocating tachycardia or from other mechanisms such as atrial (muscle) tachycardia or AV nodal tachycardia [60,61]. Finally, ventricular tachycardia must be considered in the differential diagnosis of wide-QRS tachycardia [11,60].

Technical limitations of the ECG in children involve the recording problems in active young children and infants. Artifact-free recordings are essential in eliciting maximum data. This problem is resolved at the University of Nebraska Medical Center by using at least two ECG technicians occasionally assisted further by attention diverting nurses. Because of the fast tachycardia rates in pediatric patients, recording at twice standard amplitude and at speeds faster than the standard 25 mm/sec are used often to measure intervals accurately. Moreover, simultaneous continuous leads are essential in measuring intervals and assessing morphology because abrupt changes may go undetected if single channel or noncontinuous recordings are obtained.

AMBULATORY ECG (HOLTER) MONITORING

Data obtained from Holter monitoring aids in the evaluation of the pediatric patient in several areas. Valuable information is gained by noting the degree of preexcitation with variation in heart rates. Although the effect of heart rate on degree of preexcitation is discussed further later in this chapter (Exercise Testing), Holter monitoring is valuable in young patients in whom exercise testing is not feasible. Also, intermittent preexcitation at any age may be detected by Holter monitoring. When intermittent preexcitation is found without a change in *p* wave axis, it suggests a prolonged accessory AV connection refractory period in patients who have the WPW syndrome (Figure 18–4) [67]. It is helpful to record two limb leads with nearly perpendicular axis (e.g., Lead I and II) because a change in the site of atrial rhythm is best detected in this manner. Atrial activation influences the degree of preexcitation and, therefore, the interpretation of antegrade accessory AV connection conduction characteristics may be incorrect if change in atrial activation (e.g., wandering atrial rhythm) is the cause of changing preexcitation rather than variable heart rate.

Characteristics of accessory AV connection conduction in the antegrade direction also can be derived by Holter monitoring when premature beats are found. If the premature beats are atrial and the beats occur at variable coupling intervals and during variable heart rates, antegrade effective refractory periods of the accessory AV connection can be calculated during different states of activity (Figure 18–5).

Holter monitoring is most helpful when the patient has frequent, recurrent signs/symptoms suggestive of tachycardia. Documentation of the rate, type, and mechanism of arrhythmia (e.g., paroxysmal, repetitive, reciprocating tachycardia and/or atrial flutter-fibrillation) is important in the evaluation because decisions regarding further testing to a large degree depend on the type of arrhythmia (Figure 18–5).

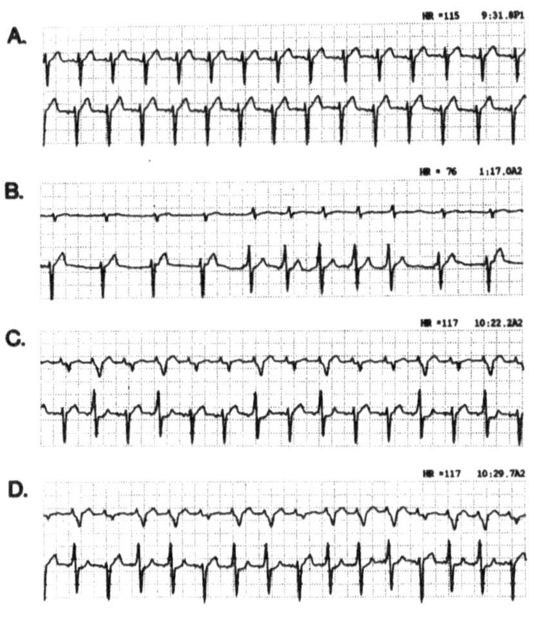

FIGURE 18–4. Intermittent preexcitation is shown in Holter monitor ECG recordings (CardioData, Northboro, Mass.) from an 11-month-old child who also has transposition of the great arteries. The baby had normal QRS tachycardia initially during preoperative cardiac catheterization. Subsequent preoperative electrophysiologic study disclosed a paraseptal accessory AV connection that only conducted in the retrograde direction. Holter ECG recordings at that time were normal without signs of preexcitation. Early postoperative (age 9 months) rapid paroxysmal reciprocating tachycardia (270 bpm) was controlled with overdrive atrial pacing and propranolol. This subsequent postoperative recording showed: (A), sinus rhythm (115 bpm) without preexcitation; (B), junctional rhythm (76 bpm) without preexcitation followed by 5 sinus beats (90 bpm) with preexcitation; (C) and (D), intermittent preexcitation. (The two ECG channels are recorded simultaneously in each A–D and represent limb leads I and II, top-bottom.)

Finally, correlation of symptoms with absence of arrhythmia is extremely useful in patient management, since it permits reassurance of the concerned parent and child.

Successful Holter recordings are obtained from children of every age. We have found several practical aids in attaining maximum benefit from the Holter in the form of high-quality ECG recordings and patient acceptance/compliance. After prepping the skin with alco-

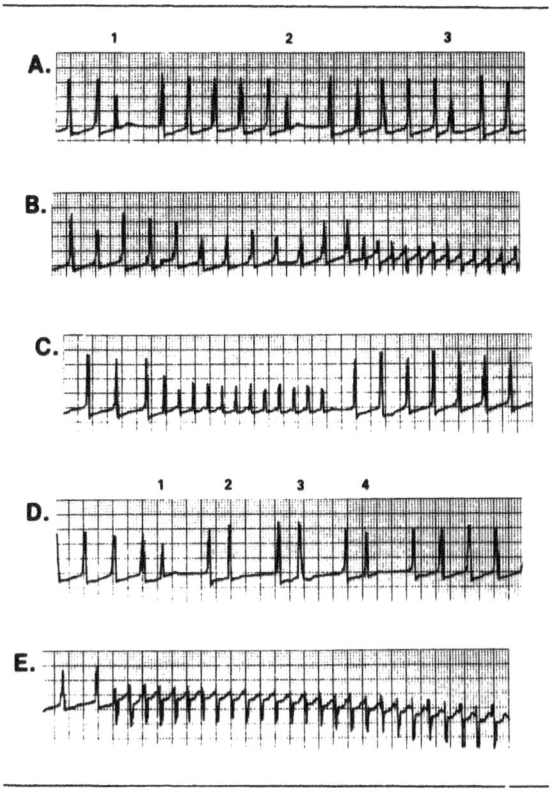

FIGURE 18–5. Five (A–E) Holter ECG (Lead I) recordings in a 4-month-old girl with preexcitation syndrome show the range of data obtained during various activity. In (A) at 1:12 pm during napping, 3 premature beats (labeled 1–3), spontaneously occur. In the first two, the effective antegrade refractory period of the accessory AV connection is reached (because the QRS is normal) but no tachycardia is induced. (A less likely but possible alternative explanation: the normal QRS beats are junctional in origin.) In the third the premature beat is preexcited. While awake at 7:30 pm (B) tachycardia (300 bpm) is induced after a spontaneous premature beat occurs during sinus rhythm (150 bpm). Nonsustained normal QRS tachycardia at 300 bpm (C) also is induced later (8:35 pm). In (D) during sleep (9:22 pm), tachycardia is not induced after any of the four (1–4) premature beats. Similar to the findings in (A), nonpreexcited premature beats (1–4) fail to result in tachycardia. Because *p* waves are not visualized, it cannot be determined where the conduction fails in the reentry circuit. It is appealing to speculate that conduction did not proceed through the AV node based on the likely vagotonia during sleep. This speculation is not supported however, by the recording in (E), also during sleep (1:39 am) showing induction of tachycardia (300 bpm). Note that in (B) and (E) the QRS during tachycardia is abberrant suggesting right bundle branch block but the rate appears unchanged. It is emphasized however, that at this fast rate, slight changes in cycle lengths during bundle branch block only may be detected by faster paper speed recordings and no conclusions should be made regarding location of the accessory AV connection (see Figure 18–29).

hol and fine sand paper, the resistance of each applied electrode is checked to assure maximum quality ECG recordings. Small recorders have decreased tape malfunction problems, but in the extremely active toddler lead/tape malfunction cannot be eliminated. In the shy or appearance-conscious older child/adolescent, most often elective Holter monitoring is carried out during weekends or vacations rather than during school. However, in any child with suspected life-threatening arrhythmia, Holter monitoring with telemetry is carried out as an inpatient in the hospital.

Caution should be exercised with most of the new total computer and computer aided Holter systems. Only a few of these new Holter systems (e.g., CardioData, Northboro, Mass) adequately detect and analyze tachyarrhythmias in infants and young children, whereas other systems are designed for the adult with slower heart rates, obviously fewer heart beats per day, and so on.

TELEPHONIC TRANSMISSION OF ECG RHYTHM

Transmission of ECG rhythm via the telephone is a productive and inexpensive technique for documenting tachyarrhythmias that occur infrequently (Figure 18–6) [68–70]. The newer units often have memory capacity (differences relate to specific manufacturer). This permits the patient or adult observer to record the ECG rhythm by placing the device on the chest or by using arm bracelet or finger leads and then activating the memory recorder. After a recording (differences in duration depend upon the specific manufacturer), the recorder beeps, signaling termination of the recording period. At a convenient later time, the stored ECG rhythm is transmitted to the receiving unit by telephone.

The limitations of the memory telephonic transmitter relate to age and to the practical aspect of immediate accessiblity to the device. In the infant and young nonverbal child, it is often difficult to detect intermittent signs of

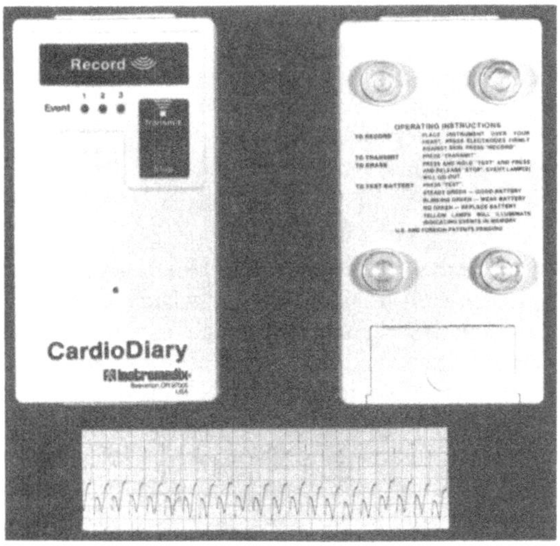

FIGURE 18–6. Display of transtelephonic unit with record/memory capability. This particular unit is referred to as CardioDiary (Instromedix[R], Beaverton, Oregon). The front of the unit is shown on the left and the back with its four electrodes and its instructions is shown on the right. The ECG recording at the bottom was transmitted by a 14-year-old boy who had palpitations and a pulse "too fast to count" during basketball practice and games. Treadmill exercise and Holter monitor recording were normal. Tachycardia successfully was documented at a rate of 200 bpm during the first week of Cardio Diary use.

tachycardia. Therefore, the device is of greater practical value in the older child and adolescent. Accessiblity to the device is a problem at any age but it can be a particularly troublesome problem in the active and more independent older child and adolescent. If symptoms of tachyarrhythmia develop, for example, while the child is at school, involved in neighborhood play, or at athletic events, it is impractical for the patient to carry the device or to have close access to it. If the duration of the symptoms/arrhythmia is sufficiently long, the success of recording the ECG rhythm is increased. When symptoms progress beyond the expected palpitations (e.g., dizziness/near-syncope), it usually implies a more serious arrhythmia. In this situation, the device is valuable because usually the parent or adult observer has access to it and usually this person is nearer than the ECG machine in the physician's office or emergency room. However, a major limitation involves its use in the patient who has near-syncope or syncope. Certainly with impending or sudden unconsciousness, the patient is unable to apply the device to himself or herself. The only success in this situation is obtained when an accompanying observer has access to the unit and records the patient's rhythm (see Chapter by Pritchett).

EXERCISE TESTING

The productivity of exercise testing probably has been underestimated in the noninvasive evaluation of the cooperative pediatric patient who has the preexcitation syndrome. Although several studies have been reported in adults [71–75], only recently Bricker et al. [76] reported the utility of exercise testing in children with WPW syndrome. These investigators found that changes or disappearance of the delta wave with increased heart rates during exercise correlated with long (360–390 ms) antegrade effective refractory period of the accessory AV connection determined during catheter electrophysiology study. This finding is illustrated in Figure 18–7.

Tachycardia often occurs in the active, athletic child/adolescent who has symptomatic preexcitation syndrome. Although a history of exercise-induced tachycardia is common at all ages, the frequency with which tachycardia is elicited during exercise testing has been disappointing in reported series of adults. Similarly, only two of the 17 children in the study of Bricker et al. had tachycardia during exercise testing [76]. No data are given regarding the clinical correlation of exercise tachycardia in these 2 patients or in the 15 patients who did not have tachycardia during testing.

To increase the sensitivity of exercise testing in reproducing clinical tachyarrhythmias, it behooves the investigator to use a flexible protocol. For example, if a patient has symptoms of tachyarrhythmia with bursts of exercise activity, the exercise protocol needs to be altered accordingly. Despite maximal effort of observer and patient, the success with which exercise testing reproduces clinically suspected tachyarrhythmia is considerably less than 100%. The success is disappointing, especially when an individual patient with preexcitation syndrome has frequent symptoms and signs of tachyarrhythmia with exercise, but exercise testing fails to reproduce the problem (Figure 18–6).

The technical limitations of exercise testing relate to age and cooperation of the pediatric

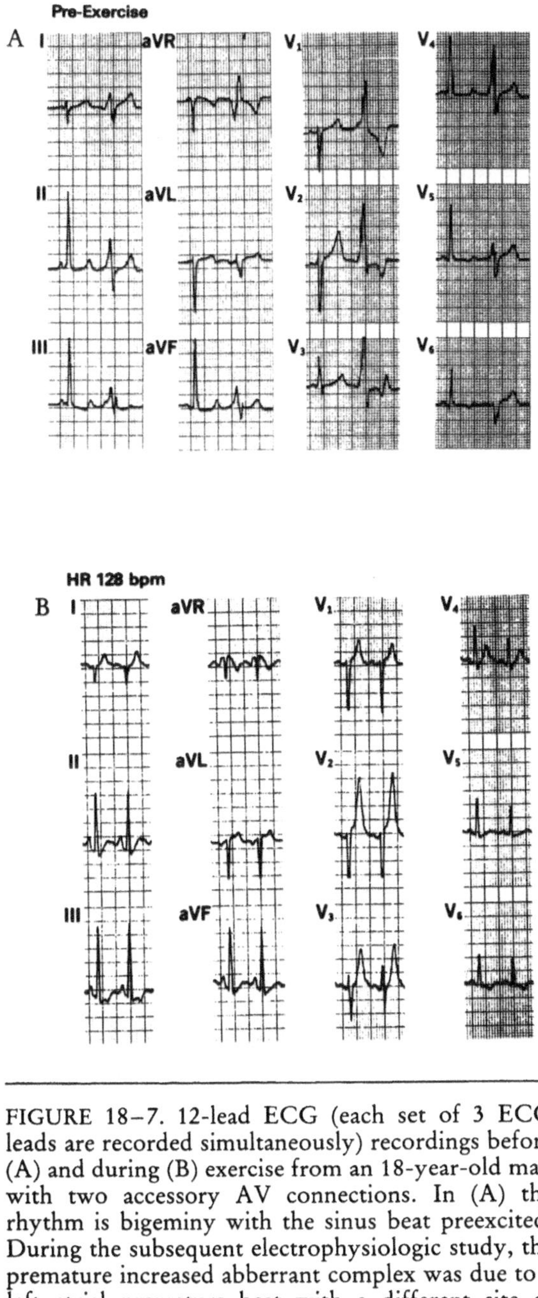

FIGURE 18–7. 12-lead ECG (each set of 3 ECG leads are recorded simultaneously) recordings before (A) and during (B) exercise from an 18-year-old man with two accessory AV connections. In (A) the rhythm is bigeminy with the sinus beat preexcited. During the subsequent electrophysiologic study, the premature increased abberrant complex was due to a left atrial premature beat with a different site of preexcitation. In (B) no preexcitation is evident at a heart rate of 128 bpm suggesting that the patient does not have accessory AV connection(s) with short antegrade effective refractory period. During electrophysiology study, antegrade effective refractory period of left lateral accessory AV connection was long (540 ms at 600 ms cycle length) and the paraseptal accessory AV connection conducted only retrograde.

patient. Cooperation and successful completion of exercise tests is best in children older than 6 years of age. Occasionally, successful testing is carried out in children 4–5 years old. Maximal exercise duration is difficult to attain without patient cooperation. Therefore, great effort may be required of the physician to encourage continuation of exercise to exhaustion.

Other minor technical problems concern the methods of exercise testing in children (e.g., skin preparation, bicycle vs. treadmill, etc.). These are reviewed elsewhere [77,78]. Every effort should be made to obtain the highest quality ECG recordings because detection of preexcitation can be subtle — especially during exercise and high heart rate (Figure 18–8) (see Chapter 8 by Levy).

TRANSESOPHAGEAL ECG AND ATRIAL PACING

The transesophageal technique of ECG recording and atrial pacing in evaluating and treating patients who have tachyarrhythmias recently has been repopularized [79–84]. The resurgence of the technique, its refinement within the past 5 years, and its application to patients who have the preexcitation syndrome is reviewed in the chapter in this volume by Chung and Kerr. However, additional review of the appication to the pediatric patient is given in this chapter.

Benson and associates [85–89] and Dick et al. [90] have evaluated transesophageal recording and pacing in pediatric patients. From these studies, the characteristics of transesophageal atrial pacing threshold, pulse width, catheter interelectrode spacing, and catheter insertion depth may be determined for the pediatric patient. To summarize the technical studies of Benson et al, the effective atrial pacing threshold and pulse width were reached at average values of 10 ms and 10–15 mA (depending on study) respectively. Flexible silicone rubber-coated bipolar pacing catheters with 15, 22, and 28 mm interelectrode spacing were used. No difference in effectiveness was found with the variable interelectrode distances.

The transesophageal technique of recording elicits separation of atrial and ventricular depolarization of ECG during tachycardia (Figure 18–9). This permits analysis of valuable data leading to the determination of the tachycardia mechanism. Confirming the work of Benditt et al., primarily in adults [91], Benson and associates found the measurement of ventriculoatrial

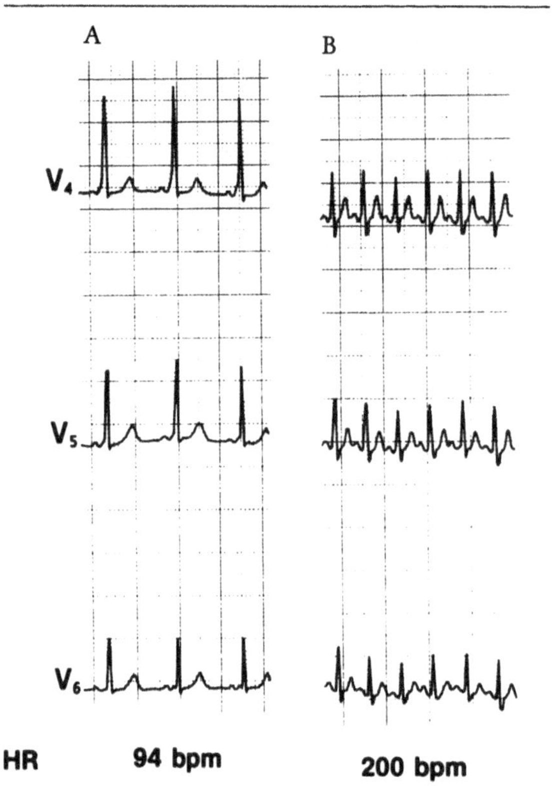

FIGURE 18–8. Two sets of three simultaneous ECG recordings during (A) preexercise and (B) maximum treadmill exercise in a 14-year-old girl. During preexercise as well as during maximum exercise, preexcitation persists (best noted in V4). This finding suggests that the patient does not have a long antegrade refractory period of the accessory AV connection. However, with a maximum heart rate of 200 bpm (300 ms cycle length), the refractory period may not be dangerously short (e.g., if the HR was 210 bpm or 285 ms cycle length, preexcitation may disappear). At subsequent electrophysiology study, the antegrade effective refractory period was 280 ms and the functional was 250 ms during atrial flutter-fibrillation and isoproterenol.

conduction time of >70 ms during tachycardia in 14 infants to be consistent with the presence of an accessory AV connection [86]. Moreover, they distinguished this mechanism from other tachycardia by the following explanations [86]. Although intracardiac electrophysiologic studies were not carried out for definite confirmation, the logical addition of conduction time supports this conclusion. Because the base of the ventricle is depolarized before any retrograde accessory AV connection conduction can occur during reciprocating tachycardia and the average duration of QRS in infants is 55 ms, it follows that if retrograde accessory AV connection conduction occurs, the total ventriculoatrial conduction time is longer than 55 ms, approaching a minimum of 70 ms. Furthermore, the major other type of reciprocating tachycardia, reentry within the AV node, has short ventriculoatrial conduction times and atrial depolarization is usually initiated before ventricular depolarization is completed. Using this logical explanation, Benson et al. concluded that transesophageal measurement of ventriculoatrial intervals during tachycardia will reveal the presence of an AV accessory connection participating in tachycardia in a greater number of infants than presently suspected by some investigators.

Moreover, in patients without ECG evidence of preexcitation during sinus rhythm, the presence of an accessory AV connection (so-called concealed because it conducts only in retrograde direction) is difficult to determine noninvasively. With only retrograde conducting properties, the connection can be detected noninvasively by measuring the ventriculoatrial interval. Rarely this is possible by noting visible *p* waves during tachycardia on surface ECG. Transesophageal ECG recording however, permits the distinct recording of atrial and ventricular depolarization (Figure 18–9). Therefore, if transesophageal recording was carried out and ventriculoatrial conduction time measured during tachycardia in all infants, the detection of concealed accessory AV connections would be much greater. Thus transesophageal data recorded during tachycardia appears to have great potential in the evaluation of the pediatric patient.

Transesophageal recording and stimulation technique is also useful in evaluation of the conduction characteristics of the accessory AV connection. For example, by transesophageal atrial pacing utilizing decremental extra stimuli in the manner described later in the chapter (see "Intracardiac Electrophysiology Study"), the refractory period of the accessory connection in the antegrade direction can be determined. One limitation to the technique however, concerns the restriction of pacing at a single site. Therefore, the determination of antegrade refractory period of, for example, a right lateral accessory AV connection may not be obtained accurately. In the study of Critelli et al. in adults, atrial

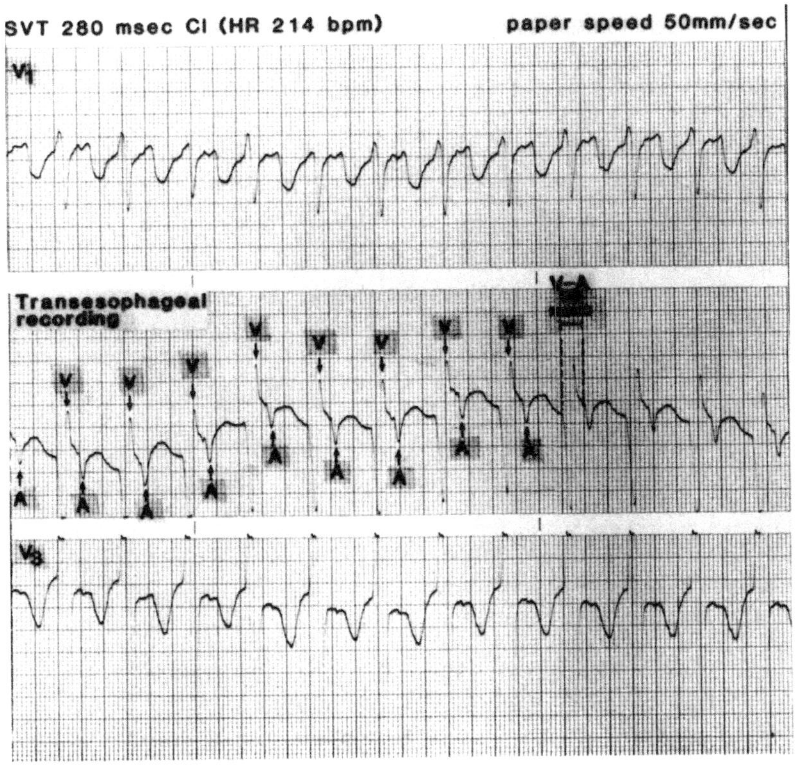

FIGURE 18–9. Simultaneous V1, (*top*), transesophageal (*middle*), and V3 (*bottom*) ECG recordings (at 50 mm/sec paper speed) in a 7-year-old boy who had tachycardia (see Figure 18–3). With separation of ventricular (V) and atrial (A) depolarizations, the VA interval is measured at 90 ms during transesophageal recording suggesting the presence of an accessory AV connection. A left-lateral accessory AV connection was verified during subsequent electrophysiology study.

flutter-fibrillation was induced by transesophageal pacing [84]. Characteristics of accessory AV connection conduction then was studied by measuring the shortest and average VV interval.

Details of treatment are discussed in the chapter by Benson and Dunnigan. However, it is useful to mention here that early results suggest prognostic evaluation is feasible by transesophageal pacing [85,88,89,92]. A recent study by Benson et al. in 24 infants best illustrates its potential use in pediatric patients [89]. These investigators predicted digoxin failure by inducing tachycardia using transesophageal pacing following digoxin administration. These investigators earlier also reported quinidine treatment failures in two patients who had tachycardia induced by esophageal pacing [85]. Studies in a larger number of pediatric patients are necessary before final conclusions are made but it appears that transesophageal pacing has excellent potential in predicting the success of chronic antiarrhythmic treatment in the pediatric patient.

The technical limitations of transesophageal recording and pacing in the evaluation of the pediatric patient who has the preexcitation syndrome comprise three major areas: (1) patient discomfort, (2) equipment availability, and (3) operator inexperience. Although the transesophageal technique is noninvasive by the definition that applies to cardiac procedures involving intravascular techniques, it is invasive by the strict sense that an electrode catheter is used "inside" the body. In the older infant and young pediatric patient, sedation is required frequently. Meperidine and diazepam were administered intravenously in the early studies reported by Benson et al. [85,86]. No sedation was required in the recent young infant study by the same investigators [89]. Similarly, we find sedation unnecessary in the neonate. However, in the older infant and child, intramuscular meperidine (2 mg/kg) and promethazine (1 mg/kg) are given. If further sedation is required, ketamine (2 mg/kg) or diazepam (0.2 mg/kg) is administered intramuscularly. In most pediatric patients because of the sedation requirement, inpatient hospitalization is required for at least a few hours. Some patients who are lightly sedated or have no sedation complain of discomfort expressed as "burning" during pacing — especially with pacing stimulus amplitude greater than 15 mA. Even in the most uncooperative child, adequate studies can be obtained by using sufficient sedation.

There is a paucity of commercially available transesophageal recording and pacing equipment. We use the catheter (Medtronic Model 6902) and custom-made stimulator (University of Minnesota) recommended by Benson and co-workers (Figure 18–10). The usual commercially available cardiac stimulators are unusable in transesophageal pacing because maximum pulse width and, in some units amplitude, are inadequate. As transesophageal cardiac stimulation increases in popularity, more commercially available equipment may become available. Moreover, operator experience will increase and result in increased technical success.

CHEST ROENTGENOGRAM

The chest X-ray film is useful only when evaluating underlying heart disease and/or severity of congestive heart failure. Without the presence of these related problems, the chest X-ray does not help in the evaluation of the pediatric patient with preexcitation syndrome.

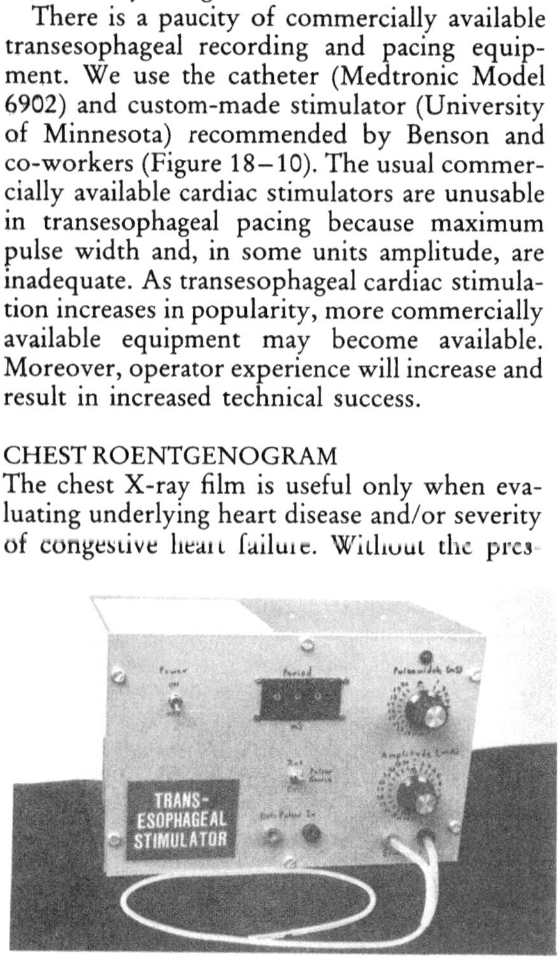

FIGURE 18–10. Photograph of custom-made stimulator (designed and manufactured by Department of Bioengineering, University of Minnesota Hospitals) with accompanying esophageal lead (Medtronic 6902) with 15 mm interelectrode distance.

ECHOCARDIOGRAPHY

Presently, the utility of echocardiography lies primarily in determining the presence and severity of underlying heart disease. However, a word of caution is indicated regarding echocardiographic measurement of left ventricular function in patients who have preexcitation of the ventricle. When ventricles are preexcited, myocardial contraction is eccentric in many patients and therefore indices such as % fractional shortening and ejection fraction are affected from the eccentric ventricular activation.

Recently, 2–D echocardiography studies of ventricular preexcitation have been carried out to determine whether or not the site of the accessory AV connection can be localized. Armstrong et al. were successful in predicting the site (confirmed by intracardiac study) of preexcitation in 18 of 20 patients [93]. An example from a 16-year-old boy is illustrated in Figure 18–11. No large studies or studies in children have been reported. The clinical value of 2–D echocardiography in predicting the site of the accessory AV connection is unknown but early results are encouraging.

NUCLEAR PHASE ANALYSIS

Another new method, similar to echocardiography, of noninvasively determining the location of the accessory AV connection is by gated nuclear studies [94,95]. No studies have been reported in children, also, the technique is too new to determine its present clinical value. (See chapter 5 by Botvinick et al.)

Invasive Evaluation

Intracardiac electrophysiology studies have contributed considerably to the understanding of the preexcitation syndromes. The technique has also been invaluable in the management of patients who have tachyarrhythmias and who have the preexcitation syndrome. Young patients of virtually any age or size may undergo electrophysiologic study to evaluate the preexcitation syndromes. However, there are age-related variations of the technique. First in this section of the chapter, specific applications of these techniques in infants and children are

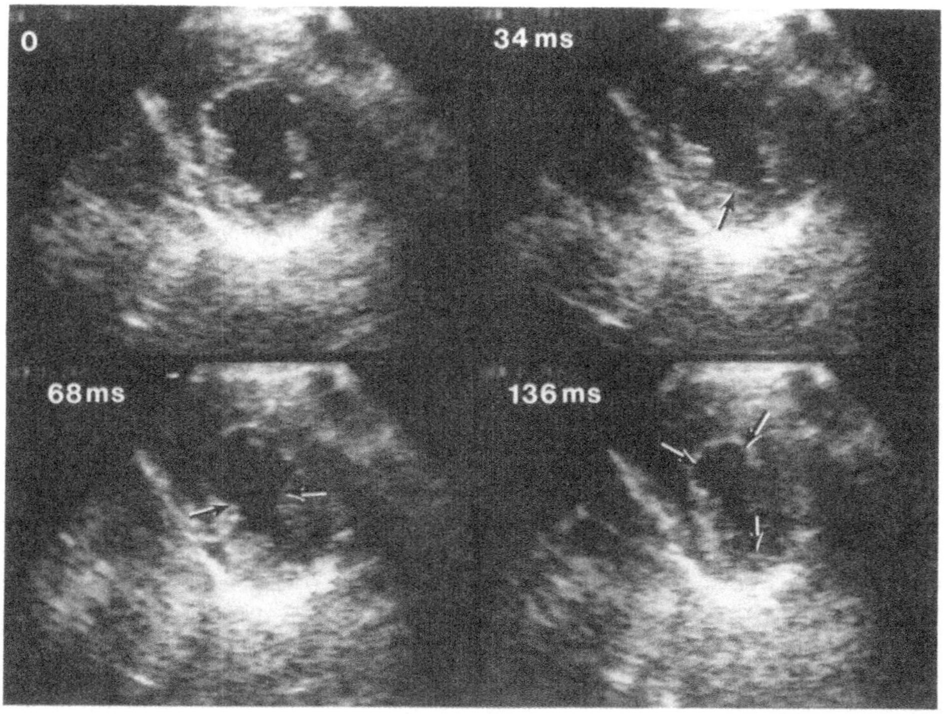

FIGURE 18–11. Series of four still frame photographs from a parasternal short axis 2-dimensional echocardiogram in a 16-year-old boy who has preexcitation. Each photograph is taken after the onset of systole (timing is triggered from R wave, not shown). At 34 ms an inward motion of the left ventricular lateral wall is shown by the arrow. At 68 ms the posterior septum and anterior wall are moving inward (*arrows*) and at 136 ms the septum and right ventricular wall are moving inward (*top arrows*) while the lateral posterior wall is now relaxing (*bottom arrow*). These findings suggest the presence of a left-lateral accessory AV connection because the initial ventricular contraction arises from the left lateral area. Subsequent electrophysiologic study confirmed the echo-predicted site of the accessory AV connection. (Photograph courtesy of Windle JR, Armstrong WF, Feigenbaum H, Miles WM, Prystowsky EN, Krannert Institute of Cardiology, Indiana University School of Medicine.)

discussed. Next, the recording and stimulation protocol for evaluation of preexcitation is reviewed as it relates to children.

Before discussing the details of the technique, it is necessary to outline the general information derived from the invasive catheter studies. The major objectives during the study of patients with preexcitation syndrome includes the following: (1) document diagnosis of preexcitation syndrome and determine cause of preexcitation (e.g., accessory AV connection and/or nodofascicular connection), (2) determine whether or not life-threatening arrhythmias exist or potentially exist (e.g., this includes isoproterenol administration during atrial flutter-fibrillation), (3) determine mechanism of tachycardia (e.g., assure that the accessory connection participates in the tachycardia reentry circuit, (4) exclude other arrhythmias (e.g., ventricular tachycardia), (5) localize the site(s) of the accessory connection(s), (6) determine modes of onset and termination, and (7) assess response to antiarrhythmic drug(s) including digitalis when digoxin is considered for chronic treatment. Thus these studies establish the diagnosis and permit definition of the treatment options.

TECHNIQUE

Educational and Emotional Preparation.

Preparation of the pediatric patient is essential to a successful and complete electrophysiology study. Beginning with age-related explanations to the patient and parents by the pediatric electrophysiologist, the educational and emotional support is continued by pediatric cardiology electrophysiology nurses and technicians before and throughout the study. This often overlooked aspect of the study is emphasized here because the long duration of the electrophysiology procedure can be a major factor contributing toward exaggeration of the usual anxieties of pediatric patients undergoing cardiac catheterization. If patients are not prepared properly and a patient is uncooperative or anxious during the study, this inhibits data collection and interferes with completion of a successful procedure.

Sedation. The use of sedation is an important, necessary adjunct in the preparation of the pediatric patient for electrophysiology study. We use meperidine 2 mg/kg and promethazine 1 mg/kg, administered intramuscularly 30–45 minutes before the procedure. During the study, if further sedation is required either meperidine (1 mg/kg) or promethazine (0.5 mg/kg) or both are given intravenously. Occasionally when this is ineffective or when DC cardioversion/defibrillation is required, additional sedation using intravenous diazepam (0.2 mg/kg) is given. The other commonly used sedative, chlorpromazine (and related drugs), is avoided because of its reported conduction system effects in puppies [96]. Furthermore, chlorpromazine may have antiarrhythmic action. This is further based on data from the new phenothiazine-related antiarrhythmia agents [97]. Because meperidine, promethazine, and diazepam separately or in combination may have effects on the conduction system, there is little choice other than to standardize sedation drugs and technique. This is not only important within a medical center but also preferable among institutions involved with carrying out extensive electrophysiologic studies in children.

Preparation of Patient in Cardiac Catheterization Laboratory. Initial patient preparation in the laboratory involves placement of surface ECG leads, cardioversion/defibrillator pads, and positioning of the patient for local infiltration of lidocaine. Placement for surface ECG electrodes is important because constant comparison is necessary between intracardiac electrograms and the QRS morphology. Orthogonal surface limb leads 1 and AVF are routinely used in combination with chest leads V_1 and/or V_6. If another lead or leads display preexcitation better, then this lead(s) replaces one or more of the above "routine" leads. It may be argued that only one chest lead, V_1 or V_6, is necessary. However, occasional multiform beats or transitional beats during the study provide a challenge that simultaneous V_1 and V_6 recordings help solve. Furthermore, each lead confirms the other's morphology.

The availability of the disposable defibrillator pad and lead system, has greatly enhanced the defibrillating and cardioverting technique [98]. Preparation includes placement of the Apex-Posterior R_2 Corotin pads (R_2 Corporation, Skokie, Illinois) appropriately sized to the pediatric patient. Moreover, the synchronizing system is checked and the energy level calculated and set at 1.0 joule/kg (maximum 50 joules) for possible use during the study.

Final preparation includes precise positioning of the patient for local lidocaine infiltration of the groins. (Neck and arm are not infiltrated initially unless groin is inaccessible from previous study.) This step often receives little attention and is especially important in the pediatric patient who undergoes a multiple catheter study to evaluate the preexcitation syndrome. Variable sheath/catheter introduction techniques are used among pediatric cardiologists. With each technique the correct, precise position of the patient appropriately facilitates effort and maximizes success. The initial step of local anesthetic infiltration is emphasized because when not performed correctly, success rates of sheath placement decrease. In small patients (<10 kg), these preparation steps are critical because the success of the percutaneous sheath technique is compromised by patient (i.e. vessel) size. One rather than 2% lidocaine is used because potentially therapeutic serum concentrations of lidocaine have been documented in patients undergoing study after groin infiltration of lidocaine. If the patient complains or is suspected of having groin discomfort during the procedure, the infiltration is repeated.

Sheath Placement. Percutaneous sheath placement is carried out in each groin using the technique by Neches et al. [99]. If the coronary sinus is inaccessible by manipulating a catheter from the femoral vein, the percutaneous technique also is used in the left arm (modified by Hesslein et al. [100]) or either side of the neck (modified by Latson et al. [101]). In the groin, multiple sheaths are placed in the femoral veins.

The maximum number of sheaths in each

femoral vein is limited by patient size and catheter/sheath size. In the older child and adolescent (>40 kg), three #6 French or two #6 French and one #7–8 French sheaths (Cook, Inc., Bloomington, Indiana) are placed easily and maintained in each femoral vein. With the latter combination, the larger sheath has a "side-arm" to enable infusion of intravenous drugs during the study thus avoiding removal of the catheter (Figure 18–12). Administration of fluid or drugs via the side-arm is facilitated when a smaller catheter (e.g., #6 French) is used within the sheath (e.g., #7–8 French).

In the younger child and older infant (<5.5 kg), the maximum number of sheaths varies between two and three in each femoral vein. The largest side-arm sheath in these smaller patients varies between #5.5 and #6.5 French size. When the arm approach is necessary, the #5.0 French sheath is the largest sheath placed regardless of patient size. Similarly, the #5.0 French sheath is used most often in the neck; however, if necessary, a #6 French sheath is easily introduced in the jugular vein.

In patients of all ages, the femoral artery pressure is continuously monitored during the study. This is valuable when life-threatening arrhythmias are induced and when administering drugs that have effects on blood pressure. The femoral artery pressure is monitored either by a plastic cannula (Quik-Cath^{R}, Travenol Laboratories, Deerfield, 1L) or by a side-arm from a sheath (each placed by percutaneous technique). In the absence of an atrial communication, the arterial sheath is required in some patients because left ventricular pacing is necessary (discussed later).

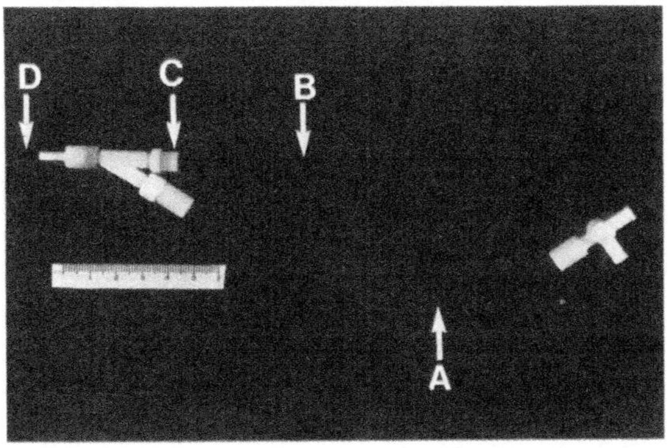

FIGURE 18–12. Photograph of a side-arm sheath used during electrophysiology study. The side-arm (A) provides access for intravenous administration of fluids and drugs during the study. Free flow of fluid is facilitated by using one French size smaller electrode catheter (B) then the French size of the catheter (e.g., a #7 French side-arm sheath with a #6 French catheter). Leaking of administrated fluid is prevented in the sheath (D) and side-arm system by screw-tightening the end (C) at the entrance of the sheath (Cook, Inc.).

After all sheaths are introduced, heparin (70 units/kg, maximum 5000 units) is administered to decrease the risk of thromboembolic complications. At the end of the procedure, the anticoagulation is one-half corrected with protamine sulfate.

ELECTRODE CATHETERS

Choice of electrode catheter size, number of electrodes, number of catheters, and manipulation/placement are discussed next.

Catheter Size. The size of electrode catheters utilized in pediatric patients include #4, #5, or #6 French (Figure 18–13). A combination of #5 French and #6 French catheters are used in the older child and adolescent. The actual size of catheter utilized depends on the area/chamber of catheter placement. In most older children, #6 French catheters are placed in the high right atrium (HRA), other areas in the right atrium for mapping, and across the tricuspid valve to record low septal right atrial (LSRA), His, and right ventricular inflow/septal area (RVI). Either #5 or #6 French catheters are employed in this age group in the coronary sinus, the left ventricle, and the right ventricular apex (RVA) or outflow tract (RVO).

In the younger child and older infant, #5 French catheters are used, but in the small infant or neonate, a combination of #4 French and #5 French catheters are utilized. In the young infant the decision of whether to use a #4 French or #5 French depends on the area/chamber of catheter placement. Presently, most manufacturers do not produce #4 French catheters with four electrodes (quadrapolar) and tripolar #4 French catheters are not a satisfactory substitute.

Catheter Electrodes. Ideally, quadrapolar electrode catheters are utilized in areas where simultaneous pacing and recording are carried out. When bipolar or tripolar electrode catheters are employed, simultaneous recording and

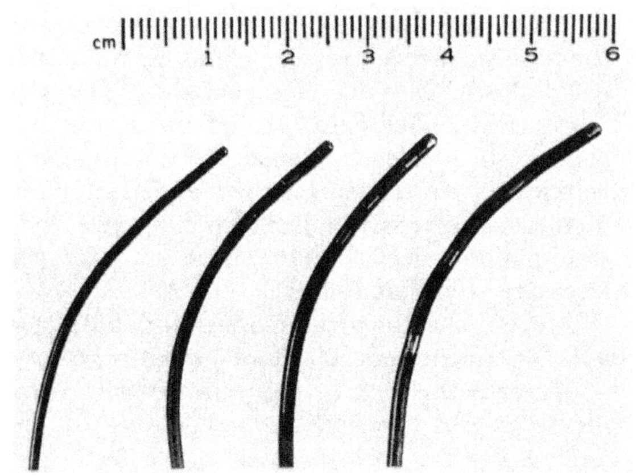

FIGURE 18–13. Photograph of examples of electrode catheters used in pediatric patients. From left to right the catheters are: (1) #4 French tripolar USCI (U.S. Catheter Inc., Billerica, Mass.) with 5 mm interelectrode distance. (2) #5 French quadrapolar Elecath (Electro-Catheter Corporation, Rahawy, N.J.) with 3 mm interelectrode distance between the two proximal and the two distal electrodes and 5 mm between the second and third electrodes. (3) #6 French USCI quadripolar catheter of modular construction with 2 mm interelectrode distance between the two distal electrodes and 3 mm between the two proximal electrodes with 5 mm separating the second and third electrodes. (4) #6 French USCI woven dacron quadrapolar with 10 mm distance between each electrode. The first three catheters are custom made and the fourth is not.

pacing cannot be accomplished because an electrode cannot be connected to pacing and recording concomitantly.

Every effort is made to record and pace between electrodes of small interelectrode distance. This is especially important in the smaller pediatric patient. With short interelectrode distances of 1, 2, 3, and 5 mm, recordings are more discreet without "noise" but equally important, during mapping the localization of the earliest activation greatly is enhanced by recording between short-distance electrodes at the catheter tip. Most manufacturers of electrode catheters are responsive to custom orders of individualized specifications (Figure 18–13).

Number of Catheters. The number of electrode catheters employed during a study depends first on the size of the pediatric patient. This is dictated by the number of sheaths permissible within the femoral veins and to the number of catheters within the heart to allow safe, accurate, and easy manipulation. Ideally, five electrode catheters are utilized when evaluating the pediatric patient who has the preexcitation syndrome. These are advanced and positioned in the right atrium for mapping coronary sinus, high right atrium, across the tricuspid valve for His bundle recording, and the right ventricular apex. When left ventricular stimulation is required (see Protocol), a sixth catheter is introduced and in some older patients who have wide-QRS and/or ventricular tachycardia a seventh catheter is advanced to the RVO area (Figure 18–14).

Certainly, the evaluation of a pediatric patient who has preexcitation syndrome also can be accomplished with fewer catheters. However, the disadvantages of fewer catheters appear to outweigh the potential problems of more catheters. The major disadvantages of using fewer catheters involves the requirement of frequent catheter manipulation during the study and decreased number of simultaneous intracardiac recordings. When three catheters are utilized, frequent catheter manipulation involves using the catheter in the HRA to also pace/record in one of the ventricles as well as to carry out mapping. The catheters across the tricuspid valve and in the coronary sinus are not changed at any time. When four catheters are employed, separate catheters are placed in HRA and right ventricular apex, thus eliminating this manipulation. However, one of these catheters is needed for mapping. Each time a catheter is manipulated and changed from its initial position, problems may develop. A major problem involves returning the catheter to its original position. Therefore, consistency of the electrograms is compromised. This includes the manipulated catheter but also the other catheters that may be moved slightly or dislodged while manipulating the catheter. Moreover, during atrial mapping an additional catheter in the HRA is valuable because reciprocating tachycardia occasionally terminates during mapping. In this case, tachycardia is reinduced more quickly when the HRA catheter is already present and connected to the stimulator rather than switching between atrial mapping and stimulator when only a single catheter is employed. Also, duration of the study is prolonged with increased catheter manipulation and, frequent catheter manipulation may arouse the otherwise satisfactorily sedated child.

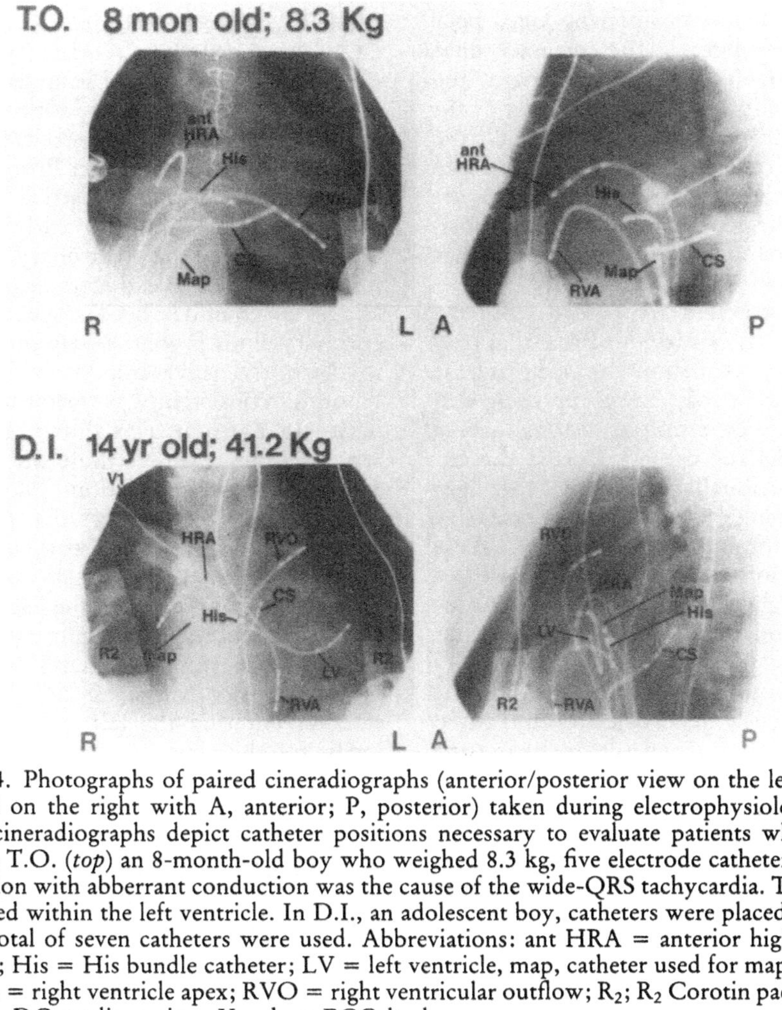

FIGURE 18–14. Photographs of paired cineradiographs (anterior/posterior view on the left with R, right; L, left and lateral on the right with A, anterior; P, posterior) taken during electrophysiologic studies in two patients. The cineradiographs depict catheter positions necessary to evaluate patients who have wide-QRS tachycardia. In T.O. (*top*) an 8-month-old boy who weighed 8.3 kg, five electrode catheters were used. Atrial flutter-fibrillation with abberrant conduction was the cause of the wide-QRS tachycardia. Therefore, a catheter was not required within the left ventricle. In D.I., an adolescent boy, catheters were placed within the LV and RVO, thus a total of seven catheters were used. Abbreviations: ant HRA = anterior high right atrium; CS, coronary sinus; His = His bundle catheter; LV = left ventricle, map, catheter used for mapping atrium and/or ventricle; RVA = right ventricle apex; RVO = right ventricular outflow; R_2; R_2 Corotin pads (R_2 Corporation, Skokie, IL) for DC cardioversion; V_1, chest ECG lead.

While there are major advantages to employing at least five catheters in the evaluation of the small infant, it is not as practical for the size-related reasons cited. The minimal number is one catheter, but extensive manipulation as well as multiple assumptions are necessary. The reliance on surface ECG changes is important because the assumptions are based on the correlation with intracardiac electrogram. For example, the assumptions include the absence of any intracardiac change when surface ECG is unchanged or, to the contrary, specific intracardiac change when surface ECG changes.

For these reasons, within the limitations discussed above, we utilize the maximum number of catheters when carrying out complete electrophysiologic study in pediatric patients who have the preexcitation syndromes. The internal jugular route has provided additional catheter access. Therefore in the small infant, at least three catheters are utilized: one in each femoral vein and one in the internal jugular. When each femoral vein can accomodate two sheaths/catheters (usually when child is >5.5 kg), four or five catheters (the latter if internal jugular vein used) are employed during the study.

Catheter Manipulation and Placement. Catheter manipulation and placement is more difficult in the small pediatric patient. Merely advancing two or more catheters from the left femoral vein can be fraught with difficulty, especially at the iliac vein-inferior vena caval junction. However, because the coronary sinus is the most difficult catheter placement and catheter manipulation is less difficult from the right side, one catheter usually is advanced from the right femoral vein first and manipulated into the coronary sinus. Next, the catheters are advanced from the left femoral vein and positioned in areas where no further catheter change is planned (e.g., HRA, RVA). Lastly, the remainder of the catheters are passed from the right femoral vein and situated in areas that may require further/repeat manipulation during the procedure. The latter may entail replacing dislodged catheters. For example, during pacing and/or tachycardia the catheter across the tricupsid valve occasionally retracts to the right atrium. The mapping catheter requires extensive manipulation during the study. For these reasons, a high priority exists for using the three catheters in the right femoral vein for the coronary sinus, His, and right atrial mapping. After the catheters are positioned, a Luer-Lock^R (Cook, Inc.) prevously placed by threading the catheter through the Luer-Lock hole and fitted onto the sheath, is tightened thus securing the catheter to the sheath (Figure 18–15). This minimizes catheter movement and dislodgement from the intended positions.

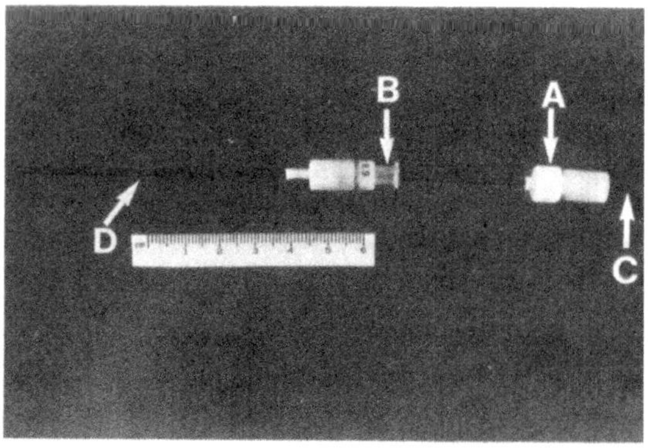

FIGURE 18–15. Photograph of the Luer-Lock^R (Cook, Inc.) method of securing catheter (C) within a sheath (D). The catheter is advanced through the Luer-Lock^R (A) and then through the sheath. The Luer-Lock^R fits securely onto the proximal end of the sheath (B) and is screw-tightened to maintain catheter position as well as to prevent back-flow bleeding.

LEFT ATRIAL RECORDING/STIMULATION: CORONARY SINUS CATHETERIZATION

Left atrial recording and stimulation is essential when carrying out an electrophysiologic study in a patient who has preexcitation syndrome (see Recording-Stimulation Protocol). The best method of recording left atrial electrograms is by placing a quadrapolar catheter within the coronary sinus [102]. Coronary sinus cannulation is preferred to catheters directly within the left atrial chamber because the course of the coronary sinus is consistently directly posterior to the mitral valve annulus with its orifice or "mouth" consistently posterior to the AV node in the right atrium. This allows precision during atrial mapping to determine the location of an accessory AV connection. Moreover, when attempting to detect accessory AV connection depolarization, a stable catheter position is essential within the coronary sinus [103,104]. Catheter positions within the left atrial chamber can be variable and difficult to document because of the size and shape of the chamber [105,106]. Also, the angle and position of the catheter entering the left atrium is influenced easily by the type of approach or site at the atrial septum (e.g., patent foramen ovale, atrial septal defect, transseptal) [105, 106].

Passing an electrode catheter into the coronary sinus can be difficult and is especially challenging in infants, small children, and obese older children and adolescents. Three sites of catheter introduction (left arm, internal jugular, and femoral) provide the opportunity for variations in the technique of gaining catheter access to the coronary sinus (Figure 18–16). The passing of the catheter from the right atrium into the coronary sinus probably is easier from the superior vena caval approach. This may be accomplished via internal jugular vein, left brachial vein, or left subclavian vein.

One disadvantage of the superior vena caval approach is increased patient discomfort. The discomfort especially is manifested when the arm is used because it may be necessary to delay complete local infiltration of lidocaine (avoiding spasm and/or decreased ability to palpate vein) until after gaining initial needle access to the vein [100]. Furthermore, this approach requires prolonged arm extention during the long procedure. Arm extension may complicate the use of biplane fluoroscopy and cineradiography. Many of these problems may be minimized by utilizing a subclavian vein or internal jugular

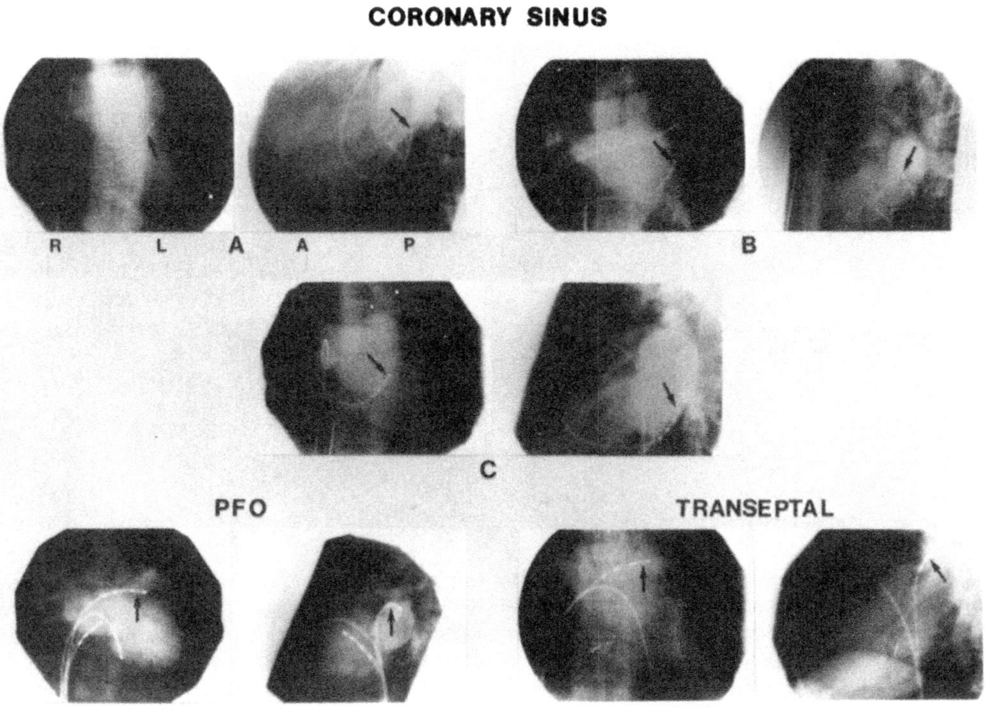

FIGURE 18–16. Photographs of five pairs of cineradiographs (same anterior/posterior, lateral positions and abbreviations as in Figure 18–14) depicting five different methods of catheter access to left atrial recording/stimulation. Three different catheter approaches to the coronary sinus are shown at the top (A and B) and middle (C). In (A), the superior vena caval approach (jugular, left subclavian, or left brachial vein) is shown. In (B) and (C) the catheter is advanced from the right femoral vein. In (B) the catheter is directly passed from right atrium to coronary sinus while in (C) the catheter is "looped" within the right atrium (see Figure 18–17). In the bottom row of cineradiographs, direct left atrial access is accomplished by a catheter advanced through the patent foramen ovale (PFO) or by a catheter advanced through a sheath placed in the left atrium by the Mullins transeptal technique.

vein approach [101]. However, with any catheter approach via the superior vena cava, the recording (electrode junction unit) and stimulation (pacing isolation unit) equipment must be moved or duplicated; it can be inconvenient to install stationary equipment between the groin and neck/arm locations.

Due to the disadvantages of the superior vena caval approach, we prefer to pass the catheter from the right femoral vein to the coronary sinus. This is accomplished by using two techniques usually using a #5 French quadrapolar catheter (Electro Catheter-Corporation, Rahawy, NJ): (1) directly from right atrium (Figure 18–16b) and, (2) looping the catheter in the right atrium (Figures 18–16c, 18–17). During the past two years, the coronary sinus has been entered with a catheter passed from the femoral vein in 19 of 29 children and young adults (age 8 months to 27 years) in whom the attempt was made. In the 10 patients in whom this technique was unsuccessful, the left atrial recording was obtained by passing the catheter through a transseptal Mullin's sheath (6 patients), patent foramen ovale (3 patients), or coronary sinus by the superior vena caval approach (1 patient).

In the obese patient, it often is difficult to manipulate the catheter into the coronary sinus, especially using the looping technique or the superior vena caval approach. The catheter struggle usually is due to the obesity-related superiorly displaced diaphragm causing alteration of the inferior border of the right atrium, an important factor in the success of the technique. Occasionally, a deep breath corrects this problem but often we find that the transseptal Mullin's sheath is necessary [106].

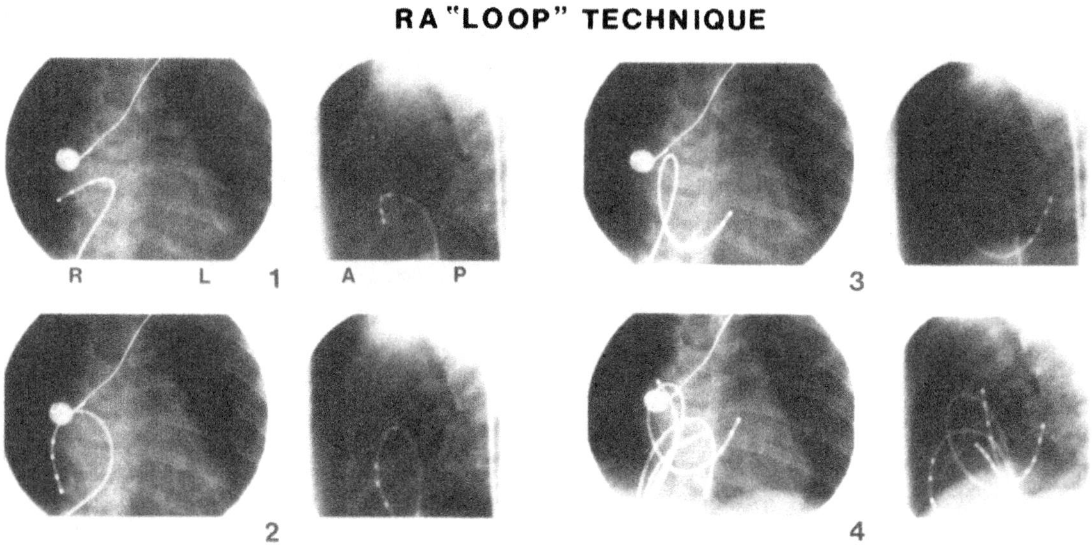

FIGURE 18–17. Chronologic series (1–4) of photographs depicting catheter manipulations required when passing an electrode catheter from the right atrium (RA) to coronary sinus by "looping" the catheter within the RA. In this 4-year-old boy, a #5 French Elecath quadrapolar catheter is first positioned against the lateral low-mid RA wall forming an inverted "J." In (2), the end of the catheter is positioned in the low-lateral RA wall. By advancing the catheter and by counterclockwise torque it is directed posteriorly (lateral view). With continued application of counterclockwise motion, the catheter is advanced into the coronary sinus as shown in (3). After verifying the catheter position within the coronary sinus by catheter movement on biplane fluoroscopy, other electrode catheters are positioned as shown in (4). Refer to Figures 18–14, 18–16 for abbreviations and explanation of anterior/posterior and lateral views.

When the coronary sinus is not accessible for left atrial recordings, the transseptal Mullin's sheath technique is valuable. For example, in the patient who has undergone surgical division of left-sided accessory AV connection the coronary sinus anatomy may be altered making it even more difficult to gain access to the coronary sinus (Figure 18–16).

RECORDING AND STIMULATION TECHNIQUE

After catheters are positioned, paired electrode terminals are connected to either the recording junction unit or to the stimulator isolation unit. The quadrapolar catheters involved with simultaneous recording and stimulation usually are connected by using the distal pair of electrodes for pacing and the proximal for recording. Only the distal electrodes with the smallest interelectrode distance (usually 1, 2, or 3 mm) on the mapping catheter are used for recording. Combinations of electrode connections can be employed from the quadrapolar catheter across the tricuspid valve to obtain the highest quality of His bundle electrogram.

Before beginning the stimulation protocol at each intracardiac site, the stimulation threshold is measured to assure standard stimulation protocol, within each patient as well as among patients. This is accomplished by pacing at a rate slightly faster than the patient's heart rate followed by slowly decreasing the mA until loss of capture occurs. The current then is increased slightly to regain capture, thus defining the threshold. The final stimulation is carried out at twice the threshold mA. This is usually below 1.0 mA and virtually always below 2.0 mA. The threshold is determined in each area of stimulation as well as after interventions such as drugs.

There is no standard method or order of displaying and recording the electrograms on the oscilloscope and paper. In our laboratory, the surface ECG leads are displayed at the top followed by the intracardiac electrograms from right atrium, left atrium/coronary sinus, His bundle, and right ventricle (Figure 18–18). The

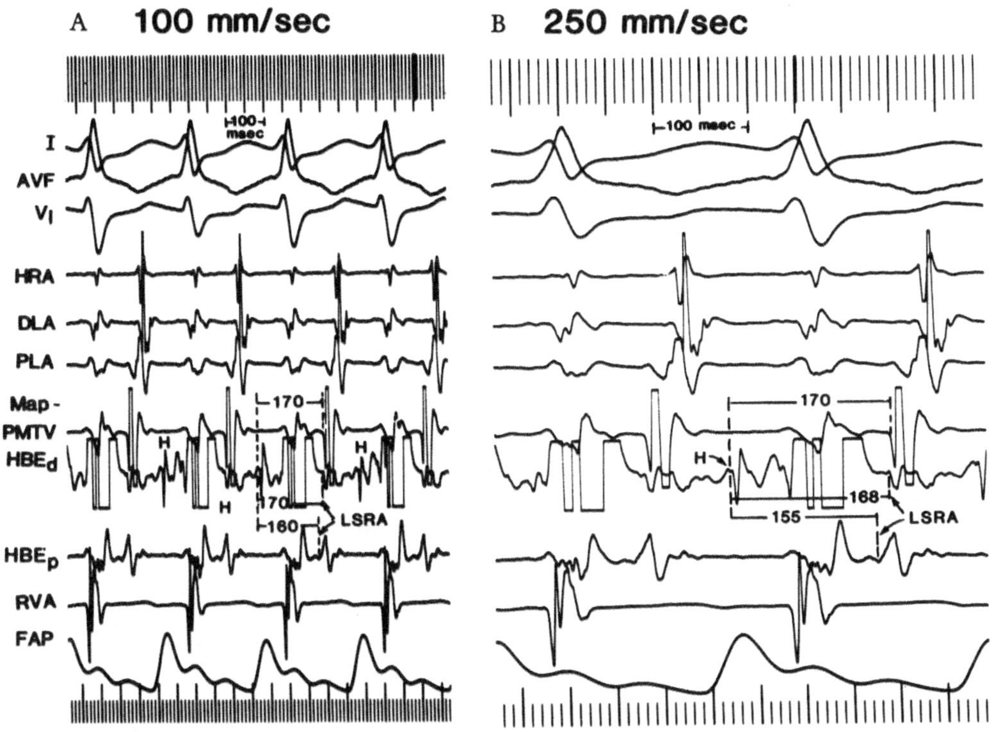

FIGURE 18–18. Simultaneous surface and intracardiac electrograms recorded in a 12-year-old girl with preexcitation syndrome during reciprocating tachycardia (255 ms cycle length), demonstrate better delineation of intervals during fast paper speed (250 mm/sec) recording (B) than at the slower 100 mm/sec paper recording (A). Although it is shown during 100 mm/sec that the earliest retrograde atrial activation occurs at 160 ms after His depolarization in the proximal low septal right atrium (LSRA), it is better and more clearly delineated (155 ms) during 250 mm/sec paper recording. In this patient who had a right posterior paraseptal accessory AV connection, the distal electrodes on the catheter across the tricuspid valve recorded the LSRA area slightly later (170 and 168 ms in (A) and (B) respectively) than the proximal electrodes (160 and 155 ms, respectively). Fast paper speed recordings are even more important in children with faster tachycardia. Additional abbreviations from top to bottom: I, AVF, and V1, surface ECG leads; HRA = high right atrium; DLA and PLA = distal and proximal left atrium, respectively; Map – PMTV, mapping catheter at the posterior mid-tricuspid valve area; HBE d and HBE p = distal and proximal His (H) bundle electrograms, respectively; RVA = right ventricular apex; FAP = femoral artery pressure.

femoral arterial pressure is recorded at the bottom. By the directive of the electrophysiologist and controlled by foot pedal, the photographic paper (Kodak Linagraph 1930, Rochester, NY) is recorded at 100 mm/sec or at 250 mm/sec. Fast paper speed is essential to separate close electrograms in pediatric patients because of the fast tachycardia rates (Figure 18–18).

Protocol decisions based on elicited data are made continually during the study. Consequently, a method of reviewing the information immediately after recordings are obtained is essential. An oscilloscope with "freeze-screen" capability is utilized in our laboratory (Tektronix, Inc., Overland Park, Kansas) and is favored over direct heat sensitive paper recordings. The freeze-screen oscilloscope offers instantaneous viewing of multiple simultaneous recordings displayed on a grid to facilitate accurate measurements. The onset of each oscilloscope sweep is triggered by the preselected external stimulus (e.g., eighth S_1). After the preselected extrastimulus trigger, the subsequent beats are displayed at adjustable time-base sweep speeds.

When review is completed, and after erasure, the freeze-screen oscilloscope is reset for the next drive train of stimuli.

A magnetic tape recorder also is valuable in the laboratory. Turned on at the outset of each study and continuously run during the study, the tape provides a back-up system if the paper recording (and/or developing of photographic paper) system malfunctions. Also, during paper changing or between protocol steps, occasional spontaneous rhythm changes may develop when the paper recorder is inactive. Thus the tape recorder does not allow any changes in rhythm to go unrecorded.

Electrophysiology technicians are invaluable during study. At the University of Nebraska Medical Center after sheath/catheter introduction, a minimum of two technicians assist during the study. One technician is stationed at the physiologic monitor/recorder constantly observing the cathode ray tube to assure unchanged and high-quality recordings. This technician automatically records chronologically pertinent data. The technician also activates the paper recorder as needed. The electrophysiologist is positioned at the freeze-oscilloscope and stimulator. The second technician is stationed near the patient's head. This technician responds to the patient's needs and also assures continued availability and operation of the synchronized cardioverter/defibrillator.

BASIC PROTOCOL FOR ELECTROPHYSIOLOGIC STUDY

Baseline Recording. At the outset of the study, baseline recording is carried out for a variable duration. The duration of recording is determined by the underlying rhythm. If continuous sinus rhythm with constant preexcitation at a constant rate is present, only a 10–20 sec recording is necessary. However, when a variable rate and rhythm exists, much longer continuous recordings are required. Moreover, when spontaneous changes in rhythm are noted at any time during the study, a recording is obtained. As described earlier, the magnetic tape provides invaluable back-up because the onset of the spontaneous changed rhythm often is important and only obtainable when a tape system is employed.

In addition to the usual baseline recordings of the areas already described, Prystowsky et al. [103] and Jackman et al. [104] have shown that it is possible to directly record an accessory AV connection depolarization. The presence of a detectable accessory connection electrogram may be more common that previously appreciated. However, considerable attention to recording technique together with use of custom electrode catheters and fastidious catheter manipulation (see Chapter by Jackman et al.). It is as yet unclear whether or not the required extra time and effort to record the accessory AV connection depolarizaion is essential.

Stimulation and Mapping Protocol. The order of the protocol is individualized to the patient's underlying arrhythmia(s) and to the rhythm present at the outset of the study (Table 18–1). For example, if atrial flutter-fibrillation has been documented or is suspected, every effort is made to avoid induction of atrial flutter-fibrillation. If atrial flutter-fibrillation is induced, DC cardioversion may be required because most other parts of the procotol cannot be carried out during atrial flutter-fibrillation. Thus multiple DC cardioversions are eliminated when induction of atrial flutter-fibrillation is avoided until later in the protocol. However, when atrial flutter-fibrillation inadvertently occurs, for example, during initial catheter manipulation or spontaneous conversion during reciprocating tachycardia it is often advantageous to carry out some of the evaluation of atrial flutter-fibrillation (see protocol steps #8, #9).

Similarly, reciprocating tachycardia is frequently induced during initial catheter placement or later manipulation. The study protocol must be flexible enough to permit evaluation of

TABLE 18–1. EPS stimulation and mapping protocol

1. Premature ventricular stimuli during ventricular paced rhythm.
2. Single ventricular stumulus during reciprocating tachycardia.
3. Atrial pacing at multiple rates and sites.
4. Premature atrial stimuli during sinus, atrial paced, and reciprocating tachycardia rhythms.
5. Localization of the accessory AV connection.
6. Search for multiple accessory AV connections.
7. Modes of tachycardia termination.
8. Induction of atrial flutter-fibrillation.
9. Isoproterenol infusion.
10. Digitalis administration (repeat 1–4; 6–8).
11. Antiarrhythmia drug administration (repeat 1–8).

the tachycardia at that time. Atrial mapping, single ventricular stimuli induced during the tachycardia, isoproterenol infusion, modes of termination such as premature atrial stimuli or overdrive atrial pacing (each discussed in greater detail later), are carried out during reciprocating tachycardia whenever it occurs. If these techniques are postponed and not performed when tachycardia first is noted, occasionally later the reciprocating tachycardia either is not easily induced or is not sustained, thus making it difficult to assess completely.

Premature Ventricular Stimuli during Ventricular Paced Rhythm. This technique is carried out by introducing a single right ventricular stimulus at progressively earlier intervals (S_1S_2) into a right ventricular paced rhythm (after the last beat of an eight beat drive). The ventricular drive cycle length (S_1S_1) must be shorter than the patients sinus cycle length. To start, S_1S_1 usually is 500 ms and after reaching the ventricular muscle refractory period, the S_1S_2 stimulation is repeated at another shorter cycle length, 400 ms. In infants it is common to start with S_1S_1 of 400 or 350 ms and then to use 350 or 300 ms cycle length.

Ventricular premature stimulation is used not only to determine ventricular muscle refractory periods but, more importantly, to aid in defining the conduction characteristics of the accessory AV connection in the retrograde direction. Retrograde conduction via accessory AV connection usually results in atrial depolarization with minimal delay [107]. After the single (S_1S_2) premature ventricular stimuli part of the protocol is completed, double (S_2S_3) and then triple (S_3S_4) premature ventricular stimuli protocol is carried out. The latter procedure is performed in our laboratory because patients who have preexcitation syndrome may have ventricular arrhythmias. Ventricular arrhythmia evaluation is essential in patients who have syncope and/or sudden death and/or wide-QRS tachycardia — regardless of other electrophysiologic data (Figure 18–19) [60,61,108]. However, as suggested by preliminary data from Milstein et al., the induction of ventricular tachycardia may not be clinically relevant [109].

Single Premature Ventricular Stimuli during Reciprocating Tachycardia. The major purpose of this technique is to determine whether or not the accessory AV connection participates as a necessary link in the reentry circuit [3,5]. The single progressively premature (usually by 10 ms decrements) ventricular stimuli are introduced after sensing every eighth tachycardia beat. If the ventricular extrastimulus occurs nearly simultaneously with His bundle depolarization, and if retrograde conduction proceeds to the atrium shortening the A_1A_2 (with unchanged retrograde activation), then this supports the concept that an accessory AV connection exists and participates in the reentry circuit. However, as emphasized by Benditt and associates, interventricular conduction delay can prevent this technique from demonstrating the finding when standard right ventricular stimuli are introduced in a patient who has a left-sided accessory AV connection [110]. Therefore, left ventricular stimulation during reciprocating tachycardia may be necessary in order to make this demonstration (Figure 18–20).

Atrial Pacing at Multiple Rates and Sites. Atrial pacing is carried out for approximately 30 sec at a rate slightly faster than the sinus rate. In between pacing periods, the rate is increased by increments of 10 bpm. During each pacing episode, close observation of QRS morphology and HV interval reveals valuable information. If the pacing site is near the site of an accessory AV connection, the degree of preexcitation may increase during increased pacing rates manifested by increased delta wave/QRS abberrancy and short stimulus to delta interval with decreased HV interval [3,5]. Increased preexcitation with incremental atrial pacing occurs because conduction velocity decreases through the AV node and is unchanged through the accessory AV connection. When nonpreexcited beats (i.e., normal QRS) are found during atrial pacing, the antegrade refractory period of the accessory AV connection is reached. Furthermore, as illustrated in Figure 18–21, it has been well documented that atrial pacing at multiple sites may be necessary in order to document the area producing the greatest preexcitation as well as to exclude the presence of additional accessory connections (see "*Search for Multiple Accessory Connections*") [3,5,111–113]. Incremental atrial pacing at each site is continued until block within the accessory connection(s) and AV node and/or His-purkinje system occurs. Determination of the latter is especially important because patients who have

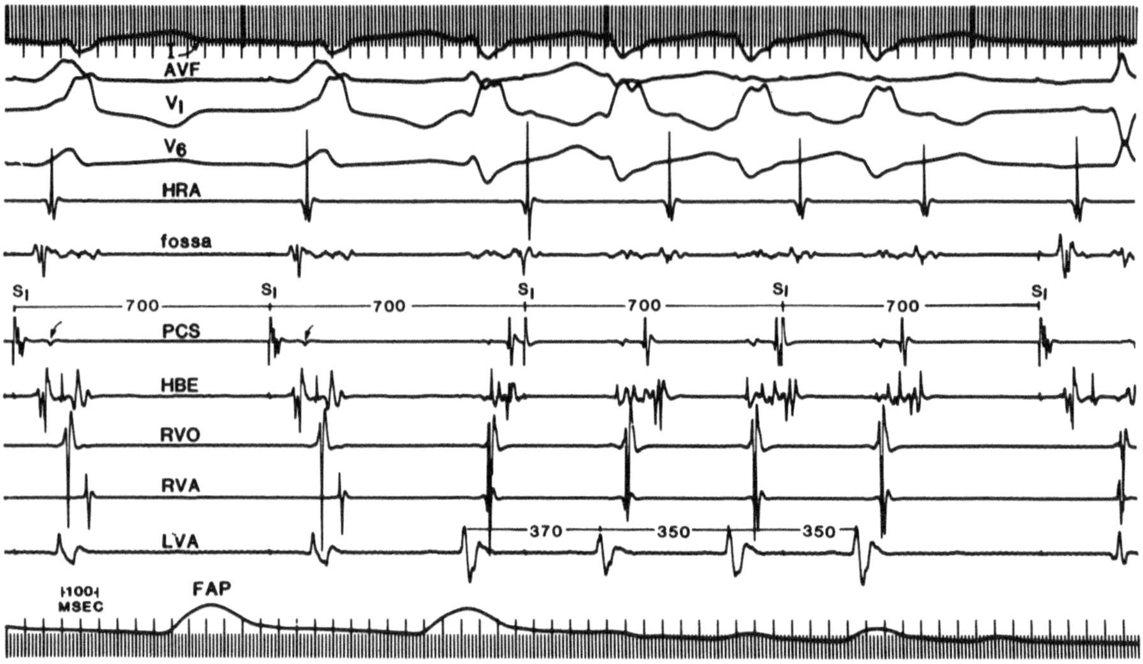

FIGURE 18–19. Simultaneous surface and intracardiac electrograms recorded in an 18-year-old man with preexcitation syndrome, syncope and wide-QRS tachycardia after exercise, show four beats of ventricular tachycardia during continuous atrial pacing (700 ms cycle length) in the distal coronary sinus. The first two-paced beats (S_1) in the recording demonstrate left atrial capture with delta wave and preexcitation. The third and fourth S_1 fail to capture the atrium because four beats of spontaneous ventricular tachycardia (350–370 ms cycle length) occur originating from the left ventricle (LV) as shown by the LV apex (LVA) recording. The morphology of other ventricular beats during the study were identical when the catheter within the LV was withdrawn, thus assuring that this catheter was not an iatrogenic cause of the ventricular beats. Abbreviations are the same as in Figure 18–18 with the following additions: V6, surface ECG lead; fossa, fossa ovalis; PCS, proximal coronary sinus; RVO, RV outflow tract.

preexcitation syndrome also may have enhanced AV nodal function (see Chapter 12 by Benditt). The enhanced AV nodal conduction must be considered a potential abnormality accounting for arrhythmias and/or symptoms (see later Atrial Flutter-Fibrillation discussion). Normal values of atrial pacing rates producing Mobitz I and II second degree AV nodal block are not precisely known. It is generally accepted however, that the range in adolescents is 140–200 bpm. In normal younger children and infants the range of atrial pacing rate resulting in second degree AV block is faster: 170–250 bpm.

Atrial pacing is useful in delineating other causes of a short HV interval. For example, the His electrogram may be in fact, the right bundle electrogram. This misrepresentation often is detected easily in patients who do not have the preexcitation syndrome because the right bundle electrogram–ventricle interval is short (less than 30 ms). However, in patients who have the preexcitation syndrome, the expected finding of a short HV interval makes it more difficult to exclude a right bundle electrogram. As illustrated in Figures 18–22, 18–23, measurement of the interval during atrial pacing and then during reciprocating tachycardia together with slow withdrawal of the catheter aids in delineating the His from right bundle electrogram.

The presence of a fasiculoventricular accessory connection may also result in a short HV interval [64]. In patients who have the nodofas-

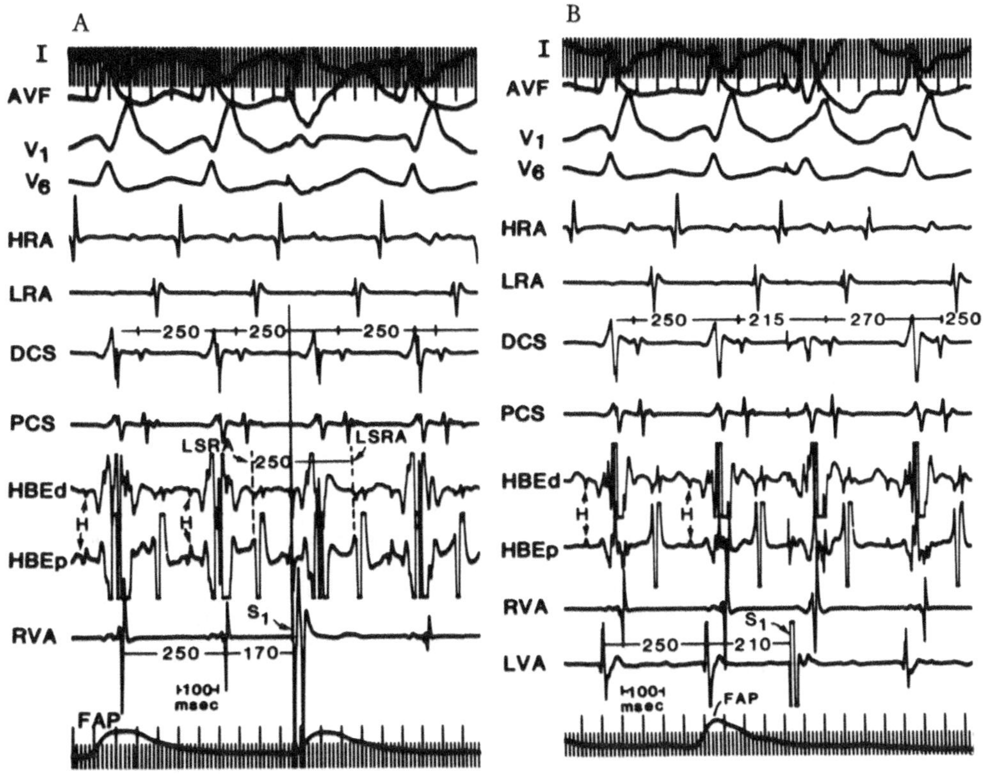

FIGURE 18–20. Two sets (A and B) of simultaneous surface ECG and intracardiac recordings during reciprocating tachycardia (250 ms cycle length) are shown in a 14-year-old girl with a left lateral accessory AV connection. These recordings illustrate the importance of introducing single premature ventricular stimuli (S_1) from the LV (B) when RV stimuli (A) fail to preexcite the left atrium. In (A), the S_1 is introduced 170 ms after the last spontaneous RVA depolarization and immediately after His depolarization (noted best in HBEp). All other S_1 delivered within the RVA as well as this S_1 failed to preexcite either the right atrium or the distal coronary sinus (DCS) because the atrial cycle length in all areas is unchanged. In (B), the S_1 is introduced in LVA 210 ms after the last LVA depolarization and again immediately after the His depolarization. Because the site of delivered S_1 now is nearer the left lateral accessory AV connection, there is no interventricular conduction delay and the left atrium is preexcited (DCS-DCS 215 ms). Abbreviations are the same as in previous figures.

cicular type of accessory connection, progressive left bundle branch block is found with incremental atrial pacing. Moreover, in these patients, greater degree of left bundle branch abberrancy is produced by right atrial compared to left atrial pacing. The AH prolongs and the HV shortens during incremental atrial pacing in patients who have the nodofasicular type of accessory connection (see Chapter 10 by Gallagher).

Premature Atrial Stimuli. The major objectives of the premature atrial stimulus technique in patients who have the preexcitation syndrome involves determining the refractory periods of the accessory connection, AV node, His–Purkinje system, and atrial muscle. Since refractory periods are rate-dependent, in our laboratory the premature stimuli are introduced during sinus rhythm and two paced cycle lengths (usually 500 and 400 ms). In small children and infants, shorter basic cycle lengths are required. Additionally, determination of refractory periods of the accessory AV connec-

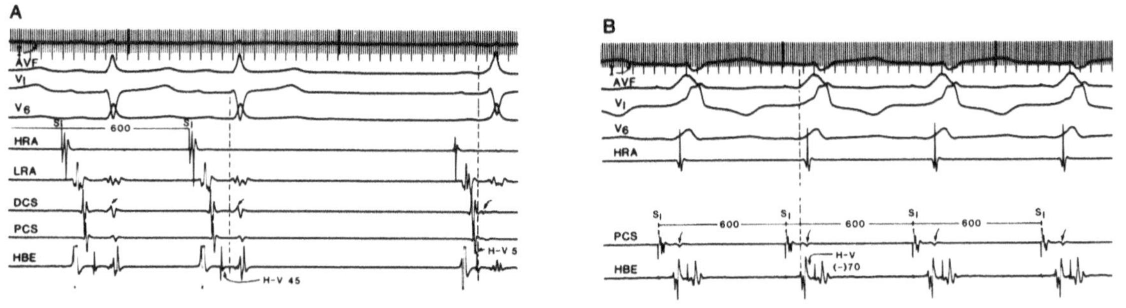

FIGURE 18–21. Two sets (A and B) of recorded simultaneous surface and intracardiac electrograms are shown in a 18-year-old man who has preexcitation syndrome. The recordings demonstrate the importance of atrial pacing at different sites to reveal maximum preexcitation. In (A), HRA pacing at 600 ms cycle length (CL) reveals no evidence of preexcitation because no delta wave is present and HV is normal (45 ms). In (B), atrial pacing in the distal coronary sinus at the same cycle length but near the left lateral accessory AV connection produces maximal preexcitation manifested by large delta wave in surface ECG leads and by HV of negative 70 ms. Also note that in (B) and with preexcited sinus beat in (A), the His depolarization clearly is recorded. While the His often is not recorded during preexcitation in patients with paraseptal or right-sided accessory AV connections, a recorded His is not uncommon in patients who have preexcitation with a left, lateral accessory AV connection and normal or enhanced AV nodal conduction. The finding is illustrated here: the ventricular prexcitation is first noted in the LV (depicted by arrows on coronary sinus recordings) but the RV inflow area is not depolarized until later by fusion from normal antegrade ventricular conduction and from conduction resulting from LV preexcitation. Abbreviations are the same as in previous figures.

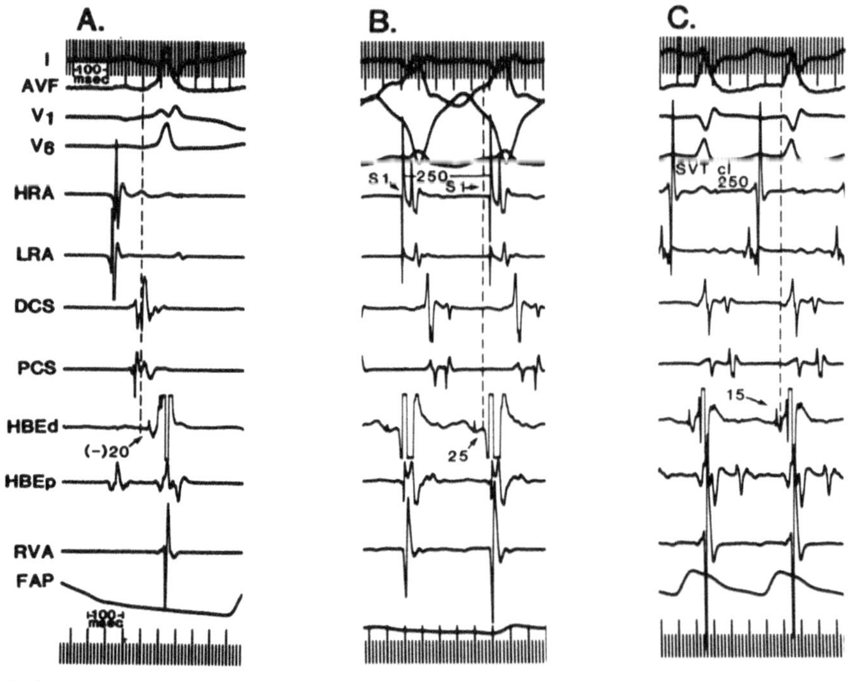

FIGURE 18–22.

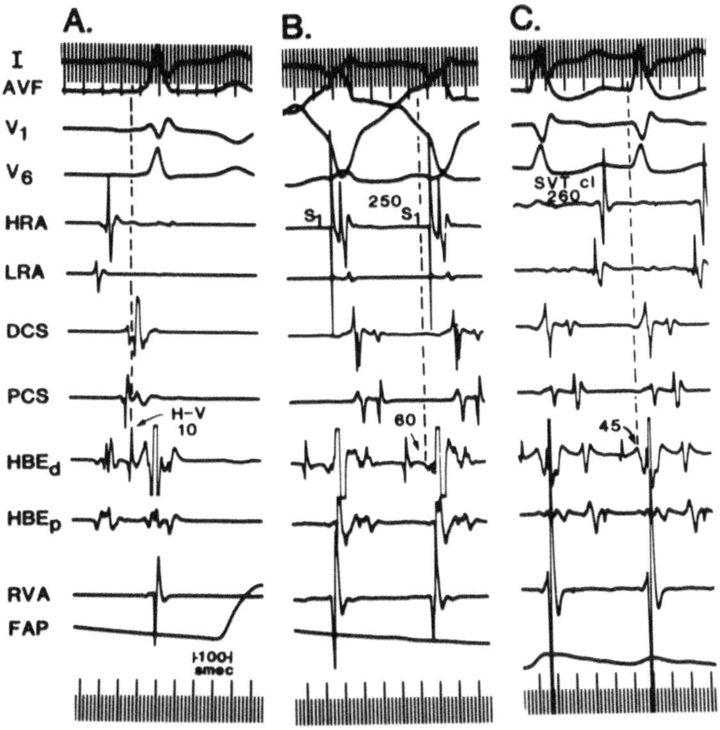

FIGURE 18–23.

FIGURE 18–22 and 18–23. Two figures of simultaneous surface and intracardiac electrograms in a 14-year-old girl illustrate the problem of distinguishing the right bundle from the His bundle electrogram in a patient with preexcitation syndrome. In both Figures 18–22 and 18–23, the three sets of recordings (A, B, and C) and during sinus rhythm, HRA pacing, and reciprocating tachycardia (SVT), respectively. In Figure 22A, a negative 20 ms interval is measured from the electrogram on the HBEd (depicted by arrow) to the onset of the delta wave on surface ECG (best shown in AVF and illustrated by dashed line). With the expectation that a negative H-V is found in patients with preexcitation sydrome and with the finding of adequate low septal RA depolarization (directly under the label "20" on HBEp), HRA pacing was carried out (B). In Figure 18–22B, the interval from the apparent H to ventricle increases but remains short (25 ms). Left bundle branch block (LBBB) and short H-V suggests different preexcitation as does the shorter HV (15) finding in Figure 18–22C during reciprocating tachycardia. However, in Figure 18–22C no preexcitation is noted on surface ECG because a normal QRS tachycardia is noted. Findings in Figure 18–22B and 18–22C prompted 5 mm withdrawal of the electrode catheter across the tricuspid valve because the apparent His electrogram was probably a right bundle electrogram. This suspicion was confirmed as illustrated by the recordings in Figure 18–23. Preexcitation again is noted during sinus beats 23A but the positively identified H now reveals the HV as 10 ms. In 23B, the HRA pacing induced-LBBB produces no preexcitation manifested by a slightly prolonged HV of 60 ms. Moreover, during normal-QRS reciprocating tachycardia, the HV is normal. Refer to previous figures for abbreviations.

tions may depend on the stimulation site; thus, stimulation should be performed from the both right and left atria.

Similar to the data obtained in adults by Tonkin et al. [3] Gillette and his coworkers [51] found that the antegrade refractory period of the accessory AV connection was longer than that of the AV node in 18 of 20 children and adolescents. However, the absolute mean value for the pediatric group was longer than reported for adults. In view of the fact that refractory periods of normal cardiac conduction tissues are usually shorter in children than in adults, this finding was surprising. As alluded to earlier in this chapter (see "Evaluation by History and Physical Examination: Adolescent"), the explanation may in part lie in the clinical presentation of patients (i.e., reciprocating tachycardia

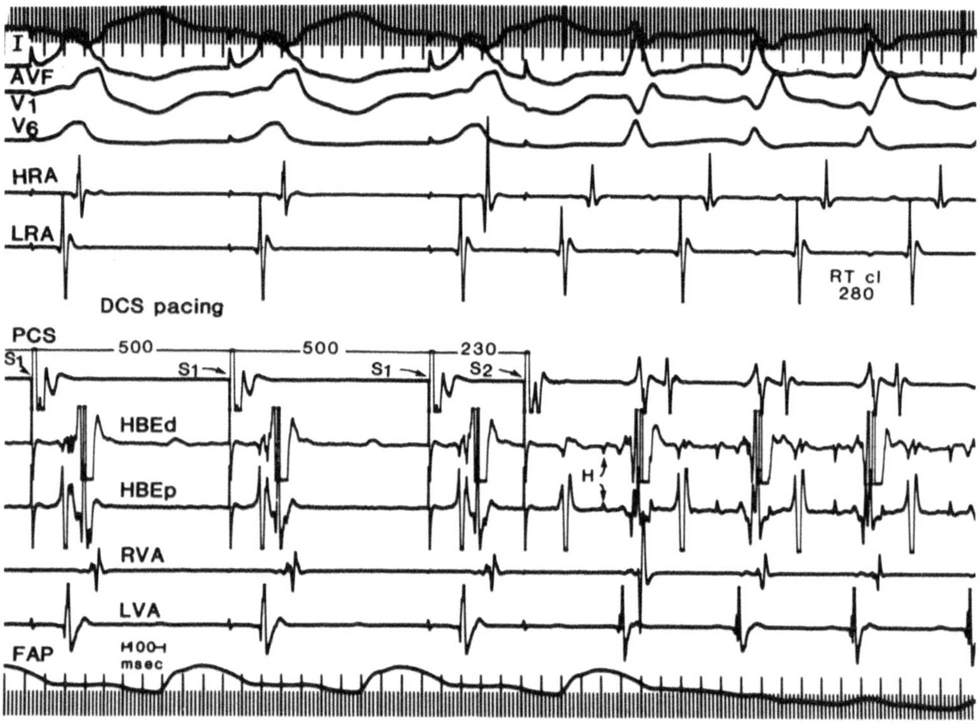

FIGURE 18–24. Simultaneous surface and intracardiac electrograms recorded in a 14-year-old girl with preexcitation due to a left lateral accessory AV connection, show the induction of reciprocating tachycardia (RT) at a cycle length (CL) of 280 ms. Eight beats of left atrial pacing in the DCS at S_1S_1 500 ms is followed by a premature stimulus at S_1S_2 of 230 ms. Note preexcitation during S_1S_1 but after S_2, preexcitation disappears (loss of delta with AH and HV now recorded in HBEd and HBEp). After antegrade conduction only through the AV node/His–Purkinje system with sufficient delay allows the left, lateral accessory AV connection to recover, retrograde conduction proceeds to the left atrium (depicted here by early LA activation in PCS). Because the AV node/His–Purkinje system permits continued antegrade conduction and the accessory AV connection allows retrograde conduction, sustained RT at 280 ms persists. Refer to previous figures for abbreviations.

versus atrial flutter-fibrillation). Patients presenting with short antegrade accessory AV connection refractory periods tend to be older since they would more likely present with atrial flutter-fibrillation, and the occurrence of atrial flutter-fibrillation increases with older age. Even within the pediatric age group, atrial flutter-fibrillation is more common in adolescents. (Also see Chapter 2 by Dunnigan.)

The premature atrial stimulus technique is valuable in inducing reciprocating tachycardia and atrial flutter-fibrillation or other atrial tachycardia (Figures 18–24, 18–25). When the effective refractory period of the accessory AV connection is reached, reciprocating tachycardia is induced if sufficient delay occurs in the antegrade (AV node/His–Purkinje) direction to allow recovery in the accessory AV connection and atria. The delay usually is found in the AV node (Figure 18–24) but may occur within the His–Purkinje system (Figures 18–26a, b). Thus after ventricular activation (via AV node/His–Purkinje), returns to the atrium by conduction in the retrograde direction (VA) via the accessory AV connection. Thereafter, if antegrade AV nodal/His–Purkinje system conduction continues together with retrograde VA conduction via accessory AV connection, reciprocating tachycardia continues. Occassionally, the AV node or His–Purkinje system does not permit further conduction after one or two beats (reciprocal or "echo" beats).

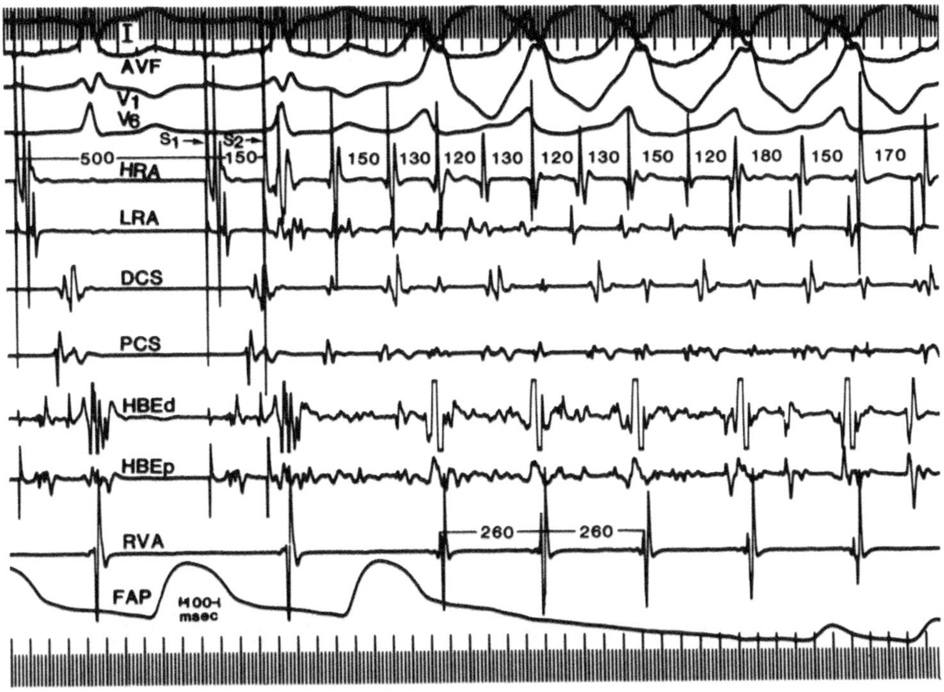

FIGURE 18–25. Simultaneous surface and intracardiac electrograms recorded in a 14-year-old girl with preexcitation syndrome show the induction of atrial flutter-fibrillation by the single premature atrial stimulus technique. After the eighth beat of HRA pacing (S_1S_1) at 500 ms, a premature atrial stimulus (S_2) is introduced at a cycle length of 150 ms. Sustained atrial flutter-fibrillation is induced resulting in preexcited beats with shortest VV of 260 ms shown here. Refer to previous figures for abbreviations.

Vagotonic effects from sleep or sedation may prevent the AV node from sustaining tachycardia. The administration of atropine and/or isoproterenol aids the induction of sustained reciprocating tachycardia in these patients. Isoproterenol has the advantage of a relatively short-lived effect, whereas the vagolytic effect of atropine may influence data for the duration of the study.

Localization of the Accessory AV Connection: Atrial Mapping; Bundle Branch Block during Reciprocating Tachycardia; Analysis of Delta Waves; Others. Although the general location of the accessory AV connection is surmised by several other techniques discussed below, endocardial mapping of the left and right atrium is essential to determine the precise site of the accessory AV connection (Figure 18–18) [3,5].

Since the retrograde atrial activation during orthodromic reciprocating tachycardia usually occurs via the accessory AV connection, the site of earliest atrial activation localizes the accessory AV connection. The possible sites of accessory AV connections include virtually the entire tricuspid valve anulus and septal area as well as the posterior and lateral mitral valve anulus. Mapping of retrograde atrial activation is also carried out during continuous ventricular pacing. This technique is performed using the same principle of earliest atrial activation localizing the accessory connection to that site. However, retrograde fusion with VA conduction via the His bundle – AV node axis may complicate interpretation of the map.

The most precise atrial mapping is obtained in small hearts when the distal electrodes on the mapping catheter are used and where they are separated by a short distance (e.g., 1, 2, or 3

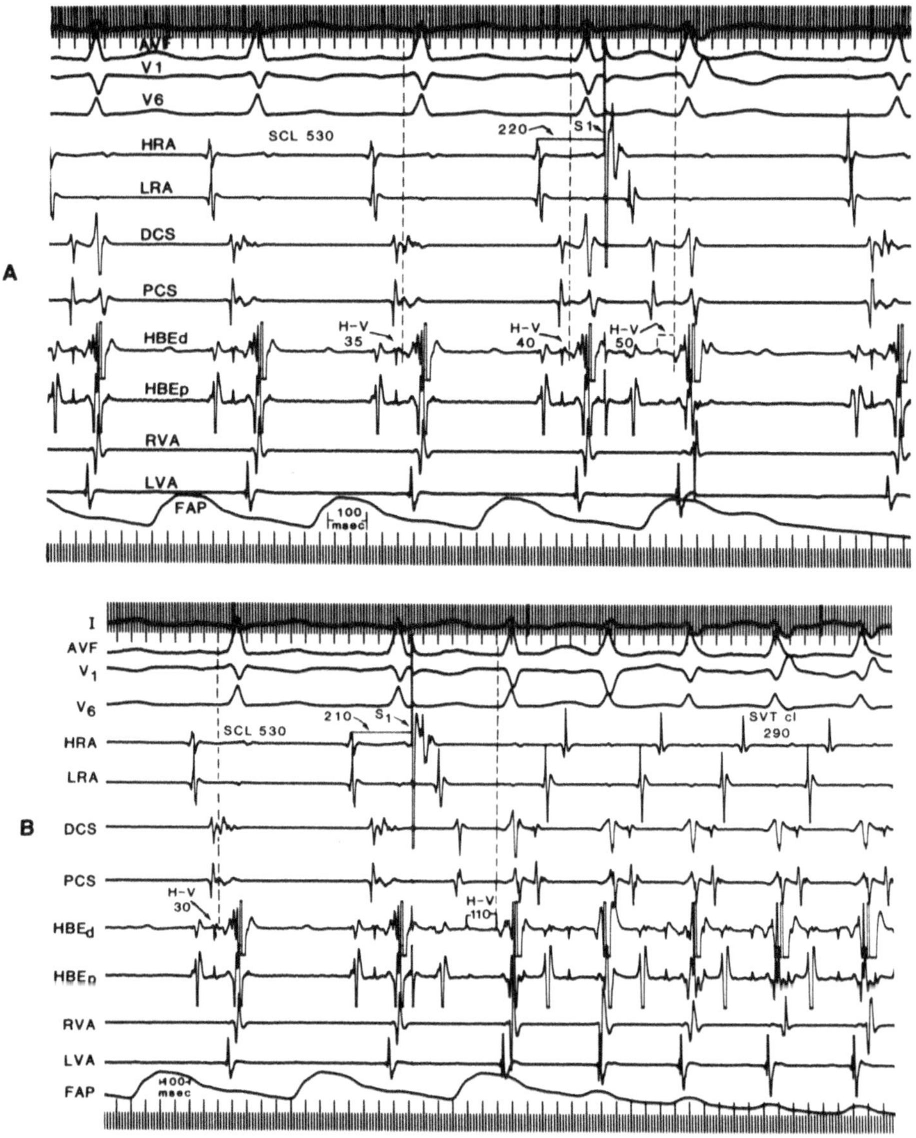

FIGURE 18–26A Two sets (A,B) of electrograms in a 14-year-old girl who had preexcitation syndrome illustrate that delay in the His–Purkinje system rather than the AV node may account for inducibility of reciprocating tachycardia. During pre-drug stimulation, reciprocating tachycardia was induced when antegrade effective refractory period of the left lateral accessory AV connection was reached and conduction also was delayed within the AV node (Figure 18–24). Procainamide was administered (25 mg/kg during 1 hr; 16.6 mcg/ml serum concentration 30 min later) to determine its efficacy and safety. In both Figure 18–26A and B a single premature HRA stimulus is introduced after procainamide during sinus cycle length (SCL) of 530 ms. (Note only minimal intermittent preexcitation with low amplitude delta wave and borderline short HV during sinus rhythm.) In Figure 18–26A, the S_1S_2 of 220 results in prolonging the HV and no conduction proceeds through the accessory AV connection. Although the AH prolongs compared to previous beats, the procainamide indirect effect of AV nodal conduction acceleration does not permit a longer AV nodal delay. In 26B, S_1S_2 of 210 ms results in His–Purkinje system delay (HV 110 ms), allowing the accessory AV connection sufficient time to recover (from antegrade block) thus retrograde conduction back to the atrium occurs and reciprocating tachycardia is induced. Refer to previous figures for abbreviations.

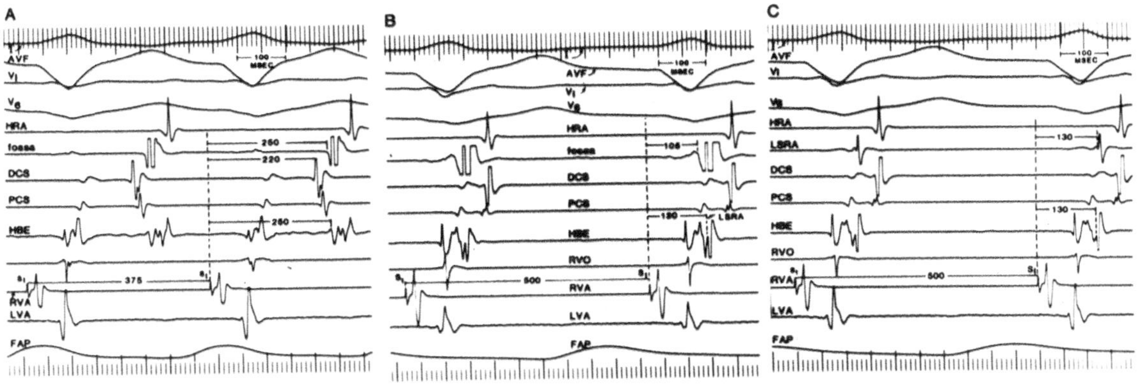

FIGURE 18–27. Three sets (A,B,C) of electrograms (recorded at 250 mm/sec) in an 18 year old show the value of atrial mapping during different cycle lengths of ventricular pacing. In (A) during RVA pacing at 375 ms CL, the earliest retrograde depolarization is found in the DCS (S_1–A, 220 ms). In (B) during RVA pacing at 500 ms CL, the earliest atrial depolarization is found in the atrial septum at the posterior fossa (ovalis), S_1–A = 105 ms. Because the onset of the LSRA was difficult to determine on the HBE (fusion of terminal RV inflow depolarization recorded by same electrodes across the tricuspid valve), the mapping catheter was moved from the fossa to the LSRA (C). At the same RVA pacing CL (500 ms), the S_1–LSRA was confirmed at 130 ms; thus the earliest retrograde atrial depolarization was correctly identified in (B) at the posterior septal (fossa) area. From these recordings, it is apparent that at a shorter ventricular cycle length, no conduction was demonstrated through the septal accessory AV connection but conduction was present through the left, lateral accessory AV connection. Refer to previous figures for abbreviations.

mm) (Figure 18–13). In our laboratory, precision is enhanced by recording at paper speeds of 250 mm/sec (Figures 18–18, 18–27) and by documenting catheter-electrode position on short bursts of cineradiograms (Figure 18–28). After the accessory AV connection is localized to an area, repeat simultaneous recordings and cineradiographs are carried out for more definitive and confirmatory data.

Patients who have a septal or paraseptal accessory AV connection provide a particular mapping challenge. The onset of earliest retrograde atrial activation in these patients is often difficult to detect by the electrodes on the catheter in the His region because of superimposition with the terminal portion of the ventricular electrogram (Figures 18–18, 18–27). The use of the mapping catheter with its distal short interelectrode distance enhances and verifies detection of the earliest retrograde atrial activation in the paraseptal area (Figures 18–18, 18–27). This is carried out during tachycardia as well as during right and left ventricular pacing at several cycle lengths.

Other techniques are also helpful to distinguish retrograde conduction through the normal AV node/His bundle from paraseptal accessory connection. Some of these techniques have been discussed elsewhere in this chapter and involve eliciting characteristics of conduction that distinguish AV nodal conduction from accessory connection conduction.

One method of distinguishing reentry within the AV node from reciprocating tachycardia using an accessory connection is by measuring VA conduction during reciprocating tachycardia. This measurement was found valuable by Benditt and coworkers [91]. These investigators noted the VA interval was virtually always greater than 70 ms when adult patients had reciprocating tachycardia and the retrograde conduction was through the accessory connection. However, during AV nodal reentry tachycardia the VA interval was less than 70 ms and most often less than 60 ms. A similar intracardiac study has not been reported in children. However, Benson et al. have found comparable measurements in children by using transesophageal recordings [86]. Although documentation of an accessory AV connection was not carried out by intracardiac studies, other reasoning (see "Transesophageal Recording and

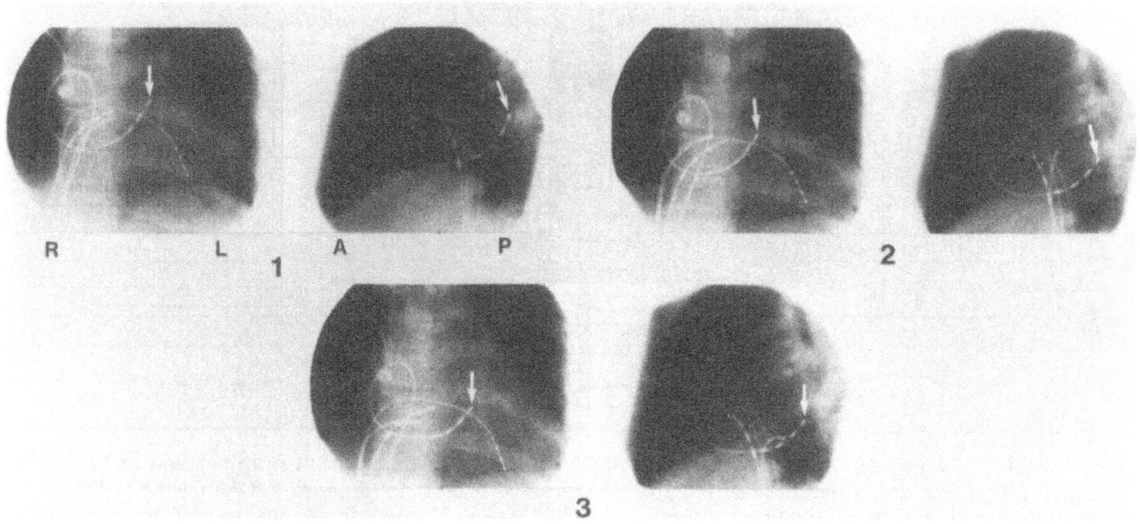

FIGURE 18–28. Consecutive chronologic series of three sets (1,2,3) of anterior/posterior and lateral cineradiograph photographs depicting left atrial mapping by stepwise withdrawal of the coronary sinus electrode catheter. In (1), the catheter is positioned in the distal coronary sinus (*arrow*). In (2), the catheter is positioned with the distal electrodes recording the midcoronary sinus area and the proximal electrodes recording the most proximal coronay sinus. In (3), the proximal electrodes are recording the mouth or os area of the coronary sinus. Refer to Figures 18–16 and 18–17 for abbreviations.

Stimulation") appears consistent and therefore, these absolute values will probably prove valid in future studies in young patients.

Bundle branch block during reciprocating tachycardia aids in localizing the accessory AV connection. Increase in the tachycardia cycle length in association with QRS morphology aberration, but without ventricular preexcitation, implies that the tachycardia circuit involves conduction through that part of the bundle branches (Figure 18–29). For example, when the cycle length prolongs left bundle branch block QRS morphology reciprocating tachycardia, and the retrograde atrial activation is unchanged, the tachycardia circuit involves conduction through the left bundle branch system (Figure 18–29).

Analysis of delta wave during atrial pacing techniques also reveals valuable information regarding the localization of the accessory AV connection. As outlined above and illustrated in Figure 18–21, the shortest atrial pacing stimulus to delta wave suggests that the accessory connection is near that atrial pacing site. Three other localizing techniques include: ventricular mapping during sinus or atrial paced rhythm [114]; VA conduction time after right ventricular premature stimulus [115]; and the preexcitation index [116]. Because of the problems of catheter manipulation and more complex ventricular preexcitation patterns of the ventricular mapping technique as well as the paucity of data with each of the methods, these are not standard techniques used in localizing accessory AV connections. However, further refinement likely will provide additional data in localizing accessory AV connections. The ventricular mapping technique especially appears valuable when the rare antidromic form of reciprocating tachycardia is found [117,118].

Search for Multiple Accessory Connections. Although this is not strictly a protocol technique, it is mentioned here because it is important to constantly search for multiple connections during the study [64,66,119–123]. Additional accessory AV connections or types of accessory connection (e.g., nodoventricular or fasciculoventricular) may be present. More than one accessory AV connection has been found in approximately 10% of patients with preexcitation syndrome [119]. Several observations reveal the presence of another connection. One simple but suprisingly often overlooked aspect

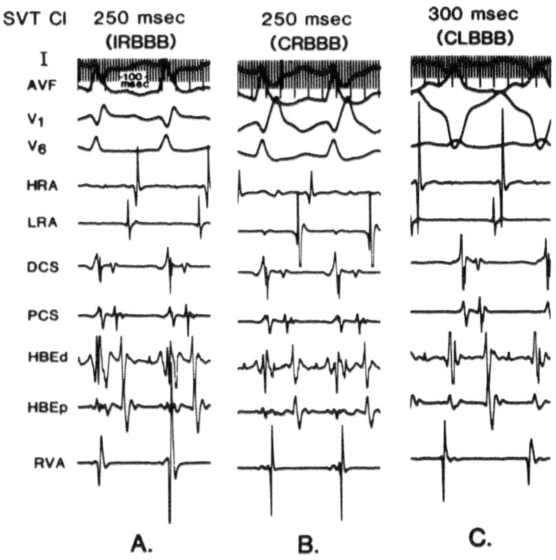

FIGURE 18–29. Three sets (A,B,C) of electrograms in a 14-year-old girl with a left lateral accessory AV connection illustrate the important finding of bundle branch block during reciprocating tachycardia. In (A), incomplete right bundle branch block (IRBBB) is found during reciprocating tachycardia at a cycle length (CL) of 250 ms. No change in CL is found in (B) when the bundle branch block is "complete" (CRBBB). However, when complete left bundle branch block (CLBBB) occurs (C) the CL prolongs, thus indicating the left-sided His–Purkinje system is a necessary part of the reentry circuit. This finding is evidence that a left-sided accessory AV connection is present and that it participates in the reentry tachycardia circuit. Note the slight prolonged HV (best recorded in HBEd) in (C) compared to (A) and (B). Also note the earliest atrial depolarization occurs in the distal coronary sinus in each recording also localizing the accessory AV connection to the left side. Refer to previous figures for other abbreviations.

involves detecting changes in delta wave morphology during atrial fibrillation or atrial pacing. When the QRS morphology changes with loss of one type of delta wave but another delta wave appears together with short stimulus to delta or short AH intervals, a second accessory AV connection is suspected. When a second delta wave is found or the delta wave never changes with earlier atrial premature stimuli but the AH prolongs and HV show no change, a fasiculoventricular connection is suspected [64]. In the nodoventricular type of accessory connection, a variable response of the AH and HV intervals is found. When the combination of an accessory AV connection and nodoventricular connection exist, Ebstein's anomaly may be also found [28].

A second accessory AV connection may be identified and distinguished from a fasciculoventricular connection by premature atrial stimuli introduced into the reciprocating tachycardia. Alternatively, during administration of ventricular extrastimuli (S_1S_2), the A_1A_2 is measured in right and left atrial sites. Sudden changes in earliest eccentric atrial activation site and/or cycle length indicates retrograde block in the accessory AV connection, thus suggesting a second accessory AV connection. When the new atrial activation appears earliest in the low septal right atrial area, further evaluation is necessary to determine whether this represents a paraseptal accessory AV connection, normal retrograde conduction via His–Purkinje–AV node, or another type of preexcitation (e.g., nodofasicular or fasciculoventricular connection). Ventricular pacing at different cycle lengths aids in delineating retrograde conduction through two or more pathways. In this manner, retrograde block may develop at one site (e.g., accessory AV connection) and the earliest retrograde conduction may localize to a different site (e.g., through a second accessory AV connection) (Figure 18–27). For these reasons, regardless of whether or not retrograde atrial mapping is carried out successfully during reciprocating tachycardia, atrial mapping also is necessary during ventricular pacing.

When reciprocating tachycardia is induced and the QRS remains preexcited, further investigation is necessary to determine whether or not multiple connections exist. After assurance that the His electrogram is indeed the His depolarization and not the right bundle electrogram (Figures 18–22, 18–23), evaluation is focused on the possibilities of another accessory connection. In patients who have a nodoventricular connection, the QRS morphology virtually always is left bundle branch block with left axis deviation [64,66]. The HV is variable depending where the connection leaves the AV node and inserts in a fascicle or the ventricular myocardium. In patients who have a fasciculoventricular connection the HV and QRS morphology are unchanged if this connec-

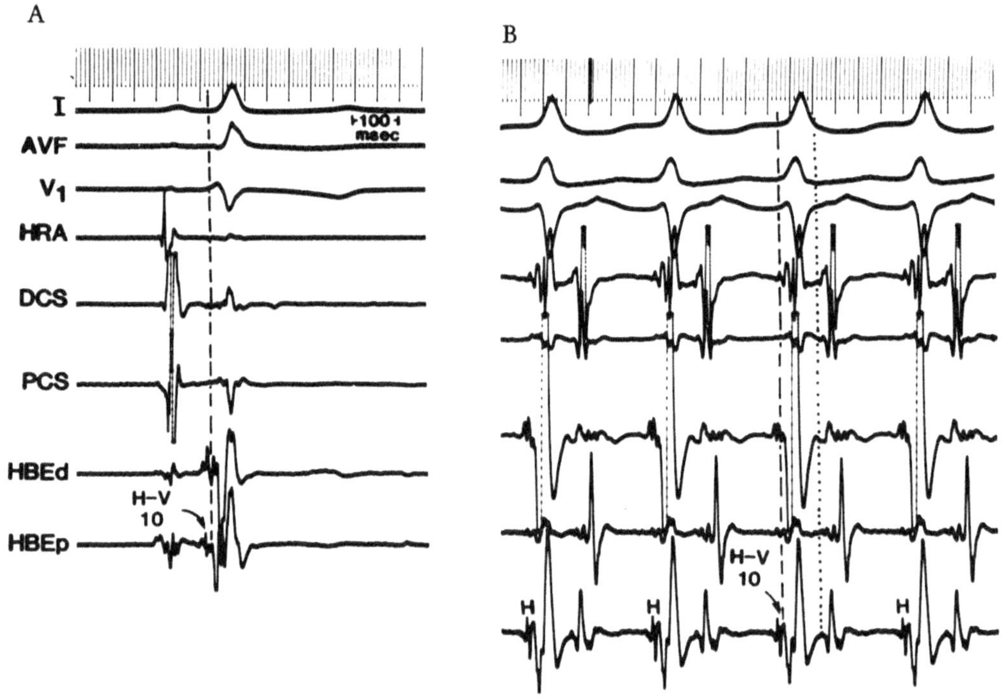

FIGURE 18–30. Two sets of electrograms in a 14-year-old boy show preexcitation during sinus rhythm (A) as well as during reciprocating tachycardia (B). In (A), the small delta wave is positive in V1, negative in AVF and probably isoelectric in I. The HV is short (10 ms). During reciprocating tachycardia (B), the QRS morphology changes slightly most notably in AVF as a negative deflection is not present. However, the H-V does not change, thus preexcitation also is found during tachycardia. The earliest atrial activation during reciprocating tachycardia at times was localized to the anterior medial HRA (*dotted line*) and during other recordings to the os of the coronary sinus (not shown). During all atrial pacing and extra stimulation, as well as atrial flutter-fibrillation, the HV also was unchanged, thus the presence of a fasiculoventricular accessory connection was confirmed. Thus, the likely reentry circuit involved antegrade AV node/His/fascicle directly to ventricular myocardium (bypassing bundle branches), retrograde via an accessory AV connection(s) located in the paraseptal area anterior and/or posterior. Refer to previous figures for abbreviations.

tion is solely responsible for the preexcitation during sinus and atrial paced rhythm. However, in patients in whom a fasciculoventricular connection and an accessory AV connection with antegrade conducting properties in both exist, the type of preexcitation and QRS morphology changes if the accessory AV connection now participates in the retrograde direction during the reciprocating tachycardia (Figure 18–30) [64].

Modes of Tachycardia Termination. The determination of the mechanisms during termination of reciprocating tachycardia is important because of therapeutic implications. During spontaneous termination of orthodromic reciprocating tachycardia, termination may occur because of failure to conduct through the antegrade limb (AV node or His–Purkinje system) or retrograde limb (accessory AV connection), or in between the limbs in either the atrial or ventricular mycoardium. When the termination of tachycardia is found in the accessory AV connection or at the ventricular insertion, or at/before the atrial insertion of the connection, the final recorded electrogram during tachycardia is the ventricular depolarization. However, with the new techniques of recording the accessory connection depolarization, the exact site of block within the retrograde limb is possible. Site of block is easier to identify in the antegrade limb because whether or not the His depolarization is recorded delineates the block to the AV node (most common) or to the His–Purkinje system.

When tachycardia terminates in the retrograde limb, the clinical therapeutic implication is that drugs with conduction slowing effects in the accessory AV connection (e.g., Type I agents) may be effective chronically. Conversely, when conduction is slow or fails through the AV node, propranolol or verapamil may be effective. The determination of termination mode is important after drug administration because occasionally characteristics change. For example, if procainamide causes enhanced AV nodal conduction with His–Purkinje delay, the beneficial retrograde suppressive effect on the accessory AV connection may be overruled by the detrimental His–Purkinje effect resulting in failure of control or exacerbation of the tachycardia (Figures 18–26a, b).

In nonspontaneous termination of reciprocating tachycardia, it is important to define fully the specific termination techniques. Details include cycle lengths when using overdrive atrial and/or ventricular pacing and when using premature atrial and/or ventricular stimuli. These data are important when considering antitachycardia pacemaker implantation (see Chapter 23 by Peters).

Induction of Atrial Flutter-Fibrillation. Bursts of rapid atrial pacing are carried out if atrial flutter-fibrillation is neither induced during any of the stimulation techniques described (Figure 18–25) nor occurs spontaneously (usually during reciprocating tachycardia or during catheter manipulation). It is important to induce atrial flutter-fibrillation to assess AV conduction characteristics because rapid conduction during this atrial arrhythmia may be life-threatening [124–127]. Therefore, repeated bursts of atrial pacing in the coronary sinus/left atrium and in several areas of the right atrium are carried out at cycle lengths near the atrial muscle refractory period. If all techniques are unsuccessful, AV conduction assessment is similarly made during continuous atrial pacing at rates as rapid as possible.

Measurements of AV conduction during atrial flutter-fibrillation are directed toward finding the shortest and average VV interval and the presence/degree of preexcitation (Figures 18–31, 18–32) [53,126]. The shortest VV during preexcited beats approximates the antegrade functional refractory period of the accessory AV connection. This value represents the shortest VV during resting atrial flutter-fibrillation and, if short, has been used by some investigators to indicate whether or not the patient is at risk for resulting life-threatening ventricular arrhythmias. However, as alluded to earlier in the chapter the definition of "short" has not been determined. The problem relates to the paucity of data including the relation of refractory period values to specific signs and symptoms. Furthermore, the values have been determined during rest/sleep and sedation. Therefore, the true or clinically relevant values perhaps have not been obtained. These limitations have prompted the use of isoproterenol during study (see "*Isoproterenol Infusion*").

The clinical significance of inducing atrial flutter-fibrillation during electrophysiologic study is not well known. Moreover, the definition of "sustained" atrial flutter-fibrillation is not well-defined, especially regarding correlation with documented clinical arrhythmia and symptoms [50,127–130]. Baurenfeind [50], in adult patients with documented spontaneous atrial flutter-fibrillation (but without preexcitation syndrome), defined atrial flutter-fibrillation induced during electrophysiologic study exceeding 30 sec as sustained. In another study, Bauernfeind and associates [130] found that documented atrial fibrillation was significantly more common in adult patients who had inducible reciprocating tachycardia and underlying heart disease or both. Klein et al. [49] also showed that patients who have multiple accessory AV connections also have a greater chance of atrial fibrillation and moreover ventricular fibrillation. A similar study of pediatric patients who have the preexcitation syndrome and atrial flutter-fibrillation has not been reported.

Isoproterenol Infusion. The importance of the catecholamine enhancing effect on antegrade conduction through the accessory AV connection was reported first by Weisfogel et al. in 1979 [2]. Independently thereafter Przybylski [131], Wellens [132], Cosio [133], German [129], and their coworkers showed that isoproterenol significantly shortened the antegrade accessory AV connection refractory period. Moreover, Cosio et al. [133] found that iso-

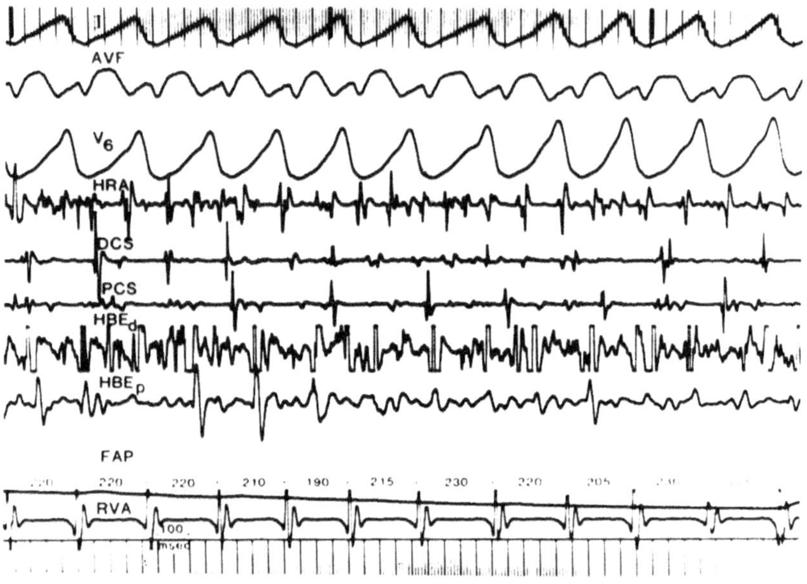

FIGURE 18–31. Simultaneous electrograms recorded in an 18-year-old man who had preexcitation syndrome and who presented with syncope, show fast conduction through an accessory AV connection during atrial fibrillation. Soon after induction of atrial fibrillation, the preexcited beats occur at a short cycle length. The shortest VV was 195 ms (RVA, *bottom*) and the average V-V was 215 ms. Refer to previous figures for abbreviations.

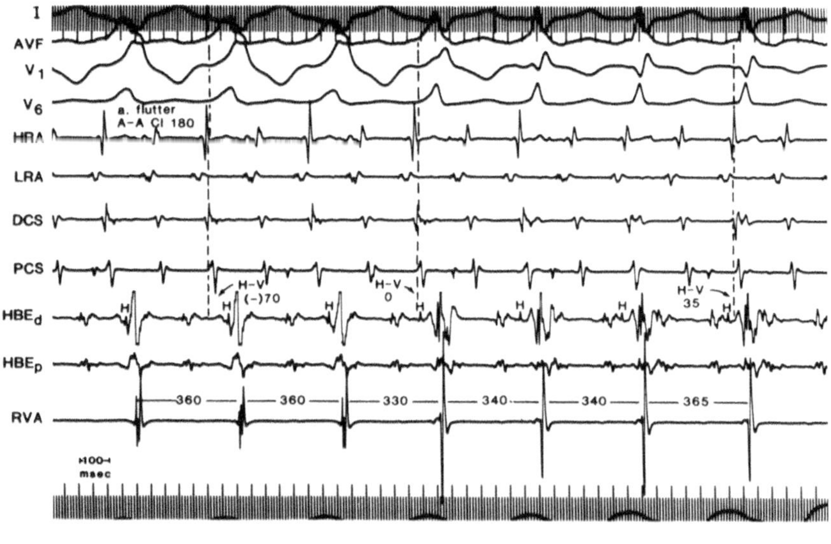

FIGURE 18–32. Simultaneous electrograms recorded in a 14-year-old girl with preexcitation syndrome during atrial flutter. The first four beats show preexcitation (delta wave with negative HV of 70 ms) and the last two beats show little evidence of preexcitation. The VV does not appreciably change during the variable degree of preexcitation indicating little difference between AV conduction via the two routes (normal AV node/His–Purkinje and abnormal accessory AV connection). Refer to previous figures for abbreviations.

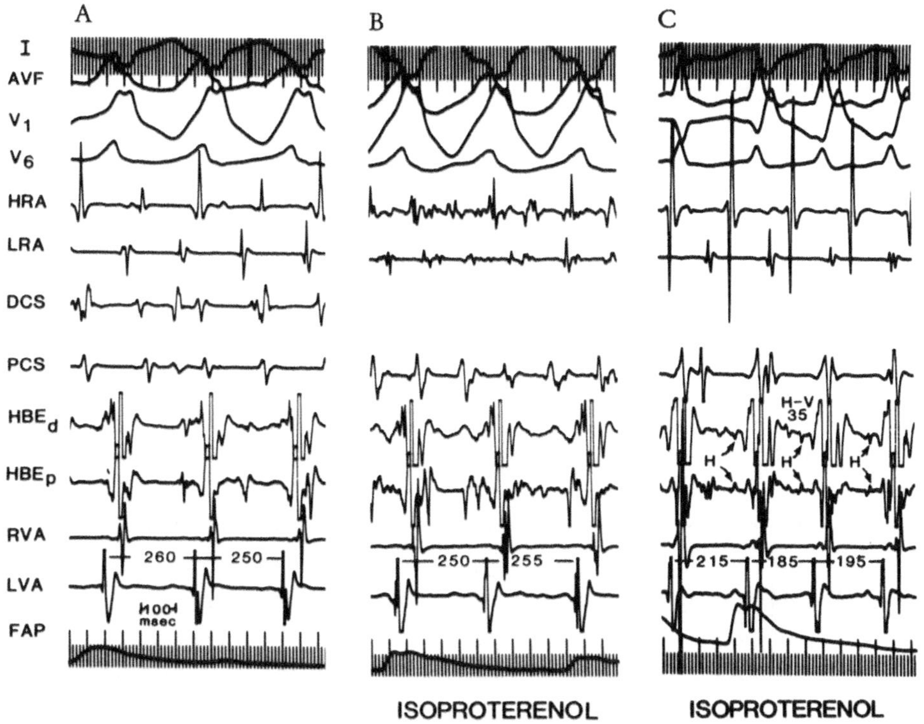

FIGURE 18–33. Three sets (A,B,C) of simultaneous electrograms in a 14-year-old girl with preexcitation syndrome due to a left lateral accessory AV connection, show the effects of isoproterenol during atrial flutter-fibrillation. Before isoproterenol (A), the conduction of atrial flutter beats through the accessory AV connection is shown by preexcited beats with the shortest VV of 250 ms. During isoproterenol infusion and atrial fibrillation (B), no further shortening of the VV interval occurs (shortest V-V, 250 ms) during preexcited beats. Shortly later during continued isoproterenol (C), little preexcitation is noted, manifested by HV of 35 ms but the VV decreases (shortest VV, 185 ms). Therefore, the effect of isoproterenol appears greatest within the normal AV node/His–Purkinje system rather than the accessory AV connection. This finding is clinically important because if treatment is focused on slowing or preventing AV conduction through the accessory connection, treatment failure may be encountered. Refer to previous figures for abbreviations.

proterenol unmasked otherwise undetected ventricular fibrillation in a 18-year-old youth who presented with sudden cardiac arrest. In the latter patient, the shortest PR interval between preexcited beats during induced atrial fibrillation shortened from 270 ms in the resting drug-free state to 180 ms during isoproterenol.

It also is important to note whether or not the short VV beats are preexcited. In some patients, fast ventricular rates result from the acceleration of AV nodal/His-Purkinje system conduction in addition to or rather than through the accessory AV connection (Figure 18–33C). This distinction has critical therapeutic implications (Figure 18–33 and Chapter 22 by Benson and Dunnigan).

By administering isoproterenol during atrial flutter-fibrillation, it appears that clinical correlation of symptoms is enhanced and may better approximate correlation of or prediction of clinically significant life-threatening symptoms than correlation of electrophysiologic data obtained during the resting/sedated state. The results from a large number of adult or pediatric patients have not been reported but the preliminary studies suggest that isoproterenol infusion during atrial flutter-fibrillation is a necessary part of electrophysiologic protocol in patients who have the preexcitation syndrome (see Chapters 8 by Levy et al. and 17 by German et al.).

In addition to giving isoproterenol during

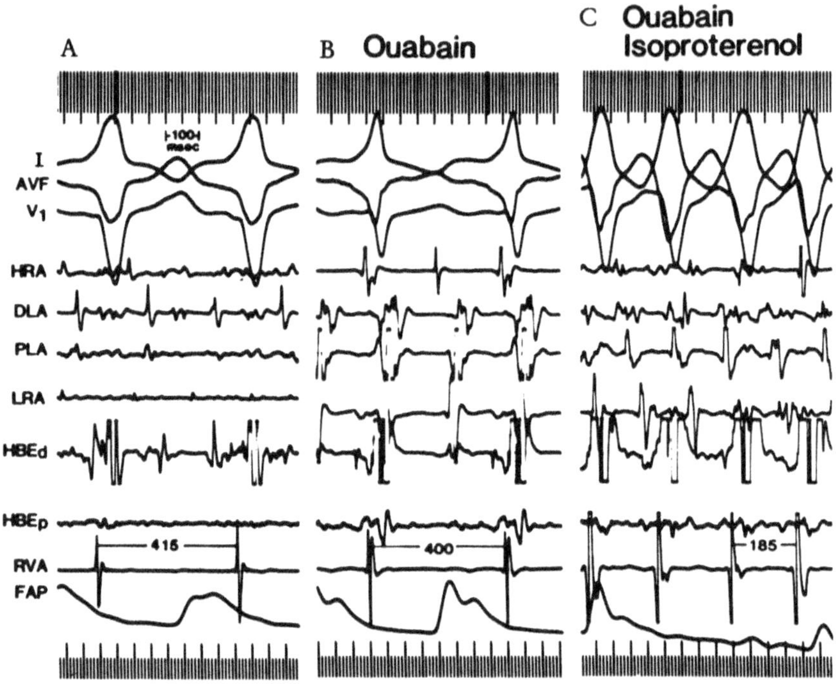

FIGURE 18–34. Three sets (A,B,C) of simultaneous electrograms in a 12-year-old girl with preexcitation syndrome show the effects of ouabain alone (B) and isoproterenol after ouabain (C) during atrial flutter-fibrillation. Before drugs (A), preexcited beats are demonstrated during atrial fibrillation but the shortest VV is only 415 ms. Forty-five minutes after intravenous ouabain (750 mcg), the shortest preexcited VV was essentially unchanged during atrial flutter (B). During isoproterenol after ouabain, the VV shortened to 185 ms, thus demonstrating that the combination of ouabain and increased catecholamines potentially is life-threatening. Refer to previous figures for abbreviations.

atrial flutter-fibrillation, it also is important to administer the drug during reciprocating tachycardia (see earlier discussion), during rapid atrial pacing and when determining antegrade accessory AV connection refractory periods. The latter two techniques are particularly helpful when atrial flutter-fibrillation is not inducible.

In our laboratory, the dose of isoproterenol ranges from 0.01 to 0.1 mcg/kg/min, and most commonly it is given at 0.05 mcg/kg/min. This dose usually results in increasing a normal resting heart rate by 20–50% and correlates with the reported doses used in the adult studies (1–5 mcg/min).

Isoproterenol infusion is also valuable after antiarrhythmic drug testing (Figure 18–34). In this manner, repeat stimulation protocol during isoproterenol infusion provides additional information regarding the efficacy of the antiarrhythmic drug(s) during a simulated increased catecholamine state.

Digitalis Administration. When digitalis is considered as therapy for a patient who has preexcitation syndrome, it is advantageous to administer the drug during electrophysiologic study to determine its effects. It is well known that digitalis may decrease the antegrade refractory period of accessory AV connections in some patients [4,5,10]. Jedeikin and associates [10] studied 21 children (average age 10 years) and found the antegrade effective refractory period decreased in 9 (43%) and was unchanged in 10 (48%). Moreover, Byrum et al. [6] and Mehta et al. [7] have reported pediatric patients with fast conduction via the accessory AV connection and who were treated with digoxin before life-threatening episodes.

Because digitalis has a potentially deleterious effect, it is important that it be administered during electrophysiologic study. Moreover, isoproterenol infusion also is indicated to determine the catecholamine enhancing effect on accessory AV connection conduction in the presence of digitalis (Figure 18–34). Digitalis administration has the disadvantage of the time required to await digitalis effect. Now that the short-acting ouabain preparation is not commerically available, intravenous digoxin is used. However, waiting 45–60 min following administration is required to assure digitalis effect.

Antiarrhythmic Drug Administration. Administration of antiarrhythmic drugs during electrophysiologic studies has proven useful not only in determining the safety and efficacy of the drugs acutely but also in predicting the long-term results of drug therapy [126,134–137]. Electrophysiologic studies to assess antiarrhythmic drug efficacy were pioneered in patients with life-threatening ventricular arrhythmias but have proved valuable in patients with supraventricular arrhythmias. Recently, the techniques were refined in pediatric patients by Kugler et al. [137]. These investigators also found drug studies productive in managing young patients who had ventricular and/or atrial arrhythmias. Kugler and coworkers found drug studies useful in four children who had WPW syndrome. In each of the four, no arrhythmias occurred after therapeutic drug concentrations were achieved during chronic treatment. Three other children with WPW syndrome were treated with a drug not acutely tested and two had recurrences in spite of therapeutic drug concentrations.

Similar results were obtained by Morady et al. [126] in 20 adults who had WPW syndrome and atrial fibrillation. These investigators found only one patient failed chronic medical treatment based on results of drug studies.

The choice of drug is based on several factors. These include data generated during the predrug stimulation (Table 18–1, protocol steps 1–9 or 10), presenting arrhythmia, history of symptoms, history of previous subtherapeutic or therapeutic doses/concentrations of antiarrhythmic drugs, and age. Generally, one or more of the drugs are administered intravenously after baseline data are obtained. A second drug is given either during the same study or one to two days later, when sufficient time has allowed for clearance of the unsuccessful drug. In our laboratory, the most commonly used drugs in patients who have the preexcitation syndrome are: procainamide 25–30 mg/kg IV during 1 hr; propranolol 0.15–0.20 mg/kg IV during 10–20 min; digoxin 20 mcg/kg IV during 1 min; verapamil 0.1 mg/kg IV bolus, repeated 5–10 min after first dose; or quinidine 25–35 mg/kg/24 hr orally. Blood is withdrawn at appropriate intervals after drug administration for determination of drug concentration when the stimulation protocol is repeated (Table 18–1, protocol 1–4, ±5, 6–9). If the sustained arrhythmia(s) is controlled completely or is nonsustained and no life-threatening side effects occur, the drug is considered successful. If long term drug therapy is recommended, the dose and achieved serum concentrations are based on the findings during the drug study.

COMPLICATIONS OF INTRACARDIAC ELECTROPHYSIOLOGIC STUDY

The major disadvantage of electrophysiologic studies relates to the test's being invasive. Although the mortality risk is low (0/325 total studies, July 1976–January 1985 at the University of Nebraska Medical Center), minor morbidity is high when the ubiquitous complaint of mild groin (and/or neck/arm) discomfort during the study, and for 2–3 days after the long procedure, is included. Other problems of moderate severity include acute side effects from drugs (45/94 trials, 48%) [137], discomfort from cardioversion or defibrillation (18 times in 13/61 patients undergoing drug studies) [137], dizziness from hypotension during pacing and tachyarrhythmias (approximately 25% of all electrophysiologic studies). More serious problems can occur; venous thrombosis (2/325 total electrophysiologic studies); cerebral vascular accident (1/325 total studies); perforation (0/325 total studies). Combined, the serious morbidity is less than 0.1% of patients undergoing electrophysiologic studies.

It might appear that electrophysiologic studies are not cost effective. However, it has been shown that when noninvasive studies together with empiric therapy are carried out, the disadvantages of incomplete data, cost of more noninvasive evaluation and follow-up, are outweighed by the small risks and increased benefits of invasive studies [138]. With further refinements of noninvasive evaluation, this may not hold true in the future.

Noninvasive or Invasive Evaluation Relative to Age and Sign/Symptom

Indications for proceeding with evaluation, as well as indications for the specific type of evaluation, in the pediatric patient who has the preexcitation syndrome are discussed in this part of the chapter. First, the degree of evaluation (noninvasive versus invasive) is presented according to the age and specific type of signs and symptoms. Later, the extent of evaluation is discussed relative to the asymptomatic pediatric patient. The data presented earlier in this chapter provide the background for the recommendations here. Although brief references to this data are necessary, detailed explanations are not repeated.

Throughout this discussion, it must be remembered that these recommendations are based on more opinion than factual data (see also Chapter 28 by Benditt and Benson).

SYMPTOMATIC PATIENTS (TABLE 18–2)

Infants. Most symptomatic infants who have the preexcitation syndrome have signs and symptoms that warrant only noninvasive testing. (In this discussion, transesophageal recording/pacing is considered noninvasive.) Rarely are life-threatening signs and symptoms found (Table 18–2) and, therefore, it is uncommon for infants to undergo complete electrophysiologic studies. However, as alluded to in the chapters by Benson and Dunnigan and by Benditt and Benson, there is a controversy regarding the use of digitalis for chronic treatment. It has been the view of some that electrophysiologic studies be carried out to determine whether or not digoxin is safe, prior to initiating treatment. Gillette has advocated invasive study with a single catheter to determine whether or not the antegrade refractory period of the accessory AV connection shortens following digoxin administration to an abnormal value (arbitrarily chosen as abnormal if less than 220 ms) [24]. It is unknown whether the advantages of the one catheter study are worth the risk, albeit small, of the invasive procedure. Furtheremore, opponents argue against the need because they believe the natural history of successful digoxin treatment does not warrant any further testing. The proponents of digoxin evaluation believe even the low risk of digoxin-related sudden death in infancy justifies the risk and cost of testing.

A complete multiple catheter study is indicated in the rare infant in whom surgical division of the accessory AV connection is contemplated. This possibility is most common in infants who have underlying congenital heart disease requiring intracardiac operations. In such patients, postoperative life-threatening arrhythmias may occur despite absence of significant preexcitation related symptoms preoperatively [27]. Thus it is worth the small risk of intracardiac study and the extra intraoperative time to divide the accessory AV connection [27,30–32].

The major problem facing the clinician who elects only noninvasive testing is to decide which test or tests to use. Since many symptomatic infants with preexcitation syndrome present with signs/symptoms of congestive heart failure, each of the noninvasive tests are useful. Commonly, the question of whether or not underlying disease exists provides the impetus to use the chest X-ray film and echocardiography. Holter monitoring is very helpful and probably underutilized in the intensive care setting. Too often the infant in the intensive care unit or infant on a telemetry system is assessed only by routine rate alarm screening with automatic recordings obtained only when a fast or slow rate occurs. It is easy to miss important rhythm information if monitoring with continuous surveillance is not carried out. Examples include otherwise undetected short bursts of paroxysmal tachycardia or pauses with pertinent information relating to onset and termination of these events.

In the infant who has infrequent nonsustained tachycardia and no other sign or symptom, it may be argued that no evaluation is necessary beyond history, physical examination, and ECG. However, to decide whether or not treatment is indicated, data derived from full noninvasive evaluation are helpful. For example, it is possible that the infant has paroxysmal atrial flutter-fibrillation with fast wide-QRS tachycardia only detected by Holter monitoring and/or by transesophageal recording/pacing. In such an infant, indications for further testing and management is different than in the infant who has nothing more than a few episodes of normal-QRS tachycardia lasting only several seconds each.

It is difficult at the present time to definitively define the role of transesophageal recording/stimulation in the symptomatic infant. The

TABLE 18–2. Preexcitation syndrome noninvasive vs. invasive evaluation of symptomatic patients

Infants	
Noninvasive*	Invasive**
Frequent or repetitive tachycardia	Near-miss SIDS
CHF/hydrops fetalis	Unexplained seizure
Underlying heart disease	Ventricular fibrillation
Determine drug efficacy	Atrial flutter-fibrillation
Frequent tachycardia	Any wide-QRS tachycardia
	Medically refractory tachycardia
	Underlying CHD requiring operation
	Determine antegrade RP before and after digitalis
Children and Adolescents	
Noninvasive*	Invasive**
Palpitations	Syncope/near-syncope
Mild chest discomfort	Angina
Underlying heart disease	Unexplained seizure
Fatigue	Ventricular fibrillation
Mild dizzyness	Atrial flutter-fibrillation
Determine drug efficacy	Any wide-QRS tachycardia
	Medically refractory tachycardia
	Underlying CHD requiring operation
	Determine antegrade RP before and after digitalis
	Determine drug efficacy/safety
	Exercise paroxysmal tachycardia

* Includes transesophageal recording/stimulation.
** Includes noninvasive and invasive.

Abbreviations: CHD — congenital heart disease; CHF — congestive heart failure; RP — antegrade refractory period of AV accessory connection; SIDS — sudden infant death syndrome.

major problem relates to unfamiliarity with the technique. With further studies as well as refinement and increased availability of equipment, it is likely that the pediatric cardiologist will find the transesophageal technique tremendously valuable in the evaluation of the infant with preexcitation syndrome. Particularly promising is the ability to determine efficacy of acute treatment, and the use of these data to predict chronic treatment [85,89]. Additional studies may show that the technique is effective in determining and predicting the safety of digoxin (or other drugs) in infants with the preexcitation syndrome.

Children and Adolescents. The recommendations outlined above in infants apply to children and adolescents with a few modifications. Exercise testing in the cooperative patient is an important adjunct to noninvasive evaluation for reasons specified earlier (see "Noninvasive Testing — Exercise Testing").

In this age group with preexcitation syndromes, a major dilemma facing clinicians involves whether or not to carry out invasive study. No problems exist in reaching an affirmative decision in the patient who has a documented life-threatening arrhythmia or who has experienced life-threatening symptoms. However, recommendations are less clear cut in patients with other problems (e.g., exercise-induced paroxysmal tachycardia in an otherwise asymptomatic patient). Also there is a dilemma regarding whether or not to recommend electrophysiology study when the electrophysiologist is confronted with a patient in whom chronic medical therapy, particular digoxin may be indicated.

In the symptomatic child or adolescent who has preexcitation syndrome and exercise-induced paroxysmal tachycardia, a strong argument for invasive testing is made when exercise testing reveals the likelihood of a short accessory AV connection refractory period. This particularly is true in an adolescent because the risk of developing atrial flutter-fibrillation increases with age. However, a middle-of-the-road approach is to recommend invasive testing when non-life-threatening signs/symptoms are interrupting the patient's and/or family's lifestyle. This approach must be individualized. In some patients one episode is too much, in another patient one episode per day is tolerable. After reassurance based on noninvasive testing, no further evaluation (or treatment) usually is carried out.

There is not uniform agreement in whether or not to carry out invasive testing to evaluate the child or adolescent in whom it has been recommended to begin chronic medical treatment. Two related factors are involved. One concerns the use of digitalis and the other concerns the use of any antiarrhythmic agent. The digitalis controversy is discussed further in the chapters by Benditt and Benson and by Prystowsky. Briefly, advocates of invasive testing believe because digoxin can be deleterious to the extreme of causing sudden death, it should not be recommended unless it is evaluated and found safe during the study — including testing during isoproterenol infusion (Figure 18–34).

The recommendation of invasive study to evaluate the response to any chronically planned antiarrhythmia drug is based on the reasons cited earlier in "Invasive Testing, Antiarrhythmic Drug Administration." To emphasize these points, the advantages of successful prediction of chronic therapy and of detecting adverse effects appear to outweigh the disadvantages of the invasive procedure. It is possible that future studies will show that the transesophageal technique may be equally effective in selected patients.

Asymptomatic patients (Table 18–3). Decisions are particularly difficult regarding extent of evaluation in the asymptomatic patient with preexcitation syndromes of any age. Usually in the infant or small child without sings/symptoms of arrhythmias, the preexcitation syndrome is detected when an ECG is performed to evaluate congenital heart disease. Full evaluation including invasive study is indicated before intracardiac operations because of reasons already presented [27,30–32].

In the asymptomatic infant or child who has infrequent or frequent tachycardia detected incidentally, noninvasive evaluation is indicated. Echocardiography is helpful to evaluate underlying heart disease and to determine if adverse effects (chamber enlargement) have resulted from chronic tachycardia. Holter monitoring and/or memory-telephonic recording are indicated to document the tachyarrhythmia. If none of these tests reveal needed information, transesophageal stimulation then can be carried out.

In the asymptomatic older adolescent, we advise full evaluation by noninvasive testing because of the potential for developing atrial flutter-fibrillation. Although transesophageal testing may become an important adjunct in the future, presently the noninvasive testing (especially exercise testing) need not include routine transesophageal evaluation unless the pertinent information is unobtainable by the other noninvasive evaluation. The athlete also is considered a special asymptomatic patient because exhaustion and bursts of activity may result in life-threatening arrhythmias.

In any asymptomatic pediatric patient in whom wide-QRS tachycardia is found, further evaluation by invasive electrophysiologic study is recommended. During particular situations (e.g., fright or other sudden catecholamine or autonomic changes), patients may become symptomatic and the first symptoms may be sudden death from ventricular arrhythmia related to the preexcitation syndrome [3,53]. Therefore, invasive testing is justified in asymptomatic patients who have wide-QRS tachycardia.

Family history of sudden death warrants at least noninvasive evaluation. It is rare to find a positive family history of unexplained sudden death in patients who have preexcitation syndrome. If a positive family history is elicited, investigation is first focused on associated heart disease such as hypertrophic cardiomyopathy, mitral valve prolapse, or other arrhythmias [36–39]. Invasive testing may be indicated in selected patients. These may include patients who have a family history of multiple sudden unexplained cardiac or arrhythmia deaths. Although only one family has been reported relating family history of multiple sudden death to the preexcitation syndrome [16], because of

TABLE 18-3. Preexcitation syndrome evaluation of asymptomatic patients

Noninvasive*	Invasive**
Frequent or infrequent tachycardia	Underlying heart disease requiring intracardiac operation
Adolescent	Wide-QRS tachycardia
Athlete	± Family history sudden death
Family history of sudden death	
?All patients	

* Includes transesophageal recording/stimulation.
** Includes noninvasive and invasive.

the possibility of sudden death in these patients, invasive testing appears justified in this specific situation.

Although lack of data does not allow a firm recommendation here, a case can be made to carry out minimal noninvasive evaluation — especially Holter and exercise testing — in all young asymptomatic patients who have preexcitation syndrome. In addition to gathering natural history data that presently is incomplete, reassurance may be possible for some patients. On the other hand, possible life-threatening problems may be found in others.

Summary

In this chapter, evaluation of the patient with preexcitation syndrome has included the essentials of historical data with the most common presentations relative to age of the pediatric patient. This data in combination with the discussion of the advantages and limitations of noninvasive testing and the details of the invasive electrophysiologic study pertinent to the age of the pediatric patient, provided the background for evaluation indications. It is anticipated that further refinement of present techniques, the development of new methods in the future, and correlation of data among the techniques while working closely with our adult electrophysiology colleagues, will furnish the pediatric electrophysiologist with the needed impetus to continue advancements in evaluation of the pediatric patient.

Acknowledgments

I thank Bob West, Lynn Rozler, Stacey Froemming, and Jane Pillen for their expert assistance in the Electrophysiology Cardiac Catheterization Laboratory. Also, I thank Joan Steffensmeier, Candy Heston, Janet Rau, Melodie Barnett, and Jim Griess for assuring high standards in developing and processing of film and photographic paper, and Margaret Marsh and Sheila Urbach for assuring high-quality Holter monitor ECG analysis and recording.

I thank Cathy Blodgett, RN, BSN; Cynthia Foreman, RN, BSN; Stephanie Goodrich; and especially Jeanine Armitage for their invaluable time and effort in preparing the manuscript. Also, I wish to express appreciation to Carl Gumbiner, M.D., for his review of the chapter.

References

1. Benson DW Jr, Benditt DG, Anderson RW, Dunnigan A, Pritzker MR, Kulik TJ, Zavoral JH: Cardiac arrest in young, ostensibly healthy patients: Clinical, hemodynamic, and electrophysiologic findings. *Am. J. Cardiol.* 52:65, 1983.
2. Weisfogel GM, Stein RA, Fernaine A, Krasnow N: Increasing pre-excitation during exercise and isoproterenol infusion. Evidence for a catecholamine sensitive bypass tract. *J. Electrocardiol.* 12(3):315, 1979.
3. Gallagher JJ, Gilbert M, Svenson RH, Sealy WC, Kasell J, Wallace AG: Wolff-Parkinson-White Syndrome: The problem, evaluation, and surgical correction. *Circulation* 51:767, 1975.
4. Sellers TD, Bashore TM, Gallagher JJ: Digitalis in the Pre-excitation Syndrome: Analysis during atrial fibrillation. *Circulation* 56:260, 1977.
5. Gillette PC, Garson A Jr, Kugler JD: Wolff-Parkinson-White Syndrome in Children: Electrophysiologic and pharmacologic characteristics. *Circulation* 60:1487, 1979.
6. Mehta AV, Pickoff AS, Raptoulis A, Wolff GS, Garcia OL, Tamer DF, Ferrer PL, Gelband H: Atrial flutter and atrial fibrillation associated with Wolff-Parkinson-White Syndrome in childhood. *Pediatr. Cardiol.* 1:197, 1980.
7. Byrum CJ, Wahl RA, Behrendt DM, Dick M:

Ventricular fibrillation associated with use of digitalis in a newbrom infant with Wolff-Parkinson-White Syndrome. *J. Pediatr.* 101:400, 1982.
8. Rowland TW: Augmented ventricular rate following verapamil treatment for atrial fibrillation with Wolff-Parkinson-White Syndrome. *Pediatrics* 72:245, 1983.
9. Gulamhusein S, Ko P, Klein GJ: Ventricular fibrillation following verapamil in the Wolff-Parkinson-White Syndrome. *Am. Heart J.* 106:145, 1983.
10. Jedeikin R, Gillette PC, Garson A Jr., Porter CJ, Beder S, Baron P, Zinner AJ, III: Effect of ouabain on the anterograde effective refractory period of accessory atrioventricular connections in children. *J. Am. Coll. Cardiol.* 1:869, 1983.
11. Lloyd EA, Hauer RN, Zipes DP, Heger JJ, Prystowsky EN: Syncope and ventricular tachycardia in patients with ventricular pre-excitation. *Am. J. Cardiol.* 52:79, 1983.
12. Surawicz B, Knoebel SB: Long QT: good, bad or indifferent? *J. Am. Coll. Cardiol.* 4:398, 1984.
13. Bricker JT, Garson A Jr., Gillette PC: A family history of seizures associated with sudden cardiac deaths. *Am. J. Dis. Child.* 138:866, 1984.
14. Mclntire MS, Freed AE: The Wolff-Parkinson-White Syndrome. *AMA Am. J. Dis.* 9:743, 1955.
15. Gillette, PC, DeBow F, McNamara D: A proposed autosomal dominent method of inheritance of the Wolff-Parkinson-White Syndrome and supraventricular tachycardia. *J. Pediatr.* 93:257, 1978.
16. Gallagher JJ, Sealy WC, Cox JL, Kasell JH: Results of surgery for preexcitation in 200 consecutive cases. In *Cardiac Arrhythmias From Diagnosis to Therapy* Levy S, Scheinman MM (eds.). Mount Kisco, Futura, 1984, p. 323.
17. Byrum CJ, Kavey RE, Deal BJ, Keane J, Safee B, Mueller W: Wolff-Parkinson-White Syndrome and supraventricular tachycardia presenting in the first four months of life: A multicenter investigation. (Submitted for publication.)
18. Engle MA: Wolff-Parkinson-White Syndrome in infants and children. *Am. J. Dis. Child.* 84:692, 1952.
19. Swiderski J, Lees MH, Nadas AS: The Wolff-Parkinson-White Syndrome in infancy and childhood. *Br. Heart J.* 24:561, 1962.
20. Giardina ACV, Ehlers KH, Engle MA: Wolff-Parkinson-White syndrome in infants and children. *Br. Heart J.* 34:839, 1972.
21. Wolff GS, Han J, Curran J: Wolff-Parkinson-White Syndrome in the neonate. *Am. J. Cardiol.* 41:559, 1978.
22. Garson A Jr, Gillette PC, McNamara DG: Supraventricular tachycardia in children: Clinical features, response to treatment, and long-term follow-up in 217 patients. *J. Pediatr.* 98:875. 1981.
23. Garson A Jr, Gillette PC: Electrophysiologic studies of supraventricular tachycardia in children. I. Clinical-electrophysiologic correlations. *Am. Heart J.* 102:233, 1981.
24. Gillette P: The Preexcitation Syndromes. In *Pediatric Cardiac Dysrhythmias*, Gillette PC and Garson A, Jr (eds.). New York, New York, Grune and Stratton, 1981, p. 153.
25. Deal BJ, Keane JF, Gillette PC, Garson A Jr: Wolff-Parkinson-White Syndrome and supraventricular tachycardia during infancy: Management and follow-up. *J. Am. Coll. Cardiol.* 5:130, 1985.
26. Kastor JA, Goldreyer BN, Josephson ME, Perloff JK, Scharf DL, Manchester JH, Shelburne JC, Hirshfeld JW Jr: Electrophysiologic characteristics of Ebstein's anomaly of the tricuspid valve. *Circulation* 52:987. 1975.
27. Kugler JD, Gillette PC, Duff DF, Cooley DA, McNamara DG: Elective mapping and surgical division of the bundle of Kent in a patient with Ebstein's anomaly who required tricuspid valve replacement. *Am. J. Cardiol.* 41:602, 1978.
28. Smith WM, Gallagher JJ, Kerr CR, Sealy WC, Kasell JH, Benson Jr DW, Reiter MJ, Sterba R, Grant AO: The electrophysiologic basis and management of symptomatic recurrent tachycardia in patients with Ebstein's anomaly of the tricuspid valve. *Am. J. Cardiol.* 49:1223, 1982.
29. Benson DW Jr, Gallagher JJ, Oldham HN, Sealy WC, Sterba R, Spach MS: Corrected transposition with severe intracardiac deformities with Wolff-Parkinson-White Syndrome in a child. *Circulation* 61:1256, 1980.
30. Gillette PC, Garson A Jr, Kugler JD, Cooley DA, Zinner A, McNamara DG: Surgical treatment of supraventricular tachycardia in infants and children. *Am. J. Cardiol.* 46:281, 1980.
31. Dick II M, Behrendt DM, Byrum CJ, Sealy WC, Stern AM, Hees P, Rosenthal A: Tricuspid atresia and the Wolff-Parkinson-White Syndrome: Evaluation methodology and successful surgical treatment of the combined disorders. *Am. Heart. J.* 101:496, 1981.
32. Benson DW Jr, Gallagher JJ, Spach MS, Barr RC, Edwards SB, Oldham HN, Kasell J: Accessory atrioventricular pathway in an infant: Prediction of location with body surface maps and ablation with cryosurgery. *J. Pediatr.* 96:41, 1980.
33. Rosenberg HS, Klima T, McNamara DG, Leachman RD: Atrioventricular communication in the Wolff-Parkinson-White Syndrome. *Am. J. Clin. Pathol.* 56:79, 1971.
34. Frais MA, Manyari DE, Duff HJ, Wyse DG, White AVM, Mitchell LB: Coexistent arrhyth-

mogenic right ventricular dysplasia and Wolff-Parkinson-White syndrome. *Am. J. Cardiol.* 53:632, 1984.
35. Bharati S, Strasberg B, Bilitch M, Salibi H, Mandel W, Rosen KM, Lev M: Anatomic substrate for preexcitation in idiopathic myocardial hypertrophy with fibroelastosis of the left ventricle. *Am. J. Cardiol.* 48:47, 1981.
36. Chen S, Fagan LF: Wolff-Parkinson-White syndrome in Marfan's syndrome. (Letter to the editor.) *J. Pediatr.* 84:301, 1974.
37. Chen WWC, Wong PHC, Chow JSF: Mitral valve prolapse and pre-excitation *PACE* 5:773, 1982.
38. Drake CE, Hodsden JE, Sridharan MR, Flowers NC: Evaluation of the association of mitral valve prolapse in patients with Wolff-Parkinson-White type ECG and its relationship to the ventricular activation pattern. *Am. Heart J.* 109:83, 1985.
39. Krikler DM, Davies MJ, Rowland E, Goodwin JF, Evans RC, Shaw DB: Sudden death in hypertrophic cardiomyopathy: associated accessory atrioventricular pathways. *Br. Heart J.* 43:245, 1980.
40. Belhassen B, Pauzner D, Blieden L, Sherez J, Zinger A, David M, Muhlbauer B, Laniado S: Intrauterine and postnatal atrial fibrillation in the Wolff-Parkinson-White Syndrome. *Circulation* 66:1124, 1982.
41. Epstein ML, Stone FM, Benditt DG: Incessant atrial tachycardia in childhood: Association with rate-dependent conduction in an accessory atrioventricular pathway. *Am. J. Cardiol.* 44:498, 1979.
42. Epstein ML, Benditt DG: Long-term evaluation of persistent supraventricular tachycardia in children: Clinical and electrocardiographic features. *Am. Heart J.* 102:80, 1981.
43. Kugler JD, Baisch SD, Cheatham JP, Latson LA, Pinsky, WW, Norberg W, Hofschire PJ: Improvement of left ventricular dysfunction after control of persistent tachycardia. *J. Pediatr.* 105:543, 1984.
44. Anderson RH, Bouton J, Burrow CT, Smith A: Sudden death in infancy: A study of cardiac specialized tissue. *Br. Med. J.* 20:135, 1974.
45. Montague TJ, Finley JP, Mukelabai K, Black SA, Rigby SM, Spencer CA, Horacek BM: Cardiac rhythm, rate and ventricular repolarization properties in infants at risk for sudden infant death syndrome: Comparison with age- and sex-matched control infants. *Am. J. Cardiol.* 54:301, 1984.
46. Kugler JD: Electrical instability. In *Cardiovascular Complications of Exercise*, edited by McManus B. Chicago, Year Book (in press, 1986).
47. Weissler AM, Warren JV: Vasodepressor syncope. *Am. Heart J.* 57:786, 1959.
48. Epstein SE, Stampler M, Beiser GD: Role of the capacitance and resistance vessels in vasovagal syncope. *Circulation* 37:524, 1968.
49. Klein GJ, Bashore TM, Sellers, TD, Pritchett ELC, Smith WW, Gallagher JJ: Ventricular fibrillation in the Wolff-Parkinson-White Syndrome. *N. Engl. J. Med.* 301:1080, 1979.
50. Bauernfeind RA, Wyndham CR, Swiryn SP, Palileo EV, Strasberg B, Lam W, Westveer D, Rosen KM: Paroxysmal atrial fibrillation in the Wolff-Parkinson-White Syndrome. *Am. J. Cardiol.* 47:562, 1981.
51. Tonkin AM, Miller HC, Svenson RH, Wallace AG, Gallagher JJ: Refractory periods of the accessory pathway in the Wolff-Parkinson-White Syndrome. *Circulation* 52:563, 1975.
52. Tonkin AM, Wagner GS, Gallagher JJ, Cope GD, Kasell J, Wallace AG: Initial forces of ventricular depolarization in the Wolff-Parkinson-White Syndrome: Analysis based upon localization of the accessory pathway by epicardial mapping. *Circulation* 52:1030, 1975.
53. Gallagher JJ, Pritchett ELC, Sealy WC, Kasell J, Wallace AG: The preexcitation syndromes. *Prog. Cardiovasc. Dis.* 20:285, 1978.
54. Rosenbaum FF, Hecht HH, Wilson FN, Johnson FD: The potential variations of the thorax and the esophagus in anomalous atrioventricular excitation (Wolff-Parkinson-White Syndrome). *Am. Heart J.* 29:281, 1945.
55. Prystowsky EN, Miles WM, Heger JJ, Zipes DP: Preexcitation Syndromes. *Med. Clin. N. A.* 68:831, 1984.
56. Garson A Jr, Gillette PC: Electrophysiologic studies of supraventricular tachycardia in children. II. Prediction of specific mechanism by noninvasive features. *Am. Heart J.* 102:383, 1981.
57. Wellens HJJ, Brugada P, Heddle WF: Value of the 12 lead electrocardiogram in diagnosing type and mechanism of a tachycardia: A survey among 22 cardiologists. *J. Am. Coll. Cardiol.* 4:176, 1984.
58. Bar FW, Brugade P, Dassen WRM, Wellens HJJ: Differential diagnosis of tachycardia with narrow QRS complex (shorter than 0.12 second). *Am. J. Cardiol.* 54:555, 1984.
59. Green M, Heddle B, Dassen W, Wehr M, Abdollah H, Brugada P, Wellens HIJ: Value of QRS alternation in determining the site of origin of narrow QRS supraventricular tachycardia. *Circulation* 68:368, 1983.
60. Benditt DG, Pritchett ELC, Gallagher JJ: Spectrum of regular tachycardias with wide QRS complexes in patients with accessory atrioventricular pathways. *Am. J. Cardiol.* 42:828, 1978.
61. Benson DW Jr, Smith WM, Dunnigan A, Sterba R, Gallagher JJ: Mechanisms of regular,

wide QRS tachycardia in infants and children. *Am. J. Cardiol.* 49:1778, 1982.
62. Bardy GH, Fedor JM, German LD, Packer DL, Gallagher JJ: Surface electrocardiographic clues suggesting presence of a nodofascicular Mahaim fiber. *J. Am. Coll. Cardiol.* 3:1161, 1984.
63. Dongas J, Lehmann MH, Mahmud R, Denker S, Soni J, Akhtar M: Value of preexisting bundle branch block in the electrocardiographic differentiation of supraventricular from ventricular origin of wide QRS tachycardia. *Am. J. Cardiol.* 55:717, 1985.
64. Gallagher JJ, Smith WM, Kasell JH, Benson DW Jr, Sterba R, Grant AO: Role of Mahaim fibers in cardiac arrhythmias in man. *Circulation* 64:176, 1981.
65. Sung RJ, Castellanos A, Mallon SM, Bloom MG, Gelband H, Myerburg RJ: Mechanisms of spontaneous alternation between reciprocating tachycardia and atrial flutter-fibrillation in the Wolff-Parkinson-White syndrome. *Circulation* 56(3):409, 1977.
66. Bardy GH, Packer DL, German LD, Gallagher JJ: Preexcited reciprocating tachycardia in patients with Wolff-Parkinson-White syndrome: Incidence and mechanisms. *Circulation* 70:377, 1984.
67. Klein GJ, Gulamhusein SS: Intermittent preexcitation in the Wolff-Parkinson-White Syndrome. *Am. J. Cardiol.* 52:292, 1983.
68. Williams RL: Use of transtelephonic electrocardiography in patients with symptoms suggesting cardiac arrhythmia. *Pediatrics* 61:493, 1978.
69. Dick M II, McFadden D, Crowley D, Rosenthal A: Diagnosis and management of cardiac rhythm disorders by transtelephonic electrocardiography in infants and children. *J. Pediatr.* 94:612, 1979.
70. Kugler JD, Yabek SM: Sick sinus syndrome: Clinical features and noninvasive evaluation. In *The Sinus Node in Pediatrics*, Yabek SM, Gillette PC, Kugler JD (eds.). London, Churchill Livingstone, 1984, p. 48.
71. Lamb LE: Multiple variations of WPW conduction in one subject. Intermittent normal conduction and a false positive exercise test. *Am. J. Cardiol.* 4:346, 1959.
72. Ahlborg B, Atterhog JH, Ekelund LG, Ericsson G: Pre-excitation in young men. *Acta Med. Scand.* 196:275, 1974.
73. Strasberg B, Ashley WW, Wyndham CRC, Bauernfeind RA, Swiryn SP, Dhingra RC, Rosen KM: Treadmill exercise testing in the Wolff-Parkinson-White Syndrome. *Am. J. Cardiol.* 45:742, 1980.
74. Force T, Graboys TB: Exercise testing and ambulatory monitoring in patients with preexcitation syndrome. *Arch. Intern. Med.* 141:88, 1981.
75. Butrous GS, Nathan AW, Bexton RS, Hellestrand KJ, Camm AJ: The effect of posture and exercise on the electrophysiological properties of direct atrioventricular accessory pathways. (Abstract.) *J. Am. Coll. Cardiol.* 3:612, 1984.
76. Bricker JT, Porter CBJ, Garson Jr A, Gillette PC, Mcvey P, Traweek M, McNamara DG: Exercise testing in children with the Wolff-Parkinson-White Syndrome. *Am. J. Cardiol.* 1985 95:1001, 1985.
77. Driscoll DJ, Heise CT, Staats BA: Techniques and goals of pediatric exercise testing. *J. Cardiovasc. Pul. Tech.* 13:6, 1983.
78. James FW, Blomquist GC, Freed MD, Miller WW, Moller JH, Nugent EW, Riopel DA, Strong WB, Wessel HU: American Heart Association Special Report, standards for exercise testing in the pediatric age group. *Circulation* 66:1377A, 1982.
79. Shafiroff BGP, Linder J: Effects of external electrical pacemaker stimuli on the human heart. *J. Thorac. Surg.* 33:544, 1957.
80. Gallagher JJ, Smith WM, Kasell J, Smith WM, Grant AO, Benson Jr DW: Use of the esophageal lead in the diagnosis of mechanisms of reciprocating supraventricular tachycardia. *PACE* 3:440, 1980.
81. Prystowsky EN, Pritchett ELC, Gallagher JJ: Origin of the atrial electrogram recorded from the esophagus. *Circulation* 61:1017, 1980.
82. Gallagher JJ, Smith WM, Kerr CR, Kasell J, Cook L, Reiter M, Sterba R, Harte M: Esophageal pacing: A diagnostic and therapeutic tool. *Circulation* 65:336, 1982.
83. Andersen HR, Pless P: Trans-esophageal pacing. *PACE* 6:674, 1983.
84. Critelli G, Grassi G, Perticone F, Coltorti F, Monda V, Condorelli M: Transesophageal pacing for prognostic evaluation of preexcitation syndrome and assessment of protective therapy. *Am. J. Cardiol.* 51:513, 1983.
85. Benson DW Jr, Dunnigan A, Sterba R, Benditt DG: Atrial pacing from the esophagus in the diagnosis and management of tachycardia and palpitations. *J. Pediatr.* 102:40, 1983.
86. Benson DW Jr, Dunnigan A, Benditt DG, Pritzker MR, Thompson TR: Transesophageal study of infant supraventricular tachycardia: Electrophysiologic characteristics. *Am. J. Cardiol.* 52:1002, 1983.
87. Benson DW Jr, Sanford M, Dunnigan A, Benditt DG: Transesophageal atrial pacing threshold: Role of interelectrode spacing, pulse width and catheter insertion depth. *Am. J. Cardiol.* 53:63, 1984.
88. Benson Jr DW, Dunnigan A, Schneider SP, Schiff J, Johnson W: Follow-up of infant paroxysmal atrial tachycardia: Transesophageal study. (Abstract.) *Circulation* 70 (suppl 11):11–

206, 1984.
89. Benson DW Jr, Dunnigan A, Benditt DG, Thompson TR, Narayan A, Boros S: Prediction of digoxin treatment failure in infants with supraventricular tachycardia: Role of transesophageal pacing. *Pediatrics* 75:288, 1985.
90. Dick II M, Campbell RM, Jenkins JM: Thresholds for transesophageal atrial pacing. *Cathet. Cardiovasc. Diagn.* 10:507, 1984.
91. Benditt DG, Pritchett ELC, Smith WM, Gallagher JJ: Ventriculoatrial intervals: Diagnostic use in paroxysmal supraventricular tachycardia. *Ann. Intern. Med.* 91:161, 1979.
92. Gonzalez MD, Guillen RH, Pellizzon OA, Raimondi EC: Study of Wolff-Parkinson-White Syndrome by transesophageal pacing and assessment of long-term amiodarone therapy. *Am. J. Cardiol.* 55:852, 1985.
93. Armstrong WF, Windle JR, Miles WM, Feigenbaum H, Prystowsky EN: Digital continuous looped two-dimensional echocardiographic analysis of the site of ventricular activation comparison with electrophysiologic mapping. (Abstract.) *Clin. Res.* 33(2):166A, 1985.
94. Botvinick E, Frais M, O'Connell W, Faulkner D, Scheinman M, Morady F, Sung R, Shosa D, Dae M: Phase image evaluation of patients with ventricular preexcitation syndromes. *J. Am. Coll. Cardiol.* 3:799, 1984.
95. Nakajima K, Bunko H, Tada A, Tonami N, Hisada K, Misaki T, Iwa T: Nuclear tomographic phase analysis: Localization of accessory conduction pathway in patients with Wolff-Parkinson-White Syndrome. *Am. Heart J.* 109:809, 1985.
96. Clapp SA, Driscoll DJ, Mitrani I, Lewis RM: Comparative effects of age and sedation on sinus node automaticity and AV node conduction. *Dev. Pharmacol. Ther.* 2:180, 1981.
97. Chazov EI, Shugushev KK, Rosenshtraukh LV: Ethmozin I. Effects of intravenous drug administration on paroxysmal supraventricular tachycardia in the ventricular preexcitation syndrome. *Am. Heart J.* 108:475, 1984.
98. Kerber RE, Martins JB, Kelly KJ, Ferguson DW, Kouba C, Jensen SR, Newman B, Parke JD, Kieso R, Melton Jeffrey: Self-adhesive preapplied electrode pads for defibrillation and cardioversion. *J. Am. Coll. Cardiol.* 3:815, 1984.
99. Neches WH, Mullins CE, Williams RL, Vargo TA, McNamara DG: Percutaneous sheath cardiac catheterization. *Am. J. Cardiol.* 30:378, 1972.
100. Hesslein PS, Mullins CE, Kugler JD, Gillette PC: Percutaneous sheath brachial vein cardiac catheterization in children. *Cathet. Cardiovasc. Diagn.* 6:197, 1980.
101. Latson L, Cheatham J, Kugler J, Hofschire P, Gumbiner C: Cardiac catheterization via the internal jugular vein in infants and children. Second World Congress of Pediatric Cardiology. (Abstracts) Springer-Verlag, New York, NY., 1985, p. 98.
102. Josephson ME, Scharf DL, Kastor JA, Kitchen JG: Atrial endocardial activation in man. Electrode catheter technique for endocardial mapping. *Am. J. Cardiol.* 39:972, 1977.
103. Prystowsky EN, Browne KF, Zipes DP: Intracardiac recording by catheter electrode of accessory pathway depolarization. *J. Am. Coll. Cardiol.* 1:468, 1983.
104. Jackman WM, Friday KJ, Scherlag BJ, Dehning MM, Schechter E, Reynolds DW, Olson EG, Berbari EJ, Harrison LA, Lazzara R: Direct endocardial recording from an accessory atrioventricular pathway: localization of the site of block, effect of antiarrhythmic drugs, and attempt at nonsurgical ablation. *Circulation* 68:906, 1983.
105. Shapiro JB, Kaltman AJ: Left atrial electrograms recorded through the patent foramen ovale. *Cathet. Cardiovasc. Diagn.* 6:89, 1980.
106. Mullins CE: Transseptal left heart catheterization: Experience with a new technique in 520 pediatric and adult patients. *J. Pediatr. Cardiol.* 4:239, 1983.
107. Klein, GJ, Prystowsky EN, Pritchett ELC, Davis D, Gallagher JJ: Atypical patterns of retrograde conduction over accessory atrioventricular pathways in the Wolff-Parkinson-White Syndrome. *Circulation* 60:1477, 1979.
108. Lloyd EA, Hauer RN, Zipes DP, Heger JJ, Prystowsky EN: Syncope and ventricular tachycardia in patients with ventricular preexcitation. *Am. J. Cardiol.* 52:79, 1983.
109. Milstein S, Klein GJ, Sharma AD: Nonclinical ventricular tachycardia in Wolff-Parkinson-White syndrome: A common, nonspecific phenomenon. (Abstract.) *Circulation* 70 (suppl 11):11–339, 1984.
110. Benditt DG, Benson DW Jr, Gornick CC, Dunnigan A: Effect of ventricular extrastimulus site on inducibility of atrial preexcitation during reciprocating tachycardia. (Abstract.) *Circulation* 70 (suppl 11):11–339, 1984.
111. Denes P, Wyndham CR, Amat-Y-Leon F, Wu D, Dhingra RC, Miller RH, Rosen KM: Atrial pacing at multiple sites in the Wolff-Parkinson-White Syndrome. *Br. Heart J.* 39:506, 1977.
112. Garcia OL, Castellanos A, Sung RJ, Gelband H: Exposure of concealed right bundle branch block in Wolff-Parkinson-White type B by pacing from the vicinity of the A-V node. *Am. Heart J.* 96:662, 1978.
113. Gillette PC, Garson A Jr, Cooley DA, McNamara DG: Prolonged and decremental antegrade conduction properties in right anterior

accessory connections: Wide QRS antidromic tachycardia of left bundle branch block pattern without Wolff-Parkinson-White configuration in sinus rhythm. *Am. Heart J.* 103:66, 1982.

114. Mitchell LB, Mason JW, Scheinman MM, Winkle RA, Burchell HW: Recordings of basal ventricular preexcitation from electrode catheters in patients with accessory atrioventricular connections. *Circulation* 69:233, 1984.
115. Weiss J, Brugada P, Roy D, Bar FWHM, Wellens HJJ: Localization of the accessory pathway in the Wolff-Parkinson-White Syndrome from the ventriculo-atrial conduction time of right ventricular apical extrasystoles. *PACE* 6:260, 1983.
116. Miles WM, Klein G, Zipes DP, et al.: The preexcitation index: A new method for determining accessory pathway location. (Abstract.) *Circulation* 68 (suppl 111):111–11, 1983.
117. Inoue H, Matsuo H, Takayanagi K, Ishimitsu T, Murao S: Antidromic reciprocating tachycardia via a slow Kent bundle in Ebstein's anomaly. *Am. Heart J.* 106:147, 1983.
118. Kuck KH, Brugada P, Wellens HJJ: Observations on the antidromic type of circus movement tachycardia in the Wolff-Parkinson-White Syndrome. *J. Am. Coll. Cardiol.* 2:1003, 1983.
119. Gallagher JJ, Sealy WC, Kasell J, Wallace AG: Multiple accessory pathways in patients with the pre-excitation syndrome. *Circulation* 54:571, 1976.
120. Cinca J, Valle V, Gutierrez L, Figueras J, Rius J: Reciprocating tachycardia using bilateral anomalous pathways: Electrophysiologic and clinical implications. *Circulation* 62:657, 1980.
121. Kaku T, Fukatani M, Kiya F, Hashiba K: Wolff-Parkinson-White syndrome with bilateral accessory pathways both exhibiting antegrade and retrograde conduction. *Am. Heart J.* 102:296, 1981.
122. Heddle WF, Brugada P, Wellens HJJ: Multiple circus movement tachycardias with multiple accessory pathways. *J. Am. Coll. Cardiol.* 4:168, 1984.
123. Morady F, Scheinman MM, DiCarlo Jr LA, Winston SA, Davis JC: Coexistent posteroseptal and right-sided atrioventricular bypass tracts: A previously unrecognized association. (Abstract). *Circulation* 70 (suppl 11):11–340, 1984.
124. Campbell RW, Smith RA, Gallagher JJ, Pritchett EL, Wallace AG: Atrial fibrillation in preexcitation syndrome. *Am. J. Cardiol.* 40:514, 1977.
125. Dreifus LS, Wellens HJJ, Watanabe Y, Kimbiris D, Truex R: Sinus bradycardia and atrial fibrillation associated with the Wolff-Parkinson-White Syndrome. *Am. J. Cardiol.* 38:149, 1976.
126. Morady F, Sledge C, Shen E, Sung RJ, Gonzales R, Scheinman MM: Electrophysiologic testing in the management of patients with the Wolff-Parkinson-White Syndrome and atrial fibrillation. *Am. J. Cardiol.* 51:1623, 1983.
127. Kugler JD, Pinsky WW, Cheatham JP, Hofschire PJ: Atrial muscle tachydysrhythmia in the young. (Abstract.) *J. Am. Cardiol.* 1:614, 1983.
128. Josephson ME, Seides SF: *Clinical Cardiac Electrophysiology: Techniques and Interpretations.* London, Henry Kimpton Publishers, 1979, p. 194.
129. German LD, Gallagher JJ, Broughton A, Guarnieri T, Trantham, JL: Effects of exercise and isoproterenol during atrial fibrillation in patients with Wolff-Parkinson-White syndrome. *Am. J. Cardiol.* 51:1203, 1983.
130. Bauernfeind RA, Swiryn SP, Strasberg B, Palileo E, Scagliotti D, Rosen KM: Electrophysiologic drug testing in prophylaxis of sporadic paroxysmal atrial fibrillation: Technique, application, and efficacy in severely symptomatic preexcitation patients. *Am. Heart J.* 103 (6):941, 1982.
131. Przybylski J, Chiale PA, Halpern MS, Nau GJ, Elizari MV, Rosenbaum MB: Unmasking of ventricular preexcitation by vagal stimulation or isoproterenol administration. *Circulation* 61:1030, 1980.
132. Wellens HJJ, Brugada P, Roy D, Weiss J, Bar FW: Effect of isoproterenol on the anterograde refractory period of the accessory pathway in patients with the Wolff-Parkinson-White Syndrome. *Am. J. Cardiol.* 50:180, 1982.
133. Cosio FG, Benson DW Jr, Anderson RW, Hession WT, Pritzker MR, Kriett JM, Benditt DG: Onset of atrial fibrillation during antidromic tachycardia: Association with sudden cardiac arrest and ventricular fibrillation in a patient with Wolff-Parkinson-White Syndrome. *Am. J. Cardiol.* 50:353, 1982.
134. Wu D, Amat-Y-Leon F, Simpson Jr RJ, Latif P, Wyndham CRC, Denes P, Rosen KM: Electrophysiological studies with multiple drugs in patients with atrioventricular re-entrant tachycardias utilizing an extranodal pathway. *Circulation* 56:727, 1977.
135. Bauernfeind RA, Swiryn S, Petropoulos AT, Coelho A, Gallastegui J, Rosen KM: Concordance and discordance of drug responses in atrioventricular reentrant tachycardia. *J. Am. Coll. Cardiol.* 2:345, 1983.
136. Wu D, Kou HC, Yeh SJ, Lin FC, Hung JS: Effects of oral verapamil in patients with atrioventricular reentrant tachycardia incorporating an accessory pathway. *Circulation* 67:426, 1983.
137. Kugler JD, Bansal AM, Cheatham JP, Pinsky WW, Mooring PK, Hofschire PJ: Drug-

electrophysiology studies in infants, children and adolescents. *Am. Heart J.* (In press, August 1985.)

138. Ferguson D, Saksena S, Greenberg E, Craelius W: Management of recurrent ventricular tachycardia: Economic impact of therapeutic alternatives. *Am. J. Cardiol.* 53:531, 1984.

19. NEW CATHETER TECHNIQUES FOR RECORDING ACCESSORY AV PATHWAY ACTIVATION

Warren M. Jackman

Few aspects of clinical electrophysiology are more intriguing than the variability in conduction properties of accessory AV pathways [1–6] and their unusual responses to antiarrhythmic agents [7–16]. Although potential mechanisms have been proposed [17], one of the greatest limitations to testing these hypotheses has been the inability to determine the location of conduction delay and block — that is, whether block occurs within the body of the accessory pathway or at the atrial or ventricular interface. Recently developed catheter techniques for recording accessory pathway activation [18–20] have provided useful tools for determining characteristics of impulse propagation across accessory pathways [19,21–23]. This chapter describes these new recording techniques and discuss some of their limitations.

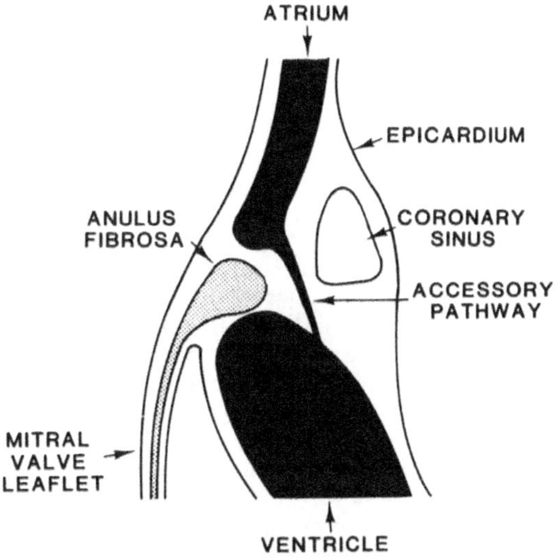

FIGURE 19–1. Diagrammatic cross-sectional view of the mitral anulus illustrating the typical course of left free-wall accessory AV pathways. Note the proximity of the accessory pathway to the coronary sinus or great cardiac vein. (Modified from Becker AE, Anderson RH, Durrer D, Wellens HJJ: The anatomical substrates of Wolff-Parkinson-White syndrome *Circulation* 57:870, 1978.)

Left Accessory AV Pathway Recordings

Left free-wall accessory AV pathways usually course on the epicardial side of the anulus fibrosa, close to the coronary sinus or great cardiac vein, connecting the epicardial surfaces of the left atrium and left ventricle [24,25] (Figure 19–1). Despite the proximity, there are no prior reports of accessory pathway potentials being recorded from catheter electrodes in the coronary sinus. The inability to identify discrete accessory pathway potentials may have

Supported by the American Heart Association, Oklahoma Affiliate, Young Investigator Award

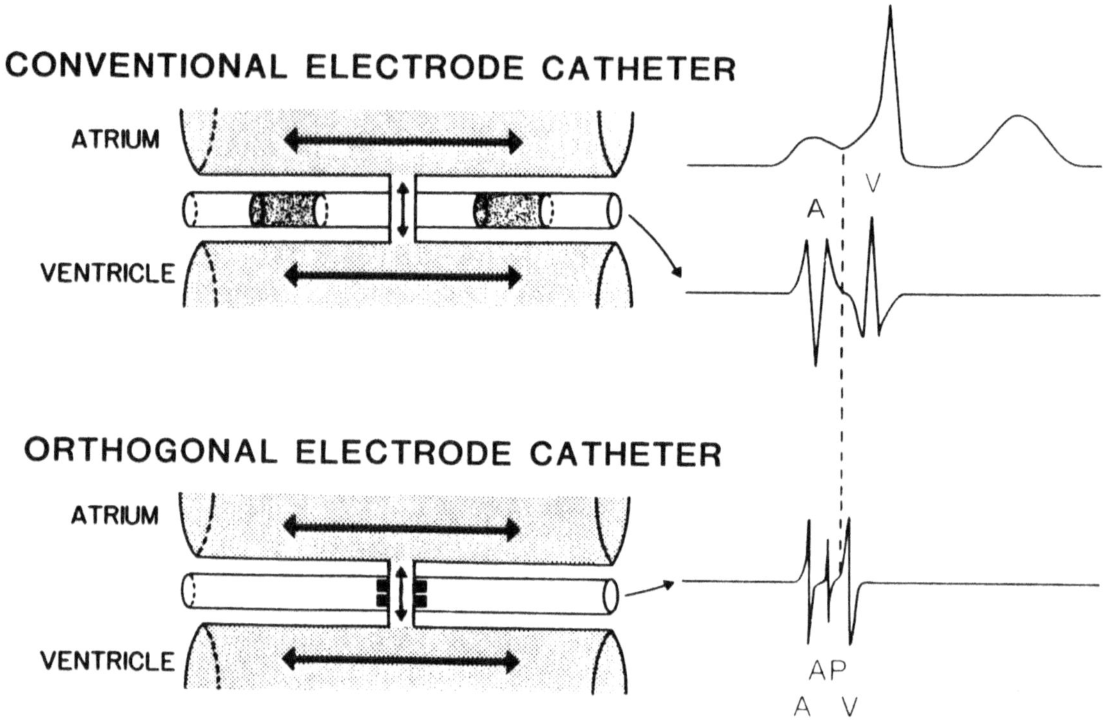

FIGURE 19–2. Schematic representation of the relationship between left-sided accessory AV pathways and catheter electrodes in the coronary sinus, as viewed from the endocardial surface of the left free-wall. Coarsely stippled areas represent atrial and ventricular myocardium and the myocardium of the accessory pathway (*unlabeled*). Arrows indicate the predominant direction(s) of electrical wavefronts traversing these regions of the base of the heart. Unfilled horizontal cylinder represents a catheter in the coronary sinus and the finely stippled or filled regions represent electrodes. (*Upper panel*) Conventional bipolar catheter electrode consisting of two ring electrodes separated usually by 5–10 mm. This relatively large electrode records atrial and ventricular activation from distant sites as well as locally, producing wide atrial (A) and ventricular (V) potentials (*right*). Combined with filtering artifact, these wide potentials tend to obscure local phenomena. Electrogram resolution (the ability to discriminate between two closely timed potentials) is decreased by increasing the interelectrode distance or by increasing the recording gain. (*Lower panel*): Orthogonal bipolar electrode arrangement consisting of two small electrodes aligned circumferentially such that the recording dipole is perpendicular to the long axis of the catheter and parallel the accessory pathway. When recorded at very low gain (<1 cm/mV), the close electrode spacing and orthogonal orientation minimize far field sensing and produce narrow, discrete local atrial and ventricular potentials which should not overlap the potential (AP) produced by activation of the accessory pathway (*right*). The dotted vertical line at right denotes the onset of the delta wave.

been a result of the recording techniques used. Conventional catheter bipolar electrograms are recorded between widely spaced (5–10 mm) ring electrodes with the recording dipole oriented parallel to the catheter. This electrode arrangement in the coronary sinus enhances the relatively large atrial and ventricular potentials propagating parallel to the catheter and minimizes the relatively small accessory pathway potentials propagating perpendicular to the catheter (Figure 19–2, upper panel). Unipolar electrodes also record activation from relatively large regions of atrial and ventricular myocardium, overshadowing accessory pathway activation. Consequently, it seemed reasonable to assume that low amplitude accessory pathway potentials could be enhanced while minimizing higher amplitude atrial and ventricular

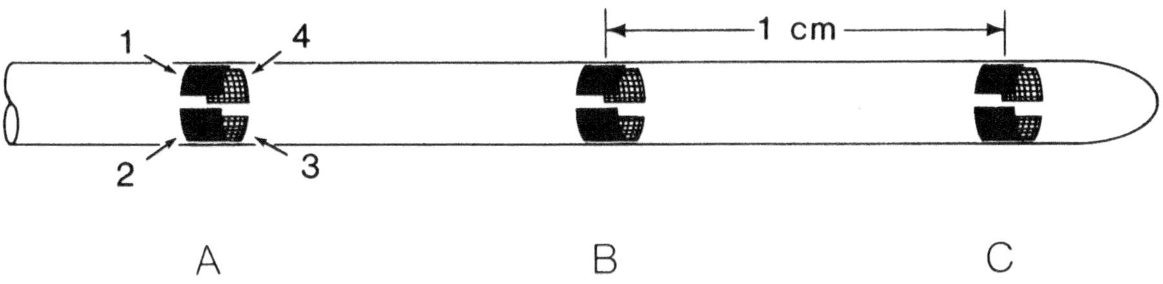

FIGURE 19–3. Schematic representation of the orthogonal electrode catheter used to record accessory pathway activation from the coronary sinus and great cardiac vein. Darkened areas represent electrodes, and *A*, *B*, and *C* mark the proximal, middle, and distal group or ring of electrodes. Each ring is composed of four separate electrodes spaced equally around the circumference of the catheter (interelectrode distance = 1.5 mm, center-to-center). The rings of electrodes are spaced at 1–cm intervals, center-to-center.

potentials by recording between closely spaced electrodes aligned across the circumference of the catheter. This creates a recording dipole oriented perpendicular to the long axis of the catheter and parallel to the accessory pathway (Figure 19–2, lower panel). An electrode catheter for recording in this manner was custom designed and fabricated by Webster Laboratories (Baldwin Park, California), [18]. This #6 French orthogonal catheter contains 12 small rectangular electrodes in three groups or rings of four electrodes. The four electrodes of each ring are spaced equally around the circumference of the catheter with an interelectrode distance of 1.5 mm, center-to-center (Figure 19–3). The longitudinal distance between rings of electrodes is 10 mm, center-to-center.

The orthogonal electrode catheter was utilized in the electrophysiologic studies of 18 patients with left accessory AV pathways. The catheter was inserted percutaneously into the left subclavian vein under local anesthesia and advanced via the coronary sinus into the distal great cardiac vein. Coronary sinus catheterization was facilitated by fluoroscopic imaging in the left anterior oblique projection. Three #6 French multipolar electrode catheters were inserted percutaneously into the right femoral vein and advanced to the right ventricular apex, His bundle region, and across the lateral endocardial surface of the right AV ring. The latter catheter was used to identify the location and record activation from right accessory AV pathways as described in the next section. The left AV ring was mapped during sinus rhythm or atrial pacing and during atrioventricular reentrant tachycardia or ventricular pacing by recording two orthogonal bipolar electrograms (for example, electrodes 1–2 and 2–3 in Figure 19–3) from each of the three electrode rings (A, B, and C). The catheter was slowly withdrawn from an initial position in the anterior great cardiac vein (when possible) to a proximal position where electrode ring A lies within the right atrium, outside of the coronary sinus os. The electrode positions along the coronary sinus and great cardiac vein were identified by fluoroscopic imaging in the left anterior oblique projection, using the His bundle and right ventricular electrodes to identify the septum. The coronary sinus electrograms were recorded at very low gain (usually <1 cm/mV) using a filter bandpass of 30–500 Hz. Accessory pathway potential amplitudes were measured from unfiltered electrograms (0.04–5000 Hz).

The improvement in electrogram resolution obtained by using the orthogonal electrode arrangement and recording at low gain is illustrated in Figure 19–4. The upper and lower coronary sinus electrograms (fourth and sixth tracings from the top, respectively) were recorded between longitudinal pairs of electrodes, mimicking the conventional electrode configuration. Despite the very low recording gain (0.5 cm/mV), the atrial and ventricular potentials are relatively wide and contain multiple components. This pattern suggests that the potentials contain signals of activation from relatively large regions of myocardium. The middle coronary sinus electrogram (fifth tracing from the top) was recorded between two adjacent orthogonal electrodes at the same low

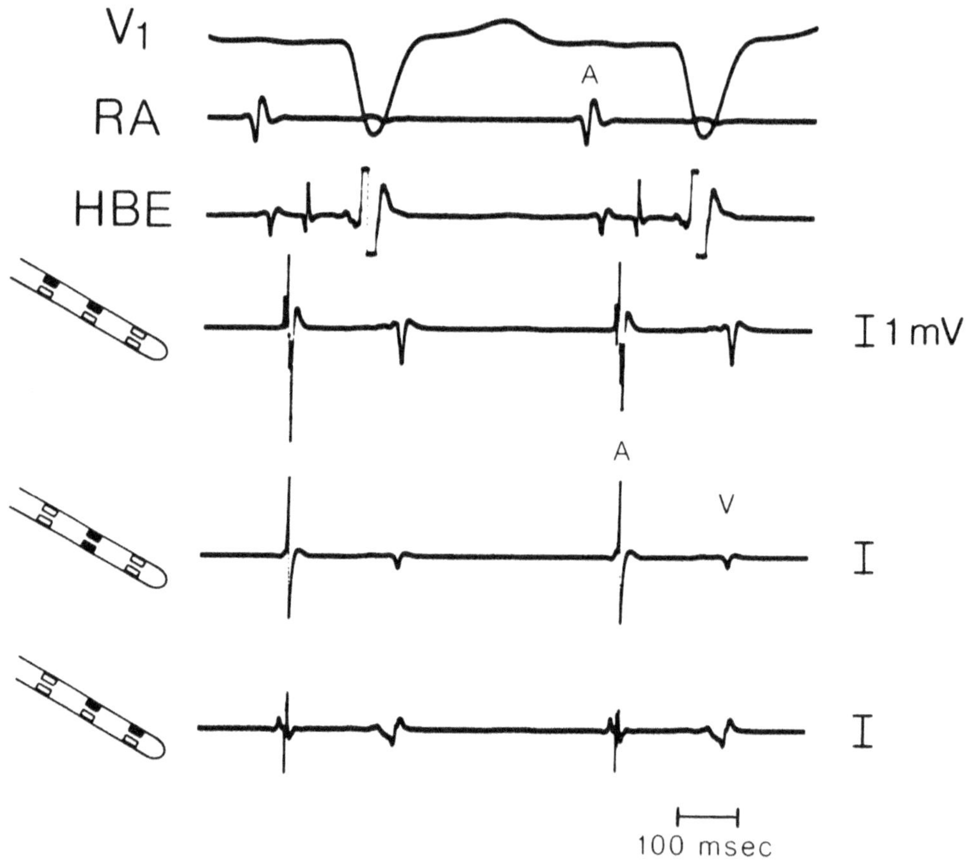

FIGURE 19–4. Resolution of low gain, orthogonal recordings from the coronary sinus in a patient who does not have an accessory pathway. Tracings from the top are ECG leads V_1, right atrial electrogram (RA), His bundle electrogram (HBE), and three electrograms recorded from the posterolateral coronary sinus. In this and all subsequent figures, a catheter symbol in the left margin indicates the electrogram was recorded from the coronary sinus using an orthogonal catheter, and the filled electrode symbols indicate which electrodes were used to record the tracing. All intracardiac electrograms in this and subsequent figures were recorded using a filter bandwidth of 30–500 Hz, unless labeled otherwise.

The middle coronary sinus electrogram (fifth tracing from the top) was recorded orthogonally at a recording gain of only 0.5 cm/mV. Note the brief, discrete atrial (A) and ventricular (V) potentials. The upper and lower coronary sinus electrograms (fourth and sixth tracings) were recorded from longitudinal bipolar electrodes (10 mm interelectrode distance) located just proximal and distal to the orthogonal electrode (one electrode was common to all three bipolar electrodes). Despite the same low recording gain, the atrial and ventricular potentials are wider and contain multiple components. The RA and HBE electrograms were recorded at low gain from conventional bipolar catheter electrodes (two ring electrodes separated by 5 mm). See text for discussion.

gain. This electrogram exhibits atrial and ventricular potentials which are discrete and narrow, implying that these tracings represent myocardial activation only in the immediate vicinity of the electrode. This restricted field of view allows two wavefronts passing close to the electrode less than 20 ms apart to be recorded as separate, discrete potentials.

These principles can be applied to record left free-wall accessory AV pathway activation. At some point during pullback of the coronary sinus catheter, one of the orthogonal electrodes will be positioned close to the midbody of the accessory pathway. During sinus rhythm or atrial pacing, the atrial wavefront propagates quickly through the restricted field of view of the electrode. Atrial activation is no longer being recorded 10–30 ms later when the accessory pathway (AP) potential is being inscribed. The result is two discrete, identifiable potentials (Figure 19–5, bottom two tracings). As the electrode position approaches the atrial insertion of the accessory pathway, the atrial and AP potentials occur too close in time to be inscribed as separate, discrete potentials (Figure 19–5, third tracing from top).

The same phenomena occur during AV reentrant tachycardia with retrograde conduction via an accessory AV pathway. A low gain recording from an orthogonal electrode close to the midbody of the accessory pathway records discrete ventricular, AP, and atrial potentials (Figure 19–6, bottom tracing). This is done while an electrode close to the atrial insertion of the accessory pathway records fused or indiscriminate AP and atrial potentials (Figure 19–6, fourth tracing from top). However, even in fused potentials the AP component can often be discerned by following the AP potential from the midbody region to the atrial insertion of the accessory pathway (Figures 19–5 and 19–6). Fused or indiscriminate potentials are usually seen only within 2–3 mm of the atrial or ventricular insertions (Figure 19–6).

After identifying discrete potentials near the sites of earliest retrograde atrial activation or earliest antegrade ventricular activation, the accessory pathway origin of the potential can be verified by excluding the likelihood that the potential represents either atrial or ventricular activation. During sinus rhythm or atrial pacing, the antegrade AP potential can be dissociated from atrial activation by the occurrence of block between the atrial and AP potentials as illustrated in Figures 19–7A and 19–8. In the absence of A–AP block, the antegrade AP potential can be dissociated from the atrium by introducing a ventricular extrastimulus which, by retrograde activation of the accessory pathway, advances the AP potential without affecting the atrial potential (Figures 19–7B and 19–9). During AV reentrant tachycardia or ventricular pacing, the retrograde AP potential can be dissociated from atrial activation by observing retrograde block between the AP and atrial potentials, as illustrated in Figure 19–7C. Retrograde AP potential can also be dissociated from atrial activation by introducing an atrial extrastimulus which advances atrial activation without affecting the retrograde AP potential (Figures 19–7D and 19–10A–C).

The antegrade AP potential can be dissociated from ventricular activation by the occurrence of block distal of the AP potential (Figures 19–11A and 19–12C), or by delivering a ventricular extrastimulus which advances ventricular activation without affecting the antegrade AP potential (Figures 19–11B and 19–9E). The retrograde AP potential can be dissociated from ventricular activation by the occurrence of block proximal to the AP potential (Figures 19–11C and 19–13), or by delivering an atrial extrastimulus which advances the AP potential without affecting the ventricular potential or the QRS complex (Figures 19–11D and 19–10D).

Further evidence that the AP potential actually represents accessory pathway activation results from the use of the orthogonal catheter for intraoperative mapping in five patients [26]. During normothermic cardiopulmonary bypass, the orthogonal catheter was inserted into the coronary sinus through a right atriotomy. The catheter was manipulated through the length of the coronary sinus and great cardiac vein during AV reentrant tachycardia or left ventricular pacing, until the retrograde AP potential was recorded from an orthogonal electrode at the catheter tip (this occurred in four of the five patients). A bipolar fingertip electrode was placed on the epicardium directly overlying the catheter tip with the electrodes oriented perpendicular to the AV groove and parallel to the orthogonal catheter electrodes. The epicardial electrode recorded

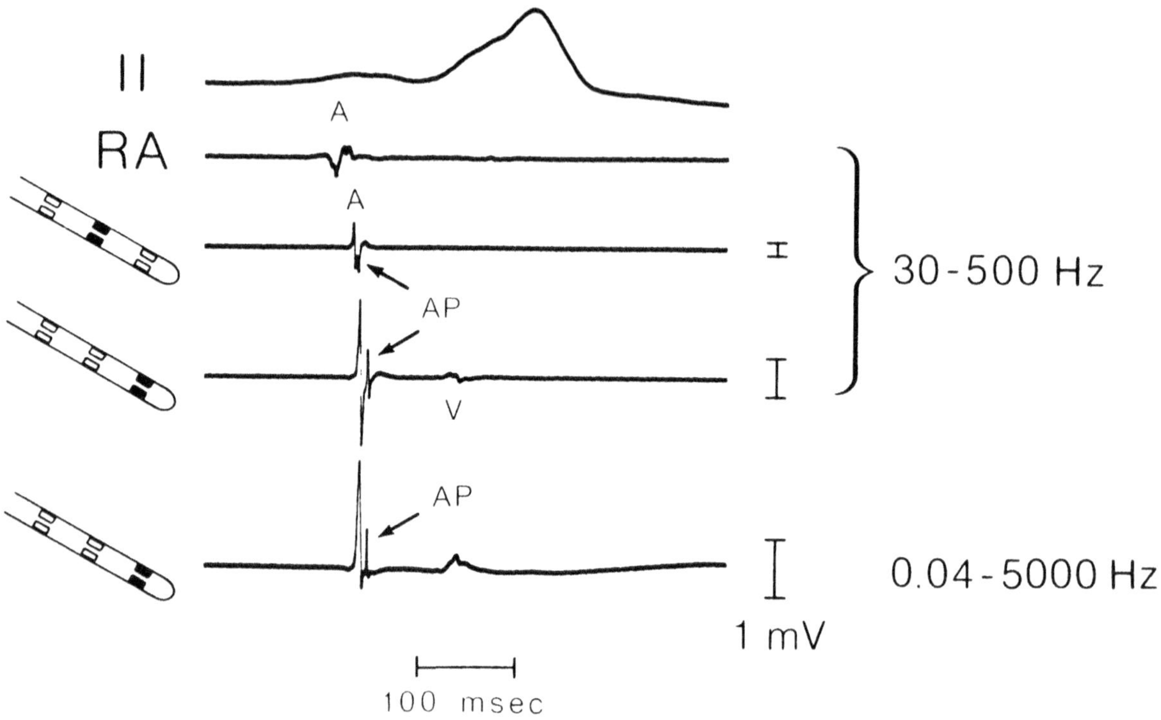

FIGURE 19–5. Orthogonal electrograms recorded from the *posterior* coronary sinus during sinus rhythm in a patient who has at least three left-sided accessory AV pathways, an overt anterior pathway and two pathways capable of antegrade conduction only intermittently, located at the posterior and lateral AV groove. Tracings from the top are ECG lead II, right atrial electrogram, orthogonal electrogram recorded from the middle electrode ring, orthogonal electrogram recorded from the distal electrode ring, and the same distal orthogonal electrogram recorded unfiltered (filter bandwidth 0.04–5000 Hz). The catheter was positioned close to the left posterior accessory AV pathway which was responsible for retrograde conduction during AV reentrant tachycardia. At the time of this recording the left posterior accessory pathway failed to excite the ventricle, and the delta wave evident in ECG lead II resulted from antegrade conduction via the left anterior accessory AV pathway.

The upper coronary sinus electrogram, recorded near the atrial insertion of the accessory pathway, reveals a single potential containing both atrial and accessory pathway (AP) components separated by less than 10 ms. The second coronary sinus electrogram, recorded near the mid-body of the accessory pathway, reveals separate, discrete atrial and AP potentials less than 15 ms apart. The greater time differential between the two potentials in this electrogram results from more rapid propagation *in the lateral direction* of the atrial wavefront as compared to that of the accessory pathway. The failure of this accessory pathway to activate the ventricular myocardium is reflected in the long interval (80 ms) between the AP potential and the local ventricular potential (V), and the finding that the local ventricular potential is inscribed after, rather than preceding, the onset of the delta wave. Unfiltered recordings are less likely to introduce artifactual components to the potentials, and occasionally provide easier separation of atrial, AP, and ventricular potentials (bottom tracing). The unfiltered AP potential amplitude = 0.8 mV.

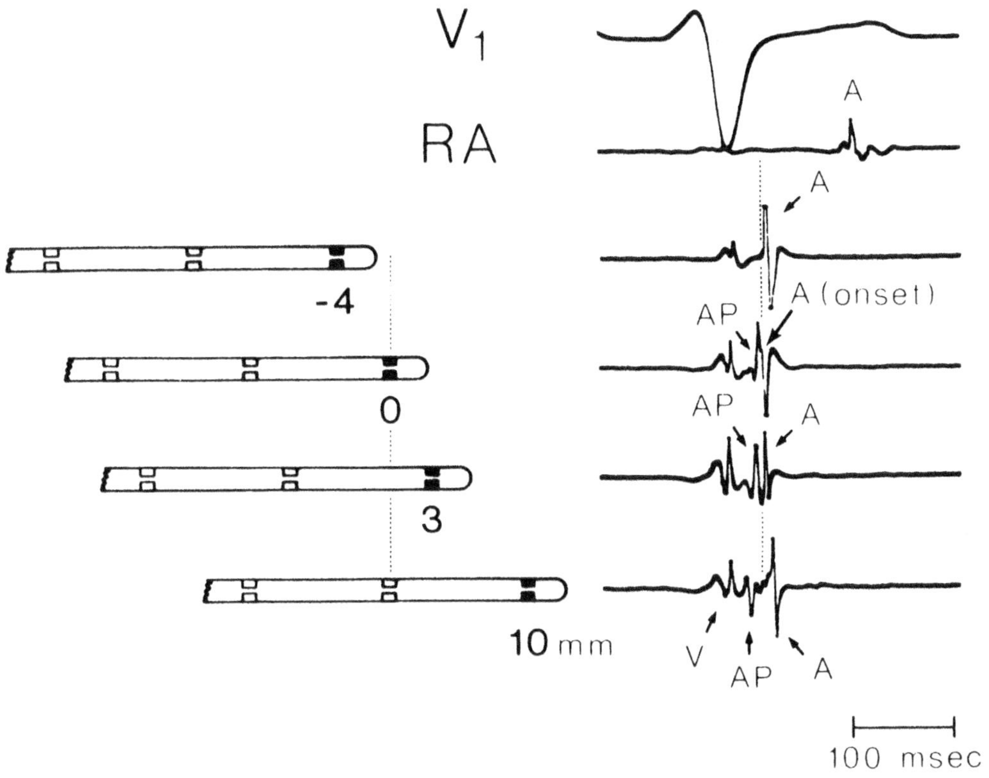

FIGURE 19–6. Orthogonal coronary sinus electrograms recorded during AV reentrant tachycardia in a patient with a concealed left lateral accessory AV pathway. The lower four tracings were recorded from the same orthogonal electrode during pullback of the catheter in the lateral coronary sinus. The catheter symbols at the left represent the relative location of the electrode in the coronary sinus at the time the tracing was recorded, and the numbers represent the distance in millimeters from the electrode site closest to the atrial insertion of the accessory pathway. These distances are estimated by interpolating the electrogram patterns as described later in the text.

The bottom tracing, recorded 10 mm distal (anterior) to the atrial insertion and close to the midbody of the accessory pathway, reveals discrete ventricular, retrograde AP, and retrograde atrial potentials. Retrograde AP and atrial potentials are still separable only 3 mm distal to the location recording fused AP and atrial potentials, presumably representing the atrial insertion of the accessory pathway (third and second coronary sinus electrograms). The vertical dotted line and the large arrow in the second coronary sinus electrogram identify an inflection point in the fused potential which probably represents the onset of retrograde atrial activation.

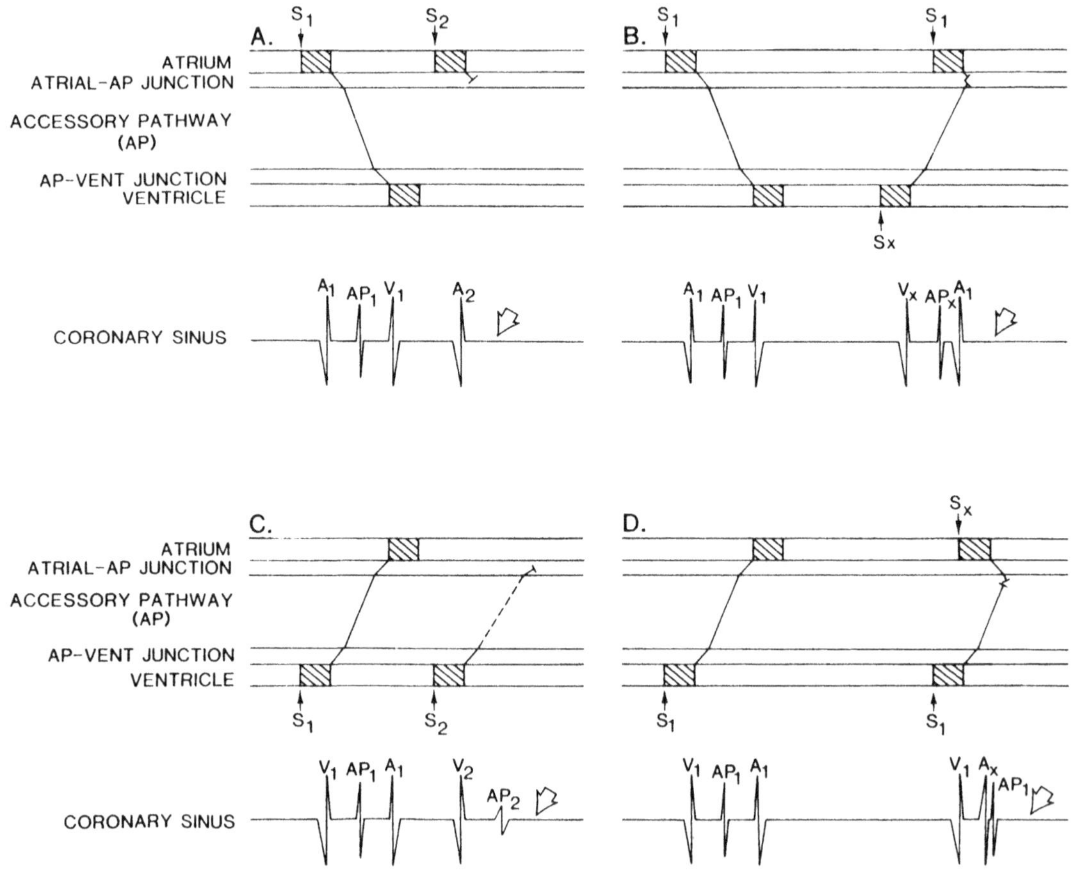

FIGURE 19–7. Programmed stimulation techniques used to verify that the AP potential does not represent activation of the atrial myocardium. The timing of activation of the accessory pathway and the adjacent atrial and ventricular myocardium is represented schematically in a ladder diagram and as an orthogonal electrogram recorded from the coronary sinus. Electrical stimuli are represented by vertical arrows labeled S. (A) Rapid atrial pacing or atrial extrastimulus (S_2) results in an atrial impulse (A_2) which fails to excite the accessory pathway. The absence of the AP potential (*unfilled arrow*) without loss of the local atrial potential (A_2) strongly suggests that the atrial and AP potentials result from activation of physiologically separate, if not anatomically separate, myocardial structures. (B) Ventricular extrastimulus (S_x) is introduced relatively late during atrial pacing (S_1) at constant cycle length, such that the resulting premature ventricular impulse (V_x) activates the accessory pathway in the retrograde direction, advancing the AP potential (AP_x) without altering the timing or morphology of the atrial impulse (A_1). The unfilled arrow marks the time the AP potential would have occurred if the accessory pathway had not been activated prematurely by the ventricular impulse. Since the field of view of the orthogonal electrode in the coronary sinus is probably far less than 1 cm, the ability to advance the AP potential by 15–20 ms without altering the atrial potential is probably sufficient evidence to establish that the atrial and AP potentials result from activation of separate structures. (C) During rapid ventricular pacing or the delivery of a ventricular extrastimulus (S_2), the loss of retrograde atrial activation (*unfilled arrow*) without the loss of the retrograde AP potential (AP_2) provides strong evidence that the retrograde AP and atrial potentials result from activation of separate structures. (D) Introduction of a late atrial extrastimulus (S_x) during ventricular pacing (S_1) at constant cycle length, advancing atrial activation (A_x potential) without altering the timing or morphology of the retrograde AP potential (AP_1). The unfilled arrow indicates the time the retrograde atrial potential would occur in the absence of the atrial extrastimulus. Advancing the atrial impulse (A_x) by 15–20 ms without altering the retrograde AP potential (AP_1) is probably sufficient to establish that these two potentials result from activation of different structures.

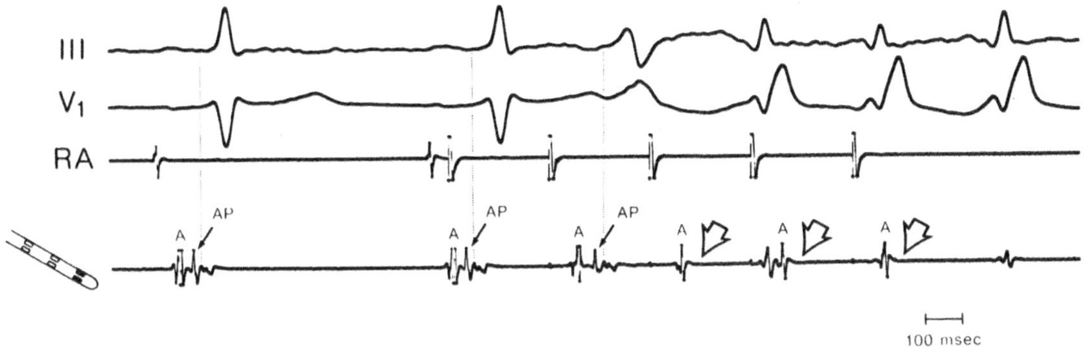

FIGURE 19–8. Use of rapid right atrial pacing to dissociate the atrial and AP potentials by producing conduction block at the atrial-accessory pathway interface. Small arrows mark the antegrade AP potentials and the large unfilled arrows mark the time the AP potential would have occurred had the final three atrial potentials (A) been successful in exciting the accessory pathway. The loss of the AP potential (associated with loss of ventricular preexcitation) without the loss of the local atrial potential, suggests that the atrial and AP potentials result from activation of separate structures. Note, in the presence of ventricular preexcitation, the onset of local ventricular activation (vertical dotted lines) precedes the onset of the delta wave in ECG leads III and V_1.

the AP potential in only two of the four patients. In all four patients, light pressure on the epicardial electrode resulted in loss of the AP potential in the catheter orthogonal electrograms and complete antegrade and retrograde block in accessory pathway conduction (Figure 19–14). Manipulation of the epicardial electrode at locations other than directly over the catheter electrodes recording the AP potential had no effect on accessory pathway conduction. Mechanically induced accessory pathway conduction block was always associated with loss of the AP potential.

There are at least two major pitfalls in identifying AP potentials from the coronary sinus. The first relates to the probability that many (if not all) of the left free-wall accessory pathways course laterally as well as vertically between the atrium and ventricle [22]. The atrial insertion of the accessory pathway is typically 10–15 mm medial or posterior to the ventricular insertion (closer to the coronary sinus os). Figure 19–15, recorded from the same patient as Figure 19–10, is a composite of five orthogonal electrograms recorded during the same episode of AV reentrant tachycardia. The top and second coronary sinus electrograms were recorded simultaneously from orthogonal electrodes on the proximal and middle rings, respectively. Coronary sinus electrograms 3 and 4 were recorded simultaneously from the proximal and middle rings, respectively, while the catheter was positioned approximately 14 mm distal to the position recording electrograms 1 and 2. The lowermost coronary sinus electrogram was recorded from the distal ring while the catheter was positioned 20 mm distal to the position recording electrograms 1 and 2. The relative location of each electrode is estimated by interpolating the timing and morphology of the potentials recorded from that electrode, between those recorded from the proximal, middle, and distal electrodes at some reference catheter position. For example, in Figure 19–15, the electrode distances are referenced to the middle electrode while the catheter was positioned to record the top and second coronary sinus electrograms (left vertical dotted line). When the catheter was positioned to record the third and fourth coronary sinus electrograms, the timing and morphology of the ventricular potential recorded from the proximal electrode was intermediate between those recorded from the middle and distal reference electrodes and slightly closer to that of the middle, placing this electrode approximately 4 mm distal to the middle reference electrode. When the catheter was positioned to record the lowermost electrogram, the potentials recorded from the proximal electrode were identical to those in the distal reference electrogram and intermediate between those of the proximal and middle electrodes

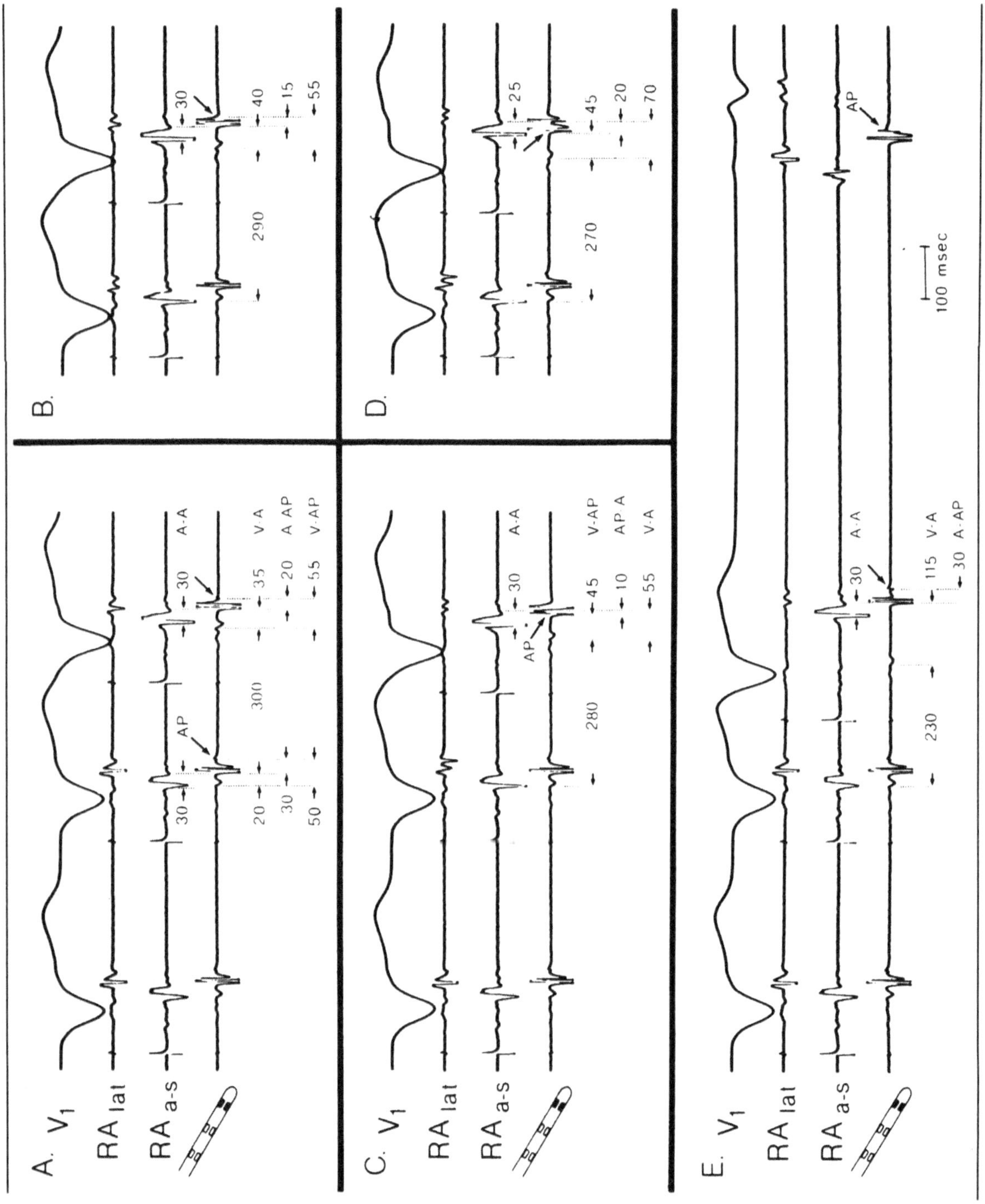
A. V1
RA lat
RA a-s
AP
30
300
A-A
V-A
A-AP
V-AP
B.
290
C. V1
RA lat
RA a-s
AP
280
V-AP
AP-A
V-A
D.
270
E. V1
RA lat
RA a-s
AP
230
115 V-A
30 A-AP
100 msec

FIGURE 19–9. Use of ventricular extrastimuli to dissociate the antegrade AP potential from atrial activation. Tracings from the top are ECG lead V_1, low lateral right atrial electrogram, anteroseptal right atrial electrogram (recorded close to the His bundle), and the orthogonal electrogram recorded from the coronary sinus in a patient with a left lateral accessory AV pathway. The first right ventricular pacing stimulus in panels B and D and the first two stimuli in panels A, C, and E are the last of ten drive stimuli at cycle length 400 ms. (A) During the right ventricular driving cycles the atrium is activated retrogradely via the AV node, and the atrial impulse is conducted to the left lateral AV groove before the pacing-induced ventricular impulse reaches the accessory pathway. Therefore, the accessory pathway is activated antegradely from the atrium. The antegrade AP potential, occurring 30 ms following the atrial potential in the coronary sinus electrogram, is identified by the first angled arrow. The ventricular extrastimulus (coupling interval = 300 ms) is associated with prolongation of the retrograde AV nodal conduction time, causing the atrial impulse to arrive near the coronary sinus electrode 35 ms after arrival of the ventricular impulse (V–A), compared to only 20 ms during the ventricular drive cycles. The accessory pathway was activated in the retrograde direction causing the AP potential (*arrow*) to be inscribed only 20 ms following the local atrial potential (A–AP). (B) Shortening the extrastimulus coupling interval to 290 ms results in further retrograde AV nodal conduction delay, causing the atrial impulse to arrive near the coronary sinus electrode 40 ms after the ventricular impulse. The accessory pathway is activated retrogradely by the ventricular impulse and the *end* of the AP potential (*arrow*), which is barely perceptible at the end of the local atrial potential, is inscribed 55 ms following the local ventricular potential. (C) Shortening the ventricular extrastimulus coupling interval to 280 ms results in further retrograde AV nodal conduction delay, causing the atrial impulse to arrive at the coronary sinus electrode 55 ms following arrival of the ventricular impulse (VA), an increase from 40 ms in panel B. The retrograde AP potential (*arrow*), *beginning* 45 ms following the ventricular potential, is now visible as a separate potential, preceding the arrival of the local atrial potential by 10 ms (AP–A). Note that the atrial potential is only 10 ms in duration. Since this potential has the same morphology and timing (30 ms following the atrial potential in the anteroseptal RA electrogram) as the preceding atrial potentials, it is likely that this potential represents the true atrial potential and the multiple components at the middle and end of the preceding atrial potentials may represent antegrade activation of other components of the accessory pathway apparatus. (D) Shortening the extrastimulus coupling interval to 270 ms results in further retrograde AV nodal conduction delay. The onset of the retrograde AP potential is unchanged from panel C at 45 ms following the local ventricular potential (V–AP). The local atrial potential now arises from retrograde activation via the accessory pathway as reflected by shortening of the A–A interval to 25 ms and change in the morphology of the atrial potential. (E) Further shortening of the ventricular extrastimulus coupling interval to 230 ms results in block of retrograde accessory pathway conduction while the atria continue to be activated retrogradely via the AV node. Retrograde accessory pathway block was associated with reappearance of the antegrade AP potential (*arrow*) 30 ms following local atrial activation (A–AP).

In Panels A–C, the 40 ms advance in timing of the AP potential, without altering the timing or initial morphology of the local atrial potential, strongly suggests that the atrial and AP potentials result from activation of separate structures. In Panel E, the abrupt increase in the interval from the local ventricular potential to the AP potential demonstrates that the ventricular and AP potentials must result from activation of separate structures. Since the AP potential represents neither atrial nor ventricular activation, it must by exclusion result from activation of the accessory pathway.

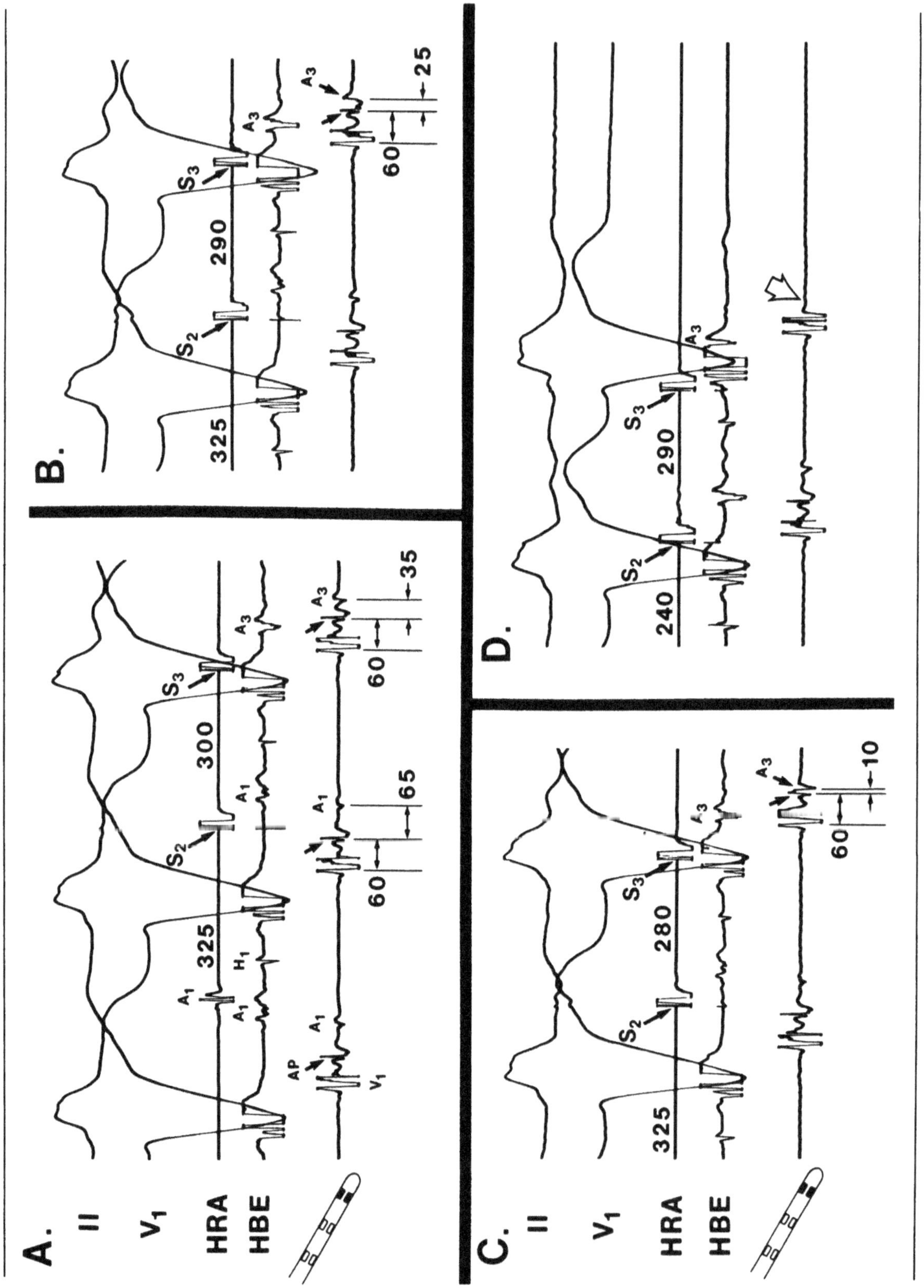
A.
II
V1
HRA
HBE
AP
V1
A1
H1
325
S2
300
S3
A3
60
65
35
B.
325
S2
290
S3
A3
60
25
C.
II
V1
HRA
HBE
325
S2
280
S3
A3
60
10
D.
240
S2
290
S3
A3

FIGURE 19–10. Use of atrial extrastimuli during AV reentrant tachycardia to dissociate the retrograde AP potential from both atrial and ventricular activation, in a patient with a concealed left lateral accessory AV pathway. (*A*) Two extrastimuli (S_2 and S_3) are delivered to the right atrium at coupling intervals of 325 ms and 300 ms. The first atrial extrastimulus does not alter the timing of atrial activation (A_1) in the His bundle or coronary sinus electrograms, and the retrograde AP potential (*arrow*) continues to follow the local ventricular potential by 60 ms and precede the local atrial potential by 65 ms. The second atrial extrastimulus (S_3) results in early antegrade atrial activation (A_3), shortening the interval between the AP and atrial potentials without affecting the timing or morphology of the AP potential (*arrow*). (*B*) and (C) As the coupling interval of the second atrial extrastimulus (S_2–S_3) is shortened to 290 ms and 280 ms, the interval between the AP (*arrow*) and atrial potentials is shortened to 25 ms and 10 ms, respectively, without affecting the timing or morphology of the AP potential. Since local atrial activation could be advanced 55 ms (AP–A interval shortened from 65 ms to 10 ms) without affecting the AP potential, it is unlikely that the AP potential represents atrial activation. (D) Shortening both right atrial extrastimulus coupling intervals to 240 ms and 290 ms results in antegrade activation of the accessory pathway, advancing the AP potential to within the ventricular potential. The unfilled arrow marks the absence of the retrograde AP potential. Since the AP potential could be displaced without affecting the timing or morphology of the local ventricular potential or the QRS complex (leads II and V_1), it is unlikely that the AP potential represents activation of the ventricular myocardium. Since the AP potential represents neither atrial activation nor ventricular activation, by exclusion the AP potential must represent activation of the accessory pathway. The long V–AP and AP–A conduction times are primarily a result of the long skewed (lateral) course of the accessory pathway (see Figure 19–15), but may also reflect residual amiodarone effects. Chronic amiodarone therapy was discontinued 6 weeks prior to study.

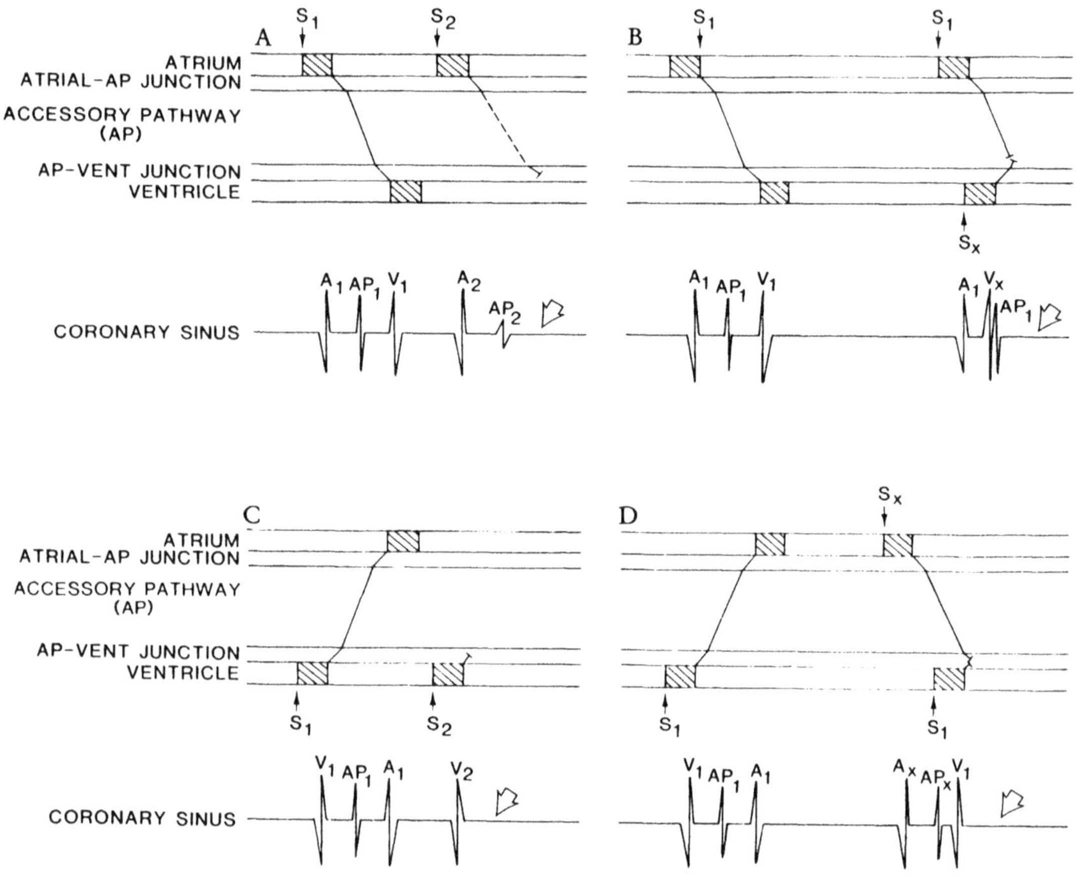

FIGURE 19–11. Programmed stimulation techniques used to verify that the AP potential does not represent activation of the ventricular myocardium. Format same as Figure 19–7. (A) During rapid atrial pacing or the delivery of an atrial extrastimulus (S_2) the absence of ventricular activation (*unfilled arrow*) without the loss of the AP potential (AP_2) provides strong evidence that the AP and ventricular potnetials result from activation of separate structures. (B) Delivering a late ventricular extrastimulus (S_x) during atrial pacing (S_1) at constant cycle length advances ventricular activation (V_x) without altering the timing or morphology of the antegrade AP potential (AP_1). The unfilled arrow indicates the time the antegrade ventricular potential would have occurred without the ventricular extrastimulus. Advancing the ventricular potential (V_x) by 15–20 ms without altering the antegrade AP potential (AP_1) is probably sufficient to establish the separate origin of the AP and ventricular potentials. (C) Rapid ventricular pacing or ventricular extrastimulus (S_2) results in a ventricular impulse (V_2) which fails to excite the accessory pathway. The absence of the AP potential (*unfilled arrow*) without loss of the local ventricular potential (V_2) strongly suggests separate origins for the ventricular and AP potentials. (D) Atrial extrastimulus (S_x) introduced relatively late during ventricular pacing (S_1) at constant cycle length results in early antegrade activation of the accessory pathway, advancing the AP potential (AP_x) without altering the timing or morphology of the ventricular impulse (V_1). The unfilled arrow marks the time the retrograde AP potential would occur in the absence of the atrial extrastimulus. The ability to advance the AP potential by 15–20 ms without altering the ventricular potential is probably sufficient evidence to establish separate origins for the AP and ventricular potentials.

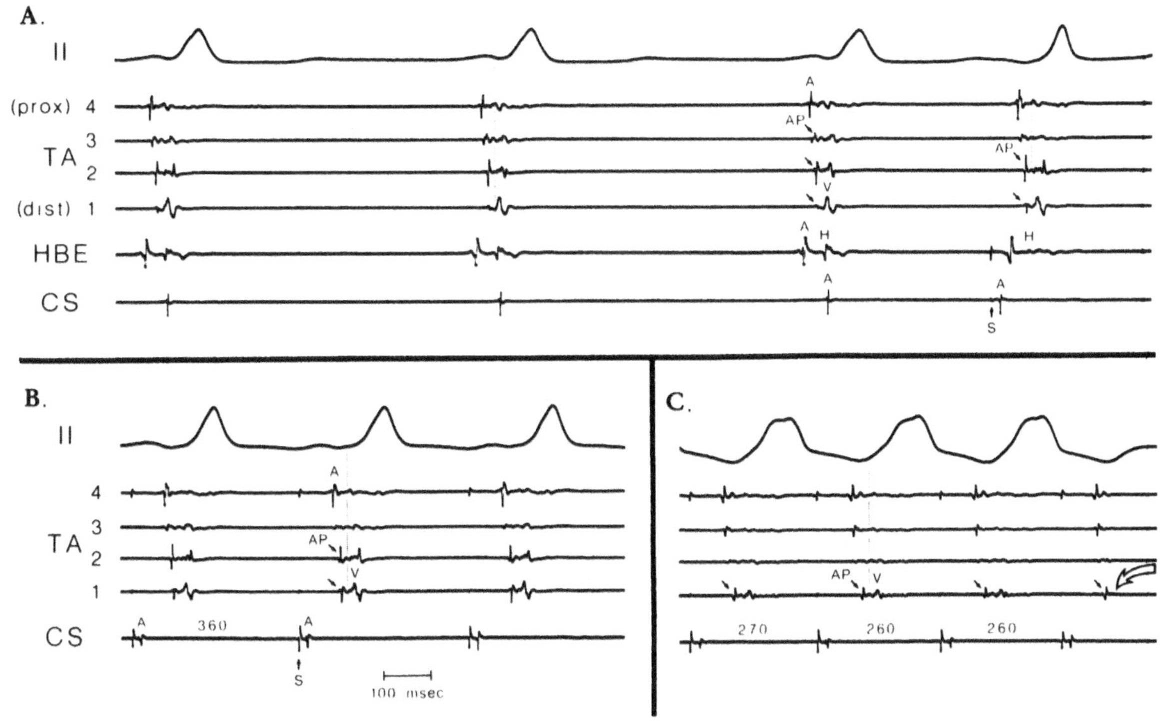

FIGURE 19–12. Use of rapid atrial pacing to dissociate the antegrade AP potential from ventricular activation in a patient with a right anterior accessory AV pathway. The four tricuspid anulus electrograms (TA) were recorded from a catheter with eight conventional ring electrodes spaced at 2 mm intervals, center-to-center (1 mm edge-to-edge). The catheter was positioned against the endocardial surface of the anterior tricuspid anulus, 1 cm anterior and lateral to the catheter recording the His bundle electrogram (which was also recorded at low gain between 2 mm spaced electrodes). Note the electrogram recorded between the two most proximal electrodes (TA-4) exhibits predominantly an atrial potential (A) while the electrogram recorded between the two most distal electrodes (TA-1) exhibits predominantly a ventricular potential (V). The coronary sinus electrogram was recorded at low gain from an orthogonal electrode in the posterolateral coronary sinus. (A) Sinus rhythm and, at the end of the tracing, a single left atrial pacing stimulus (S) delivered from the coronary sinus catheter. The antegrade AP potential (*arrow*) is seen emerging from the atrial potential in electrogram TA-3, propagating distally towards the ventricle in electrograms TA-2 and TA-1, and merging with the local ventricular potential (V) in electrogram TA-1. The vertical dotted line, which marks the onset of ventricular activation in TA-1, substantially precedes the onset of the delta wave in ECG lead II. (B) and (C) were recorded during decremental left atrial pacing (via the coronary sinus) and demonstrate the typical small increase in interval between local atrial activation and the AP potential, while the interval between the AP potential and the onset of local ventricular activation (*dotted line*) remains relatively constant. As the atrial pacing cycle length is shortened to 260 ms, antegrade block in accessory pathway occurs. The unfilled arrow in Panel C marks the absent ventricular potential. The persistence of the AP potential (*small filled arrow*) despite the loss of ventricular activation, verifies the AP potential does not represent ventricular activation. Note that each of the four TA electrograms exhibits discrete patterns, different from the adjacent electrograms, even though all four are recorded over a distance of only 14 mm. Further, slight changes in catheter position result in significant changes in each of the electrograms. This is illustrated by comparing Panels B and C, which were recorded during the same decremental atrial pacing run. In Panel C, the catheter had advanced slightly towards the ventricle, and electrogram TA-1 closely resembles electrogram TA-2 in Panel B, electrogram TA-2 resembles electrogram TA-3 in Panel B, and electrogram TA-3 resembles electrogram TA-4 in Panel B. These observations suggest that the closely spaced ring electrodes record myocardial activation only within a several millimeter distance of the electrode when recording at very low gain.

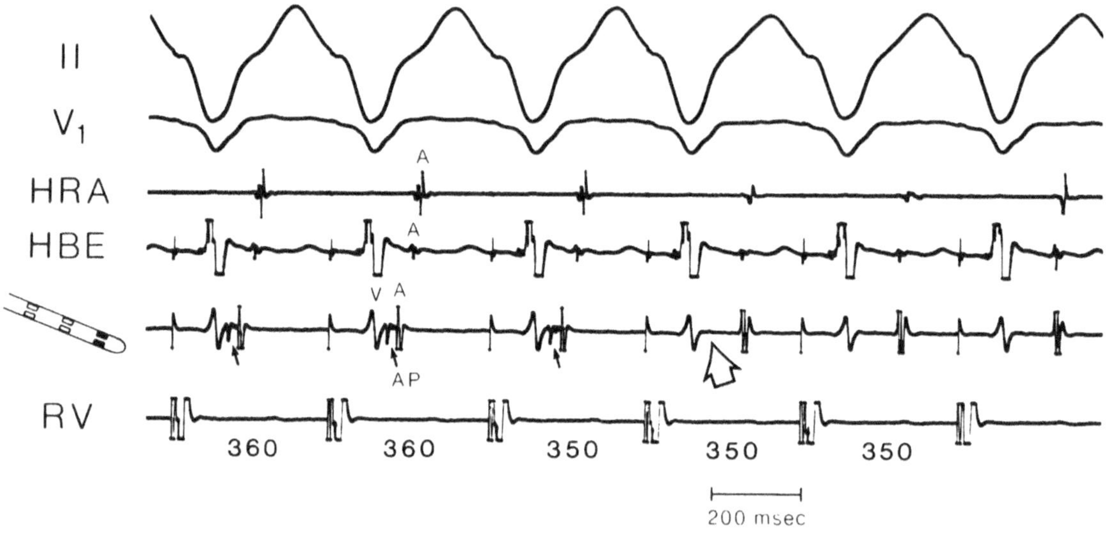

FIGURE 19–13. Use of rapid right ventricular pacing to dissociate the retrograde AP potential from ventricular activation in a patient with a left posterior accessory AV pathway (same patient as in Figure 19–8; however, this tracing was recorded following procainamide administration). As the ventricular pacing cycle length is shortened from 360 ms to 350 ms, retrograde block of accessory pathway conduction occurs, reflected by an abrupt increase in the VA interval and change in the retrograde atrial activation sequence. Note that retrograde accessory pathway block is associated with loss of the AP potential (*unfilled arrow*) without change in the timing or morphology of the local ventricular potential or the QRS complex. The loss of the AP potential without change in ventricular activation provides strong evidence that the AP potential does not represent activation of ventricular myocardium.

(slightly closer to the middle) when the catheter was positioned to record the third and fourth coronary sinus electrograms.

The resolution of this interpolation technique is estimated at 3–4 mm, because at least 3 discrete electrogram patterns are usually recorded from an electrode during catheter pullback before the electrogram mimicks the electrogram originally recorded 10 mm proximally (i.e., until the electrogram recorded from electrode C in Figure 19–3 mimicks the electrogram recorded initially from electrode B). In Figure 19–15, the retrograde AP potential is recorded earliest in the fourth coronary sinus electrogram. This electrode position is, presumably, the point along the coronary sinus which is closest to the ventricular insertion of the accessory pathway. As accessory pathway conduction proceeds in the retrograde direction, the AP potential is recorded from electrodes at progressively more medial locations until it merges with the earliest retrograde atrial potential in the second coronary sinus electrogram. Note that this electrode position, presumably the closest to the atrial insertion of the accessory pathway, is approximately 14 mm medial to the ventricular insertion site. Since retrograde atrial activation emanates from the site at which the AP and atrial potentials are fused, atrial activation is recorded *later* in the electrograms displaying the isolated AP potentials (electrograms 3 and 4). If one were to assume the accessory pathway traverses the AV groove exactly perpendicular to the coronary sinus, the AP potential would be sought only in the electrogram recording the earliest retrograde atrial potential (electrogram 2). Due to the limits of resolution of this technique (2–4 mm), a discrete AP potential, separate from the atrial potential, may not be identified in that electrogram. The actual AP potentials recorded more distally might be assumed to represent fragmented or delayed ventricular activation.

Another pitfall in identifying AP potentials is the small, often insignificant appearance of the atrial and ventricular potentials produced by these recording techniques. Although the position of the coronary sinus and great cardiac vein

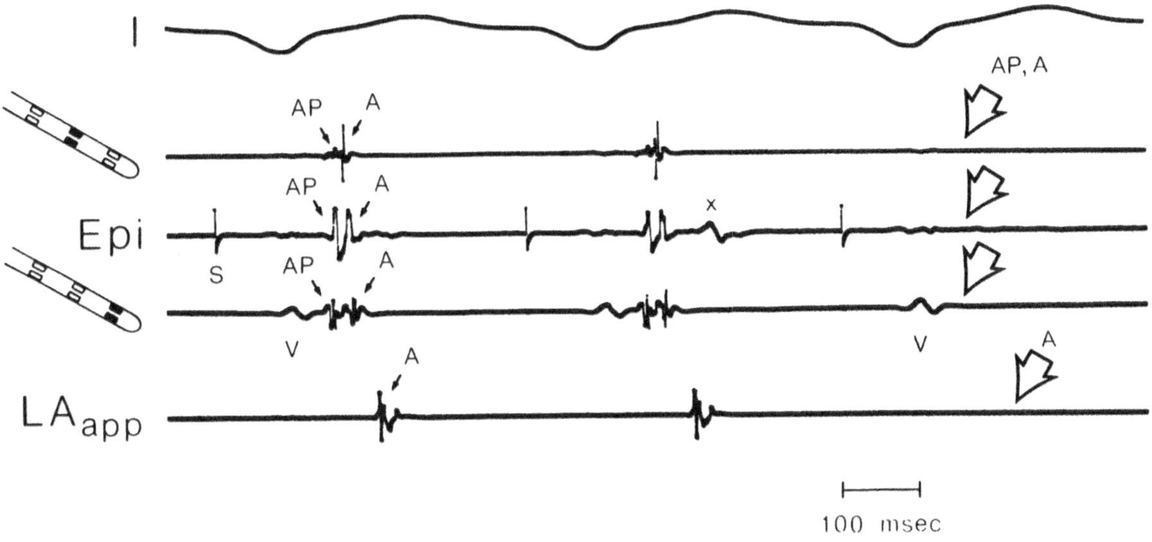

FIGURE 19–14. Intraoperative use of the orthogonal catheter to validate the accessory pathway origin of the AP potentials. These tracings were recorded during normothermic cardiopulmonary bypass in a patient with a left posterolateral accessory AV pathway, while pacing the left ventricular apex at cycle length 400 ms via an epicardial plaque electrode. The catheter was positioned in the posterolateral coronary sinus such that an orthogonal electrode on the distal ring (*fourth tracing from the top*) recorded potentials from the midbody of the accessory pathway, while an orthogonal electrode from the middle ring (*second tracing from the top*) recorded potentials close to the atrial insertion of the accessory pathway. A close bipolar roving electrode, placed on the epicardial surface of the AV groove directly over the catheter tip (*third tracing from the top*), also records accessory pathway activation (AP). The timing of the AP and atrial potentials in the epicardial electrogram (Epi) is intermediate between those recorded from the middle and distal orthogonal electrodes suggesting the epicardial electrode was located between the two catheter electrodes. The bottom tracing is a reference atrial electrogram recorded from a plaque electrode on the epicardial surface of the left atrial appendage. Note that the motion artifact (*X*) in the epicardial electrogram is followed by loss of retrograde atrial activation and the retrograde AP potential (*unfilled arrows*). The development of retrograde conduction block in the accessory pathway from light pressure on the epicardial electrode implies a very close relationship between the locations of the epicardial electrode and the accessory pathway. Further, the loss of the AP potential without change in the timing or morphology of the local ventricular potential (V) or the QRS complex, strongly suggests the AP potential does not represent activation of local ventricular myocardium (similar to Figures 19–11C and 19–13).

in the AV groove fatpad is variable, the coronary sinus tends to lie closer to the atrial myocardium near the os whereas distally the vein may lie closer to the ventricular myocardium. Because of very close electrode spacing and low recording gain, the ventricular potentials recorded from the proximal coronary sinus tend to be diminished (Figures 19–4, 19–5, 19–8, 19–9, and 19–14), whereas distally the atrial potentials tend to be greatly reduced (Figures 19–10 and 19–15). Since the AP potentials are enhanced by these recording techniques, they may be mistaken for the ventricular potential proximally or the atrial potential distally. For example, in Figure 19–10 the large retrograde AP potential might be mistaken for retrograde atrial activation, ignoring the small true atrial potential 65 ms later. The actual identity of the various potentials, however small, can be determined by the programmed stimulation techniques outlined in Figures 19–7 and 19–11. In Figure 19–10, the timing of the small late potential is advanced by the right atrial extrastimuli. This confirms an atrial origin.

Orthogonal electrode maps of the coronary sinus and great cardiac vein in the 18 patients identified the presence of *at least* 24 separate left-sided (≥5 mm distal to coronary sinus os) accessory AV pathways. The catheter could not be advanced far enough into the great cardiac

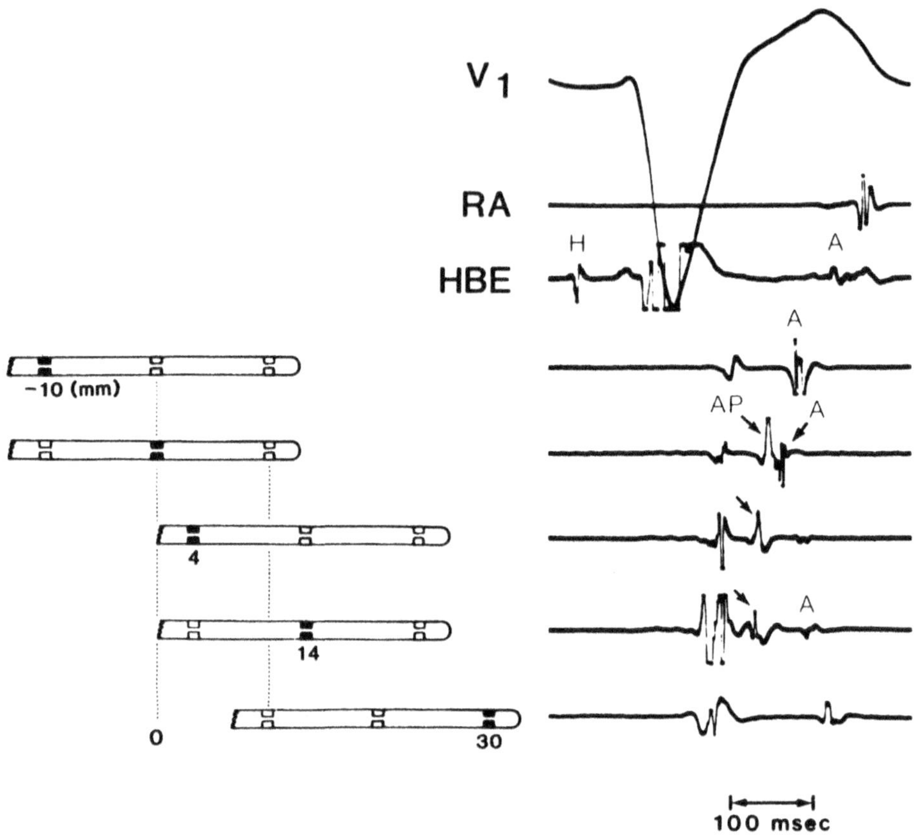

FIGURE 19–15. Composite of coronary sinus electrograms recorded during AV reentrant tachycardia in a patient with a concealed left lateral accessory AV pathway, demonstrating a substantial lateral component (14 mm) in the course of the accessory pathway between ventricle and atrium. The catheter symbols at the left margin indicate the relative position along the coronary sinus of the recording sites (distances listed in millimeters). Arrows on the left identify the retrograde AP potentials. See text for discussion.

vein to cross two lateral and two anterior pathways. Antegrade and retrograde AP potentials were recorded and could be dissociated from atrial and ventricular activation in 18 of the 20 accessible pathways, six of which demonstrated conduction only in the retrograde direction. The ability to record accessory pathway activation was independent of pathway location, as AP potentials were recorded from 6 of 7 posterior, 9 of 10 lateral, and all 3 anterior pathways crossed by the catheter. Fusion of the atrial and AP potentials (Figures 19–5, 19–6, 19–14, and 19–15), presumably representing the atrial insertion site, was recorded in the majority of patients. However, in several patients, fusion of the AP and ventricular potentials (Figure 19–8) was not recorded from any location in the coronary sinus. The inability to record activity from the ventricular insertion site may be explained by the histologic observations of Becker, Anderson, and coworkers. They found that while the atrial insertion of left free-wall accessory AV pathways is usually close to the anulus fibrosa (and the coronary sinus), the ventricular insertion is often some distance apically from the anulus [24,25] (Figure 19–1). These observations are supported electrophysiologically by Gallagher et al., who recorded and traced the AP potential from a left posterior pathway at surgery using a hand-held epicardial electrode [27] (Figure 19–16). The accessory pathway potential merged with the earliest ventricular potential on the epicardial surface of the ventricle, approximately 1 cm apical to the AV ring.

Right Accessory AV Pathway Recordings

The principles used for recording activation of left-sided accessory AV pathways are also applicable to right-sided pathways, namely: (1) closely spaced bipolar electrodes; (2) orienting the electrodes perpendicular to the anulus fibrosa; and (3) very low recording gain. However, the right AV ring is explored from the endocardial surface, using a catheter that lies across the tricuspid anulus. Since the catheter is oriented perpendicular to the anulus, the recording dipole of the electrodes should be parallel to the catheter. The author uses a #6 French catheter with eight conventional ring electrodes spaced at 2 mm, center-to-center (Webster Laboratories, Baldwin Park, California). The catheter is inserted percutaneously into the right femoral vein and advanced across the lateral right AV ring. Simultaneous tracings from four 2 mm spaced bipolar electrodes (electrodes 1–2, 3–4, 5–6, and 7–8), spanning a distance of only 14 mm, are recorded at very low gain (<1 cm/mV). Apposition of the electrode group to the endocardial surface of the tricuspid anulus is achieved when the proximal bipolar electrode records a sharp, discrete atrial potential with a diminutive, low frequency ventricular potential, while the distal electrode records a distinct ventricular potential with little or no atrial potential (Figure 19–12). All four electrograms are recorded during atrial pacing and during AV reentrant tachycardia (or ventricular pacing) as the catheter is advanced around the right AV ring in increments of less than 5 mm. The right AV ring is visualized fluoroscopically in the left anterior oblique projection, using the His bundle electrode and coronary sinus catheters as the principal septal landmarks. The origin of potentials arising near the sites of earliest antegrade ventricular activation or earliest retrograde atrial activation can be determined using the programmed stimulation techniques outlined in Figures 19–7 and 19–11.

Table 19–1 lists the results obtained using this approach in 17 patients with right-sided accessory AV pathways. AP potentials were identified in all seven patients with right septal accessory AV pathways, including one patient

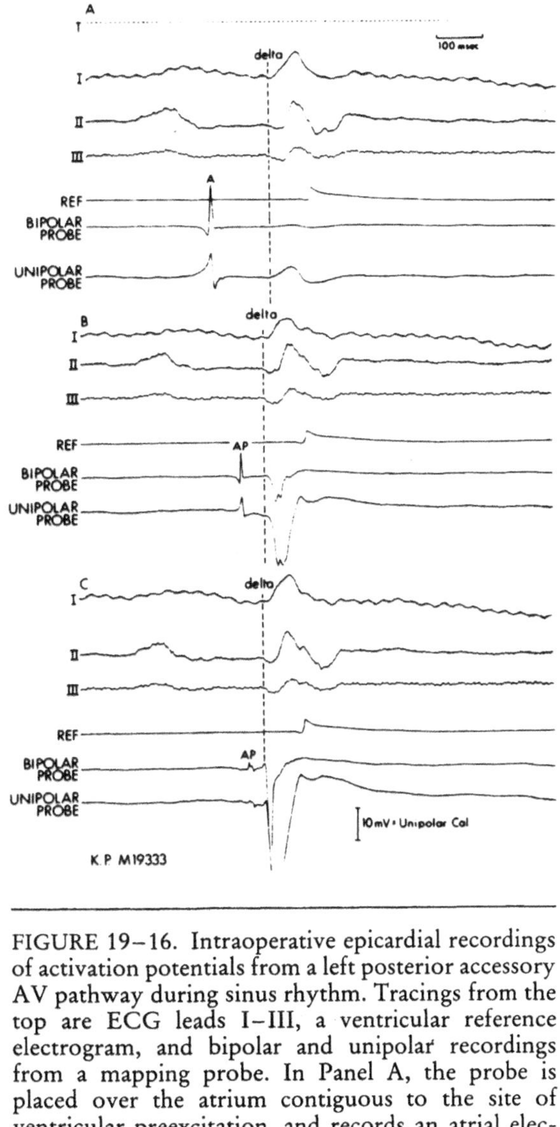

FIGURE 19–16. Intraoperative epicardial recordings of activation potentials from a left posterior accessory AV pathway during sinus rhythm. Tracings from the top are ECG leads I–III, a ventricular reference electrogram, and bipolar and unipolar recordings from a mapping probe. In Panel A, the probe is placed over the atrium contiguous to the site of ventricular preexcitation, and records an atrial electrogram (A). In Panel B, the probe is placed on the ventricular side of the AV groove and records a distinct AP potential. In Panel C, the probe is moved 1 cm distal (apical) to the AV ring and that electrode records the merging of the AP and local ventricular potentials, presumably representing the ventricular insertion of the accessory pathway. (Reproduced by permission from Gallagher JJ, Sealy WC, Anderson RW, Kasell J, Millar R, Campbell RWF, Harrison L, Pritchett ELC, Wallace AG: Cryosurgical ablation of accessory atrioventricular connections: a method for correction of the pre–excitation syndrome. *Circulation* 55:471, 1977.)

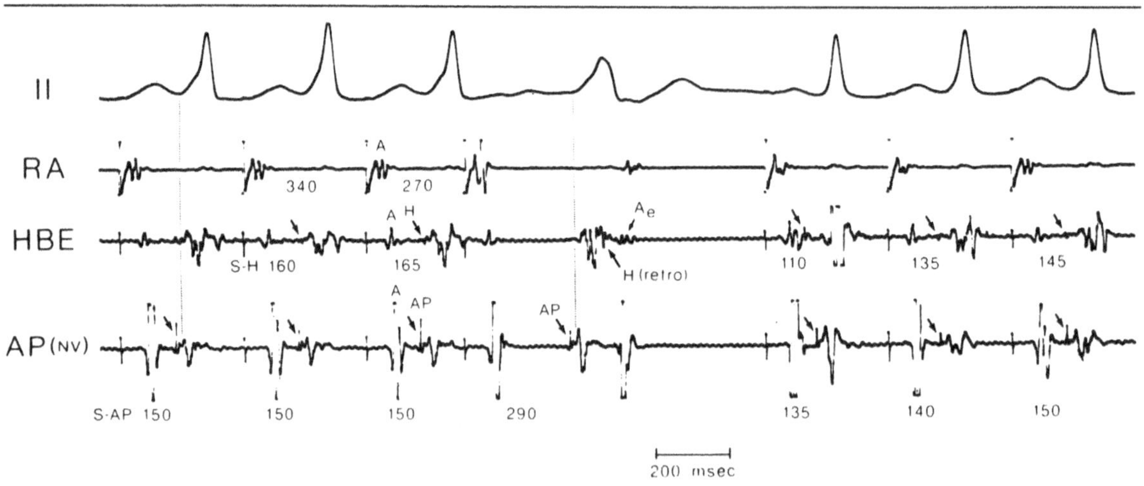

FIGURE 19–17. Direct recording of nodoventricular (NV) Mahaim fiber activation during atrial extrastimulus testing. The bottom electrogram, exhibiting the nodoventricular fiber potentials (*arrows, labeled AP*), was recorded from a bipolar catheter electrode (3 mm spacing, center-to-center) on the right ventricular endocardium approximately 7 mm apical and slightly inferior to the electrode recording the His bundle electrogram (HBE). Numbers below the AP electrogram indicate the interval from the right atrial pacing stimulus to the onset of the AP potential (SAP). The arrows above the HBE electrogram mark the His bundle potential (H), and the numbers below represent the interval from the right atrial pacing stimulus to the onset of the His bundle potential (S–H). The atrial extrastimulus results in an increase in S–AP interval from 150 ms to 290 ms which is followed by retrograde activation of the His bundle and an atrial echo complex. Note the AP potential always precedes local ventricular activation (*vertical dotted line*) by 25 ms which, in turn, always precedes the onset of the delta wave in ECG lead II.

with a nodoventricular (Mahaim) tract (Figure 19–17). Anteroseptal pathways were defined as those in which the AP potential was recorded in the immediate vicinity of the His bundle electrode. Two prior case reports demonstrated accessory pathway potentials recorded on the His bundle electrogram [28,29]. Midseptal accessory pathways were defined as those in which the AP potential was recorded posterior to the His bundle electrode and anterior to the coronary sinus os. Septal pathways recorded posterior to the coronary sinus os were labeled posteroseptal. In this small group of patients, no AP potentials were recorded from within the coronary sinus os (first 5 mm).

Activation potentials were recorded from 5 of 10 right free-wall accessory pathways (Table 19–1). The inconsistency of recording AP potentials in this group may result from several factors. Like left-sided pathways, some right free-wall pathways course on the epicardial side of the anulus fibrosa [25]. The endocardial electrodes may be too far from the accessory pathway to allow resolution between the AP and surrounding atrial and ventricular potentials. Another significant problem is the difficulty maintaining catheter contact with the free-wall. Modifying the catheter with a central lumen to accept a semirigid stylet is helpful in this regard [30]. Despite these limitations, Kuck and coworkers have had substantial success in identifying right free-wall accessory pathway activation potentials [20,23].

Summary

Potentials resulting from electrical activation of left free-wall accessory AV pathways can be recorded consistently from catheter electrodes in the coronary sinus by using closely spaced bipolar electrodes oriented perpendicular to the long axis of the coronary sinus and very low recording gain. Activation of right septal and free-wall accessory pathways can also be recorded from endocardial catheter electrodes, although not consistently. Again, close electrode spacing and low recording gain are important to prevent the overshadowing of the acces-

TABLE 19-1. Accessory pathway activation recorded from the right AV ring

Pathway location	Patients studied	AP potentials recorded
Septum		
anteroseptal	3*	3
midseptal	1	1
posteroseptal	3	3
Anterior wall	3	2
Lateral wall	5	2
Posterior wall	2	1
Total	17	12

* Includes 1 patient with a nodoventricular fiber.

sory pathway potential by surrounding atrial and ventricular activity. These techniques are beginning to allow the study of accessory pathway conduction in greater depth, much as His bundle electrocardiography facilitated study of the normal AV conduction system. From a clinical perspective, these techniques improve the localization of the pathways and increase the likelihood that the presence of multiple, closely spaced accessory pathways will be disclosed preoperatively. These factors should facilitate the surgical management of the Wolff-Parkinson-White syndrome and aid in the development of effective percutaneous catheter ablative techniques.

References

1. Coumel PH, Attuel P: Reciprocating tachycardia in overt and latent preexcitation. Influence of functional bundle branch block on the rate of tachycardia. *Eur. J. Cardiol.* 1:423, 1974.
2. Zipes DP, DeJoseph RL, Rothbaum DA: Unusual properties of accessory pathways. *Circulation* 49:1200, 1974.
3. Spurrell RAJ, Krikler DM, Sowton E: Retrograde invasion of the bundle branches producing aberration of the QRS complex during supraventricular tachycardia studied by programmed electrical stimulation. *Circulation* 50:487, 1974.
4. Neuss H, Schlepper M, Thormann J: Analysis of re-entry mechanisms in three patients with concealed Wolff-Parkinson-White syndrome. *Circulation* 51:75, 1975.
5. Wellens HJJ, Durrer D: The role of an accessory atrioventricular pathway in reciprocal tachycardia. Observations in patients with and without the Wolff-Parkinson-White syndrome. *Circulation* 52:58, 1975.
6. Tonkin AM, Gallagher JJ, Svenson RH, Wallace AG, Sealy WC: Antegrade block in accessory pathways with retrograde conduction in reciprocating tachycardia. *Eur. J. Cardiol.* 3:143, 1975.
7. Wellens HJJ, Bar FW, Dassen WRM, Brugada P, Vanagt EJ, Farre J: Effect of drugs in the Wolff-Parkinson-White syndrome: importance of initial length of effective refractory period of the accessory pathway. *Am. J. Cardiol.* 46:665, 1980.
8. Wellens HJJ, Durrer D: Effect of digitalis on atrioventricular conduction and circus movement tachycardias in patients with Wolff-Parkinson-White syndrome. *Circulation* 47:1229, 1973.
9. Dhingra RC, Palileo EV, Strasberg B, Swiryn S, Baurenfeind R, Wyndham C, Rosen KM: Electrophysiological effects of ouabain in patients with preexcitation and circus movement tachycardia. *Am. J. Cardiol.* 47:139, 1981.
10. Jedeikin R, Gillette PC, Garson A, Porter CJ, Beder S, Baron P, Zinner AJ: Effect of ouabain on the antegrade effective refractory period of accessory atrioventricular connections in children. *J. Am. Coll. Cardiol.* 1:869, 1983.
11. Rinkenberger RL, Prystowsky EN, Heger JJ, Troup PJ, Jackman WM, Zipes DP: Effects of intravenous and chronic oral verapamil administration in patients with supraventricular tachyarrhythmias. *Circulation* 62:996, 1980.
12. Gulamhusein S, Ko P, Carruthers SG, Klein G: Acceleration of the ventricular response during atrial fibrillation in the Wolff-Parkinson-White syndrome after verapamil. *Circulation* 65:348, 1982.
13. Hamer A, Peter T, Platt M, Mandel WJ: Effects of verapamil on supraventricular tachycardia in patients with overt and concealed Wolff-Parkinson-White syndrome. *Am. Heart J.* 101:600, 1981.
14. Harper RW, Whitford E, Middlebrook K, Federman J, Anderson S, Pitt A: Effects of verapamil on the electrophysiologic properties of the accessory pathway in patients with the Wolff-Parkinson-White syndrome. *Am. J. Cardiol.* 50:1323, 1982.
15. Barrett PA, Laks MM, Mandel WJ, Yamaguchi I: The electrophysiologic effects of intravenous lidocaine in the Wolff-Parkinson-White syndrome. *Am. Heart J.* 100:23, 1980.
16. Akhtar M, Gilbert CJ, Shenasa M: Effect of lidocaine on atrioventricular response via the accessory pathway in patients with Wolff-Parkinson-White syndrome. *Circulation* 63:435, 1981.
17. de la Fuente D, Sasyniuk B, Moe GK: Conduction through a narrow isthmus in isolated canine atrial tissue: a model of the W-P-W syndrome. *Circulation* 44:803, 1971.
18. Jackman W, Friday K, Bizouati G, Schechter E,

Olson E, Berbari E, Harrison L, Scherlag B, Lazzara R: New catheter system for recording accessory accessory AV pathway potentials from the coronary sinus. (Abstract). *J. Am. Coll. Cardiol.* 3:512, 1984.
19. Jackman WM, Friday KJ, Scherlag BJ, Dehning MM, Schechter E, Reynolds DW, Olson EG, Berbari EJ, Harrison LA, Lazzara R: Direct endocardial recording from an accessory atrioventricular pathway: localization of the site of block, effect of antiarrhythmic drugs, and attempts at nonsurgical ablation. *Circulation* 68:906, 1983.
20. Kunze K, Kuck K: Transvenous ablation of accessory pathways in patients with incessant atrioventricular tachycardia. (Abstract.) *Circulation* 70 (Suppl II): II–412, 1984.
21. Jackman W, Beck B, Aliot E, Friday K, Lazzara R: Basis for concealed accessory AV pathways. (Abstract.) *Circulation* 70 (Suppl II):II–337, 1984.
22. Jackman W, Friday K, Aliot E, Beck B, Lazzara R: Spatial orientation of atrial and ventricular insertions in left free-wall accessory AV pathways. (Abstract.) *J. Am. Coll. Cardiol.* 5:400, 1985.
23. Kuck K, Kunze K, Costard A: Further evaluation of intermittent Wolff-Parkinson-White syndrome by direct accessory pathway recording. (Abstract.) *Circulation* 70 (Suppl II):II–337, 1984.
24. Becker AE, Anderson RH, Durrer D, Wellens HJJ: The anatomical substrates of Wolff-Parkinson-White syndrome: a clinicopathologic correlation in seven patients. *Circulation* 57:870, 1978.
25. Becker AE, Anderson RH: The Wolff-Parkinson-White syndrome and its anatomical substrates. *Anat. Rec.* 201:169, 1981.
26. Harrison L, Jackman W, Friday K, Aliot E, Beck B, Lazzara R: Specialized catheter facilitates intraoperative mapping during WPW surgery. (Abstract.) *J. Am. Coll. Cardiol.* 5:399, 1985.
27. Gallagher JJ, Sealy WC, Anderson RW, Kasell J, Millar R, Campbell RWF, Harrison L, Pritchett ELC, Wallace AG: Cryosurgical ablation of accessory atrioventricular connections: a method for correction of the pre-excitation syndrome. *Circulation* 55:471, 1977.
28. Bharati S, Strasberg B, Bilitch M, Salibi H, Mandel W, Rosen KM, Lev M: Anatomic substrate for preexcitation in idiopathic myocardial hypertrophy with fibroelastosis of the left ventricle. *Am. J. Cardiol.* 48:47, 1981.
29. Prystowsky EN, Browne KF, Zipes DP: Intracardiac recording by catheter electrode of accessory pathway depolarization. *J. Am. Coll. Cardiol.* 1:468, 1983.
30. Gallagher JJ, Pritchett ELC, Benditt DG, Tonkin AM, Campbell RWF, Dugan FA, Bashore TM, Tower A, Wallace AG: New catheter techniques for analysis of the sequence of retrograde atrial activation in man. *Eur. J. Cardiol.* 6:1, 1977.

V. TREATMENT

20. PRACTICAL MANAGEMENT OF THE WOLFF-PARKINSON-WHITE SYNDROME

Edward L.C. Pritchett

The Wolff-Parkinson-White (WPW) syndrome is the arrhythmia syndrome that is understood best. It holds a special fascination for cardiologists interested in patients with arrhythmias. Speculation and deduction by electrocardiographers about the mechanisms of tachycardia in these patients have largely been confirmed by elegant studies done during the past 15 years using intracardiac recording and programmed stimulation with electrode catheters [1,2]. Intraoperative mapping of epicardial activation and successful operative treatment of these patients have further enhanced our understanding of this interesting syndrome [3,4].

Electrode catheter studies also have been used to measure the effect of antiarrhythmic drugs on conduction and refractoriness in the accessory atrioventricular (AV) connections and in the normal specialized conduction tissues of patients with the WPW syndrome. In the day-to-day management of specific patients, however, these studies add disappointingly little useful information. Precise knowledge of arrhythmia mechanism beyond what can be inferred from scalar electrocardiography is simply not necessary for most management; and objective changes in conduction times and refractory periods measured while a patient is taking antiarrhythmic drugs are not readily translatable into objective measures of drug efficacy.

While electrode catheter studies of these patients provided important information, they have attracted attention away from serious studies of antiarrhythmic therapy utilizing objective measures of chronic efficacy. There is a paucity of information from controlled clinical trials, and treatment remains largely based on anecdotal and uncontrolled clinical experience. The recommendations in this chapter have evolved over several years of treating patients referred to the Duke University Medical Center [5]. The present practice for patients being seen in this clinic is to initiate therapy based on electrocardiographic diagnosis of tachycardia and to change therapy based on electrocardiographic documentation of treatment failure. Patients with WPW syndrome may have more than one tachycardia. The only information required to initiate treatment of most patients with the WPW syndrome is electrocardiographic recordings during normal sinus rhythm and during each symptomatic tachycardia.

Documenting Tachycardia

An electrocardiogram recorded during tachycardia is the single most important piece of information that can be obtained for planning treatment. The first electrocardiogram showing a tachycardia is commonly recorded from these

Ann Clayton patiently coached the author in the challenging task of word-processing, and ultimately she transformed the text into a real manuscript. Patricia Hodgson edited the manuscript.

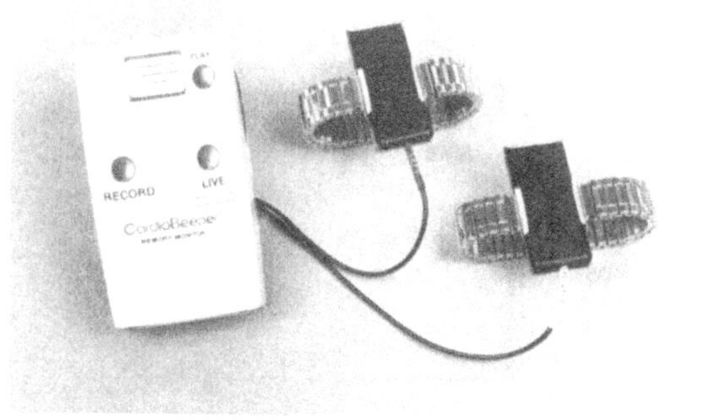

FIGURE 20–1. Transmitting device for sending electrocardiograms over the telephone. The black plates attached to the wrist bands are recording electrodes. This unit has a memory and may be used to record electrocardiograms for playback at a later time.

patients when they develop sustained symptoms of their arrhythmia and go to an emergency room. Emergency room physicians rarely provide continuing follow-up for patients treated acutely. Patients usually are referred to an internist or cardiologist for consultation and longterm management. It is the responsibility of this consultant to retrieve the electrocardiograms recorded during the patient's tachycardia. There is no possible way that a rational treatment program can be devised without precise knowledge of the arrhythmias and their associated symptoms that occur spontaneously; and there is simply no substitute for electrocardiographic documentation during each symptomatic tachycardia.

If a patient referred because of symptoms of tachycardia (e.g., palpitations) has not already had an electrocardiogram recorded during tachycardia, we now use telephone transmission of the electrocardiogram to document the cardiac rhythm during symptoms [6]. The transmitters are small, battery-operated devices about the size of a cigarette package (Figure 20–1). Several different models are available. We currently prefer a unit that has a memory, allowing patients to record their electrocardiogram in any remote location and to play it back over the telephone when convenient. The recording electrodes are small plaques that allow a selection of electrocardiogram leads depending on electrode placement. Most commonly, our patients use wrist bands to record electrocardiogram lead I.

The transmitting device modulates the electrocardiogram into an audible tone that is stored in a digital memory. The tone can then be played back over any convenient telephone and transmitted to our laboratory where it is received by a 24-hour-per-day, toll-free, answering device. The answering device demodulates the tone back into a scalar electrocardiogram rhythm strip of extremely high diagnostic quality.

The diagnostic quality achieved with this system is demonstrated by comparing an electrocardiogram that was made using a standard hospital recording instrument with electrocardiograms that were made using the telephone device (Figures 20–2 and 20–3). The 12-lead electrocardiogram recorded with a standard three-channel instrument shows normal sinus rhythm (Figure 20–2); a small Q wave in lead I is the delta wave. Figure 20–3 shows three electrocardiogram rhythm strips that were made using the telephone system. Panel A shows normal sinus rhythm; the small delta wave is present. Panel B shows orthodromic reciprocating tachycardia; the Q wave is missing because atrioventricular conduction is using the atrioventricular node exclusively. Panel C shows atrial fibrillation. The delta wave was missing also during this arrhythmia, which is recognized by the irregularly irregular rhythm. The beats showing an S wave in Panel C probably are the result of atrioventricular conduction over the atrioventricular node and aberrant intraventricular conduction.

We withhold therapy until the exact symptomatic arrhythmia has been confirmed by electrocardiogram. For most patients, it should be possible to document an arrhythmia within three months. If no tachycardia is recorded in that period, there seems little point in extending the observation time. Once an arrhythmia has been diagnosed, the patient can be treated according to the principles outlined below.

Ventricular Fibrillation

Fortunately ventricular fibrillation is an uncommon event in patients with the WPW syndrome. However, it is discussed first here because the spectre of it colors the discussion of all other arrhythmias that occur in this syndrome. Klein et al. reported 31 patients with the WPW syndrome and ventricular fibrillation who were referred to Duke University Medical Center for electrophysiology study between 1970 and 1979

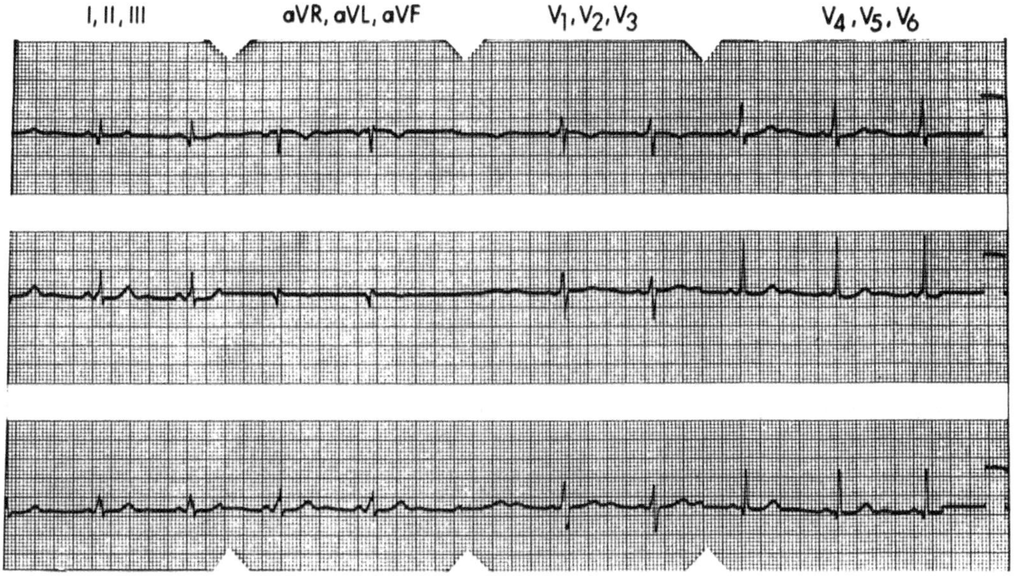

FIGURE 20–2. Twelve-lead electrocardiogram from a patient with the Wolff-Parkinson-White syndrome. The delta wave is seen as a small Q wave in lead I. Rhythm strips from this patient are shown in Figure 20–3.

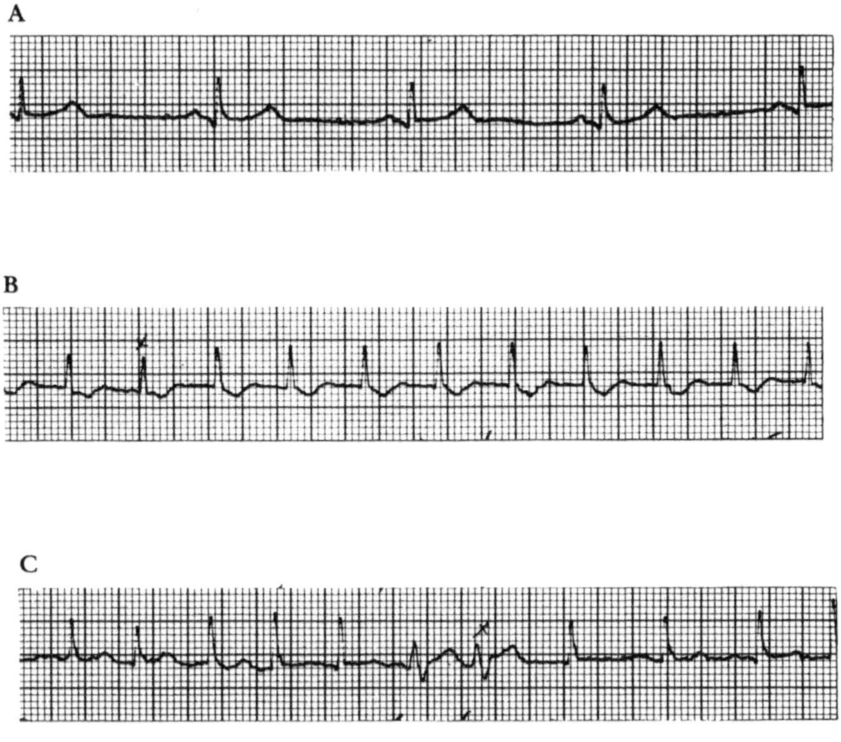

FIGURE 20–3. Electrocardiogram rhythm strips recorded from a patient with the Wolff-Parkinson-White syndrome. (A) shows normal sinus rhythm; the small Q wave is the delta wave (compare with lead I of the electrocardiogram from the same patient shown in Figure 20–2). The other two rhythm strips show orthodromic reciprocating tachycardia (B) and atrial fibrillation (C). These electrocardiograms were recorded using our telephone transmitting and recording system.

[7]. Ventricular fibrillation was thought to have resulted from atrial fibrillation in 25 of these patients. Factors predisposing to ventricular fibrillation were: (1) a history of both atrial fibrillation and orthodromic reciprocating tachycardia, (2) rapid ventricular rates measured during induced atrial fibrillation, and (3) presence of multiple accessory atrioventricular connections. Probably most of these 25 patients had orthodromic reciprocating tachycardia as their primary arrhythmia. This reentrant arrhythmia precipitated atrial fibrillation, during which there was rapid conduction to the ventricles over the accessory atrioventricular connection (or connections) leading to ventricular fibrillation. In general, all patients who have ventricular fibrillation as a result of their accessory atrioventricular connections should be considered candidates for surgical treatment and should be referred for study to a center where surgery is performed.

Atrial Fibrillation

LONG TERM MANAGEMENT

Atrial fibrillation is more common than ventricular fibrillation and less common than orthodromic reciprocating tachycardia. Many patients develop atrial fibrillation during the course of an attack of orthodromic reciprocating tachycardia; one-fifth of all patients with this reentrant tachycardia may develop atrial fibrillation at some time [8–10]. In addition, some patients whose accessory AV connections conduct exclusively in the antegrade direction develop atrial fibrillation as a primary arrhythmia when they get older [11]. These latter patients are not subject to reciprocating tachycardia because their accessory connections do not conduct in the retrograde direction.

The QRS complexes that are recorded during atrial fibrillation may be all preexcited, all normal, or a mixture of preexcited and normal. To have all normally conducted beats is uncommon; most patients have some or all preexcited beats [4]. The mix in population of QRS morphologies is due to concealed penetration of some impulses into the accessory AV connection in both the antegrade and retrograde directions [12].

Klein and Gulamhusein have suggested that accessory AV connections that lack the ability to conduct rapidly in the antegrade direction during atrial fibrillation can be identified by a distinctive electrocardiographic finding. This finding is sudden block of conduction in the antegrade direction during normal sinus rhythm [13]. Klein and Gulamhusein found that any patient demonstrating this finding on scalar electrocardiogram was not at risk for rapid ventricular rates during atrial fibrillation. However, they emphasized the importance of examining several electrocardiogram leads and the importance of showing that repolarization as well as depolarization was altered (Figure 20–4). In the upper panel of Figure 20–4 the PR interval is .16 sec, the QRS morphology is normal, and the slope of the ST segment is upward. In the lower panel the PR interval is .08 sec, the QRS morphology is preexcited, and the slope of the ST segment is downward. Thus these electrocardiograms recorded with the telephone system permit clear distinction between the normal and the abnormal AV conduction. The patient from whom these electrocardiograms were recorded would not be at risk for rapid conduction in the antegrade direction during atrial fibrillation.

Wellens et al. have attempted to use pharmacologic challenge with procainamide or ajmaline to demonstrate accessory atrioventricular connections that were not likely to pose a risk of rapid conduction in the antegrade direction during atrial fibrillation [14]. They found that procainamide (10 mg/kg) given intravenously produced complete conduction block in the antegrade direction (the delta wave disappeared from the QRS complex recorded during normal sinus rhythm) in 19 of 20 patients whose accessory connections had effective refractory periods equal to or greater than 270 ms. Conversely, the delta wave persisted in 18 of 19 patients in whom this refractory period was equal to or less than 260 ms.

For practical management it is unnecessary to use these indirect methods to infer the conduction properties of an accessory atrioventricular connection once a patient has had atrial fibrillation. One simply uses the electrocardiogram recorded during atrial fibrillation as a guide to therapy. If the patient has any preexcited ventricular beats during atrial fibrillation, a drug should be prescribed that has therapeutic effects on both the accessory connection and the myocardium. Fortunately, many drugs combine

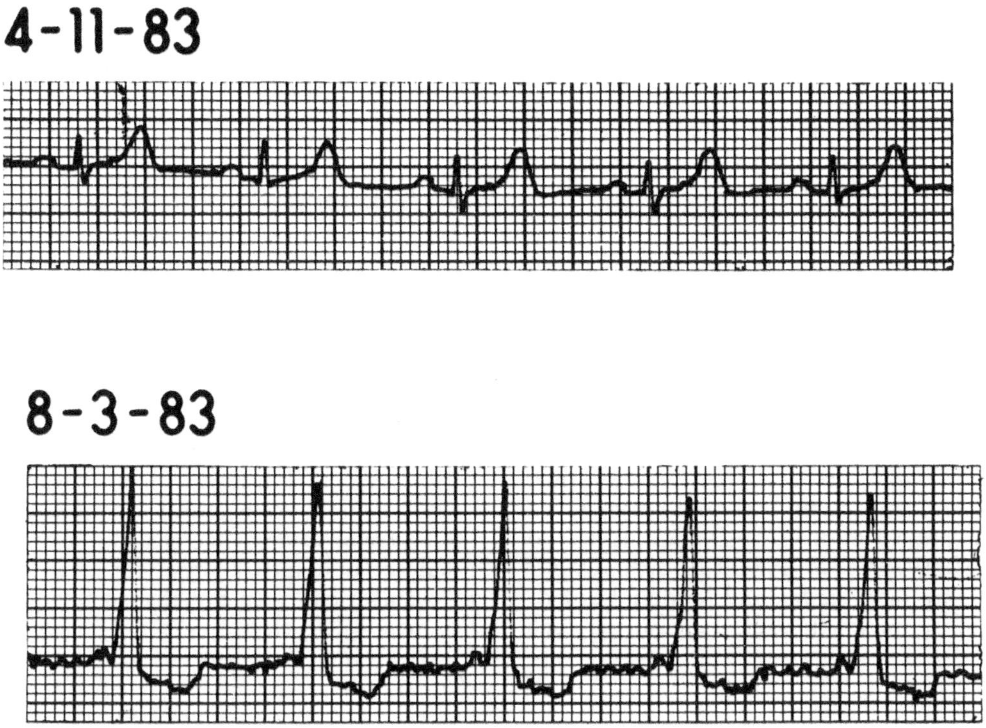

FIGURE 20–4. Electrocardiogram rhythm strips recorded from a patient with the Wolff-Parkinson-White syndrome. Both panels show normal sinus rhythm. On April 11, 1983 the PR interval was .16 sec, the QRS morphology was normal, and the slope of the ST segment was upward (*upper panel*). On August 3, 1983, the PR interval was .08 sec, the QRS morphology was preexcited, and the slope of the ST segment was downward (*lower panel*). These electrocardiograms were recorded using our telephone transmitting and recording system.

these properties.

Among the drugs that possess these properties are quinidine, procainamide, disopyramide, flecainide, and amiodarone. These drugs probably have at least three salutary effects in patients with atrial fibrillation: (1) preventing atrial fibrillation, (2) stabilizing the ventricle so that ventricular fibrillation is less likely to occur, and (3) slowing the rate that impulses are conducted to the ventricle during atrial fibrillation. Unfortunately, the only one of these effects that is directly measurable is the third.

Quinidine is an attractive first choice for the treatment of atrial fibrillation [15]. It is almost universally available, and most practitioners are familiar with its use. Quinidine sulfate 300 mg every six hours is our usual initial dose. Plasma quinidine levels drawn at the end of a dosing interval should be at least 4.0 mg/dl to provide reassurance that a favorable effect could be present. Procainamide and disopyramide are very acceptable alternatives from the point of view of their therapeutic spectrum; however, side effects of these latter two agents make them less desirable as the first choice [15,16]. Flecainide and amiodarone have been used in some European countries, but their use in the United States has been limited to investigational protocols until recently [17–20].

Since many patients develop atrial fibrillation during an episode of orthodromic reciprocating tachycardia, one may ask whether it is reasonable to treat them for their reentrant tachycardia in hope of preventing both arrhythmias. For example, would verapamil, which prevents orthodromic reciprocating tachycardia by blocking AV nodal conduction, also prevent atrial fibrillation? In theory this is logical treatment; but we still prefer the added reassurance that comes from using drugs like quinidine that have more direct antifibrillatory effects and more direct effects on the accessory atrioventricular connections.

Digitalis compounds should never be given parenterally to a patient who has rapid conduction in the antegrade direction over an accessory AV connection. Digitalis may increase the ventricular rate during atrial fibrillation and may precipitate ventricular fibrillation [7,21]. In the report of Klein et al., ventricular fibrillation occurred within a short interval of the time that digitalis was intravenously administered acutely to six of their patients who were in atrial fibrillation [7]. Digitalis is thus contraindicated in a patient with a history of atrial fibrillation and conduction in the antegrade direction over an accessory connection. It should not be given for the treatment of atrial fibrillation, it should not be given for the treatment of orthodromic reciprocating tachycardia, and it should not be given for the treatment of heart failure in such patients.

ACUTE MANAGEMENT

The patient in atrial fibrillation with rapid conduction in the antegrade direction over an accessory connection is a medical emergency. Mean ventricular rates in this setting may reach 400 beats/min, resulting in hypotension, syncope, or hemodynamic collapse. Ventricular fibrillation may result, and acute treatment must be delivered quickly. All pharmacologic therapy is too slow for the patient who is unconscious or has hemodynamic collapse. The treatment of choice is immediate DC-cardioversion. If equipment for cardioversion is not immediately available, the best pharmacologic treatment is intravenous procainamide.

Intravenous administration of procainamide is tedious because it must be given slowly to avoid aggravating the hypotension that is invariably present due to the rapid heart rate. For this reason its use is reserved for those patients who have no signs of low cardiac output or for those situations where DC-cardioversion is not immediately available. Customarily we give 100 mg every five minutes to a maximum dose of 1.2 grams. Each 100 mg dose should be pushed into a running intravenous line over a period of two to three minutes. The blood pressure should be checked after each bolus; if the systolic pressure has decreased by more than 20%, drug administration should be stopped while the blood pressure is restored with intravenous fluids or while preparations are made for DC-cardioversion.

Orthodromic Reciprocating Tachycardia

Orthodromic reciprocating tachycardia is the most common tachycardia in patients with WPW syndrome. It is a reentrant rhythm that uses the atrioventricular node for conduction in the antegrade direction and an accessory AV connection for conduction in the retrograde direction (Figure 20–5, panel A). It is called by a variety of synonyms for everyday use. "Orthodromic reciprocating tachycardia" and "AV reciprocating tachycardia" are good, accurate, descriptive terms for use when the mechanism has been established unequivocally by intracardiac electrophysiology study.

When the diagnosis has been made by electrocardiogram and the mechanism of the tachycardia has not been established by electrophysiologic study, the terms *paroxysmal atrial tachycardia, paroxysmal supraventricular tachycardia*, or *paroxysmal junctional tachycardia* are used commonly. These terms are more general and recognize that tachycardia due to reentry within the AV node may masquerade as orthodromic reciprocating tachycardia in an occasional patient with WPW syndrome. In this chapter we will use the term *orthodromic reciprocating tachycardia* to conform with the editors' style for this book.

LONG TERM MANAGEMENT

Not every patient with orthodromic reciprocating tachycardia requires treatment since the arrhythmia is usually not intrinsically dangerous. In young people with normal myocardium and normal coronary arteries it does not cause heart attacks, strokes, renal failure, or any of the other sequelae associated with ventricular tachycardia in patients with coronary artery disease. Orthodromic reciprocating tachycardia mostly makes patients uncomfortable when they have it; symptoms resolve when the tachycardia stops. Palpitations are the predominant symptom during attacks, and frequently they are the only symptom. Patients who have infre-

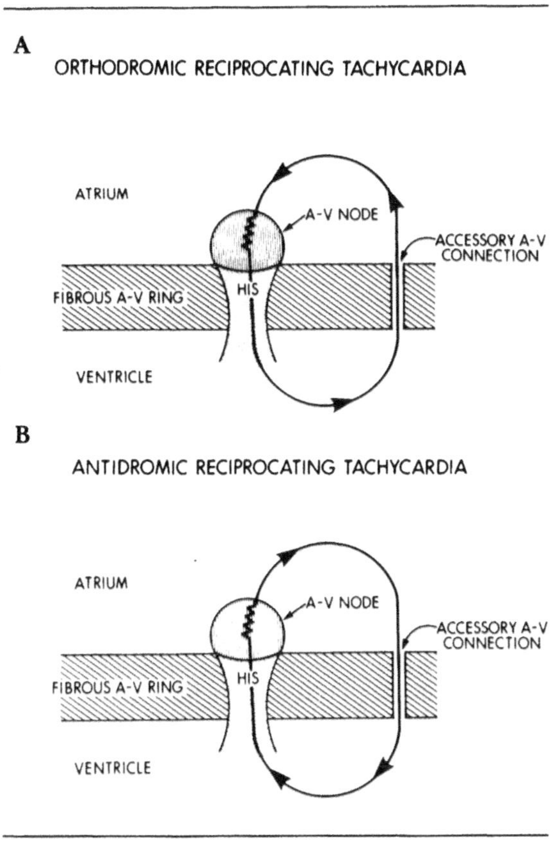

FIGURE 20–5. Mechanism of reciprocating tachycardias. Orthodromic reciprocating tachycardia (A) is a very common reentrant rhythm that uses the atrioventricular node for conduction in the antegrade direction and an accessory atrioventricular connection for conduction in the retrograde direction. Antidromic reciprocating tachycardia (B) is a very uncommon arrhythmia that uses an accessory atrioventricular connection for conduction in the antegrade direction and the atrioventricular node for conduction in the retrograde direction.

quent, brief, self-terminating attacks may take no prophylactic medication and deal with each attack when it comes. The decision to initiate therapy should be made jointly by the patient and the physician and should be based on agreement that the nuisance of the attacks is worse than the nuisance, cost, and risks of treatment.

Drugs that slow AV nodal conduction are excellent choices for patients with orthodromic reciprocating tachycardia. These drugs include two of the calcium channel blocking drugs, verapamil and diltiazem; all the beta-adrenergic blocking compounds and all the digitalis compounds. Among the calcium channel blocking drugs, verapamil is used most widely as an antiarrhythmic drug. The initial dose is 120 mg three times daily; and the dose can be increased to 120 mg four times daily if the patient's response is not satisfactory [21,22]. A big advantage of verapamil is the low incidence of side effects in patients taking it; the major disadvantage is the inconvenience of having to take it several times daily.

Among the beta-adrenergic blocking drugs, propranolol has been used most as an antiarrhythmic agent. A very low does such as 40 mg per day is effective therapy for orthodromic reciprocating tachycardia in some patients. Propranolol is given four times daily, unless a specific long-acting formulation is used. If the initial dose of propranolol is ineffective, the daily dose is doubled to 80, 160, and then 320 mg per day. Side effects limit using higher doses.

Atenolol, another beta-adrenergic blocking drug, is an excellent alternative to propranolol because it can be given once daily. The initial dose is 50 mg per day, which can be increased to 100 mg per day. All the beta-adrenergic blocking drugs are probably useful in the treatment of orthodromic reciprocating tachycardia, but experience with the others is extremely limited.

Digitalis compounds have been used for many years to treat orthodromic reciprocating tachycardia. They are attractive antiarrhythmic drugs because they are convenient to take and inexpensive. Most practitioners are familiar with their use. However, in recent years concern has been expressed about the role of digitalis in precipitating ventricular fibrillation in patients with atrial fibrillation [7]. Certainly, digitalis should never be given to a patient with atrial fibrillation and rapid conduction in the antegrade direction over an accessory AV connection. Probably it is best to reserve digitalis for initial therapy of patients with infrequent orthodromic reciprocating tachycardia. If the arrhythmia is not abolished completely by digitalis, a calcium channel blocker or a beta adrenergic blocker should be used; the digitalis should be stopped.

Antiarrhythmic drugs with local anesthetic properties, such as quinidine, procainamide, and disopyramide, are also excellent drugs for the management of orthodromic reciprocating tachycardia. These drugs probably exert a therapeutic effect by suppressing premature atrial beats and premature ventricular beats that initiate reciprocating tachycardia. They are usually not used as initial therapy because they require dosing three or four times daily and because their side effects are more troublesome than those of the calcium channel blockers, beta-adrenergic blockers, and digitalis. These local anesthetic drugs are particularly attractive therapy for patients with both orthodromic reciprocating tachycardia and atrial fibrillation.

ACUTE MANAGEMENT

Many attacks of orthodromic reciprocating tachycardia terminate spontaneously or can be terminated by the patient doing a Valsalva maneuver. Patients should be taught the Valsalva maneuver so that they can treat themselves. If a patient is taking a calcium channel blocker or a beta-adrenergic blocker, we recommend taking an extra dose of medication at the onset of an attack. This extra dose will terminate many attacks.

Some patients with very infrequent attacks of tachycardia may prefer to treat their attacks when they occur rather than to take regular prophylactic medication. Verapamil 120 mg given by mouth can be used to terminate attacks of tachycardia in these patients because it is absorbed very rapidly after oral administration. Most attacks terminate within one hour after a single dose (Figures 20-6 and 20-7). If the first dose does not achieve the desired therapeutic effect, a second dose may be given after one hour. We encourage the patient to lie down while doing this because a brief sinus pause may occur when the tachycardia stops.

Occasional patients require physician intervention for attacks of tachycardia. Some of these attacks can be terminated by a well-coached Valsalva maneuver, our recommended initial step. If the Valsalva maneuver does not work, carotid sinus massage is the next step. If neither vagal procedure is effective, verapamil given intravenously is the treatment of choice [23]. The electrocardiogram should be monitored continuously and the drug should be given into a running intravenous line. The initial dose is 5 mg; if this is ineffective, a second dose of 10 mg may be given after 30 minutes. Verapamil given in this way should terminate almost 90% of orthodromic reciprocating tachycardia.

Antidromic Reciprocating Tachycardia

Antidromic reciprocating tachycardia is an unusual rhythm that uses an accessory atrioventricular connection for conduction in the antegrade direction and the atrioventricular node for conduction in the retrograde direction (Figure 20-5, panel B) [24,25]. On electrocardiogram it is recognized as a rapid, regular tachycardia. The QRS morphology is preexcited; the vector of the delta wave during tachycardia is the same as during normal sinus rhythm. Because the arrhythmia is so unusual, there is a particular shortage of information to guide its management. However, quinidine and drugs with similar actions should be helpful.

It is not unreasonable to refer most patients with antidromic reciprocating tachycardia to a center where electrophysiology studies are performed so that appropriate studies can be done to confirm the diagnosis. Potentially more dangerous arrhythmias with similar electrocardiographic appearance include ventricular tachycardia and atrial flutter with 1:1 conduction in the antegrade direction over an accessory AV connection [25].

Asymptomatic Subjects Whose Electrocardiograms Show Delta Waves

Electrocardiograms are recorded so routinely as screening procedures that delta waves are found in many patients who have no arrhythmia symptoms. These patients should be told that their electrocardiogram shows this common variant and that some patients with this variant develop episodes of rapid heart beating. No further diagnostic tests and no treatment are required.

References

1. Scherlag BJ, Lau SH, Helfant RM, Stein E, Berkowitz WD, Damato AN: Catheter technique for recording His bundle activity in man. *Circulation* 39:13, 1969.
2. Durrer D, Schoo L, Schuilenburg RM, Wellens HJJ: The role of premature beats in the initiation and termination of supravenatricular tachycardia in the Wolff-Parkinson-White syndrome. *Circulation* 36:644, 1967.
3. Cobb FR, Blumenschein SD, Sealy WC, Boineau JP, Wagner GS, Wallace AG: Successful surgical

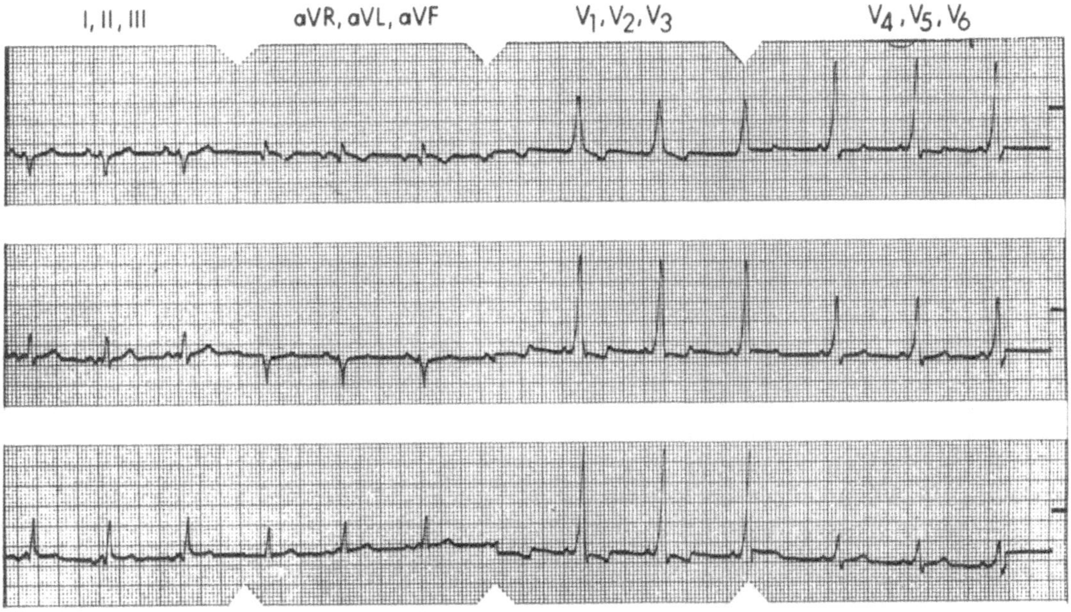

FIGURE 20–6. Twelve-lead electrocardiogram from a patient with the Wolff-Parkinson-White syndrome. Rhythm strips from this patient are shown in Figure 20–7.

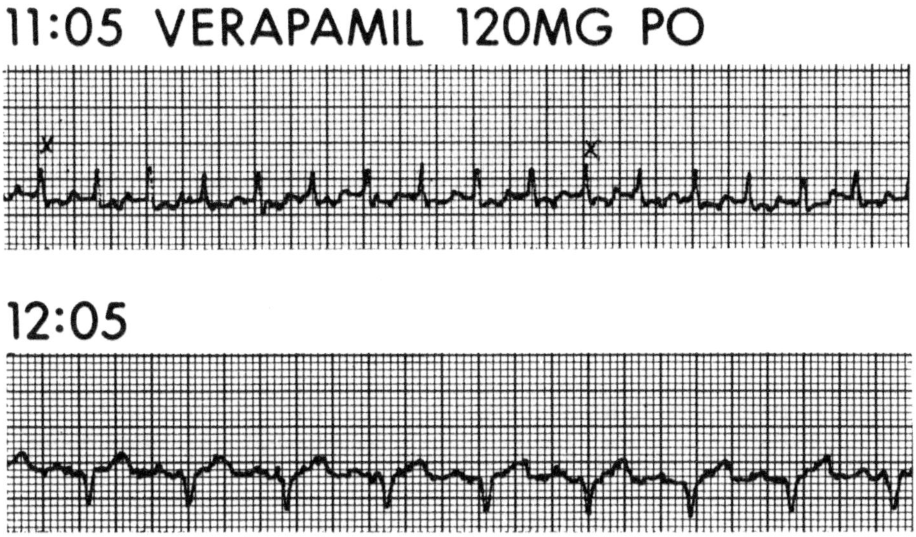

FIGURE 20–7. Electrocardiogram rhythm strips recorded from a patient who was taking no antiarrhythmic medication. Orthodromic reciprocating tachycardia was recorded at 11:05 A.M. (*upper panel*). The patient then took a single tablet of verapamil 120 mg. Normal sinus rhythm was restored by 12:05 P.M. (*lower panel*). These electrocardiograms were recorded using our telephone transmitting and recording system.

interruption of the bundle of Kent in a patient with Wolff-Parkinson-White syndrome. *Circulation* 38:1018, 1968.

4. Pritchett ELC, Gallagher JJ, Sealy WC, Anderson R, Campbell RWF, Seller TD, Jr, Wallace AG: Supraventricular tachycardia dependent upon accessory pathways in the absence of ventricular preexcitation. *Am. J. Med.* 61:214, 1978.
5. Pritchett ELC: *Office Management of Arrhythmias*, Saunders, Philadelphia, 162 pages, 1982.
6. Pritchett ELC, Zimmerman JM, Hammill KF, Reiter MJ, Hammill SC: Electrocardiogram recording by telephone in antiarrhythmic drug trials. *Chest* 81:473, 1982.
7. Klein GJ, Bashore TM, Sellers TD, Pritchett ELC, Smith WM, Gallagher JJ. Ventricular fibrillation in the Wolff-Parkinson-White syndrome. *N. Engl. J. Med.* 30:1081, 1979.
8. Campbell RWF, Smith RA, Gallagher JJ, Pritchett ELC, Wallace AG: Atrial fibrillation in the preexcitation syndrome. *Am. J. Cardiol.* 40:514, 1977.
9. Bauerfeind RA, Wyndham CR, Swiryn SP, Palileo E, Strasberg B, Lam W, Westveer D, Rosen KM: Paroxysmal atrial fibrillation in the Wolff-Parkinson-White syndrome. *Am. J. Cardiol.* 47:562, 1981.
10. Roark SF, McCarthy EA, Lee KL, Pritchett ELC: The incidence of atrial fibrillation in patients with paroxysmal atrial tachycardia. *Circulation.* (in. press).
11. Hammill SC, Pritchett ELC, Klein GJ, Smith WM, Gallagher JJ: Accessory atrioventricular pathways that conduct only in the antegrade direction. *Circulation* 62:1335, 1980.
12. Klein GJ, Yee R, Sharma AD: Concealed conduction in accessory pathways: an important determinant of the expression of arrhythmias in patients with Wolff-Parkinson-White syndrome. *Circulation* 70:402, 1984.
13. Klein GJ, Gulamhusein SS: Intermittent preexcitation in the Wolff-Parkinson-White syndrome. *Am. J. Cardiol.* 52:292, 1983.
14. Wellens HJJ, Braat S, Brugada P, Gorgels APM, Bar FW: Use of procainamide in patients with the Wolff-Parkinson-White syndrome to disclose a short refractory period of the accessory pathway. *Am. J. Cardiol.* 50:1087, 1982.
15. Sellers TD Jr, Campbell RWF, Bashore TM: Effects of procainamide and quinidine sulfate in the Wolff-Parkinson-White syndrome. *Circulation* 55:15, 1977.
16. Kerr CR, Prystowsky EN, Smith WM, Cook L, Gallagher JJ: Electrophysiological effects of disopyramide phosphate in patients with Wolff-Parkinson-White syndrome. *Circulation* 65:869, 1982.
17. Hellestrand KJ, Nathan AW, Bexton RS, Spurrell RAJ, Camm AJ: Cardiac electrophysiologic effects of flecainide acetate for paroxysmal reentrant junctional tachycardias. *Am. J. Cardiol.* 51:770, 1983.
18. Neuss H, Buss J, Schlepper M, Berthold R, Mitrovic V, Kramer A, Musical WJ: Effects of flecainide on electrophysiological properties of accessory pathways in the Wolff-Parkinson-White syndrome. *Eur. Heart J.* 4:347, 1983.
19. Rosenbaum MB, Chiale PA, Ryba D, Elizari MV: Control of tachyarrhythmias associated with Wolff-Parkinson-White syndrome by amiodarone hydrochloride. *Am. J. Cardiol.* 34:215, 1974.
20. Ward DE, Camm AJ, Spurrell RAJ: Clinical antiarrhythmic effects of amiodarone in patients with resistant paroxysmal tachycardias. *Br. Heart J.* 44:91, 1980.
21. Mauritson DR, Winniford MD, Walker WS, Rude RE, Cory JR, Hillis LD: Oral verapamil for paroxysmal supraventricular tachycardia. A long-term, double-blind randomized trial. *Ann. Intern. Med.* 96:409, 1982.
22. Pritchett ELC, Hammill SC, Reiter MJ, Lee KL, McCarthy EA, Zimmerman JM, Shand DG: Life table methods for evaluating antiarrhythmic drug efficacy in patients with paroxysmal atrial tachycardia. *Am. J. Cardiol.* 52:1007, 1983.
23. Waxman HL, Myerburg RJ, Appel R, Sung RJ: Verapamil for control of ventricular rate in paroxysmal supraventricular tachycardia and atrial fibrillation and flutter. *Ann. Intern. Med.* 94:1, 1981.
24. Bardy GH, Packer DL, German LD, Gallagher JJ: Preexcited reciprocating tachycardia in patients with Wolff-Parkinson-White syndrome: incidence and mechanisms. *Circulation* 70: 377, 1984.
25. Benditt DG, Pritchett ELC, Gallagher JJ: Spectrum of regular tachycardias with wide QRS complexes in patients with accessory atrioventricular pathways. *Am. J. Cardiol.* 42:828, 1978.

21. ANTIARRHYTHMIC DRUG THERAPY IN PATIENTS WITH PREEXCITATION SYNDROMES

Eric N. Prystowsky

Patients with preexcitation syndromes may exhibit a variety of tachyarrhythmias [1]. The accessory pathway(s) associated with a particular preexcitation syndrome may be used as part of an atrioventricular (AV) reentrant tachycardia circuit (i.e., orthodromic or antidromic reciprocating tachycardia), or in certain arrhythmias such as atrial fibrillation the accessory pathway may not be needed to sustain tachycardia but is utilized to conduct impulses to the ventricle. Patients with preexcitation syndrome also may have tachycardias that do not involve conduction over the accessory pathway, such as ventricular tachycardia [2].

It is important to discuss a therapeutic "philosophy" before examining the potential benefits of individual antiarrhythmic agents. As is the case with many disorders, the most difficult decision is often not which drug to use but rather whether treatment is necessary. For example, patients who have ventricular preexcitation may have no or only occasional tachyarrhythmias. If these tachyarrhythmias occur infrequently and are not associated with significant symptoms, the patient may require no therapy. If a patient has frequent episodes of tachyarrhythmias and/or the arrhythmias cause significant symptoms, therapy should be instituted to control these arrhythmias. Although antiarrhythmic drugs suppress or modify tachycardia in most patients, certain patients may be candidates for alternative forms of therapy such as surgical or catheter ablation of the accessory pathway or electrical treatment with implantable pacemakers.

An interesting problem has arisen concerning identification of the asymptomatic patient with ventricular preexcitation who may be at risk for developing life-threatening arrhythmias. During atrial fibrillation, a rapid ventricular response may occur as a result of conduction over the accessory pathway and, in these patients, atrial fibrillation may degenerate into ventricular fibrillation [3,4]. If it were possible to identify which patients were susceptible to rapid preexcited ventricular responses during atrial fibrillation, then therapy to prevent atrial fibrillation or alter conduction over the accessory pathway might theoretically benefit these patients.

Previous investigations [5,6] have demonstrated that the shortest interval between two

Supported in part by the Herman C. Krannert Fund, Indianapolis, Indiana; by Grants HL-06308, and HL-07182 from the National Heart, Lung and Blood Institute of the National Institutes of Health, Bethesda, Maryland; and by the Attorney General of Indiana Public Health Trust and by the Roudebush Veterans Administration Medical Center, Indianapolis, Indiana; and by a Grant-In-Aid from the American Heart Association, Indiana Affiliate, Inc., Indianapolis, Indiana.

I am very appreciative of the expert secretarial assistance of Nancy S. Lineback, who helped in the preparation of this manuscript.

Benditt, D.G. and Benson, D.W., Cardiac Preexcitation Syndromes.

preexcited QRS complexes (shortest RR interval) during atrial fibrillation correlated well with the antegrade accessory pathway effective refractory period (APERP) obtained during atrial pacing. Two studies suggest that noninvasive data may identify patients with short antegrade APERP [7,8]. Wellens et al. [7] administered intravenously both ajmaline (≤50 mg) and at a later time procainamide (≤10 mg/kg given over 5 minutes) to 39 patients with ventricular preexcitation (Figure 21–1). Responses to the drugs were concordant, and loss of conduction over the accessory pathway occurred in 20 patients of whom 19 had an antegrade APERP ≥270 ms (<300 msec in 10/20); the antegrade APERP was <260 ms in 17 of 19 patients in whom conduction over the accessory pathway persisted. In another study, Klein and Gulamhusein [8] showed that patients with spontaneous loss of conduction over the accessory pathway during sinus rhythm (intermittent preexcitation) tended to have longer antegrade APERP than patients with persistent ventricular preexcitation. During induced atrial fibrilla-

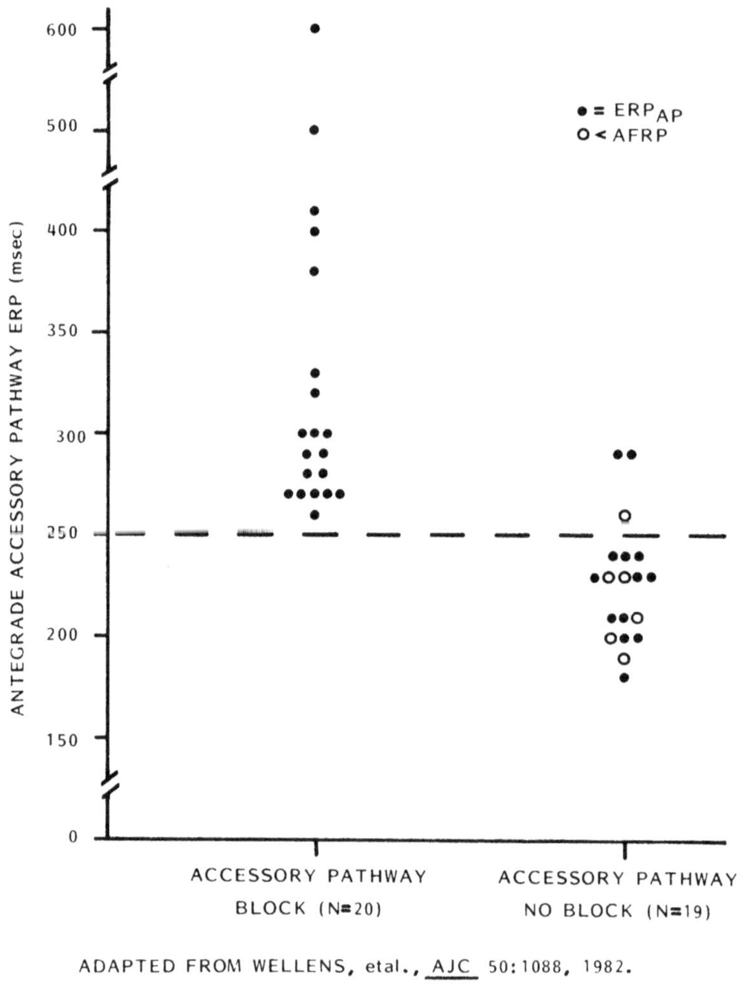

FIGURE 21–1. Correlation of accessory pathway antegrade effective refractory period with response to intravenous procainamide/ajmaline test. When drug administration produced block in accessory pathway conduction in the antegrade direction the effective refractory period (ERP) of the pathway was >250 ms. AFRP = atrial functional refractory period. See text for details.

tion the shortest RR interval was <250 ms in only 4 of 26 patients with intermittent preexcitation.

There are several problems with the preceding observations: (1) some investigators have not noted a correlation between the shortest RR interval during atrial fibrillation and the antegrade APERP [9]; (2) intermittent preexcitation does not preclude a rapid preexcited ventricular response during atrial fibrillation (Figure 21–2); and (3) no specific value of the antegrade APERP appears to discriminate between patients with ventricular preexcitation with and without a history of ventricular fibrillation [4]. Thus, determination of antegrade APERP does not appear to be a reliable method to predict the patient *potentially* at risk for development of ventricular fibrillation. Rather, it would be preferable to induce atrial fibrillation and measure the shortest preexcited RR interval , which was ≤250 ms in all patients with a history of ventricular fibrillation, although 66% of patients without a history of ventricular fibrillation had similar values [4]. Isoproterenol significantly shortens the preexcited intervals during atrial fibrillation [10] and its use may provide further insight into this problem in selected patients [11].

In my opinion, attempts to identify the asymptomatic patient with ventricular preexcitation who is potentially at risk for subsequent sudden death is investigational and should be done only as a prospective natural history study of the Wolff-Parkinson-White (WPW) syndrome. Possible exceptions might be individuals involved in competitive athletics or certain employment situations, for example airline pilots, or in patients in whom digitalis therapy is considered (see below).

Drug Therapy

In patients with accessory AV pathways, reentrant tachycardia most commonly utilizes the

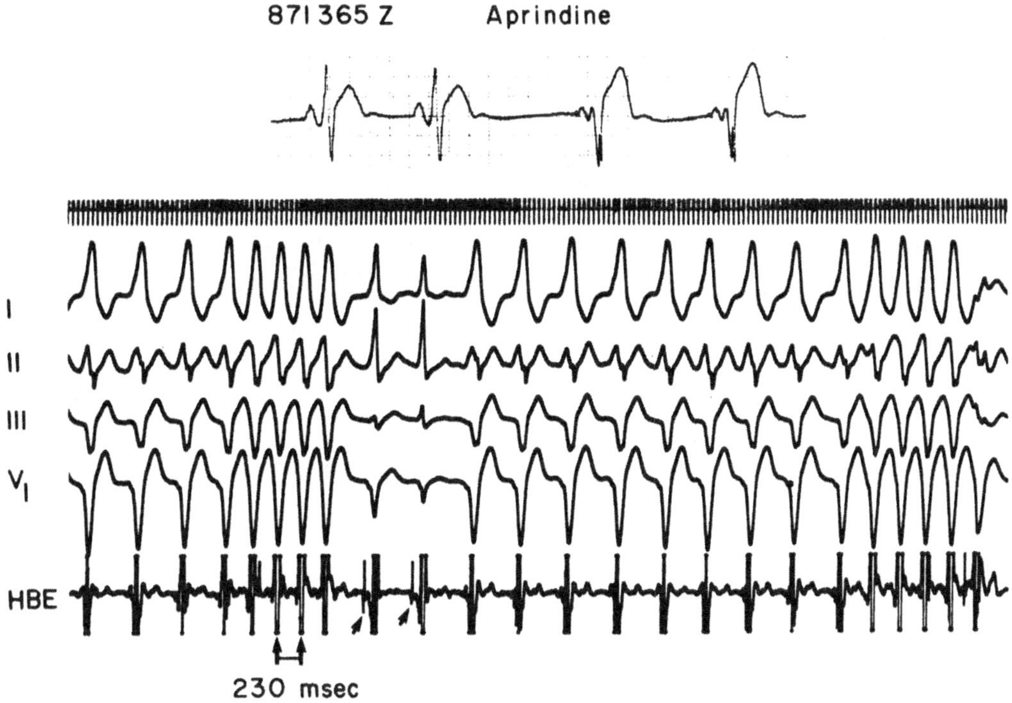

FIGURE 21–2. Intermittent conduction via the accessory pathway during aprindine therapy, and preexcited ventricular response during induced atrial fibrillation. HBE = His bundle electrogram. Arrows point to His deflections of nonpreexcited QRS complexes.

normal AV conduction system for conduction in the antegrade direction and the accessory pathway for conduction in the retrograde direction. Drugs that increase refractoriness and slow conduction in the accessory pathway and/or AV node may suppress spontaneous episodes of reentrant tachycardia. It is not possible at present to predict which drug(s) will be most effective for each patient. For example, quinidine may produce conduction block in both the antegrade and retrograde directions in the accessory pathway and prevent occurrence of reentrant tachycardia. In another patient, quinidine may cause only conduction block in the antegrade direction in the accessory pathway, may widen the tachycardia echo zone (i.e., a greater range of premature atrial coupling intervals may initiate tachycardia), and may increase the frequency of arrhythmias. Further, drugs that modify electrophysiologic properties of the AV node but do not affect conduction or refractoriness in accessory bypass tracts are not useful, and may be harmful (see below) in treating patients with atrial fibrillation and predominantly preexcited ventricular complexes.

In this chapter I have divided drugs into three categories based on their antiarrhythmic effects on accessory pathways and the normal AV conduction system [12]. Utilization of this approach enables one to formulate rational single or combined drug therapy for patients with tachycardia involving accessory pathways.

Drugs with Primarily Antiarrhythmic Effects on the AV Node

DIGITALIS

There is considerable concern and controversy over the use of digitalis in patients with ventricular preexcitation due to accessory AV pathways. The problem is that digitalis can shorten both antegrade APERP as well as the closest coupled preexcited RR interval during atrial fibrillation [13,14,15], and it has been implicated as a contributory factor in the occurrence of ventricular fibrillation [3,14,16] (an issue discussed below). The antiarrhythmic effects of digitalis presumably occur because of its alteration of AV nodal physiology, either directly or indirectly via modification of autonomic nervous system activity, especially enhanced vagal effects.

Digitalis slows conduction and increases refractoriness of the AV node [17] and is used often for the treatment of AV reciprocating tachycardia. Wellens and Durrer [15] performed electrophysiologic studies before and during ouabain therapy (0.75 to 1.5 mg given intra-atrially) in six patients with preexcitation. AV nodal refractoriness was measured in five patients, and increased after ouabain administration from 30 to 70 ms in 5/5 patients. Ouabain prolonged AV nodal conduction time in 6/6 patients. In two patients ouabain prevented induction of AV reentrant tachycardia. Of note, ouabain shortened the APERP in the antegrade direction from 10 to 50 msec in all patients.

Dhingra et al. [18] investigated the antiarrhythmic actions of intravenous ouabain (0.01 mg/kg) in patients with AV reentrant tachycardia. Ouabain prevented induction of tachycardia in 2/19 patients, and the tachycardia cycle length minimally increased from 320 ± 6.7 to 340 ± 8.1 ms ($p < .01$) in the presence of ouabain. No statistically significant change in antegrade APERP occurred during ouabain therapy when data were analyzed for all patients. However, antegrade APERP decreased 10 to 65 ms in five patients, increased 10 to 30 ms in three patients, and was unchanged in two patients.

The primary concern with the use of digitalis is its ability to increase the preexcited ventricular rate during atrial fibrillation, an effect that can culminate in ventricular fibrillation. Dreifus et al. [3] administered intravenous digoxin to a patient who had atrial fibrillation with preexcited ventricular complexes and this was followed by ventricular fibrillation. Digoxin was given again with similar results. Sellers et al. [14] evaluated the effect of digitalis during atrial fibrillation in two groups of patients with WPW syndrome. Twelve patients with relatively long antegrade APERP were given digoxin after the shortest preexcited RR interval had been determined during induced atrial fibrillation. Ten patients received 0.75 to 1.0 mg of intravenous digoxin, 7 of whom were retested during oral digoxin (0.25 mg daily) therapy; two patients were tested only while receiving oral digoxin. The shortest preexcited RR interval during intravenous digoxin shortened by 20 to 65 ms (mean 45) in 3/10 patients, lengthened by 20 to 100 ms (mean 63) in 6/10 patients, and was unchanged in one patient. Of particular importance, the authors were unable to predict the results obtained during oral therapy from the changes noted with intravenous drugs. An additional nine patients were studied who had a spontaneous episode of ventricular fibrillation while taking digitalis [14]. Seven of these patients had ECG evidence of atrial fibrillation degenerating into ventricular fibrillation following intravenous digitalis in 4 patients and during oral therapy in 3 of 5 patients. At electrophysiologic study in the absence of digitalis the shortest preexcited RR interval during induced atrial fibrillation was <220 ms in all nine patients.

Survival data in infants with WPW syndrome who received oral digoxin therapy for the control of their arrhythmias are disturbing [16]. During a mean follow-up period of 6.5 years sudden cardiac death occurred in 2 of 55 patients who received digoxin alone, a frequency higher than expected; the authors [16] suggest that it might be better to use alternative forms of therapy unless the electrophysiologic properties of the accessory pathway are known.

In summary, the findings summarized above demonstrate that during electrophysiologic testing digitalis only uncommonly prevents initiation of reciprocating tachycardia utilizing an accessory AV pathway, and, when initiated, minimally slows the rate of tachycardia. Regardless of these findings, clinical experience suggests that digitalis will prevent the occurrence of spontaneous reciprocating tachycardia in many patients. Since digitalis can shorten antegrade APERP and has been implicated in the conversion of atrial fibrillation to ventricular fibrillation, digitalis should not be used as a single agent to treat patients with ventricular preexcitation unless the antegrade electrophysiologic properties of the accessory pathway are known, or the pathway is capable of retrograde conduction only. My preference is to evaluate the preexcited ventricular response during induced atrial fibrillation in the absence of drug therapy and not to rely on noninvasive or invasive estimates of antegrade APERP.

BETA-ADRENERGIC BLOCKERS

Propranolol has been the beta-adrenergic blocker most extensively studied in patients with WPW syndrome, although preliminary data suggest a potential salutary effect of prindolol [19], atenolol [20], metoprolol [21], timolol [22], and nadolol [23] on AV reentrant tachycardia. The parasympathetic and sympathetic nervous system exert a balanced effect on the human AV node in the resting state [24] and under these conditions propranolol slows conduction and prolongs refractoriness in the AV node [24,25]. In contrast, propranolol, given intravenously in a dose of 0.1 mg/kg, exerts minimal effects on electrophysiologic properties of accessory pathways. Denes et al. [26] showed no change in either antegrade or retrograde APERP following propranolol administration. Further, 10 of 14 patients still had tachycardia induced during propranolol therapy, and the tachycardia cycle length increased only a small amount from 328 ± 18 ms to 352 ± 19 ms ($p < .01$).

Barrett et al. [27] found that although propranolol increased antegrade APERP from 273 ± 14 ms to 291 ± 11 ms ($p < .01$), there was no change in the shortest atrial pacing cycle length maintaining 1:1 conduction over the accessory pathway. Also, there was no effect of propranolol on retrograde APERP. Seven patients had orthodromic reciprocating tachycardia induced before and during propranolol treatment, and the tachycardia cycle length increased only 12%, from 311 ± 14 ms to 347 ± 19 ms ($p < .008$).

The preceding studies suggest that propranolol as a single agent would be a minimally effective antiarrhythmic drug to treat AV reentrant tachycardia in patients with WPW syndrome, and would not be useful at all to slow the preexcited ventricular rate in patients who have atrial fibrillation. However, this reasoning negates the potential antiarrhythmic effects of beta-adrenergic blockers during heightened sympathetic tone [10,11]. Increased sympathetic tone facilitates AV nodal conduction, and recent data demonstrate that isoproterenol infusion can improve conduction and shorten refractoriness over the accessory pathway [28,29]. Thus, beta-adrenergic blockers potentially could exert substantial antiarrhythmic effects on both the AV node and accessory pathway if enhanced sympathetic tone were present, or if the onset of tachycardia were related to exercise. Regarding the latter point, beta-blockers can prevent recurrence of tachycardia in a patient with exercise-induced reciprocating tachycardia (Figure 21–3).

SLOW CHANNEL BLOCKERS

Existing experimental data suggest that cells in the AV node are slow channel-dependent, and

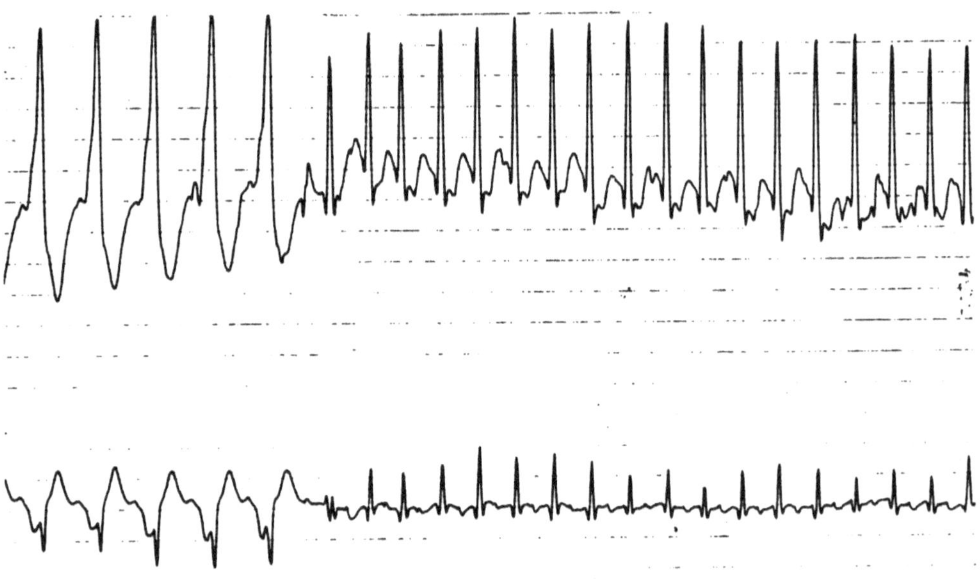

FIGURE 21–3. Exercise-induced reciprocating tachycardia utilizing an accessory pathway. During treadmill exercise testing, conduction proceeded over the accessory pathway (first five QRS complexes) until block over the pathway occurred (sixth complex). This unidirectional block allowed reciprocating AV reentrant tachycardia to occur. Beta-blocker therapy prevented episodes of tachycardia. (From Prystowsky, E.N., et al.: *Med. Clin. North Am.*, 68: 831, 1984. Reproduced with permission from W.B. Saunders Publishing Company.)

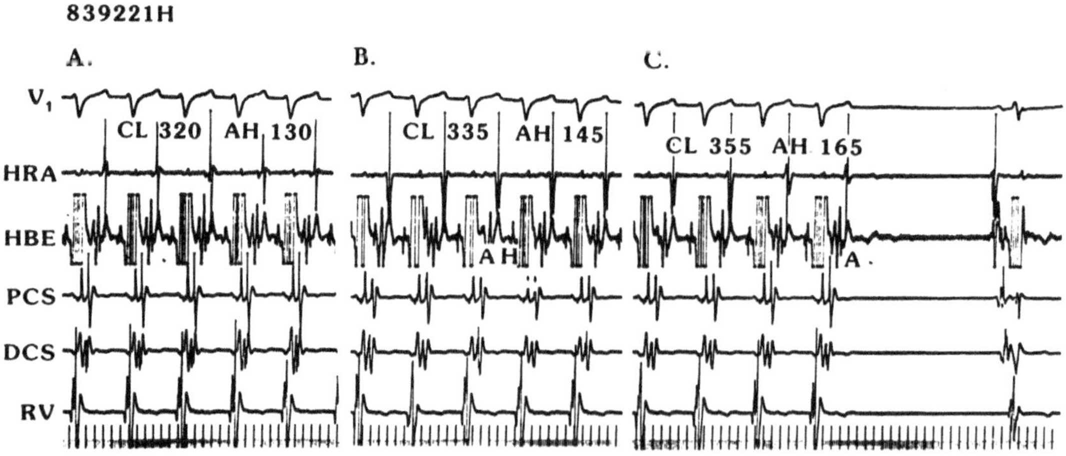

FIGURE 21–4. Effect of verapamil on orthodromic reciprocating tachycardia. (A) Control tachycardia cycle length is 320 ms with an AH interval of 130 ms. (B) Verapamil, 10 mg intravenously, was given and after approximately 30 seconds the tachycardia cycle length prolongs 15 ms due to AV nodal delay. (C) Prior to termination, AH interval prolongs more and tachycardia ends with antegrade block in the AV node — that is, atrial deflection without a His deflection. (From Prystowsky, EN, et al.: *Med. Clin. North Am.*, 68:831, 1984. Reproduced with permission from WB Saunders Publishing Company.)

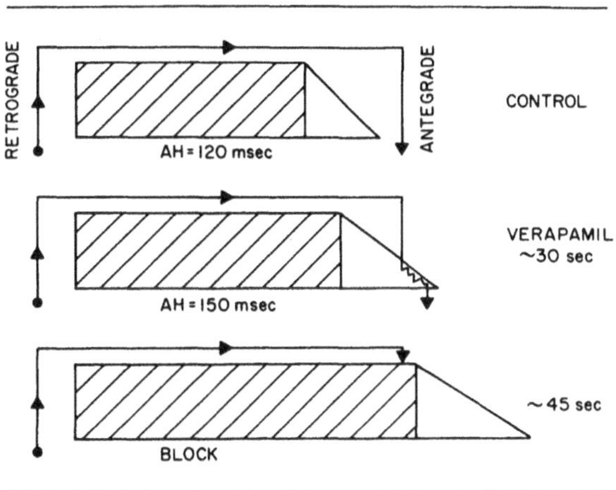

FIGURE 21-5. Schematic of mechanism of tachycardia termination with infusion of verapamil. Retrograde conduction is over the accessory pathway and is not affected by verapamil (*left*). Antegrade conduction is over the AV node and His-Purkinje system (*right*). The center hatched rectangle represents AV nodal effective refractory period, and the triangle AV nodal relative refractory period. During control, the assumption is made that antegrade conduction does not encroach on AV nodal refractoriness. After 30 seconds of verapamil infusion, AV nodal effective and relative refractoriness increase, and AH interval and tachycardia cycle length prolong because antegrade conduction encroaches on AV nodal relative refractory period. At about 45 seconds, the AV nodal effective refractory period lengthens sufficiently to block antegrade conduction and terminate tachycardia. (From Prystowsky, EN, et al.: *Med. Clin. North Am.* 68: 831, 1984. Reproduced with permission from WB Saunders Publishing Company.)

that AV nodal conduction can be slowed or blocked and refractoriness prolonged by agents that interfere with the slow inward current [30-32]. Verapamil exerts such an action [33] and is very effective (particularly when given intravenously) in terminating AV reciprocating tachycardia (Figures 21-4 and 21-5) [34-40], as are other slow channel blocking drugs [41-46].

Verapamil. Verapamil is the prototype of the slow channel blockers and is very useful in terminating reciprocating tachycardia when given intravenously as well as preventing recurrence of tachycardia during oral therapy. Recently, Klein et al. [34] demonstrated that antiarrhythmic results obtained during electrophysiologic testing with intravenous verapamil predicted efficacy of long-term therapy with oral verapamil. Thus, if sustained reciprocating tachycardia could not be induced during intravenous verapamil administration, oral verapamil, 80 mg every 6 hours, also prevented induction of tachycardia and these patients remained asymptomatic after hospital discharge.

Verapamil usually has minimal but variable effects on conduction and refractoriness of accessory pathways [36,38]. For example, eight patients were given 10 mg of intravenous verapamil and APERP in the antegrade direction increased 5 to 40 ms in four, decreased 5 to 35 ms in three, and did not change in one patient [38]. APERP in the retrograde direction was assessed in four patients and increased 80 ms in one patient and was unchanged in three patients. Nevertheless, administration of intravenous verapamil can increase the ventricular rate during atrial fibrillation by increasing the number of preexcited ventricular complexes [36, 47-49]. In one study [47] two patients required direct current cardioversion because of hemodynamic deterioration associated with an accelerated ventricular rate after verapamil administration. Petri et al. [50] showed that oral verapamil does not appear to increase the number of preexcited ventricular complexes during atrial fibrillation. At present, administration of intravenous verapamil is contraindicated in patients with atrial fibrillation associated with predominantly preexcited ventricular complexes.

Diltiazem. Diltiazem is under investigation by the U.S. Food and Drug Administration for the treatment of arrhythmias. However, studies suggest that it is effective in the treatment of reciprocating tachycardia [42-44]. Yeh et al. [43] studied 24 patients with AV reciprocating tachycardia before and after 270 mg of oral diltiazem. All 24 patients had sustained reciprocating tachycardia induced before drug therapy but diltiazem prevented induction of tachycardia in 17 patients and 3 additional patients had only initiation of nonsustained tachycardia.

Bepridil. Bepridil is a new investigational agent that affects both slow and fast inward currents, has proven efficacy in the treatment of angina pectoris, and appears to have salutary effects on both supraventricular and ventricular tachyarrhythmias [45,46].

Minimal data are available on the effects of bepridil on supraventricular tachycardia. Rowland et al. [46] compared the effects of intravenous bepridil (2 mg/kg) with verapamil (0.15 mg/kg) in 9 patients with AV nodal reentrant tachycardia, and with ajmaline (0.75 mg/kg) in 8 patients with reciprocating tachycardia associated with WPW syndrome. Both bepridil and verapamil terminated AV nodal reentrant tachycardia in all 9 patients. On the other hand, while ajmaline restored sinus rhythm in all WPW patients, bepridil failed to terminate tachycardia in 3 of these 8 patients. Twelve patients received a total of 1500 mg of oral bepridil and were restudied three days after initiation of therapy. In 6 patients tachycardia could not be induced, and in the other 6 patients the rate of tachycardia was stated to be slower. The authors do not mention whether antiarrhythmic efficacy with oral bepridil was different for AV nodal reentry versus reentrant tachycardia utilizing accessory AV pathways. Since bepridil can block conduction over the accessory pathway as well as over the AV node [45], it might be an excellent drug to treat patients with atrial fibrillation and ventricular preexcitation.

PURINES

Purinergic receptors are present in cardiac tissue and intravenous injection of adenosine triphosphate (ATP), or adenosine depresses AV nodal conduction and is antiarrhythmic [51–53]. Adenosine may have an advantage over ATP because of fewer side effects [53]. Di Marco et al. [52] terminated AV reentrant tachycardia within 20 sec after peripheral injection of adenosine due to AV nodal block, and there were no episodes of sinus bradycardia or AV block after termination of tachycardia. These agents may be used more frequently in the future to treat certain supraventricular tachyarrhythmias.

Drugs with Primarily Antiarrhythmic Effects on Accessory Pathways

Drugs that depress conduction and increase refractoriness of accessory pathways may be used to prevent, slow, or terminate AV reentrant tachycardia, as well as to decrease the maximum preexcited ventricular response occurring during atrial fibrillation or flutter. Some of these drugs also prolong AV nodal conduction time and refractoriness and will be discussed in a separate section (see below).

Wellens et al. [54] compared the change in APERP during antiarrhythmic drug therapy with the control APERP in 59 patients. They divided their patients into those in whom the control APERP was ≥270 ms (group I) or <270 ms (group II). Drugs produced antegrade complete conduction block over the accessory pathway in 84% of group I patients, but no group II patients developed block during drug therapy. Drug-induced prolongation of the retrograde APERP was less, regardless of the initial retrograde APERP. Complete retrograde conduction block over the accessory pathway occurred in only 6 (10%) patients, 3 in group I, and 3 in group II. These interesting results demonstrate the importance of evaluating electrophysiologic and antiarrhythmic effects of drugs in patients who have accessory pathways with similar initial electrophysiologic properties. The discrepant results of antiarrhythmic efficacy noted below in investigations that used the same or different drugs may be explained, in part, by patient selection.

LIDOCAINE

Rosen et al. [55] noted that intravenous lidocaine depressed accessory pathway antegrade conduction in four patients who had conduction block over the accessory pathway at a mean atrial pacing cycle length of 409 ms before lidocaine was given. In contrast, lidocaine exerted minimal effects on accessory pathway conduction in two patients with relatively rapid antegrade conduction over the accessory pathway in the control state. Josephson et al. [56] administered 100 mg of intravenous lidocaine to a patient who had atrial fibrillation with a mean preexcited ventricular rate of 190/min and abolished conduction over the accessory pathway.

More recent data suggest that lidocaine offers minimal benefit and may even be harmful when given to patients with WPW syndrome [57,58]. Barrett et al. [57] administered 1 mg/kg of intravenous lidocaine to 12 patients with accessory pathways and noted no significant change in antegrade or retrograde APERP, nor any antiarrhythmic efficacy. In another study Akhtar et al. [58] suggested cautious use of lidocaine during atrial fibrillation in patients who have accessory pathways with relatively rapid antegrade conduction characteristics. These authors studied 10 patients before and during lidocaine therapy (2 mg/kg intravenous bolus followed by 3 to 4 mg/min constant intravenous infusion). In patients with antegrade APERP ≤300 ms, lidocaine generally had no significant effect or accelerated the preexcited ventricular response during atrial fibrillation. In fact, in 2 of 8 patients acceleration of ventricular rate after lidocaine administration was associated with hemodynamic deterioration, necessitating direct current cardioversion in 1 patient. Thus, it appears that lidocaine should not be used as first line therapy to terminate or slow the tachycardia rate in patients who have arrhythmias with conduction over an accessory pathway.

AJMALINE

Ajmaline is an investigational antiarrhythmic drug that is commonly given intravenously (usually 50 mg over three minutes). It affects conduction and refractoriness of the accessory pathway and decreases the number of preexcited ventricular complexes during atrial flutter or fibrillation [54,59–62]. Ajmaline prolongs antegrade conduction and refractoriness over the accessory pathway most markedly if the control antegrade APERP is ≥270 ms [54]. For example, following ajmaline administration complete antegrade conduction block over the accessory pathway occurred in eight of nine patients with control APERP ≥270 ms, and in none of nine patients with control APERP <270 ms. In the latter group APERP increased in five patients and did not change in four patients after ajmaline was given. Ajmaline had less effect on accessory pathway retrograde conduction.

Chang et al. [63] treated 14 patients who had AV reentry with N-propylajmaline, an oral agent similar to ajmaline, at a dose of 60–80 mg daily. Initiation of AV reentrant tachycardia at electrophysiologic study was prevented in 7 of 14 patients and the tachycardia rate was slowed in the remaining 7 patients during drug treatment. The effective refractory period of the accessory pathway increased significantly from 285 ± 24 ms to 350 ± 22 ms.

Wellens et al. [61] administered 50 mg of intravenous ajmaline to 59 patients with WPW syndrome. Complete antegrade pathway conduction block occurred in 32 patients (mean control APERP = 327 ± 70 ms) and conduction persisted in 27 patients (mean control APERP = 233 ± 28 ms). These authors suggested that "the use of ajmaline intravenously is ... a reliable and rapid procedure for identifying those patients with the WPW syndrome who have a short refractory period of the accessory pathway and are possibly at risk of circulatory insufficiency or sudden death if atrial fibrillation supervenes" [61]. However, two points deserve comment. First, ajmaline caused accessory pathway conduction block in patients with antegrade APERP as short as 230 ms, and 7 patients who developed conduction block had antegrade APERP ≤270 ms. These patients would have been classified as having a "long" antegrade APERP based on the results of ajmaline administration. Second, no prospective data exist at present to suggest that patients who have a "short" antegrade APERP are at increased risk of sudden death (see above). Since ajmaline administration rarely may result in patient death [64], and loss of preexcitation may occur in patients with a relatively short APERP, use of this test is discouraged.

QUINIDINE, PROCAINAMIDE, AND DISOPYRAMIDE

These drugs have local anesthetic properties and, in various circumstances, can depress conduction and prolong refractoriness of accessory pathways [54,62,65–69]. Wellens et al. [54] showed that when the pre-drug antegrade APERP was ≥270 ms, complete antegrade conduction block over the accessory pathway occurred in four of five patients given quinidine and in six of seven patients given procainamide. When control antegrade APERP was <270 ms, neither drug blocked conduction over the accessory pathway and quinidine and procainamide insignificantly increased mean APERP by 18 and 31 ms, respectively. Regardless of the initial retrograde APERP, procainamide and quinidine prolonged retrograde APERP less than antegrade APERP. The antiarrhythmic properties of quinidine and procainamide were investigated in another study [62]. Administration of procainamide prevented initation of AV reentrant tachycardia in three of four patients, and quinidine prevented tachycardia induction in two of four patients.

Sellers et al. [67] evaluated the electrophysiologic effects of procainamide and quinidine on accessory pathways. When the APERP could be determined prior to drug therapy, the antegrade APERP was <270 ms in 24 patients and ⩾270 ms in 4 patients, and the retrograde APERP was <270 ms in 20 patients and ⩾270 ms in 3 patients. These authors noted only modest effects of procainamide and quinidine to decrease the preexcited ventricular response during induced atrial fibrillation in this group of patients with predominantly short APERP. For example, the shortest preexcited RR interval increased 20 to 70 ms in 15 of 21 patients, and did not significantly change in 6 of 21 patients receiving procainamide. Results were somewhat better during quinidine therapy, and the shortest preexcited RR interval increased 20 to 170 ms in 16 of 16 patients. In contrast with the above study, procainamide treatment resulted in antegrade conduction block over the accessory pathway in 10 of 13 patients, most of whom had antegrade APERP >270 ms [66]. Further procainamide prevented AV reentrant tachycardia induction in 6 of 9 patients [66].

Kerr et al. [65] investigated the electrophysiologic and antiarrhythmic effects of intravenous and oral disopyramide in patients with the WPW syndrome. The shortest preexcited RR interval during atrial fibrillation was used to assess antegrade APERP. Before drug therapy the mean shortest RR interval was 169 ± 18 ms. Intravenous disopyramide prolonged the shortest RR interval to 226 ± 24 ms ($p < .0001$) and oral disopyramide prolonged the shortest RR interval to 248 ± 36 ms ($p < .0001$). After oral disopyramide therapy, the episodes of atrial fibrillation were shorter and self-terminating. Atrioventricular reciprocating tachycardia was initiated in ten patients before and during oral disopyramide therapy, and the tachycardia cycle length significantly increased from 331 ± 53 ms at control to 370 ± 68 ms during drug therapy. The prolonged tachycardia cycle length resulted mainly from an increase in the ventriculoatrial interval during tachycardia.

In summary, as single agents quinidine and procainamide have substantial antiarrhythmic properties in patients who have accessory pathways with "relatively long" effective refractory periods. Disopyramide appears more effective in patients who have accessory pathways with "relatively short" effective refractory periods. Further, disopyramide is well suited for chronic oral therapy in young patients with WPW syndrome who usually have neither myocardial dysfunction nor urinary obstructive problems. In patients with atrial fibrillation, intravenous procainamide is useful to block antegrade conduction over the accessory pathway as well as to terminate atrial fibrillation in a substantial number of patients (Figure 21–6 A and B).

MEXILETINE

Preliminary data suggest that mexiletine may be useful therapy to treat orthodromic reciprocating tachycardia [70,71]. Attempts to induce tachycardia were performed in 14 patients with reciprocating tachycardia utilizing an accessory AV pathway before and during intravenous mexiletine (10 mg/min, total 300–400 mg) infusion, and in 6 patients mexiletine prevented initiation of sustained tachycardia [70]. Further, mexiletine prolonged ventriculoatrial conduction time from 133 ± 72 ms to 163 ± 100 ms ($p < .05$). More studies are needed to define the role of mexiletine in patients with WPW syndrome.

Drugs with Antiarrhythmic Effects on the AV node and Accessory Pathway

Several drugs depress conduction and increase refractoriness in both the AV node and accessory pathway. These agents often are very effective therapy for AV reentry for they modify the electrophysiologic properties of multiple tissues in the tachycardia circuit. Further, during atrial tachyarrhythmias these drugs can decrease the ventricular response by blocking impulses over the accessory pathway as well as over the normal AV conducting system.

ENCAINIDE

In my opinion, encainide is one of the most effective antiarrhythmic drugs available to treat AV reentrant tachycardia. We [72] showed that oral encainide therapy significantly depressed AV nodal conduction and lengthened atrial and ventricular effective refractory period. Because encainide altered electrophysiologic properties of both the AV node and cardiac muscle, we hypothesized that it might exert important antitachycardia effects in patients who had AV reentrant tachycardia or atrial fibrillation. Electrophysiologic studies were performed in 19 patients with accessory AV pathways, 5 with

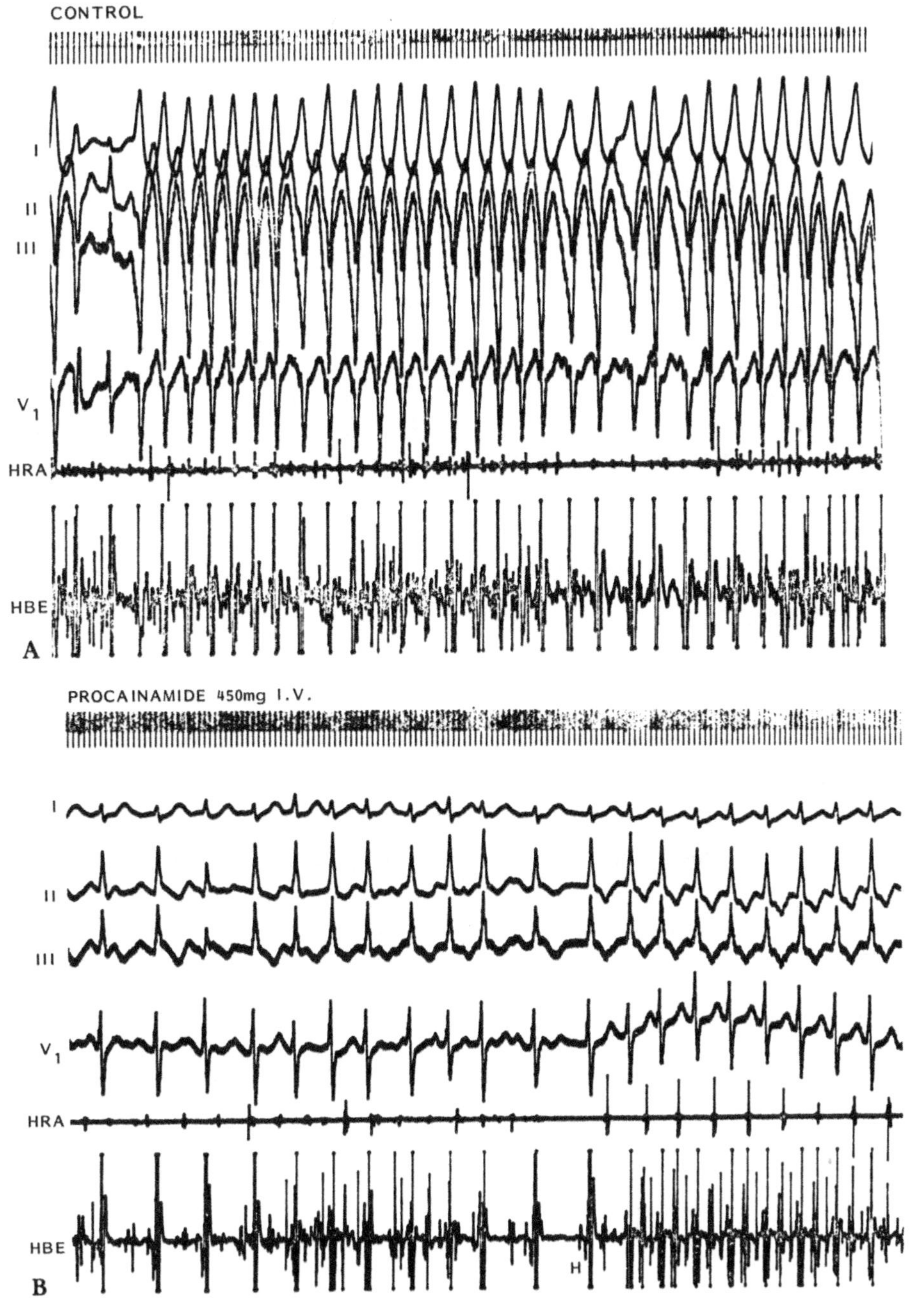

FIGURE 21–6. Effect of intravenous procainamide on preexcited ventricular response during atrial fibrillation. (A) Atrial fibrillation with rapid ventricular response due to preexcited QRS complexes. All but the second and third QRS complexes are preexcited. The shortest RR interval is 180 ms (333 beats per minute), and the mean RR interval is 207 ms (290 beats per minute). (B) Termination of atrial fibrillation with intravenous procainamide administration. Procainamide blocked conduction over the accessory pathway and then terminated atrial fibrillation. Note that a junctional complex (H) following atrial fibrillation initiates AV reentrant tachycardia. (From Prystowsky, EN, et al. *Med. Clin. North Am.* 68: 831, 1984. Reproduced with permission from WB Saunders Publishing Company.)

concealed conduction, before and during oral encainide therapy (mean dose, 197 mg per day) [73]. AV reentrant tachycardia had been present for a mean of 15.8 years, and 3.6 drug trials per patient had failed to prevent recurrence of tachycardia. Encainide caused complete antegrade conduction block in 8 of 14 patients, three of whom had an initial APERP <270 ms. The effects of encainide on retrograde accessory pathway conduction and refractoriness were more marked than those reported for any other drug, including amiodarone. Retrograde conduction could be evaluated in 14 patients, and block in the accessory pathway occurred in 7 patients, (5 with initial retrograde APERP <270 ms). Encainide prevented induction of reciprocating tachycardia in 10 of 19 patients. When initiated, the cycle length of orthodromic reciprocating tachycardia increased from 313.9 ± 53 ms to 418 ± 80.9 ms ($p < 0.0001$) (Figure 21–7). Currently, more than 30 patients, 2 with nodoventricular pathways, have been discharged receiving encainide therapy; only a few have had recurrence of tachycardia during follow-up.

Other investigators [74,75] corroborated our findings on the electrophysiologic effects of oral encainide therapy. Although they noted it to be useful in the treatment of tachyarrhythmias associated with accessory pathways, their overall success rate was less than our results. The discrepancy may be explained in large part by differences in doses of encainide employed in the different studies [73–75]. We have noted

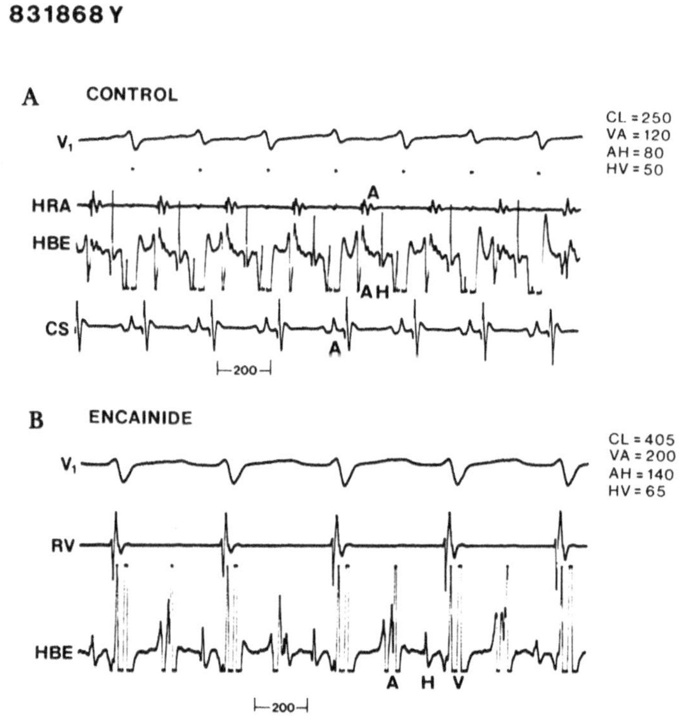

FIGURE 21–7. Orthodromic reciprocating tachycardia before and during encainide therapy. (A) Initial cycle length of tachycardia is 250 ms. (B) Encainide treatment did not prevent initiation of tachycardia during electrophysiologic study, but prolonged the cycle length of tachycardia to 405 ms as a result of an increase in VA interval of 80 ms, in AH interval of 60 ms, and in HV interval of 15 ms. (From Prystowsky, EN, Klein, GJ, Rinkenberger, RL, et al.: Clinial efficacy and electrophysiologic effects of encainide in patients with the Wolff-Parkinson-White syndrome. *Circulation* 69: 278, 1984. Reproduced with permission of the American Heart Association.)

that maximal therapeutic efficacy is usually achieved at encainide dosages of approximately 200 mg daily, and if patients tolerate the drug at the time of hospital discharge they usually do not have emergence of long-term side effects. In one study [74], repeat electrophysiologic testing was done during encainide treatment at 75 to 200 mg daily (mean 147 mg), and in the other investigation [75] oral encainide was given at a mean dose of 156 mg daily.

AMIODARONE

Amiodarone has become one of the most frequently used drugs to treat patients with supraventricular or ventricular tachycardia, even though significant side effects occur in many patients [76,77]. As yet, the "best" dosing schedule and duration of time after beginning treatment to judge therapeutic efficacy have not been well defined. In addition to the antiarrhythmic effects of amiodarone exerted on the AV node and accessory pathway, amiodarone is one of the most efficacious drugs used to prevent recurrence of paroxysmal atrial fibrillation [78]. Thus, amiodarone will usually either prevent recurrence of AV reciprocating tachycardia or atrial fibrillation, or slow the ventricular rate of the tachycardia [77,79–85]. Rosenbaum et al. [80] administered amiodarone, 300 to 600 mg/day, to 6 patients with reciprocating tachycardia utilizing an accessory AV pathway tachycardia and 5 patients with atrial fibrillation or flutter. In all patients the arrhythmias were totally controlled for periods ranging from 2 to 8 months. In another study, the electrophysiologic and antiarrhythmic properties of amiodarone were evaluated in 15 patients with WPW syndrome [84]. Electrophysiologic testing was performed before and after 14 days of drug therapy (600 mg/day for days 1 to 7 and 300 mg/day for days 8 to 14). Antegrade APERP lengthened in all patients, but retrograde APERP increased in only 8 of 15 patients. During amiodarone therapy AV reentrant tachycardia no longer could be induced in 5 of 15 patients, and in the other 10 patients drug-induced slowing of tachycardia rate occurred. Seven patients had initiation of atrial fibrillation before and during amiodarone treatment, and the mean ventricular rate decreased from 180–270/min to 130–240/min. Amiodarone, like other antiarrhythmic drugs (see above), prolongs APERP more if the initial APERP is ≥270 ms [54].

Rowland and Krikler [81] treated 13 patients with WPW syndrome and arrhythmias with amiodarone in a dose of 600 mg/day for the first month, 400 mg/day for the second month, and 200 mg/day maintenance if the response to therapy was satisfactory. Four patients who were treated for paroxysmal atrial fibrillation had atrial fibrillation induced at electrophysiologic study before and 3 months after start of therapy. Analysis of their data during atrial fibrillation show that the shortest RR interval increased a mean of 76 ms, and the mean RR interval increased a mean of 164 ms. In 9 patients AV reentrant tachycardia cycle length increased a mean of 119 ms during amiodarone treatment. However, amiodarone successfully controlled clinical arrhythmias in only 4 of 9 patients with AV reentry. Ward et al. [77] noted better antiarrhythmic results of amiodarone therapy in their patients, most of whom had AV reentrant tachycardia. In their series drug success was judged by subjective symptoms. Total and partial suppression of arrhythmias occurred in 59% and in 23% of patients, respectively [77].

PROPAFENONE

Propafenone therapy depresses AV nodal conduction and prolongs the effective refractory period of accessory pathways [86–88]. Breithardt et al. [87] evaluated the antiarrhythmic efficacy of propafenone in 47 patients with accessory pathways. Of patients undergoing electrophysiologic evaluation before and during drug therapy, propafenone was associated with an increase in antegrade APERP (238 to 322 ms, $p < .02$) and retrograde APERP (245 to 295 ms, $p < .01$); the shortest RR interval during atrial fibrillation increased from 232 to 303 ms ($p < .05$); and when reciprocating tachycardia could still be induced the tachycardia cycle length increased from 324 to 395 ms ($p < .01$). During a follow-up period of 2 to 3 years, 35 of 43 patients had no or only rare recurrences of symptomatic supraventricular tachycardia.

FLECAINIDE

Neuss et al. [89] investigated the electrophysiologic and antiarrhythmic properties of intravenous flecainide (100 mg) in 12 patients with WPW syndrome. Flecainide increased antegrade and retrograde APERP and prolonged AV nodal conduction time. When given during orthodromic reciprocating tachycardia, flecainide terminated tachycardia in 8 of 9 patients.

Nine patients were given oral flecainide at daily dosages of 200 to 500 mg and 5 patients had no recurrence of tachycardia during follow-up.

Recently, we had the opportunity to study the effect of flecainide in a child with the permanent form of AV reciprocating tachycardia, alternatively labeled PJRT. Dosage was initially 2 mg/kg daily but was titrated up to approximately 8 mg/kg daily. As the plasma drug level increased there were progressively longer tachycardia-free intervals until only sinus rhythm prevailed. During a 4-month follow-up period only isolated echo beats have been observed during repeated 24-hour ECG recordings.

SOTALOL

Sotalol is a beta-adrenergic antagonist that also prolongs refractoriness in myocardial cells [90,91]. Bennet [90] administered 1.5 mg/kg of intravenous sotalol to 15 patients with accessory pathways and noted an increase in the effective refractory period of the atria, ventricles, and accessory pathways. Both the cycle length of AV reentry and shortest preexcited RR interval during atrial fibrillation were increased. Of note, the shortest preexcited RR interval prolonged from 268 ± 77 ms to 351 ± 63 ms ($p < .002$).

Nathan et al. [91] noted the effects of 0.4 mg/kg of intravenous sotalol in 13 patients with WPW syndrome. The antegrade APERP increased from 317 ± 88 to 350 ± 81 ms ($p < .02$), and the retrograde APERP prolonged from 296 ± 40 to 371 ± 139 ms ($p < .05$). Sotalol terminated AV reentry in 5 of 12 patients, and the cycle length of tachycardia overall increased significantly from 355 ± 64 to 413 ± 54 ms.

LORCAINIDE

Preliminary data show potential antiarrhythmic efficacy for lorcainide in patients with WPW syndrome [92]. Kasper et al. [92] administered intravenous lorcainide (2 mg/kg) to 20 patients with accessory pathways. Retrograde conduction over the accessory pathway was blocked in 5 of 18 patients and antegrade conduction was blocked in 6 patients. The shortest preexcited RR interval during atrial fibrillation increased from 228 ± 35 to 304 ± 103 ms ($p < .05$).

Drug Selection

A plethora of new drugs have demonstrated efficacy in the treatment of supraventricular tachyarrhythmias in patients with WPW syndrome. The choice of a specific antiarrhythmic agent to treat patients with tachycardia utilizing accessory pathways is discussed in detail elsewhere in this volume and depends on many factors. Some of these factors include patient age, myocardial function, presence of other medical disorders, integrity of peripheral vascular tone, and type and frequency of occurrence of arrhythmia. For example, I avoid giving verapamil or disopyramide to patients with substantial ventricular myocardial dysfunction and prefer not to administer procainamide to young patients because of its known effects on the autoimmune system. Assuming that: (1) all pertinent factors about the patient and arrhythmia have been evaluated, (2) the patient is hemodynamically stable, and (3) all drugs are available for use, my present initial choices of therapy are:

1. intravenous verapamil to terminate AV reentry,
2. intravenous procainamide to block antegrade conduction over the accessory pathway during atrial fibrillation,
3. oral digitalis, a drug that can be given once a day, to treat patients with AV reentry involving a concealed accessory pathway or an accessory pathway with a known "long" antegrade effective refractory period, and
4. encainide to treat patients with AV reentry in whom the antegrade accessory pathway ERP is unknown or "short".

References

1. Prystowsky EN, Miles WM, Heger JJ, Zipes DP: Preexcitation syndromes. *Med. Clin. N. A.* 68:831, 1984
2. Lloyd EA, Hauer RN, Zipes DP, Heger JJ, Prystowsky EN: Syncope and ventricular tachycardia in patients with ventricular preexcitation. *Am. J. Cardiol.* 52:79, 1983.
3. Dreifus LS, Haiat R, Watanabe Y, Arriaga J, Reitman N: Ventricular fibrillation. A possible mechanism of sudden death in patients with Wolff-Parkinson-White syndrome. *Circulation* 43:520, 1971.
4. Klein GJ, Bashore TM, Sellers TD, Pritchett ELC, Smith WM, Gallagher JJ: Ventricular fibrillation in the Wolff-Parkinson-White syndrome. *N. Engl. J. Med.* 301:1080, 1979.
5. Wellens HJ, Durrer D: Wolff-Parkinson-White

syndrome and atrial fibrillation. Relation between refractory period of accessory pathway and ventricular rate during atrial fibrillation. *Am. J. Cardiol.* 34:777, 1974.
6. Tonkin AM, Miller HC, Svenson RH, Wallace AG, Gallagher JJ: Refractory periods of the accessory pathway in the Wolff-Parkinson-White syndrome. *Circulation* 52:563, 1975.
7. Wellens HJJ, Braat S, Brugada P, Gorgels APM, Bar FW: Use of procainamide in patients with the Wolff-Parkinson-White syndrome to disclose a short refractory period of the accessory pathway. *Am. J. Cardiol.* 50:1087, 1982.
8. Klein GJ, Gulamhusein SS: Intermittent preexcitation in the Wolff-Parkinson-White syndrome. *Am. J. Cardiol.* 52:292, 1983.
9. Rowland E, Curry P, Fox K, Krikler D: Relation between atrioventricular pathways and ventricular response during atrial fibrillation and flutter. *Br. Heart J.* 45:83, 1981.
10. German LD, Gallagher JJ, Broughton A, Guannieri T, Trantham JL: Effects of exercise and isoproterenol during atrial fibrillation in patients with Wolff-Parkinson-White syndrome. *Am. J. Cardiol.* 51:1203, 1983.
11. Cosio FG, Benson DW Jr, Anderson RW, Hession WT, Pritzker MR, Kreit JM, Benditt DG: Onset of atrial fibrillation during antidromic tachycardia: Association with sudden cardiac arrest and ventricular fibrillation in a patient with Wolff-Parkinson-White syndrome. *Am. J. Cardiol.* 50:353, 1982.
12. Prystowsky EN: Pharmacologic therapy of tachyarrhythmias in patients with Wolff-Parkinson-White syndrome. *Herz* 8:133, 1983.
13. Jedeikin R, Gillette PC, Garson A, Porter CJ, Beder S, Baron P, Zinner AJ III: Effect of ouabain on the anterograde effective refractory period of accessory atrioventricular connections in children. *J. Am. Coll. Cardiol.* 1:869, 1983.
14. Sellers TD, Bashore TM, Gallagher JJ: Digitalis in the preexcitation syndrome. Analysis during atrial fibrillation. *Circulation* 56:260, 1977.
15. Wellens HJJ, Durrer D: Effect of digitalis on atrioventricular conduction and circus-movement tachycardia in patients with Wolff-Parkinson-White syndrome. *Circulation* 47:1229, 1973.
16. Deal BJ, Keane JF, Gillette PC, Garson A: Wolff-Parkinson-White syndrome and supraventricular tachycardia during infancy: management and follow-up. *J. Am. Coll. Cardiol.* 5:130, 1985.
17. Damato AN, Caracta AR, Akhtar M, Lau SH: The effects of commonly used cardiovascular drugs on AV conduction and refractoriness. In *His Bundle Electrocardiography and Clinical Electrophysiology*, Narula OS (ed.), Philadelphia, Davis Publishing Co., 1975, pp. 105–125.
18. Dhingra RC, Palileo EV, Strasberg B, Swiryn S, Bauernfeind R, Wyndham C, Rosen KM: Electrophysiologic effects of ouabain in patients with preexcitation and circus movement tachycardia. *Am. J. Cardiol.* 47:139, 1981.
19. Vrhovac B, Bakran I, Durakovic Z, Gjurasin M, Francetic I, Mohacek I: The effect of propranolol, prindolol, practolol and verapamil versus placebo on exercise induced tachycardia in patients with ventricular preexcitation. *Int. J. Clin. Pharmacol.* 14:132, 1976.
20. Hombach V, Braun V, Hopp H-W, Gil-Sanchez D, Behrenbeck DW, Tauchert M, Hilger HH: Antiarrhythmic effects of acute beta-blockade with atenolol on supraventricular tachycardias at rest and during exercise. *Klin. Wochenschr.* 59:123, 1981.
21. Gmeiner R, Ng CK: Metoprolol in the treatment and prophylaxis of paroxysmal reentrant supraventricular tachycardia. *J. Cardiovasc. Pharmacol.* 4:5, 1982.
22. Skale BT, Heger JJ, Zipes DP, Prystowsky EN: Timolol: electrophysiologic and antiarrhythmic evaluation in ventricular and supraventricular tachycardia. (Submitted for publication.)
23. Chang M-S, Sung RJ, Tai T-Y, Lin S-L, Liu P-H, Chiang BN: Nadolol and supraventricular tachycardia: an electrophysiologic study. *J. Am. Coll. Cardiol.* 2(5):894, 1983.
24. Prystowsky EN, Jackman WM, Rinkenberger RL, Heger JJ, Zipes DP: Effect of autonomic blockade on ventricular refractoriness and atrioventricular nodal conduction in man. Evidence supporting a direct cholinergic action on ventricular muscle refractoriness. *Circ. Res.* 49:511, 1981.
25. Berkowitz WD, Wit AL, Lau SH, Steiner C, Damato AN: The effects of propranolol on cardiac conduction. *Circulation* 40:855, 1969.
26. Denes P, Cummings JM, Simpson R, Wu D, Amta-y-Leon R, Dhingra R, Rosen KM: Effects of propranolol on anomalous pathway refractoriness and circus movement tachycardias in patients with preexcitation. *Am. J. Cardiol.* 41:1061, 1978.
27. Barrett PA, Jordan JL, Mandel WJ, Yamaguchi I, Laks MM: The electrophysiologic effects of intravenous propranolol in the Wolff-Parkinson-White syndrome. *Am. Heart J.* 98:213, 1979.
28. Przybylski J, Chiale PA, Halpern S, Nau GJ, Elizari MV, Rosenbaum MB: Unmasking of ventricular preexcitation by vagal stimulation or isoproterenol administration. *Circulation* 61:1030, 1980.
29. Wellens HJJ, Brugada P, Roy D, Weiss J, Bar FW: Effect of isoproterenol on the antegrade refractory period of the accessory pathway in patients with the Wolff-Parkinson-White syndrome. *Am. J. Cardiol.* 50:180, 1982.

30. Wit AL, Cranefield PF: Effect of verapamil on the sinoatrial and atrioventricular nodes of the rabbit and the mechanism by which it arrests reentrant atrioventricular nodal tachycardia. *Circ. Res.* 35:413, 1974.
31. Zipes DP, Fischer JC: Effects of agents which inhibit the slow channel on sinus node automaticity and atrioventricular conduction in the dog. *Circ. Res.* 34:124, 1974.
32. Zipes DP, Mendez C: Action of manganese ion and tetrodotoxin on atrioventricular nodal transmembrane potentials in isolated rabbit hearts. *Circ. Res.* 32:447, 1973.
33. Singh BN, Vaughan Williams EM: A fourth class of antidysrhythmic action? Effect of verapamil on ouabain toxicity, on atrial, and ventricular intracellular potentials, and on other features of cardiac function. *Cardiovasc. Res.* 6:109, 1972.
34. Klein GJ, Gulamhusein S, Prystowsky EN, Carruthers SG, Donner AP, Ko PT: Comparison of the electrophysiological effects of intravenous and oral verapamil in patients with paroxysmal supraventricular tachycardia. *Am. J. Cardiol.* 49:117, 1982.
35. Krikler DM, Spurrell RAJ: Verapamil in the treatment of paroxysmal supraventricular tachycardia. *Postgrad. Med.* 50:447, 1974.
36. Rinkenberger RL, Prystowsky EN, Heger JJ, Troup PJ, Jackman WM, Zipes DP: Effects of IV and chronic oral verapamil administration in patients with a variety of supraventricular tachyarrhythmias. *Circulation* 62:996, 1980.
37. Schamroth L, Krikler DM, Garrett C: Immediate effects of intravenous verapamil in cardiac arrhythmias. *Br. Med. J.* 1:660, 1972.
38. Spurrell RAJ, Krikler DM, Sowton E: Effects of verapamil on electrophysiological properties of anomalous atrioventricular connexion in Wolff Parkinson-White syndrome. *Br. Heart J.* 36:256, 1974.
39. Wellens HJJ, Tan SL, Bar FW, Duren DR, Lie KI, Dohmen HM: Effect of verapamil studied by programmed electrical stimulation of the heart in patients with paroxysmal reentrant supraventricular tachycardia. *Br. Heart J.* 39:1058, 1977.
40. Hamer A, Peter T, Platt M, Mandel WJ: Effects of verapamil on supraventricular tachycardia in patients with overt and concealed Wolff-Parkinson-White syndrome. *Am. Heart J.* 101:600, 1981.
41. Prystowsky EN, Gilmour RF Jr: Role of slow channel blockers in the treatment of arrhythmias: Basic considerations and clinical applications. In *Pharmacological Treatment of Cardiovascular Diseases*, Kostis JB, Defelice EA (eds.), New York, Medical Examination Publishing Co., 1985 (in press).
42. Rozanski JJ, Zaman L, Castellanos A: Electrophysiologic effects of Diltiazem Hydrochloride on supraventricular tachycardia. *Am. J. Cardiol.* 49:621, 1982.
43. Yeh SJ, Kou HC, Liov FC, Hung JS, Wu D: Effects of oral Diltiazem in paroxysmal supraventricular tachycardia. *Am. J. Cardiol.* 52:271, 1983.
44. Betriu A, Chaitman BR, Bourassa MG, Brevers G, School JM, Bruneau P, Gagne P, Chabot M: Beneficial effect of intravenous Diltiazem in the acute management of paroxysmal supraventricular tachyarrhythmias. *Circulation* 67:88, 1983.
45. Prystowsky EN: Electrophysiologic and antiarrhythmic properties of bepridil. *Am. J. Cardiol.* 55(7):59C, 1985.
46. Rowland E, McKenna W, Krikler DM: Comparative electrophysiological effects of novel antiarrhythmic drug, bepridil. (Abstract.) *Br. Heart J.* 48:87, 1982.
47. Gulamhusein S, Ko P, Carruthers SG, Klein GJ: Acceleration of the ventricular response during atrial fibrillation in the Wolff-Parkinson-White syndrome after verapamil. *Circulation* 65:348, 1982.
48. Petri H, Kafka W, Hall D, Rudolph W: Potential acceleration of the ventricular rate in Wolff-Parkinson-White syndrome with atrial fibrillation after verapamil. (Abstract.) *Circulation* 62:262, 1980.
49. Harper RW, Whitford E, Middlebrook K, Federman J, Anderson S, Pitt A: Effects of verapamil on the electrophysiologic properties of the accessory pathway in patients with the Wolff-Parkinson-White syndrome. *Am. J. Cardiol.* 50:56, 1982.
50. Petri H, Kafka W, Rudolph W: Discrepant effects of oral and intravenous verapamil on A-V conduction in patients with ventricular preexcitation and atrial fibrillation. *Herz* 8:144, 1983.
51. Puech P, Sassine A, Munoz A, Masse C, Zettelmaier F, Leenhardt A, Yoshimura H: Electrophysiologic effects of purines; Clinical applications. In *Cardiac Electrophysiology and Arrhythmias*, New York, Grune and Stratton, 1985, pp. 443–450.
52. DiMarco JP, Sellers TD, Berne RM, West GA, Belardinelli L: Adenosine: electrophysiologic effects and therapeutic use for terminating paroxysmal supraventricular tachycardia. *Circulation* 68:1254, 1983.
53. Belhassen B, Pelleg A: Acute management of paroxysmal supraventricular tachycardia: Verapamil, adenosine triphosphate or adenosine? *Am. J. Cardiol.* 54:225, 1984.
54. Wellens HJJ, Bar FW, Dassen WRM, Brugada P, Vanagt EJ, Farre J: Effect of drugs in the Wolff-Parkinson-White syndrome. Importance of initial length of effective refractory period of the accessory pathway. *Am. J. Cardiol.* 46:665, 1980.
55. Rosen KM, Barwolf C, Ehsani A, Rahimtoola

SH: Effects of lidocaine and propranolol on the normal and anomalous pathways with preexcitation. *Am. J. Cardiol.* 30:801, 1972.
56. Josephson ME, Kastor JA, Ketchen JG: III: Lidocaine in Wolff-Parkinson-White syndrome with atrial fibrillation. *Ann. Intern. Med.* 84:44, 1976.
57. Barrett PA, Laks MM, Mandel WJ, Yamaguchi I: The electrophysiologic effects of intravenous lidocaine in the Wolff-Parkinson-White syndrome. *Am. Heart J.* 100:23, 1980.
58. Akhtar M, Gilbert CJ, Shenasa M: Effect of lidocaine on atrioventricular response via the accessory pathway in patients with Wolff-Parkinson-White syndrome. *Circulation* 63:435, 1981.
59. Puech P, Latour H, Hertault J, Grolleau R: L'ajmaline injectable dans les tachycardies paroxystiques et le syndrome de Wolff-Parkinson-White. Comparison avec le procainamide. *Arch. Mal Coeur* 2:897, 1964.
60. Selarovsky S, Kracoff OH, Strasberg B, Lewin RF, Agmon J: Paroxysmal atrial flutter and fibrillation associated with preexcitation syndrome: treatment with ajmaline. *Am. J. Cardiol.* 48:929, 1981.
61. Wellens HJJ, Bar FW, Gorgels AP, Vanagt EJ: Use of ajmaline in patients with the Wolff-Parkinson-White syndrome to disclose short refractory period of the accessory pathway. *Am. J. Cardiol.* 45:130, 1980.
62. Wellens HJJ, Durrer D: Effect of procaine amide, quinidine, and ajmaline in the Wolff-Parkinson-White syndrome. *Circulation* 50:114, 1974.
63. Chang M-S, Tai D-Y, Chiang BN, Sung RJ: Efficacy and antiarrhythmic mechanism of N-propyl Ajmaline in the treatment of paroxysmal supraventricular tachycardia. *J. Am. Coll. Cardiol.* 5:479, 1985.
64. Wellens HJJ, Bar FW, Vanagt EJ: Death after ajmaline administration. *Am. J. Cardiol.* 45:905, 1980.
65. Kerr CR, Prystowsky EN, Smith WM, Cook L, Gallagher JJ: Electrophysiologic effects of disopyramide phosphate in patients with Wolff-Parkinson-White syndrome. *Circulation* 65:869, 1982.
66. Mandel WJ, Laks MM, Obayashi K, Hayakawa H, Daley W: The Wolff-Parkinson-White syndrome: Pharmacologic effects of procainamide. *Am. Heart J.* 90:744, 1975.
67. Sellers TD Jr, Campbell RWF, Bashore TM, Gallagher JJ: Effects of procainamide and quinidine sulfate in the Wolff-Parkinson-White syndrome. *Circulation* 55:15, 1977.
68. Spurrell RAJ, Thorburn CW, Camm J, Sowton E, Deuchar DC: Effects of disopyramide on electrophysiological properties of specialized conduction system in man and on accessory atrioventricular pathway in Wolff-Parkinson-White syndrome. *Br. Heart J.* 37:861, 1975.
69. Bennett DH: Disopyramide in patients with the Wolff-Parkinson-White syndrome and atrial fibrillation. *Chest* 74:624, 1978.
70. Benditt DG, Pool-Schneider S, Dunnigan A, Gornick CC, Benson DW Jr: Suppression of paroxysmal supraventricular tachyarrhythmias with intravenous mexiletine. (Abstract.) *PACE* 8:302, 1985.
71. Touboul P, Gressard A, Kirkorian G, Atallah G: Effects of mexiletine in the Wolff-Parkinson-White syndrome. *Arch. Mal Coeur* 74:1315, 1981.
72. Jackman WM, Zipes DP, Naccarelli GV, Rinkenberger RL, Heger JJ, Prystowsky EN: Electrophysiology of oral encainide. *Am. J. Cardiol.* 49:1270, 1982.
73. Prystowsky EN, Klein GH, Rinkenberger RL, Heger JJ, Naccarelli GV, Zipes DP: Clinical efficacy and electrophysiologic effects of encainide in patients with the Wolff-Parkinson-White syndrome. *Circulation* 69:278, 1984.
74. Kunze K-P, Kuck K-H, Schluter M, Kuch B, Bleifeld W: Electrophysiologic and clinical effects of intravenous and oral encainide in accessory atrioventricular pathway. *Am. J. Cardiol.* 54:323, 1984.
75. Abdollah H, Brugada P, Green M, Wehr M, Wellens HJJ, with the technical assistance of Paulussen G: Clinical efficacy and electrophysiologic effects of intravenous and oral encainide in patients with accessory atrioventricular pathways and supraventricular arrhythmias. *Am. J. Cardiol.* 54:544, 1984.
76. Heger JJ, Prystowsky EN, Jackman WM, Naccarelli GV, Warfel KA, Rinkenberger RL, Zipes DP. Amiodarone: clinical efficacy and electrophysiology during long-term therapy for recurrent ventricular tachycardia or ventricular fibrillation. *N. Engl. J. Med.* 305:539, 1981.
77. Ward DE, Camm AJ Spurrell RAJ: Clinical antiarrhythmic effects of amiodarone in patients with resistant paroxysmal tachycardias. *Br. Heart J.* 44:91, 1980.
78. Yee KG, Heger JJ, Prystowsky EN, Miles WM, Zipes DP: Predictors of clinical efficacy for amiodarone in supraventricular tachyarrhythmias. (Abstract.) *Circulation* 70:II–438, 1984.
79. Chamberlain DA, Clark ANG: Atrial fibrillation complicating Wolff-Parkinson-White syndrome treated with amiodarone. *Br. Med. J.* 2:1519, 1977.
80. Rosenbaum MB, Chiate PA, Ryba D, Elizari MV: Control of tachyarrhythmias associated with Wolff-Parkinson-White syndrome by amiodarone hydrochloride. *Am. J. Cardiol.* 34:215, 1974.
81. Rowland E, Krikler DM: Electrophysiological assessment of amiodarone in treatment of resis-

tant supraventricular arrhythmias. *Br. Heart J.* 44:82, 1980.
82. Touboul P, Porte J, Huerta F, Delahaye J-P: Effets electrophysiologiques de l'amiodarone dans le syndrome de Wolff-Parkinson-White. *Arch. Mal Coeur* 69:855, 1976.
83. Waleffe A, Bruninx P, Kulbertus HE: Effects of amiodarone studied by programmed electrical stimulation of the heart in patients with paroxysmal re-entrant supraventricular tachycardia. *J. Electrocardiol.* 11:253, 1978.
84. Wellens HJJ, Lie KI, Bar FW, Wesdrop JC, Dohmen HJ, Duren DR, Durrer D: Effect of amiodarone in Wolff-Parkinson-White syndrome. *Am. J. Cardiol.* 38:189, 1976.
85. Kappenberger LJ, Fromer MA, Steinbrunn W, Shenasa M: Efficacy of amiodarone in the Wolff-Parkinson-White syndrome with rapid ventricular response via accessory pathway during atrial fibrillation. *Am. J. Cardiol.* 54:330, 1984.
86. Chilson DA, Heger JJ, Zipes DP, Browne KF, Prystowsky EN: Electrophysiologic effects and clinical efficacy of oral propafenone therapy in patients with ventricular tachycardia. *J. Am. Coll. Cardiol.* 5(6):1407, 1985.
87. Breithardt G, Borggrefe M, Wiebringhaus E, Seipel L: Effect of propafenone in the Wolff-Parkinson-White syndrome: Electrophysiologic findings and long-term follow-up. *Am. J. Cardiol.* 54:29D, 1984.
88. Waleffe A, Mary-Rabine L, de Rijbel R, Soyeur D, Legrand V, Kulbertus HE: Electrophysiological effects of propafenone studied with programmed electrical stimulation of the heart in patients with recurrent paroxysmal supraventricular tachycardia. *Eur. Heart J.* 2:345, 1981.
89. Neuss H, Buss J, Schlepper M, Berthold R, Mitrovic V, Kramer A, Musial J: Effects of flecainide on electrophysiological properties of accessory pathways in the Wolff-Parkinson-White syndrome. *Eur. Heart J.* 4:347, 1983.
90. Bennett DH: Acute prolongation of myocardial refractoriness by sotalol. *Br. Heart J.* 47:521, 1982.
91. Nathan AW, Hellestrand KJ, Bexton RS, Ward DE, Spurrell RAJ, Camm AJ: Electrophysiological effects of sotalol — just another beta blocker? *Br. Heart J.* 47:515, 1982.
92. Kasper W, Treese N, Meinertz T, Jahnchen E, Pop T: Electrophysiologic effects of lorcainide on the accessory pathway in the Wolff-Parkinson-White syndrome. *Am. J. Cardiol.* 51:1618, 1983.

22. TREATMENT OF PEDIATRIC PATIENTS WITH PREEXCITATION SYNDROMES

D. Woodrow Benson, Jr.
Ann Dunnigan

For young patients with preexcitation syndromes the associated tachycardias and available treatment options are virtually identical to those discussed in other chapters in this book. However, the symptomatic expression of tachycardia may be quite different in young patients with preexcitation syndromes. The role of age-related changes in autonomic tone, morphologic-functional changes in the atrioventricular (AV) node or accessory connection, or changes in the initiating event of tachycardia in serially determining the presence or absence and severity of symptoms in patients with preexcitation syndromes is poorly understood. Nevertheless, age-related differences in symptom expression must be considered in treatment of the young patient. For example, unless associated heart disease is present, an otherwise healthy child may have surprisingly few symptoms from tachycardias even when the rate is rapid. Additionally, death or sudden cardiac arrest in patients with preexcitation syndromes has rarely been documented in the first decade [1–3], possibly because atrial fibrillation (the arrhythmia most closely associated with sudden death in preexcitation syndrome patients) has been reported rarely during the first decade of life [4,5]. Finally, time is often an ally, since young patients may cease having episodes of tachycardia for many years [6–8]. This phenomenon is poorly understood, and emphasizes our incomplete knowledge about the natural history of preexcitation syndromes in affected patients (see Chapter 2 by Dunnigan).

Benditt, D.G. and Benson, D.W., Cardiac Preexcitation Syndromes.

Approach to Treatment

Once a decision to institute therapy has been reached, then the successful treatment of the neonate, infant, or child with one of the preexcitation syndromes requires a logical approach to the specific rhythm disturbance presented. Until recently, the treatment of rhythm disturbances associated with the preexcitation syndromes, especially in infants and children, was empiric. This was partly due to a paucity of methods for defining tachycardia characteristics, and partly due to a limited number of treatment options. However, improved methods for better defining the electrophysiologic characteristics of tachycardias have become available, and knowledge about electrophysiologic characteristics of tachycardias has permitted a more rational approach to a considerably increased number of treatment choices. For example, while orthodromic reciprocating tachycardia is believed to be the most frequently occurring tachycardia in patients with preexcitation syndromes, the observation that 10 to 50% of tachycardia episodes in infants with preexcitation exhibit a prolonged (wide) QRS complex [6,9] raises the possibility that the occurrence of antidromic tachycardia, orthodromic tachycardia with bundle branch block, or tachycardia with an accessory nodoventricular connection are more common than previously recognized in young patients [10]. These distinctions have important implications for the likelihood of successful tachycardia treatment with available medical, surgical, or pacemaker options.

The current approach to the management of the young patient with preexcitation stems from the idea that management can be individualized, rather than "one drug fits all." Thus, in planning treatment for the young patient with arrhythmia and preexcitation it is important to define or at least establish a differential diagnosis of the mechanism of tachycardia. For consideration of subsequent treatment, it is important to assess the frequency, duration, and mode of onset of tachycardia episodes as well as the severity of tachycardia related symptoms. For example, the approach to treatment in a patient who infrequently had symptomatic tachycardia episodes which lasted many hours might be quite different than for a patient who had several episodes per day of symptomatically equivalent tachycardia each lasting seconds to minutes. Similarly, treatment considerations would be different in a mildly symptomatic patient who only suffered from the sensation of rapid heart beating as opposed to a patient who experienced syncope or cardiac arrest due to tachycardia.

In some young patients with preexcitation syndromes, no treatment is indicated. When treatment is indicated, the traditional approach has usually relied on prophylactic medication administered several times daily; however, it is now known that some patients do well when medication is taken following tachycardia onset (periodic treatment). Additionally, recent developments in permanent antitachycardia pacing provide suitable pacemaker treatment in very select patients. Finally, a major breakthrough in the management of patients with preexcitation syndromes has been the development of techniques for ablation of accessory AV connections, thereby resulting in "cure" of preexcitation syndromes in some patients. In this chapter, the management of young patients with preexcitation syndromes will be considered from the standpoint of immediate treatment following tachycardia onset (established episode) and treatment to prevent tachycardia recurrence.

Tachycardias Associated with Preexcitation Syndromes

Tachycardia mechanisms associated with preexcitation syndromes are discussed in detail elsewhere in this book (see Chapters 9 by Sung and Tai, 6 by Morady, and 18 by Kugler). Assessment of the ECG during tachycardia should permit establishing a differential diagnosis of tachycardia (Figure 22–1). Special attention should be directed to whether tachycardia is regular or irregular and whether QRS duration is normal or prolonged (wide QRS) and whether the morphology is normal or due to bundle branch block or preexcitation. Critical observation of QRS duration is required since for patients in the first decade of life, average QRS duration is less than 65 ms and a QRS duration of 85 ms is at the 98th percentile of normal [11].

In the preexcitation syndromes, regular tachycardia with a normal QRS is commonly documented; this tachycardia usually results from depolarization of the ventricles via the normal conduction system and atrial depolarization resulting from retrograde excitation of the accessory connection (orthodromic reciprocating tachycardia). The reentrant circuit may sometimes be reversed resulting in regular tachycardia with a prolonged QRS duration and preexcited QRS morphology (antidromic reciprocating tachycardia) [10]. During atrial fibrillation, other primary atrial tachycardias, or reentry within the AV node — any of which may occur coincidentally in patients who also happen to have accessory connections — regular or irregular wide QRS tachycardias with rapid ventricular rate may occur as the result of ventricular activation due primarily to antegrade conduction of the atrial impulse via the accessory connection.

In this chapter an attempt has been made to refer to tachycardias by specific mechanisms when possible (e.g., orthodromic reciprocating tachycardia). When the mechanism is unknown, tachycardia with prolonged or wide QRS is referred to descriptively. Regular tachycardias with a normal QRS duration and no evidence of AV dissociation are referred to descriptively or else by a specific mechanism.

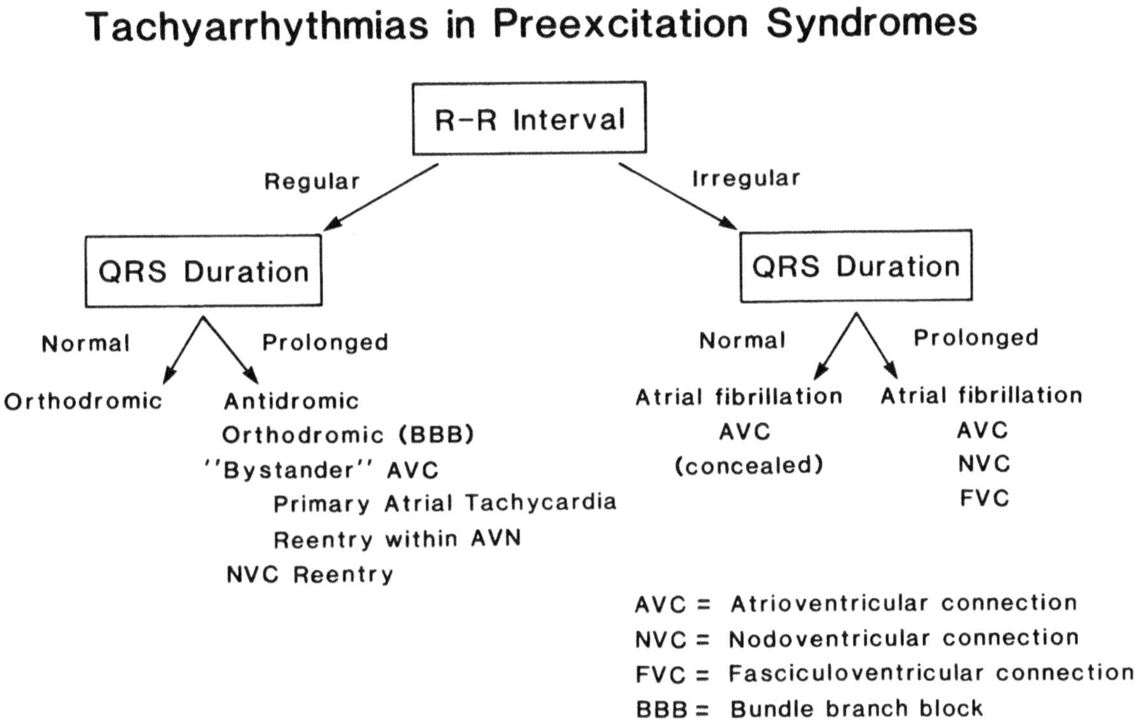

FIGURE 22–1. ECG diagnosis of tachyarrhythmias in preexcitation syndromes.

In a simple way, reciprocating tachycardias associated with preexcitation syndromes may be considered in terms of their antegrade and retrograde limbs. Refractoriness or conduction characteristics, or both, of the cardiac tissues comprising the antegrade or retrograde limbs of the reentrant circuit may affect the initiation or maintenance of tachycardia. As assessed during catheter electrophysiologic study, most antiarrhythmic agents can be demonstrated to affect one or the other limb of the reentrant circuit. For example, disopyramide, quinidine and procainamide [12–15] usually prolong refractoriness in accessory AV connections, whereas verapamil [16–18] primarily affects the AV node. Thus, while verapamil may be effective in orthodromic reciprocating tachycardia, it does not slow and may actually increase the ventricular rate during atrial fibrillation [19]. On the other hand, amiodarone [20,21] and encainide [22,23] may have salutory effects for tachycardia termination and prevention on both limbs of the reentrant circuit. Finally, it is well recognized that some antiarrhythmic drugs do not have the same effects on conduction and refractoriness on antegrade and retrograde limbs of the reentrant circuit [13].

Treatment of Established Tachycardia

DIGITALIS DERIVATIVES

These ancient compounds have been the mainstay of tachycardia management for many decades. Their efficacy has been widely touted. However, digitalis derivatives may be hazardous when parenterally administered for treatment of some tachycardias associated with preexcitation syndromes, while other therapeutic avenues to be discussed offer many advantages over digitalis in the acute treatment of established tachycardia. Consequently, we no longer recommend use of digitalis derivatives for acute treatment of established tachycardia.

REFLEX VAGAL STIMULATION

Since early in this century, maneuvers that reflexly increase vagal tone have been used to terminate tachycardia. These maneuvers are

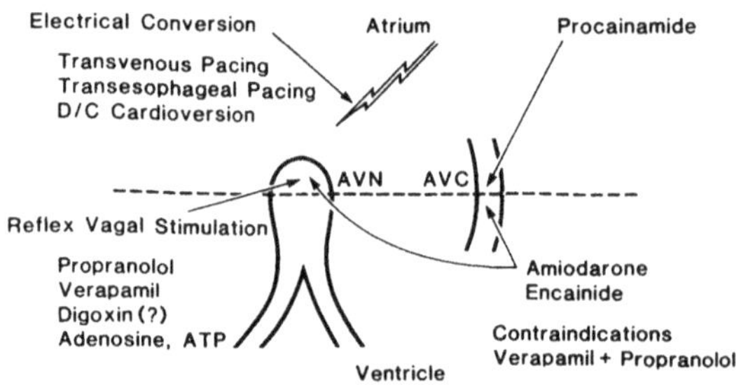

FIGURE 22–2. Treatment options for established regular tachycardia with a normal QRS.

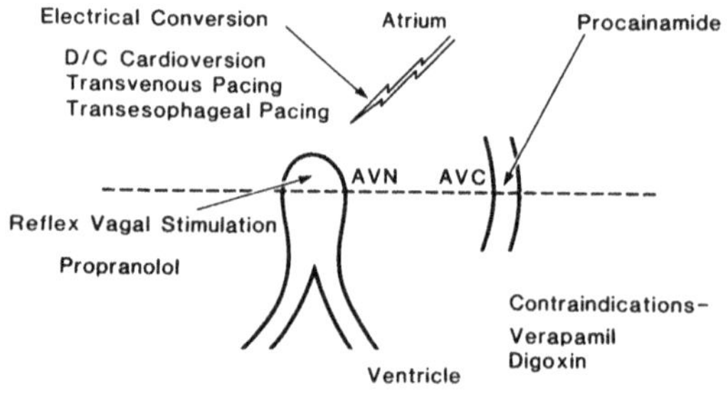

FIGURE 22–3. Treatment options for established tachycardia with a prolonged (wide) QRS.

thought to act by inducing neural-mediated interference with AV node conduction (Figures 22–2 and 22–3). However, since the report by Nadas et al. [24], it has been widely stated that reflex vagal stimulation for tachycardia termination in the very young is not only ineffective but may be hazardous. On the other hand, reflex vagal stimulation has not been as systematically studied in the very young as it has in the older patient. For example, the studies of Waxman et al. [25] nicely summarize the results of reflex vagal stimulation in 68 consecutive cases of either orthodromic reciprocating tachycardia or reciprocating tachycardia due to reentry within the AV node in patients 14 to 74 years old. In these studies, carotid sinus massage, carotid massage plus edrophonium, valsalva and phenylephrine infusion were used as graded forms of reflex vagal stimulation. Waxman et al. [25] found reflex vagal stimulation to be highly successful in tachycárdia termination, but an increase in background sympathetic tone or muscarinic receptor blockade with atropine interfered with or eliminated the therapeutic effect.

Bisset et al. [26] reported uniform success of tachycardia conversion in 10 patients 1 day to 15 years of age when an ice bag applied to the face was used to stimulate the "diving reflex." These investigators interpreted their findings as indicating that the diving reflex provided intense reflex vagal stimulation in young patients. Studies by Sperandeo et al. [27] reported similar success in 10 infants less than six months of age. In anectdotal reports, other forms of reflex vagal stimulation, e.g. assuming upside-down position and induction of hypertension with alpha adrenergic agonists have been reported to be successful in producing reflex vagal stimulation to effect tachycardia termination.

ELECTRICAL CONVERSION

Most available antiarrhythmic drugs interfere with cardiac function and/or vascular tone such that hypotension occurs as a common side effect. If drug administration results in tachycardia conversion, then the side effect is often well tolerated. However, if tachycardia persists, life-threatening symptoms may develop following antiarrhythmic administration. The situation may become more critical if additional anti-arrhythmic medications are acutely administered. Such complications may be avoided by use of electrical conversion (Figures 22–2 and 22–3).

Electrical conversion of tachycardia is the treatment of choice when the mechanism of tachycardia is unknown or when the patient is critically ill. Synchronized direct electrical current cardioversion using 1–2 joules/kg has been a highly effective and safe form of treatment for acute termination of tachycardia in young patients with preexcitation syndromes. Alternatively, the use of temporary pacing with transvenous (28–30) or transesophageal catheters (31–33) has been particularly useful for tachycardia conversion in young patients especially when tachycardia recurrences are frequent (Figures 22–4 and 22–5). Electrical conversion may mistakenly be interpreted as being ineffective. In this situation, it may be possible to observe that electrical stimulation terminates tachycardia, but that spontaneous reinitation occurs following a few sinus beats. When this

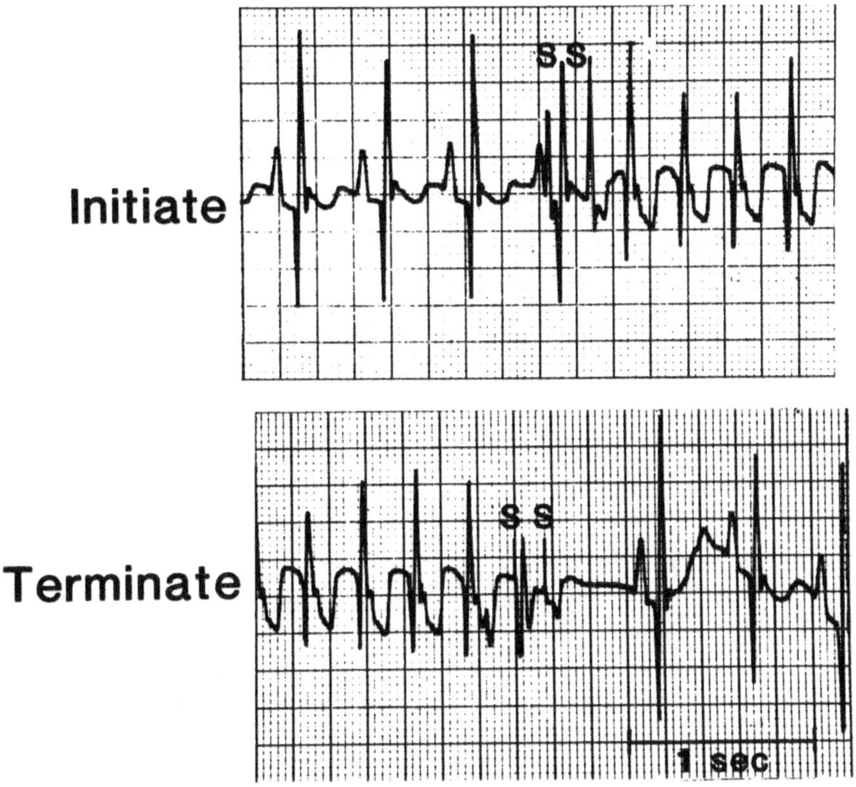

FIGURE 22–4. Use of transesophageal pacing to initiate and terminate tachycardia. Tachycardia cycle length is 285 ms in this one-week-old infant. Tachycardia is initiated (*top panel*) and terminated (*lower panel*) with two synchronized stimuli(s). Reproduced with permission of publisher [90].

occurs, it may be necessary to use antiarrhythmic drugs prior to electrical conversion.

VERAPAMIL (INTRAVENOUS)

In recent years, verapamil, a prototypical "slow channel" blocking drug, has been demonstrated to be an effective agent which rapidly terminates orthodromic reciprocating tachycardia when administered intravenously [16,17,34]. Its principal usefulness as an antiarrhythmic drug is related to its negative dromotropic effect on the AV node. The chief side effects from its use are hypotension and bradycardia. However, Weiss et al. [35] and Roguin et al. [36] showed that the hypotensive effect could be minimized by pretreatment with intravenous calcium. Symptomatic hypotension is most likely to occur when verapamil administration during tachycardia fails to restore normal rhythm. The importance of recognizing the type of tachycardia prior to use of verapamil is illustrated further by the studies of Gulamhuseim et al. [19] who noted that verapamil accelerated the ventricular rate during atrial fibrillation in patients with preexcitation. Thus, verapamil is specifically contraindicated when atrial fibrillation is suspected in a patient with preexcitation syndrome. Following tachycardia termination, bradycardia resulting from verapamil administration will respond well to administration of isoproterenol, if necessary to improve hemodynamic status. Special precautions are required when verapamil is used in conjunction with beta adrenergic antagonists [37]. Recently Reiter et al. [38] demonstrated safety and efficacy of a continuous intravenous infusion of verapamil; con-

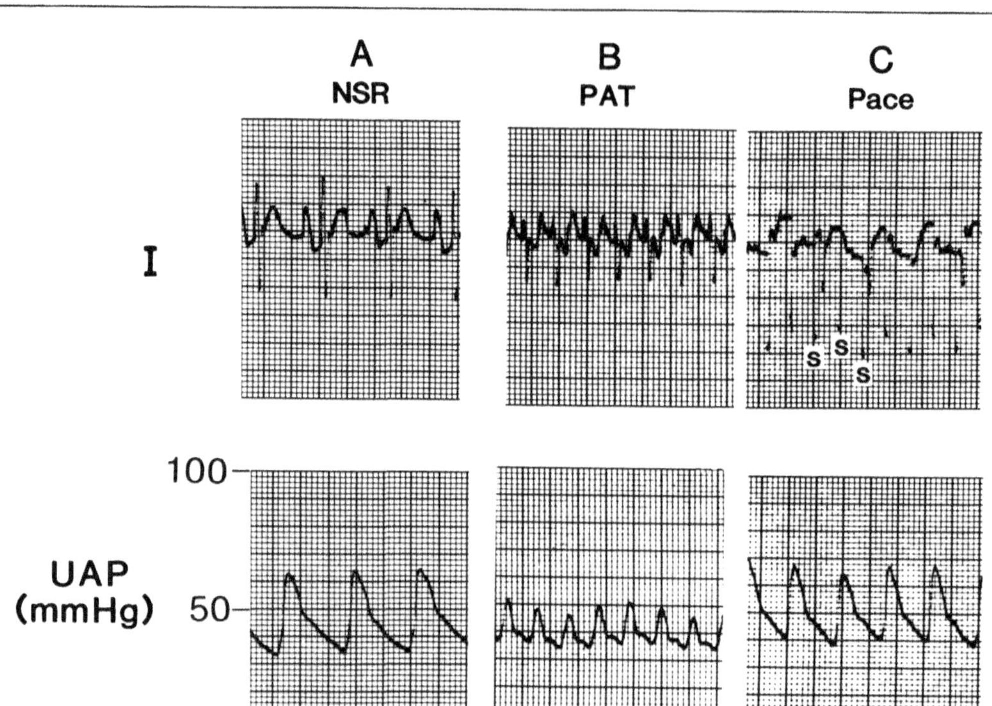

FIGURE 22–5. Use of transesophageal pacing in the treatment of tachycardia. In this 1200-gm premature infant tachycardia could be terminated by pacing. However, sinus rhythm (NSR, *Panel A*) only lasted seconds prior to spontaneous reinitiation of tachycardia (PAT, *Panel B*). The occurrence of tachycardia was associated with marked fall in umbilical artery pressure (UAP). Therefore continuous transesophageal atrial pacing was performed at cycle length 174 ms (350 beats/minute). This resulted in 2:1 block and restored blood pressure to normal (Pace, *Panel C*). After 48 hours the pacing could be stopped since therapeutic concentration of antiarrhythmic medication was achieved.

tinuous infusion may be useful for the short-term management of hospitalized patients with frequent tachycardia recurrences.

ATP AND ADENOSINE (INTRAVENOUS)

Adenosine-5′-triphosphate (ATP) is not available as an antiarrhythmic drug in the United States. However, ATP has been used in Europe for termination of tachycardia. For example, Greco et al. [34] compared acute treatment of regular, normal QRS tachycardia using intravenous digitalis, ATP and verapamil in 62 children ages 4 days to 12 years. Acute tachycardia termination in 1 to 2 minutes was noted in about 90% of patients treated with ATP or verapamil. Digitalis (lantoside C) was only effective in 60–70% and took as long as two hours to result in tachycardia conversion. Belhassen et al. [39] also reported successful use of ATP in rapid conversion of regular, normal QRS tachycardia. Their studies in older patients, 25 to 72 years, were complicated by the transient occurrence of second and third degree block.

Adenosine is an intermediate metabolite in many important biochemical pathways. Di Marco et al. [40] showed that the human sinus and AV nodes are sensitive to physiologic doses of adenosine, and then demonstrated that adenosine could be used safely and effectively to terminate acute episodes of orthodromic reciprocating tachycardia or tachycardia due to reentry within the AV node. Adenosine did not terminate any primary atrial tachycardias but transiently slowed the ventricular response by increasing AV block.

At the present time adenosine and ATP are investigational agents. These agents have an extremely short half life and appear to be potent for transiently impairing AV node conduction. Few studies have assessed their effects on conduction in accessory connections. However, Belhassen et al. [39] noted a lack of an effect of ATP on conduction in accessory connections in the retrograde direction and Di Marco et al. [40] noted a lack of an effect of adenosine on conduction in the antegrade direction.

PROPRANOLOL (INTRAVENOUS)

The intravenous dose of propranolol, for tachycardia conversion, has not been extensively studied. Denes et al. [41] and Barrett et al. [42] found that propranolol (0.1 mg/kg) slowed but seldom terminated orthodromic reciprocating tachycardia. The antiarrhythmic actions of propranolol are complex, but the principal usefulness of propranolol in the treatment of orthodromic reciprocating tachycardia is related to its negative dromotropic effect on the AV node. In our laboratory, 0.2 mg/kg of propranolol has been safely administered and occasionally effective in terminating tachycardia when infused over 5 to 10 minutes (Figures 22–2 and 22–3). In patients with functionally normal hearts, no symptoms have resulted from its intravenous use. However, systemic arterial blood pressure should be monitored during the infusion. The dose of 0.2 mg/kg intravenously is identical to that utilized to treat hypercyanotic spells in patients with tetralogy of Fallot [43], as well as to accomplish beta-adrenergic blockade [44].

PROCAINAMIDE (INTRAVENOUS)

In young patients procainamide is underutilized as an antiarrhythmic drug for termination of tachycardia in patients with preexcitation syndromes. When uncertainty exists about the type of tachycardia, e.g., when prolonged QRS is present, it is probably the drug of choice for safe intravenous administration (Figures 22–2 and 22–3). In patients with preexcitation, procainamide acts principally by impairment of conduction in the accessory connection in the antegrade and/or retrograde direction. Procainamide may be administered intravenously in a dose of 15 mg/kg at a rate of 1 mg/kg/min delivered by an infusion pump [45]. Systemic arterial blood pressure should be carefully monitored during infusion since hypotension occasionally occurs, but usually reverses upon slowing the infusion rate. At the end of the 15-minute infusion, the peak procainamide serum concentrations range from 6 to 30 mg/l in patients of all ages. Even in patients with mild symptoms of heart failure, infusion of procainamide with this protocol has not resulted in symptomatic hypotension. This regimen should not be used in critically ill patients, especially if hepatic function has been compromised.

PERIODIC ANTIARRHYTHMIC DRUG TREATMENT

The traditional treatment of paroxysmal tachycardia has utilized chronic oral antiarrhythmic drug prophylaxis to prevent tachycardia recurrences. Utilizing a prophylactic regimen, one or more antiarrhythmic drugs are taken on a scheduled basis, one or more times a day, in order to prevent paroxysmal tachycardia which may occur relatively infrequently. The risk of adverse side effects and the cumulative expense of medication are recognized disadvantages of chronic prophylactic therapy in young patients. Margolis et al. [46] proposed use of intermittent drug therapy in which a combination of antiarrhythmic drugs in the form of a "cocktail" was taken only following the onset of an episode of tachycardia. Subsequently, Yet et al. [47] demonstrated in adolescents and young adults with orthodromic reciprocating tachycardia that a single dose of diltiazem and propranolol terminated tachycardia. Benson et al. [45] demonstrated that a single dose of procainamide terminated tachycardia in selected patients, a regimen termed *periodic procainamide*. In patients with orthodromic reciprocating tachycardia in whom intravenous procainamide (15 mg/kg at 1 mg/kg/minute) terminated the tachycardia, a single dose of oral procainamide (25 mg/kg) was very successful in terminating subsequent tachycardia episodes within 30 to 60 minutes in most patients (Figure 22–6).

Periodic therapy is best suited for patients with infrequent but sustained episodes of non-life-threatening tachycardia. The periodic regimens described to date have required 30 to 60 minutes before terminating tachycardia. Success of a periodic regimen depends on the pharmacodynamic properties of the anti-

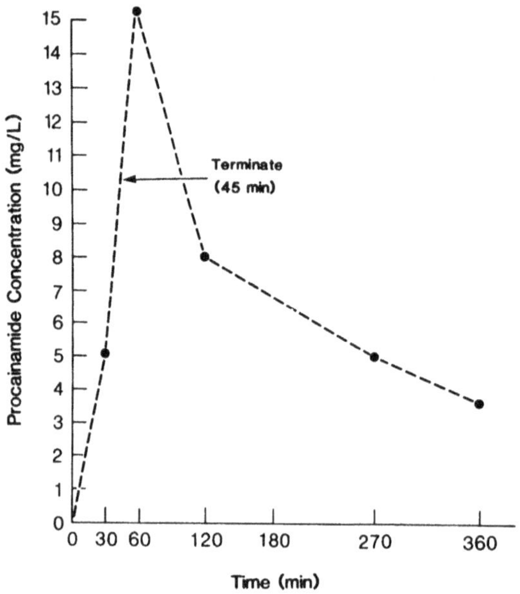

FIGURE 22–6. Procainamide for periodic use. In this example, a five year old with recurrent orthodromic reciprocating tachycardia was administered 750 mg (26 mg/kg) of procainamide orally at time 0. Peak procainamide concentration was detected at 60 minutes. Tachycardia terminated at 45 minute following ingestion of procainamide.

arrhythmic drug and the pharmacokinetics following oral administration in a particular patient.

TRANSPLACENTAL TREATMENT

Even though available evidence is convincing that preexcitation syndromes are congenital, there is no general way to screen for their presence in utero unless tachycardia occurs. Fetal ultrasound is useful for detecting the presence of tachycardia, establishing the AV relationship during tachycardia and determining whether tachycardia is regular or irregular [48]. The association of tachycardia in the fetus with severe congestive heart failure in utero (hydrops fetalis) and death has been well documented [48,49]. Based on electrocardiographic analysis following delivery, it is apparent that tachycardia associated with preexcitation can occur in utero [4,49–52].

The approach to the in utero treatment of tachycardia has been administration of digoxin [49,51,53–55] propranolol [54,56] procainamide [50,54], quinidine [51], and verapamil [55,57,58], either alone or in combination to the mother in dosages that are nontoxic to the mother and hopefully therapeutic to the fetus (Figure 22–7). These reports of tachycardia treatment in the fetus have been largely in the form of isolated cases. Tachycardia in the fetus has not been reported prior to the 24th week of pregnancy [48, 57, 58]. At this stage of gestation major organogenesis is complete and the principal adverse antiarrhythmic drug effects would be expected to manifest as interference with fetal growth and development. These considerations have been reviewed recently [59]. Use of amiodarone has not been reported to treat a fetus with tachycardia, but its use during the last seven weeks of pregnancy in a mother with an accessory AV connection was described by McKenna et al. [60]. In this case the infant suffered no apparent side effects from amiodarone.

Treatment to Prevent Tachycardia Recurrence

ELECTROPHYSIOLOGIC TESTING OF ANTIARRHYTHMIC DRUG EFFICACY

A major difficulty in assessing antiarrhythmic drug efficacy is the lack of a generally agreed-upon definition of efficacy. A number of reports have attested to the successful use of a variety of treatments in neonates, infants and children with preexcitation syndromes. Chronic use of orally administered digitalis derivatives [6,24,61], verapamil [17], propranolol [62], amiodarone [63,64], and quinidine [65] has been reported. The use of electrical stimulation to test for the prevention of reinitiation of tachycardia, although well established as a means of selecting treatment in the older patient, has rarely been performed in the young patient [61,65] (Figure 22–4).

When electrical stimulation is used for drug testing, the antiarrhythmic agents are often given intravenously during laboratory study. If effective intravenously, a conversion is made to chronic oral use. This raises important questions. First, is the acute effect of a drug administered intravenously indicative of the chronic effect of that drug administered orally? The answer may be affirmative for verapamil [66] and procainamide [45], but Alboni et al. [67]

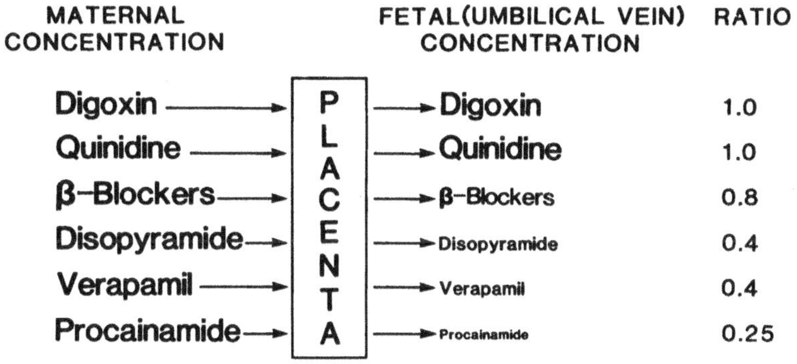

FIGURE 22–7. Treatment options for transplacental treatment of fetal tachyarrhythmias associated with preexcitation syndromes. The relationship between maternal drug concernation and that in cord blood of the fetus at delivery is illustrated.

found for amiodarone that a change in the inducibility of tachycardia after intravenous administration had a negative predictive value for the response following chronic oral administration. An additional question is whether the results of drug studies can be extrapolated to predict the action of drugs that effect the same limb of the tachycardia circuit. Bauernfeind et al. [68] found that there were similar effects of drugs that increased refractoriness in the antegrade limb (propranolol, ouabain) as well as similar effects of drugs that increased refractoriness in the retrograde limb (procainamide, quinidine, disopyramide) in patients with orthodromic reciprocating tachycardia.

LONG TERM PROPHYLAXIS

For many years digitalis derivatives were the mainstay of tachycardia management in young patients. In recent years their use in terminating established tachycardias has diminished, but they continue to be widely recommended for chronic prophylaxis. However, Swiderski et al. [69] commented on the relative lack of effect of digitalis in young patients with preexcitation. Additionally, for the past decade concern has been expressed about the effect of digitalis on conduction in the accessory AV connection during atrial fibrillation [70]. Thus, concerns about the effectiveness and safety of digitalis derivatives, and the relatively high incidence of toxicity [71] suggest that other agents should be considered for chronic prophylaxis.

One difficulty in the evaluation of chronic antiarrhythmic drug efficacy in young patients with preexcitation is that there is no quantitative description of either the clinical course or the severity of tachycardia episodes. That is, tachycardia occurs as sporadic attacks of variable duration that may recur many times per day or be separated by weeks, months or years. As recently emphasized by Pritchett et al. [72], this spontaneous variability makes it difficult to utilize objective methods to describe the clinical course for purposes of evaluating antiarrhythmic drug efficacy.

There have been very few pharmacologic-efficacy studies in pediatric patients [73]. While differences of pharmacokinetic and pharmacodynamic responses to some antiarrhythmic drugs have been demonstrated in the neonate versus adult animal [74,75], the clinical relevance of observed differences is unknown. Since beneficial effects, similar in all ages, can be achieved by adjusting drug dosage, the general approach to utilization of antiarrhythmic drugs on a chronic basis has been to administer the starting dose based on the child's size. Once steady state plasma concentration has been achieved, the dose is increased or decreased to achieve a "therapeutic" concentration. Once the desired drug concentration is achieved, the drug may be tested electrophysiologically by testing for prevention of tachycardia reinitiation or empirically by observing whether spontaneous tachycardia recurrences are prevented. This approach works well for most available drugs, but amiodarone is a notable exception.

Based on available evidence, it is not possible to recommend a single antiarrhythmic drug for treatment of tachyarrhythmias associated with preexcitation syndromes. Numerous publications give testimonial to efficacy of specific antiarrhythmic drugs in select patients. The current approach is based on the idea that treatment can be individualized.

TREATMENT TO MODIFY INITIATING EVENT

One important feature that may influence the natural history of the occurrence of tachycardia in young patients is the type and frequency of initiating events. Dunnigan et al. [76] described four types of age-related initiating events in young patients with orthodromic reciprocating tachycardia. These included atrial or ventricular extrasystoles, sinus acceleration and sinus pause with junctional escape. Atrial extrasystoles and sinus acceleration were solely responsible for tachycardia initiation in infants whereas in children, atrial and ventricular extrasystoles and sinus pause with junctional escape were responsible (Table 22–1).

TABLE 22–1. Initiating events Orthodromic Reciprocating Tachycardia

	Infants	Children
Atrial extrasystole	+	+
Ventricular extrasystole	−	+
Sinus acceleration	+	−
Sinus pause with junctional escape	−	+

+ = present.
− = absent.

Spontaneous onset of tachycardia rarely occurs during electrocardiographic monitoring (Figure 22–8), and little work has been done to formulate treatment plans based on initiating events. However, age-related differences in initiating events may be important in determining antiarrhythmic drug effectiveness in different age groups. For example, Levy and Bonazinga [77] commented that in children in whom sinus pause with junctional escape was the means of initiating tachycardia the use of digitalis derivatives and/or beta-adrenergic antagonists might actually facilitate the occurrence of tachycardia by providing more sinus pauses with junctional escape (initiating events). This consideration may not apply to infants since sinus pause with junctional escape may not be an initiating event in infants.

ANTITACHYCARDIA PACING

The use of pacing in the preexcitation syn-

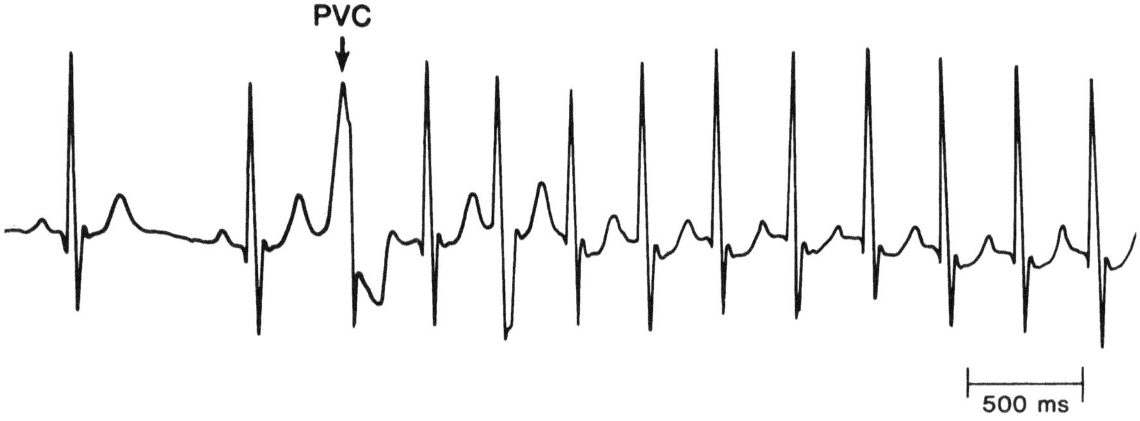

FIGURE 22–8. Onset of orthodromic reciprocating tachycardia initiated by a spontaneous ventricular extrasystole in an eight year old. Even though disopyramide did not prevent initiation by tachycardia by transesophageal atrial stimulation, disopyramide did prevent spontaneous recurrences of tachycardia. This salutory drug effect was presumably due to modification of the initiating event.

dromes is discussed in Chapter 23 by Peters in this volume, and will be reviewed here only briefly as it might relate to use in young patients. The tachycardias associated with preexcitation syndromes usually result from reentry. Therefore, there are two ways in which pacing might be theoretically useful: (1) to prevent tachycardia initiation, or (2) to terminate established tachycardia. Prevention of tachycardia initiation may be accomplished by overdrive suppression of the initiating event (e.g., atrial extrasystole), by increasing the resting heart rate, or by repetitively depolarizing a portion of the reentry circuit so as to prevent initiation of a reentrant tachycardia. Termination of established tachycardia is thought to be accomplished by invasion of the reentry circuit by a critically timed electrical stimulus so as to create refractoriness ahead of the circulating wavefront responsible for tachycardia.

Uses of pacing for control of tachycardia in children with preexcitation syndromes has been limited. Dreifus et al. [78] reported successful use of a radio frequency pacemaker in a 5-week-old infant. The unit and transvenous lead were successfully used for tachycardia control for approximately 14 months. Spurrell et al. [79] included an adolescent in a series of patients treated with an automatic scanning pacemaker.

The technical problems, morbidity, and mortality of permanent pacing for bradycardia in the young child have been well described [80, 81]. The long-term complications of antitachycardia pacing have not been well defined, e.g., inadvertent initiation of atrial fibrillation which could be catastrophic in a patient in whom conduction via an accessory connection in the antegrade direction might result in excessively rapid ventricular responses. Additionally, in the very young, the heart rates during tachycardia are quite rapid (short cycle lengths). For example in infants with orthodromic reciprocating tachycardia during the first month of life, the average cycle length during tachycardia is 222 ms, with a range of 195 to 295 ms [61]. Antitachycardia pacing modalities designed to be effective at longer cycle lengths in older patients may be ineffective in young patients.

TREATMENT BY ABLATION OF ACCESSORY AV CONNECTIONS

The details of surgical treatment of preexcitation syndromes are covered in the chapters by Tobler et al., Cox and Cain, and Guiradon et al. and catheter ablation therapy in Chapter 24 by Scheinman in this volume. There are no generally agreed-upon guidelines for ablation therapy of preexcitation in young patients. In very young patients undergoing surgical treatment of congenital heart disease, the issue of preexcitation should be addressed since it has been generally agreed that ablation be performed in this circumstance even when tachycardia has not been previously documented. This recommendation should be interpreted in light of additional risk incurred by extending the operative procedure [1,6,82–84]. Ablation of accessory AV connections for medically refractory tachycardia has rarely been reported in infants without associated congenital heart disease [85]. Tachycardia control by ablation of the AV node–His bundle has not been reported in infants, and when preexcitation is present this approach is less desirable than ablation of the accessory AV connection. Incessant forms of tachycardia may result in cardiac dysfunction, and such tachycardias should be considered for ablative therapy if medically refractory [86,87].

Adolescents and young adults require different considerations than younger patients. Patients in this age group may have cardiac arrest, presumably resulting from rapid ventricular response during atrial fibrillation, as their initial manifestion of preexcitation syndrome [88]. Ablation of the accessory connection has usually been recommended in such patients. However, Morady et al. [89] demonstrated that electrophysiological testing could identify a subgroup of these patients in whom medical therapy appeared to be a suitable alternative. At the present time, prospective selection of patients "at high risk for sudden death" based on electrophysiologic testing cannot be reliably accomplished due to incomplete natural history studies. In other adolescents and young adults, chronic prophylactic medication interferes with life-style even when effective tachycardia control results. Additionally, tachycardia recurrences in this age group may interfere with life-style since they are often associated with physical activity. Activity restriction in this physically active group of patients is poorly accepted. Thus in the adolescent-young adult patient, the indications for accessory AV connection ablation may involve special consideration for non-life-threatening tachycardias. In this group of patients, the cumulative risk and cost of medical therapy for indefinite periods of time make ablative techniques an attractive alternative.

Summary

Treatment of tachycardia in young patients with preexcitation syndromes can be approached from the standpoint of terminating established tachycardia versus prevention of tachycardia recurrence. In young patients with preexcitation syndromes ECG documentation of tachycardia is essential prior to treatment. Based on ECG assessment a differential diagnosis of tachycardia should be established. The latter assessment is important since certain forms of treatment may be contraindicated for some tachycardias associated with the preexcitation syndromes. Specific knowledge regarding tachycardia frequency, duration, initiating event, mechanism, and associated symptoms are essential in order to make rational use of available pharmacologic, pacing, and ablative techniques.

References

1. Benson DW, Jr, Gallagher JJ: Electrophysiologic evaluation and surgical correction of Wolff-Parkinson-White Syndrome in children. *Clin. Pediat.* 19:575, 1980.
2. Fasth A: Wolff-Parkinson-White Syndrome. A fatal case in a girl with no other heart disease. *Acta Paediatr. Scand* 64:138, 1975.
3. Brechenmacher C, Courtadon M, Jourde M, Yermia JC, Cheynel J, Voegtlin R: Syndrome de Wolff-Parkinson-White par association de fibres atriohissiennes et de fibres de Mahaim. *Arch. Mal Coeur* 69:1275, 1976.
4. Belhassen B, Pauzner D, Blieden L, Sherez J, Zinger A, David M, Muhlbauer B, Laniado S: Intrauterine and postnatal atrial fibrillation in the Wolff-Parkinson-White syndrome. *Circulation* 66:1124, 1982.
5. Mehta AV, Pickoff AS, Raptoulis A, Wolff GS, Garcia OL, Tamer DF, Ferrer PF, Gelband H: Atrial flutter and atrial fibrillation associated with Wolff-Parkinson-White syndrome in childhood. *Pediatr. Cardiol.* 1:197, 1980.
6. Mantakas ME, McCue CM, Miller WM: Natural history of Wolff-Parkinson-White syndrome discovered in infancy. *Am. J. Cardiol.* 41:1097, 1978.
7. Lundberg A: Paroxysmal atrial tachycardia in infancy: Long-term follow-up study of 49 subjects. *Pediatrics* 70:638, 1982.
8. Benson DW Jr, Dunnigan A, Benditt DG, Schneider SP: Follow-up of infant paroxysmal atrial tachycardia: Transesophageal study. (Abstract.) *Circulation* 70:II, 1984.
9. Giardina ACV, Ehlers KH, Engle MA: Wolff-Parkinson-White syndrome in infants and children: A long term follow-up study. *Br. Heart J.* 34:839, 1972.
10. Benson DW Jr, Smith WM, Dunnigan A, Sterba R, Gallagher JJ: Mechanisms of regular, wide QRS tachycardia in infants and children. *Am. J. Cardiol.* 49:1778, 1982.
11. Dauvignon A, Rautaharju P, Boisselle E, Soumis F, Megelas M, Choquette A. Normal ECG standards for infants and children. *Pediatr. Cardiol.* 1:123, 1979/80.
12. Sellers TD Jr, Campbell RFW, Bashore TM, Gallagher JJ: Effects of procainamide and quinidine sulfate in the Wolff-Parkinson-White syndrome. *Circulation* 55:15, 1977.
13. Wellens HJJ, Bar FW, Dassen WRM, Brugada P, Vanagt EJ, Farre J: Effect of drugs in the Wolff-Parkinson-White syndrome: Importance of initial length of effective refractory period of the accessory pathway. *Am. J. Cardiol.* 46:665, 1980.
14. Kerr CR, Prystowsky EN, Smith WM, Cook L, Gallagher JJ: Electrophysiologic effects of disopyramide phosphate in patients with Wolff-Parkinson-White syndrome. *Circulation* 65:869, 1982.
15. Swiryn S, Bauernfeind R, Wyndham CRC, Dhingra RC, Palileo E, Strasberg B, Rosen KM: Effects of oral disopyramide phosphate on induction of paroxysmal supraventricular tachycardia. *Circulation* 64:169, 1981.
16. Soler-Soler J, Sagrista-Sauleda J, Dabrera A, Sauleda-Pares J, Iglesias-Berengue J, Permanyer-Miralda G, Roca-Llop J: Effect of verapamil in infants with paroxysmal supraventricular tachycardia. *Circulation* 59:876, 1979.
17. Porter CJ, Gillette PC, Garson A Jr, Hesslein PS, Karpawich PP, McNamara DG: Effects of verapamil on supraventricular tachycardia in children. *Am. J. Cardiol.* 48:487, 1981.
18. Wu D, Keu HC, Yeh SJ, Lin FC, Hung JS: Effects of oral verapamil in patients with atrioventricular tachycardia incorporating an accessory pathway. *Circulation* 67:426, 1983.
19. Gulamhusein S, Ko P, Carruthers SG, Klein GJ: Acceleration of the ventricular response during atrial fibrillation in the Wolff-Parkinson-White syndrome after verapamil. *Circulation* 65:348, 1982.
20. Zipes DP, Prystowsky EN, Heger JJ: Amiodarone: Electrophysiologic actions, pharmacokinetics and clinical effects. *J. Am. Coll. Card.* 3:1059, 1984.
21. Wellens HJJ, Brugada P, Abdolla AH: Effect of amiodarone in paroxysmal supraventricular tachycardia with or without Wolff-Parkinson-White syndrome. *Am. Heart J.* 106:876, 1983.

22. Prystowsky EN, Klein GJ, Rinkenberger RL, Hager JJ, Naccarelli GV, Zipes DP: Clinical efficacy and electrophysiologic effects of encainide in patients with Wolff-Parkinson-White syndrome. *Circulation* 69:278, 1984.
23. Jackman WM, Zipes DP, Naccarelli GV, Rinkenberger RL, Heger JJ, Prystowsky EN: Electrophysiology of oral encanide. *Am. J. Cardiol.* 49:1270, 1982.
24. Nadas AS, Daeschner CW, Roth A, Blumenthal SL: Paroxysmal tachycardia in infants and children — Study of 41 cases. *Pediatics* 9:167, 1952.
25. Waxman MB, Wald RW, Sharma AD, Huerta F, Cameron DA: Vagal techniques for termination of paroxysmal supraventricular tachycardia *Am. J. Cardiol.* 46:655, 1980.
26. Bissett GS, Gaum W, Kaplan S: The ice bag: A new technique for interruption of supraventricular tachycardia. *J. Pediatr.* 97:593, 1980.
27. Sperandeo V, Pierri D, Palazdo P, Donzelli M, Spataro G: Supraventricular tachycardia in infants: Use of the "diving reflex." *Am. J. Cardiol.* 51:286, 1983.
28. Massumi RA, Kisten AD, Tawakkel AA: Termination of reciprocal tachycardia by atrial stimulation. *Circulation* 36:637, 1967.
29. Durrer D, Schoo L, Schuilenburg RM, Wellens JJ: The role of premature beats in the initiation and the termination of supraventricular tachycardia in the Wolff-Parkinson-White syndrome. *Circulation* 36:644, 1967.
30. Sugre DD, McLaran C, Hammill SC, Gersh BJ, Mair DD, Holmes DR Jr: Refractory supraventricular tachycardia in the neonate: Treatment with temporary antitachycardia pacing. *Mayo Clin. Proc.* 60:169, 1985.
31. Gallagher JJ, Smith WM, Kerr CR, Kasell J, Cook L, Reiter M, Sterba R, Harte M: Esophageal pacing: A diagnostic and therapeutic tool. *Circulation* 65:336, 1982.
32. Kerr CR, Gallagher JJ, Smith WM, Sterba R, German LD, Cook L, Kasell JH: The induction of atrial flutter and fibrillation and the termination of atrial flutter by esophageal pacing. *PACE* 6:60, 1983.
33. Benson DW Jr, Dunnigan A, Benditt DG, Schneider SP: Transesophageal cardiac pacing: History, application, technique. *Clin. Prog. Pac. Electrophysiol.* 2:360, 1984.
34. Greco R, Musto B, Arienzo V, Alborino A, Garofalo S, Marsico F: Treatment of paroxysmal supraventricular tachycardia in infancy with digitalis, adenosine-5′-triphosphate, and verapamil: A comparative study. *Circulation* 66:504, 1982.
35. Weiss AT, Lewis BS, Halon DA, Hasin Y, Gotsman MS: The use of calcium with verapamil in the management of supraventricular tachyarrhythmias. *Int. J. Cardiol.* 4:275, 1983.
36. Roguin N, Shapir Y, Blazer S, Zeltzer M, Berant M: The use of calcium gluconate prior to verapamil in infants with paroxysmal supraventricular tachycardia. *Clin. Cardiol.* 7:613, 1984.
37. Yee R, Gulamhusein SS, Klein GJ: Combined verapamil and propranolol for supraventricular tachycardia. *Am. J. Cardiol.* 53:757 1984.
38. Reiter MJ, Shand DG, Aanonsen LM, Wagoner R, McCarthy E, Pritchett ELC: Pharmacokinetics of verapamil: Experience with a sustained intravenous infusion. *Am. J. Cardiol.* 50:716, 1982.
39. Belhassen B, Pelleg A, Shoshani D, Geva B, Laniado S: Electrophysiologic effects of adenosine-5′-triphosphate on atrioventricular reentrant tachycardia. *Circulation* 68:827, 1983.
40. DiMarco JP, Sellers TD, Berne RM, West GA, Belardinelli L: Adenosine: electrophysiologic effects and therapeutic use for terminating paroxysmal supraventricular tachycardia. *Circulation* 68:1254, 1983.
41. Denes P, Cummings JM, Simpson R, Wu D, Amat-Y-Leon F, Dhuigra R, Rosen KM: Effects of propranolol on anomalous pathway refractoriness and circus movement tachycardias in patients with preexciation. *Am. J. Cardiol.* 41:1061, 1978.
42. Barett PH, Jordan JL, Mandel WJ, Yamaguchi I, Laks MM: The electrophysiologic effects of intravenous propranolol in the Wolff-Parkinson-White syndrome. *Am. Heart J.* 98:213, 1979.
43. Ponce FE, Williams LC, Webb HM, Riopel DA, Hohn AR: Propranolol palliation of tetralogy of Fallot: Experience with long-term drug treatment in pediatric patients. *Pediatrics* 52:100, 1973.
44. Cumming GR, Mir GH: Heart rate and haemodynamics after autonomic blockade in infants and children. *Br. Heart J.* 32:766, 1970.
45. Benson DW Jr, Dunnigan A, Green TP, Benditt DG, Schneider SP: Periodic procainamide for paroxysmal tachycardia. *Circulation.* 72:147, 1985.
46. Margolis B, De Silva RA, Lown B: Episodic drug treatment in the management of paroxysmal arrhythmias. *Am. J. Cardiol.* 45:621, 1980.
47. Yeh SJ, Lin FC, Chou YY, Hung JS, Wu D: Termination of paroxysmal supraventricular tachycardia with single oral dose of diltiazem and propranolol. *Circulation* 71:104, 1985.
48. Kleinman CS, Donnerstein RL, Jaffe CC, DeVore GR, Weinstein EM, Lynch DC, Talner NS, Berkowitz RL, Hobbins JC: Fetal echocardiography: A tool for evaluation of in utero cardiac arrhythmias and monitoring of in utero therapy: Analysis of 71 patients. *Am. J. Cardiol.* 51:237, 1983.
49. Newburger JW, Keane JF: Intrauterine supraventricular tachycardia. *J. Pediatr.* 95:780, 1979.
50. Given BD, Phillippe M, Sanders SP, Dzau VJ:

Procainamide cardioversion of fetal supraventricular tachyarrhythmia. *Am. J. Cardiol.* 53:1460, 1984.
51. Spinnato JA, Shaver DC, Flinn GS, Sibai BM, Watson DL, Marin-Garcia J: Fetal supraventricular tachycardia: In utero therapy with digoxin and quinidine. *Obstet. Gynecol.* 64:730, 1984.
52. Valerius NH, Jacobson JR: Intrauterine supraventricular tachycardia. *Acta Obstet. Gynecol. Scand.* 57:407, 1978.
53. Harrigan JT, Kangos JJ, Sikka A, Spisso KR, Natarajan N, Rosenfeld D, Leiman S, Korn D: Successful treatment of fetal congestive heart failure secondary to tachycardia. *N. Engl. J. Med.* 304:1527, 1981.
54. Dumesic DA, Silverman NH, Tobias S, Golbus MS: Transplacental cardioversion of fetal supraventricular tachycardia with procainamide. *N. Engl. J. Med.* 307:1128, 1982.
55. Wolff F, Breuker KH, Schlensker KH, Bolte A: Prenatal diagnosis and therapy of fetal heart rate anomalies: With a contribution on the placental transfer of verapamil. *J. Perinat. Med.* 8:203, 1980.
56. Teuscher A, Bossi E, Imhof P, Erb E, Stocker FP, Weber JW: Effect of propranolol on fetal tachycardia in diabetic pregnancy. *Am. J. Cardiol.* 42:304, 1978.
57. Allan LD, Crawford DC, Anderson RH, Tynan M: Evaluation and treatment of fetal arrhythmias. *Clin. Cardiol.* 7:467, 1984.
58. Crowley DC, Dick M, Rayburn WF, Rosenthal A: Two-dimensional and M-mode echocardiographic evaluation of fetal arrhythmia. *Clin. Cardiol.* 8:1, 1985.
59. Rotmensch HH, Elkayam U, Frishman W: Antiarrhythmic drug therapy during pregnancy. *Ann. Int. Med.* 98:487, 1983.
60. McKenna WJ, Harris L, Rowland E, Whitelaw A, Storey G, Holt D: Amiodarone therapy during pregnancy. *Am. J. Cardiol.* 51:1231, 1983.
61. Benson DW Jr, Dunnigan A, Benditt DG, Thompson TR, Narayan A, Boros S: Prediction of digoxin treatment failure in infants with supraventricular tachycardia: Role of transesophageal pacing. *Pediatrics* 75:288, 1985.
62. Pickoff AS, Zies L, Ferrer PL, Tamer D, Wolff G, Garcia O, Gelband H: High-dose propranolol therapy in the management of supraventricular tachycardia. *J. Pediatr.* 94:144, 1979.
63. Coumel P, Fidelle J: Amiodarone in the treatment of cardiac arrhythmias in children: One hundred thirty-five cases. *Am. Heart J.* 100:1063, 1980.
64. Shahar E, Frand M, Feigel A: Amiodarone in control of sustained tachyarrhythmias in children with Wolff-Parkinson-White Syndrome. *Pediatrics* 72:813, 1983.
65. Benson DW Jr, Dunnigan A, Sterba R, Benditt DG: Atrial pacing from the esophagus in the diagnosis and management of tachycardia and palpitations. *J. Pediatr.* 102:40, 1983.
66. Klein GJ, Gulamhusein S, Prystowsky EN, Carruthers SG, Donner AP, Ko PT: Comparison of the electrophysiologic effects of intravenous and oral verapamil in patients with paroxysmal supraventricular tachycardia. *Am. J. Cardiol.* 49:117, 1982.
67. Alboni P, Shantha N, Pirani R, Baggioni F, Scarfo S, Tomasi AM, Masoni A: Effects of amiodarone on supraventricular tachycardia involving bypass tracts. *Am. J. Cardiol.* 53:93, 1984.
68. Bauernfeind RA, Swiryn S, Petropoulos AT, Coelho A, Gallastegui J, Rosen KM: Concordance and discordance of drug responses in atrioventricular reentrant tachycardia. *J. Am. Coll. Cardiol.* 2:345, 1983.
69. Swiderski J, Lees MH, Nadas AS: The Wolff-Parkinson-White syndrome in infancy and childhood. *Br. Heart J.* 24:561, 1962.
70. Sellers TD Jr, Bashore TM, Gallagher JJ: Digitalis in the pre-excitation syndrome: Analysis during atrial fibrillation. *Circulation* 56:260, 1977.
71. Hastreiter AR, Van der Horst RL, Chow-Tung E: Digitalis toxicity in infants and children. *Pediatr. Cardiol.* 5:131, 1984.
72. Pritchett ELC, Hammill SC, Reiter MJ, Lee KL, McCarthy E, Zimmerman JM, Shand DM: Life-table methods for evaluating antiarrhythmic drug efficacy in patients with paroxysmal atrial tachycardia. *Am. J. Cardiol.* 52:1007, 1983.
73. Singh S, Gelband H, Mehta AV, Kesslerk, Casta A, Pickoff AS: Procainamide elimination kinetics in pediatric patients. *Clin. Pharmacol. Ther.* 32:607, 1982.
74. Ezrin AM, Epstein K, Bassett AL, Myerburg RJ, Gelband H: Effects of procainamide on cellular electrophysiology of neonatal and adult dog myocardium. *Dev. Pharmacol. Ther.* 1:352, 1980.
75. Pickoff AS, Singh S, Flinn CJ, Torres E, Ezrin AM, Gelband H: Dose-dependent electrophysiologic effects of amiodarone in the immature canine heart. *Am. J. Cardiol.* 52:621, 1983.
76. Dunnigan A, Benditt DG, Benson DW Jr: Modes of onset ("initiating events") of paroxysmal atrial tachycardia in infants and children. *Am. J. Cardiol.* (In Press, June 1986).
77. Levy AM, Bonazinga BJ: Sudden sinus slowing with junctional escape: A common mode of initiation of juvenile supraventricular tachycardia. *Circulation* 67:84, 1983.
78. Dreifus LS, Arriaga J, Watanabe Y, Downing D, Haiat R, Morse D: Recurrent Wolff-Parkinson-White tachycardia in an infant: Successful treatment by a radio-frequency pacemaker. *Am. J.*

Cardiol. 28:586, 1971.
79. Spurrell RAJ, Nathan AW, Bexton RS, Hellestrand KJ, Nappholz T, Camm AJ: Implantable automatic scanning pacemaker for termination of supraventricular tachycardia. *Am. J. Cardiol.* 49:753, 1982.
80. Furman S, Young D: Cardiac pacing in children and adolescents. *Am. J. Cardiol.* 39:550, 1977.
81. Simon AB, Dick M II, Stern AM, Behrendt DM, Sloan H: Ventricular pacing in children. *PACE* 5:836, 1982.
82. Kugler JD, Gillette PC, Duff DF, Cooley DA, McNamara DG: Elective mapping and surgical division of the bundle of Kent in a patient with Ebstein's anomaly who required tricuspid valve replacement. *Am. J. Cardiol.* 41:602, 1978.
83. Benson DW Jr, Gallagher JJ, Spach MS, Barr RC, Edwards SB, Oldham HN, Kasell J: Accessory atrioventricular pathway in an infant: Prediction of location with body surface maps and ablation with cryosurgery. *J. Pediatr.* 96:41, 1980.
84. Benson DW Jr, Gallagher JJ, Oldham HN, Sealy WC, Sterba R, Spach MS: Corrected transposition with severe intracardiac deformities and Wolff-Parkinson-White syndrome in a child: Electrophysiological investigation and surgical correction. *Circulation* 61:1256, 1980.
85. Byrum CJ, Wahl RA, Behrendt, Dick M: Ventricular fibrillation associated with the use of digitalis in a newborn infant with Wolff-Parkinson-White syndrome. *J. Pediatr.* 101:400, 1982.
86. Gallagher JJ, Sealy WC: The permanent form of junctional reciprocating tachycardia: Further elucidation of the underlying mechanism. *Eur. J. Cardiol.* 8:413, 1978.
87. Epstein ML, Benditt DG: Long term evaluation of persistent supraventricular tachycardia in children: Clinical and electrocardiographic features. *Am. Heart J.* 102:80, 1981.
88. Cosio FG, Benson DW Jr, Anderson RW, Hession WT, Pritzker MR, Benditt DG: Onset of atrial fibrillation during antidromic tachycardia: Association with sudden cardiac arrest and ventricular fibrillation in a patient with Wolff-Parkinson-White syndrome. *Am. J. Cardiol.* 50:353, 1982.
89. Morady F, Sledge C, Shen E, Sung RJ, Gonzales R, Scheinman MM: Electrophysiologic testing in the management of patients with the Wolff-Parkinson-White syndrome and atrial fibrillation. *Am. J. Cardiol.* 51:1623, 1983.
90. Benson DW Jr, Dunnigan A, Benditt DG, Pritzker MR, Thompson TR: Transesophageal study of infant supraventricular tachycardia: Electrophysiologic characteristics. *Am. J. Cardiol.* 52:1002, 1983.

23. PACEMAKER TECHNIQUES FOR MANAGEMENT OF TACHYCARDIAS ASSOCIATED WITH PREEXCITATION SYNDROMES

Robert W. Peters

With the recent explosion in pacemaker technology, there has been increasing interest in the use of pacing techniques for the management of patients with tachycardia involving accessory atrioventricular (AV) connections. In this chapter I will review the theoretical rationale for the use of pacing in these patients, the types of pacemakers that are currently available, and the clinical experience that has accumulated to date.

General Principles of Tachycardia

There are thought to be three basic mechanisms underlying the tachyarrhythmias seen in clinical medicine.

AUTOMATICITY

Cells within the specialized conduction system possess automaticity, a property that allows them to depolarize spontaneously rather than being dependent upon an external stimulus. Ordinarily, cells within the sinoatrial node have the most rapid rate of spontaneous depolarization and thus initiate the heartbeat. Under abnormal circumstances, the rate of the sinoatrial node may be exceeded by that of cells from lower areas of the specialized conduction system due to an increased rate of automatic depolarization (or perhaps, by automaticity developing in cells outside the conduction system), thus producing an ectopic tachycardia. Enhanced or abnormal automaticity is not believed to be a common cause of tachycardia and would not be expected to be amenable to pacemaker therapy. Ectopic foci may be temporarily suppressed by pacing but regain their automaticity once pacing is terminated.

TRIGGERED AUTOMATICITY

A delayed after-depolarization generated by an action potential may, under certain circumstances, achieve threshold and cause repetitive beating, producing a tachycardia. This repetitive beating is termed *triggered automaticity* and is thought to be responsible for the tachyarrhythmias associated with digitalis intoxication. There has been insufficient experience to determine whether this mechanism is associated with clinically important tachycardias or whether pacing techniques can reliably terminate arrhythmias due to triggered automaticity.

REENTRY

Reentry is by far the most common mechanism of tachycardia encountered in patients with the preexcitation syndromes. The presence of an accessory AV connection and an intact AV node provide the anatomic substrate for reentry. In the vast majority of cases, the accessory AV connection has a relatively long refractory

Benditt, D.G. and Benson, D.W., Cardiac Preexcitation Syndromes.

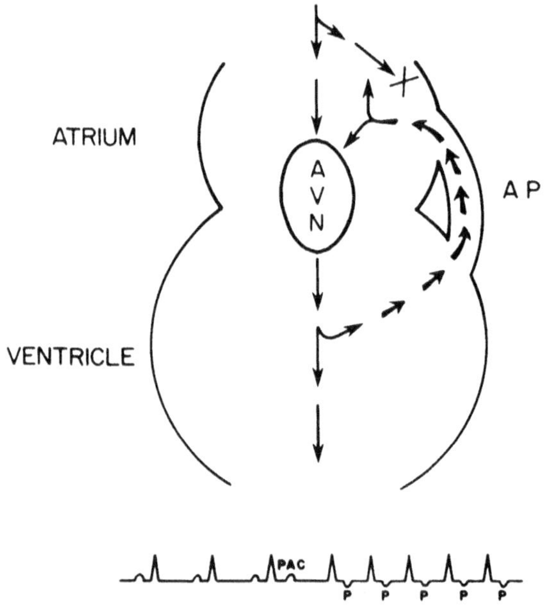

FIGURE 23-1. A schematic diagram of the heart with the accompanying rhythm strip shown below. A premature atrial contraction (PAC) is blocked in the AV accessory connection (AP) and proceeds down the AV Node (AVN) and up the accessory AV connection initiating a narrow QRS complex AV reciprocating tachycardia. P = *p* waves.

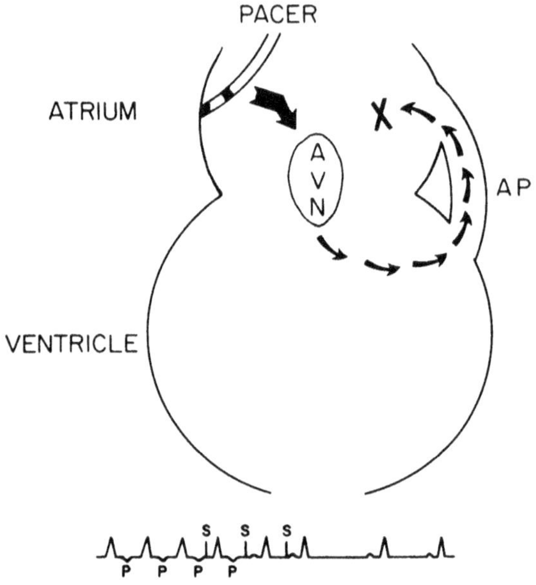

FIGURE 23-2. A schematic diagram of the heart with the accompanying rhythm strip revealing AV reciprocating tachycardia shown below. Rapid pacing is initiated from the right atrium and the third pacing stimulus(s) is able to capture part of the reentrant pathway. The reentrant impulse finds the area around the AV node refractory on its next circuit and the tachycardia is terminated. P = *p* waves, AVN = AV node, AP = Accessory AV connection.

period. Thus, a premature atrial depolarization will be likely to conduct in the antegrade direction through the AV node–His bundle and subsequently conduct in the retrograde direction in the accessory AV connection, resulting in a reciprocating tachycardia with a normal QRS (Figure 23-1). Less commonly, conduction proceeds in the antegrade direction over the accessory AV connection, producing a preexcited QRS complex tachycardia. These AV reciprocating tachycardias (AVRT) are well suited for pacemaker intervention because: (1) they are usually easily inducible in the electrophysiology laboratory allowing repeated testing to ascertain the most effective pacing modality for tachycardia termination, and (2) the large reentry circuit facilitates timing of a pacing stimulus such that it is able to capture part of the reentry loop and interrupt tachycardia (Figure 23-2).

Application of Pacing to Reciprocating Tachycardia

Pacing techniques have been employed to prevent tachycardia, to terminate episodes of tachycardia, and — if neither of these is possible — to decrease the ventricular response in patients with excessively rapid atrial rates. This last aim is primarily palliative and is rarely needed in this era of experimental antiarrhythmic drugs and ablative techniques. Accordingly, my discussion will be limited to the prevention and/or termination of tachycardia by pacing.

PREVENTION OF TACHYCARDIA BY PACING

There has been considerable interest in prevention of tachycardia by pacemakers since Zoll and coworkers demonstrated that it was possible to suppress ventricular tachycardia by pacing at a rate faster than that of the sinus node [1]. There are a variety of theoretical reasons why pacing might prevent tachycardia, including membrane effects upon ionic flux, and upon phase four depolarization, thereby decreasing the frequency of ectopic beats, a reduction in the dispersion of refractoriness, and hemodynamic factors related to the increase in heart rate [2–5].

Any intervention which reduces the incidence of extra beats (which initiate tachycardia) or alters conduction velocity and/or refractoriness within the reentry circuit may be effective in preventing the arrhythmia.

Most of the clinical studies dealing with prevention of tachycardia by means of pacing have involved dual chamber stimulation. The initial work of Coumel and associates showed that simultaneous stimulation of atria and ventricles was effective in preventing reentrant arrhythmias, presumably because the collision of impulses within the AV junction produced refractoriness within the reentry circuit [6]. More recently, Akhtar et al. found that simultaneous or sequential AV pacing either narrowed the zone in which premature beats could induce tachycardia (tachycardia induction zone) or prevented tachycardia induction during electrophysiologic study in three patients [7]. Similarly, Sung and associates totally abolished the tachycardia induction zone in four patients with tachycardia using automatically triggered simultaneous AV stimulation [8]. Using an early version of an AV sequential pacemaker, in which fixed rate atrial and demand ventricular pacing were triggered by bradycardia, Field and coworkers reported successful control of tachycardia with temporary and permanent pacing in a large group of patients with recurrent tachycardia (some with AVRT) [9]. An atrial synchronous pacemaker was employed by Spurrell and Sowton in a 51-year-old patient with recurrent PSVT [10]. A sensed atrial premature beat triggered a ventricular response following a delay of 30 ms, presumably preventing tachycardia initiation by capturing, and thus making refractory, part of the reentrant circuit. Levy et al. used dual demand (activated by both bradycardia and tachycardia) AV sequential pacing in three patients with drug resistant tachycardia, two of whom had AVRT [11]. Their pacing unit consisted of a sensing circuit (triggered by a five beat run of tachycardia at a cycle length <395 ms) which activated pacing at a rate of 77 beats/min and an AV delay of 60 ms. In the 6–16 month follow-up period, no further episodes of tachycardia were detected, although two of the three patients remain on antiarrhythmic drugs. A similar type of pacemaker was employed by Medina-Ravell and associates in 23 patients with drug-resistant PSVT, 16 of whom had AVRT [12]. Their unit had the advantage of programmability and functioned successfully without apparent adverse effects over the 1–31 month follow-up period. Curry et al. used dual chamber pacing to produce "permanent preexcitation" (with electrodes placed to produce the largest possible delta waves) as a means of increasing refractoriness in the accessory AV connection, thereby reducing the frequency of episodes of AVRT [13].

Despite considerable promise, the use of pacing to prevent AVRT is still relatively new. Although complications and/or adverse effects of preventive pacing were not described in the above-mentioned reports, all are limited by relatively small numbers and relatively short follow-up. Some of the potential disadvantages of prophylactic dual chamber pacing (Table 23–1) include the possibility of premature ventricular stimulation because of a sensed premature atrial depolarization or the development of a rapid ventricular rate in response to an atrial tachyarrhythmia. Although both of these problems are theoretically preventable by programming the pulse generator to a long atrial refractory period, this alteration may limit efficacy because some of the early atrial premature beats capable of initiating PSVT may not be sensed. In addition, failure to sense an atrial premature beat may cause the pacemaker to fire during the repolanzation phase of the spontaneous premature beat and actually initiate tachycardia. Another potential difficulty is that AV sequential pacing with a short AV delay may adversely affect the patients' hemodynamic status.

TERMINATION OF TACHYCARDIA BY PACING

Most of the clinical experience with pacing in the preexcitation syndromes has dealt with termination of, rather than prevention of, tachycardia. The ability of one or more pacing stimuli to interrupt a reciprocating tachycardia is dependent upon a variety of factors (Table 23–2). Of particular importance are electrophysiologic properties (conduction velocity, refractoriness, etc.) of the myocardium located between the

TABLE 23–1. Pacing techniques currently being used in the management of AV reciprocating tachycardia

Pacing technique	Advantages	Limitations
1. Underdrive	Uncomplicated technology	Ineffective at "high rate" tachycardia
a. Dual demand (demand pacing activated by bradycardia and tachycardia)	Low incidence atrial fibrillation; adds bradycardia mode	Ineffective at "high rate" tachycardia
b. Dual Chamber	May be more effective than single chamber underdrive pacing; may prevent PSVT	Equipment more complicated; expensive; relatively new and untested
2. Overdrive (burst)	Effective for "high rate" tachycardia	High incidence atrial fibrillation
a. Patient initiated	Uncomplicated technology; easily reprogrammable; battery easily changed	Patient must be reliable Inconvenient if tachycardia is frequent Cannot be used if tachycardia has "explosive" onset
b. Automatic	Convenient; does not rely on patient	Over/under sensing is frequent
3. Cycle scanning	Lower incidence atrial fibrillation	Complicated technology; may need frequent reprogramming; may take longer to terminate tachycardia

TABLE 23–2. Factors affecting the ability of pacing to terminate PSVT

Size of reentrant circuit
Location of stimulating electrodes
Pacing techniques
Tachycardia rate
Electrophysiologic properties of myocardium

tachycardia circuit and the electrodes [14] (see Table 23–2). Specifically, there must be an "excitable gap" between the head and tail of the tachycardia circuit, that is, an interval during which a part of the circuit is no longer refractory from the leading impulse, but has not yet been depolarized by the return impulse. This interval is termed the *termination* or *capture zone* (Figure 23–3). According to this principle, a very rapid tachycardia with a reentrant circuit covering a small area of myocardium with a high degree of refractoriness will be almost impossible to terminate by pacing. Conversely, AVRT is particularly well suited for pacemaker therapy because of the large size of the reentry circuit.

The pacing technique is an important determinant of success in terminating tachycardia. In general, the closer the stimulating electrodes are to the reentrant circuit, the greater the number of stimuli employed and the closer the interval between stimuli, the greater the likelihood of terminating the tachycardia. In a series of 32 patients with tachycardia, Wellens reported that tachycardia rates below 160 beats/min always responded to one or two extrastimuli, while faster rates usually required three or more extrastimuli to terminate the tachycardia [14]. Conversely, the greater the number of extrastimuli employed and the closer the interval between them, the greater the chance of a pacing stimulus reinitiating tachycardia immediately following a "successful" termination. It is therefore logical to review in greater detail the various pacing techniques employed clinically to terminate AVRT.

Underdrive Pacing. Underdrive pacing consists of the introduction of a train of pacing stimuli at a rate below that of the tachycardia. In general, this form of pacing is useful only in those patients in whom it has previously been demonstrated that single stimuli can reproducibly terminate the tachycardia. Since the pacing rate is independent of the tachycardia cycle length, eventually a stimulus falls within the

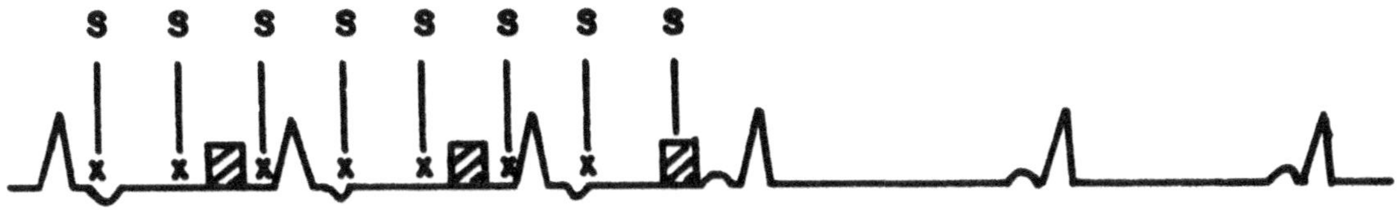

FIGURE 23–3. A schematic rhythm strip showing AV reciprocating tachycardia being treated with overdrive atrial pacing (*the arrows represent pacing stimuli*). The sixth stimulus falls within the capture zone (*crosshatched area*) and terminates the tachycardia.

termination zone, terminating the tachycardia and allowing normal sinus rhythm to resume. Underdrive pacing has the advantage of requiring relatively unsophisticated pacing technology and, in theory, should have a low likelihood of inducing atrial fibrillation and flutter (because of the low pacing rate employed). In its simplest form, underdrive pacing consists of a single chamber unit that is patient-activiated by means of a magnet. Despite early reports of success, simple underdrive pacing seems to be relatively ineffective in the majority of patients. Thus, Ward et al. evaluated a variety of pacing techniques in patients with AVRT by electrophysiologic study and found that brief periods (15 seconds) of atrial or ventricular underdrive pacing were the least successful [15]. More recently, there has been increased interest in dual demand underdrive pacing. Dual demand pacemakers have a sensing circuit and are activated automatically when the heart rate exceeds (tachycardia mode) or drops below (bradycardia mode) preset levels. At least two pacing units that are commercially available can be programmed to a dual demand mode by increasing the refractory period to its maximum (437 ms) so that fixed rate pacing occurs when the patient's heart rate exceeds 137 beats/min. Curry and associates described the use of permanent dual demand pacing in six patients with drug-resistant AVRT [16]. Pacing electrodes were placed at the site where the arrhythmia was terminated most easily and reproducibly during electrophysiologic study. All patients routinely received therapeutic doses of beta blockers or verapamil to decrease tachycardia frequency and to prevent unit activation by sinus tachycardia. During the 11–47 month follow-up period, pacing was completely effective in three patients but became ineffective at rapid tachycardia rates in one; two patients developed sensing difficulties, limiting the usefulness of the unit.

The advent of dual chamber pacemakers has provided a new and potentially more effective means of applying underdrive pacing to patients with PSVT. In theory, stimulation of both atrium and ventricle should provide a statistically greater chance of depolarizing part of the reentrant circuit or, perhaps, inducing bidirectional block. Medina-Ravell et al. implanted dual demand dual chamber pacemakers in 16 patients with recurrent AVRT [17]. The pacing unit was programmable with a ventricular pacing rate from 63–109 beats/min and an AV delay of 125–250 ms. During a follow-up period of 1–31 months, there were no sustained episodes of tachycardia although Holter recordings revealed brief runs successfully terminated by pacing. Less favorable results were described by Sowton et al. who found that the tachycardia rate, the pacing rate, and the relationship between them were important determinants of success [18]. The benefits and disadvantages of underdrive pacing are summarized in Table 23–1.

Overdrive (Burst) Pacing. The use of a rapid burst of pacing stimuli decreases the refractory period at the site of stimulation and enhances the likelihood of being able to capture part of the reentrant circuit (Figure 23–4). Thus, overdrive pacing is particularly applicable to patients with rapid tachycardia rates in whom underdrive pacing is not likely to be successful. The type of overdrive permanent pacemakers employed most frequently have been patient-activated radiofrequency units with implanted receivers and external pulse generators which are carried by the patient. Alternatively, a tachycardia mode has been incorporated into a demand pacemaker and is either activated by means of a magnet or automatically activated

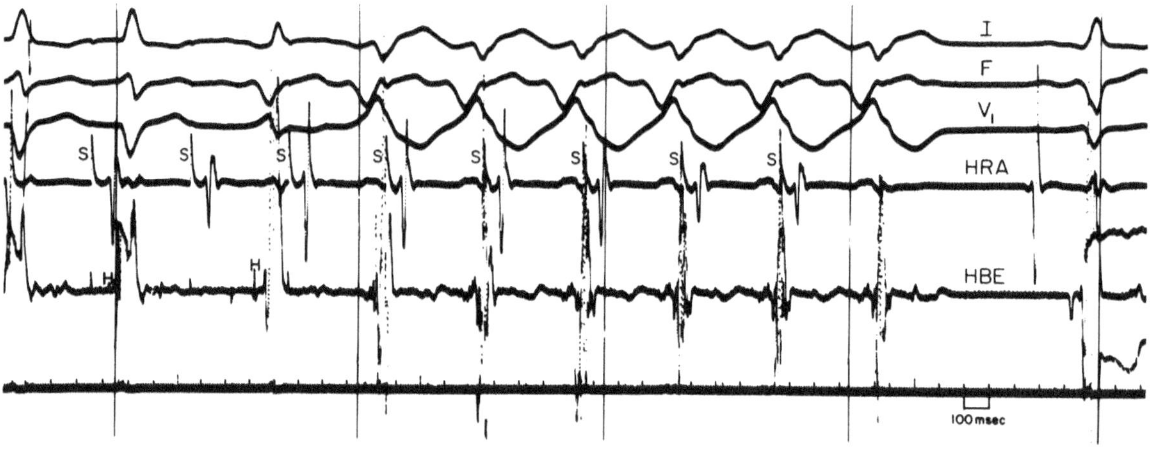

FIGURE 23–4. AV reciprocating tachycardia at a cycle length of approximately 450 ms terminated by right atrial overdrive pacing at a cycle length of 410 ms. The fourth pacing stimulus affects QRS morphology and all subsequent paced beats are preexcited indicating pacemaker capture. Note the loss of the His bundle depolarization (H) during the preexcited beats (it is buried within ventricular depolarization). Paper recording speed = 100 mm/second and the large vertical time lines are spaced one second apart I, F, and V_1 = surface ECG leads I, AVF, and V_1; HRA = high right atrial electrogram; HBE = His bundle electrogram.

through a sensing circuit. Prior to implantation, the efficacy and safety of burst pacing should be tested repeatedly in the electrophysiology laboratory and the pulse generator set at the lowest rate which consistently terminates the tachycardia. Numerous case reports and some studies have documented the efficacy of burst pacing in terminating tachycardia over relatively short time periods, but in longer-term studies complications have developed. Peters et al. described a follow-up of up to 10 years in five patients with drug-resistant AVRT in whom radiofrequency activated burst pacemakers were implanted [19]. Despite the ability to repeatedly terminate AVRT by pacing prior to implantation and the absence of other tachyarrhythmias on prolonged electrocardiographic monitoring, four of the five patients ultimately developed spontaneous and/or pacing-induced atrial fibrillation or flutter, necessitating alternative forms of therapy (Figure 23–5). Similar problems were encountered by Nathan and associates who also found psychological and social difficulties associated with long-term pacemaker use [20].

A modification of burst pacing for drug-resistant AVRT was described by Mandel and coworkers who used a magnet-activated unit in which the initial rate of 165 beats/min increases to a maximum of 300 beats/min over a two-minute period [21]. The authors theorize that the gradual increase in rate shortens atrial refractoriness, perhaps producing a corresponding decrease in the atrial vulnerable period. A similar unit that is activated automatically was employed by Nathan et al. in the electrophysiology laboratory in 20 patients with recurrent tachycardia, 12 of whom had AVRT [22]. Atrial fibrillation or flutter was not seen using this "autodecremental pacing" while these arrhythmias occurred frequently with standard burst pacing. Griffin and associates report the successful use, over an unspecified follow-up period, of an automatic burst pacemaker in five patients with recurrent PSVT [23]. Their unit has the advantage of programmability of sensitivity, pulse duration, sensing criteria, as well as burst rate and duration. The authors emphasized the need for such programmability because they found that in a given patient, tachycardia termination requirements vary considerably between the controlled environment of the electrophysiology laboratory and everyday existence in the outside world.

Cycle Scanning Pacemaker. The use of programmed, synchronized premature stimulation to terminate reentrant arrhythmias was attempt-

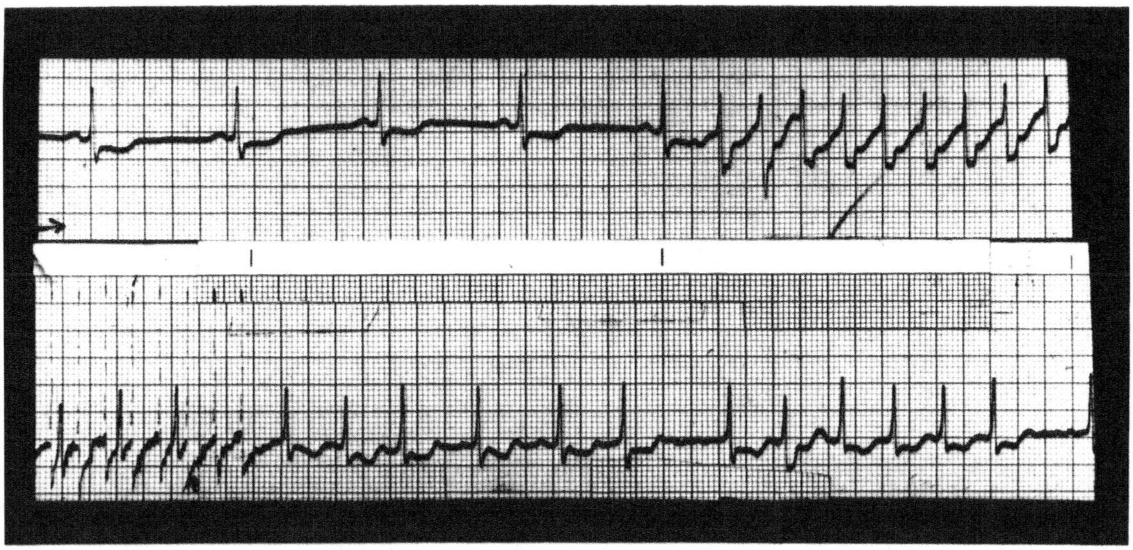

FIGURE 23–5. Standard ECG lead 2 showing the initiation of an episode of AVRT (*top strip*) by a premature atrial beat (*the notch deforming the T wave on the fifth sinus beat*). Rapid right atrial pacing is initiated (*left side of bottom strip*) producing atrial fibrillation.

ed intially in the electrophysiology laboratory and has recently been applied to permanent pacing for tachyarrhythmias. Single or double extrastimuli have been shown to be capable of terminating the majority of episodes of tachycardia [14]. Theoretically, programmed stimuli should produce a lower incidence of atrial fibrillation or flutter but location of the stimulating electrodes close to the reentrant circuit and exact timing of the premature beats may be more important than with burst pacing, especially at faster tachycardia rates. Spurrell and Sowton, using programmed premature stimulation to terminate tachycardia in the electrophysiology laboratory, found that appropriately timed single stimuli could interrupt the tachycardia in four patients while three patients required double extrastimuli [24]. Of particular importance is that the termination zone varied from episode to episode within the same patient, perhaps due to minor changes in cycle length, refractoriness, or antonomic tone. Thus, it appears that the ability to scan the cardiac cycle during each tachycardia episode may be a necessary feature for this type of pacemaker. Nathan et al. describe their experience in the electrophysiology laboratory using an adaptive cycle scanning unit in 16 patients with recurrent tachycardia, 12 of whom had AVRT [25]. Their pacing system consists of a sensing circuit (designed to recognize four consecutive beats within an adjustable range of rates as tachycardia), a pulse generator which can deliver up to 15 premature stimuli with varying coupling intervals, and a memory which will automatically utilize the setting from the preceding successful use for the next tachycardia episode. In the 12 patients with AVRT, single or double extrastimuli successfully terminated the tachycardia in all and no unwanted arrhythmias were induced. The authors also describe the use of this unit on a permanent (implanted) basis in 7 patients with AVRT. During a 1 to 6-month follow-up period, no episodes of pacing-resistant tachycardia have occurred, although most patients required beta-blockers to prevent misinterpretation of exercise-related sinus tachycardia as AVRT. An implanted cycle-scanning pacemaker was also employed by den Dulk et al. in 9 patients with drug-resistant AVRT [26]. The device consisted of an implanted pulse generator that had both a demand mode and a patient-activated tachycardia mode which delivers up to 99 stimuli at various coupling intervals if the arrhythmia fulfills preset rate criteria. The unit also contains a memory, is programmable, and can produce a wide variety of pacing modes, although reprogramming currently must be done at the factory. During a follow-up period of 7–26 months, the vast

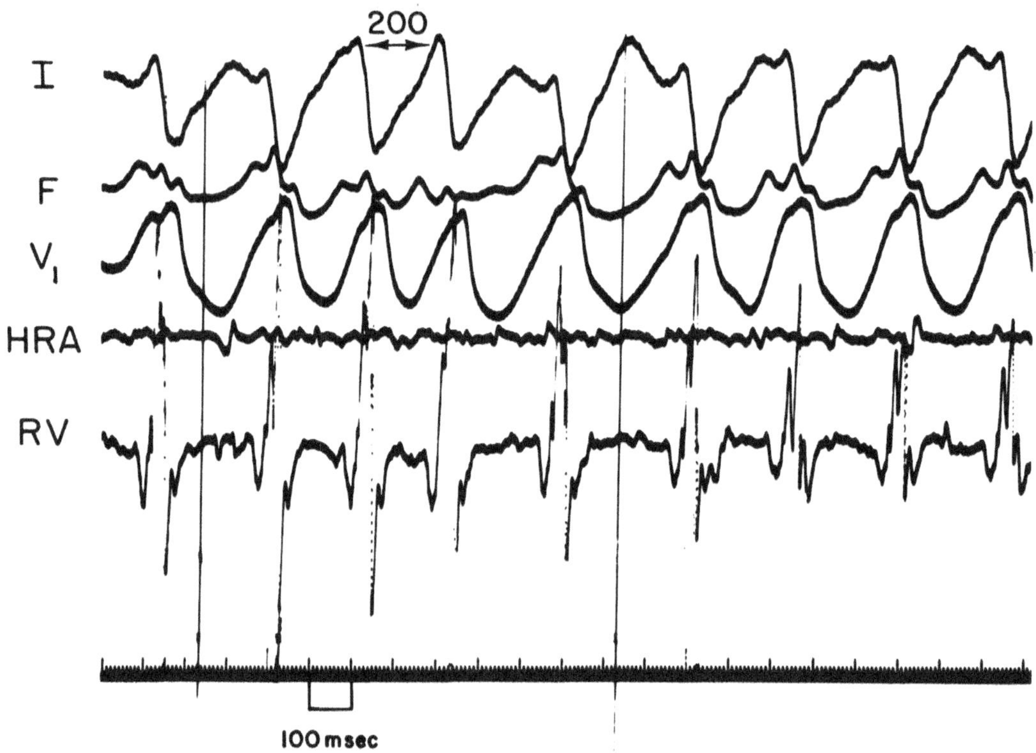

FIGURE 23–6. Three simultaneous ECG leads (I, AVF, and V_1, from top to bottom) and two intracardiac leads (high right atrial and right ventricular leads) in a patient with ventricular preexcitation and rapid atrial fibrillation. The shortest RR interval of 200 ms represents a potential ventricular rate of 300 beats/min and has been associated with an increased incidence of sudden death. Paper recording speed = 100 mm/sec, and the large vertical time lines are spaced one second apart.

majority of tachycardia episodes were terminated without difficulty, although most patients continued to receive antiarrhythmic drugs and some units had to be reprogrammed.

Indications for Pacing and Specific Pacing Techniques in Patients with the Preexcitation Syndrome (Table 23–3)

With the advent of new and more potent antiarrhythmic drugs, the increasing applicability of ablative techniques and the development of more sophisticated pacing techniques, the role of pacing in the management of patients with recurrent AVRT needs to be better defined. In light of the relatively high complication rate encountered in some of the long-term studies, it is mandatory that all patients being considered for pacemaker implantation undergo prolonged continuous electrocardiographic monitoring and complete electrophysiologic evaluation including repeated induction and termination of the tachycardia (by means of pacing) as well as the attempted induction of atrial fibrillation. In patients found to have spontaneous atrial fibrillation, those capable of very rapid antegrade conduction through the accessory AV connection (Figure 23–6), those individuals in whom pacing does not consistently and easily terminate the tachycardia, and those patients who experience syncope or seizures at the onset of their arrhythmia, pacing is not recommended and they should be advised to seek alternative forms of therapy. Other candidates in whom alternate treatment forms should be sought include individuals with psychiatric disorders and

TABLE 23-3. Prerequisities for pacemaker management in AVRT

Recurrent tachycardia.
Tachycardia resistant to drugs and/or drugs cause intolerable side effects.
Tachycardia reproducibly terminated by pacing.
No spontaneous atrial fibrillation or flutter.
Pacing does not produce unwanted arrhythmia or other adverse effects.
Accessory AV connection not capable of rapid antegrade conduction.
Patient emotionally stable.
Symptomatic tachycardia episodes not extremely frequent.

those with very frequent symptomatic episodes of tachycardia, in whom frequent use of the pacemaker may be incompatible with a normal life-style. Pacing should not necessarily be considered a permanent solution for recurrent AVRT, since a substantial number of patients either become refractory or develop atrial fibrillation on long-term follow-up. Neither should it be looked upon as a means of avoiding chronic antiarrhythmic therapy since the majority of patients in the clinical studies referred to above needed to continue taking antiarrhythmic drugs. In summary, the "ideal" candidate for pacing should be an individual with drug-resistant AVRT who is emotionally stable, whose arrhythmia occurs infrequently and is hemodynamically well tolerated, and in whom neither atrial fibrillation nor flutter is demonstrable despite prolonged electrocardiographic monitoring. During electrophysiologic study, the arrhythmia should be reproducibly and safely terminated by pacing, and the AV node and accessory AV connection should be demonstrated to have relatively long refractory periods so that if atrial fibrillation should occur, the ventricular response will not be excessively rapid.

Once the decision has been made to use permanent pacemaker therapy in a patient with recurrent AVRT, the clinician is faced with a bewildering assortment of pacing techniques, each with its advantages and drawbacks [27,28] (Table 23-1). Thus, underdrive pacing causes unwanted arrhythmias infrequently but is relatively ineffective, especially in patients with rapid tachycardia rates. Dual demand pacing has the advantage of having a bradycardia mode, making it especially effective in patients with alternating bradycardia and tachycardia. In addition, dual demand units offer the convenience of automatic activation although this may be somewhat of a mixed blessing because sensing problems are frequent and most patients require large doses of beta or calcium blockers to prevent activation of the tachycardia mode by exercise-mediated sinus tachycardia. The sensing difficulties seen with automatically activated pacemakers are well illustrated by the experience of Lerman et al. in three patients with recurrent tachycardia, one of whom had AVRT [29]. Despite repeated testing of the units following implantation, all three developed problems with over and/or undersensing shortly after hospital discharge, necessitating extensive reprogramming or removal of the unit. Recently, Arzbacher and coworkers have developed a computer system to be incorporated into permanent pacemakers that can supposedly differentiate between AVRT and sinus tachycardia, which they hope will improve sensing capabilities [30]. Dual chamber pacemakers have added a promising new dimension to antitachycardia pacing, especially in the realm of tachycardia prevention, but they are relatively complicated devices. Long-term follow-up has not yet been reported. Overdrive (burst) pacing tends to be highly effective in terminating PSVT but is associated with a relatively high incidence of atrial fibrillation and flutter, plus the potential of transmission of very rapid paced rates to the ventricles. The newer cycle-scanning pacemaker promises to be both effective and have a low incidence of unwanted arrhythmias although further experience with these units is needed to document efficacy. Currently available scanning units have the disadvantage that cycle-scanning may be a relatively lengthy procedure, allowing the patient to remain symptomatic during this period of time.

A variety of newer techniques are being developed which promise to eliminate some of the difficulties encountered with current antitachycardia pacemakers [31]. These new techniques include: a program to scan the cardiac cycle much more rapidly, the use of higher current levels of increase efficacy, tachycardia entrainment combined with cycle scanning (which may cause a lower incidence of atrial fibrillation than with burst pacing), underdrive pacing at rates just below that of the tachycardia, or at certain proportions of the tachycardia cycle length, short bursts of very high frequency pacing (e.g., 800 beats/min) initiated during the refractory period, and very rapid subthreshold burst pacing. These techniques are all experimental and await detailed clinical testing.

Conclusion

In conclusion, AVRT is potentially manageable by pacing techniques in selected patients. With available devices concurrent antiarrhythmic medication is usually necessary. Early studies have confirmed the efficacy of certain types of pacing, but all have their limitations and adverse effects. New and promising techniques are currently under investigation. Further studies are needed to fully assess their safety and efficacy.

References

1. Zoll PM, Linenthal AJ, Zarsly LRN: Ventricular fibrillation: treatment and prevention by external electric currents. *N. Engl. J. Med.* 262:105, 1960.
2. Lange G: Action of driving stimuli from intrinsic and extrinsic sources or in situ cardiac pacemaker tissues. *Circ. Res.* 27:449, 1965.
3. Han J, Moe GK: Nonuniform recovery of excitability in ventricular muscle. *Circ. Res.* 24:44, 1964.
4. Han J, Millet D, Chizzonitti B, Moe GK: Temporal dispersion of recovery of excitability in atrium and ventricle as a function of heart rate. *Am. Heart J.* 71:481, 1966.
5. Han J, Detraglia J, Millet D, Moe GK: 1966. Incidence of ectopic beats as a function of basic rate in the ventricle. *Am. Heart J.* 72:632, 1966.
6. Coumel P, Cabrol C, Fabiato A, Gourgon R, Slama R: Tachycardia permanente par rhythme reciproque. *Arch. Mal Coeur* 60:1830, 1967.
7. Akhtar M, Gilbert CJ, Al-Nouri M, Schmmidt DH: Electrophysiologic mechanisms for modification and abolition of atrioventricular junctional tachycardia with simultaneous and sequential atrial and ventricular pacing. *Circulation* 60:1443, 1979.
8. Sung RJ, Styperek JL, Castellanos A: Complete abolition of the reentrant supraventricular tachycardia zone using a new modality of cardiac pacing with simultaneous atrioventricular stimulation. *Am. J. Cardiol.* 45:72, 1980.
9. Fields J, Berkovits BV, Matloff JM: Surgical experience with temporary and permanent A-V sequential demand pacing. *J Thorac. Cardiovasc. Surg.* 66:865, 1973.
10. Spurrell RAJ, Sowton E: Pacing techniques in the management of supraventricular tachycardias: Part 2. *J. Electrocardiol.* 9:89, 1976.
11. Levy S, Berkovits B, Mandel W, Broustet JP, Obel IWF, Dricand H: Refractory supraventricular tachycardias: successful therapy with double demand sequential pacing. (Abstract.) *Am. J. Cardiol.* 45:457, 1980.
12. Medina-Ravell V, Castellanos A, Portillo-Acosta B, Maduro-Maytin C, Rodriguez-Salas L, Hernandez-Arenas M, LaSalle-Toro R, Mendozo-Mujica I, Ortega-Maldonado M, Berkovitz BV: 1983. Management of tachyarrhythmias with dual-chamber pacemaker. *PACE* 6:333, 1983.
13. Curry PVL, Davies DW, Bucknall MB: 1984. Anti-tachycardia prophylaxis: permanent paced pre-excitation. (Abstract.) *J. Am. Coll. Cardiol.* 3:473, 1984.
14. Wellens HJJ, den Dulk K, Brugada P: Pacemaker management of cardiac arrhythmias. *Cardiovasc. Clin.* 14:165, 1983.
15. Ward DE, Camm AJ, Spurrell RAJ: The response of regular reentrant supraventricular tachycardia to right heart stimulation. *PACE* 2:586, 1979.
16. Curry PVL, Rowland E, Krikler DM: Dual-demand pacing for refractory atrioventricular re-entry tachycardia. *PACE* 2:137, 1979.
17. Medina-Ravell V, Maduro C, Mejias J, Portillo B, Portillo-Leon V, Berkovitz BV, Castellanos A, Rodriguez-Salas L: Use of dual-demand AV sequential (DVI, MN) pacemaker in the management of supraventricular tachycardias. *Cardiovasc. Clin.* 14:227, 1983.
18. Sowton E, O'Keeffe DB, Curry PVL: Use of a multiprogrammable pacemaker in the dual-demand mode: influence of pacing rate on termination of tachycardia. *Eur. Heart J.* 1:165, 1980.
19. Peters RW, Shafton E, Frank S, Thomas AN, Scheinman MM: Radiofrequency-triggered pacemakers: uses and limitations: a long-term study. *Ann. Intern. Med.* 88:17, 1978.
20. Nathan AW, Hellestrand K, Bexton RS, Spurrell RAJ, Camm AJ: Problems with longterm radiofrequency rapid atrial pacing for tachycardia. *PACE.* (In press.)
21. Mandel WJ, Laks MM, Yamaguchi I, Fields J, Berkovitz B: Recurrent reciprocating tachycardia in the Wolff-Parkinson-White syndrome: control by the use of a scanning pacemaker. *Chest* 69:769, 1976.
22. Nathan A, Hellestrand K, Ward D, Spurrell R, Camm J: Rate-related accelerating (autodecremental) atrial pacing for reversion of paroxysmal supraventricular tachycardia. J Electrocardial 15:77, 1982.
23. Griffin JC, Mason JW, Calfec RV: A programmable tachycardia terminating pacemaker for the treatment of arrhythmias. In *Cardiac arrhyth-*

mias: a decade of progress. D. Harrison (ed.). Boston, Mass., GK. Hall Medical Publishers, 1981, p. 383.
24. Spurrell RAJ, Sowton E: Pacing techniques in the management of supraventricular tachycardias. J Electrocardial 8:287, 1975.
25. Nathan A, Hellestrand K, Bexton R, Nappholz T, Spurrell R, Camm J: Clinical evaluation of an adaptive tachycardia intervention pacemaker with automatic cycle length adjustment. *PACE* 5:201, 1982.
26. Dan Dulk K, Bertholet M, Brugada P, Dar FW, Demoulin JC, Waleffc A, Bakels N, Lindemans F, Bourgeois I, Kulbertus HE, Wellens HJJ: Clinical experience with implantable devices for control of tachyarrhythmias. *PACE* 7:548, 1984.
27. German LD, Strauss HC: Electrical termination of tachyarrhythmias by discrete pulses. *PACE* 7:514, 1984.
28. Echt DS: Potential hazards of implanted devices for the electrical control of tachyarrhythmia. *PACE* 7:580, 1984.
29. Lerman B, Waxman HC, Buxton AE, Sweeney M, Josephson ME: Tachyarrhythmias associated with programmable automatic atrial antitachycardia pacemakers. *Am. Heart J.* 106:1029, 1983.
30. Arzbacher R, Bump T, Jenkins J, Glick K, Munkenbeck F, Brown J, Nandhakumar N: Automatic tachycardia recognition. *PACE* 7:541, 1984.
31. Camm J, Ward D: New modes and new pacemakers for tachycardia termination. In *Pacing for tachycardia control.* London, Telectronics 1983, p. 97.

24. CATHETER ABLATION FOR PATIENTS WITH VENTRICULAR PREEXCITATION SYNDROMES

Melvin M. Scheinman

The newly introduced method of catheter electrocoagulation of the atrioventricular (AV) [1,2] junction or accessory pathway [3,4] has provided a new treatment modality for patients with cardiac arrhythmias involving accessory pathways. Techniques for catheter electrocoagulation of the AV junction were introduced almost four years ago, while specific catheter techniques for accessory pathway ablation were introduced only two years ago. While the introduction of these techniques offers great promise for patients with tachycardia utilizing an accessory pathway, the experience, to date, is limited and the follow-up is short. Therefore, definitive recommendations are not possible. In this chapter, we lean heavily on our own experience with the ablative techniques since available reports of these procedures are sparse [3–7]. The purpose is to describe the currently available catheter ablative techniques and explore use of these techniques in the management of patients with recurrent tachycardias associated with accessory pathways in whom tachyarrhythmia has proved refractory to antiarrhythmics and/or antitachycardia devices (Table 24–1).

AV Junctional Ablation: Technical Approach

Most ablative procedures have been performed using a standard 6 French or 7 French USCI quadripolar or tripolar catheter. Studies by Fisher et al. [8] have shown that not all commercially available electrode catheters are suitable for ablative procedures. This is an important consideration due to the enormous amounts of electrical energy discharged through the catheter. The catheter is inserted into the femoral vein and positioned to record the largest bipolar His bundle electrogram; then each of the electrode poles are coupled to ground in order to record unipolar potentials. It is assumed that the catheter electrode closest to the His bundle will show the largest deflection, since previous clinical studies during open-heart surgical mapping have shown a steep exponential decline in the amplitude of the His bundle deflection as the electrode probe is moved away from the common bundle [9]. In addition, it should be appreciated that most of the amplitude of a bipolar His deflection is generated from only

TABLE 24–1. Possible uses of catheter ablative techniques in patients with accessory pathways

A. Accessory AV pathways
   1. Posteroseptal
   2. Free wall
B. AV junctional ablation
   1. AV reentrant arrhythmias
   2. Nodoventricular connections with the AV junction as a necessary component of the tachycardia circuit

Benditt, D.G. and Benson, D.W., Cardiac Preexcitation Syndromes. Copyright © 1986, Martinus Nijhoff Publishing.

one of the electrodes; the other acts largely as a "remote" indifferent electrode.

Prior to delivery of shocks to the AV junction, an additional electrode catheter should be positioned within the right ventricle and checked to be certain that its position is stable and that it has a suitable threshold for ventricular stimulation. The latter point is especially important since the shock may result in transient periods of both AV block as well as ventricular asystole. A catheter is also inserted into a peripheral artery to allow for continuous monitoring of the arterial pressure. Such monitoring is desirable both during administration of a short acting anesthetic agent as well as in the period immediately after delivery of the shocks. In our experience, additional hemodynamic monitoring, including use of a Swan-Ganz catheter, has not added to the safety of this procedure and has been deleted from our protocol.

Once all catheters are in place, the catheter recording the His bundle potential is manipulated in order to obtain the largest possible atrial and His bundle potentials. The amplitude of these potentials are measured in relationship to standardized calibration markers. It is preferable to deliver the shocks to the atrial portion of the His bundle in order to avoid delivery of shocks to the summit of the ventricular septum. If one cannot obtain a unipolar His bundle electrogram of suitable amplitude (>150 mV), our current practice is to manipulate the catheter so that the largest bipolar His bundle electrogram is obtained. The two electrodes are then coupled and used as the cathode for delivery of shocks. In the event that the latter procedure is necessary, we tend to apply larger shocks, 300–400 joules; while if large unipolar His bundle signals are obtained, we tend to use lesser energies (200 joules). The electrode(s) showing the largest His bundle deflection is used as the cathode (current source) while a patch positioned over the left scapula becomes the anode (current sink). The electrode patch-system is connected to a direct-current defibrillator and one or more discharges are applied. Our practice has been to use at least two shocks, even if complete AV block is achieved with the first shock. The reason for this approach is related to the fact that the His bundle deflection may become difficult or impossible to find after the first shock, so that the best opportunity for producing chronic complete AV block is often during the initial portion of the procedure. After the first shock, both the catheter position and intracardiac signals are carefully checked before delivery of the second shock.

The patient should be monitored in the catheterization laboratory for at least 30 minutes after delivery of the shocks. Immediately postshock, complete AV block with ventricular asystole is the rule and, therefore, ventricular pacing is required. Patients with atrial fibrillation or flutter will usually revert to sinus rhythm after the shock and postshock induction of ventricular arrhythmias has been reported [10]. The patient is then tested with ventricular pacing at varying paced rates to be certain that retrograde ventriculoatrial (VA) conduction has been interrupted. Atropine may be given in order to determine whether AV conduction resumes.

It should be emphasized that AV node–His bundle ablation procedure be done only by physicians skilled in performing cardiac electrophysiologic studies. An anesthesiologist should be in attendance for administration of the anesthetic agents prior to shock and a cardiac surgeon should be on call for possible emergent problems. When the procedure is completed the patient is then transferred to an intensive care monitoring area with the right ventricular pacing catheter in place and monitored for at least 24 hours. The paced rate may be intermittently and gradually slowed in order to characterize the escape pacemaker. If AV conduction does not resume within 24–48 hours, then a permanent pacemaker is inserted. In any event, the patient should be observed and the ECG monitored for an additional three days in a telemetered area prior to hospital discharge.

Ablation of Posteroseptal Accessory AV Pathways

TECHNICAL APPROACH

In the catheterization laboratory, electrode catheters are inserted transvenously and positioned in the right ventricle, into the coronary sinus, and across the tricuspid valve for His bundle recordings. An arterial catheter is inserted, allowing for continuous monitoring of the arterial pressure. In patients with orthodromic reciprocating tachycardia, the arrhythmia is induced and the sequence of retrograde atrial excitation should confirm that the atrial electrogram recorded from the coronary sinus os precedes the atrial electrogram recorded from any other atrial site. Subsequently, the coronary sinus catheter is manipulated so that the distal electrode poles of the coronary sinus catheters are placed just within the os of the coronary sinus and the proximal electrode pairs are positioned just outside the os. The proximal electrodes are coupled and used as the cathode while a patch positioned over the sternum is used as the anode. Two shocks of 200 to 400 joules each are delivered from the proximal electrode pair to the patch using a direct-current defibrillator. After delivery of the shock, a transient period of complete AV block with ventricular asystole may occur and, therefore, right ventricular pacing may be required.

In our experience, AV block has been transient and sinus rhythm with conduction over AV node–His bundle axis supervenes within minutes of the shock. In addition, junctional rhythms are common and the operator should not interprete the finding of abolition of preexcitation due to emergence of a junctional rhythm as being due to direct damage to the accessory pathway. It is our policy to repeat the shock even if the first shock results in complete disruption of conduction in both the antegrade and retrograde direction over the accessory pathway. After delivery of the shocks and assurance of hemodynamic stability, the right ventricle is paced and the pattern of retrograde atrial excitation is determined. The most common postshock finding is ventriculoatrial (VA) dissociation even at the slowest feasible ventricular paced rates. Following shock, the patient is monitored for 30 minutes in the catheterization laboratory and repeated atrial pacing is used both to exclude the possibility of resumption of antegrade conduction over the accessory pathway and to assess antegrade conduction characteristics over the AV node–His bundle axis. After demonstration of a stable sinus rhythm with normal AV conduction, all catheters are removed and the patient transferred to a unit where continuous electrocardiographic monitoring can be performed. The patient is allowed to ambulate the following day during continuous electrocardiographic monitoring. If a 24-hour Holter recording three days following delivery of shocks shows stable sinus rhythm without evidence of preexcitation, the patient is discharge from the hospital. Follow-up exercise treadmill testing, a 24-hour ambulatory electrocardiographic monitoring, and repeat electrophysiologic testing is performed 3 months after the procedure to assess completeness of accessory pathway interruption.

EXPERIENCE

To date, we have applied the above-described technique to seven patients with posteroseptal accessory pathways. A detailed electrophysiologic study prior to ablation is mandatory both for precise pathway localization as well as to exclude additional pathways and to define the mechanism(s) of the arrhythmia(s). Our experience with patients with posteroseptal pathways, for example, has shown a high incidence of associated right-sided accessory pathways [11]. The electrocardiogram during maximum preexcitation is an excellent guide to the possible presence of a posteroseptal pathway [11–13]. The classic findings include a negative delta wave in leads II, III, and aVF and a slightly positive or negative (isoelectric) delta wave in V_1, together with marked positive delta waves in the other precordial leads (V_2–V_6).

Five of the seven patients who underwent attempted catheter ablation of a posteroseptal accessory pathway demonstrated complete conduction block in both the antegrade and retrograde directions over the accessory pathway, but our follow-up time is short. Coronary arteriography in two patients studied three and six months after successful ablation showed no evidence of coronary arterial or coronary sinus lesions. One patient with two accessory pathways required subsequent surgical interruption of a right anterior accessory pathway. Direct inspection showed no gross lesions in the region previously exposed to electrode catheter shock.

An illustrative case example of catheter ablation of a posteroseptal accessory pathway is detailed in Figures 24–1 to 24–6. The patient was a 28-year-old white male with the Wolff-Parkinson-White (WPW) syndrome (Figure 24–1) and paroxysmal atrial fibrillation associated with very rapid ventricular response (Figure 24–2). Electrophysiologic studies showed that the shortest preexcited RR interval during atrial fibrillation was 180 ms and this was not changed by intravenous procainamide infusion. Figure 24–3 shows ventricular preexcitation with the His bundle deflection occurring within the QRS complex. During right ventricular pacing earliest atrial activation was recorded

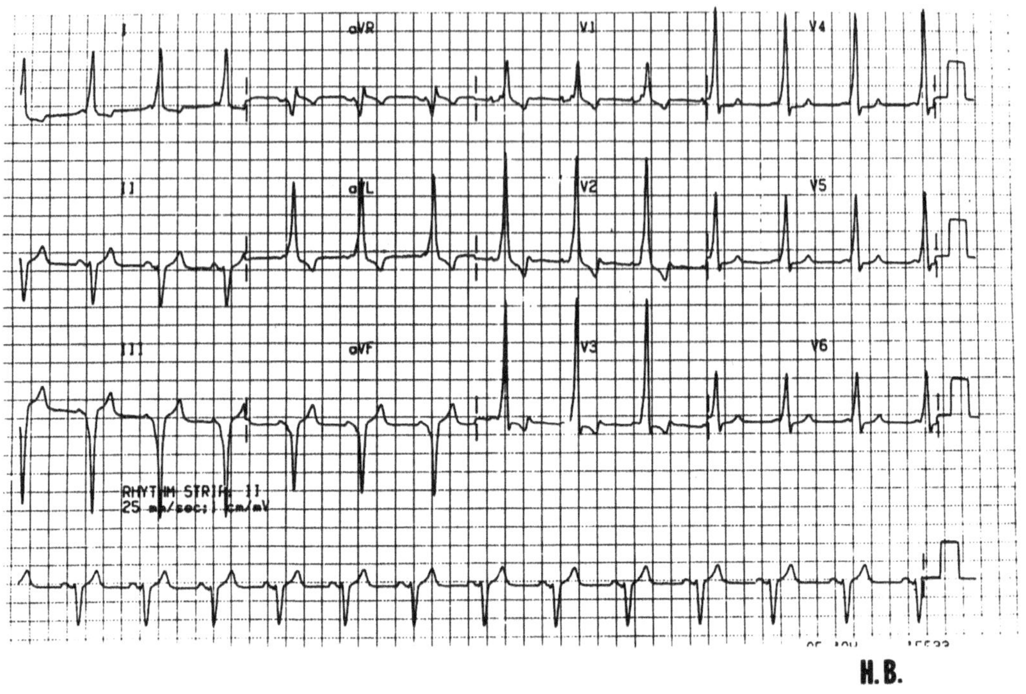

FIGURE 24–1. Standard 12-lead ECG of a patient with a posteroseptal accessory pathway. The atypical feature of this ECG is the positive delta wave in V_1.

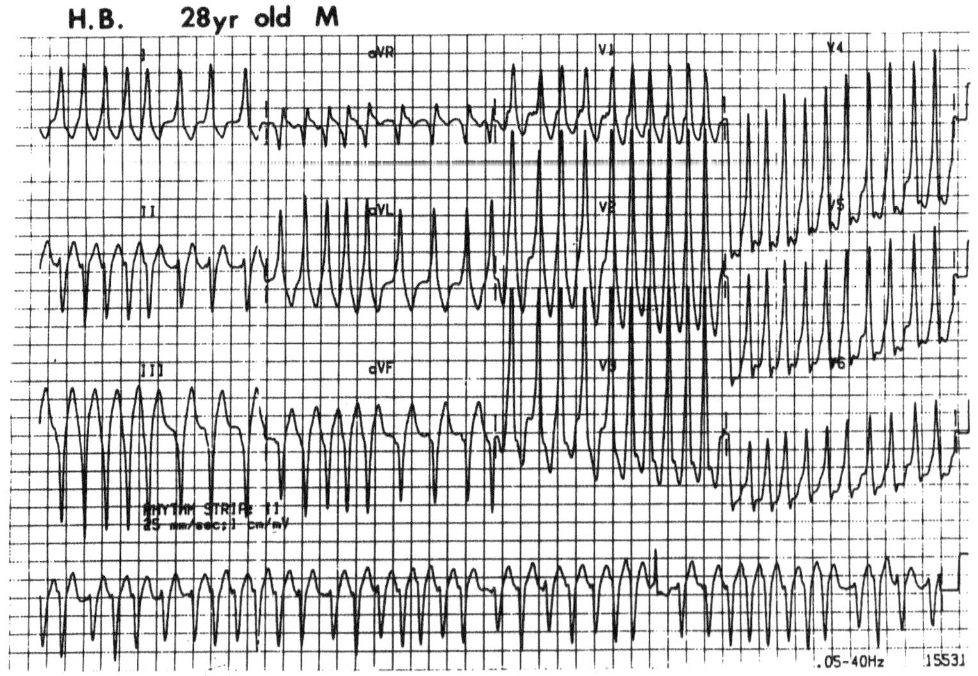

FIGURE 24–2. Twelve-lead ECG of a patient with a posteroseptal accessory pathway and atrial fibrillation with rapid ventricular response. The 12-lead ECG during sinus rhythm is shown in Figure 24–1.

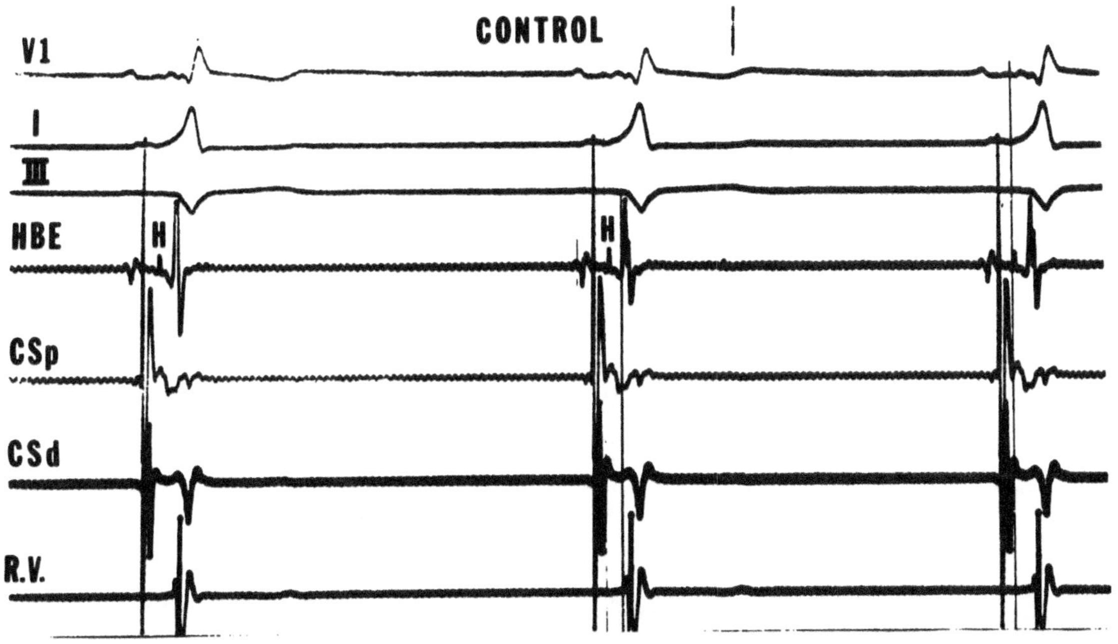

FIGURE 24–3. Control recordings of patients with a posteroseptal accessory pathway whose 12-lead ECGs are shown in Figures 24–1 and 24–2. Simultaneous surface leads V_1, I, and III are recorded with the His bundle electrogram (HBE) as well as recordings from the proximal (CS_p) and distal (CS_d) electrode pairs of a catheter inserted into the coronary sinus. The recordings from an electrode catheter in the right ventricular apex (RV) is shown at the bottom of the tracing. In this tracing, the initial delta wave is flat in V_1 in contrast to that recorded in Figures 24–1 and 24–2 and is perhaps related to slight variation in the positioning of the V_1 electrode. The His bundle deflection (H) occurs within the delta wave.

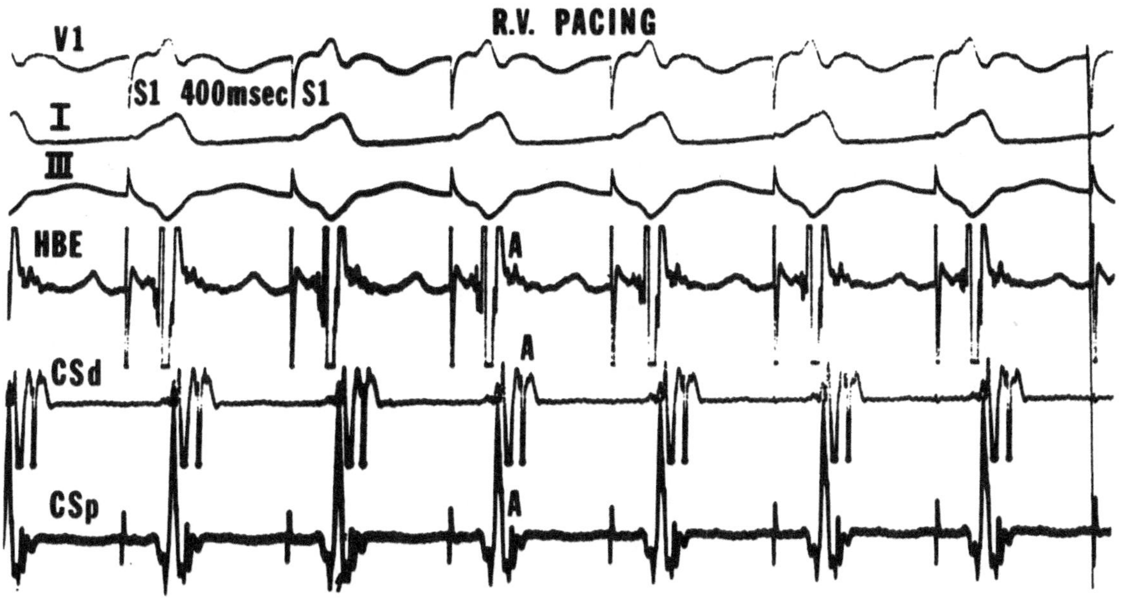

FIGURE 24–4. The abbreviations are the same as in Figure 24–3. Right ventricular overdrive pacing at a cycle length of 400 ms shows that the atrial electrogram recorded from the region of the os of the coronary sinus precedes that from the more distal coronary sinus recording as well as the septal atrial electrogram.

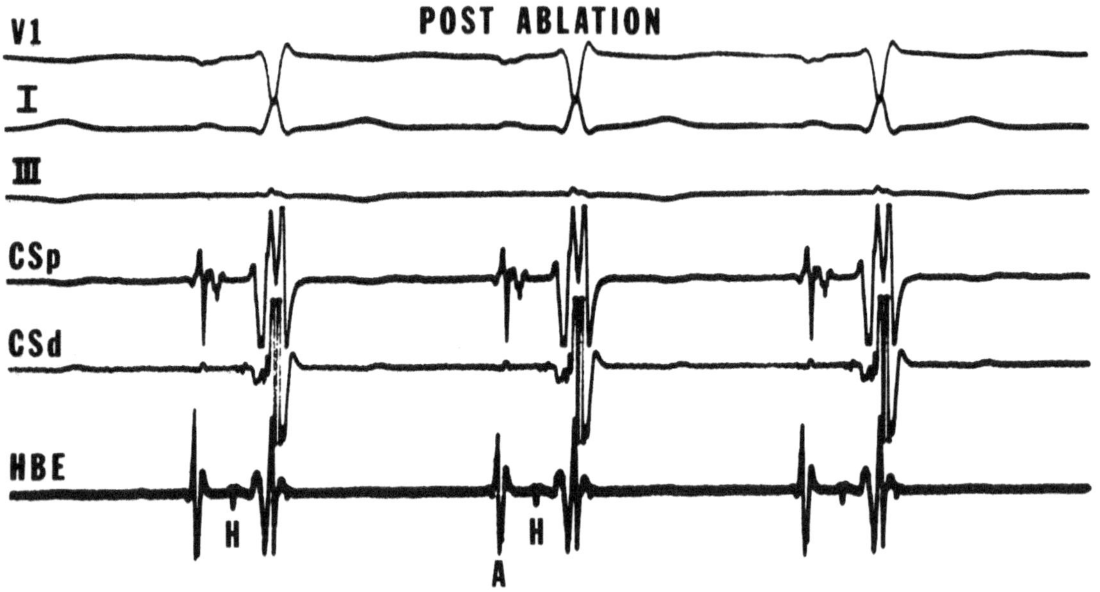

FIGURE 24–5. Abbreviations as in Figure 24–3. After delivery of two shocks of 300 joules to electrodes positioned just outside the coronary sinus, sinus rhythm with normal AV conduction is present.

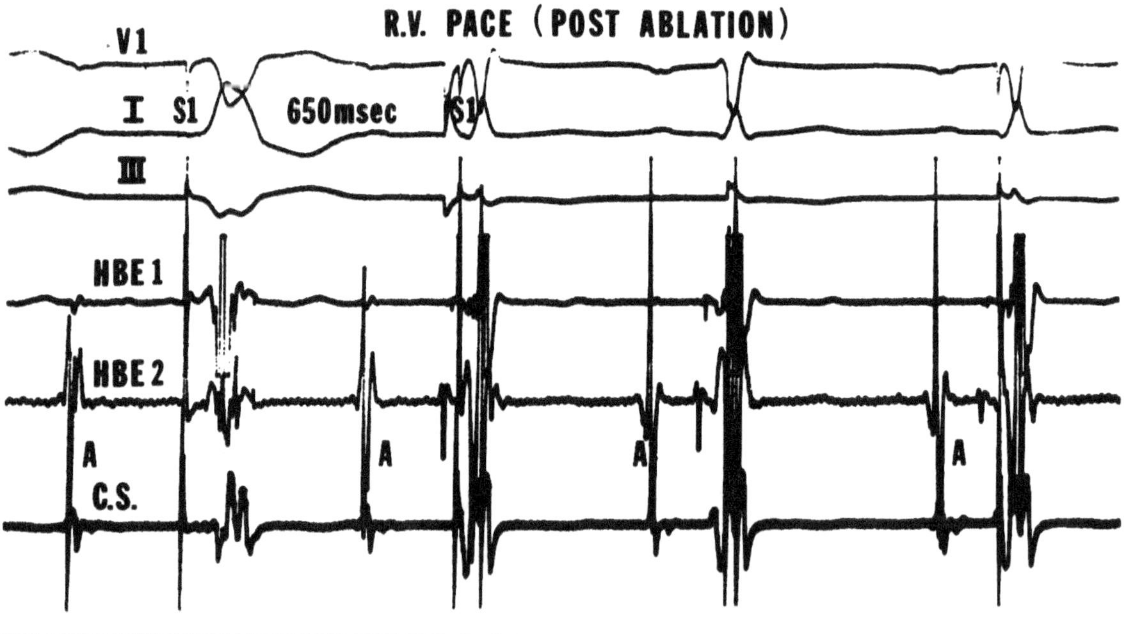

FIGURE 24–6. Abbreviations as in Figure 24–3. Right ventricular pacing at a cycle length of 650 ms after ablation shows AV dissociation.

from the coronary sinus os (Figure 24–4). In this patient, atrial mapping during induced orthodromic reciprocating tachycardia proved difficult since the arrhythmia rapidly deteriorated into atrial fibrillation. Sinus rhythm after the ablation procedure showed no evidence of ventricular preexcitation (Figure 24–5). In addition, during right ventricular pacing at cycle length 650 ms, VA dissociation was present (Figure 24–6). Thus postshock, AV node conduction in the antegrade direction was present, and there was no evidence of either antegrade or retrograde conduction over the accessory pathway.

Ablation of Free Wall Accessory Pathways

Only preliminary reports are available describing attempted ablation of free wall accessory pathways [3,6,7]. Fisher et al. [5] have recently detailed their experience with attempted electrical ablation of left free wall accessory pathways by delivery of multiple shocks within the coronary sinus immediately adjacent to the accessory pathway. In each patient, disruption of accessory pathway conduction in the antegrade direction occurred only transiently and eventually resumed. However, modification of antegrade accessory pathway conduction was found in several patients. One patient developed cardiac tamponade (requiring pericardiocentesis) following apparent disruption of the coronary sinus after shock.

Preliminary experience suggests that ablation of free wall accessory pathways is seldom effective and probably of higher risk than either AV junction or posteroseptal accessory pathway ablation. Jackman et al. [14] have described use of a catheter with orthogonal electrode array for direct recording of the accessory pathway potentials. Conceivably, this innovation coupled with safer systems to deliver energy in closer proximity to the accessory pathway may improve safety and efficacy of catheter ablation of free wall accessory pathways.

Ablation of Concealed Accessory Pathways

It is well recognized that in a subset of patients with recurrent paroxysmal supraventricular tachycardia, the arrhythmia circuit may involve a concealed accessory pathway. It is well to remember that these pathways may occur anywhere around the cardiac anulus or septum (including the posteroseptal area). This is important since some patients with drug refractory tachycardia may never manifest overt preexcitation but may have an accessory pathway which is amenable to catheter ablation. Figures 24–7 to 24–9 illustrate use of this technique in a patient with a concealed posteroseptal accessory pathway.

A 24-year-old white female had recurrent syncopal episodes owing to rapid ventricular response during supraventricular tachycardia. She failed trials of all conventional antiarrhythmic drugs and also proved unresponsive to propafenone. Multiple electrocardiographic recordings showed no evidence of ventricular preexcitation. Figure 24–7 shows a recording during orthodromic reciprocating tachycardia. Earliest atrial activation during tachycardia was localized to the os of the coronary sinus. Atrial pacing from the os of the coronary sinus showed no evidence of ventricular preexcitation (Figure 24–8). Postshock, atrial pacing at a cycle length of 350 ms showed AV nodal Wenckebach conduction (Figure 24–9). Ventricular pacing at cycle length of 600 ms showed VA dissociation (Figure 24–10).

Ablation of the AV Junction in Patients with AV Reciprocating Tachycardia

Catheter ablation of the AV junction will prevent tachycardia in those patients with reciprocating tachycardia utilizing the AV junction as a necessary component of the tachycardia circuit. However, this form of treatment should be approached cautiously. Patients with accessory pathways that permit rapid ventricular response during atrial fibrillation may receive little benefit since antegrade conduction over the accessory pathway is usually intact following AV junctional ablation. Further, a permanent ventricular pacemaker is recommended since the long-term stability of antegrade accessory pathway conduction is unknown. Figures 24–11 and 24–12 illustrate intracardiac recordings prior to and following AV junction ablation in a woman with left posterior free wall accessory pathway and recurrent orthodromic reciprocating tachycardia refractory to drug therapy There was no prior history of atrial fibrillation.

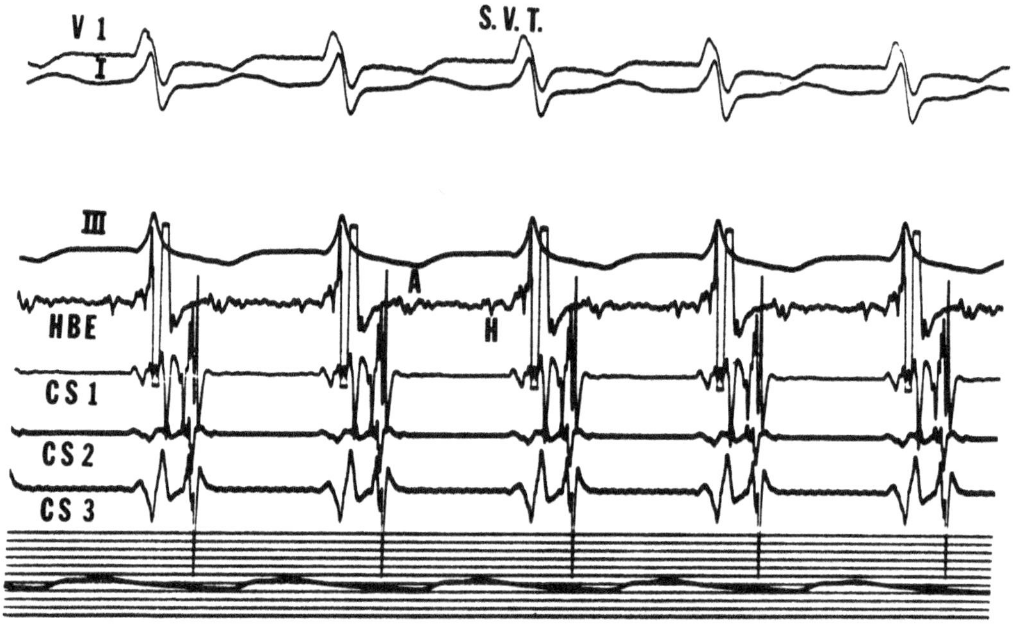

FIGURE 24–7. Simultaneous surface leads V_1, I, and III together with His bundle recordings (HBE) and recordings from distal (CS_1-coronary os) and more proximal coronary sinus sites (CS_2, CS_3). The arterial pressure is recorded on the bottom of the tracing. During tachycardia, the coronary sinus os atrial electrogram preceded those from all other atrial sites.

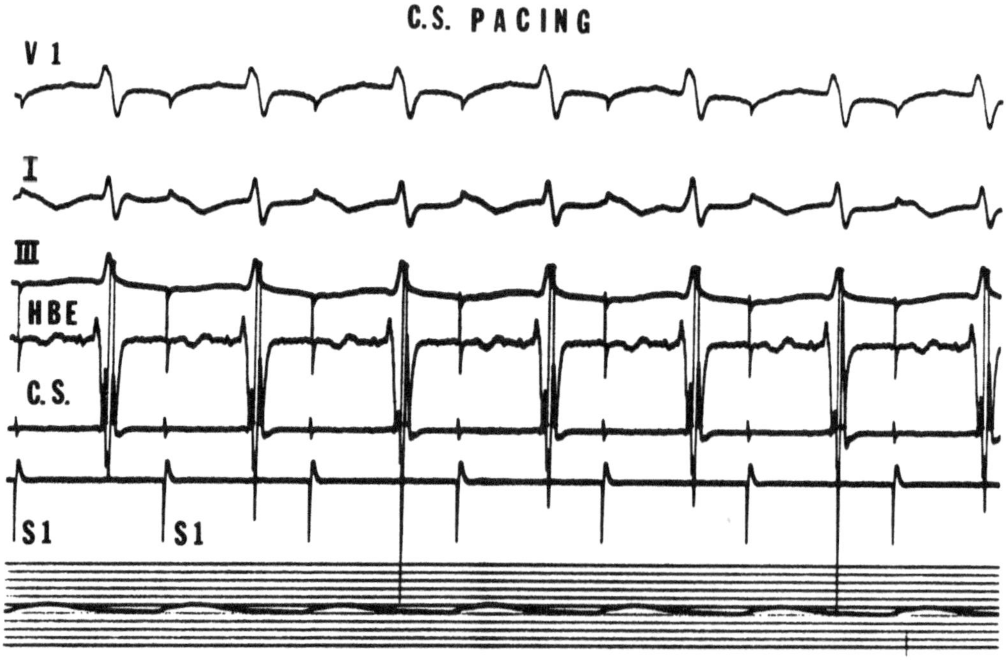

FIGURE 24–8. Abbreviations as in Figure 24–7. Atrial overdrive pacing from the coronary sinus os shows no evidence of ventricular preexcitation.

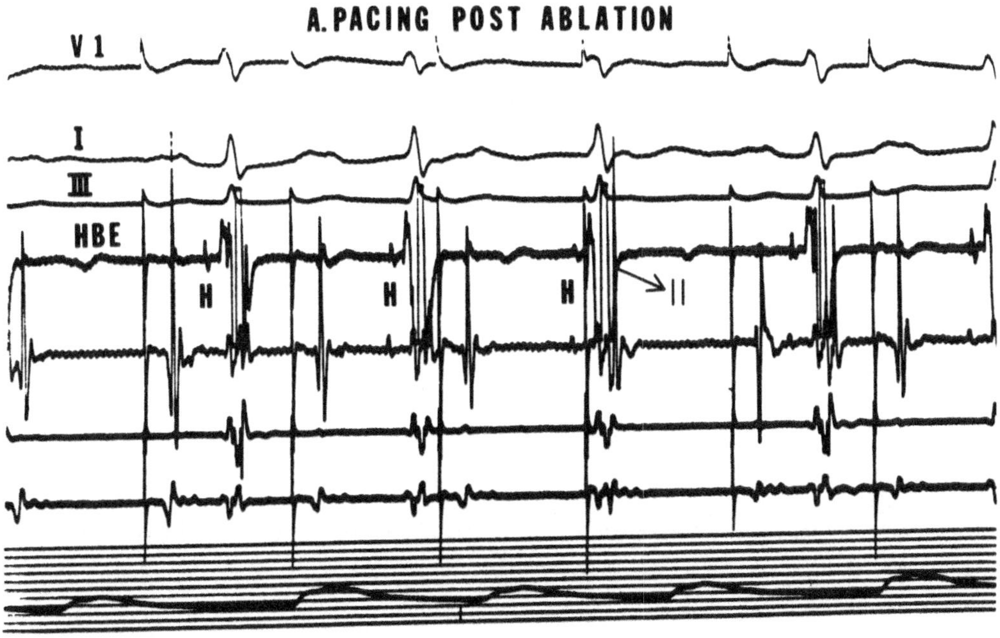

FIGURE 24–9. Atrial pacing at a paced cycle length of 350 ms after ablation shows AV nodal Wenckebach conduction. Abbreviations as in Figure 24–7.

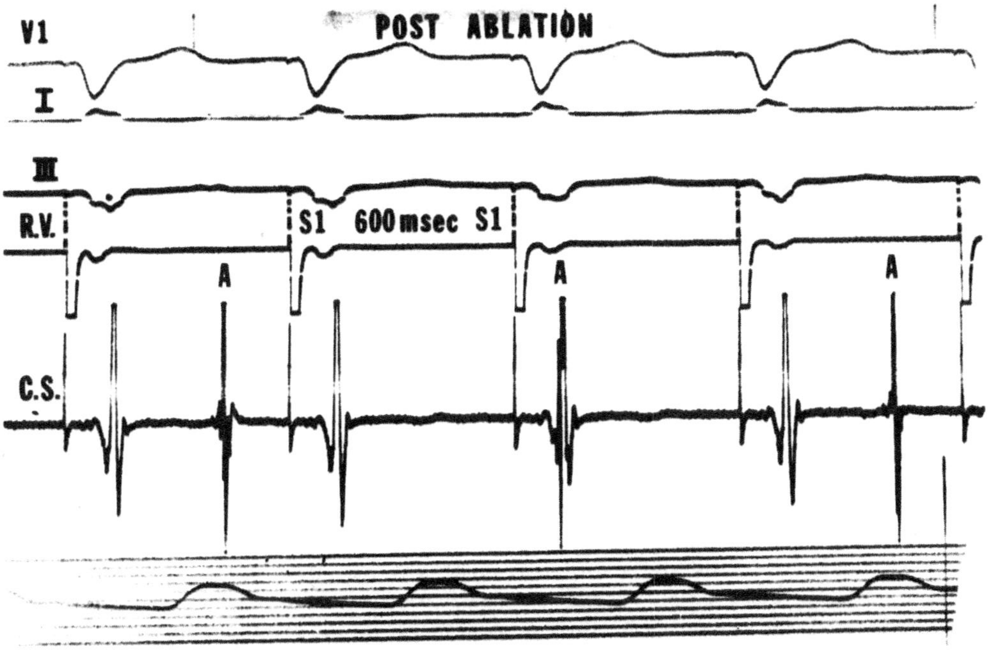

FIGURE 24–10. Ventricular pacing at a paced cycle length of 600 ms shows AV dissociation.

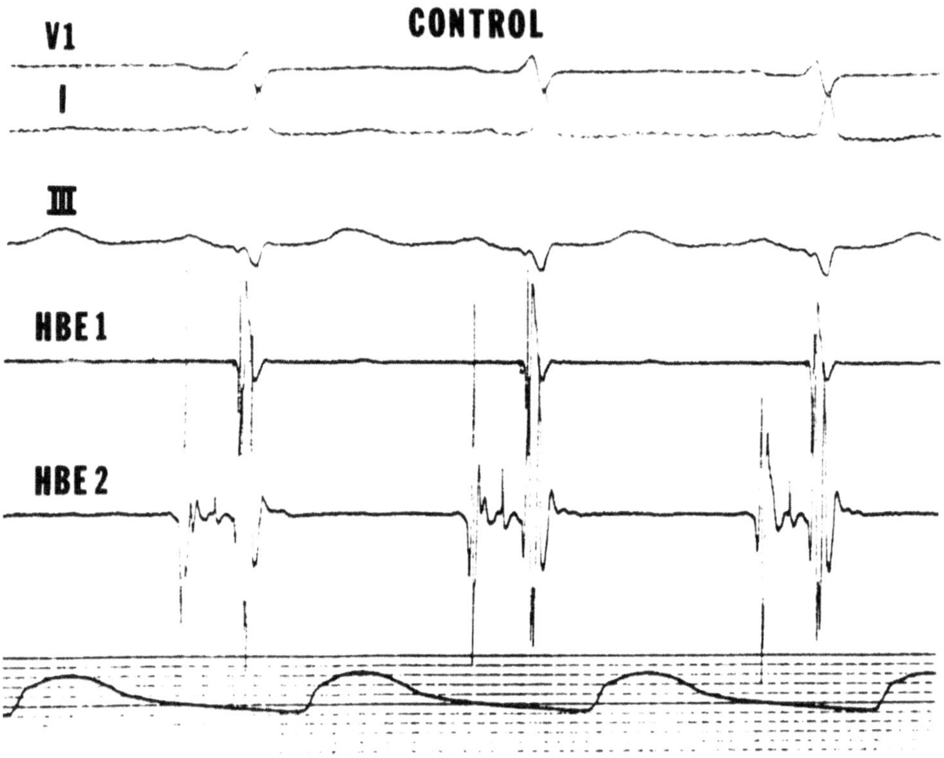

FIGURE 24–11. Simultaneous recordings of surface leads V_1, I, and III together with His bundle recordings from a multipolar electrode catheter (HBE_1 and HBE_2) prior to AV junctional ablation. Control recordings show no evidence of pre-excitation. Endocardial mapping during orthodromic tachycardia showed earliest atrial preexcitation in the region of postrior free wall of the left atrium.

She was not a candidate for antitachycardia pacing since her tachycardia could not be consistently terminated with either burst or premature atrial stimulation.

In Figure 24–11 the control recording shows evidence of minimal ventricular preexcitation. Electrophysiologic studies showed evidence of a posterior free wall accessory AV pathway with an effective refractory period of 310 ms (determined at an atrial paced rate of 120 per minute). Figure 24–12 shows simultaneous surface leads and intracardiac electrograms after catheter induced ablation of the AV junction. Note that the complexes are fully preexcited and no His bundle deflection could be recorded. Right ventricular pacing resulted in 1:1 retrograde conduction over the accessory pathway with no evidence for retrograde conduction through the AV junction. A "backup" VVI pacemaker was inserted.

Ablation in Patients with Nodoventricular Connections

Patients with nodoventricular connections may suffer from recurrent episodes of paroxysmal tachycardia [15,16]; those who cannot be managed with conventional medical therapy may be candidates for catheter ablation of the AV junction. The precise role of the nodoventricular connection in supporting tachycardia has not been established [15,17]. A technique (either surgical or catheter) for direct ablation of the nodoventricular connection has yet to be described (see Cox et al. this volume). These patients must be carefully studied to be sure that an additional accessory AV pathway is not present. In addition, dependence of tachycardia on maintenance of AV conduction must be demonstrated. Successful arrhythmia control in a patient with a nodoventricular connection by

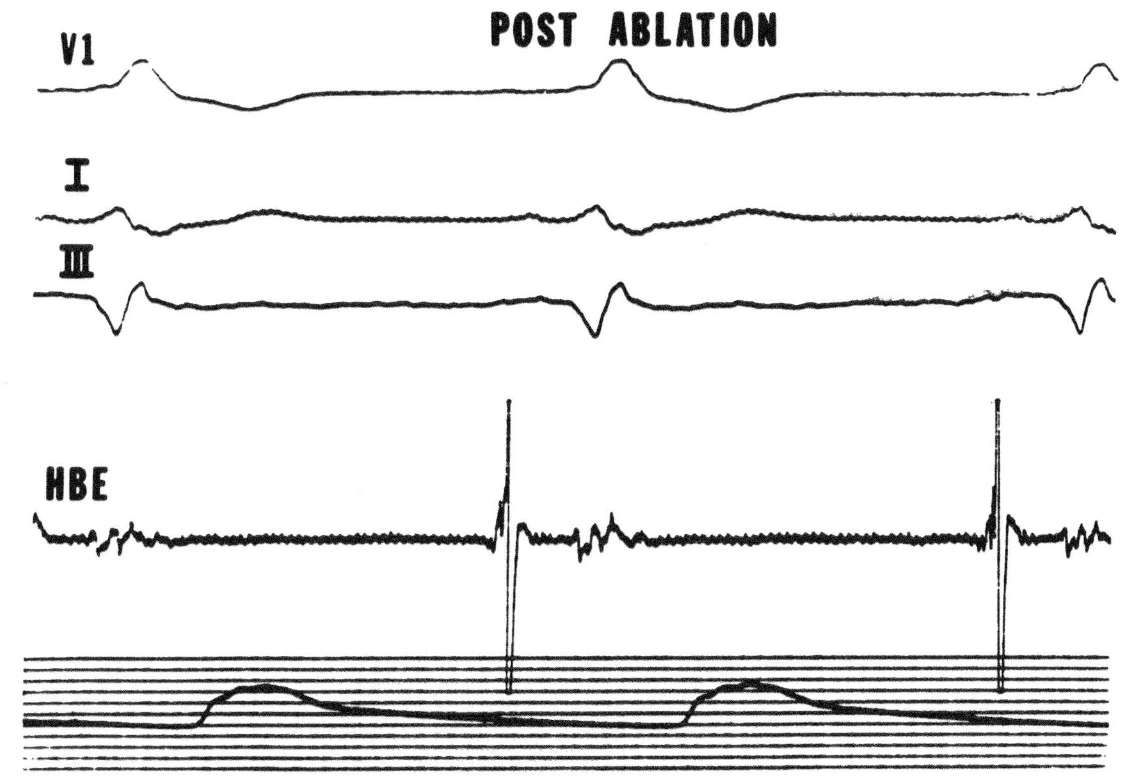

FIGURE 24–12. After AV junctional ablation, maximal preexcitation is recorded and no His bundle deflection is recorded.

means of catheter ablation of the AV junction has been reported [18].

Accessory Pathway Ablation in Patients with the Permanent Form of Junctional Reciprocating Tachycardia

Currently available data suggest that the mechanisms of permanent junctional reciprocating tachycardia (PJRT) involve antegrade conduction over the normal AV conducting system and retrograde conduction over an accessory AV pathway with AV node-like function. In one case, the pathway was identified anatomically as a tortuous bundle which winds around the proximal portion of the coronary sinus [19]. (See Critelli et al. this volume) Thus these patients (whose tachycardias often prove to be drug resistant) may be treated with catheter ablative techniques. An inital report showed that catheter ablation of the AV junction allowed for both arrhythmia control as well as unmasking of antegrade conduction over the bypass tract [19,20]. More recent reports have shown that direct catheter ablation of the accessory pathway is possible by means of applying shocks via an electrode catheter in the proximal portion of the coronary sinus [21]. Ablative procedures may prove especially important for these patients who are plagued with incessant cardiac arrhythmias.

Pacemaker Therapy

Both the presence of a pacemaker unit prior to the ablation procedure as well as the choice of permanent cardiac pacemaker therapy after catheter ablation merits serious consideration. In our experience, patients with previously implanted VVI pacemakers may safely undergo

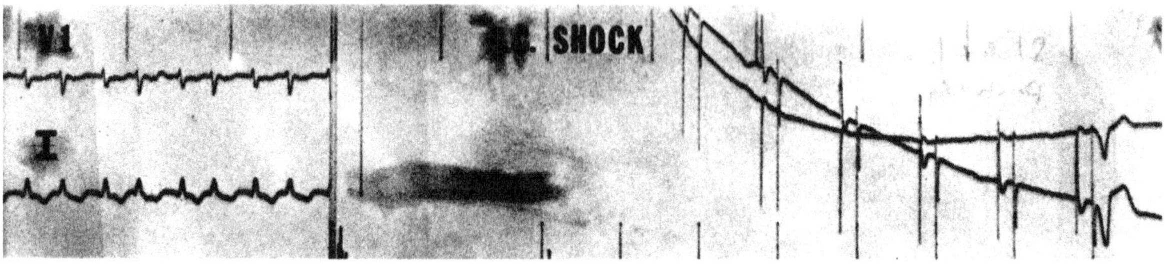

FIGURE 24–13. Simultaneous recording of surface leads V_1 and I during administration of a 300 joules shock to a catheter in the region of the AV junction. The patient had previously undergone insertion of a permanent DVI pacemaker for sinus node dysfunction. After shock, there is a transient period of lack of ventricular capture. After a follow-up period of six months, there was no evidence of pacemaker malfunction.

catheter ablative procedures. However, we have noted spontaneous reprogramming of a DDD pacemaker as well as transient failure to capture after delivery of shock (Figure 24–13). For these reasons, temporary ventricular pacing is mandatory even in those patients with previously implanted well functioning units and pacemaker function should be carefully assessed after the completion of the procedure. We are not aware of any long-term pacemaker failure following shock.

In subjects who have undergone successful ablation of the accessory pathway, chronic cardiac pacing is not usually required since the patient is left with an intact AV junction. One must, in addition, assess AV conduction after ablation to exclude either shock-induced or underlying dysfunction of the AV node–His axis. In patients with accessory pathways undergoing AV junctional ablation, permanent cardiac pacing is recommended since the natural history of accessory pathway conduction in the antegrade direction is not known. A standard VVI pacemaker should suffice for this purpose. AV junctional ablation of patients with concealed accessory pathways poses special problems in terms of pacemaker choice. A standard VVI pacemaker may be sufficient for some, but in those patients in whom rate-responsiveness is deemed desirable, careful consideration should be given to the choice of settings for dual-chamber pacemakers. The atrial refractory period, for example, should be of sufficient length to account for retrograde (VA) conduction time, since VA conduction resulting in pacemaker mediated tachycardia is possible via the intact accessory pathway. Finally, two of our patients with accessory pathways also had ectopic atrial tachycardias. A VVI or DVI pacemaker would avoid the problem of atrial sensing and ventricular tracking of the atrial tachycardia inherent in the use of a DDD pacemaker. The ultimate decision with regard to use of DDD pacing in such a patient would depend on the need for rate-responsiveness versus the rate of the atrial tachycardia. One patient, for example, with an accessory pathway who underwent AV junctional ablation because of recurrent drug refractory tachycardia, had infrequent and asymptomatic episodes of atrial tachycardia. A trial of DDD pacing was instituted with the expectation that either reprogramming to a DVI or VVI mode or drug therapy might be required to suppress the atrial tachycardia. The considerations governing pacemaker use are summarized in Table 24–2.

Summary

The introduction of catheter ablative techniques have provided the clinician with major new options in the management of patients with arrhythmias incorporating an accessory bypass tract. These techniques may prove valuable in the management of patients whose arrhythmias prove resistant to conventional therapy or in those patients who do not choose life-long drug dependency for arrhythmia control. In most patients with accessory pathways, the mechanism of the arrhythmia involves antegrade conduction over the AV junction and the retrograde conduction over the pathway. Current ablative techniques allow for fashioning an ablative prescription which produces permanent block either at the site of the AV junction or in selected patients at the site of the accessory

TABLE 24-2. Pacemaker therapy

A. Chronic pacemaker therapy following AV junctional ablation for patients with pathway-mediated tachycardias.
1. Intact accessory pathway conduction – VVI backup pacing
2. Poorly conducting or concealed accessory pathway – VVI or DDD for younger patients.
B. Accessory pathway ablation unmasking defective condution over the AV node-His axis-DDD pacing in suitable patients.

pathway. The latter approach is clearly more desirable since it leaves the normal AV conducting system intact and obviates the need for chronic pacemaker therapy.

It should be emphasized that the catheter ablative techniques for patients with accessory pathways should only be performed by individuals well experienced in the use of invasive electrophysiologic testing. Obviously, the choice of the optimal ablative technique will depend on proper identification of both the site(s) of the accessory pathway as well as precise definition of the arrhythmia mechanism. It must be appreciated that catheter ablation is associated with physical complications, including the risk of death [10]. Therefore, this technique should be considered only in those patients with life-threatening or disabling arrhythmias which do not respond to conventional drug therapy. While catheter ablative techniques are still considered experimental, the available data suggest that the catheter technique may supplant the surgical approach as the initial ablative approach for patients with refractory AV reentrant arrhythmias incorporating a posteroseptal accessory pathway. Finally, catheter ablation of the AV junction is an alternative to surgery in selected patients with refractory orthodromic tachycardia who are high-risk surgical candidates.

References

1. Scheinman MM, Morday F, Hess DS, Gonzalez R: Catheter-induced ablation of the atrioventricular junction to control refractory supraventricular arrhythmias. *JAMA* 7:851, 1982.
2. Gallagher JJ, Svenson RH, Kasell JH, German LD, Bardy GH, Broughton A, Critelli G: Catheter technique for a closed chest ablation of the atrioventricular conduction system. A therapeutic alternative for the treatment of refractory supraventricular tachycardia. *N. Engl. J. Med.* 306:194, 1982.
3. Morady F, Scheinman MM: Transvenous catheter ablation of a posteroseptal accessory pathway in a patient with the Wolff-Parkinson-White syndrome. *N. Engl. J. Med.* 310:705, 1984.
4. Weber H. Schmitz L, Wesselhoeft H: A new technique of mapping for localization and closed-chest ablation of reentry pathways. (Abstract.) *Circulation* 68:III–175, 1983.
5. Fisher JD, Brodman R, Kim SG, Matos JA, Brodman E, Wallerson D, Waspe LE: Attempted nonsurgical electrical ablation of accessory pathways via the coronary sinus in the Wolff-Parkinson-White syndrome. *J. Am. Coll. Cardiol.* 4:685, 1984.
6. Kunz KP, Kuck KH: Transvenous ablation of accessory pathways in patients with incessant atrioventricular tachycardia. (Abstract.) *Circulation* 70:II–412, 1984.
7. Nathan AW, Davies DW, Creamer JE, Butrons GS, Camm JA: Successful catheter ablation of abnormal atrioventricular pathways in man. (Abstract.) *Circulation* 70:II–99, 1984.
8. Fisher JD, Brodman R, Johnston DR, Waspe LE, Kim SG, Matos JA, Scavin G: Nonsurgical electrical ablation of tachycardias: importance of prior in vitro testing of catheter leads. *PACE* 7:74, 1984.
9. Dick M II, Antar RE, Hoffman BF, Bowman Fo Jr, Malm JR, Krongrad E: Sensitivity of His bundle (HB) recording technique during open heart surgery in man. (Abstract.) *Circulation* 50:III–81, 1974.
10. Scheinman MM, Evans-Bell T and the Executive Committee of the Percutaneous Cardiac Mapping and Ablation Registry: Catheter ablation of the atrioventricular junction: A report of the percutaneous mapping and ablation registry. *Circulation* 70:1024, 1984.
11. Morady F, Scheinman MM, DiCarlo LA Jr, Winston SA, Davis JC: Coexistent posteroseptal and right-sided atrioventricular bypass tracts: A previously unrecognized association. (Abstract.) *Circulation* 70:II–340, 1984.
12. Gallagher JJ, Svenson RH, Sealy WC, Wallace AG: The Wolff-Parkinson-White syndrome and the preexcitation dysrhythmias. Medical and surgical management. *Med. Clin. N. A.* 60:101, 1976.
13. Scheinman MM: The AJC in September. *Am. J. Cardiol.* 54:702, 1984.
14. Jackman WM, Friday KJ, Scherlag BJ, Dehning MM, Schecter E, Reynolds DW, Olson EG, Berbari EJ, Harrison LA, Lazzara R: Direct endocardial recording from an accessory atrioventricular pathway: Localization of the site of block, effect of antiarrhythmic drugs and

attempt at nonsurgical ablation. *Circulation* 68:906, 1983.
15. Gallagher JJ, Smith WM, Benson DW: Role of Mahaim fibers in cardiac arrhythmias in man. *Circulation* 64:176, 1981.
16. Ward DE, Camm AJ, Spurrell RAJ: Ventricular preexcitation due to anomalous nodo-ventricular pathways. *Eur. J. Cardiol.* 49:995, 1982.
17. Morady F, Scheinman MM, Gonzalez R, Hess DS: His-ventricular dissociation in a patient with reciprocating tachycardia and a nodo-ventricular bypass tract. *Circulation* 67:674, 1983.
18. Bhandari A, Morady F, Shen EN, Schwartz AB, Botvinick E, Scheinman MM: Catheter-induced His bundle ablation in a patient with reentrant tachycardia associated with a nodo-ventricular tract. *J. Am. Coll. Cardiol.* 4:611, 1984.
19. Critelli G, Gallagher JJ, Monda V, Coltorti F, Scherillo M, Rossi L: Anatomic and electrophysiologic substrate of the permanent form of junctional reciprocating tachycardia. *J. Am. Coll. Cardiol.* 4:601, 1984.
20. Critelli G, Perticone F, Coltorti F, Monda V, Gallagher JJ: Antegrade slow bypass conduction after closed chest ablation of the His bundle in permanent junctional reciprocating tachycardia. *Circulation* 67:687, 1983.
21. Gallagher JJ: Personal communication.

25. TECHNIQUES FOR INTRAOPERATIVE MAPPING OF TACHYARRHYTHMIAS IN PREEXCITATION SYNDROMES

H. Gareth Tobler
Robert W. Anderson
W. Steves Ring
David G. Benditt

Advances in both cardiac surgery and the technology of recording and displaying electrical signals from biologic tissues have contributed to the evolution of intraoperative electrophysiologic evaluation in patients with preexcitation syndromes. As early as 1930, Barker [1] demonstrated the feasibility of epicardial electrogram recordings in the human heart and reported activation times at ventricular epicardial sites in a patient with a chronically open chest wound (Figure 25–1). In 1967, Durrer and Roos [2] obtained activation times determined from unipolar ventricular electrograms and demonstrated very early excitation at the lateral aspect of the base of the right ventricle in a patient with atrial septal defect and Wolff-Parkinson-White (WPW) syndrome. In that same year Burchell et al. [3] utilized ventricular activation times to evaluate ventricular excitation during sinus rhythm, and atrial activation times to evaluate atrial excitation during tachycardia in a patient with atrial septal defect and WPW syndrome. Even though the attempt to interrupt the accessory connection in this patient was unsuccessful, demonstration of the proximity of the site of early ventricular activation during preexcitation to the early site of atrial activation during tachycardia was important in establishing and defining the role of intraoperative electrophysiologic recordings in localizing the site of surgical exploration or accessory connection ablation (Figure 25–2). In 1968, a report from Duke University described the successful surgical ablation of an accessory connection [4]; the localization of the accessory connection was determined from the ventricular epicardial excitation sequence (isochrone map).

The isochrone map [5], which is constructed from local activation times has become the standard for characterizing total heart electrical activity, and during the past decade has been extensively utilized to evaluate cardiac excitation in a variety of circumstances in patients undergoing surgery [6–11].

This work was supported in part by NHLBI NRSA #HL 06593 (HGT), HL 22152 (RWA) and HL 29460 (DGB) from the National Institutes of Health, Bethesda, Maryland, and was completed during Dr. Benditt's tenure as an Established Investigator of the American Heart Association, Dallas, Texas

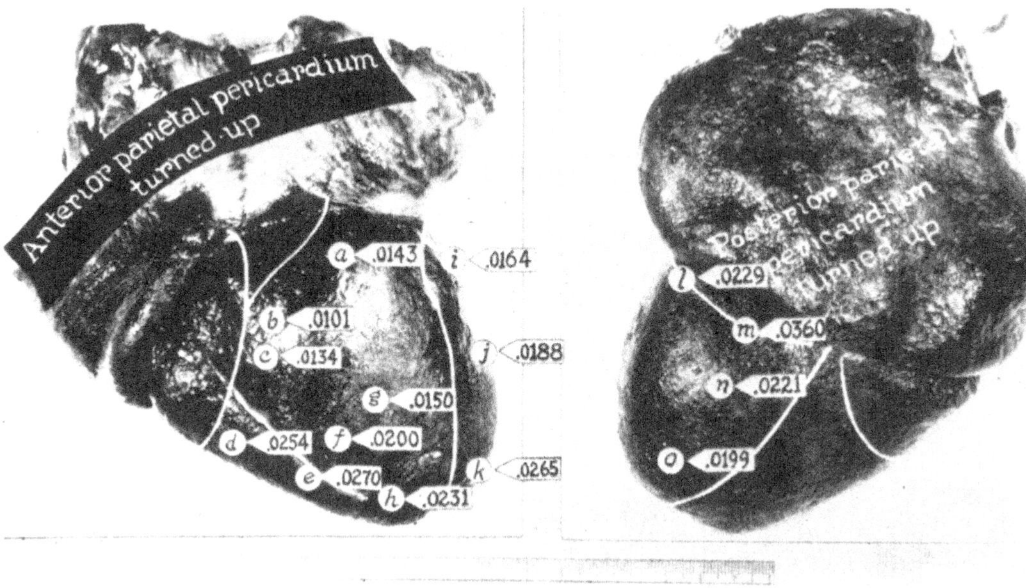

FIGURE 25–1. Postmortem photograph of heart and recording sites mapped by Barker et al. The times of local activation with respect to the R wave of lead II are shown for the areas from which recordings were made. Reproduced with permission from Barker [1].

The objective of this chapter is to outline the procedure for obtaining activation times and constructing isochrone maps. We will discuss essential equipment and instrumentation, approaches to data acquisition and analysis and provide examples of the utilization of this technique in the operative treatment of preexcitation syndromes.

The Preoperative Catheterization Laboratory Study

Clinical electrophysiologic studies in the cardiac catheterization laboratory have become more sophisticated and continue to achieve greater accuracy in assessing cardiac activation sequences during a variety of arrhythmias [12–14]. The study in the catheterization laboratory permits an overall assessment of the nature of anomalous conduction in the patient with preexcitation. The primary characteristics of the accessory connection(s) are determined: the capability of the accessory connection(s) to conduct in both antegrade and retrograde direction, the number of accessory connections, their location, and their participation in tachycardia and the effects of pacing site on preexcitation and arrhythmia initiation.

In patients who go to operative ablation of accessory connection(s), the epicardial activation sequence map obtained in the operating room complements the endocardial recordings from the catheterization procedure, and in many instances the operative map will improve the overall precision of accessory connection localization. Several factors distinguish intracavitary electrode catheter studies from intraoperative mapping procedures. Consequently, each technique contributes essential and unique information to the assessment of the accessory connection. In the catheterization laboratory, the patient is awake and free of the influence of general anesthesia which may alter susceptibility to arrhythmias, create hemodynamic instability, and limit the time available for detailed study. Multiple extrastimulus sequences and pacing sites can be evaluated in order to determine the optimal means for initiation of tachyarrhythmias, providing the most efficient pacing sequences for subsequent use in the operating room. The area of the heart from which the endocardial electrograms are recorded can be accurately estimated from biplane fluoroscopic visualization of endocardial catheter electrodes, and the various recording sites

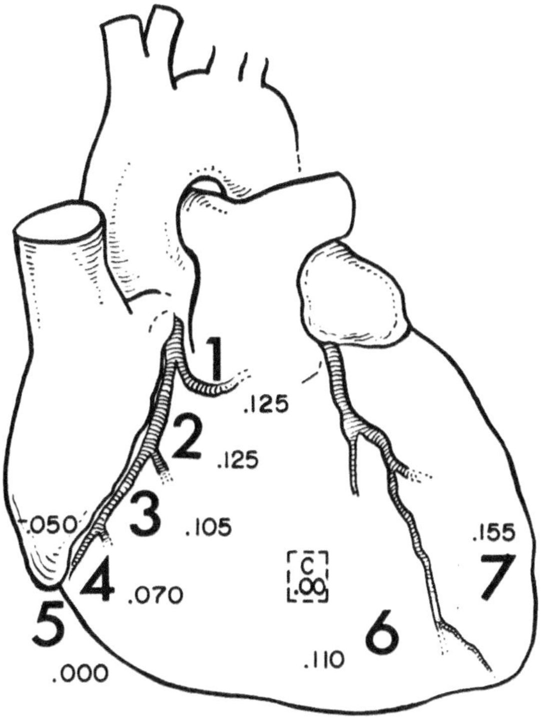

FIGURE 25–2. Diagram of heart used by Burchell. Values shown are times of local activation with respect to right ventricular border near AV groove (marked .000). Reproduced by permission from Burchell and by permission of the Americal Heart Association, Inc. [3].

may be documented as needed by cinefluoroscopy. In the operating room, although there is limited time to obtain epicardial activation sequences, a detailed study can be obtained if conditions are optimal. Often, the point at which an accessory connection crosses the atrioventricular (AV) groove can be localized to within a centimeter. As a result, intraoperative mapping tends to provide greater precision of accessory connection localization than is obtained by catheter technique. Further, secondary accessory connections, not identified during the catheter study, but which could become clinically significant when the most prominent connection is transected, may become apparent in the operating room. Importantly, since the cardiac activation sequence recorded intraoperatively is obtained directly from the epicardial (and in some cases the endocardial) surface of the heart using standardized localization schemes (Figure 25–3), it is possible to compare findings among patients more precisely than can be achieved with endocardial catheter studies. Further, since mapping can be carried out, if necessary, during normothermic cardiopulmonary bypass, activation sequences can be obtained during tachycardias that are too rapid or hemodynamically unstable to permit evaluation in the catheterization laboratory. Finally, in the case of operative ablation of accessory connections, it has been possible to obtain recordings from the accessory connection itself thereby substantiating the precision of the techniques [15]. Only recently have analogous recordings been obtained in a few patients with electrode catheter techniques [16]. The technique for obtaining the latter recordings is described in more detail in the chapter by Jackman in this volume.

From the point of view of surgical personnel and anesthesia team, the intraoperative mapping procedure may seem quite tedious and time-consuming. Indeed, some suggest that the patient is unnecessarily jeopardized by the prolonged anesthetic time. Nonetheless, a well-planned concise mapping procedure can yield important information in a minimal amount of time. Therefore, since localization information obtained by intraoperative mapping is of value in confirming findings obtained in the catheterization laboratory, and since comparisons between "pre-ablation" and "post-ablation" maps are particularly helpful to assess the success of attempted surgical ablation of accessory connections, intraoperative mapping will remain extremely valuable.

Intraoperative Mapping Equipment

OVERVIEW

The primary components of an intraoperative cardiac arrhythmia mapping system are illustrated in Figure 25–4. The three essential recordings are: (1) surface ECG, (2) a reference electrogram, and (3) one or more recording or "probe" electrograms. The recording capabilities in the operating room are a critical factor in determining the manner in which epicardial activation sequence data is obtained and subsequently analyzed. The larger the number of recording channels available, the more simultaneous electrograms one is able to record,

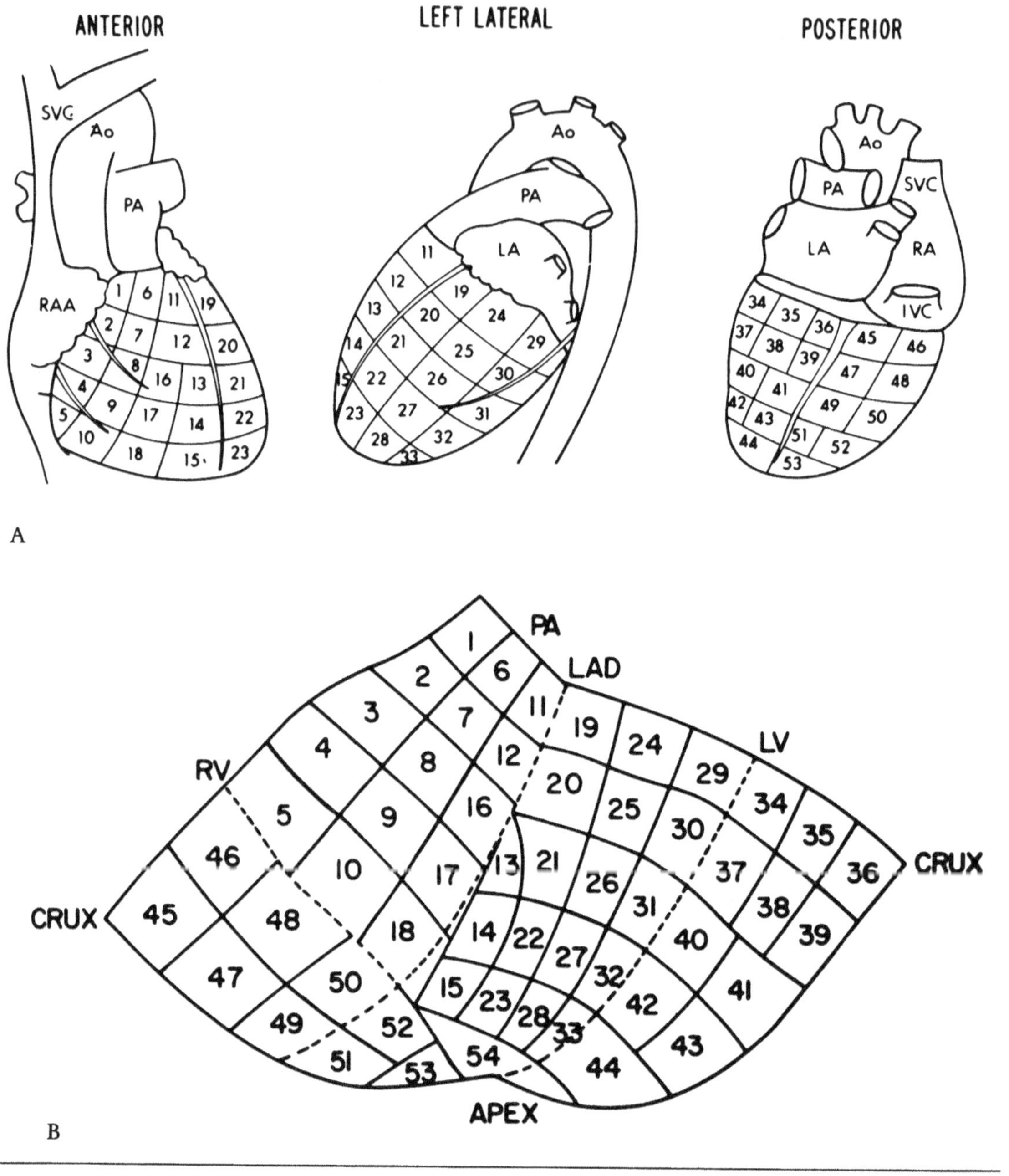

FIGURE 25–3. Two epicardial grid drawings. (A) is a three-view representation showing the epicardial areas from anterior, left lateral, and posterior views. Surface landmarks help to place the boundaries of areas and allow a point of reference for communication between the operating and mapping team. (B) is a single view of a folded-out surface of the ventricular epicardium. Sites on the two grids are essentially equivalent. Both modified after maps used at Duke University Medical Center.

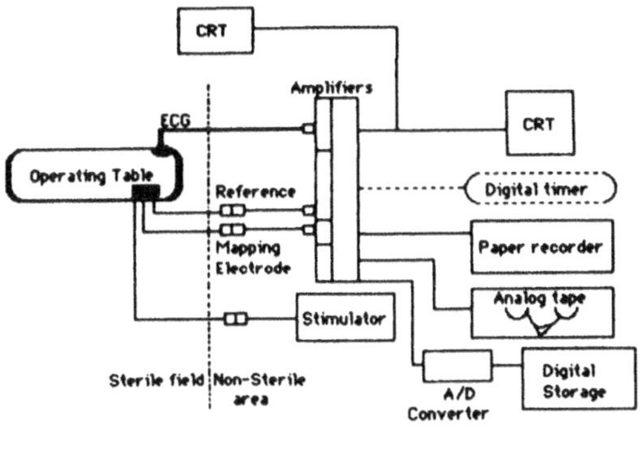

FIGURE 25–4. Components of a typical single probe mapping system. Surface ECG leads, reference electrode pairs and recording electrode pairs are connected to the amplifier system. The recordings are displayed on a visual display unit (CRT) as well as being recorded on paper and/or magnetic media (Analog and/or digital storage). A digital timer can be used to obtain an instantaneous readout of local activation time for a single area. Pacing electrodes are connected to a stimulator. Two-part cables separate the sterile field from the recording equipment.

thereby either shortening the time it takes to complete the procedure or increasing the detail of the information accumulated. For each ECG lead and electrogram being recorded simultaneously there must be both an amplifier and a recording channel (paper and/or magnetic tape, etc.) available, as well as the ability to display the recordings during acquisition by means of an oscilloscope or other display device. Multiplexing can increase the number of "simultaneous" electrograms acquired, but each multiplexed channel must be displayed and recorded. The data analysis and display system should be adjacent to the operating suite to permit rapid data analysis turnaround.

SURFACE ECG

The surface ECG serves as the common point of reference in all electrophysiologic studies. In the operating room setting, at least two orthogonal surface leads are essential. Additional leads would be helpful since any single lead may become isoelectric as a result of manipulation of the heart during the mapping procedure. Further, multiple ECG leads permit comparison of an induced tachycardia with its appearance on a preoperative ECG, thereby helping verify that the arrhythmia induced in the operating room is the "clinical" arrhythmia of interest in that patient. Finally, some patients are known to have more than one spontaneous arrhythmia; multiple ECG leads are useful to distinguish among various types. A set of frontal plane ECG leads is usually used.

Interfacing the ECG with the operating room environment may be a difficult problem depending on the manufacturers of the mapping equipment and the equipment routinely used in the operating room for patient monitoring. An interface to record from the same ECG electrodes used by the anesthesia team would be helpful, but in some cases it may be necessary to record an independent surface ECG to insure a reliable high quality signal. Placement of the surface electrodes in a safe posterior position and covering them with a protective drape or tape will prevent loss of signal due to perspiration and skin preparation solutions, a not uncommon problem. Assessing ECG quality prior to skin preparation and draping is critical and may save time later in the procedure.

BIPOLAR VERSUS UNIPOLAR RECORDINGS

Most often, cardiac mapping studies utilize bipolar electrode recordings since timing of local activation at the electrode site is the principal objective. Unipolar electrodes, using an indifferent surface lead as the reference, record the potential difference between the surface electrode and the recording electrode. Cardiac depolarization is recorded by the unipolar electode as an increasing potential difference or positive waveform as the excitation wave approaches, and as a decreasing or negative potential difference as the activation wave front passes the recording site (Figure 25–5). A second adjacent unipolar electrode would generate an almost identical waveform as the first electrode but the electrogram recorded by the second electrode would be slightly out of phase (i.e., slightly delayed in time) from the first. Consequently, a bipolar recording, which effectively records the difference between two closely spaced unipolar recordings, tends to eliminate far field signals and primarily identifies the timing of electrical activity as it passes between the two adjacent electrodes. Thus, for purposes of local activation timing, bipolar electrograms lend to provide the more "noise-free" signals and the peak of the bipolar electrogram

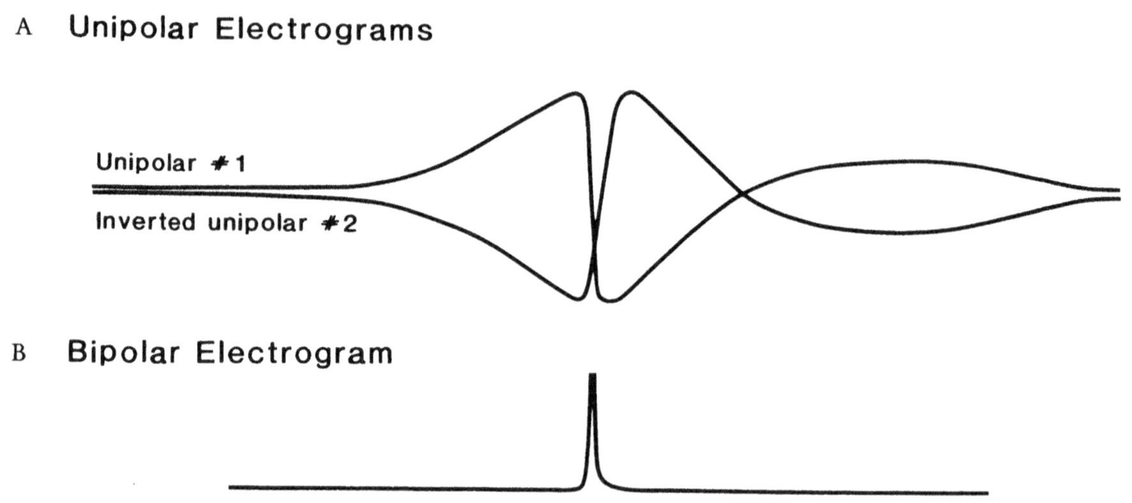

FIGURE 25–5. Unipolar electrograms and Bipolar electrogram. Recordings from two adjacent unipolar electrodes (A). The electrogram from electrode #2 is inverted. The bipolar electrogram in (B) results from the electrical difference between unipolar electrodes #1 and #2.

appears to provide the best representation of true local activation at the recording site.

EPICARDIAL ELECTRODES: DESIGN

Electrodes capable of recording high-quality noise-free signals are relatively simple to manufacture. For example, a triad or tetrad of brass or copper electrodes can be embedded in a plaque of dental epoxy or other resin. We have found that if the electrodes project somewhat from the surface of the plaque (1–2 mm), surface contact and signal stability seem to improve (Figure 25–6). Using a triad or tetrad electrode, bipolar electrogram detection can be optimized by switching between the various electrodes and choosing the most effective pair, without moving and/or resuturing the plaque. Holes pre-drilled on the sides of the electrode plaques permit suturing to the heart. Alternatively, the electrode plaque can be backed with silastic sheeting through which sutures are placed (Figure 25–7).

Reference electrodes. A basic element of epicardial mapping procedures is the need for stable stationary reference electrodes sewn to the heart, usually in both atrial and ventricular positions. When the heart is lifted from the chest, surface ECG leads may become isoelectric, presumably due to the lack of contact of the heart with the rest of the body. Additionally, the slow rise time of the delta wave in patients with preexcitation or the QRS in patients without preexcitation prevents their use as accurate and reproducible references. The epicardial reference electrograms provide stable points of reference from which to measure local activation times at sites being scanned by the roving probe (Figure 25–8). The atrial reference electrode may be placed anywhere, but care should be taken to avoid the site of cannula insertion. Similarly, the ventricular reference may be placed wherever desired, but is commonly placed over the midportion of the anterior right ventricular free wall, the zone often associated with earliest epicardial activation during normal ventricular activation. The latter position is generally "out of the way" (particularly in the case of surgery for ventricular tachycardia where the dissection is usually within the left ventricle) and activates relatively early in the QRS when ventricular activation is normal. Thus the activation times of ventricular areas activated before the normal sequence of activation will be negative with respect to the reference electrogram.

Pacing electrodes. Electrodes for atrial and

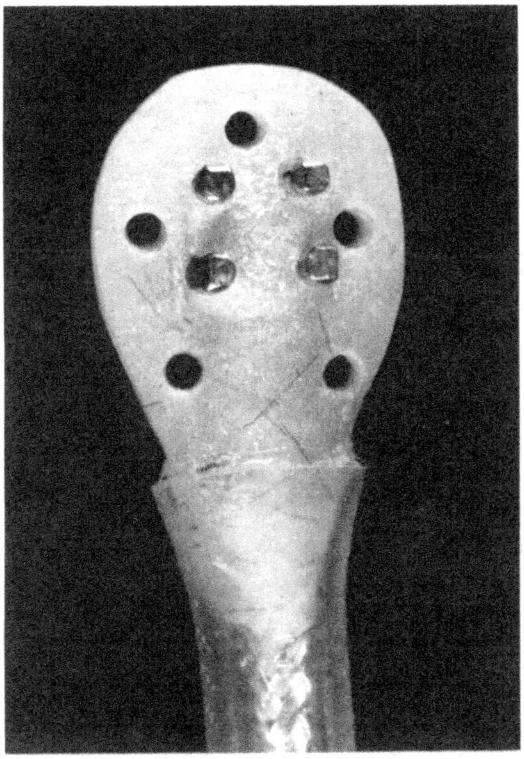

A

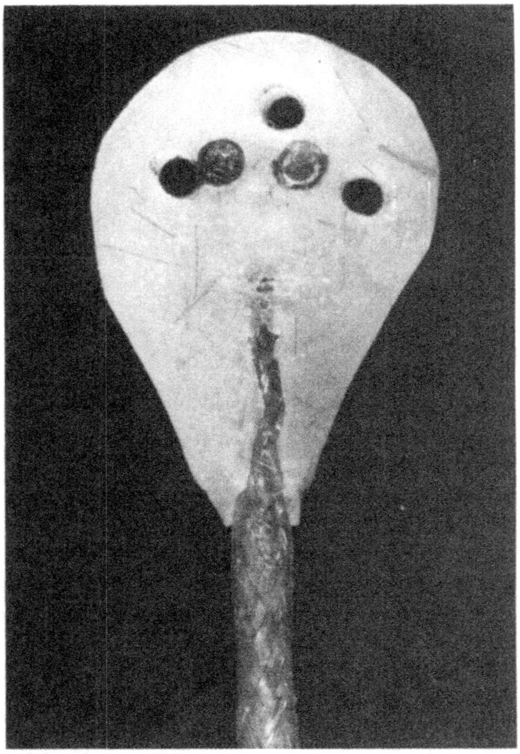

C

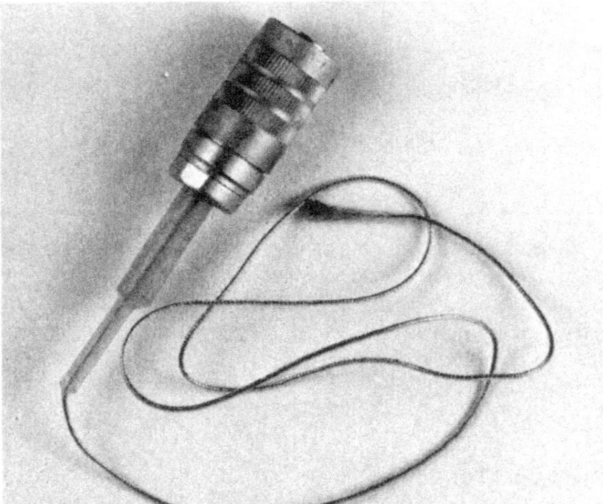

B

FIGURE 25–6. (A,B) Quadripolar reference electrode which is sewn to the epicardial surface. Any two electrode pairs can be selected to obtain the best bipolar electrogram. (C) Bipolar epicardial pacing electrode pair.

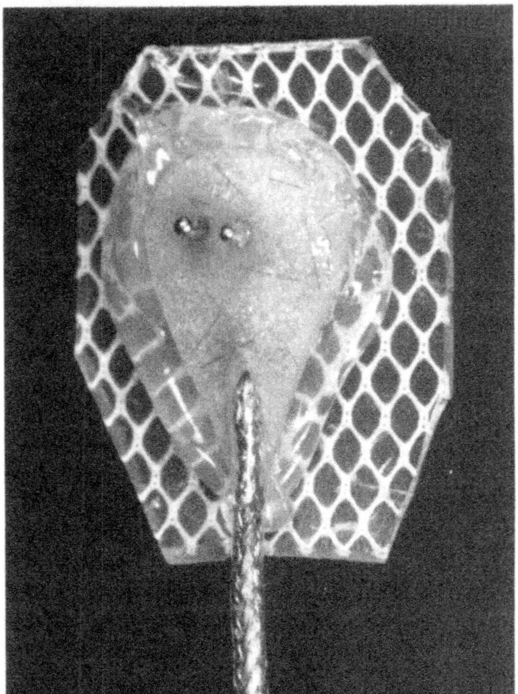

FIGURE 25–7. Silastic backed reference or pacing electrode pair. Sutures can be placed through the silastic allowing simple placement.

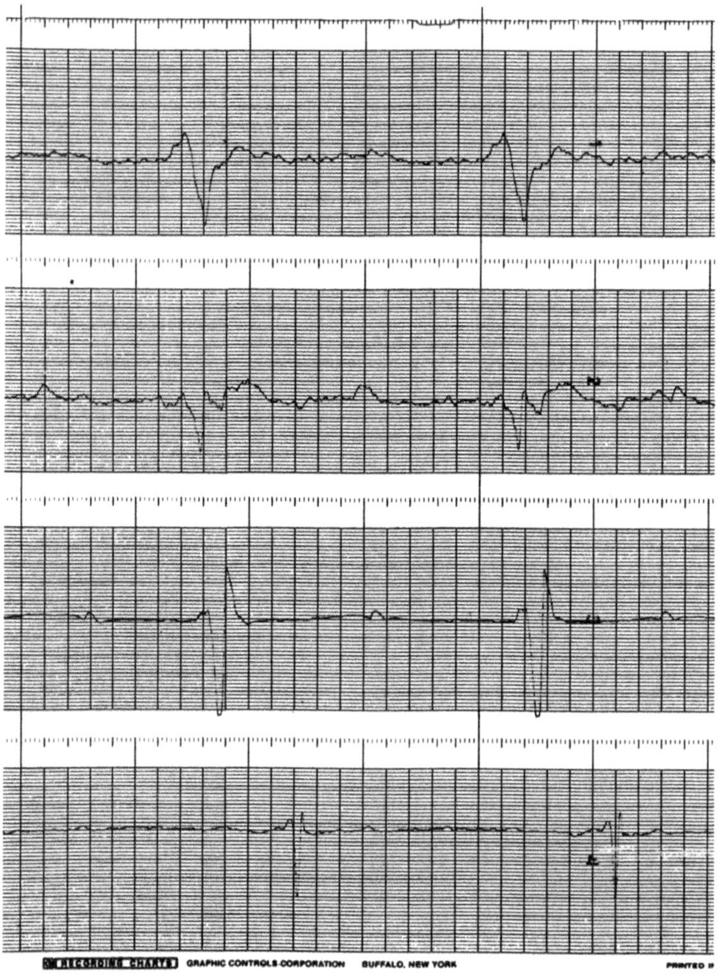

FIGURE 25–8. Intraoperative recordings obtained at different times during the mapping procedure. The four simultaneous traces from the top are surface leads I, AVF, right ventricular reference electrogram, and electrograms from the roving electrode pair. The position of the surface lead and reference electrode pair are the same for the first and the second panel. The roving electrode pair electrograms are recorded from different sites on the epicardium. Note that the surface electrograms have changed significantly from the first panel to the second panel while the reference electrogram has not significantly changed.

ventricular pacing are similar in design to the reference electrodes except that a bipolar configuration is usually sufficient (Figure 25–6C). It is helpful to mark the pacing electrodes in some way to prevent confusion with the reference electrodes. For example, we use different connectors for pacing and recording electrode plaques in order to distinguish the types. Nonetheless, it is possible to pace through the reference electrode by use of a special adapter. Atrial pacing electrodes are usually placed near the site of the suspected accessory connection in order to accentuate preexcitation. In this manner the ventricular epicardial activation sequence map obtained during atrial pacing is more distinctive than would be the case if the mapping procedure were carried out during sinus rhythm. Similarly, the ventricular pacing electrode is placed near the presumed ventricular insertion of the accessory connection in order to accentuate retrograde conduction over the accessory connection during ventricular pacing. The eccentric atrial activation sequence achieved by atrial pacing near the accessory connection

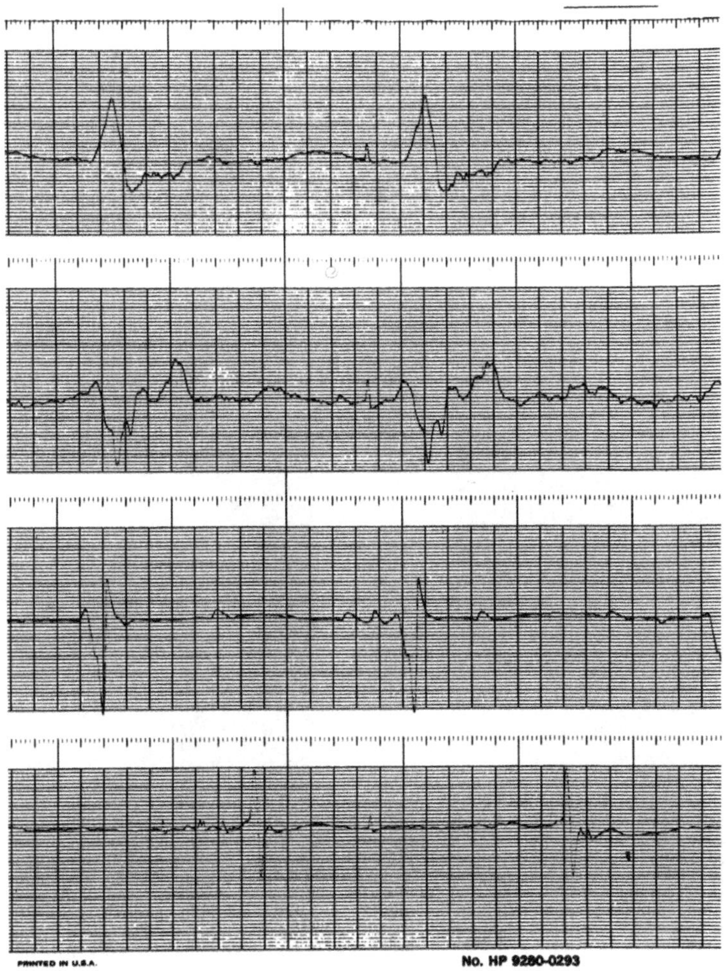

can be useful in conjunction with atrial mapping during reciprocating tachycardia, to identify the site of atrial insertion of the accessory connection.

Recording electrodes. There are two basic methods of recording electrograms for intraoperative mapping: (1) recording from a single roving probe moved from one location on the heart to the next in sequence and (2) recording from two or more electrode pairs simultaneously. The method used for epicardial recordings will depend upon available data acquisition capacity. In the case where the overall epicardial activation sequence is to be constructed from a series of single recordings (single point method), a "roving" bipolar probe is used. A "roving" probe, positioned at the tip of a wand can be useful in order to record from most locations on the heart (Figure 25–9). However, the wand electrode probe has limitations in certain difficult to reach areas such as the crux of the heart. Consequently, alternative probe designs such as the fingertip ring electrode (Figure 25–10) should be available in the operating room. The latter electrode can be positioned on the heart wherever the surgeon is able to place a finger, although confirming the exact electrode position is often limited by inability to visualize the recording site adequately.

When multiple recordings can be obtained simutaneously, several approaches have been used. One option consists of the use of a flexible mesh sock containing multiple bipolar electrode pairs arranged to record from equally spaced epicardial sites. The sock is designed to fit snugly over the epicardial surface of both ventricles and a large number of electrograms re-

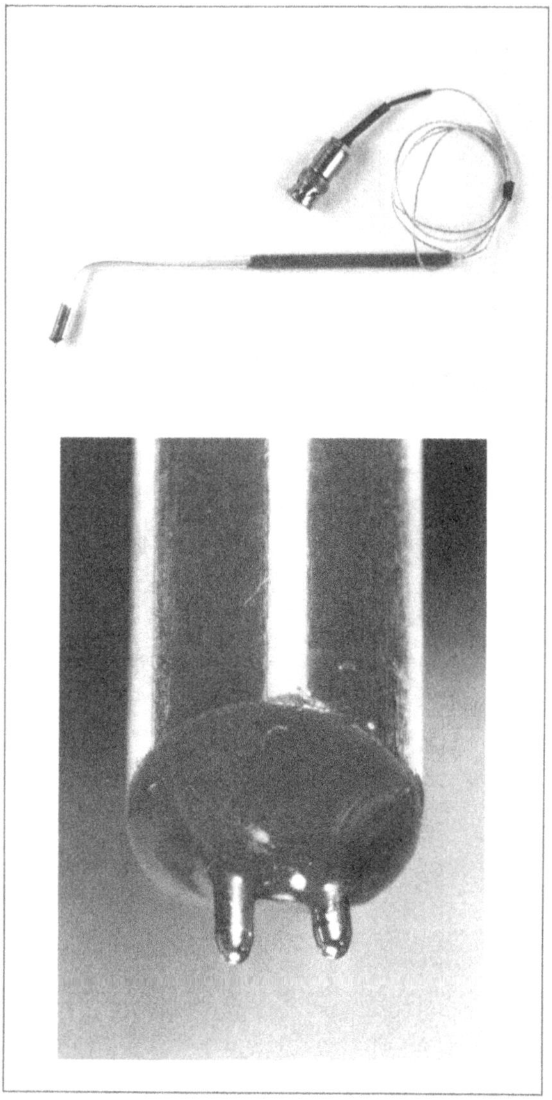

FIGURE 25–9. Wand type mapping electrode pair. Electrodes are placed 2–3 mm apart and embedded in epoxy with the tips of the electrodes protruding to facilitate good surface contact.

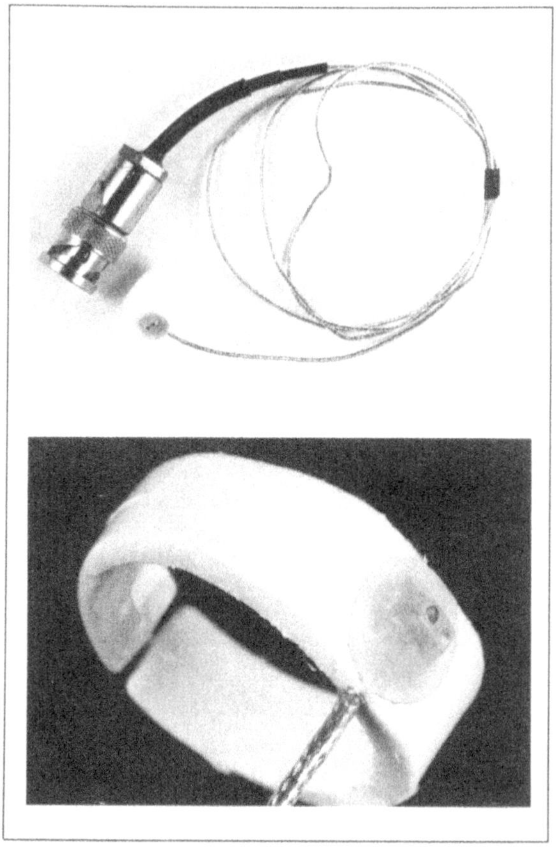

FIGURE 25–10. Fingertip ring electrode pair. Electrograms can be recorded from inferior, posterior and lateral surfaces using this ring electrode placed over the tip of the finger with minimal displacement of the heart.

corded simultaneously [17] (Figure 25–11). Optimally, the sock technique permits a complete epicardial activation map to be obtained in one beat. Witowski et al. [18] have described use of a strip of 16 electrodes placed adjacent to the AV groove to record simultaneous epicardial electrograms from each of 16 areas. In the case of preexcitation mapping, the strip electrode technique has the advantage of concentrating the recordings at the area of maximum interest (i.e., in the vicinity of the AV groove). However, a potential disadvantage is failure to recognize abnormal ventricular activation sequences which become obvious only when activation sequence recordings are obtained several centimeters below the AV groove (Figure 25–12). In the latter instance, epicardial "breakthrough" associated with a "deep" accessory atrioventricular connection may not be as clearcut at the base of the heart immediately adjacent to the AV groove as it is in a slightly more apical position. Consequently, it is important to move the recording electrode away from the AV groove, recording from several additional "epicardial layers" in an apical direction. In addition to epicardial recordings, needle electrodes have been used to obtain midwall and endocardial recordings to determine more precisely the site of accessory connections since they may cross the AV groove at different depths. Needle elec-

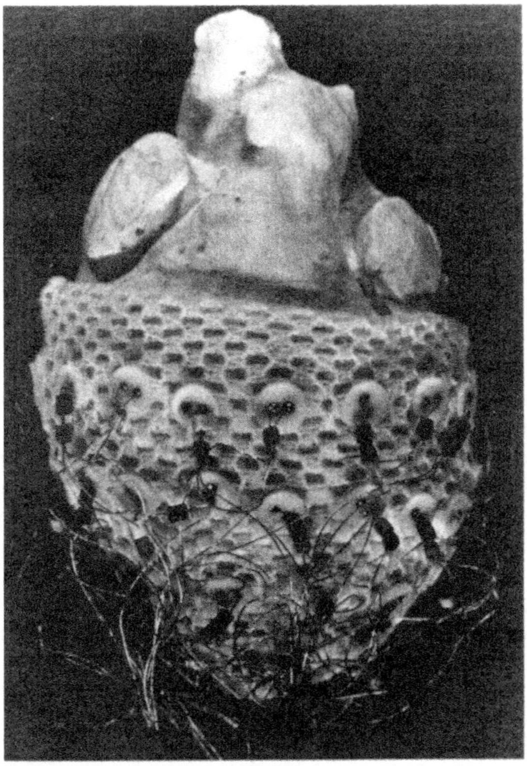

FIGURE 25–11. The sock electrode array shown on a latex model of a canine heart. Pairs of bipolar electrodes dispersed over the surface of the ventricular allow simultaneous recording from 52 representative areas of the epicardial surface. Reproduced with permission from Harrison et al. [17].

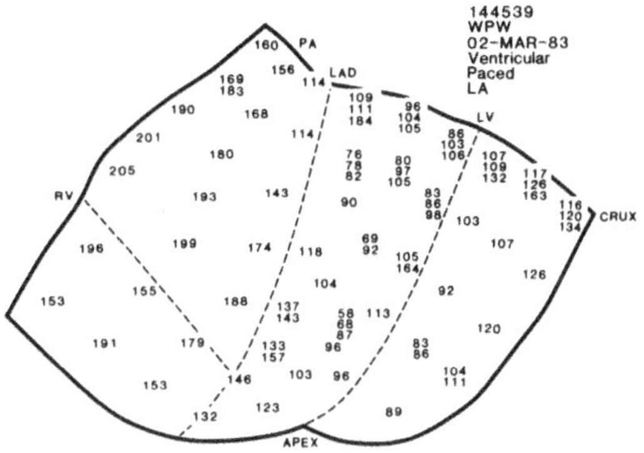

FIGURE 25–12. Ventricular epicardial activation sequence map of a patient with preexcitation during atrial pacing. The shortest activation times are shown in the shaded area which is one row beyond sites adjacent to the AV groove.

trodes may be especially useful in septal locations [19].

A two-piece set of cables allows a convenient interface between the sterile operative field and the recording system (Figure 25–4). The electrodes within the sterile field are connected by flexible wire to a junction box on the edge of the operating table with cables extending away from the sterile field. These cables are connected to a second set of cables connected to the amplifier system. Using this configuration, easy connections can be made and the minimum amount of equipment needs sterilization.

AMPLIFIERS

A high-quality amplifier system incorporates several features which increase the ease of obtaining quality recordings and also provide patient safety. In order to record cardiac electrograms accurately, yet with a minimum of extraneous electrical interference, amplifiers should have both a high input impedance (typically of the order of 10^{11} ohms) and the capability to filter out high- and low-frequency noise. In general such amplifiers must be able to accommodate a variety of signal strengths, ranging from 0.1 mV to 200 mV. The low cutoff filter minimizes baseline drift while the high cutoff filter prevents high-frequency noise from entering into the recordings. The low cutoff is usually set to about 30 Hz and the high cutoff is set to 1000 Hz. Optical isolation is desirable to minimize the potential for leakage currents reaching the patient.

ENVIRONMENT

The recording of high-fidelity electrophysiologic signals is susceptible to extraneous noise from many sources, especially in electrically "noisy" situations such as the modern operating room. Often a considerable amount of time can be wasted in searching for and eliminating sources of electrical noise in an effort to obtain the highest quality signals. Some general measures, both to minimize susceptibility of the recording equipment to noise and to reduce the obvious sources of electrical noise, will minimize tedious trial and error searches for its source. First, all cables and electrodes should be shielded and grounded. Deficiencies in the latter areas, and inadequacy of simple electrical connections, are simple yet elusive sources of noise.

Second, operating room equipment such as electrocautery, bloodwarmers, and fibrillators are often turned on only in anticipation of need, and can be turned off during the activation sequence mapping procedure. Operation of other equipment, such as the heating blanket, can be temporarily suspended. Certain pieces of equipment such as defibrillators, the cardiopulmonary bypass pump, and cardiac monitors, are potential sources of electrical noise, but cannot be readily dispensed with. Consequently, it is advantageous whenever possible to complete as much of the mapping procedure as possible before initiating cardiopulmonary bypass.

RECORDING

The amplifying and recording system should be able to record a minimum of four channels simultaneously: two surface ECG leads, an epicardial reference electrogram (atrial or ventricular as appropriate) and an electrogram from the moveable "mapping" or recording electrode. Most available direct-writing paper recording systems are able to respond rapidly enough to record cardiac electrograms. However, the maximum resolution for hand digitizing electrograms with either a graphics tablet or a millimeter ruler is about +1 mm or +10 ms at a paper speed of 100 mm/sec. A minimum resolution of 10 ms is usually sufficient to define the epicardial activation sequence adequately. Consequently, a minimum paper speed of 100 mm/sec is required. The relationship between paper speed and resolution of local activation holds over most paper speeds, however at faster speeds the frequency response of a mechanical pen motor system may decrease the accuracy of the recordings. FM analog tape recording is an efficient means of storing cardiac signals during the operating room procedure. Alternatively, analog signals may be converted to digital form as they are obtained, stored temporarily in a data buffer and then transferred to a permanent storage device or written directly to digital magnetic tape. To obtain a satisfactory representation of a cardiac electrogram, an analog-to-digital (A/D) converter sampling rate of at least 1,000 samples per second per channel is recommended [20].

OTHER EQUIPMENT

A stimulator capable of both pacing over a wide range of cycle lengths as well as inserting extrastimuli during intrinsic rhythm and paced trains is required for intraoperative mapping procedures. Optimally, a CRT (cathode ray tube) display in the operating room permits the surgeon to view the electrograms during the operative procedure and thereby allows him to adjust electrode orientation and positioning to optimize electrogram quality.

DATA ANALYSIS

Regardless of the type of recording system used, the data analysis must be performed rapidly so that the course of surgery is not unnecessarily prolonged. The analysis system may be portable for use in one or more operating rooms or dedicated to use in a specific operating room assigned for electrophysiologic procedures. In either case, provision must be made for storing, retrieving and displaying the raw data in an easy and readily understandable form.

Analog recordings (i.e., ECGs and electrograms) are analyzed by measuring the time of local activation at each of the sites from which electrograms are recorded with respect to the appropriate reference electrode. The reference electrode is standardized to the onset of the surface QRS at the beginning of the analysis procedure. In practice, a QRS to reference interval is obtained and that number is added to the result of the measurement from the reference electrogram to the probe electrogram. The same reference electrogram can be used as long as the rhythm being evaluated and the QRS morphology remain unchanged. The resulting activation time at each site is then expressed in milliseconds before or after the onset of the surface QRS. A/D conversion can be done at several points in the process. In the simplest situation, ECG and electrogram recordings are measured directly from the multichannel recordings obtained in the operating room and activation times determined by hand using a ruler with millimeter divisions. A simple but significant advance in this process has been the introduction of the "electronic ruler," the graphics tablet. The graphics tablet is connected to a computer that can interactively perform the repetitive subtraction and milliseconds per millimeter calibrations rapidly, returning the measured interval in milliseconds (Figure 25–13). This system is limited mostly by the speed of the operator in locating the next point and by the capabilities of the software that processes, stores and displays the results. A computer graphics tablet system that can per-

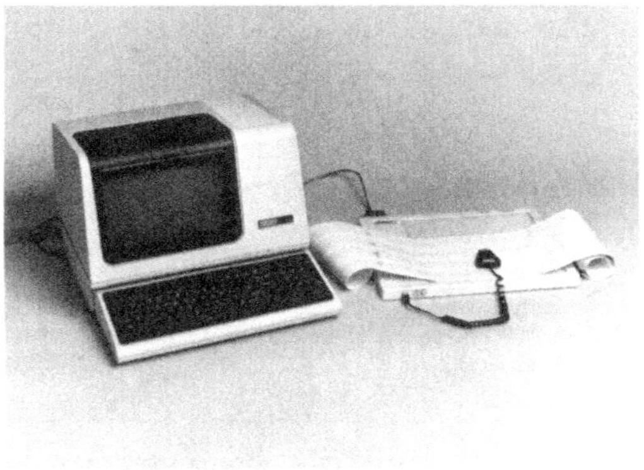

FIGURE 25–13. Computer terminal and graphics tablet.

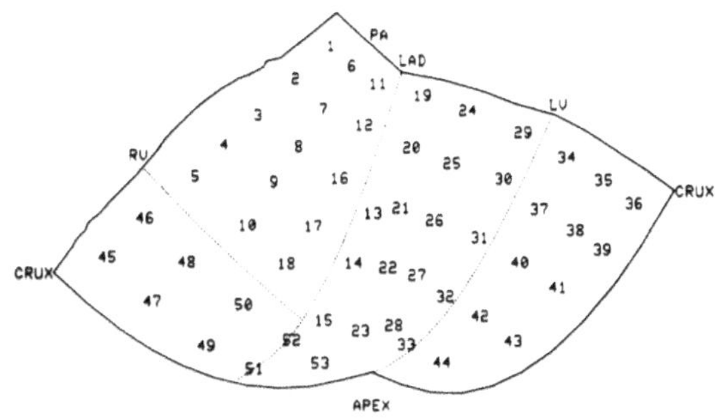

FIGURE 25–14. Folded out ventricular epicardial surface map. Fifty-three recording sites are interspersed over the ventricular epicardium. Their relative positions are located with respect to surface landmarks.

form these simple tasks is certainly worth the investment. An alternative to the manual process is to have analog signals (i.e., electrograms) digitized directly by an on-line A/D converter and local activation times determined by available computer algorithms. However, even with the most sophisticated software, operator supervision and interaction will be required to verify the determination of local activation. A technique that has been used as a supplement to recording systems is an analog device based on the circuitry used in cardiac monitors to sense the QRS. Coupled with a delay and digital timer this device can, if triggered appropriately on the electrogram to be measured, provide an instantaneous readout of the local activation time [21]. Inappropriate triggering may often be a problem, particularly during atrial or ventricular pacing.

Although automation of local activation time determination could streamline activation sequence mapping and electrophysiologic procedures considerably, cautious user input and verification is still advisable to insure accuracy. Further, as complexity of the system increases, capital cost and maintenance expenses multiply.

DISPLAYING RESULTS

Activation times, coupled with a representation of the area from which the electrogram was measured are best displayed using a visual format on a CRT screen. As activation time measurements are generated, either by hand or by the computer program controlling the process, the results can be displayed on a copy of whichever grid system the mapping team has chosen to employ. Thus, the most critical results of the measurements are depicted for both the surgeon and mapping team to review. Using the graphics capability of our system, we have displayed a projection of the ventricular surface folded out as described initially by Fontaine et al. [22] (Figure 25–14). On this map, local activation times are displayed as they are measured from the graphics tablet and stored in the computer. Further, the computer program can reproduce this map whenever called upon, and the map can be printed and placed in the patient's chart (Figure 25–15). For convenience, atrial activation sequence maps are represented by using numbers of corresponding ventricular areas across the AV groove (Figure 25–16). Smith and Ideker [23] utilized simultaneous acquisition of 32 channels, displaying results in a table arranged by activation times and mapping sites (Figure 25–17). This table allowed quick visualization of the earliest sites of activation, and provided an idea of the sequence in which the wave of activation proceeded. Isochronous maps may also be generated using grid systems such as the ones described above (Figure 25–18). Recently, Witowski et al. [18] have used a multichannel high speed A/D conversion in conjunction with a data storage system and high resolution display to measure local activation times, code areas of earliest activation by color and display color-coded isochronous maps. Parson and Downar [25] have reported an on-line analog system which records 116 simultaneous electrograms from a sock electrode. The analog electrogram signals are recorded on

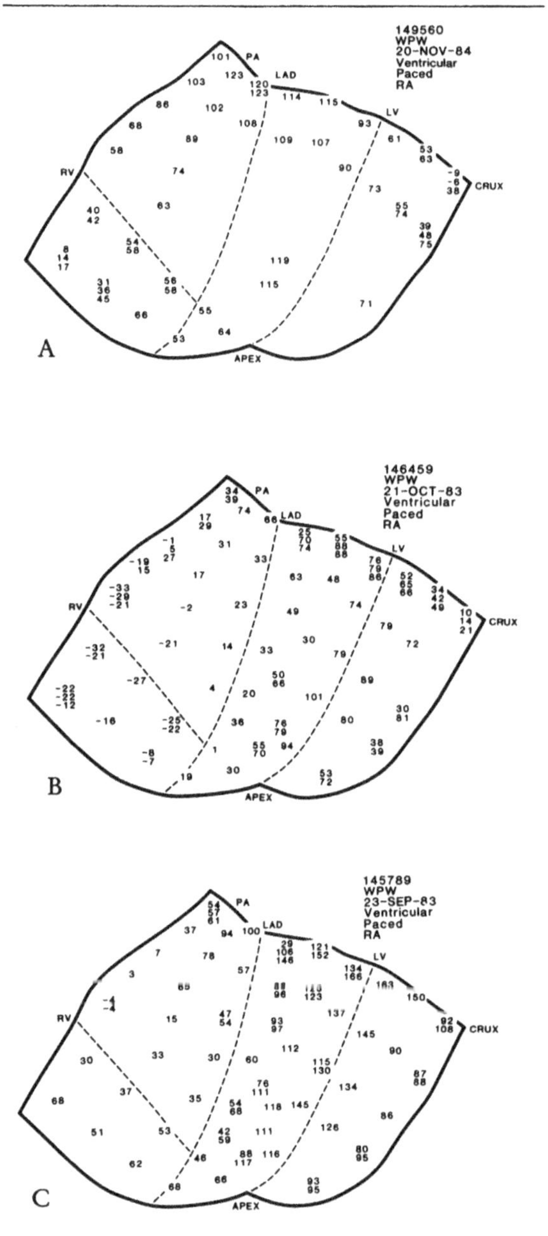

FIGURE 25–15. Ventricular epicardial surface activation sequence maps. One to three measured local activation times are displayed at each site. (A) shows a map of a patient with a posterior septal accessory connection. The negative numbers on the left posterior basal LV near the crux represent areas activated before the onset of the QRS. (B) shows a ventricular activation sequence map of a patient with a right lateral accessory connection with a broad area of ventricular attachment. (C) shows a ventricular activation sequence map of a patient with a right lateral accessory connection with a more localized insertion.

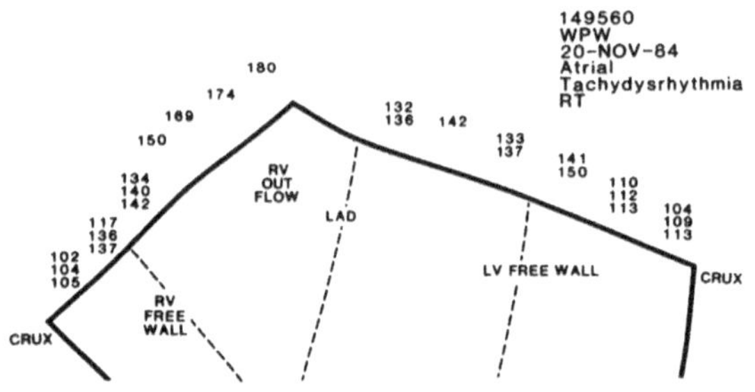

FIGURE 25–16. Atrial activation sequence map of a patient with a posterior septal accessory connection recorded during reciprocating tachycardia. The shortest activation times are recorded on each side of the map indicating the crux as the probable ventricular attachment of the accessory connection.

video tape. Local activation is determined using realtime differentiation and displayed on a radial representation of the heart using a video monitor (Figure 25–19). While the acquisition system is attractive due to its relatively low cost per recording channel and rapid graphic representation, the radial ventricular display does not lend itself easily to display of atrial mapping results. The advantage of each of these levels of sophistication is the ability to acquire the mapping data as quickly as possible, represent the results clearly so that the areas of interest can be easily visualized, and obtain the greatest resolution in localizing the suspected accessory connection(s).

DATA STORAGE

If ECG and electrograms are recorded using a multichannel paper recorder, representative electrograms can be stored in a patient's chart. FM tape can also be used to store analog data quite inexpensively and can be played back for subsequent analysis by any of the methods described above. With on-line A/D conversion, data can be stored temporarily in computer memory and then transferred to permanent storage media after collection of a series of electrograms [26] or recorded as digital signals directly on magnetic tape [27]. There are a variety of types of digital storage media available (floppy disk, magnetic tape in several formats, fixed and removable hard disk, etc.), some of which are quite affordable and others of which allow rapid storage and retrieval of large volumes of data. In general, digital storage of

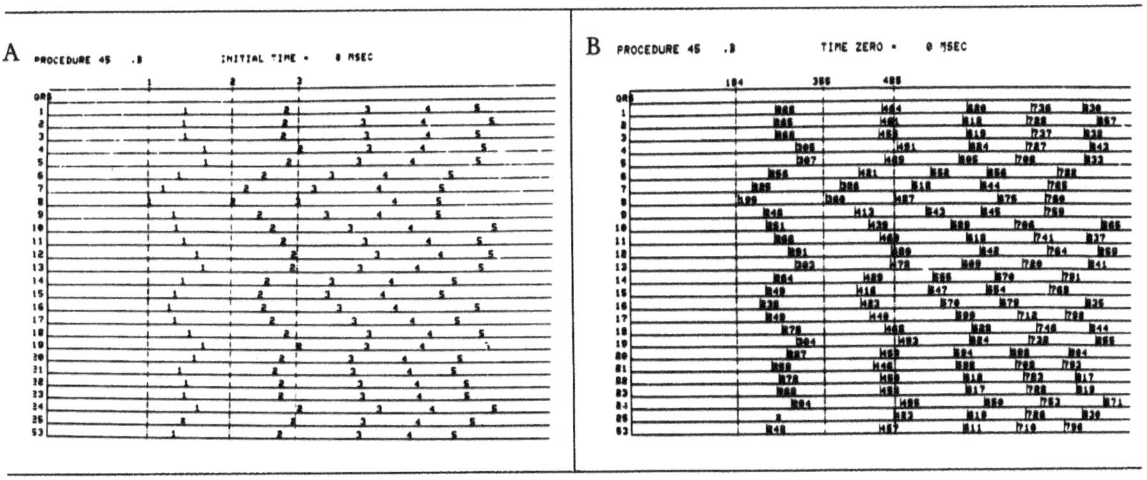

FIGURE 25–17. Table of activation times. On the left of the table are the areas from which electrograms were recorded. Each row represents the time of activation of that epicardial area for the several beats displayed. Activation times are staggered left to right to represent the activation of that area with respect to the other areas; earliest activation times are the farthest to the left. In Panel A, the activation is represented only by beat number, while Panel B shows the actual local activation times. Reproduced by permission from Smith and Ideker [23].

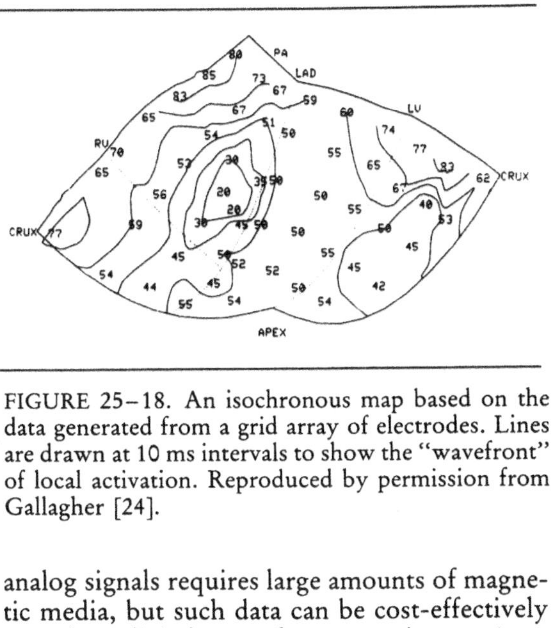

FIGURE 25–18. An isochronous map based on the data generated from a grid array of electrodes. Lines are drawn at 10 ms intervals to show the "wavefront" of local activation. Reproduced by permission from Gallagher [24].

analog signals requires large amounts of magnetic media, but such data can be cost-effectively stored on digital or analog magnetic tape (e.g., video or FM tape) [24,28] for storage and retrieval.

Operative considerations

ANESTHESIA

The primary anesthetic concern in patients with preexcitation syndromes, as in patients undergoing any cardiac surgical procedure, has been avoidance of myocardial depression and dysrhythmias. However, in the setting of intraoperative mapping of all forms of tachyarrhythmias, the latter concern has been somewhat reversed since reproducing the tachycardia is desired. Consequently, halothane which has been advocated because it suppresses catecholamine release and has been used successfully to prevent dysrhythmias in patients with preexcitation syndrome should be avoided [29]. Similarly, the butyrophenones (e.g., droperidol) are potent alpha-blockers and have been used to suppress dysrhythmias in patients with preexcitation [30,31]. On the other hand, both ethrane and fentanyl exhibit minimal myocardial depressant activity, and do not tend to inhibit tachycardia induction. Both of these agents have been used successfully in mapping procedures.

Approach to the Mapping Procedure

The strategy employed for intraoperative study of patients undergoing operative ablation of accessory conduction tissue depends on the characteristics of the accessory connection as determined by the preoperative studies. (Table 25–1).

BIDIRECTIONAL ACCESSORY CONNECTION

The most common situation consists of an accessory connection known to conduct in both antegrade and retrograde directions. In this

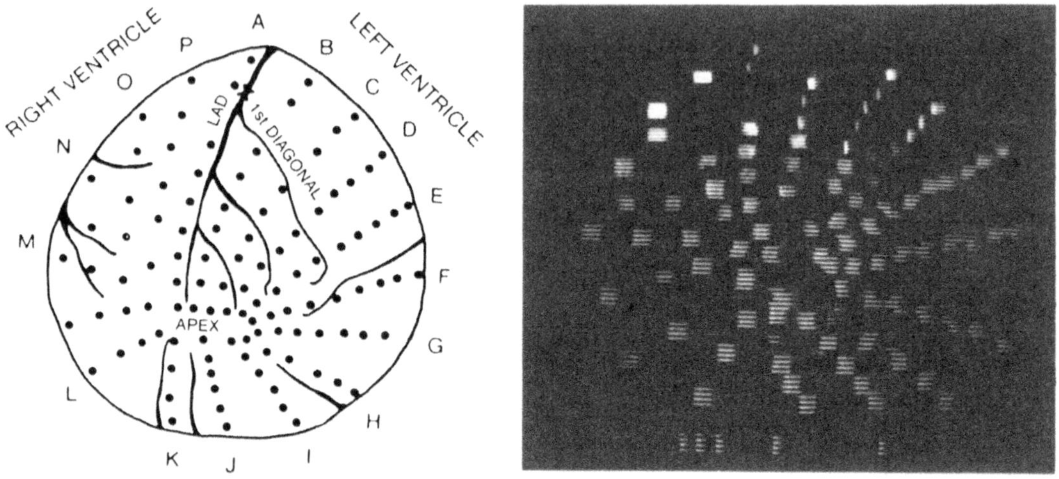

FIGURE 25–19. Radial electode distribution and video matrix image. In left panel is a "polar" projection of the heart showing the distribution of unipolar electrode buttons on the epicardial surface. The right panel shows the video matrix corresponding to the electrode positions. The rectangles become bright as the areas they represents are activated. All 116 areas are bright in this photograph for demonstration purposes. Reproduced with permission from Parson and Downar [24].

TABLE 25–1. Intraoperative Mapping Strategy

Type of Preexcitation	Approximate Incidence	Most Common Presentation	ECG	Intraoperative Activation Sequence
Accessory AV connection capable of conduction in both AV and VA directions	82%	RT or AF or VF	Delta Wave	1. Atrial — during orthodromic RT 2. Atrial — during V pacing 3. Ventricular — during atrial pacing
Accessory AV connection capable of only VA conduction (concealed)	14%	RT	no delta wave	1. Atrial — during RT 2. Atrial — during V pacing
Accessory AV connection capable of only AV conduction	4%	AF with rapid Ventricular response	Delta wave	1. Ventricular — during atrial pacing 2. Ventricular — during antidromic RT (rarely)

Definitions: V = Ventricular, AV = atrioventricular, VA = vetriculoatrial, AF = Atrial fibrillation, VF = Ventricular fibrillation, RT = Reciprocating tachycardia.

setting, intraoperative mapping is designed to localize both the atrial and ventricular insertions of the accessory connection during atrial and venticular pacing, as well as during reciprocating tachycardia (usually orthodromic reciprocating tachycardia). As a rule the first step is to induce orthodromic reciprocating tachycardia and record from right and left atrial sites at various points along the AV groove The atrial map permits identifying the point(s) of earliest atrial activation as conduction proceeds in the retrograde direction from ventricle to atrium over the accessory connection during tachycardia. When a single recording probe is being used, the operating surgeon places the probe on an atrial area and identifies the area to the recording team — usually using a predetermined grid system (Figure 25–20). In our ex-

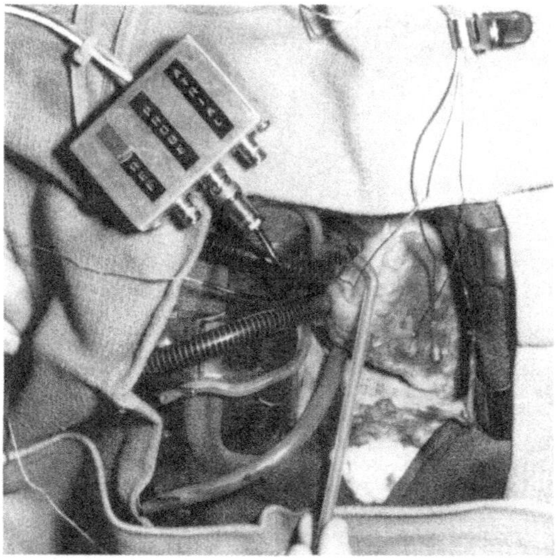

FIGURE 25–20. Atrial activation sequence mapping. Wand type roving probe is placed on the right atrial appendage. Ventricular pacing electrode pair and quadripolar reference plaque are shown sewn to the right ventricle.

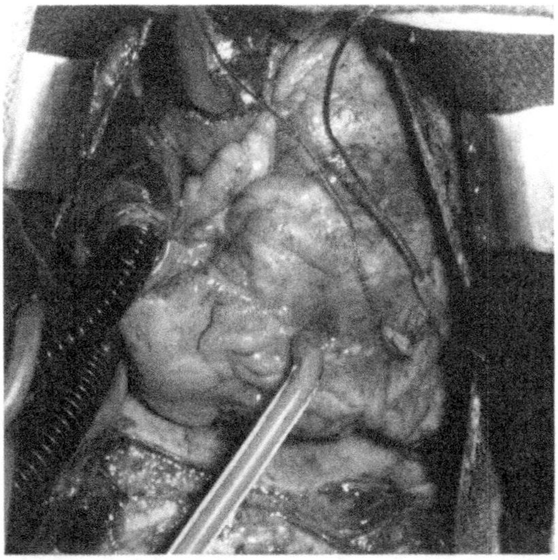

FIGURE 25–21. Ventricular activation sequence mapping. Wand type roving probe is placed on the right ventricle.

perience we have found that a cotton glove on one hand can help to hold the heart during the mapping procedure to obtain a stable signal. When a recording of good quality has been verified, the electrode is moved to the next site. A series of recording from atrial sites adjacent to the atrioventricular groove can be obtained in this fashion in a relatively short period of time. Similarly, a series of atrial recordings during ventricular pacing (pacing near the presumed accessory connection) may be desirable, particularly if sustained tachycardia cannot be induced. Conduction through the accessory connection is accentuated by proximity of the pacing site. It is often useful to increase the number of measurements obtained within a 2–4 cm area closest to the presumed site of the accessory connection. One can often recognize the area from which electrograms are recorded earliest with respect to the reference electrogram during a cursory examination of the recordings as they are made. Following this initial confirmation of the site for dissection, the operative division could proceed, if necessary, while the data is formally measured.

The second mapping stage usually consists of defining the ventricular activation sequence during atrial pacing (Figure 25–21). A series of ventricular recordings obtained while pacing is preferred to mapping during sinus rhythm since preexcitation can often be accentuated by placing the pacing electrode near the suspected site of the accessory connection. An eccentric ventricular epicardial activation sequence identifies the site along the AV groove where abnormal ventricular activation is initiated, thereby defining the ventricular insertion of the accessory connection.

Although the atrial and ventricular data obtained in this fashion may appear to be just two ways of confirming the same data, the information obtained from these maps is often not as clear as one would hope. The puzzle can result in the revelation of additional accessory connections in the vicinity of the clinically significant connection.

ACCESSORY AV CONNECTIONS CAPABLE OF CONDUCTION ONLY IN THE RETROGRADE DIRECTION

In the case where the accessory connection conducts only in the retrograde direction there is no preexcitation (i.e., no delta wave on the surface electrogram). Consequently, intraoperatively, a series of atrial recordings is obtained after induction of reciprocating tachycardia and then again while pacing the ventricle (from a site close to the site of the suspected connection).

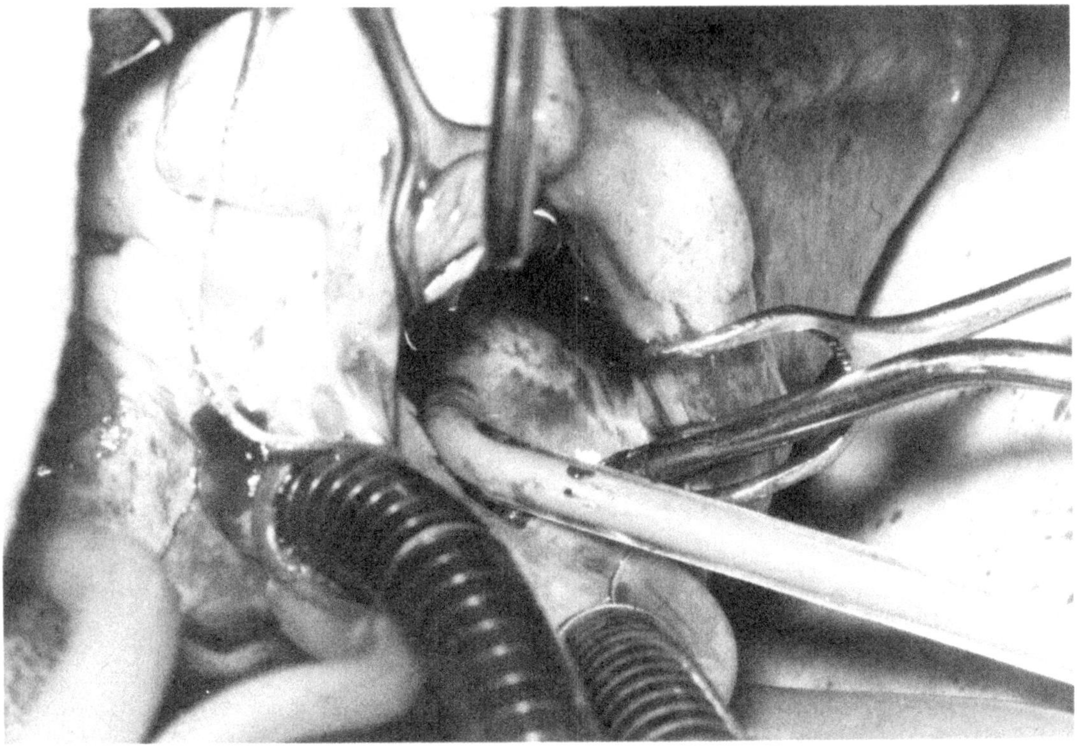

FIGURE 25–22. Endocardial atrial activation sequence mapping. Wand type roving probe is placed through a right atriotomy. Electrograms are recorded from various areas on the atrial septum to identify the His bundle and AV node in order to avoid injury to these structures.

ACCESSORY AV CONNECTIONS CAPABLE OF CONDUCTION ONLY IN THE ANTEGRADE DIRECTION

In the rare case of the accessory connection that conducts only in the antegrade direction, a ventricular series is recorded during atrial pacing. Since there is no orthodromic reciprocating tachycardia in these patients, atrial mapping during that tachycardia cannot be obtained. However, in rare cases it may be possible to map the ventricular epicardial surface during antidromic tachycardia, thereby confirming participation of the accessory connection in that tachycardia.

SUSPECTED POSTERIOR SEPTAL ACCESSORY AV CONNECTIONS

Accessory AV connections in areas such as the posterior septum may make epicardial maps difficult to interpret since the connection may be deep to the epicardial surface of the AV groove and may insert at a distance from the groove. It is important to record from areas beyond those adjacent to the AV groove and to recognize the 3-dimensional relationships in this area. A discrete nonnecrosing cryolesion may aid in confirming the location of the accessory connection by temporarily obliterating conduction through the connection.

Further, right atrial endocardial mapping of the normal AV conduction system is often helpful so that dissection can be done in close proximity without causing damage to normal conduction (Figure 25–22).

POSTABLATION STUDY

When the ablative procedure has been completed and sinus rhythm has been reestablished, the absence of a delta wave on the ECG is the first test of the success of the procedure in patients with previously known preexcitation. If a prominent delta wave was present prior to ablation, the absence of the delta wave is the first indication of successful ablation. Attention is then directed at demonstrating that conduction through the accessory connection has been interrupted. An atrial series of recordings may be performed during ventricular pacing, similar to the map recorded preoperatively. A postresection atrial map will show earliest atrial activation to be consistent with retrograde conduction through the AV node-His bundle axis. Similarly, a ventricular map obtained during atrial pacing when compared with the preablation map should show activation times consistent with normal AV conduction (unless other coexisting accessory connections are present). Additional confirmatory evidence can be obtained by attempting to demonstrate the point at which 1:1 ventriculoatrial (VA) conduction ceases. With the recording electrode placed on the atrium, the ventricle is paced at increasingly shorter pacing cycle lengths until second degree VA block is recorded. If the ablation has been successful, second degree VA block will be noted at cycle lengths consistent with retrograde conduction through the AV node (i.e., commonly cycle lengths <350 ms).

REOPERATION

An accessory connection that has been damaged, but not completely transected, may appear to have been ablated in the immediate postoperative period. If the tissue is able to recover, the delta wave may reappear postoperatively. Indeed, the irritability of the postoperative heart may precipitate orthodromic reciprocating tachycardia, or atrial fibrillation with conduction in the antegrade direction through the recovered accessory connection. As a rule, early reoperation is indicated. Although the anatomy may be distorted and landmarks may be difficult to identify, a patient detailed mapping procedure taking care to examine any areas that may have been missed at the first procedure is essential.

FUTURE GOALS AND PROSPECTS

Recording electrograms and measuring activation times with greater accuracy in shorter time will increase the success rate and decrease the morbidity and mortality of the procedure. Improvement in the accuracy with which the site of an accessory connection is identified will likewise improve the success rate of the surgical procedure. Similarly, greater accuracy of accessory connection localization will allow more localized ablative procedures. The ability to record multiple data channels simultaneously will decrease the time required to obtain the necessary recordings while rapid automated data analysis and detailed graphical display will present the results quickly and accurately. The technology and expertise for all of these improvements presently exist; their implementation will take place as they become more readily available and cost-effective.

References

1. Barker PS, Macleod AG, Alexander J: The excitatory process observed in the exposed human heart. *Am. Heart J.* 5:720, 1930.
2. Durrer D, Roos JP: Epicardial excitation of the ventricles in a patient with Wolff-Parkinson-White syndrome (type B). *Circulation* 35:15, 1967.
3. Burchell HB, Frye RL, Anderson MW, McGoon DC: Atrioventricular and ventriculoatrial excitation in Wolff-Parkinson-White syndrome (type B): Transitory ablation at surgery. *Circulation* 36:663, 1967.
4. Cobb FR, Blumenschein SD, Sealy WC, Bioneau JP, Wagner GS, Wallace AG: Successful surgical interruption of the bundle of Kent in a patient with Wolff-Parkinson-White syndrome. *Circulation* 38:1018, 1968.
5. Scher AM, Young AC: The pathway of ventricular depolarization in the dog. *Circ. Res.* 4:461, 1956.
6. Horowitz LN, Alexander JA, Edmunds LH: Postoperative right bundle branch block: Identification of three levels of block. *Circulation* 62:2, 1980.
7. Wyndham MB, Smith T, Meeran MK, Mammana R, Levitsky S, Rosen KM: Epicardial activation in patients with left bundle branch block. *Circulation* 61:4, 1980.
8. Wyndham CR, Meeran MK, Smith T, Engelman RM, Levitsky S, Rosen KM: Epicardial activation in human left anterior fascicular block. *Am. J. Cardiol.* 44:638, 1979.
9. Gallagher JJ, Kasell J, Sealy WC, Pritchett ELC, Wallace AG: Epicardial Mapping in the Wolff-Parkinson-White Syndrome. *Circulation* 57:5, 1978.
10. Waldo AL, Pacifico AD, Bargeron LM Jr, James TN, Kirklin JN: Electrophysiologic delineation of the specialized A-V conduction system in patients with corrected transposition of the great vessels and ventricular septial defect. *Circulation* 52:435, 1975.
11. Krongrad E, Malm JR, Bowman FO, Jr, Hoffman BF, Kaiser GA, Waldo AL: Electrophysiologic delineation of the specialized atrioventricular conduction system in patients with congenital heart disease. *J. Thorac Cardiovasc. Surg.* 67:875, 1974.

12. Gallagher JJ, Pritchett ELC, Sealy WC, Kasell J, Wallace AG: The Preexcitation Syndromes. *Prog. Cardiovasc. Dis.* 20:285, 1978.
13. Gallagher JJ, Pritchett ELC, Benditt DG, Tonkin AM, Campbell RWF, Dugan FA, Bashore TM, Wallace AG: New catheter techniques for analysis of the sequence of antegrade atrial activation in man. *Eur. J. Cardiol.* 6:1, 1977.
14. Kupersmith J: Electrophysiologic mapping during open heart surgery. *Prog. Cardiovasc. Dis.* 23:167, 1976.
15. Gallagher JJ, Sealy WC, Kasell J, Millar R, Campbell RWF, Harrison L, Pritchett ELC, Wallace AG: Cryosurgical ablation of accessory atrioventricular connections: a new technique for correction of the preexcitation syndrome. *Circulation* 44:471, 1977.
16. Jackman W, Beck B, Aliot E, Friday K, Lazzara R: Basis for concealed accessory AV pathways. (Abstract.) *Circulation* 70:II–337, 1984.
17. Harrison L, Ideker RE, Smith WM, Klein GJ, Kasell J, Gallagher JJ: The sock electrode array. A tool for determining global epicardial activation during unstable arrhythmias. *PACE* 3:531, 1980.
18. Witowski FX, Corr PB: An automated, simultaneous transmural cardiac mapping system. *Am. J. Physical.* 247 (Heart Circ Physical): H661, 1984.
19. Meijne NG, Mellink HM, van Dam RT, Durrer D: Surgical treatment of ventricular preexcitation. *J. Thor. Cardiovasc. Surg.* 14:232, 1973.
20. Barr RC, Spach MS: Sampling rates required for digital recording of intracellular and extracellular cardiac potentials. *Circulation* 55:40, 1977.
21. Kasell J, Gallagher JJ: A digital timer for on-line interval measurement. *PACE* 4:497, 1981.
22. Fontaine G, Guiraudon G, Frank R, Coutte R, Dragodanne C: Epicardial mapping and surgical treatment in six cases of resistant ventricular tachycardia not related to coronary artery disease. In *The Conduction System of the Heart*, Wellens HJJ, Lie KI, Janse MJ (eds.). The Netherlands, Martinus Nijhoff, 1976, pp. 543–563.
23. Smith WM, Ideker RE: Computer techniques for epicardial and endocardial mapping. *Prog. Cardiovasc. Dis.* 26:15, 1983.
24. Gallagher JJ, Kasell JH, Cox JL, Smith WM, Ideker RE, Smith WM: Techniques of intraoperative electrophysiologic mapping. *Am. J. Cardiol.* 49:221, 1982.
25. Parson I, Downar E: Clinical Instrumentation for the Intra-operative mapping of ventricular arrhythmias. *PACE* 7:683, 1984.
26. Janse MJ, van Capelle FJL, Marsink H, Kleber AG, Wilms-Schapman F, Cardinal R, D'Alnoncourt CN, Durrer D: Flow of "injury" current and patterns of excitation during early ventricular arrhythmias in acute regional myocardial ischemia in isolated porcine and canine hearts: Evidence for two different arrhythmogenic mechanisms. *Circ. Res.* 47:151, 1980.
27. Wyatt RF, Lux RL: Application of multiplexing techniques in the collection of body surface maps from single complexes. *Adv. Cardiol.* 10:26, 1974.
28. Mendler P, Parson I, Downar E: Multichannel recording of cardiac potentials. *Med. Biol. Eng. Comput.* 18:617, 1980.
29. Sadowski AR, Moyers JR: Anesthetic Management of the Wolff-Parkinson-White Syndrome. *Anesthesiology* 51:553, 1979.
30. van der Starre PJA: Wolff-Parkinson-White syndrome during anesthesia. *Anesthesiology* 48:369, 1978.
31. Katz J Kadis L: *Anesthesia and Uncommon Diseases*. Philadephia, WB Saunders, 1973.
32. Hammill SC, Pritchett ELC Klein GJ, Smith WM, Gallagher JJ: Accessory atrioventricular pathways that conduct only in the antegrade direction. *Circulation* 62:1335, 1980.

26. SURGERY FOR PREEXCITATION SYNDROMES

James L. Cox
Michael E. Cain

The majority of patients who experience cardiac arrhythmias associated with preexcitation syndromes can be treated satisfactorily by nonsurgical methods. When these arrhythmias cannot be controlled medically or when they are potentially lethal, surgical intervention may be required. By far, the most common of the preexcitation syndromes requiring surgery is Wolff-Parkinson-White (WPW) syndrome in which the ventricles are preexcited because of accessory atrioventricular (AV) connections [1]. Recently, surgical procedures have also been applied clinically to control life-threatening arrhythmias associated with presumed accessory atriofascicular [atrio-Hisian] bypass tracts [2] and accessory nodoventricular connections.

Candidates for surgical treatment of preexcitation syndromes should first undergo thorough electrophysiologic evaluation, a subject that is discussed in detail elsewhere within this text. Prior to surgery, electrophysiology study in patients with preexcitation syndromes should document the basis of preexcitation, and the location and conduction characteristics of the accessory connection(s). In some patients, an accessory connection may be demonstrated to permit a rapid, potentially life-threatening response during spontaneous atrial flutter or fibrillation. Such patients, as well as those with medically refractory reciprocating tachycardia and/or drug intolerance represent indications for surgery. In patients with the WPW syndrome, life-threatening tachycardias are uncommon, and the most common indications for surgery are medically refractory reciprocating tachycardia and drug intolerance [3]. We have also liberalized indications for surgery in the WPW syndrome to include young, otherwise healthy individuals who experience any significant symptoms or who require more than minimal medical therapy to prevent recurrent episodes of reciprocating tachycardia. Indications for surgery are also discussed in the next chapter in this volume.

Operative Approach in Patients with WPW Syndrome

INTRAOPERATIVE ELECTROPHYSIOLOGIC EVALUATION

The preoperative electrophysiologic evaluation is of special importance in patients who are to undergo surgery for the WPW syndrome. Once the diagnosis has been established by the preoperative study, it is important to determine the number of accessory AV connections and to localize them to one of four regions around the AV groove: (1) right sided free-wall, (2) left sided free-wall, (3) posterior septal, (4) anterior septal (Figure 26–1) [4]. Preoperative localization of the site of the AV connection is helpful not only in situations where intraoperative identification is impossible, but it also dictates

Supported by NIH Grant HL-32257.

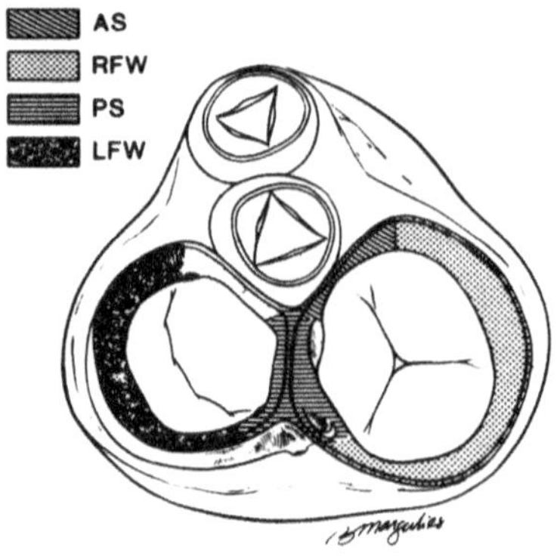

FIGURE 26–1. The heart with the atria cut away (the two anuli viewed from above), showing the boundaries upon which the classification of the accessory AV connections associated with the WPW syndrome is based. AS = anterior septal; PS = posterior septal; LFW = left free-wall; RFW = right free-wall. (Reproduced by permission from Sealy [4].)

the venous cannulation technique for cardiopulmonary bypass [5]. In patients with left free-wall accessory AV connections, the superior and inferior vena cavae are cannulated through separate purse-string sutures in the right atrium. In patients with right free-wall, posterior septal, and most anterior septal pathways, the superior vena cava is cannulated through a purse-string suture in the right atrial appendage and the inferior vena cava is cannulated through a venotomy in the saphenous vein bulb to gain entrance to the deep femoral vein in the groin. The latter venous cannulation technique is necessary because the surgical approach to right free-wall, posterior septal, and anterior septal pathways is via a right atriotomy. If the inferior vena cava cannula is placed through the right atrium, it interferes with the exposure necessary for proper dissection of the AV groove structures required to ablate these accessory connections.

Although the preoperative electrophysiology study is of obvious importance in patients who are to undergo surgery for the WPW syndrome, the intraoperative electrophysiology study is perhaps even more important. For several years it was not uncommon to discover, intraoperatively, that patients had multiple accessory AV connections despite a preoperative electrophysiology study that had identified only one accessory connection [1]. Although this discrepancy has now become extremely rare, its potential occurrence continues to represent the major indication for intraoperative mapping in patients with the WPW syndrome.

Perhaps the most common intraoperative problem encountered during the early years of surgery for the WPW syndrome was the inability to perform adequate intraoperative mapping because of blocked antegrade and/or retrograde conduction across the accessory AV connection at the time of surgery. A variety of factors may be responsible for changes in the conduction characteristics of accessory connections intraoperatively, including general anesthesia, alterations in circulating catecholamine levels and in autonomic stimulation of the heart, exposure of the heart to room temperature, cannulation for cardiopulmonary bypass, alterations in cardiac geometry, and cardiac manipulation, the latter being particularly important [6].

Inability to obtain accurate intraoperative electrophysiologic data in patients undergoing surgery for the WPW syndrome has a major detrimental effect on the overall results of surgery. This problem may be circumvented in most patients if they have had complete and accurate preoperative electrophysiology studies. However, surgical dissection based on the preoperative study in those patients who have been identified to have a single accessory connection but who, in fact, have multiple accessory connections may be inadequate. Moreover, some patients exhibit only intermittent ventricular preexcitation and others have associated atrial fibrillation, both conditions making performance and interpretation of preoperative and intraoperative electrophysiology studies more difficult, leading to less satisfactory surgical results. Prolonged cardiopulmonary bypass in patients who are unusually difficult to map intraoperatively also increases the risk associated with the operation.

In an effort to overcome the problems associated with obtaining accurate intraoperatively electrophysiologic data, a computerized intraoperative mapping system was developed at our institution [7]. Although the system is capable of recording up to 160 separate data channels simultaneously for use in ventricular tachyarrhythmia surgery, we record only 16 channels simultaneously in patients undergoing surgery for the WPW syndrome [8]. A flexible band electrode incorporating 16 bipolar pairs is placed around the ventricular side of the AV groove and atrial pacing is initiated to effect maximal ventricular preexcitation (Figure 26–2). Data from the 16 bipolar electrodes are digitized, transmitted to a digital tape recorder via a fiberoptic cable, processed by a specially designed computer program, and displayed on a color graphics terminal in the operating room within 120 seconds of recording. The band electrode is then placed around the atrial side of the AV groove and either reciprocating tachycardia or ventricular pacing is initiated to accentuate conduction in the retrograde direction across the accessory AV connection so that the atrial activation sequence adjacent to the AV groove can be assessed. The data are processed as described above and are displayed within 120 seconds of the time of recording.

Although this intraoperative mapping system has greatly reduced the time required for intraoperative localization of accessory AV connections, the major advantage of the system is that both the ventricular and atrial maps are measured during a single cardiac cycle. Therefore, patients who exhibit only intermittent conduction via the accessory connection intraoperatively, can be mapped quite accurately by evaluating only those cardiac cycles in which conduction via the accessory connection was present [9]. The ability to determine activation sequences during a single cardiac cycle facilitates evaluation of patients with atrial fibrillation as well as those suspected of having multiple accessory connections.

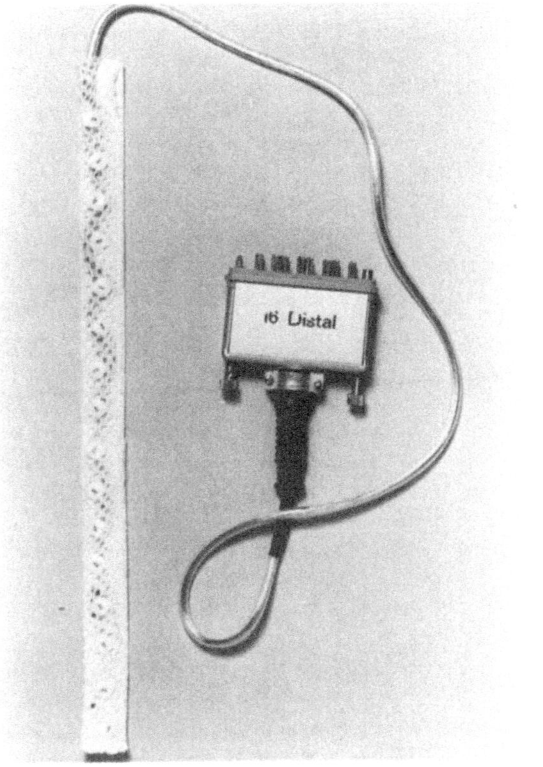

FIGURE 26–2. Band electrode employed for the intraoperative mapping of patients undergoing surgery for the WPW syndrome (see text for further discussion).

ENDOCARDIAL SURGICAL APPROACH

A median sternotomy is performed regardless of the suspected position of the accessory AV connection prior to surgery. Once the atrial and ventricular insertions of the accessory AV connection have been identified by intraoperative mapping, cardiopulmonary bypass is instituted. Accessory AV connections located in the *right free-wall* position are approached initially by performing a right atriotomy. The area of the anulus fibrosis corresponding to the site of the accessory AV connection is identified and a supraanular incision is placed approximately 2 mm above the anulus of the tricuspid valve, exposing the AV groove fat pad encompassing the right coronary artery and vein. Generally, the incision is extended 2 cm on each side of the previously determined location of the accessory connection. The AV groove fat pad containing the coronary vessels is separated from the top of the external wall of the ventricle to the level of the ventricular epicardial reflection throughout the length of the supraanular incision (Figure 26–3) [2]. The extension of this incision anteromedially to the anterior aspect of the membranous septum is occasionally necessary in order to divide anterior septal pathways passing through the fat pad between the right fibrous trigone and the site of insertion of the right coronary artery into the AV groove. This fat pad lies just anterior to the membranous portion of the interatrial septum between the pericardial reflection of the ascending aorta and the medial wall of the right atrium. After completion of the AV groove dissection, a sharp nerve hook or knife is used to divide any remaining fibers between the atrium and ventricle at the level of the tricuspid valve anulus. This last manuever results in the ability to visualize the tricuspid valve annulus throughout the length of the supraanular incision which is then closed

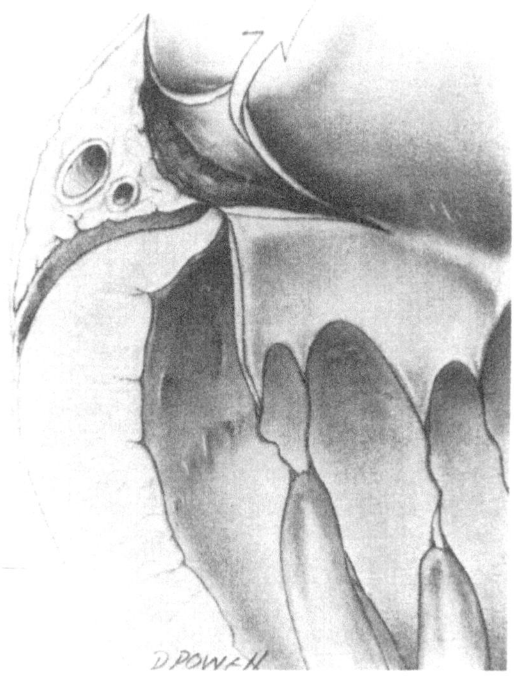

FIGURE 26–3. Illustrated is the appropriate plane of dissection to be established beneath the AV groove fat pad for surgical ablation of an accessory AV connection. The endocardial incision is made slightly above the valve anulus and a plane of dissection is established between the external *ventricular* wall and the AV groove fat pad. This plane of dissection is carried from the level of the endocardial incision all the way to the epicardial reflection off the ventricular wall onto the AV groove fat pad. Such extensive dissection between the AV groove fat pad and the external *atrial* wall is no longer performed but the cut edge of the atrial wall is dissected for a few millimeters to allow safe closure of the supraanular incision. (Reproduced by permission from Cox [2].)

with a continuous 4-0 nonabsorbable suture.

Exposure of *left free-wall* AV connections is accomplished via a left atriotomy in the manner routinely used to expose the mitral valve. All patients with left free-wall pathways undergo the same surgical dissection regardless of the precise location of the left free-wall pathway. A supraanular incision is placed 2 mm above the posterior mitral valve anulus from the left fibrous trigone to the posterior interventricular septum. A plane of dissection is established between the underlying AV groove fat pad and the top of the posterior left ventricle throughout the length of the supraanular incision. This plane of dissection is carried to the epicardium as it reflects off the posterior left ventricle onto the AV groove fat pad throughout the length of the supraanular incision. A sharp nerve hook or knife is then used to divide any remaining fibers connecting the atrium to the ventricle at the level of the posterior mitral valve anulus, and the supraanular incision is closed with a 4-0 nonabsorbable suture.

The most difficult accessory AV connections to interrupt surgically are those located posteriorly in the region of the crux (*posterior septal* pathways). A right atriotomy is performed in these patients prior to arresting the heart with cold potassium cardioplegia. The His bundle is identified with a handheld probe that is used to map the lower right interatrial septum. Once the His bundle has been identified, a supraanular incision is placed just posterior to the site of the His bundle and extended in a counterclockwise direction onto the posterior right atrial free-wall. A plane of dissection is established between the fat pad and the top of the posterior interventricular septum. All dissection that is to be accomplished in the region of the His bundle is performed during either atrial pacing or reciprocating tachycardia in an effort to avoid injury to the AV node–His bundle complex. Once dissection in that area has been completed, the heart is arrested with cold potassium cardioplegic solution and the remainder of the posterior pyramidal space overlying the posterior interventricular septum is dissected. This dissection is carried medially to the level of the mitral valve anulus and posteriorly to the epicardial reflection off the posterior ventricular surface. Particular attention is paid to dissection of the left corner of the pyramidal space overlying the posterior superior process of the left ventricle at the site where the posterior interventricular septum is juxtaposed to the posterior free-wall of the left ventricle. Once dissection has been completed, the supraanular incision is closed with a continuous 4-0 nonabsorbable suture.

In the first 200 patients undergoing surgery for the WPW syndrome at Duke University Medical Center, surgical division of the accessory AV pathway was successful in 98% of right free-wall connections, 92% of left free-wall pathways, and 77% of posterior septal connections [10]. The technique that had evolved during the course of treatment of those patients was modified in August 1981 to include several additional important aspects: (1) 2.5 power optical magnification, (2) exclusive use of the endocardial approach under cardioplegic arrest, (3) wider margins of surgical dissection, (4) sharp dissection of the involved valve anulus, (5) division of only the ventricular insertion of the accessory AV connection, and (6) internal identification of the ventricular epicardial peel in all regions of dissection [11]. Using these modifications 148/149 accessory connections have been divided successfully in the last 118 consecutive patients. In comparison to the initial 200 patients, the modified surgical technique has resulted in an increase in the overall success rate from 86% to 99.3%, a decrease in the reoperation rate from 19.5% to 0% and a decrease in the incidence of heart block from 10.5% to 0.8%. Associated abnormalities in these patients included Ebstein's anomaly (12%), other arrhythmias (34%), coronary artery disease (6%), cardiomyopathy (6%), and other congenital heart disease (22%). Twenty percent of patients had multiple (2–4) accessory connections, accounting for the total of 149 connections being present in the 118 patients.

EPICARDIAL SURGICAL APPROACH

Recently an external closed heart approach for the division and/or cryoablation for the division of epicandial accessory connections has been reported by Klein et al. [11]. This surgical technique is quite similar to that employed by Sealy in the first 40 patients in the Duke series. This technique was abandoned because of serious hemorrhagic complications that frequently arose in patients with friable epicardial peels that would not hold sutures adequately and in the presence of an intramural coronary artery or coronary sinus. These complications were fatal in two elderly patients. The group of patients recently reported to have undergone the external approach combined with cryosurgery [11] does not represent the spectrum of patients incorporated in the Duke or St. Louis experience [8]. For example, the mean age of Guiraudon's patients was 29 years, none of the patients had coexisting heart disease, only one patient had multiple (two) accessory connections, and none had septal pathways. Thus, in our opinion, the endocardial approach continues to be the procedure of choice for the surgical treatment of the WPW syndrome.

Surgical Approaches to Reentry within the AV node, Atriofascicular (Atrio–Hisian) Bypass Tracts, and Accessory Nodoventricular Connections

The most common abnormality involving the AV node and peri-AV nodal tissues leading to paroxysmal reciprocating tachycardia is reentry within the AV node believed to be on the basis of "dual AV node physiology." While this abnormality does not result in ventricular preexcitation and therefore is not classified as a type of preexcitation syndome, its frequency of occurrence and occasional refractoriness to medical therapy dictated that a surgical procedure be designed specifically for the treatment of tachycardias using this mechanism. During the course of developing a procedure for the treatment of this reentrant arrhythmia, it became apparent that the same technique might be applied to ablate atriofascicular (atrio–Hisian) bypass tracts. The danger of atriofascicular bypass tracts lies in their ability to bypass the normal protective effects of the AV node against atrial tachyarrhythmias and thereby permit excessively rapid ventricular responses during atrial flutter or fibrillation.

Prior to 1981, the only surgical therapy available for patients with medically refractory tachycardia due to reentry within the AV node was elective cryoablation of the bundle of His [12]. In 1981, a closed chest technique was described for permanent His bundle ablation in which direct-current electrical shock is delivered through an electrode catheter positioned in the vicinity of the His bundle [13,14]. This procedure effectively replaced cryoablation of the His bundle for the treatment of medically refractory primary atrial tachycardias or reciprocating tachycardia due to reentry within the AV node because it did not require a formal cardiac surgical operation.

Since both cryoablation and catheter ablation of the bundle of His require placement of permanent pacemaker systems, we developed a new surgical technique for the treatment of reentry within the AV node in which discrete cryosurgical lesions are created around the borders of the AV node in an effort to alter the functional characteristics of the AV node and its input pathways [15]. The AV node is located anatomically within the confines of the Triangle of Koch (Figure 26–4) [16]. This anatomic triangle is bounded superiorly by the Tendon of Todaro which extends from the upper rim of the os of the coronary sinus to the membranous portion of the interatrial septum. The inferior border of the Triangle of Koch is formed by the posterior medial tricuspid valve anulus extending from the membranous portion of the interatrial septum posteriorly to the level of the os of the coronary sinus. The posterior boundary of the Triangle of Koch is formed by a straight line connecting the os of the coronary sinus to the tricuspid valve anulus immediately beneath the coronary sinus. In performing the discrete cryosurgical procedure, as many as nine separate 3 mm lesions are placed around the borders of the Triangle of Koch (Figure 26–5) [2]. The discrete cryolesions are applied until there occurs either a temporary block of AV conduction or a permanent prolongation of the AV interval, at which time the cryothermic application is discontinued (Figure 26–6) [15].

The ability of this surgical procedure to limit the ventricular response rate to spontaneous atrial flutter was first demonstrated in a dog with spontaneous atrial flutter at 6 and 14 weeks after the animal had undergone discrete cryosurgical modification of the AV node (Figure 26–7) [2]. This documentation that the ventricular response rate to spontaneous atrial flutter could be manipulated surgically ultimately led to the application of discrete cryosurgery of the AV node in an attempt to

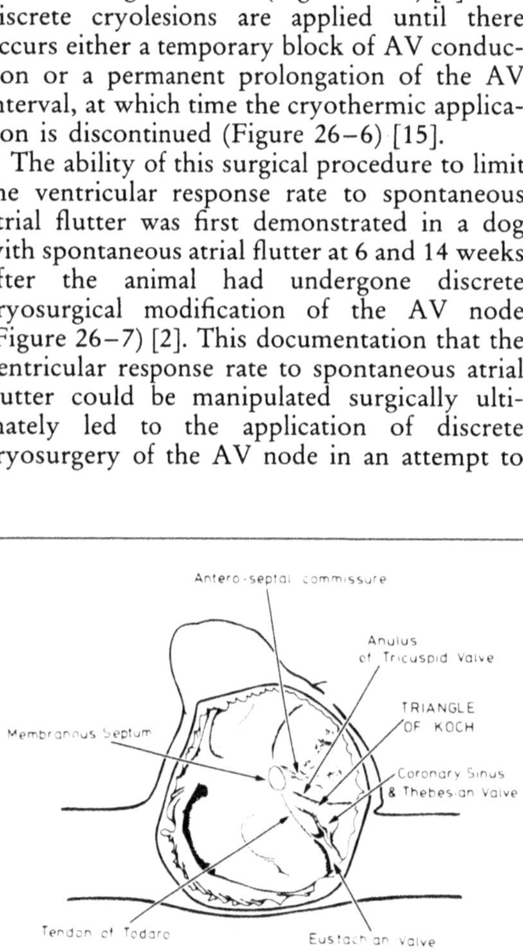

FIGURE 26–4. Landmarks of the Triangle of Koch that contain the AV node. (Reproduced by permission from Anderson and Becker [16].)

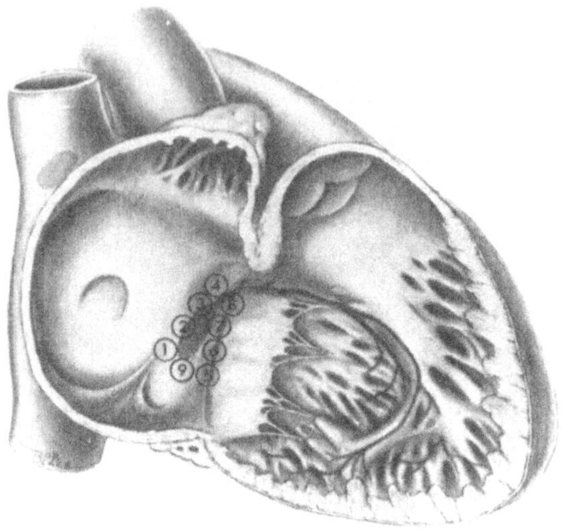

FIGURE 26–5. Discrete cryosurgery of the AV node. The sites of the nine cryolesions are shown in relation to the AV node–His bundle, coronary sinus, and tricuspid valve annulus. Mapping of the His bundle at the time of surgery confirms the location of the specialized conduction system prior to the application of the cryolesions. (Reproduced by permission from Cox [2].)

ablate both accessory atriofascicular (atrio–Hisian) bypass tracts and accessory nodoventricular connections.

The first clinical application of the discrete surgical procedure for AV node reentry tachycardia was performed in a 35-year-old female on August 13, 1982 [2]. Three other patients have undergone the procedure for reciprocating tachycardia due to reentry within the AV node, three patients for accessory nodoventricular connections, and one patient for an accessory atriofascicular bypass tract. The procedure has been uniformly successful in these eight patients without the necessity for pacemaker implantation.

Summary and Conclusions

The safety and efficacy of surgical therapy for the treatment of the WPW syndrome has been documented. Although several different surgical techniques may be employed, the endocardial approach that has evolved during the past 17 years continues to be the procedure of choice in our hands. Recently, the ability to apply small cryolesions to the peri-AV nodal tissues to alter

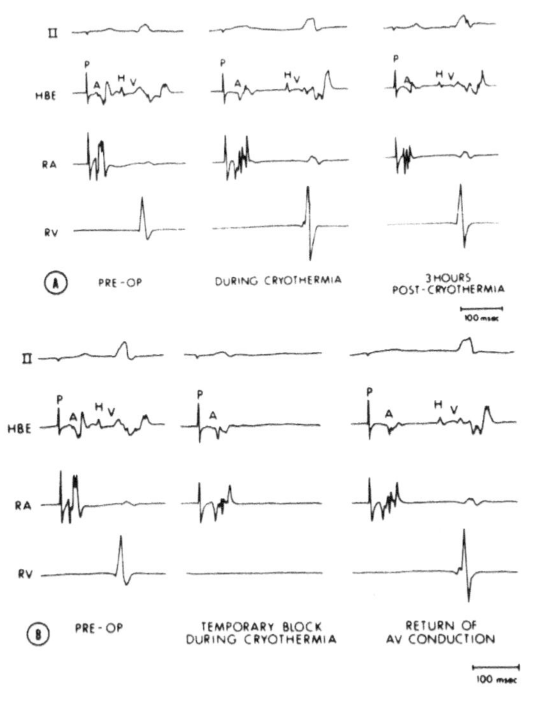

FIGURE 26–6. (A) Typical electrophysiologic changes during application of cryothermia. The AH interval prolongs to a maximal value at the termination of the cryolesion and shows persistent prolongation three hours postoperatively. (B) Third degree heart block occurring in the AV node region as shown by the loss of the H and V complexes during the cryothermic exposure. This block is only temporary if the cryothermic exposure is promptly terminated. P = pacing artifact; A = atrial depolarization; H = His bundle depolarization; V = ventricular depolarization; II = limb-lead II; HBE = His bundle electrogram; RA = right atrial bipolar electrograms; RV = right ventricular bipolar electrogram. (Reproduced by permission from Holman et al. [15].)

abnormal AV conduction without creating heart block has provided a means of surgically modifying AV node conduction properties and ablating accessory connections in and around the AV node in a manner that has proven to be as selective as the procedures employed for the interruption of accessory AV connections associated with the WPW syndrome. Thus our clinical experience indicates that, if necessary, any type of preexcitation syndrome can be treated surgically with success rates approaching 100%.

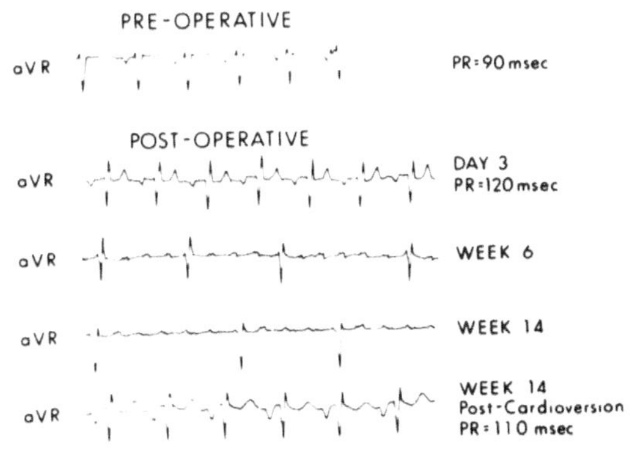

FIGURE 26–7. Decrease in the ventricular response rate to spontaneous atrial flutter at 6 and 14 weeks after this animal had undergone discrete cryosurgery at the AV node. The usual response in dogs to spontaneous atrial flutter is 2:1 AV conduction block resulting in a ventricular response rate of 150 beats per minute. Following discrete cryosurgery of the AV node, this animal demonstrated 5:1 and 6:1 AV conduction block during spontaneous atrial flutter despite the fact that normal 1:1 AV conduction with only slight prolongation of the PR interval was present during normal sinus rhythm. (Reproduced by permission from Cox [2].)

References

1. Gallagher JJ, Sealy WC, Cox JL, German LD, Kasell JH, Bardy GH, Packer DL: Results of surgery for pre-excitation caused by accessory atrioventricular pathways in 267 consecutive cases. In *Tachycardias: Mechanisms, Diagnosis, and Treatment* Josephson ME, Wellens HJJ (eds.). Lea & Febiger, Philadelphia, 1984, pp. 259–269.
2. Cox JL: Surgery for cardiac arrhythmias. *Current Problems in Cardiology*. Yearbook Medical Publishers, Chicago, VIII, No. 4, July 1983.
3. Cox JL: Status of surgery for cardiac arrhythmias *Circulation* 71:413, 1985.
4. Sealy WC: The surgical treatment of arrhythmias caused by accessory pathways of atrioventricular conduction. In *Cardiac Arrhythmias, a Decade of Progress* Harrison DC (ed.). GK Hall Medical Publishers, Boston, 1981, pp. 431–445.
5. Cox JL: Surgical management of cardiac arrhythmias. In Gibbon's *Surgery of the Chest* (4th Ed.), Sabiston DC, Jr, Spencer FC (eds.). WB Saunders Company, Philadelphia, pp. 1552–1584, 1983.
6. Gallagher JJ, Kasell JH, Cox JL, Smith WM, Ideker RE, Smith WM: The techniques of

intraoperative electrophysiologic mapping, *Am. J. Cardiol.* 49:221, 1982.

7. Witkowski FX, Cain ME, Corr PB: A system for true simultaneous isochronic and isovoltaic mapping of the myocardium. (Abstract.) *Circulation* 68 (Supp II):360, 1983.
8. Cox JL, Gallagher JJ, and Cain ME: Experience with 118 consecutive patients undergoing operation for the Wolff-Parkinson-White syndrome. *J. Thorac. Cardiovasc. Surg.* 90:490, 1985.
9. Kramer JB, Corr PB, Cox JL, Witkowski FX, Cain ME: Simultaneous computer mapping to facilitate intraoperative localization of accessory pathways in patients with Wolff-Parkinson-White syndrome. *Am. J. Cardial* 56:571, 1985.
10. Gallagher JJ, Sealy WC, Cox JL, Kasell JH: Results of surgery for pre-excitation in 200 Cases. (Abstract.) *Circulation* 64 (Suppl II):545, 1981.
11. Klein GJ, Guiraudon G, Perkins DG, Jones DL, Yee R, Jarvis E: Surgical correction of the Wolff-Parkinson-White syndrome in the closed heart using cryosurgery: A simplified approach. *J. Am. Coll. Cardiol.* 3:405, 1984.
12. Sealy WC, Gallagher JJ, and Kasell JH: His bundle interruption for control of inappropriate ventricular responses to atrial arrhythmias: *Ann. Thorac. Surg.* 32:429, 1981.
13. Scheinman M, Morady F, Hess DS, Gonzalez R: Catheter-induced ablation of the atrioventricular junction to control refractory supraventricular arrhythmias *JAMA* 7:851, 1982.
14. Gallagher JJ, Svenson RH, and Kasell JH, German LD, Bardy GH, Broughton A, Critelli G: Catheter technique for closed chest ablation of the atrioventricular conduction system. A therapeutic alternative for the treatment of refractory supraventricular tachycardia. *N. Engl. J. Med.* 306:194, 1982.
15. Holman WL, Ikeshita M, Lease JG, Smith PK, Ferguson TB, Jr, Cox JL: Elective prolongation of atrioventricular conduction by multiple discrete cryolesions. A new technique for the treatment of paroxysmal supraventricular tachycardia. *J. Thorac. Cardiovasc. Surg.* 84:554, 1982.
16. Anderson RH, Becker AE: Cardiac anatomy for the surgeon. In Sabiston DC, Jr (ed.). *Lewis Practice of Surgery, Cardiovascular Surgery Volume*, Harper & Row, Maryland, 1979, p. 29.

27. SURGICAL TREATMENT OF WOLFF-PARKINSON-WHITE SYNDROME: THE EPICARDIAL APPROACH

Gerard M. Guiraudon
George J. Klein
Arjun D. Sharma
Douglas L. Jones

The Wolff-Parkinson-White (WPW) syndrome provides us with the most lucid model of cardiac arrhythmias amenable to surgery. The mechanism of arrhythmias [1] and the underlying anatomic substrates [2] are well understood and the localization of accessory pathways can be accurately achieved in the electrophysiology laboratory [3–4]. The first successful ablation of an accessory atrioventricular (AV) pathway by W.C. Sealy provided the critical evidence for the role of the accessory pathway as the basis for preexcitation syndrome [5].

Surgery for WPW syndrome was developed using an endocardial approach [6] which necessitates cardiopulmonary bypass, myocardial preservation with cold cardioplegia, opening of cardiac chambers, and dissection of the AV fat pad through an atrial endocardial incision along the AV anulus. This technique yielded a high success rate with low mortality [7], although a significant incidence of inadvertent AV block was observed following attempted ablation of septal accessory AV pathways [8]. Recently, we developed an epicardial approach for the ablation of left free wall accessory pathway [9]. The technique combines the mobilization of the AV fat pad from the epicardial side and the exposure and cryoablation of the AV junction at the site of the accessory pathway on the normal, beating heart (Figure 27–1). This approach does not require opening of the heart, avoids cross-clamping of the aorta and myocardial preservation, and often obviates need for cardiopulmonary bypass. The latter may decrease surgical risk, especially that related to aortic cross-clamping [10–11] and also enables continuous monitoring of accessory pathway function until the instant of ablation. The latter allows instant assessment of the efficacy of ablation without the need for rewarming and closing the heart. Since our initial experience with free wall pathways, we have extended the use of the technique to the posteroseptal pathway. Anteroseptal pathways still require an endocardial approach because of their endocardial location and proximity to the His bundle [12].

Supported in part by a grant from the Heart and Stroke Foundation of Ontario.

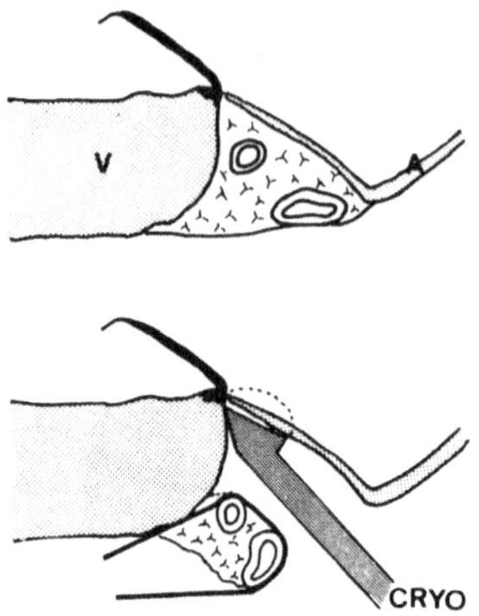

FIGURE 27–1. Rationale for epicardial approach: The upper drawing depicts a cross-section of the AV sulcus. Coronary artery and vein course along the AV sulcus. The lower drawing depicts the surgical rationale. The AV fat pad has been mobilized as well as the coronary artery and vein. The AV junction is cryoblated using a cryoprobe (−60°C, 2 min). Abbreviations: V = ventricle; A = atria; CRYO = cryoprobe.

Patient Population and Selection for Surgery

The selection of patients for surgical correction was based on clinical and electrophysiologic criteria. Consideration was given to the efficacy of drug therapy and its side effects, to the patient's acceptance of medical treatment, to the life-threatening potential of the arrhythmia, and to the impact of attacks on the patient's life-style.

The patient population was composed of 29 females and 46 males, ranging in age from 6 years to 52 with a mean of 32 ± 13. Fifty-eight patients had WPW syndrome and 17 had a concealed accessory AV pathway. All patients had palpitations, 18 patients had syncope, and 13 had been cardioverted at least once. All patients had paroxysmal tachycardia, and those patients with WPW syndrome had a mean RR interval during atrial fibrillation or flutter of 260 ms (range 140–400). Accessory AV pathway locations were left-sided in 48, posterior septal in 8, right-sided in 3, and anterior septal in 9. Three patients had multiple accessory AV pathways. Five patients had associated structural heart disease (Ebstein's anomaly of the tricuspid valve, myocardiopathy, aortic insufficiency, atrial septal defect and coronary artery disease).

OPERATIVE TECHNIQUE

The heart was exposed via a median sternotomy in all but one patient with left-sided free wall accessory pathway whose heart was approached through a left lateral thoracotomy.

Intra-operative cardiac mapping was obtained during sinus rhythm and reciprocating tachycardia [13]. When sustained reciprocating tachycardia could not be obtained, the atria were mapped during ventricular pacing. If reciprocating tachycardia was associated with low arterial pressure, cardiac mapping was carried out under the "cover" of normothermic cardiopulmonary bypass. There was an excellent correlation between preoperative and intraoperative accessory pathway localization. Normothermic cardiopulmonary bypass was used in 46 patients with a mean bypass time of 80 min (ranging from 35–240 min).

LEFT-SIDED ACCESSORY AV PATHWAYS

Left-sided accessory AV pathways were present in 42 patients. The site of the accessory pathway was closely related to the obtuse marginal region. Surgery was carried out under the cover of normothermic cardiopulmonary bypass in 41 patients. One patient with significant aortic insufficiency which did not require a surgical treatment had his left-sided free wall accessory pathway ablated via a left thoracotomy without cardiopulmonary bypass.

The left AV sulcus was exposed by dislocating the heart. Mobilization of the left AV fat pad was carried out as follows (Figure 27–2). The epicardium was incised along the atrial limit of the AV fat pad, 2–3 cm away from the coronary sinus which was always readily visible. The left atrial vein was consistently present and was divided to allow coronary sinus mobilization. There was always a clean, dry dissection plane between the coronary sinus and the left atrial wall. We never observed the "classical" myocardial fibers which are said to cover the coronary sinus [14]. Coronary sinus mobilization was the key to mobilization of the whole AV fat pad. The circumflex coronary artery was then identified. It was easily found in the upper part of the sulcus near the left appendage attachment. At that point, the AV fat pad was mobilized away from the left atrial wall, and the AV

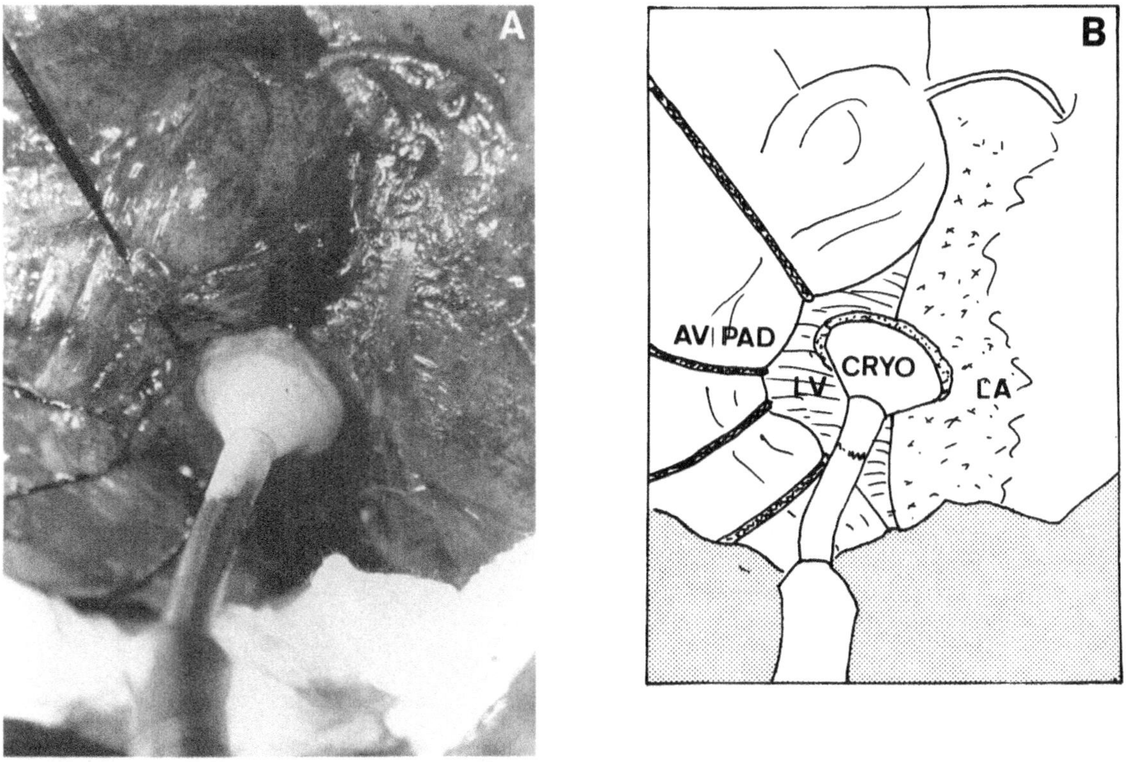

FIGURE 27–2. (A) An operative view of the left-sided free wall surgical approach. (B) Schematic drawing of the operative view: The left AV fat pad has been dissected away, and the AV sulcus is exposed. A cryoprobe 1.5 cm in diameter (−60°C, 2 min) is applied at the site of accessory AV pathway.

junction and the left ventricular wall were exposed using blunt dissection with direct visualization of the coronary sinus and coronary artery. If present, the left atrial coronary artery branch was divided. The circumflex coronary artery was intramural in seven patients. The myocardial fibers which bridge the coronary artery were severed and the coronary artery mobilized without further difficulty. Puncture of the left atrium occurred in three patients and was readily repaired. Most of the left AV fat pad was mobilized to provide an appropriate exposure of the AV junction at the site of the accessory pathway. Following surgical exposure, the AV junction was cryoablated using three overlapping applications of a probe 1.5 cm in diameter, cooled to −60°C for 2 minutes. During cryoablation, the coronary sinus and coronary arteries were kept away from the ice ball.

POSTEROSEPTAL

Posteroseptal accessory pathways were present in eight patients. Posteroseptal accessory AV pathways attach onto the posterior inferior process of the left ventricular free wall. The posterior inferior process of the left ventricle corresponds to the part of the left ventricular wall situated between the mitral valve anulus posteriorly and the muscular attachment of the tricuspid septal leaflet anteriorly. Superiorly, the posterior inferior process of the left ventricle is delineated by the inferior edge of the membranous septum which harbors part of the AV node–His bundle. Inferiorly, the posterior inferior process of the left ventricle has no well-defined limits. The inferior wall of the right atrium lays on the posterior inferior process of the left ventricle; consequently, there is an AV sulcus between the posterior inferior process of the left ventricle and the right atrium. The right atrial–left ventricular sulcus is deep. It meets anteriorly and to the right with the right AV sulcus and posteriorly and to the left with the left AV sulcus. It harbors the right coronary artery and its bifurcation. The posterior inferior process of the left ventricle and the right atrial–left ventricular junction can be exposed by mobilizing the right atrial–left ventricular fat pad which fills the right atrial–left ventricular sulcus. Then, the posterior inferior process of the left ventricle, the right atrial–left ventricular junction as well as the adjacent right and left AV junction can be cryoablated while closely monitoring AV conduction of the normothermic beating heart. The latter is critical in preventing inadvertent AV block. Epicardial ventricular mapping can determine with precision, the site of insertion of the accessory pathway either onto the posterior inferior process of the left ventricle or the adjacent right ventricle or left-sided free wall (Figure 27–3).

The same rationale as for left-sided free wall accessory pathways is used to mobilize the right atrial–left ventricular fat pad. The dissection is carried out in the beating heart. The posteroseptal region can be approached without dislocating the heart. The dissection is commenced by mobilizing the paraseptal part of the right AV fat pad (Figure 27–4). The right coronary artery is identified, and the right atrial–left ventricular fat pad is mobilized. The coronary sinus is not situated in the fat pad but lies posteriorly and to the left. This approach provides good exposure of the posterior inferior process of the left ventricle and adjacent right ventricular free wall. When the exposure of the adjacent left ventricular free wall is needed (i.e., for left posteroseptal accessory pathways), this right septal approach must be combined with a "limited" paraseptal left ventricular free wall approach. The posterior superior process of the left ventricle and adjacent right ventricular and

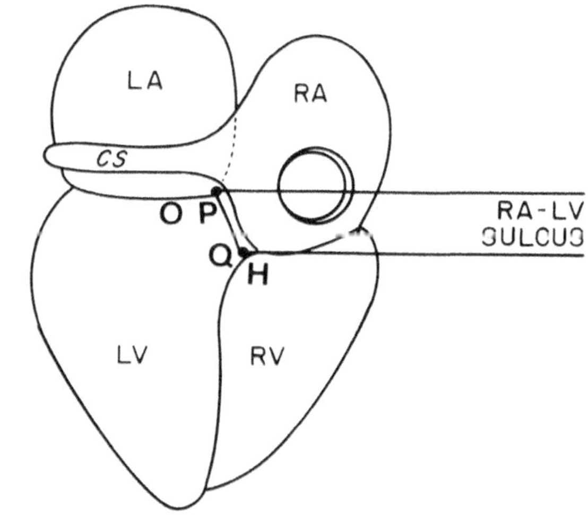

FIGURE 27–3. Epicardial mapping of the posterior septal region: The drawing depicts an inferior view of the heart. The right atrial – left ventricular sulcus is situated between the posterior inferior process of the left ventricle and the right atrial inferior wall. Sites P and Q correspond to the posterior process of the left ventricle (Posterior septal accessory pathways). Site O corresponds to the adjacent left-sided free wall (left posterior accessory pathways). Abbreviations: LA = left atrium; RA = right atrium; CS = coronary sinus; LV = left ventricle; RV = right ventricle.

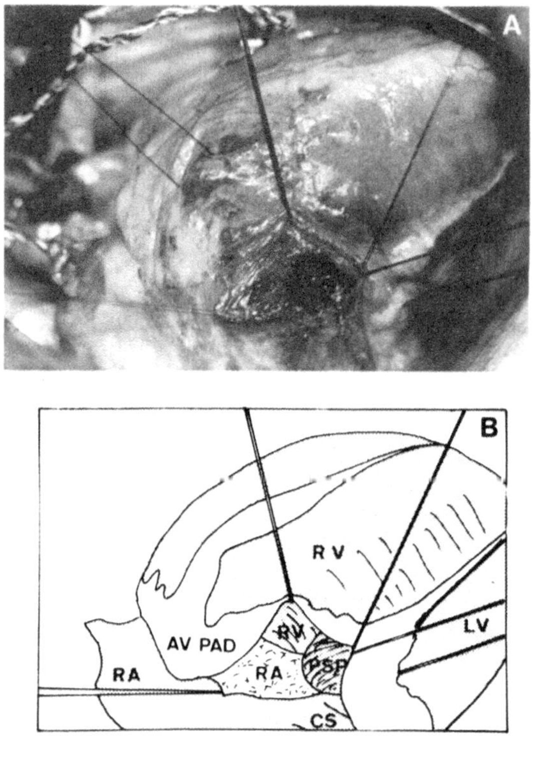

FIGURE 27–4. (A) Operative view of the posterior septal approach. (B) Schematic drawing of the operative view: The inferior wall of the heart is exposed. The right atrioventricular fat pad, and the RA-LV fat pad has been dissected and mobilized. The posterior inferior process of the left ventricle, and the adjacent right-sided free wall are exposed. Abbreviation: RA = right atrium; RV = right ventricle; AV PAD = atrioventricular fat pad; LV = left ventricle; CS = coronary sinus; PSP = posterior inferior process of the left ventricle.

left ventricular free wall are exposed and cryoablated using overlapping applications of a cryoprobe, 0.5 cm in diameter, cooled to −60°C for 2 minutes. AV conduction is monitored and freezing is abruptly terminated if AV block occurs. The posteroseptal approach may be carried out without cardiopulmonary bypass. In two patients, cardiopulmonary bypass was not used.

RIGHT-SIDED ACCESSORY AV PATHWAYS
Right ventricular free wall accessory AV pathways were ablated using a technique identical to that for left-sided free wall pathways, without cardiopulmonary bypass.

ANTEROSEPTAL ACCESSORY AV PATHWAYS
Anterior septal accessory AV pathways were present in nine patients. In all cases, atrial and ventricular activation sequence mapping resulted in a large discrepancy between the apparent ventricular and atrial insertions of the accessory pathway. Ventricular mapping suggested an insertion of the accessory pathway near the base of the infundibulum of the right ventricle, 1.5 to 2.0 cm away from the membranous septum. Conversely, atrial mapping during reciprocating tachycardia suggested an atrial insertion deep in the septum in the para–Hisian region. Observations during atrial mapping were consistent with those obtained during preoperative endocardial mapping.

A step-by-step epicardial approach was used on the normothermic, beating heart (Figure 27–5):

1. The right AV fat pad in the anterior septal region (right coronary fossa) was dissected and mobilized.
2. The right AV junction was exposed as were the aortic root and the upper part of the membranous septum.
3. The tricuspid valve anulus was identified and exposed up to its insertion onto the membranous septum. Up to that point, the delta wave was still present.
4. The cryoprobe cooled to −5° was then applied to the AV junction. The delta wave, and AV conduction through the His bundle disappeared only when the cryoprobe was applied onto the membranous septum and did so simultaneously.
5. Under normothermic cardiopulmonary bypass, the right atrial wall was incised along its insertion onto the exposed tricuspid valve anulus and the atrial portion of the membranous septum was exposed.
6. The delta wave disappeared only when the right atrial myocardial fibers covering the right side of the membranous septum were ablated, while normal conduction through the AV node–His bundle system persisted.

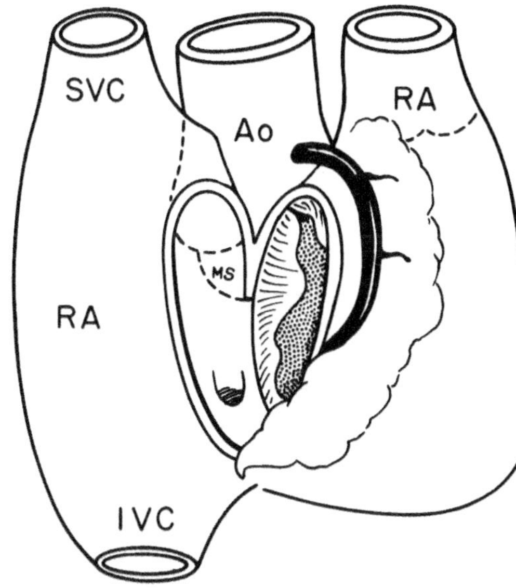

FIGURE 27–5. Schematic operative view of the surgical approach to anterior septal accessory pathways: The "septal" part of the right AV fat pad is dissected and mobilized. The right coronary artery is identified. The right atrium is opened along its attachment onto the tricuspid anulus. The atrial membranous septum is exposed. The accessory pathway is ablated when right atrial septum myocardium is incised.

This approach taught us that anteroseptal pathways are endocardial and closely related to the His bundle. The anteroseptal pathway remains the only one, necessitating an endocardial approach [12].

MULTIPLE ACCESSORY PATHWAYS
Two patients had multiple accessory AV pathways. Both had a posteroseptal accessory pathways associated with a left-sided free wall accessory pathway in one and an anterior septal accessory pathway in the other. The epicardial approach was used for the posteroseptal acces-

sory pathway at that point in our experience. In a third patient, with an accessory AV pathway conducting only in the retrograde direction, atrial mapping did not clearly localize the accessory pathway in the anterior septal or posteroseptal region. The posteroseptal region was first approached on the normothermic, beating heart using an epicardial approach to ablate the posteroseptal pathway. Afterwards, atrial mapping was repeated and clearly demonstrated the second accessory pathway in the anterior septal region. This was ablated using the epicardial approach without development of heart block. The latter patient exemplifies the advantages of the epicardial approach in patients with multiple accessory pathways; a reliable map can be obtained immediately after the completion of the first ablative procedure, thereby permitting immediate evaluation of its effectiveness.

Before the chest was closed, the absence of abnormal conduction through an accessory pathway was verified by studying anterograde and retrograde AV conduction using stimulation techniques. Pairs of temporary pacing wires were inserted over each cardiac chamber of later postoperative stimulation studies.

Operative Results

The operation was tolerated without complication in all patients, and each patient underwent electrical stimulation of the heart prior to discharge using temporary pacing electrodes. There was no evidence of conduction through an accessory pathway at these studies. Antiarrhythmic drugs were not required postoperatively. Patients have remained free from arrhythmia during a mean follow-up of 15 months.

Summary and Conclusion

The epicardial operative approach is applicable to all accessory AV pathway locations. The left sided free wall, posteroseptal and right-sided free wall accessory pathways can be ablated using a closed heart technique. The epicardial approach simplifies the ablative procedure for anterior septal accessory pathways, although an endocardial approach of the septal region is still needed using normothermic cardiopulmonary bypass.

The success rate of the epicardial approach is at least as good as the endocardial approach, (88% to 96%) [7–12]. The ablative procedure is carried out on the beating heart, allowing continuous monitoring of AV conduction which reduces likliehood of inducing inadvertent AV node–His bundle injury. The endocardial approach does not share this advantage since cross-clamping of the aorta associated with myocardial cardioplegia necessitates fibrillating the ventricles and precludes monitoring status of AV conduction. This limitation of the endocardial approach accounts in part for occurrence of postoperative transient or permanent AV block [8].

Surgical risk may be decreased using the closed heart technique since it avoids cross-clamping of the aorta. Intraoperative low output failure due to inadequate myocardial preservation, may occur even in the normal heart despite attempts to keep aortic cross-clamping time short [16]. In our experience, avoidance of aortic cross-clamping significantly decreased the incidence of atrial fibrillation in the perioperative period using the epicardial approach compared to (25%) using endocardial open heart technique ($p < .01$).

Surgical morbidity may be decreased further by avoiding cardiopulmonary bypass. Cardiopulmonary bypass is not required for the ablation of right ventricular free wall accessory pathways and can be easily avoided for posteroseptal accessory pathways. Left ventricular free wall accessory pathways may be ablated without the cover of cardiopulmonary bypass, if the left AV sulcus is approached through a left thoracotomy. However, the relative benefits of median sternotomy combined with cardiopulmonary bypass versus left thoracotomy without cardiopulmonary bypass is not established yet. Left thoracotomy is associated with poorer lung function postoperatively in terms of vital capacity and peak air flow [18]. However, this disadvantage may be offset by avoidance of the potential hazard of normothermic cardiopulmonary bypass assistance.

Surgery on the normothermic beating heart has two specific advantages: (1) AV conduction can be continuously monitored, and the risk of inadvertent AV block is decreased; (2) a reliable cardiac activation sequence map can be obtained immediately after attempting surgical ablation of the accessory pathway. Consequently, effectiveness of the ablation procedure can be assessed immediately, and the presence of additional accessory pathways can be recognized [19].

Our experience with the epicardial operative approach suggests that left ventricular free wall, posteroseptal and right ventricular free wall accessory AV pathways are epicardial structures, approachable using the closed, external approach. Anterior septal accessory pathways are deep, endocardial structures [12] but may be successfully ablated using the endocardial operative approach (see chapter by Cox and Cain, this volume).

References

1. Durrer D, Schuilenburg RM, Wellens HJJ: Preexcitation revisited. *Am. J. Cardiol.* 25:690, 1970.
2. Anderson RH, Becker AE: Stanley Kent and accessory atrioventricular connections. *J. Thorac. Cardiovasc. Surg.* 81:649, 1981.
3. Gallagher JJ, Gilbert M, Svenson RH, Sealy WC, Kasell J, Wallace AG: Wolff-Parkinson-White Syndrome. The problem, evaluation, and surgical correction. *Circulation* 51:767, 1975.
4. Klein GJ, Guiraudon GM: Surgical therapy of cardiac arrhythmias. *Cardiol. Clin.*, Arrhythmias II 1:2, 323–340, 1983.
5. Sealy WC, Hattler BG, Blumenschein SD, Cobb FR: Surgical treatment of Wolff-Parkinson-White Syndrome. *Ann. Thorac. Surg.* 8, 1:3, 1969.
6. Sealy WC, Gallagher JJ, Wallace AG: The surgical treatment of Wolff-Parkinson-White Syndrome: evolution of improved methods for identification and interruption of the kent bundle. *Ann. Thorac. Surg.* 22, 5:443, 1976.
7. Gallagher JJ, Sealy WC, Cox JL, German LD, Kasell JH, Bardy GH, Packer DL: Results of surgery for preexcitation caused by accessory atrioventricular pathways in 267 consecutive cases. *Tachycardias: Mechanisms–Diagnosis–Treatment*, by ME Josephson, HJJ Wellens, Lea & Febiger, Philadelphia, 1984, pp. 259–269.
8. Sealy WC, Gallagher JJ: The surgical approach to the septal area of the heart based on experiences with 45 patients with Kent bundles. *J. Thorac. Cardiovasc. Surg.* 79:542, 1980.
9. Guiraudon GM, Klein GJ, Gulamhusein S, Jones DL, Yee R, Perkins DG, Jarvis E: Surgical repair of Wolff-Parkinson-White syndrome: A new closed-heart technique. *Ann. Thorac. Surg.* 37, 1:67, 1984.
10. Conti VR, Bertranou EG, Blackstone EH, Kirklin JW, Digerness SB: Cold cardioplegia versus hypothermia for myocardial protection. Randomized clinical study. *J. Thorac. Cardiovasc. Surg.* 76, 5:577, 1978.
11. Miller DC, Stinson EB, Oyer PE, Jamieson SW, Mitchell RS, Reitz BA, Baumagartner WA, Shumway NE: Discriminant analysis of the changing risks of coronary artery operations: 1971–1979. *J. Thorac. Cardiovasc. Surg.* 85:197, 1983.
12. Guiraudon GM, Klein GJ, Sharma AD, Jones DL: Anteroseptal AV pathways are true septal para-Hisian structures: Verification by ice mapping. (Abstract.) *Circulation* (Supp II) 70:338, 1984.
13. Gallagher JJ, Kasell J, Sealy WC, Pritchett ELC, Wallace AG: Epicardial mapping in the Wolff-Parkinson-White syndrome. *Circulation* 57, 5:854, 1978.
14. Hollinshead WH: *Textbook of Anatomy*. 3rd Ed. Hagerstown, Maryland, Hoeber Med Div, Harper & Row, 1974, p. 531.
15. Uther JB, Johnson DC, Baird DK, et al: Surgical section of accessory atrioventricular electrical connections in 108 patients. (Abstract.) *Am. J. Cardiol.* 49:995, 1982.
16. Pennington DG, Merjavy JP, Swartz MT, Codd JE, Barner HB, Lagunoff D, Bashiti H, Kaiser GC, Willman VL: The importance of biventricular failure in patients with postoperative cardiogenic shock. *Ann. Thorac. Surg.* 39, 1:16, 1985.
17. Smith PK, Buhrman WC, Levett JM, Ferguson TB, Holman WL, Cox JL: Supraventricular conduction abnormalities following cardiac operations. A complication of inadequate atrial preservation. *J. Thorac. Cardiovasc. Surg.* 85:105, 1983.
18. Cooper JD, Nelems JM, Pearson FG: Extended indications for median sternotomy in patients requiring pulmonary resection. *Ann. Thorac. Surg.* 26, 5:413, 1978.
19. Iwa T, Magara T, Watanabe Y, Kawasuji M, Misaki T: Interruption of multiple accessory conduction pathways in the Wolff-Parkinson-White syndrome. *Ann. Thorac. Surg.* 30, 4:313, 1980.

VI. FUTURE PROSPECTS

28. UNRESOLVED ISSUES IN EVALUATION AND TREATMENT OF PREEXCITATION SYNDROMES

David G. Benditt
D. Woodrow Benson

The preexcitation syndromes have been the subject of extensive study, particularly during the last two decades. As a result, we have derived an understanding of both the anatomic substrates of the syndromes and the pathophysiology of its related tachyarrhythmias which far exceeds that of any other disorder associated with cardiac rhythm disturbances. Further, techniques for the precise analysis of the rhythm disorders associated with the preexcitation syndromes have been developed, and a relatively extensive medical and surgical armamentarium for treatment and in some instances of apparent cure of the underlying problem has resulted. Nonetheless, many aspects of the preexcitation syndromes remain to be explored and clarified. The purpose of this chapter is to highlight certain elements of these syndromes in which the final word is not yet in. The list is certainly not comprehensive. However, we hope that it will provide a stimulus for further study of a number of clinically pertinent issues, ultimately leading to both greater insight into these syndromes on the part of interested physicians and scientists and better treatment for patients.

The authors would like to thank H. Gareth Tobler M.D. and Fredrick Verhage for research assistance, and Wendy Markuson for preparing the manuscript.

Indications for Invasive Electrophysiologic Study

Electrophysiologic studies in patients with preexcitation syndromes often prove useful from both diagnostic and therapeutic points of view. However, the elements comprising an appropriate study may vary considerably from patient to patient. Such studies require careful advance planning, and should only be carried out in well-equipped dedicated electrophysiology laboratories by experienced individuals [1].

At the present time, there is no compelling reason to recommend invasive electrophysiologic studies in all patients suspected of having preexcitation syndromes. On the other hand, a consensus of opinion on reasonable indications for recommending studies has yet to be derived. To this end, Table 28–1 summarizes a proposed list of indications for study, and a corresponding list of diagnostic and therapeutic decisions to be obtained given the specific clinical circumstances. Additionally, we have attempted to provide below insight into many of the vagaries surrounding recommendations for proceeding with invasive study.

TACHYCARDIAS REFRACTORY TO EMPIRIC THERAPY

The point in time at which empiric therapy is considered to have failed is largely arbitrary, and guidelines for defining failure of empiric treatment are not readily available. At the pre-

TABLE 28–1. Indications for and Objectives of Electrophysiologic Study.

Indications for study	Principal objectives diagnostic decisions	Principal objectives therapeutic decisions
1. Recurrent regular tachycardias with normal QRS refractory to empiric therapy.	a. Establish tachycardia diagnosis. b. Define type, number, and location of AC. c. Assess participation of AC in tachycardia.	a. Determine effect of candidate antiarrhythmic drugs on AC and symptomatic tachycardia (both parenteral and oral drug studies). b. Consider suitability for AC ablation (i.e., surgical risk, AC site(s)) versus long-term drug therapy.
2. Wide QRS complex tachycardia of unknown type, but with a regular rhythm.	a. Establish tachycardia diagnosis, differentiating primary atrial tachycardias or reentry within AV node with bystander preexcitation, antidromic RT, orthodromic RT with BBB, and VT. b. Define type, number, and location of AC.	a. Determine effect of candidate antiarrhythmic drugs on AC and symptomatic tachycardia (both parenteral and oral drug studies). b. Consider suitability for AC ablation (i.e., surgical risk, AC site(s) versus long-term drug therapy.
3. Wide QRS complex tachycardia with an irregular rhythm.	a. Define type, number, and location of AC. b. Assess AC participation in tachycardia, and hemodynamic response. c. Assess potential hazard of AC by refractory period measurements supine, tilt, exercise, catecholamines, and during AF.	a. Determine effect of candidate antiarrhythmic drugs on AC and symptomatic tachycardia (both parenteral and oral drug studies). b. Consider suitability for AC ablation (i.e., surgical risk, AC site(s)) versus long-term drug therapy.
4. Previous life-threatening arrhythmia or hemodynamic collapse without documented arrhythmia with or without ECG evidence of preexcitation.	a. Define type, number, and location of AC. b. Assess potential hazard of AC, and determine whether consistent with clinical presentation (i.e., look for other possible causes) c. Assess suitability for ablation of AC (i.e., surgical risk, AC site(s)).	a. Determine effect of candidate antiarrhythmic drugs on AC and symptomatic tachycardia (both parenteral and oral drug studies). b. Consider suitability for AC ablation (i.e., surgical risk, AC site(s)) versus long-term drug therapy.
5. Other cardiac surgery planned.	a. Define type, number, and location of AC. b. Assess suitability for ablation of AC (i.e., surgical risk, AC sites(s)).	a. Consider suitability for AC ablation (i.e., surgical risk, AC site(s)) versus long-term drug therapy.

Abbreviations: AC = accessory connection; AF = atrial fibrillation; BBB = bundle branch block; RT = reciprocating tachycardia.

sent time, in the patient without life-threatening arrhythmias, failure of empiric therapy appears to most closely coincide with the point in time when usual doses of conventional antiarrhythmic agents have either been found to yield excessive side effects or have failed to prevent symptomatic tachycardia.

EVALUATION OF THE POTENTIAL HAZARD ASSOCIATED WITH ACCESSORY AV CONNECTIONS

In patients with ventricular preexcitation, documenting the electrophysiologic properties of the anatomic substrate and assessing its capacity for participating in potentially life-threatening tachyarrhythmias are widely accepted as primary goals of invasive electrophysiologic testing. However, the basic requirements for such a procedure to achieve these objectives have not been unequivocally established. Further, the interpretation of certain commonly elicited observations — in particular, measurement of effective refractory period of accessory connections and the ventricular response during stimulation-induced atrial fibrillation — have yet to be assessed critically in a prospective study capable of determining their prognostic value.

Study Requirements. The requirements for the complete electrophysiologic characterization of accessory connections have been presented in detail in preceding chapters. Nonetheless, a continued search for methods of improving the conventional electrophysiologic approach is crucial. For example, at the present time, measurement of the effective refractory period of accessory connections in the antegrade (atrioventricular [AV]) direction is considered a critical element of the assessment of the electrophysiologic hazard [2–4]. However, this assessment is typically carried out in the supine resting individual. The possible importance of examining electrophysiologic characteristics of accessory connections under a variety of pharmacological and neurohumoral conditions, such as may be achieved by graded isoproterenol infusions or by the use of exercise and tilt, has only recently begun to be studied [5–7]. Further, while the potential importance of assessing refractoriness characteristics over a wide range of basic pacing cycle lengths has been alluded to [8], particularly in the evaluation of antiarrhythmic drug effects on accessory AV connections [9,10], the possible prognostic value of such observations in the untreated patient undergoing initial evaluation has not been clearly defined.

The likelihood of an individual with preexcitation syndrome developing atrial fibrillation spontaneously has not been determined prospectively. Nonetheless assessing the ventricular response during stimulation-induced atrial fibrillation has become accepted as a necessary part of the assessment of the potential hazard associated with accessory AV connections. Concerns regarding interpretation of observations during atrial fibrillation are discussed below. However, the methodology also merits consideration. First, it is possible that atrial fibrillation induced by electrode catheter stimulation techniques may not be identical in all respects to the spontaneously occuring arrhythmia, and therefore may not adequately predict the response of the accessory connections in the nonlaboratory setting [11]. Second, the ventricular response in the resting supine patient may differ considerably from the response observed in the unsedated patient in the upright posture due to altered neurohumoral status. Finally, an analagous concern arises in the patient in whom spontaneous atrial fibrillation results in association with exercise or psychological stress; settings which are difficult to mimic accurately in the electrophysiologic laboratory.

An assessment of the hemodynamic consequences of tachyarrhythmias is among the most important pieces of information to be obtained in the evaluation of the potential hazard of an accessory connection(s) in the idividual patient. Nonetheless, continuous measurement of intraarterial pressure has yet to be considered an essential element of the electrophysiologic study. In our experience, the insights provided by such recordings have been invaluable, far exceeding the minimal risk entailed. In particular, intraarterial pressure recordings at the onset and during the initial phase of a tachycardia episode, with the patient in both the upright (which can be conveniently achieved in the catheterization laboratory by use of a tilt table) as well as the supine position, may provide valuable insight into the basis of symptoms in many instances.

INTERPRETATION OF THE LABORATORY OBSERVATIONS

In a small percentage of patients with preexcitation syndromes, life-threatening events requiring resuscitation may occur. Since ECG documentation during the event is rare in these instances, the demonstration of either the presence of an accessory AV connection with a short refractory period in the antegrade direction (typically less than 220 ms), or an exceedingly rapid ventricular response during stimulation-induced atrial fibrillation (typically a shortest RR interval less than 250 ms), has become accepted as indirect but strongly suggestive evidence implicating the accessory connection in the event. Often, under these circumstances, surgical ablation of the accessory connection(s) is advised. However, in the absence of a detailed hemodynamic evaluation in these patients (including exercise, fluid challenge, and even cardiac biopsy in some cases), the contribution of coexisting heart disease may be overlooked. Failure to recognize underlying conditions may leave apparently cured patients at risk.

Interpretation of the prognostic significance of either refractory period measurements or the ventricular response during atrial fibrillation is essentially uncharted territory, particularly in the patient who has not previously experienced a potentially lethal arrhythmia requiring resuscitation. For example, among the patients in the series reported by Klein et al. [12], shortest RR intervals less than 250 ms during atrial fibrillation were as common among patients who had not previously manifested ventricular fibrillation as those that had. The natural history of either group of patients is unknown. Therefore, while at the present time it is not uncommon for physicians to recommend treatment of such individuals with antiarrhythmic drugs or even ablation of accessory connections to reduce risk, the benefits of such advice are not yet solidly substantiated.

OPTIMIZATION OF PHARMACOLOGIC THERAPY

Electrophysiologic study is commonly recommended as a means of determining optimal antiarrhythmic drug therapy in patients with preexcitation syndromes. Indeed, clinical experience suggests that studies using parenteral antiarrhythmic drug administration, especially if followed by restudy on a short course of oral drug treatment, is useful. However, long-term follow-up comparison of arrhythmia control in patients in whom therapy was selected on an empiric basis with results in patients in whom therapy was determined by serial electropharmacologic testing is still pending. Surprisingly, there has been less interest in pursuing such studies in patients with tachyarrhythmias associated with the preexcitation syndromes than has been the case for patients with paroxysmal ventricular tachycardia. Outpatient follow-up tachniques, such as those described by Pritchett in this volume [and reference 13] will be required.

Role of Digitalis and Verapamil in Preexcitation Syndromes

DIGITALIS

The parenteral administration of digitalis has been associated with the development of ventricular fibrillation in a number of patients being treated acutely for tachyarrhythmias (most often atrial fibrillation) associated with preexcitation syndromes. Wellens and Durrer first pointed out the potential for intravenous digitalis administration to shorten the effective refractory period of accessory AV connections [14]. Subsequently, Sellers et al. [15] demonstrated that parenteral digitalis administration reduced the shortest RR interval observed during stimulation-induced atrial fibrillation in 6/22 (27%) patients. The mechanism of the apparent facilitation of conduction in the accessory connection is not known, but it has been recommended that physicians refrain from using digitalis in the preexcitation syndrome [3,4].

Several aspects of the digitalis story require clarification. Clearly there is little reason any longer to employ digitalis parenterally for the acute treatment of tachyarrhythmias including atrial fibrillation, especially in a patient whose medical history (particularly as it pertains to the possible presence of preexcitation syndrome) is not known to the treating physician. Thus, the strongest argument for avoiding the parenteral or chronic oral use of digitalis in patients with tachyarrhythmias may lie in the fact that numerous more effective therapies (including electrical cardioversion) are readily available. On the other hand, it has yet to be clearly demonstrated whether during chronic oral administration digitalis exerts the same actions on accessory AV connections as has been associated with the parenteral administration of this agent. Thus the potential hazard of digitalis in patients with preexcitation syndromes has been largely extrapolated from studies in which the parenterally administrated drug may have accentuated its central sympathomimetic effects.

VERAPAMIL

The parenteral administration of verapamil has been associated with both shortening of accessory connection effective refractory periods [16], and abbreviation of shortest preexcited RR intervals during atrial fibrillation [17,18], in patients with preexcitation. Consequently, concerns regarding the safety of verapamil in patients with preexcitation, similar to those associated with digitalis, have arisen. However, it appears likely that verapamil's potentially hazardous effects occur in response to increased circulating catecholamines resulting from drug-induced peripheral vasodilation, not as a direct effect of the drug on the accessory connection. Therefore, slow intravenous administration of verapamil, taking care to avoid hypotension, should prove to be safe and effective for treatment of paroxysmal reciprocating tachycardia. Similarly, chronic oral administration of the drug should prove safe for prophylaxis of reciprocating tachycardia in patients with preexcitation syndrome [18]. On the other hand, we have observed the development of profound hypotension as a result of excessively rapid verapamil infusion even in patients without preexcitation (especially if therapy failed to interrupt tachycardia). Furthermore, there appears to be no rationale for the administration of verapamil during atrial fibrillation in a patient in whom there is suspicion that the QRS complexes have a preexcited morphology. In the latter instance, there would appear to be little benefit to be gained, while exposing the patient to the several potential risks described above. The precise role of verapamil in patients with the preexcitation syndromes, and the appropriate doses and routes of administration for maximum safety and efficacy require further study.

OTHER SYMPATHOMIMETIC AND ANTIHYPERTENSIVE DRUGS

Given what has been learned of the possible adverse effects of digitalis and verapamil on electrophysiologic properties of accessory connections, it would be reasonable to assume that other drugs with sympathomimetic or vasodilator actions may act similarly. We are unaware that such effects have been examined systematically in patients with preexcitation syndromes.

Ablation of Accessory Connections: Indications and Techniques

The ablation of accessory AV connections represents one of the very rare instances in which cure of a tachyarrhythmia is achievable. In experienced hands, the success of operative ablation of accessory connections now approaches 100%, and is virtually independent of the site of the accessory connection(s). Furthermore, although still investigational, nonoperative techniques for ablation of accessory connections are being developed and may become particularly useful for ablation of accessory AV connections in a posteroseptal location (see Scheinman, Chapter 24). Nonetheless, although the growing enthusiasm for recommending ablation of accessory connections is readily understandable, the indications for this procedure have yet to be fully delineated, and the optimal technique for achieving ablation of accessory connections remain a source of debate (see Chapter 26 by Cox and Cain, and Chapter 27 by Guiraudon et al.).

INDICATIONS FOR ABLATION OF ACCESSORY CONNECTIONS

Life-threatening Tachycarrhythmias. The development of ventricular fibrillation or an exceedingly rapid ventricular rate resulting in hypotension, such as may occur in association with atrial fibrillation, atrial flutter, or reciprocating tachycardia in some patients with accessory AV connections, has been considered an absolute indication for recommending ablation of the accessory connection(s). However, prior to considering an ablation procedure, it is mandatory that other potentially causal factors be excluded (e.g., coronary artery disease, subtle forms of cardiomyopathy) and that as much evidence as possible be gathered to substantiate the role of the accessory connection in the event. Further, a recommendation to proceed with ablation of the accessory connection should be placed in perspective for the patient and family; namely, the natural history of patients with preexcitation syndrome who have been resuscitated following a life-threatening arrhythmia (whether untreated, treated with antiarrhythmic drugs, or treated by accessory connection ablation) has been incompletely defined.

Medically refractory tachyarrhythmias. By far the largest subgroup of patients with preexcitation syndromes who undergo ablation of accessory connections are those characterized as having failed conventional medical therapy, or in whom drug therapy resulted in intolerable side-effects and/or adverse reactions. Approximately 171 of the first 200 patients (86%) operated on the Duke University series would be so classified [19].

A crucial issue in this subset of candidates for accessory connection ablation is the definition of the term *refractory*. It has been evident for some time that the tachyarrhythmias associated with preexcitation syndromes are variable in their frequency and severity, often disappearing entirely for many years. Thus, it is conceivable that what appears to be refractory at one point in time may behave quite differently at a later date. On the other hand, it is uncertain whether it is safer to expose patients to antiarrhythmic medication for indefinite periods of time (either on a daily basis, or by use of periodic treatment regimens), or undertake the modest risk of an ablation procedure (estimated operative mortality of 1.5–2.0%, depending on the presence or absence of concomitant cardiac disease [19]).

Asymptomatic or minimally symptomatic patient. There would seem to be little justification in recommending accessory connection ablation in the patient without symptoms or the patient in whom symptoms are controlled by a single drug administered either daily or on a periodic treatment regimen [20]. However, from time to time physicians will encounter situations in which this rule may breakdown. For example, Gallagher et al. [19] reported operating on an asymptomatic patient in whom laboratory findings confirmed the potential for an exceedingly rapid ventricular response during atrial fibrillation and in whom there was a strong family history of sudden death associated with preexcitation syndromes. A similar situation may arise in the asymptomatic competitive athlete, commercial airline pilot, and so on in whom the diagnosis of preexcitation syndrome may have been made serendipitously. The appropriate direction to take in these instances is not yet clear.

Patient undergoing other cardiac surgery. A strong argument has been made for considering ablation of accessory connections known to be present in patients undergoing heart surgery for other reasons, even when there has been no documented tachyarrhythmia prior to surgery [21,22]. The case would seem particularly solid in instances where a prosthetic valve is being placed in the ipsilateral AV position. However, the added risk entailed in prolonging the operative procedure must be weighed carefully in these cases.

OPTIMAL TECHNIQUE FOR ABLATION OF ACCESSORY CONNECTIONS

Ablation of accessory AV connections can now be achieved by both operative and nonoperative (electrode catheter) techniques (see Scheinman this volume, and reference 23). By far the greatest experience at present rests with the endocardial surgical approach (see Cox and Cain, this volume). However, the epicardial technique described by Guiraudon provides a number of potentially important advantages. It is too early to compare these two operative techniques critically. Nonoperative, electrode catheter ablation of accessory AV connections is still in its developmental stages. Nonetheless, it appears that as long as the latter technique utilizes the electroshock approach it will likely be restricted in its use to connections in a posteroseptal location. Perforation of the coronary sinus during attempts to ablate leftsided accessory connections have already been observed. Alternatives to electroshock may provide a safer means of nonoperative accessory connection ablation at other sites.

Identifying Reentry Rhythms

Reciprocating tachycardias associated with preexcitation syndromes provide a model permitting development of techniques that may improve our understanding of the basis of other less-well-defined clinical tachycardias. For example, studies of entrainment in patients with accessory AV connections suggest the potential applicability of this technique for identifying the nature of other tachyarrhythmias [24].

Perplexing Problems

Many questions regarding ventricular preexcitation remain to be answered. Two particularly puzzling problems come to mind. First, even though accessory AV connections have been described at septal sites and sites along both the left and right AV groove, it is unclear why left freewall connections predominate. There has been no generally accepted hypothesis to explain the apparent nonrandom distribution of this developmental anomaly. If muscle mass alone were the explanation, one would expect right-sided predominance given the manner in which the heart develops in utero. Second, accessory AV connections with bidirectional conduction and conduction only in the retrograde (V-A) direction occur commonly, whereas accessory AV connections that conduct only in the antegrade direction are rare. Potentially, specialized recordings of electrical activity within accessory AV connections and their approaches, and further understanding of the role of concealed conduction in accessory connections, may shed light on this apparent idiosyncracy. We suspect that these and other perplexing problems will fuel the interest of investigators well into the future.

Summary

The preexcitation syndromes have proved to be a valuable accident of nature. The investigator has been provided a unique model with which to achieve greater insights into the mysteries of cardiac arrhythmias in humans. The studious physician has been provided at least this one opportunity to gain some understanding of the manner in which proposed therapies work. The surgeon has been provided a rare opportunity to effect a cure of an often-troublesome and occasionally life-threatening cardiac condition. However, the greatest gift provided by the preexcitation syndromes is an apparently inherent property which seems to drive students of biologic problems to further its understanding, yet which brings forth many more intriguing questions to be addressed as each former one is set aside. We hope that the closing remarks incorporated within this chapter will prove helpful in directing others toward a few of the multitude of queries yet to be answered.

References

1. Gettes LS, Zipes DP, Gillette PC, Josephson ME, Laks MM, Mirvis DM, Scheinman MM, Sheffield LT, Wu D: Personnel and equipment required for electrophysiologic testing. Report of the committee on electrocardiography and cardiac electrophysiology, council on clinical cardiology, The American Heart Association. *Circulation* 69:1219A, 1984.
2. Gallagher JJ, Gilbert M, Svenson RH, Sealy WC, Kasell J, Wallace AG: Wolff-Parkinson-White syndrome. The problem, evaluation, and surgical correction. *Circulation* 51:767, 1975.
3. Gallagher JJ, Pritchett ELC, Sealy WC, Kasell J, Wallace AG: The preexciation syndromes. *Prog. Cardiovasc. Dis.* 20:285, 1978.
4. Prystowsky EN, Miles WM, Heger JJ, Zipes DP: Preexcitation syndromes. Mechanisms and management. *Med. Clin. N.* 68:831, 1984.
5. Lévy S, Broustet J-P, Clementy J, Vircoulon B, Bricaud H, Gerard R: Value of noninvasive techniques in the Wolff-Parkinson-White syndrome with particular reference to exercise testing. In *Cardiac Arrhythmias: From Diagnosis to Treatment*. Lévy S, Scheinman MM, (eds.). Futura, Mont Kisco, 1984, pp. 301–312.
6. German LD, Gallagher JJ, Broughton A, Guarnieri T, Trantham JL: Effects of exercise and isoproterenol during atrial fibrillation in patients with Wolff-Parkinson-White syndrome. *Am. J. Cardiol.* 51:1203, 1983.
7. Wellens HJJ, Brugada P, Roy D, Weiss J, Bar FW: Effect of isoproterenol on the antegrade refractory period of the accessory pathway in patients with the Wolff-Parkinson-White syndrome. *Am. J. Cardiol.* 50:180, 1982.
8. Tonkin AM, Miller HC, Svenson RH, Wallace AG, Gallagher JJ: Refractory periods of the accessory pathway in the Wolff-Parkinson-White syndrome. *Circulation* 52:563, 1975.
9. Wellens HJJ, Bar FW, Dassen WRM, Brugada P, Vanagt EJ, Farre J: Effect of drugs in the Wolff-Parkinson-White syndrome. Importance of initial length of effective refractory period of the accessory pathway. *Am. J. Cardiol.* 46:665, 1980.
10. Akhtar M, Gilbert CJ, Shenasa M: Effect of lidocaine on atrioventricular response via the accessory pathway in patients with Wolff-Parkinson-White syndrome. *Circulation* 63:435, 1981.
11. Wells JL, Karp RB, Kouchoukos NT, Maclean WAH, James TN, Waldo AL: Characterization of atrial fibrillation in man: Studies following open heart surgery. *PACE* 1:426, 1978.
12. Klein GJ, Bashore TM, Sellers TD, Pritchett ELC, Smith WM, Gallagher JJ: Ventricular fibrillation in the Wolff-Parkinson-White syndrome. *N. Engl. J. Med.* 301:1080, 1979.
13. Pritchett ELC, Hammill SC, Reiter MJ, Lee KL, McCarthy EA, Zimmerman JM, Shand DG: Life table methods for evaluating antiarrhythmic drug efficacy in patients with paroxysmal tachycardias. *Am. J. Cardiol.* 52:1007, 1983.
15. Sellers TD Jr, Bashore TM, Gallagher JJ: Digitalis in the preexcitation syndrome: Analysis during atrial fibrillation. *Circulation* 56:260, 1977.
16. Spurrell RAJ, Krikler DM, Sowton E: Effects of verapamil on electrophysiological properties of anomalous atrioventricular connexion in Wolff-Parkinson-White syndrome. *Br. Heart J.* 36:256, 1974.
17. Gulamhusein S, Ko P, Carruthers SG, Klein GJ: Acceleration of the ventricular response during atrial fibrillation in the Wolff-Parkinson-White syndrome after verapamil. *Circulation* 65:348, 1982.
18. Petri H, Kafka W, Hall D, Rudolph W: Potential acceleration of the ventricular rate in Wolff-Parkinson-White syndrome with atrial fibrillation after verapamil. (Abstract.) *Circulation* 62 (Supp II):262, 1980.
19. Gallagher JJ, Sealy WC, Cox JL, Kasell JH: Results of surgery for preexcitation in 200 con-

secutive cases. In *Cardiac Arrhythmias: From Diagnosis to Therapy*. Lévy S, Scheinman MM, (eds.). Futura, Mount Kisco, 1984, pp. 323–340.
20. Benson DW, Jr, Dunnigan A, Green TP, Benditt DG, Schneider SP: Periodic procainamide for paroxysmal tachycardia. *Circulation* 72:147, 1985.
21. Kugler JD, Gillette PC, Duff DF, Cooley DA, McNamara DG: Elective mapping and surgical division of the bundle of Kent in a patient with Ebstein's anomaly who required tricuspid valve replacement. *Am. J. Cardiol.* 41:602, 1978.
22. Mantakas ME, McCue CM, Miller WM: Natural history of Wolff-Parkinson-White syndrome discovered in infancy. *Am. J. Cardiol.* 41:1097, 1978.
23. Scheinman MM, Davis JC: Catheter ablation for treatment of tachyarrhythmias: present role and potential promise. *Circulation* 73:10, 1986.
24. Waldo AL, Plumb VJ, Arciniegas JG, MacLean WAH, Cooper TB, Priest MF, James TN: Transient entrainment and interruption of the atrioventricular bypass pathway type of paroxysmal atrial tachycardia. A model for understanding and identifying reentrant arrhythmias. *Circulation* 67:73, 1983.

INDEX

Batch number: 10838292

Printed by Printforce, the Netherlands